PETERSON'S
NURSING
PROGRAMS
2014

PETERSON'S
Publishing

About Peterson's Publishing

Peterson's Publishing provides the accurate, dependable, high-quality education content and guidance you need to succeed. No matter where you are on your academic or professional path, you can rely on Peterson's print and digital publications for the most up-to-date education exploration data, expert test-prep tools, and top-notch career success resources—everything you need to achieve your goals.

For more information, contact Peterson's Publishing, 3 Columbia Circle, Suite 205, Albany, NY 12203-5158; 800-338-3282 Ext. 54229; or find us on the World Wide Web at www.petersonspublishing.com.

Bernadette Webster, Managing Editor; Jill C. Schwartz, Editor; Christine Lucas, Research Project Manager; James Ranish, Amy Weber, Research Associates; Phyllis Johnson, Software Engineer; Ray Golaszewski, Publishing Operations Manager; Linda M. Williams, Composition Manager; Carrie Hansen, Christine Lucht, Kiele Nowak, Bailey Williams, Fulfillment Coordinators

ISSN 1552-7743
ISBN-13: 978-0-7689-3752-7

Printed in the United States of America

10 9 8 7 6 5 4 3 2 1   15 14 13

Nineteenth Edition

Certified Chain of Custody

60% Certified Fiber Sourcing and
40% Post-Consumer Recycled

www.sfiprogram.org

*This label applies to the text stock.

Sustainability—Its Importance to Peterson's Publishing

What does sustainability mean to Peterson's? As a leading publisher, we are aware that our business has a direct impact on vital resources—most especially the trees that are used to make our books. Peterson's Publishing is proud that its products are certified by the Sustainable Forestry Initiative (SFI) chain-of-custody standard and that all of its books are printed on paper that is 40% post-consumer waste using vegetable-based ink.

Being a part of the Sustainable Forestry Initiative (SFI) means that all of our vendors—from paper suppliers to printers—have undergone rigorous audits to demonstrate that they are maintaining a sustainable environment.

Peterson's Publishing continuously strives to find new ways to incorporate sustainability throughout all aspects of its business.

CONTENTS

FOREWORD

The American Association of Colleges of Nursing (AACN) is proud to collaborate on *Peterson's Nursing Programs 2014.*

According to the U.S. Bureau of Labor Statistics' (BLS) Employment Projections 2010–2020 released in February 2012, the registered nursing workforce is the top occupation in terms of job growth through 2020. It is expected that the number of employed nurses will grow from 2.74 million in 2010 to 3.45 million in 2020, an increase of 712,000 or 26 percent. The projections further explain the need for 495,500 replacements in the nursing workforce, bringing the total number of job openings for nurses due to growth and replacements to 1.2 million by 2020. In March 2012, the BLS reported that job growth in the health-care sector was outpacing the growth realized in 2011, accounting for 1 out of every 5 new jobs created in that year. Hospitals, long-term care facilities, and other ambulatory-care settings added 49,000 new jobs in February 2012, up from 43,300 new jobs created in January. As the largest segment of the health-care workforce, RNs likely will be recruited to fill many of these new positions.

As registered nurses find employment beyond hospitals in such areas as home care, community health, and long-term care, newly licensed RNs must have the proper education and training to work in these settings. It is vital that those seeking to enter or advance in a nursing career find the appropriate nursing program. This guide allows readers to find the program that best fits their needs, whether beginning a new career in nursing or attempting to advance one.

According to AACN's most recent annual institutional survey, enrollment in entry-level B.S.N. programs continues to climb. Gains were reported in all parts of the country in 2012, with an overall 3.5 percent increase in enrollments nationwide.

Although the health-care environment is complex and dynamic, there continues to be a significant demand for professional-level nurses. The primary route into professional-level nursing is the four-year baccalaureate degree. The professional nurse with a baccalaureate degree is the only basic nursing graduate prepared to practice in all health-care settings, including critical care, public health, primary care, and mental health. In addition, advanced practice nurses (APNs) deliver essential services as nurse practitioners, certified nurse-midwives, clinical nurse specialists, and nurse anesthetists. APNs typically are prepared in master's degree programs, and the demand for their services is expected to increase substantially.

Higher education in nursing expands the gateway to a variety of career opportunities in the health-care field. In addition to providing primary care to patients, graduates can work as case managers for the growing numbers of managed-care companies or can assume administrative or managerial roles in hospitals, clinics, insurance companies, and other diverse settings.

The Nursing School Adviser section of this guide is instructive and invaluable. Whether you are a high school student looking for a four-year program, an RN returning to school, or a professional in another field contemplating a career change, this section will address your concerns. This information presents various nursing perspectives to benefit students from diverse backgrounds.

Peterson's effort in making this guide well organized and convenient to read cannot be overstated. Peterson's has worked with AACN in producing a publication that is comprehensive and user-friendly. Like the previous editions, this edition is a genuine collaborative work, as AACN provided input from start to finish.

AACN's dedication and achievements in advancing the quality of baccalaureate and graduate nursing education are appreciated by Peterson's. We at AACN are fortunate to work with an organization that prides itself on being the leading publisher of education search and selection.

Furthermore, this publication would not be possible without the cooperation of the institutions included in this guide. We acknowledge the time and effort of those who undertook the task of completing and returning the surveys regarding their programs. We certainly appreciate their contribution.

Peterson's Nursing Programs 2014 is the only comprehensive and concise guide to baccalaureate and graduate nursing education programs in the United States and Canada. We hope its contents will serve as the impetus for those looking for a rewarding and satisfying career in health care. AACN is proud to present this publication to the nursing profession and to those who seek to enter it.

—Jane Kirschling, PhD, RN, FAAN
President, AACN
—Geraldine D. Bednash, Ph.D., RN, FAAN
Chief Executive Officer and Executive Director, AACN

A NOTE FROM THE PETERSON'S EDITORS

For more than forty years, Peterson's has given students and parents the most comprehensive, up-to-date information on undergraduate and graduate institutions in the United States, Canada, and abroad.

Peterson's Nursing Programs 2014 provides prospective nursing students with the most comprehensive information on baccalaureate and graduate nursing education in the United States and Canada. Our goal is to help students find the best nursing program for them.

To this end, Peterson's has joined forces with the American Association of Colleges of Nursing (AACN), the national voice for America's baccalaureate-and higher-degree nursing education programs. AACN's educational, research, governmental advocacy, data collection, publications, and other programs work to establish high-quality standards for bachelor's- and graduate-degree nursing education, assist deans and directors to implement those standards, influence the nursing profession to improve health care, and promote public support of baccalaureate and graduate education, research, and practice in nursing—the nation's largest health-care profession.

For those seeking to enter the nursing profession or to further their nursing careers, *Peterson's Nursing Programs 2014* includes information needed to make important nursing program decisions and to approach the admissions process with knowledge and confidence.

The Nursing School Adviser section contains useful articles to help guide nursing education choices, with information on nursing careers today, selecting a nursing program, financing nursing education, returning to school, and more. It also includes listings that provide valuable contact information for financial aid resources and specialty nursing organizations. And if you are one of the many people interested in accelerated nursing programs, there is an article that offers an in-depth look at this increasingly popular approach to nursing education. It is a must-read for those wishing to enter an accelerated baccalaureate or generic master's degree program.

At the end of **The Nursing School Adviser** is the "How to Use This Guide" article, which explains some of the key factors to consider when choosing a nursing program. In addition, it explains how the book is organized and shows you how to maximize your use of *Peterson's Nursing Programs 2014* to its full potential.

If you already have specifics in mind, such as a particular program or location, turn to the **Quick-Reference Chart.** Here you can search through "Nursing Programs At-a-Glance" for particular degree options offered by schools, listed alphabetically by state.

In the **Profiles of Nursing Programs** section you'll find expanded and updated nursing program descriptions, arranged alphabetically by state. Each profile provides all of the need-to-know information about accredited nursing programs in the United States and Canada. Display ads, which appear near some of the institutions' profiles, have been provided and paid for by those colleges or universities that wished to supplement their profile data with additional information about their institution.

If you are looking for additional information, you can turn to the **Two-Page Descriptions** section. Here you will find in-depth narrative descriptions, with photos, of those nursing programs that chose to pay for and provide additional information.

When you turn to the back of the book, you'll find eight **Indexes** listing institutions offering *baccalaureate, master's degree, concentrations within master's degree, doctoral, post-doctoral, online,* and *continuing education* programs. The last index lists every college and university contained in the guide along with its corresponding page reference.

Peterson's publishes a full line of resources to help guide you and your family through the admission process. Peterson's publications can be found at high school guidance offices, college and university libraries and career centers, and your local bookstore or library. Peterson's guides are also available as e-books.

We welcome any comments or suggestions you may have about this publication.

Publishing Department
Peterson's, a Nelnet company
3 Columbia Circle, Suite 205
Albany, NY 12203-5158

Your feedback will help us make your educational dreams possible. The editors at Peterson's wish you great success in your nursing program search.

THE NURSING
SCHOOL ADVISER

NURSING FACT SHEET

Misconceptions about nursing have contributed to misinformation about the profession in the media. Here are the real facts:

- **Nursing is the nation's largest health-care profession, with more than 3.1 million registered nurses nationwide.** Of all licensed RNs, 2.6 million or 84.8 percent are employed in nursing.[1]

- **Registered Nurses compose one of the largest segments of the U.S. workforce as a whole and are among the highest paying large occupations.** Nearly 58 percent of RNs worked in general medical and surgical hospitals, where RN salaries averaged $66,700 per year. RNs composed the largest segment of professionals working in the health-care industry.[2]

- **Nurses compose the largest single component of hospital staff, are the primary providers of hospital patient care, and deliver most of the nation's long-term care.**

- **Most health-care services involve some form of care by nurses.** In 1980, 66 percent of all employed RNs worked in hospitals. By 2008, that number had declined slightly to 62.2 percent as more health care moved to sites beyond the hospital, and nurses increased their ranks in a wide range of other settings, including private practices, health maintenance organizations, public health agencies, primary care clinics, home health care, nursing homes, outpatient surgicenters, nursing-school-operated nursing centers, insurance and managed care companies, schools, mental health agencies, hospices, the military, industry, nursing education, and health-care research.[3]

- **Though often working collaboratively, nursing does not "assist" medicine or other fields.** Nursing operates independent of, not auxiliary to, medicine and other disciplines. Nurses' roles range from direct patient care and case management to establishing nursing practice standards, developing quality assurance procedures, and directing complex nursing care systems.

- **With more than four times as many RNs in the United States as physicians, nursing delivers an extended array of health-care services, including primary and preventive care by advanced nurse practitioners in such areas as pediatrics, family health, women's health, and gerontological care.** Nursing's scope also includes services by certified nurse-midwives and nurse anesthetists, as well as care in cardiac, oncology, neonatal, neurological, and obstetric/gynecological nursing and other advanced clinical specialties.

- **The primary pathway to professional nursing, as compared to technical-level practice, is the four-year Bachelor of Science in Nursing (B.S.N.) degree.** Registered nurses are prepared either through a B.S.N. program; a three-year associate degree in nursing; or a three-year hospital training program, receiving a hospital diploma. All take the same state licensing exam. (The number of diploma programs has declined steadily—to less than 10 percent of all basic RN education programs—as nursing education has shifted from hospital-operated instruction into the college and university system.)

- **To meet the more complex demands of today's health-care environment, the National Advisory Council on Nurse Education and Practice has recommended that at least two-thirds of the basic nurse workforce hold baccalaureate or higher degrees in nursing.**[4] Aware of the need, RNs are seeking the B.S.N. degree in increasing numbers. In 1980, almost 55 percent of employed registered nurses held a hospital diploma as their highest educational credential, 22 percent held the bachelor's degree, and 18 percent an associate degree. By 2008, a diploma was the highest educational credential for only 13.9 percent of RNs, while the number with bachelor's degrees as their highest education had climbed to 36.8 percent, with 36.1 percent holding an associate degree as their top academic preparation.[5] In 2010, 22,531 RNs with diplomas or associate degrees graduated from B.S.N. programs.[6]

- **In 2008, 13.2 percent of the nation's registered nurses held either a master's or doctoral degree as their highest educational preparation.**[7] The current demand for master's- and doctorally prepared nurses for advanced practice, clinical specialties, teaching, and research roles far outstrips the supply.

- **According to the U.S. Bureau of Labor Statistics, Registered Nursing is the top occupation in terms of the largest job growth from 2008–2018.**[8] Government analysts project that more than 581,500 new RN jobs will be created through 2018. Other projections indicate that by 2025, the U.S. nursing shortage will grow to more than 260,000 registered nurses.[9] Even as health care continues to shift beyond the hospital to more community-based primary care and other outpatient sites, federal projections say the rising complexity of acute care will see demand for RNs in hospitals climb by 36 percent by 2020.[10]

REFERENCES

1. Health Resources and Services Administration. (September 2010). *The Registered Nurse Population: Findings From the 2008 National Sample Survey of Registered Nurses.* Washington, DC: U.S. Department of Health and Human Services.

2. U.S. Bureau of Labor Statistics, (2010, May). *Occupational Employment and Wages for 2009.* Access online at **http://www.bls.gov/oes**

3. See Note 1.

4. National Advisory Council on Nurse Education and Practice. (October 1996). *Report to the Secretary of the Department of Health and Human Services on the Basic Registered Nurse Workforce.* Washington, DC: U.S. Department of Health and Human Services, Division of Nursing.

5. See Note 1.

6. American Association of Colleges of Nursing (2011). *2010–2011 Enrollment and graduations in baccalaureate and graduate programs in nursing.* Washington, DC: Author.

7. See Note 1.

8. Lacey, T. A. and B. Wright. (2010). *Occupational Employment Projections to 2018.* Washington, DC: U.S. Department of Labor, Bureau of Labor Statistics.

9. Buerhaus, P. I., D. I. Auerbach, and D. O. Staiger. (2009, July–August). The recent surge in nurse employment: causes and implications. *Health Affairs,* 28(4), w657–w668.

10. See Note 4.

CREATING A MORE HIGHLY QUALIFIED NURSING WORKFORCE

High-quality patient care hinges on having a well-educated nursing workforce. Research has shown that lower mortality rates, fewer medication errors, and positive outcomes are all linked to nurses prepared at the baccalaureate and graduate degree levels. The American Association of Colleges of Nursing (AACN) is committed to working collaboratively to create a more highly qualified nursing workforce since education enhances both clinical competency and care delivery.

Snapshot of Today's Nursing Workforce

- In September 2012, the Joint™ Statement on Academic Progression for Nursing Students and Graduates was endorsed by the American Association of Colleges of Nursing (AACN), American Association of Community Colleges, Association of Community Colleges Trustees, National League for Nursing, and the National Organization for Associate Degree Nursing. This historic agreement represents the first time leaders from the major national organizations representing community college presidents, boards, and program administrators have joined with representatives from nursing education associations to promote academic progression in nursing. With the common goal of preparing a well-educated, diverse nursing workforce, this statement represents the shared view that nursing students and practicing nurses should be supported in their efforts to pursue higher levels of education. Read the statement at www.aacn.nche.edu/aacn-publications/position/joint-statement-academicprogression

- In March 2012, the Robert Wood Johnson Foundation funded the Academic Progression in Nursing (APIN) program to advance state and regional strategies to create a more highly educated nursing workforce. A total of $4.3 million in funding was awarded to the Tri-Council for Nursing to steer this initiative. Tri-Council members include the American Association of Colleges of Nursing, National League for Nursing, American Nurses Association, and the American Organization of Nurse Executives. www.aone.org/membership/about/press_releases/2012/032312.shtml.

- According to the *2008 National Sample Survey of Registered Nurses* conducted by the Health Resources and Services Administration (HRSA), nursing is the nation's largest health-care profession, with more than 3 million registered nurses (RNs) nationwide. Of all licensed RNs, 2.6 million or 84.8 percent are employed in nursing.

- The sample survey also shows that 50 percent of the RN workforce holds a baccalaureate or graduate degree, while 36.1 percent earned an associate degree and 13.9 percent earned a diploma in nursing.

- Graduates of entry-level nursing programs (baccalaureate degree, associate degree, and diploma) sit for the NCLEX-RN® licensing examination. The fact that new nurses pass the licensing exam at the same rate does not mean that all entry-level nurses are equally prepared for practice. The NCLEX tests for *minimum technical competency* for safe entry into basic nursing practice. Passing rates *should* be high across all programs preparing new nurses. This exam does not test for differences between graduates of different programs, measure performance over time, or test for all of the knowledge and skills developed through a baccalaureate program.

- In October 2010, the Institute of Medicine released its landmark report on The Future of Nursing (http://thefutureof nursing.org), initiated by the Robert Wood Johnson Foundation, which called for increasing the number of baccalaureate-prepared nurses in the workforce to 80 percent and doubling the population of nurses with doctorates. The expert committee charged with preparing the evidence-based recommendations contained in this report state that to respond "to the demands of an evolving health-care system and meet the changing needs of patients, nurses must achieve higher levels of education."

- The National Advisory Council on Nurse Education and Practice (NACNEP), policy advisors to Congress and the Secretary for Health and Human Services on nursing issues, has urged that at least two thirds of the nurse workforce hold baccalaureate or higher degrees in nursing. For more information, visit http://bhpr.hrsa.gov/nursing/nacnep.htm.

- In March 2005, the American Organization of Nurse Executives (AONE) released a statement calling for all for registered nurses to be educated in baccalaureate programs in an effort to adequately prepare clinicians for their challenging and complex roles. AONE's statement, titled *Practice and Education Partnership for the Future*, represents the view of nursing's practice leaders and a desire to create a more highly educated nursing workforce in the interest of improving patient safety and providing enhanced nursing care. For details, visit http://www.aone.org/aone/resource/practiceandeducation.html.

Research Linking Nursing Education to Patient Outcomes

AACN and other authorities believe that education has a strong impact on a nurse's ability to practice, and that patients deserve the best educated nursing workforce possible. A growing body of research reinforces this belief and shows a connection between baccalaureate education and lower mortality rates.

- In the October 2012 issue of *Medical Care*, researchers from the University of Pennsylvania found that surgical patients in magnet hospitals had 14 percent lower odds of inpatient death within 30 days and 12 percent lower odds of failure-to-rescue compared with patients cared for in non-magnet hospitals. The study authors conclude that these better outcomes were attributed in large part to investments in highly qualified and educated nurses, including a higher proportion of baccalaureate prepared nurses.

- In an article published in *Health Services Research* in August 2008 that examined the effect of nursing practice environments on outcomes of hospitalized cancer patients undergoing surgery, Dr. Christopher Friese and colleagues found that nursing education level was significantly associated with patient outcomes. Nurses prepared at the baccalaureate level were linked with lower mortality and failure-to-rescue rates. The authors conclude that "moving to a nurse workforce in which a higher proportion of staff nurses have at least a baccalaureate-level education would result in substantially fewer adverse outcomes for patients."

- In a study released in the May 2008 issue of the *Journal of Nursing Administration* (http://jonajournal.com), Dr. Linda Aiken and her colleagues confirmed the findings from their landmark 2003 study (see below), which show a strong link between RN education level and patient outcomes. The noted nurse researchers found that every 10 percent increase in the proportion of BSN nurses on the hospital staff was associated with a 4 percent decrease in the risk of death.

- In the January 2007 *Journal of Advanced Nursing*, a study of 46,993 patients conducted by researchers at the University of Toronto found that hospitals with higher proportions of baccalaureate-prepared nurses tended to have lower 30-day mortality rates. The findings indicated that a 10 percent increase in the proportion of baccalaureate-prepared nurses was associated with 9 fewer deaths for every 1,000 discharged patients.

- In a study published in the March/April 2005 *Nursing Research*, Dr. Carole Estabrooks and her colleagues at the University of Alberta found that baccalaureate-prepared nurses have a positive impact on mortality rates following an examination of more than 18,000 patient outcomes at 49 Canadian hospitals. This study, *The Impact of Hospital Nursing Characteristics on 30-Day Mortality*, confirmed the findings from Dr. Aiken's landmark study from 2003.

- In a study published in the September 24, 2003 *Journal of the American Medical Association* (http://jama.ama-assn.org), Dr. Linda Aiken and her colleagues at the University of Pennsylvania identified a clear link between higher levels of nursing education and better patient outcomes. This extensive study found that surgical patients have a "substantial survival advantage" if treated in hospitals with higher proportions of nurses educated at the baccalaureate or higher degree level. A 10 percent increase in the proportion of nurses holding BSN degrees decreased the risk of patient death and failure to rescue by 5 percent.

For more information on the link between nursing education and patient outcomes, see www.aacn.nche.edu/media-relations/fact-sheets/impact-of-education.

Moving Toward a More Highly Educated Nursing Workforce

- The nation's magnet hospitals, which are recognized for nursing excellence and superior patient outcomes, have moved to require all nurse managers and nurse leaders to hold a baccalaureate or graduate degree in nursing by 2013. Settings applying for magnet designation must also show what plans are in place to achieve the IOM recommendation of having an 80 percent baccalaureate-prepared RN workforce by 2020. www.nursecredentialing.org

- In its October 2010 report on The Future of Nursing, the Institute of Medicine states "an increase in the percentage of nurses with a BSN is imperative as the scope of what the public needs from nurses grows, expectations surrounding quality heighten, and the settings where nurses are needed proliferate and become more complex."

- In May 2010, the Tri-Council for Nursing, a coalition of four steering organizations for the nursing profession (AACN, ANA, AONE, and NLN), issued a consensus statement calling for all RNs to advance their education in the interest of enhancing quality and safety across healthcare settings. In the statement titled Education Advancement of Registered Nurses, the Tri-Council organizations present a united view that a more highly educated nursing workforce is critical to meeting the nation's nursing needs and delivering safe, effective patient care. In the policy statement, the Tri-Council finds that "without a more educated nursing workforce, the nation's health will be further at risk." See www.aacn.nche.edu/education-resources/Tri-councilEdStatement.pdf.

- In December 2009, Dr. Patricia Benner and her team at the Carnegie Foundation for the Advancement of Teaching released a new study titled *Educating Nurses: A Call for Radical Transformation*, which recommended preparing all entry-level registered nurses at the baccalaureate level and requiring all RNs to earn a master's degree within 10 years of initial licensure. The authors found that many of today's new nurses are "undereducated" to meet practice demands across settings. Their strong support for high-quality baccalaureate degree programs as the appropriate pathway for RNs entering the profession is consistent with the views of many leading nursing organizations, including AACN.

- In the July/August 2009 issue of *Health Affairs*, Dr. Linda Aiken and colleagues call for adapting federal funding mechanisms (i.e. Title VIII and Medicare) to focus on preparing more nurses at the baccalaureate and higher-degree levels. This policy emphasis is needed to adequately address the growing need for faculty and nurses to serve in primary care and other advanced practice roles. The researchers reported that new nurses prepared in BSN programs are significantly more likely to complete the graduate-level education needed to fill nursing positions where job growth is expected to be the greatest.

- More than 630 RN-to-Baccalaureate programs are available nationwide, including more than 390 programs that are offered at least partially online. These programs build on the education provided in diploma and associate degree programs and prepare graduates for a broader scope of practice. In addition, 160 RN-to-Master's degree programs are available, which cover the baccalaureate content missing in the other entry-level programs as well as graduate-level course work.

- Articulation agreements support education mobility and facilitate the seamless transfer of academic credit between associate degree and baccalaureate nursing programs. In addition to hundreds of individual agreements between community colleges and four-year schools, statewide articulation agreements exist in many areas including Alabama, Arkansas, Connecticut, Florida, Idaho, Iowa, Maryland, Nevada, South Carolina, and Texas to facilitate educational advancement. See media-relations/fact-sheets/articulation-agreements.

References

Aiken, L.H., Cheung, R.B. & Olds, D.M. (2009, June 12). Education policy initiatives to address the nurse shortage in the United States. *Health Affairs* Web Exclusive. Accessed June 22, 2009 at http://content.healthaffairs.org/cgi/content/abstract/hlthaff.28.4.w646.

Aiken, L.H., Clarke, S.P., Sloane, D.M., Lake, E.T. & Cheney, T. (2008, May). Effects of hospital care environment on patient mortality and nurse outcomes. *Journal of Nursing Administration*, 38(5), 223-229.

Aiken, L.H., Clarke, S.P., Cheung, R.B., Sloane, D.M., & Silber, J.H. (2003, September 24). Educational levels of hospital nurses and surgical patient mortality, *Journal of the American Medical Association,* 290, 1617-1623.

American Association of Colleges of Nursing (20012). 2011-2012 Enrollment and graduations in baccalaureate and graduate programs in nursing. Washington, DC: Author.

American Organization of Nurse Executives. (2005). Practice and education partnership for the future. Washington, DC: American Organization of Nurse Executives.

Benner, P., Sutphen, M., Leonard, V. & Day, L. (2009). *Educating Nurses: A Call for Radical Transformation*. Carnegie Foundation for the Advancement of Teaching. San Francisco: Jossey-Bass.

Estabrooks, C.A., Midodzi, W.K., Cummings, G.C., Ricker, K.L. & Giovanetti, P. (2005, March/April). The impact of hospital nursing characteristics on 30-day mortality. *Nursing Research*, 54(2), 72-84.

Friese, C.R, Lake, E.T., Aiken, L.H., Silber, J.H. & Sochalski, J. (2008, August). Hospital nurse practice environments and outcomes for surgical oncology patients. *Health Services Research*, 43(4), 1145-1163.

Institute of Medicine. (2010). *The Future of Nursing: Leading Change, Advancing Health*. Washington, DC: National Academies Press.

McHugh, M.D., Kelly, L.A., Smith, H.L., Wu, E.S., Vanak, J.M. & Aiken, L.H. (2012, October). Lower Mortality in Magnet Hospitals. Medical Care, Publication forthcoming (published ahead of print).

National Advisory Council on Nurse Education and Practice (1996). *Report to the Secretary of the Department of Health and Human Services on the basic registered nurse workforce*. Washington, DC: United States Department of Health and Human Services, Health Resources and Services Administration, Bureau of Health Professions, Division of Nursing.

Tourangeau, A.E, Doran, D.M., McGillis Hall, L., O'Brien Pallas, L., Pringle, D., Tu, J.V. & Cranley, L.A. (2007, January). Impact of hospital nursing care on 30-day mortality for acute medical patients. *Journal of Advanced Nursing*, 57(1), 32-41.

Tri-Council for Nursing. (2010, May). Educational advancement of registered nurses: A consensus position. Available online at http://www.aacn.nche.edu/education-resources/TricouncilEdStatement.pdf.

Van den Heede, K., Lesaffre, E., Diya, L., Vleugels, A., Clarke, S.P., Aiken, L.H. & Sermeus, W. (2009). The relationship between inpatient cardiac surgery mortality and nurse numbers and educational level: Analysis of administrative data. *International Journal of Nursing Studies,* 46(6), 796-803.

COUNSELORS OF CARE IN THE MODERN HEALTH-CARE SYSTEM

Geraldine D. Bednash, Ph.D., RN, FAAN
Chief Executive Officer and Executive Director
American Association of Colleges of Nursing

A Different Era

The nursing profession is alive and reshaping itself. The role of nurses as those who minister exclusively to a patient's basic-care needs has changed. Much of the effectiveness and productivity of the future health-care industry will derive from the training of and services provided by nurses.

Modern nurses take a proactive role in health care by addressing health issues before they develop into problems. They oversee the continued care of patients who have left the health-care facility. Nurses are expected to make complex decisions in areas ranging from patient screening to diagnosis and education. They explore and document the effects of alternative therapies (e.g., guided imagery) and address public health problems, such as teen pregnancy. They explore and understand new technology and how it relates both to patient care and to their own job performance. They work in a variety of settings and are held accountable for their decisions. In today's health-care environment, health-care administrators must recruit nurses with a broad, well-rounded education.

Health-care providers must change the way they administer care. Instead of focusing on the treatment of illness, they must promote wellness. Nurses will oversee patient treatment and medication and must understand the repercussions of these health-care processes for the patient and his or her family.

Cost is the driving force behind this industry-wide transformation. Insurance companies have, for the most part, instigated changes in the way health-care benefits are paid. The old fee-for-service system is no longer the only option. The trend toward managed care, in which a fixed amount of money is allocated for the care of each patient, is changing the way care is provided. It seems that employers of the future will recruit nurses who understand the overall structure of the health-care industry, who possess highly developed critical-thinking skills, and who bring to their positions a well-rounded understanding of the risks and benefits of every health-care decision.

Counselors of Care

Job prospects for graduates of nursing programs are positive. Although many graduates receive associate degrees as registered nurses (RNs), hospital administrators and other employers want applicants with at least a Bachelor of Science in Nursing degree.

To practice in a fast-changing health system, entry-level RNs must understand community-based primary care and emphasize health promotion and cost-effective coordinated care—all hallmarks of baccalaureate education. In addition to its broad scientific curriculum and focus on leadership and clinical decision-making skills, a Bachelor of Science in Nursing degree education provides specific preparation in community-based care not typically included in associate degree or hospital diploma programs. Moreover, the nurse with a baccalaureate degree is the only basic nursing graduate prepared for all health-care settings—critical care, outpatient care, public health, and mental health—and so has the flexibility to practice in outpatient centers, private homes, and neighborhood clinics where demand is fast expanding as health care moves beyond the hospital to more primary and preventive care throughout the community.

Health-care administrators realize that patients are becoming more sophisticated about the care they receive, requiring an explanation and understanding of their health needs. Nurses will have to be knowledgeable care providers, working with physicians, pharmacists, and public health officials in interdisciplinary settings to satisfy these requirements.

Broader training enables graduates of baccalaureate programs to provide improved and varying types of care, and ensures stability and security in an industry now noted for its instability.

Promising Opportunities

One of the rewards of a baccalaureate education can be a competitive salary. Graduates of four-year degree programs can expect salaries starting around $37,000 per year, a figure that might fluctuate depending on geographic area and, more specifically, by the demand in that area. Obviously, the greater the need for nurses, the higher their salaries.

The baccalaureate degree also serves as a foundation for the pursuit of a master's degree in nursing, which prepares students for the role of advanced practice nurse (APN). Students can earn degrees as clinical nurse specialists in neonatology, oncology, cardiology, and other specialties or as nurse practitioners, nurse-midwives, or nurse anesthetists. Master's-prepared nurses can also enjoy rewarding careers in nursing administration and education.

These programs generally span one to two years. Graduates can expect starting salaries of approximately $50,000 annually in advanced practice nursing settings, and demand for these graduates is expected to be high over the next fifteen years. In some localities, for example, the nurse practitioner may be the sole provider of health care to a family.

Overall Transformation

The nursing field must be transformed to be compatible with the overall changes in the health-care industry. According to 2008 statistics, the average age of nurses was 46, with only 16.6 percent of nurses under the age of 35. It is projected that over the next ten years much of the nursing population will retire. Employment is projected to increase 23 percent by 2020.

The traditional career path of nurses is expected to change. More nurses will enter master's programs directly from baccalaureate programs, and more master's degree graduates will pursue doctoral degrees at a younger age. Since nurses will play a critical role in providing health care, a four-year baccalaureate degree is a crucial first step in preparing nurses to assume increased patient responsibilities within the health-care system.

RNs Returning to School: Choosing a Nursing Program

Marilyn Oermann, Ph.D., RN, FAAN, ANEF
Professor and Adult/Geriatric Health Chair
College of Nursing
The University of North Carolina at Chapel Hill

If you are thinking about returning to school to complete your baccalaureate degree or to pursue a graduate degree in nursing, you are not alone. Registered nurses (RNs) are returning to school in record numbers, many seeking advancement or transition to new roles in nursing. Over the last two decades, the number of RNs prepared initially in diploma and associate degree in nursing programs who have graduated from baccalaureate nursing degree programs has more than doubled, according to the AACN. There are expanded opportunities for nurses with baccalaureate degrees in nursing. Although the decision to return to school means considerable investment of time, financial resources, and effort, the benefits can be overwhelmingly positive.

Higher education in nursing opens doors to many opportunities for career growth not otherwise available. By continuing your education, you can do the following:

- Update your knowledge and skills, critical today in light of rapid advances in health care

- Move more easily into a new role within your organization or in other health-care settings

- Pursue a different career path within nursing

Moreover, returning to school brings personal fulfillment and satisfaction gained through learning more about nursing and the changing health-care system and using that knowledge in the delivery and management of patient care.

More Skills and Flexibility Needed

If you are contemplating returning to school, here are some facts to consider. The health-care system continues to undergo dramatic changes. These changes include hospitalized patients who are more acutely ill; an aging population; technological advances that require highly skilled nursing care; a greater role for nurses in primary care, health promotion, and health education; and the need for nurses to care for patients and families in multiple settings, such as schools, workplaces, homes, clinics, and outpatient facilities, as well as hospitals. With the nursing shortage, nurses are in great demand in hospitals. Moreover, as hospitals continue to become centers for acute and critical care, the nurse's role in both patient care and management of other health-care providers in the hospital has become more complex, requiring advanced knowledge and skills.

Because of the complexity of today's health-care environment, AACN and other leading nursing organizations have called for the baccalaureate degree in nursing as the minimum educational requirement for professional nursing practice. In fact, nurse executives in hospitals have indicated their desire for the majority of nurses on staff to be prepared at least at the baccalaureate level to handle the increasingly complex demands of patient care and management of health-care delivery. The baccalaureate nursing degree is essential for nurses to function in different management roles, move across employment settings, have the flexibility to change positions within nursing, and advance in their career. Baccalaureate nursing degree programs prepare the nurse for a broad role within the health-care system and for practice in hospitals, community settings, home health care, neighborhood clinics, and other outpatient settings where opportunities are expanding. Continuing education provides the means for nurses to prepare themselves for a future role in nursing.

The demand for nurses with baccalaureate and more advanced degrees will continue to grow. There is an excess of nurses prepared at the associate degree level, a mounting shortage of baccalaureate-prepared nurses, and only half as many nurses prepared at master's and doctoral levels as needed. Nurses with baccalaureate nursing degrees are needed in all areas of health care, and the demand for nurses with master's and doctoral preparation for advanced practice, management, teaching, and research will continue.

Identifying Strategies

The decision to return to school marks the beginning of a new phase in your career development. It is essential for you to plan this future carefully. Why are you thinking about returning to school, and what do you want to accomplish by doing so? Understanding why you want to go back to school will help you select the best program for you. Knowing what you want to accomplish will help you to focus on your goals and overcome the obstacles that could prevent you from achieving your full potential.

Even if you decide that additional education will help you reach your professional goals, you may also have a list of reasons why you think you cannot return to school—no time, limited financial resources, fear of failure, and concerns about meeting family responsibilities, among others. If you are concerned about the demands of school combined with existing responsibilities, begin by identifying strategies for incorporating classes and study time into your present schedule or consider taking an online course. Remember, you can start your program with one course and reevaluate your time at the end of the term.

Research and anecdotal evidence from adults returning to college indicate that, despite their need to balance school work with a career and often with family responsibilities, these adult learners experience less stress and manage their lives better than they had thought possible. Many of these adult learners report that the satisfaction gained from their education more than compensates for any added stress. Furthermore, studies of nurses who have returned to school suggest that while their education may create stress for them, most nurses cope effectively with the demands of advanced education.

If costs are of concern, it is best to investigate tuition-reimbursement opportunities where you are employed, scholarships from the nursing program and other nursing organizations, and loans. The financial aid officer at the program you are considering is probably the best available resource to answer your financial assistance questions.

If you are unsure of what to expect when returning to school, remember that such feelings are natural for anyone facing a new situation. If you are motivated and committed to pursuing your degree, you will succeed. Most nursing programs offer resources, such as test-taking skills, study skills, and time-management workshops, as well as assistance with academic problems. You can combine school, work, family, and other responsibilities. Even with these greater demands, the benefits of education outweigh the difficulties.

Clarifying Career Goals

Nursing, unlike many other professions, has a variety of educational paths for those who return for advanced education. You should decide if baccalaureate- or graduate-level work is congruent with your career goals. The next step in this process is to reexamine your specific career goals, both immediate and long-term, to determine the level and type of nursing education you will need to meet them. Ask yourself what you want to be doing in the next five to ten years. Discuss your ideas with a counselor in a nursing education program, nurses who are practicing in roles you are considering, and others who are enrolled in a nursing program or who have recently completed a nursing degree.

Baccalaureate degree nursing programs prepare nurses as generalists for practice in all health-care settings. Graduate nursing education occurs at two levels— master's and doctoral. Master's programs vary in length, typically between one and two years. Preparation for roles in advanced practice as nurse practitioners, certified nurse midwives, clinical nurse specialists, certified registered nurse anesthetists, nursing administrators, and nursing educators requires a master's degree in nursing. Many programs meet the needs of RNs by offering options such as accelerated course work, advanced placement, evening and weekend classes, and distance learning courses.

A trend in education for RNs is accelerated programs that combine baccalaureate and master's nursing programs. These combined programs are designed for RNs without degrees whose career goals involve advanced nursing practice and other roles requiring a master's degree. Nurses who complete these combined programs may be awarded both a baccalaureate and a master's degree in nursing or a master's degree only.

At the doctoral level, nurses are prepared for a variety of roles, including research and teaching. Doctoral programs generally consist of three years of full-time study beyond the master's degree, although some programs admit baccalaureate graduates and include the master's-level requirements and degree within the doctoral program.

Matching a Program to Your Needs

Once you have defined your career goals and the level of nursing education they will require, the next step is matching your needs with the offerings and characteristics of specific nursing programs. Some of the criteria you may want to consider in evaluating potential schools of nursing include the types of programs offered, the length of the program and its specific requirements, the availability of full-and part-time study and number of credits required for part-time study, the flexibility of the program, whether distance education courses are available, and the days, times, and sites at which classes and clinical experiences are offered as they relate to your work schedule. Take into consideration the program's accreditation status; faculty qualifications in terms of research, teaching, and practice; and the resources of the school of nursing and of the college/university, such as library holdings, computer services, and statistical consultants. You should also consider the clinical settings used in the curriculum and their relationship to your career goals, as well as the availability of financial aid for nursing students.

Carefully review the admission criteria, including minimum grade point average requirements; scores required on any admission tests, such as the Graduate Record Examinations (GRE) for master's and doctoral programs; and any requirements in terms of work experience. For students returning for a baccalaureate degree, prior nursing knowledge may be validated through testing, transfer of courses, and other mechanisms. Review these options prior to applying to a program.

While the intrinsic quality and characteristics of the program are important, your own personal goals and needs have to be included in your decision. Consider commuting distance, whether courses are offered online, costs in relation to your financial resources, program design, and flexibility of the curriculum in relation to your work, family, and personal responsibilities. While the majority of nursing programs offer part-time study, many programs also schedule classes to accommodate work situations.

Many schools offer nursing courses online, and in some places, the entire baccalaureate and master's programs are available through distance learning. The largest enrollment in nursing distance learning is in baccalaureate programs for

RNs. Distance learning allows RNs to further their education no matter where they live. Many nurses prefer online courses because they can learn at times convenient for them, especially considering competing demands associated with their jobs, families, and other commitments.

Ensure Your Success

Once you have made the decision to return to school and have chosen the program that best meets your needs, take an additional step to ensure your success. Identify the support you will need, both academic and personal, to be successful in the nursing program. Academic support is provided by the institution and may include tutoring services, learning resource centers, computer facilities, and other resources to support your learning. You should take advantage of available support services and seek out resources for areas in which you are weak or need review. Academic support services, however, need to be complemented by personal support through family, friends, and peers. With a firm commitment to pursuing advanced education, a clear choice of a nursing program to meet your goals, and support from others, you are certain to find success in returning to school.

BACCALAUREATE PROGRAMS

Linda K. Amos, Ed.D., RN, FAAN
Former Associate Vice President for Health Sciences
Dean Emerita
University of Utah

The health-care industry has continued to change dramatically over the past few years, transforming the roles of nurses and escalating their opportunities. The current shortage of nurses is caused by an increasing number of hospitalized patients who are older and more acutely ill, a growing elderly population with multiple chronic health problems, and expanded opportunities in HMOs, home care, occupational health, surgical centers, and other primary-care settings. Expanding technological advances that prolong life also require more highly skilled personnel.

The increasing scope of nursing opportunities will grow immensely as nurses become the frontline providers of health care. They are assuming important roles in the provision of managed care, and they will be responsible for coordinating and continuing the care outside traditional health-care facilities. Nurses will play a major role in educating the public and addressing the social and economic factors that impact quality of care.

Worldwide Standards

Nursing students of the future will receive a wealth of information. Understanding the technology used to manage that information will be essential to their ability to track and assess care. In this area, nurses will be able to provide care over great distances. In some areas, care is being managed by the nurse via tele-home health over the Internet. Use of the Internet and other computer-oriented systems is now an integral tool used by nurses. Nurses of the future, therefore, will have to become aware of worldwide standards of care. Nevertheless, the primary job of a nurse will be making sure that the right person is providing the right care at the right cost.

This goal will be accomplished as the industry turns away from the hospital as the center of operation. Nurses will work in a broad array of locations, including clinics, outpatient facilities, community centers, schools, and even places of business.

Much of the emphasis in health care will shift to preventive care and the promotion of health. In this system, nurses will take on a broader and more diverse role than they have in the past.

Unlimited Opportunities, Expanded Responsibilities

The four-year baccalaureate programs in today's nursing colleges provide the educational and experiential base not only for entry-level professional practice, but also as the platform on which to build a career through graduate-level study for advanced practice nursing, including careers as nurse practitioners, nurse-midwives, clinical specialists, and nurse administrators and educators. Nurses at this level can be expected to specialize in oncology, pediatrics, neonatology, obstetrics and gynecology, critical care, infection control, psychiatry, women's health, community health, and neuroscience. The potential and responsibilities at this level are great. Increasingly, many families use the nurse practitioner for all health-care needs. In almost all U.S. states, the nurse practitioner can prescribe medications and provide health care for the management of chronic non-acute illnesses and preventive care.

The health-care system demands a lot from nurses. The education of a nurse must transcend the traditional areas of study, such as chemistry and anatomy, to include health promotion, disease prevention, screening, genetic counseling, and immunization. Nurses should understand how health problems may have a social cause, such as poverty and environmental contamination, and they must develop insight into human psychology, behavior, and cultural mores and values.

The transformation of the health-care system offers unlimited opportunities for nurses at the baccalaureate and graduate levels as care in urban and rural settings becomes more accessible. According to the U.S. Bureau of Labor Statistics, employment of RNs will grow more quickly than the average employment for all occupations through 2018, due largely to growing demand in settings such as health maintenance organizations, community health centers, home care, and long-term care. The increased complexity of health problems and increased management of health problems outside of hospitals require highly educated and well-prepared nurses at the baccalaureate and graduate levels. It is an exciting era in nursing that holds exceptional promise for nurses with a baccalaureate nursing degree.

The compensation for new nurses is once again becoming competitive with that of other industries. Entry-level nurses with baccalaureate degrees in nursing can expect a salary range of about $31,000 to $46,000 per year, depending on geographic location and experience. Five years into their careers, the national average for nurses with four-year degrees is more than $50,000 per year, with many earning more than $65,000. The current shortage has prompted some employers to offer sign-on bonuses and other incentives to attract and retain staff.

Applying to College

Meeting your chosen school's general entrance requirements is the first step toward a university or college degree in nursing. Admission requirements may vary, but a high school diploma or equivalent is necessary. Most accredited colleges consider SAT scores along with high school grade point average. A strong preparatory class load in science and mathematics is generally preferred among nursing schools. Students may obtain specific admission information by writing to a school's nursing department.

To apply to a nursing school, contact the admission offices of the colleges or universities you are interested in and request the appropriate application forms. With limited spaces in nursing schools, programs are competitive, and early submission of an application is recommended.

Accreditation

Accreditation of the nursing program is very important, and it should be considered on two levels—the accreditation of the university or college and the accreditation of the nursing program itself. Accreditation is a voluntary process in which the school or the program asks for an external review of its programs, facilities, and faculty. For nursing programs, the review is performed by peers in nursing education to ensure program quality and integrity.

Baccalaureate nursing programs in the United States undergo two types of regular systematic reviews. First, the school must be approved by the state board of nursing. This approval is necessary to ensure that the graduates of the program may sit for the licensing examinations offered through the National Council of State Boards of Nursing, Inc. The second is accreditation administered by a nursing accreditation agency that is recognized by the U.S. Department of Education.

Although accreditation is a voluntary process, access to federal loans and scholarships requires it, and most graduate schools accept only students who have earned degrees from accredited schools. Further, accreditation ensures an ongoing process of quality improvement based on national standards. Canadian nursing school programs are accredited by the Canadian Association of University Schools of Nursing, and the Canadian programs listed in this book must hold this accreditation. There are two recognized accreditation agencies for baccalaureate nursing programs in the United States: the Commission on Collegiate Nursing Education (CCNE) and the National League for Nursing Accrediting Commission (NLNAC).

Focusing Your Education

Academic performance is not the sole basis of acceptance into the upper level of the nursing program. Admission officers also weigh such factors as student activities, employment, and references. Moreover, many require an interview and/or essay in which the nursing candidate offers a goal statement. This part of the admission process can be completed prior to a student's entrance into the college or university or prior to the student's entrance into the school of nursing itself, depending on the program.

In the interview or essay, students may list career preferences and reasons for their choices. This allows admission officers to assess the goals of students and gain insights into their values, integrity, and honesty. One would expect that a goal statement from a student who is just entering college would be more general than that of a student who has had two years of preprofessional nursing studies. The more experienced student would be likely to have a more focused idea of what is to be gained by an education in nursing; there would be more evidence of the student's values and the ways in which she or he relates them to the knowledge gained from preprofessional nursing classes.

Baccalaureate Curriculum

A standard basic or generic baccalaureate program in nursing is a four-year college or university education that incorporates a variety of liberal arts courses with professional education and training. It is designed for high school graduates with no previous nursing experience.

Currently, there are more than 700 baccalaureate programs in the United States. Of the 683 programs that responded to a 2009 survey conducted by the American Association of Colleges of Nursing, total enrollment in all nursing programs leading to a baccalaureate degree was 214,533.

The baccalaureate curriculum is designed to prepare students for work in the growing and changing health-care environment. As nurses take a more active role in all facets of health care, they are expected to develop critical thinking and communication skills in addition to receiving standard nurse training in clinics and hospitals. In a university or college setting, the first two years include classes in the humanities, social sciences, basic sciences, business, psychology, technology, sociology, ethics, and nutrition.

In some programs, nursing classes begin in the sophomore year; others begin in the junior year. Many schools require satisfactory grade point averages before students advance into professional nursing classes. On a 4.0 scale, admission into the last two years of the nursing program may require a minimum GPA of 2.5 to 3.0 in preprofessional nursing classes. The national average is about 2.8, but the cutoff level varies with each program.

In the junior and senior years, the curriculum focuses on the nursing sciences, and emphasis moves from the classroom to health facilities. This is where students are exposed to clinical skills, nursing theory, and the varied roles nurses play in the health-care system. Courses include nurse leadership, health promotion, family planning, mental health, environmental and occupational health, adult and pediatric care, medical and surgical care, psychiatric care, community health, management, and home health care.

This level of education comes in a variety of settings: community hospitals, clinics, social service agencies, schools, and health-maintenance organizations. Training in diverse settings is the best preparation for becoming a vital player in the growing health-care field.

Reentry Programs

Practicing nurses who return to school to earn a baccalaureate degree will have to meet requirements that may include possession of a valid RN license and an associate degree or hospital diploma from an accredited institution. Again, it is best to check with the school's admissions department to determine specifics.

Nurses returning to school will have to consider the rapid rate of change in health care and science. A nurse who passed an undergraduate-level chemistry class ten years ago would probably not receive credit for that class today because of the growth of knowledge in that and all other scientific fields. The need to reeducate applies not only to practicing nurses returning to school, but also to all nurses throughout their careers.

In the same vein, nurses with diplomas from hospital programs who want to work toward a baccalaureate degree must meet the common requirements for more clinical practice, and must develop a deeper understanding of community-based nursing practices such as health prevention and promotion.

Colleges and universities available to the RN in search of a baccalaureate give credit for previous nurse training. These programs are designed to accommodate the needs and career goals of the practicing nurse by providing flexible course schedules and credit for previous experience and education. Some programs lead to a master's-level degree, a process that can take up to three years. Licensed practical nurses (LPNs) can also continue their education through baccalaureate programs.

Nurses considering reentering school may also consider other specialized programs. For example, some programs are aimed at enabling nurses with A.D.N. degrees or LPN/LVN licenses to earn B.S.N.'s. Also, accelerated B.S.N. programs are available for students with degrees in other fields.

Choosing a Program

With more than 700 baccalaureate programs in the United States, the prospective student must do research to determine which programs match his or her needs and career objectives.

If you have no health-care experience, it might be best to gain some insight into the field by volunteering or working part-time in a care facility such as a hospital or an outpatient clinic. Talking to nurse professionals about their work will also help you determine how your attributes may apply to the nursing field.

When considering a nursing education, consider your personal needs. Is it best for you to work in a heavily structured environment or one that offers more flexibility in terms of, say, integrating a part-time work schedule into studies? Do you need to stay close to home? Do you prefer to work in a large health-care system such as a health maintenance organization or a medical center, or do you prefer smaller, community-based operations?

As for nursing programs, ask the following questions: How involved is the faculty in developing students for today's health-care industry? How strong is the school's affiliation with clinics

RN-to-Baccalaureate Programs Fact Sheet

More than 630 RN-to-baccalaureate programs are available nationwide, including programs offered in a more intense, accelerated format. Program length varies from one to two years depending upon the school's requirements, program type, and the student's previous academic achievement.

Concerns about the limited availability of RN-to-baccalaureate programs are unfounded. In fact, there are more RN-to-baccalaureate programs available than there are four-year nursing programs or accelerated bachelor's degree programs for non-nursing college graduates. Access to RN-to-baccalaureate programs is further enhanced when programs are offered completely online or on-site at various health-care facilities.

Enrollment in RN-to-baccalaureate programs is increasing in response to calls for a more highly educated nursing workforce. From 2009 to 2011, enrollments increased by 20.6 percent, marking the sixth year of increases in RN-to-baccalaureate programs.

Hundreds of articulation agreements between A.D.N. and diploma programs and four-year institutions exist nationwide (including some statewide agreements), to help students who are seeking baccalaureate-level nursing education. Before enrolling in diploma and A.D.N. programs, students are encouraged to check with school administrators to see what articulation agreements exist with baccalaureate degree–granting schools and to determine which course work will be transferable.

and hospitals? Is there assurance that a student will gain an up-to-date educational experience for the current job market? Are a variety of care settings available? How much time in clinics is required for graduation? What are the program's resources in terms of computer and science laboratories? Does the school work with hospitals and community-based centers to provide health care? How available is the faculty to oversee a student's curriculum? What kind of student support is available in terms of study groups and audiovisual aids? Moreover, what kind of counseling from faculty members and administrators is available to help students develop well-rounded, effective progress through the program?

Visiting a school and talking to the program's guidance counselors will give you a better understanding of how a particular program or school will fit your needs. You can get a closer look at the faculty, its members' credentials, and the focus of the program. It's also not too early to consider what each program can offer in terms of job placement.

Master's Programs

Kathleen Dracup, D.N.Sc., RN, FNP, FAAN
Endowed Professor in Nursing Education and Former Dean
School of Nursing
University of California, San Francisco

The transformation of the health-care system is taking place as you read this, and it can be seen even today in the most common areas:

- A mother brings her child into a clinic for treatment of an earache. Instead of a physician, a nurse practitioner provides the care.

- A patient is readied for surgery. A variety of specialists move around the surgery room, but it's not a specially trained physician administering the anesthetic—it's a certified nurse anesthetist.

- During a patient's recovery from an acute illness, it's decided that the patient no longer needs to stay in the hospital but isn't well enough to return home. The best place to continue the recovery is an intermediate-care facility. Who makes that decision? A clinical nurse specialist. Who oversees the physical and emotional rehabilitation programs at this facility? Another clinical nurse specialist.

These health-care professionals are all advanced practice nurses (APNs). All have graduate-level degrees, and they serve as proof that the demand for nurses with master's and doctoral degrees for advanced practice, clinical specialties, teaching, and research will double the supply.

Another study estimated that the U.S. could save as much as $8.75 billion annually if APNs were used appropriately in place of physicians. As more and more of the restrictions on APNs succumb to legislative or economic forces, the demand for graduate-level nurses is expected to remain high.

Educational Core for APN

A master's degree in nursing is the educational core that allows advanced practice nurses to work as nurse practitioners, certified nurse-midwives, clinical nurse specialists, and certified nurse anesthetists.

Nurse practitioners conduct physical exams, diagnose and treat common acute illnesses and injuries, administer immunizations, manage chronic problems such as high blood pressure and diabetes, and order lab services and X-rays.

Nurse-midwives provide prenatal and gynecological care, deliver babies in hospitals and private settings such as homes, and follow up with postpartum care.

Clinical nurse specialists provide a range of care in specialty areas, such as oncology, pediatrics, and cardiac, neonatal, obstetric/gynecological, neurological, and psychiatric nursing.

Nurse anesthetists administer anesthesia for all types of surgery in operating rooms, dental offices, and outpatient surgical centers.

Master's degrees in nursing administration or nursing education are also available.

There are more than 340 master's degree programs accredited by the Commission on Collegiate Nursing Education (CCNE) or by the National League for Nursing Accrediting Commission (NLNAC). The wide spectrum of programs includes the Master of Science in Nursing (M.S.N.) degree, Master of Nursing (M.N.) degree, Master of Science (M.S.) degree with a nursing major, or Master of Arts (M.A.) degree with a nursing major. The specific degrees depend on the requirements set by the college or university or by the faculty of the nursing program. There are accelerated programs for RNs, which allow the nurse with a hospital diploma or associate degree to earn both a baccalaureate and a master's degree in a condensed program. Some schools offer accelerated master's degree programs for nurses with non-nursing degrees and for non-nursing college graduates. There are joint-degree programs, such as a master's in nursing combined with a Master of Business Administration, Master of Public Health, or Master of Hospital Administration.

Master's Curriculum

The master's degree builds on the baccalaureate degree to enable the student to develop expertise in one area. That specialty can range from running a hospital to providing care for prematurely born babies, from researching the effectiveness of alternative therapies to tackling social and economic causes of health problems. It is an opportunity for the student who has assessed his or her personal career goals and matched them to individual, community, and industry needs. What students can do with their APN degrees is limited only by their imagination.

Full-time master's programs consist of eighteen to twenty-four months of uninterrupted study. Many graduate school students, however, fit their master's-level studies around their work schedules, which can extend the time it takes to graduate.

Master's-level study incorporates theories and concepts of nursing science and their applications, along with the management of health care. Research provides a foundation for the improvement of health-care techniques. Students also have the opportunity to develop the knowledge, leadership skills, and interpersonal skills that will enable them to improve the health-care system.

Classroom and clinical work are involved throughout the master's program. In class, students spend less time listening to lectures and taking notes and more time participating in student-and faculty-led seminars and roundtable discussions. Extended clinical work is generally required.

Graduate-level education in many programs includes courses in statistics, research management, health economics, health policy, health-care ethics, health promotion, nutrition, family planning, mental health, and the prevention of family and social violence. When students begin to concentrate their study in their clinical areas, any number of courses that support their chosen specialty may be included. For example, a nurse wanting to specialize in pediatrics may take courses in child development.

A clinical nurse specialist can focus on acute care, geriatrics, adult health, community health, critical care, gerontology, rehabilitation, and cardiovascular, surgical, oncology, maternity/newborn, pediatric, mental/ psychiatric, and women's health nursing. Areas of specialization in nurse practitioner programs include acute care, adult health, child care, community health, emergency care, geriatric care, neonatal health, occupational health, and primary care.

Admission Requirements

The admission requirements for master's programs in nursing vary greatly. Generally, a bachelor's degree from a school accredited by the Commission on Collegiate Nursing Education or by the National League for Nursing Accrediting Commission and a state RN license are required. Scores from the Graduate Record Examinations (GRE) or the Miller Analogies Test (MAT), college transcripts, letters of reference, and an essay are also typically required. Non-nurses and nurses with non-nursing degrees have special requirements. The profiles and in-depth descriptions of colleges and universities in this publication will give you an idea of each school's specific requirements.

It is important to remember that admissions officers look at a student's transcripts, clinical work, and letters of reference together. A low grade point average is not an automatic knockout—admissions officers are after a composite package. Also, some specialties require specific courses. Students in the nurse anesthetist program, for instance, must have taken an upper-level college course in biochemistry.

A Master's That's Best for You

Most nurses who think of entering a master's program are already practicing nurses. They have a good idea of what they want to specialize in before they apply for admission. It is crucial to know what you want to study before you enter a master's program.

The best way to ensure success in a master's program is to understand your individual strengths and career desires and then find the faculty and college setting that are best suited to help you develop those strengths. Students must make an effort to educate themselves as to the strength of the faculty in each college's master's program. That's the best thing to look for: a strong faculty in one specialty.

This can be tricky. One university's master's program may be rated reasonably high in all fields. Another program might not be rated as high overall, but its cardiovascular program, for example, may be one of the best because of its access to facilities or the fact that its faculty is in the process of developing an innovative new treatment.

This type of information is not hard for the master's candidate to discover; it just takes time. Such information is available from each school's admissions office, which should be more than happy to promote its nursing faculty and support its opinion with proof, such as the research papers that faculty members have published in journals or the number of degrees each faculty member holds.

This type of research is the best way to find a program that meets your needs. The profiles of master's nursing programs in this book should help. If you can, narrow the list to three or four graduate schools, and then write each school's admissions department for catalogs and other information. Visit the schools and take time to talk to a guidance counselor from the nursing program in each one.

Other key questions to consider when applying for a master's program are: Does the school offer financial aid, such as loans, scholarships, fellowships, or teaching posts? How much clinical work is needed? Does the clinical work meet your needs, and does the type of clinical work involved match what you understand the health-care system will be using when you graduate? Is the course work flexible? Can you work part-time and still progress toward a master's degree? This is important to know. A majority of master's program students continue to work while they pursue the degree. Therefore, master's degree programs may present a flexible offering of short courses to meet the student's schedule demands.

Some programs require a thesis, whereas others provide another type of culminating experience, such as a comprehensive examination.

The Master's Trends

Today's master's programs have increased the amount of clinical practice required by students so that graduates enter the job market ready for certification. There is also a greater emphasis on applying new research findings to methods of patient care. This might involve students' reading literature about new treatments and then incorporating the appropriate changes.

All master's program candidates should consider courses in cost-benefit analysis. As managed-care systems become more predominant in the industry, health-care workers will be asked to justify the expense of each treatment, as well as its effectiveness. This leads to the crucial issue of quality. There will always be a strong effort to minimize costs in every health-care procedure, but that cannot compromise the quality of care. It's safe to say that discharging a newborn too soon from a hospital due to shortsightedness can be quite costly.

Depending on the specialty, master's candidates entering the job market may be expected to oversee auxiliary-care providers, such as nurse aides or other unlicensed employees. They may work in a team structure, and in this capacity, the nurse specialist may be expected to manage, motivate, and steer the group. This requires team-building and other management techniques.

While everyone in the health-care facility will have a part in ensuring patient satisfaction, nurses—particularly advanced

RN-to-Master's Degree Programs Fact Sheet

Currently, there are 173 programs available nationwide to transition RNs with diplomas and associate degrees to the master's-degree level (M.S.N., M.S. or Master of Science in Nursing degree). These programs prepare nurses to assume positions requiring graduate preparation, including roles in administration, teaching, research, and as Clinical Nurse Leaders. Master's degree–prepared nurses are in high demand as expert clinicians, nurse executives, clinical educators, health policy consultants, and research assistants.

RN-to-master's programs generally take about three years to complete, with specific requirements varying by institution and the student's previous course work. Though the majority of these programs are offered in traditional classroom settings, some RN-to-M.S.N. programs are offered largely online or in a blended classroom/online format.

The baccalaureate level content missing from diploma and A.D.N. programs is built into the front-end of the RN-to-M.S.N. program. Mastery of this upper-level basic nursing content is necessary for students to move on to graduate study. Upon completion, many programs award both the baccalaureate and master's degree.

The number of RN-to-master's programs has more than doubled within the past fifteen years, from 70 programs in 1994 to 173 programs today. According to AACN's 2010 survey of nursing schools, 32 new RN-to-M.S.N. programs are in the planning stages..

growing number of patients to other types of facilities or settings. In light of this trend, it's best for the master's program student to gain experience in a variety of settings, including homes, clinics, and community-based facilities.

The demand for high-quality care will continue to grow. Medical innovations and technological advances will continue. The quality and effectiveness of health care will continue to improve, and nurses with graduate degrees will play an active role in this trend.

The Hot Employment Spots

The health-care industry has undergone such radical transformation in the last five years that administrators feel they cannot predict whether any one geographic region will have more hirings than another. Generally, nurses with master's degrees will be in demand in all regions of the country, in both the United States and Canada.

Industry trends indicate that, along with continuing opportunities in hospitals, more and more nurses will also work outside the hospital in outpatient clinics and community settings—and even in businesses. As patients spend less time in hospitals, the need grows for nurse specialists to oversee home-care settings and ensure that the quality of care is high. In this vein, some nurses are taking the initiative and running their own businesses as health-care providers, offering services as they see fit in whatever locations are appropriate.

Immediate Rewards

Advanced practice nurses right out of school can expect annual salaries ranging from $60,000 to $90,000, depending on geographic location and previous experience. However, some rural county health clinics start their nurse practitioners at salaries as low as $40,000 per year.

Certified nurse anesthetists and certified nurse-midwives, however, draw higher salaries. Nurse-midwives, for example, can draw first-year salaries as high as $90,000 per year. Areas such as the Northeast and the West Coast tend to have nurses in these fields at the higher end of the salary scale. After five years of practice, the salary range for APNs stretches from $60,000 to $100,000 a year. Again, it depends on location. After five years, nurse-midwives earn salaries ranging from $65,000 to $120,000 annually.

practice nurses—will shoulder a great deal of this load. Developing interpersonal and communication skills and having an understanding of human behavior will make it easier for the advanced practice nurse to help patients to understand modern health-care procedures, which will no doubt improve their feelings of satisfaction.

Finally, nurses at all levels should be aware of the need for flexibility. Many health-care organizations are reducing the number of beds in hospitals and transferring the care of a

THE CLINICAL NURSE LEADER

The Clinical Nurse Leader or CNL® is a rapidly emerging nursing role developed by the American Association of Colleges of Nursing (AACN) in collaboration with leaders from the nursing education and practice arenas. The national movement to advance the CNL is fueled by the critical need to improve the quality of patient care and better prepare nurses to thrive across the health-care system. The CNL role was developed following research and discussion with stakeholder groups as a way to engage highly skilled clinicians as leaders in outcome-based practices.

CNL provide lateral integration at the point of care and combine evidence-based practice with the following:

- Microsystems-level advocacy
- Centralized care coordination
- Outcomes measurement
- Risk assessment
- Quality improvement
- Interprofessional communication

In practice, the CNL oversees the care coordination of a distinct group of patients and actively provides direct patient care in complex situations. CNLs have master's degrees and are advanced generalists, evaluating patient outcomes, assessing risks, and using their authority to change care plans when necessary. CNLs are leaders in the health-care delivery system; the implementation of their roles will vary across settings.

Connecting Nursing Practice and Education

To support the creation of this new nursing role, AACN launched a national initiative involving more than 100 education-practice partnerships across the nation. Partners from schools of nursing and nursing practice sites are working together to transform care delivery by educating new CNLs and integrating them into the health delivery system.

More than seventy schools of nursing are now preparing CNLs for advanced generalist programs offered at the graduate level. Students may choose from traditional post-baccalaureate master's programs, degree completion programs for registered nurses (RNs), and accelerated programs for those seeking to make the transition into nursing. Most CNL programs are directly connected with practice sites interested in employing graduates to enhance care delivery, patient safety, and quality outcomes.

The Veterans Health Administration, the nation's largest employer of RNs, has embraced the CNL role and is planning to introduce it into all Veterans Affairs hospitals nationwide. Support for the clinical role is gaining momentum as many practice sites are reporting on the pioneering outcomes of the CNL staff.

The Key to Positive Patient Outcomes

CNLs provide efficient and cost-effective patient care services, as well as the leadership needed to repair fragmented health-care delivery systems. CNLs are having a measurable impact on the quality of nursing services with practice sites reporting that CNLs are

- quickly making significant progress on raising patient, nurse, and physician satisfaction; improving care outcomes; and realizing sizable cost-savings.

- elevating the level of practice for all nurses on the unit by promoting critical thinking and innovation in nursing care.

- constructively managing change and promoting a team-based approach to care.

- understanding the bigger picture, including outcomes and patient satisfaction, when considering next steps, needed changes, and improvements to the practice setting.

The CNL Mark of Excellence

The CNL Mark of Excellence certification is a unique credential that recognizes graduates of master's and post-master's CNL programs who have demonstrated accepted standards of practice. The CNL Mark of Excellence promotes safe, quality practice through its ongoing requirements for personal and professional growth. In 2007, AACN established a new certification commission—the Commission on Nurse Certification (CNC)—to oversee all aspects of the CNL certification program.

Becoming a CNL

Those interested in becoming a CNL are encouraged to visit the AACN Web site, www.aacn.nche.edu/CNL, to find out more about this nursing career option. Detailed information is available online, including frequently asked questions, the white paper on the CNL role, and a directory of Web links for related programs.

ACCELERATED PROGRAMS

With the Bureau of Labor Statistics projecting the need for more than 580,000 new and replacement registered nurses by the year 2018, nursing schools around the country are exploring creative ways to increase student capacity and reach out to new student populations. The challenge inherent in these efforts is to quickly produce competent nurses while maintaining the integrity and high quality of the nursing education provided.

One innovative approach to nursing education that is gaining momentum nationwide is the accelerated degree program for non-nursing graduates. Offered at both the baccalaureate and master's degree levels, these programs build on previous learning experiences and transition individuals with undergraduate degrees in other disciplines into nursing.

Shifts in the economy and the desire of many adults to make a post-September 11 difference in their work has increased interest in the nursing profession among "second-degree" students. For those with a prior degree, accelerated baccalaureate programs offer the quickest route to becoming a registered nurse, with programs generally running twelve to eighteen months long. Generic master's degrees, also accelerated in nature and geared to non-nursing graduates, generally take three years to finish. Students in these programs usually complete baccalaureate-level nursing courses in the first year followed by two years of graduate study.

Though not new to nursing education, accelerated programs have proliferated over the past fifteen years. In 1990, 31 accelerated baccalaureate programs (B.S.N.) and 12 generic master's programs (M.S.N.) were offered around the country. Today, 230 accelerated B.S.N. programs are operating and the number of generic master's programs has increased to 65. According to AACN's database on enrollment and graduations, 33 new accelerated B.S.N. programs are now in the planning stages. This number far outpaces all other types of entry-level nursing programs currently being considered at four-year nursing schools. Six new generic master's programs are also taking shape.

Graduates of accelerated programs are prized by nurse employers who value the many layers of skill and education these graduates bring to the workplace. Employers report that these graduates are more mature, possess strong clinical skills, and are quick studies on the job. Many practice settings are partnering with schools and offering tuition repayment to graduates as a mechanism to recruit highly qualified nurses.

Changing Gears: Second-Degree Students

The typical second-degree nursing student is motivated, older, and has higher academic expectations than high school–entry baccalaureate students. Accelerated students excel in class and are eager to gain clinical experiences. Faculty members find them to be excellent learners who are not afraid to challenge their instructors.

"Our accelerated students are a remarkable group," said Nancy DeBasio, Ph.D., RN, Dean of the Research College of Nursing in Kansas City. "Their mean GPA is 3.3, they come from a wide array of backgrounds, and the experiences they bring with them enrich their nursing." The compressed program format is a key motivator for this group of students. "Our exit surveys indicate that the one-year program completion time is a primary reason for enrollment in our program," Dr. Debasio explained.

Second-degree students bring new dimensions to nursing and a rich history of prior learning. "We are seeing a steady increase in applicants to our accelerated program this year, and those accepted come with backgrounds that are varied and impressive," said Janet B. Younger, Ph.D., RN, Professor Emerita of the School of Nursing at Virginia Commonwealth University. "We welcomed several Ph.D.'s, some M.D.s from other countries, and a few fine arts majors. These students excel in class and perform very well post-graduation."

Students in accelerated programs are competitive, maintain high grade point averages, and almost always pass the NCLEX-RN licensure exam on the first attempt. "Second-degree candidates are excellent students and are very likely to see the program through to graduation," said Afaf Meleis, Ph.D., DrPS(hon), FAAN, Margaret Bond Simon Dean of Nursing at the University of Pennsylvania School of Nursing. "These students are committed to their studies, are actively engaged in research, and very often involved in university organizations."

Susan M. Di Biase, CRNP, M.S.N., a faculty member at Jacksonville State University in Alabama, knows a thing or two about second-degree students. She was one. "As a nurse educator, I have taught dozens of second-degree students who often distinguish themselves as class leaders," explained Di Biase. "When I was taking classes, I thought the students were strong academically and many said nursing was harder than their first degree. My first employer made a custom of hiring second-degree students because she thought they were good thinkers and strong patient advocates."

Accelerated Baccalaureate Programs

Accelerated baccalaureate programs accomplish programmatic objectives in a shorter timeframe than traditional four-year programs, usually through a combination of bridge courses and core content. Instruction is intense, with courses offered full-time with no breaks between sessions. Students receive the same number of clinical hours as their counterparts in traditional programs. Admission standards are high with programs typically requiring a minimum of a 3.0 GPA and a thorough prescreening process.

Typically, students with a prior degree are not required to take the liberals arts content included in a four-year B.S.N. program. Accelerated programs do require prerequisites, many of which may have been completed during the student's initial degree program. "Before students can begin our program, their college transcripts are reviewed to assure that all prerequisites are met," stated Maureen C. Creegan, Ed.D., RN, Director and Professor, Division of Nursing, at Dominican College in New York. "Almost all students meet the arts and social sciences requirements; most do not meet the natural sciences requirements, including anatomy and microbiology. To assist students, we offer back-to-back prerequisite courses just prior to the start of the accelerated program."

Accelerated programs require a heavy credit load and intense clinical experiences. Identifying students who will flourish in this environment is a priority for administrators. "Due to the intensity of the program, an interview was added to the admission process to better screen students," explained Maryann Forbes, Ph.D., RN, Associate Professor and Chair, Nursing Program, Adelphi University. "Faculty members feel that the interview and ongoing mentoring are key components to student success."

"The most successful accelerated students are bright, inquisitive, and sophisticated consumers of higher education who actively pursue learning opportunities," said Harriet Feldman, Ph.D., RN, FAAN, Dean of the Lienhard School of Nursing at Pace University in New York, whose Combined Degree Program (B.S.N./M.S.) has been in existence since 1984. "As adults, these students tend to know what they need and aggressively pursue programs that best meet their needs: fast-tracked, competitive, and well respected. While some students do attend part-time, most are full-time students who want to reach their career objective as quickly and efficiently as possible."

"Our accelerated B.S.N. program attracts second-career seekers who are unable to make the time and financial commitment to a generic master's program," explained Elizabeth McGann, D.N.Sc., RN, CS, Dean of the Department of Nursing at Quinnipiac University in Connecticut. "Our program gives students the option of entering basic nursing practice now with graduate education as a potential future step."

Generic Master's Degree Programs

Having already completed a degree at the baccalaureate or graduate level, many second-degree students are attracted to the generic master's program as the natural next step in their higher education. "Why would a bachelor's prepared applicant, thinking about a career in health care, want to get a second bachelor's in nursing when they can get a professional master's or doctorate in every other health-care field?," asked Melanie Dreher, Ph.D., RN, FAAN, Dean of Rush University's College of Nursing.

"In 1974, Yale University was the first school to open its door to college graduates who were not yet nurses and instituted the Graduate Entry Prespecialty in Nursing (GEPN),"

explained Sharon Sanderson, Director of Student Recruitment for Yale's School of Nursing. "We recognized that bright, committed people without a background in nursing could be prepared as advanced practice nurses." At Marquette University in Wisconsin, students admitted into the direct-entry M.S.N. program are high achievers. "Our students are self motivated, have definite goals, demonstrate good study habits, and succeed," explained Judith Fitzgerald Miller, Ph.D., RN, FAAN, Former Interim Dean of the College of Nursing.

"Our generic M.S.N. students bring a wonderful expertise to the class," said Margery Chisholm, Ed.D., RN, CS, ABPP, Professor and Former Dean of the School of Nursing at MGH Institute of Health Professions in Boston. "We run the gamut from a 53-year-old male lawyer, students holding PhDs and master's degrees in other fields, and students fresh out of a liberal arts program. One of my past students was a horticulture major who wrote a paper on therapeutic gardens for health-care settings. As they learn from us, we also learn from them, and they learn from each other. Second-degree students are a challenging, exciting group with the potential to make significant contributions to nursing as well as to their patients, families, and communities."

Interest in generic M.S.N. programs is running high. In Chicago, the DePaul University's program grew from 20 students last year to 48 students this fall, with a minimal amount of advertising. "With little more than a one-sentence notice about the program on the school's Web site when the program was announced, we received over 100 inquiries and more than 40 applications in short order," said Kathryn Anderson, Ph.D., RN, Graduate Program Director at the Seattle University School of Nursing. "Based on this initial response, it's obvious that the most effective marketing tool is the program itself."

Many universities offer both accelerated baccalaureate and generic master's programs with opportunities for students to apply credits to both degree programs. New York University, for example, offers a dual-degree program that enables B.S.N. students to take a maximum of 9 credits at the graduate level while completing their bachelor's degree, thus accelerating the completion of an M.S.N. degree.

Education-Practice Setting Partnerships

Nurse employers recognize the value and skills second-degree students bring to the work setting as evidenced by the growing number of partnerships forming to support these graduates. "Our cooperative relationship with Poudre Valley Hospital brings the educational and practice settings closer together with clinical nurses at the hospital serving in faculty roles," explained Sandra Baird, Ed.D., B.S.N., Director of the School of Nursing at the University of Northern Colorado. The school is working to branch out and establish cooperative relationships with a wider network of health-care settings.

"Second-degree students are very attractive for any health-care institution, and many are willing to fund them in exchange for work commitments after graduation," said Cynthia Glawe Mailloux, Chair of the Nursing Department at Misericordia University. Although Creighton University in Nebraska is a private institution with a significantly higher tuition than public institutions, the reputation of its program led two Omaha health systems and four rural hospitals to offer full-tuition scholarships to accelerated nursing students in exchange for employment commitments. "Over half of the students in the accelerated baccalaureate program accepted tuition scholarships from area hospitals in return for a commitment to work in basic practice prior to going on for a master's degree," added Linda Cronenwett, Ph.D., RN, FAAN, Beerstecher-Blackwell Term Professor and Dean Emeritus of the School of Nursing at University of North Carolina–Chapel Hill.

Research College of Nursing uses both grant-funded initiatives and clinical connections to build student capacity. "Recently we received a $100,000 grant from the Helene Fuld Health Trust to support financial aid for our accelerated students," said Dean Nancy DeBasio. "Fuld had never supported this type of student before, but we were able to demonstrate that these students were economically disadvantaged, not always eligible for traditional undergraduate funding, and unable to work due to the program's intensity." The school also partners with a local health-care system to secure educational debt repayment for accelerated students in exchange for work commitments. It is projected that this arrangement will save the health system more than $3 million in nurse recruitment costs over three years.

Nursing Education in the Fast Lane

Though accelerated programs have proven to produce highly qualified nurses, the programs do present some unique challenges to nursing education. "Teaching accelerated students can be challenging because of their experience, age, and high level of inquiry," said Mary E. Pike, M.S.N., RN, faculty member at Bellarmine University in Kentucky. "Some students struggle with the transition from being a competent, worldly adult to returning to life as an undergraduate student." One key to facilitating this transition and encouraging student success is using experienced faculty members who are comfortable teaching adults.

In instances where employers are not repaying educational debt, the cost of an accelerated program can be prohibitive. "I receive many inquiries about our accelerated program, but the lack of financial aid is the major deterrent," said Arlene G. Wiens, Ph.D., RN, Nursing Department Chair at Eastern Mennonite University in Virginia.

Some find the pace of accelerated programs to be too intense and opt for more regularly paced programs offered for second-degree nursing students. "The accelerated format is taxing, and some find it too difficult to assimilate into their daily routines," said Louann Zinsmeister, D.N.Sc., M.S.N., RN, instructor at Messiah College in Pennsylvania. "These students often transfer into a more traditionally paced two-year B.S.N. program that permits them to continue working and attend to family responsibilities while completing a nursing degree."

For students who cannot accommodate full-time study, schools are looking for creative alternatives. "We are opening a part-time evening program so second-degree students and adult learners can obtain a degree while working full-time," added Cynthia Glawe Mailloux of Misericordia University. "Students attend classes two nights a week and are still able to obtain a nursing degree in two years and one semester."

Post-Graduation Success

In addition to nursing skills, second-degree students bring additional layers of education and significant work experience to their role as nurses, which enhances their clinical practice. "Initially when we began our program in 1991, our clinical partners were quite doubtful about what we could produce in one year," explained Dr. DeBasio of the Research College of Nursing. "Now they are at our doorstep each year to snap up students as they graduate." The College has tracked students through their careers and found that accelerated students move into management positions more quickly and generally excel in their roles.

"Employers of advanced practice nurses (APN) are equally pleased with graduates from both our traditional and generic M.S.N. programs," stated Linda D. Norman, D.S.N., RN, Senior Associate Dean for Academics at Vanderbilt University School of Nursing. Employers rated Vanderbilt's M.S.N. graduates who did not have a nursing background equally high in terms of level of preparation for APN positions as those who entered with a B.S.N. degree.

"We know that employers love hiring accelerated graduates because they are bright, have a track record of success, and possess an understanding of the work world not always found in younger students," said Patricia Ladewig, Ph.D., RN, Dean of the School of Health Care Professions at Regis University in Denver. "We have found that second-degree students are readily accepted by employers who understand that these graduates lacked only vacation during their academic program," confirmed Sandra S. Angell, M.L.A., RN, Associate Dean for Student Affairs at The Johns Hopkins University School of Nursing.

Growing Demand for Accelerated Programs

With a greater number of second-degree students turning to nursing, the demand for accelerated programs is growing. At the University of Pennsylvania, application trends over the past six years showed a 34 percent increase. "Within two weeks of the program's approval by the state board and without any public announcement, we received more than 50 requests for applications almost immediately," explained Marianne W. Rogers, Ed.D., RN, Chairperson for Nursing at the University of Southern Maine.

"Our program is growing very quickly, and we have seen almost a 100 percent increase in applications compared to last year," said Linda A. Bernhard, Ph.D., RN, Associate Dean for Undergraduate Studies at The Ohio State University. The 16-month Second Career/Second Degree program in nursing at Wayne State University in Michigan experienced a 25 percent increase in enrollment from Fall 2000 to Fall 2001, making it one of the school's most popular degree offerings. Enrollment in the University of Virginia's second-degree program has doubled since it was introduced in 1988.

"At this time, we are seeing an enormous increase in the numbers of applicants with bachelor's degrees applying for our new 12-month accelerated pathway to the B.S.N.," reports Christena Langley, Ph.D., RN, Assistant Dean for Undergraduate Programs at the College of Nursing and Health Science at George Mason University in Virginia. "Many of them are recent college graduates who are looking for the quickest route to the B.S.N. They are confident that they can adapt to the accelerated pace given their past success in college."

Supporting Accelerated Nursing Programs

Second-degree students bring a wealth of knowledge, experience, and energy to the nursing workforce and are highly skilled clinicians. With calls for nursing schools to produce more graduates in response to the nursing shortage, a similar call should go out to employers and legislators to increase support for accelerated nursing programs.

Hospitals, health-care systems, and other practice settings are encouraged to form partnerships with schools offering accelerated programs to remove the student's financial burden in exchange for a steady stream of new nurse recruits. Legislators on the state and federal levels are encouraged to increase scholarship and grant funding for these programs that produce entry-level nurses faster than any other basic nursing education program. These programs are ideal career transition vehicles for those segments of the labor force impacted by recent fluctuations in the economy.

"The overwhelming response to our accelerated programs demonstrates the existence of a deep pool of career changers available to nursing," said Gloria F. Donnelly, Ph.D., RN, FAAN, Dean of the College of Nursing and Health Professions at Drexel University in Philadelphia, Pennsylvania. "We need to do more to remove barriers and attract more second-degree students to the nursing profession."

"Accelerated Programs: The Fast-Track to Careers in Nursing," updated April 2008. Reprinted with permission of the American Association of Colleges of Nursing.

THE DOCTOR OF NURSING PRACTICE (DNP)

On October 25, 2004, the member schools affiliated with the American Association of Colleges of Nursing (AACN) voted to endorse the *Position Statement on the Practice Doctorate in Nursing*. This decision called for moving the current level of preparation necessary for advanced nursing practice from the master's degree to the doctorate-level by the year 2015. This endorsement was preceded by almost three years of research and consensus-building by an AACN task force charged with examining the need for the practice doctorate with a variety of stakeholder groups.

Introducing the Doctor of Nursing Practice (DNP)

- In many institutions, advanced practice registered nurses (APRNs), including Nurse Practitioners, Clinical Nurse Specialists, Certified Nurse Mid-Wives, and Certified Nurse Anesthetists, are prepared in master's-degree programs that often carry a credit load equivalent to doctoral degrees in the other health professions. AACN's position statement calls for educating APRNs and nurses seeking top systems/organizational roles in DNP programs.

- DNP curricula build on traditional master's programs by providing education in evidence-based practice, quality improvement, and systems leadership, among other key areas.

- The DNP is designed for nurses seeking a terminal degree in nursing practice and offers an alternative to research-focused doctoral programs. DNP-prepared nurses are well-equipped to fully implement the science developed by nurse researchers prepared in PhD, DNSc, and other research-focused nursing doctorates.

Why Move to the DNP?

- The changing demands of this nation's complex health-care environment require the highest level of scientific knowledge and practice expertise to assure high-quality patient outcomes. The Institute of Medicine, Joint Commission, Robert Wood Johnson Foundation, and other authorities have called for re-conceptualizing educational programs that prepare today's health professionals.

- Some of the many factors building momentum for change in nursing education at the graduate level include: the rapid expansion of knowledge underlying practice; increased complexity of patient care; national concerns about the quality of care and patient safety; shortages of nursing personnel, which demands a higher level of preparation for leaders who can design and assess care; shortages of doctorally prepared nursing faculty; and increasing educational expectations for the preparation of other members of the health-care team.

- In a 2005 report titled *Advancing the Nation's Health Needs: NIH Research Training Programs*, the National Academy of Sciences called for nursing to develop a non-research clinical doctorate to prepare expert practitioners who can also serve as clinical faculty. AACN's work to advance the DNP is consistent with this call to action.

- Nursing is moving in the direction of other health professions in the transition to the DNP. Medicine (MD), Dentistry (DDS), Pharmacy (PharmD), Psychology (PsyD), Physical Therapy (DPT), and Audiology (AudD) all offer practice doctorates.

Sustaining Momentum for the DNP

- After a two-year consensus-building process, AACN member institutions voted to endorse the *Essentials of Doctoral Education for Advanced Nursing Practice* on October 30, 2006. Schools developing a DNP are encouraged to use this document, which defines the curricular elements and competencies that must be present in a practice doctorate in nursing.

- In July 2006, the AACN Board of Directors endorsed the final report of the *Task Force on the Roadmap to the DNP,* which was developed to assist schools navigating the DNP program approval process. This report includes recommendations for securing institutional approval to transition an MSN into a DNP program; preparing faculty to teach in DNP programs; addressing regulatory, licensure, accreditation, and certification issues; and collecting evaluation data. The Roadmap report and accompanying tool kit are posted at http://www.aacn.nche.edu/dnp.

- Schools nationwide that have initiated the DNP are reporting sizable and competitive student enrollment. Employers are quickly recognizing the unique contribution these expert nurses are making in the practice arena, and the demand for DNP-prepared nurses continues to grow. According to the 2009 salary survey conducted by *ADVANCE for Nurse Practitioners* magazine, DNP-prepared NPs earned $7,688 more than master's-prepared NPs.

- The Commission on Collegiate Nursing Education (CCNE), the leading accrediting agency for baccalaureate- and graduate-degree nursing programs in the United States, began accrediting DNP programs in fall of 2008. To date, 116 DNP programs have been accredited by CCNE.

Current DNP Program Statistics

- 184 DNP programs are currently enrolling students at schools of nursing nationwide, and an additional 101 DNP programs are in the planning stages.

- DNP programs are now available in 40 states plus the District of Columbia. States with the most programs (more than 5) include Florida, Massachusetts, Minnesota, New York, Pennsylvania, and Texas.

- From 2010 to 2011, the number of students enrolled in DNP programs increased from 7,034 to 9,094. During that same period, the number of DNP graduates increased from 1,282 to 1,595.

THE NURSE PH.D.: A VITAL PROFESSION NEEDS LEADERS

Carole Anderson
Former Dean of the College of Dentistry
The Ohio State University
Past President, American Association of Colleges of Nursing

There is no doubt that education is the path for a nurse to achieve greater clinical expertise. At the same time, however, the nursing profession needs more nurses educated at the doctoral level to replenish the supply of faculty and researchers. The national shortage of faculty will soon reach critical proportions, making a significant impact on educational programs and their capacity to educate future generations of nursing students.

Although the number of doctorate programs has continued to increase, the total enrollment of students in these programs has remained fairly constant, resulting in a shortage of newly trained Ph.D.'s to renew faculty ranks. As a result, approximately 50 percent of nursing faculty possess the doctorate as a terminal degree. Furthermore, with many advances being made in the treatment of chronic illnesses, there is a continuing need for research that assists patients in living with their illness. This research requires individual investigators who are prepared on the doctoral level.

One reason there is a lack of nurses prepared at the doctoral level is that, compared to other professions, nurses have more interruptions in their careers. Many in the profession are women who work as nurses while fulfilling responsibilities as wives and mothers. As a result, many pursue their education on a part-time basis. Also, the nursing profession traditionally has viewed clinical experience as being a prerequisite to graduate education. This career path results in fewer individuals completing the doctorate at an earlier stage in their career, thereby truncating their productivity as academics, researchers, and administrators. To reverse this trend, many nursing schools have developed programs that admit students into graduate (doctoral and master's) programs directly from their undergraduate or master's programs.

Nursing Research

When nurses do research for their doctorates, many people tend to think that it focuses primarily on nurses and nursing care. In reality, nurses carry out clinical research in a variety of areas, such as diabetes care, cancer care, and eating disorders.

In the last twenty years advances in medicine have involved, for the most part, advancing treatment, not cures. In other words, no cure for the illness has been discovered, but treatment for that illness has improved. However, sometimes the treatment itself causes problems for patients, such as the unwelcome side effects of chemotherapy. Nurses have opportunities to devise solutions to problems like these through research, such as studies on how to manage the illness and its treatment, thereby allowing individuals to lead happy and productive lives.

The Curricula

Doctoral programs in nursing are aimed at preparing students for careers in health administration, education, clinical research, and advanced clinical practice. Basically, doctoral programs prepare nurses to be experts within the profession, prepared to assume leadership roles in a variety of academic and clinical settings, course work, and research. Students are trained as researchers and scholars to tackle complex health-care questions. Program emphasis may vary from a focus on health education to a concentration on policy research. The majority of doctoral programs confer the Doctor of Philosophy (Ph.D.) degree, but some award the Doctor of Nursing Science (D.N.S. or D.N.Sc.), the Doctor of Science in Nursing (D.S.N.), the Nursing Doctorate (N.D.), and the Doctor of Education (Ed.D.).

Doctoral nursing programs traditionally offer courses on the history and philosophy of nursing and the development and testing of nursing and other health-care techniques, as well as the social, economic, political, and ethical issues important to the field. Data management and research methodology are also areas of instruction. Students are expected to work individually on research projects and complete a dissertation.

Doctoral programs allow study on a full-or part-time basis. For graduate students who are employed and therefore seek flexibility in their schedules, many programs offer courses on weekends and in the evenings.

Admission Requirements

Admission requirements for doctoral programs vary. Generally, a master's degree is necessary, but in some schools a master's degree is completed in conjunction with fulfillment of the doctoral degree requirements. Standard requirements include an RN license, Graduate Record Examinations (GRE) scores, college transcripts, letters of recommendation, and an essay. Students applying for doctoral-level study should have a solid foundation in nursing and an interest in research. Programs are usually the equivalent of three to five years of full-time study.

Selecting a Doctoral Program

Selecting a doctoral program comes down to personal choice. Students work closely with professors, and thus the support and mentoring you receive while pursuing your degree is as vital as the quality of the facilities. The most important question is whether there is a "match" between your research interest and faculty research. Many of the same questions you would ask about baccalaureate and master's degree programs apply to doctoral programs. However, in a doctoral program, the contact with professors, the use of research equipment and facilities, and the program's flexibility in allowing you to choose your course of study are critical.

Other questions to consider include: Does the university consider research a priority? Does the university have adequate funding for student research? Many nurses with doctoral degrees make the natural transition into an academic career, but there are many other career options available for nurses prepared at this level. For example, nurses prepared at the doctoral level are often hired by large consulting firms to work with others in designing solutions to health-care delivery problems.

Others are hired by large hospital chains to manage various divisions, and some nurses with doctoral degrees are hired to manage complex health-care systems at the executive level. On another front, they conduct research and formulate national and international health-care policy. In short, because of the high level of education and a shortage of nurses prepared at this level, there are a number of options.

Needless to say, a doctoral education does provide individuals with a wide range of opportunities, with salaries commensurate with the type and level of responsibilities. Are there opportunities to present research findings at professional meetings? Is scholarship of faculty, alumni, and students presented at regional and national nursing meetings and subsequently published? Has the body of research done at a university enhanced the knowledge of nursing and health care?

Salaries are related to the various positions. Faculty salaries vary by the type of institution and by faculty rank, typically ranging from approximately $50,000 at the assistant professor level to above $100,000 at the professor level. Salaries of nurse executives also vary, with the lowest salaries being in small rural hospitals and the highest being in complex university medical centers. In the latter, average salaries are well above $100,000 and often reach close to $200,000 annually. Consultant salaries are wide-ranging but often consist of a base plus some percentage of work contracted. Clinical and research positions vary considerably by the type of institution and the nature of the work.

AACN INDICATORS OF QUALITY IN RESEARCH-FOCUSED DOCTORAL PROGRAMS IN NURSING

Schools of nursing must consider the indicators of quality in evaluating their ability to mount research-focused doctoral programs. High-quality programs require a large number of increasingly scarce resources and a critical mass of faculty members and students. The "AACN Indicators of Quality in Research-Focused Doctoral Programs in Nursing" represent those indicators that should be present in a research-focused program.

There is considerable consensus within the discipline that while there are differences in the purpose and curricula of Ph.D. and Doctor of Nursing/Doctor of Nursing Science programs; most programs emphasize preparation for research. Therefore, AACN recommends continuing with a single set of quality indicators for research-focused doctoral programs in nursing, whether the program leads to a Ph.D. or to a Doctor of Nursing or Doctor of Nursing Science degree.

The following indicators apply to the Doctor of Philosophy (Ph.D.) in nursing, Doctor of Nursing Science (D.N.S. or D.N.Sc.), and Doctor of Nursing (N.D.) degrees.

Faculty

I. Represent and value a diversity of backgrounds and intellectual perspectives.

II. Meet the requirements of the parent institution for graduate research and doctoral education; a substantial proportion of faculty hold earned doctorates in nursing.

III. Conceptualize and implement productive programs of research and scholarship that are developed over time and build upon previous work, are at the cutting edge of the field of inquiry, are congruent with research priorities within nursing and its constituent communities, include a substantial proportion of extramural funding, and attract and engage students.

IV. Create an environment in which mentoring, socialization of students, and the existence of a community of scholars is evident.

V. Assist students in understanding the value of programs of research and scholarship that continue over time and build upon previous work.

VI. Identify, generate, and utilize resources within the university and the broader community to support program goals.

VII. Devote a significant proportion of time to dissertation advisement. Generally, each faculty member should serve as the major adviser/chair for no more than 3 to 5 students during the dissertation phase.

Programs of Study

The emphasis of the program of study is consistent with the mission of the parent institution, the discipline of nursing, and the degree awarded. The faculty's areas of expertise and scholarship determine specific foci in the program of study. Requirements and their sequence for progression in the program are clear and available to students in writing. Common elements of the program of study are outlined below.

I. Core and related course content—the distribution between nursing and supporting content is consistent with the mission and goals of the program, and the student's area of focus and course work are included in the following:

A. Historical and philosophical foundations to the development of nursing knowledge

B. Existing and evolving substantive nursing knowledge

C. Methods and processes of theory/knowledge development

D. Research methods and scholarship appropriate to inquiry

E. Development related to roles in academic, research, practice, or policy environments

II. Elements for formal and informal teaching and learning focus on the following:

A. Analytical and leadership strategies for dealing with social, ethical, cultural, economic, and political issues related to nursing, health care, and research

B. Progressive and guided student scholarship

research experiences, including exposure to faculty's interdisciplinary research programs

C. Immersion experiences that foster the student's development as a nursing leader, scholarly practitioner, educator, and/or nurse scientist

D. Socialization opportunities for scholarly development in roles that complement students' career goals

III. Outcome indicators for the programs of study include the following:

A. Advancement to candidacy requires faculty's satisfactory evaluation (e.g., comprehensive exam) of the student's basic knowledge of elements I-A through I-E identified above

B. Dissertations represent original contributions to the scholarship of the field

C. Systematic evaluation of graduate outcomes is conducted at regular intervals

D. Within three to five years of completion, graduates have designed and secured funding for a research study, or, within two years of completion, graduates have utilized the research process to address an issue of importance to the discipline of nursing or health care within their employment setting

E. Employers report satisfaction with graduates' leadership and scholarship at regular intervals

F. Graduates' scholarship and leadership are recognized through awards, honors, or external funding within three to five years of completion

Resources

I. Sufficient human, financial, and institutional resources are available to accomplish the goals of the unit for doctoral education and faculty research.

A. The parent institution exhibits the following characteristics:

1) Research is an explicit component of the mission of the parent institution

2) An office of research administration

3) A record of peer-reviewed external funding

4) Postdoctoral programs

5) Internal research funds

6) Mechanisms that value, support, and reward faculty and student scholarship and role preparation

7) A university environment that fosters interdisciplinary research and collaboration

B. The nursing doctoral program exhibits the following characteristics:

1) Research-active faculty as well as other faculty experts to mentor students in other role preparations

2) Provide technical support for the following:

(a) Peer review of proposals and manuscripts in their development phases

(b) Research design expertise

(c) Data management and analysis support

(d) Hardware and software availability

(e) Expertise in grant proposal development and management

3) Procure space sufficient for the following:

(a) Faculty research needs

(b) Doctoral student study, meeting, and socializing

(c) Seminars

(d) Small-group work

C. Schools of exceptional quality also have the following:

1) Centers of research excellence

2) Endowed professorships

3) Mechanisms for financial support to allow full-time study

4) Master teachers capable of preparing graduates for faculty roles

II. State-of-the-art technical and support services are available and accessible to faculty, students, and staff for state-of-the-science information acquisition, communication, and management.

III. Library and database resources are sufficient to support the scholarly endeavors of faculty and students.

Students

I. Students are selected from a pool of highly qualified and motivated applicants who represent diverse populations.

II. Students' research goals and objectives are congruent with faculty research expertise and scholarship and institutional resources.

III. Students are successful in obtaining financial support through competitive intramural and extramural academic and research awards.

IV. Students commit a significant portion of their time to the program and complete the program in a timely fashion.

V. Students establish a pattern of productive scholarship, collaborating with researchers in nursing and other disciplines in scientific endeavors that result in the presentation and publication of scholarly work that continues after graduation.

Evaluation

The evaluation plan includes the following:

I.   Is systematic, ongoing, comprehensive, and focuses on the university's and program's specific mission and goals.

II. Includes both process and outcome data related to these indicators of quality in research-focused doctoral programs.

III. Adheres to established ethical and process standards for formal program evaluation, e.g., confidentiality and rigorous quantitative and qualitative analyses.

IV. Involves students and graduates in evaluation activities.

V.   Includes data from a variety of internal and external constituencies.

VI. Provides for comparison of program processes and outcomes to the standards of its parent graduate school/university and selected peer groups within nursing.

VII. Includes ongoing feedback to program faculty, administrators, and external constituents to promote program improvement.

VIII. Provides comprehensive data in order to determine patterns and trends and recommend future directions at regular intervals.

IX. Is supported with adequate human, financial, and institutional resources.

Approved by AACN Membership, November 2001.

WHAT YOU NEED TO KNOW ABOUT ONLINE LEARNING

Rosalee C. Yeaworth, Ph.D., RN, FAAN
Professor and Dean Emerita
College of Nursing
University of Nebraska Medical Center

Sue Schmidt, M.A. in Education and Human Development
Instructional Chair
Colorado Mountain College

Half a century ago, young women who graduated from high school and chose to enter a nursing program were expected to move into a "nurses' home," which housed not only dormitory-style rooms but also classrooms and faculty offices. Most of the clinical learning was done in apprenticeship style in a single hospital setting. There was no such thing as distance learning.

However, over the course of the past half-century, nursing education, like health care and education in general, has changed dramatically, creating a need for educators to implement distance education programs. The demographics of nursing students have changed. Not only is the nursing student far more likely to be a man than fifty years ago, but also the student who once was referred to as "nontraditional" is now becoming the traditional student. These students are mature, employed individuals who have complex family responsibilities and often live or work some distance from the university offering the courses they wish to take. The rapid advances in health-care knowledge and technology have increased the demand for nurses with graduate degrees. All nurses are faced with the need to enhance their knowledge through lifelong education as their roles and expectations change. In addition, a much greater effort is being made to provide education and training to residents in rural settings in the hope that they will continue to live and work in these areas.

Universities are addressing these changing educational needs by using advanced technologies and new communication capabilities. Distance learning offerings are continually enhanced by using new technologies and delivery systems such as the Internet and desktop videoconferencing. These technologies enable universities to reach beyond the boundaries imposed on them by traditional classrooms to deliver educational material to students located in different, noncentralized locations, thus allowing instruction and learning to occur independently of time and place. This model, known as "distributive learning," can be used in combination with traditional classroom-based courses and with traditional distance learning courses, or to create wholly virtual classrooms.

Tools used for distance education include the following:

E-mail: This is one of the most commonly used communication tools. It allows for a one-to-one exchange of information between the sender and receiver of the e-mail message. Course papers and draft materials may be sent, commented on, and returned as attached documents.

Listservs: This is a one-to-many communication exchange. People subscribe to listservs based on discussion topics that interest them. When a participant on a listserv sends an e-mail to the listserv, the message is copied and sent to all people who have subscribed to it. Listservs are generally free; there is no charge to subscribe.

Discussion Groups: This is a many-to-many communication exchange. E-mail and listservs deliver the messages directly to your electronic mailbox. Discussion groups, on the other hand, are retained in a specified area on the Internet. You must go to the discussion group to post your comments and read and reply to the comments of others. The advantage of a discussion group over e-mail or listservs is that the comments can be viewed easily by all and the sequence of comments and replies posted is readily apparent in its structure.

Chat Rooms: Chat is synchronous communication; the participants are online at the same time talking to each other. E-mail, listservs, and discussion groups, on the other hand, are asynchronous communication. With moderated chat, a moderator views the questions and comments posed by the participants and selects those that will be seen by all participants. After posting the comment or question, the moderator answers it. In a regular chat room, there is no management over what is or is not posted.

Streaming Video: Entire lectures can be delivered using streaming video technology. Even students accessing the material with slower modems can receive clear audio and good video images.

Desktop Videoconferencing: With a small camera mounted on top of the computer, students and faculty members are able to see and talk with each other using desktop videoconferencing software.

Virtual Reality: Student lounges can be constructed visually using virtual reality software. When students want to have a discussion with other students, they literally walk into the lounge as an avatar (a visual image of themselves they have selected) and hold live chat sessions with their fellow classmates.

Web Sites: Components of or the entire course content can be delivered via the Internet through the creation of a Web site. Any or all of the technology tools noted above can be linked through an educational Web site. Among other things, a Web site includes the syllabus, discussion groups, assignments, student lounges, faculty information, resources (including links to Web documents that enrich the course content), lecture notes, and other course components. Traditional distance education tools, such as satellite transmission, videotapes, telephone conferences, correspondence material, and CD-ROM interactive instruction, are also frequently used in conjunction with Web-delivered course material.

The key to using technology successfully is to define your goals and objectives and then decide which technology or combination of technologies will be most effective. Keep in mind that faculty members and students must have the appropriate computer equipment and user knowledge to participate in distance learning.

Even though computers today are much more user-friendly, it is important to allot some time for students to become accustomed to using the new technologies necessary for transmitting their course material. Campus information technology services should work closely with the faculty to prepare introductory manuals or self-help materials for students. Information technology specialists should be available to answer technology questions or solve problems so that faculty members can concentrate on the course content questions. Enthusiasm can be dampened if too much time must be devoted to learning the technology or dealing with technology problems.

When deciding to take distance-learning courses, other factors must be considered. What you need to participate in distance learning varies with the sophistication of the tools used by the course instructor. Sending and receiving e-mail, participating in discussion groups, and viewing online syllabi require fairly simple technology. You need a computer with a modem and an Internet service provider (ISP). When selecting an ISP, participants should consider cost, reliability of access, and speed. World Wide Web access provided through your cable provider is generally more expensive but provides significantly faster access to documents.

Video streaming and desktop videoconferencing require more sophisticated computer systems. Sometimes, in rural areas, the local telephone company or the Internet or TV provider may provide only limited services. Students may find, for example, that they have to use a teleconference line for sound with desktop videoconferencing. It is important to investigate the technology issues in your area before undertaking a course, because technical limitations can add to the cost and decrease your satisfaction and learning.

Access to the campus bookstore and library may also be a concern for students who are at considerable distance from the school offering the course. Books and supplies may be ordered online from the bookstore, and journal articles can be made available from the library through electronic reserve. Courses that use electronic reserve usually require a fee to cover copyright costs.

Some advantages of distance learning are the following:

Student-Centered versus Instructor-Directed Learning: Students take an active role in their own learning experience. They are able to select what material they need to cover more extensively and are given the opportunity for exploration through accessing linked material provided by their instructor. They are also given more opportunity to learn at their own pace and

select the time when they are more prepared to effectively view the course material.

Flexibility: Students may work at their own computers on a weekend or the middle of the night, without having to worry about library hours or driving in bad weather. Valuable time can be focused on learning rather than on the logistics of getting to class.

Accessibility: Students who would not be able to attend classes because of geographic proximity or time constraints are now able to participate.

Student Interaction Increases: Interaction increases in a distance learning environment. Students not only listen and take notes, but they also pose ideas to and ask questions of the instructor as well as other students in discussion groups. Interaction is encouraged, and the instructor has a better understanding of what and how the student is learning. In most classroom settings, it is very difficult to get students to discuss a topic. They may ask a question of or make a comment to the instructor, but they seldom interact with classmates about course topics.

Collaboration and Team Problem Solving: Using asynchronous and synchronous communication tools, students can work together on projects much more easily. It has always been difficult to bring a group together face-to-face to discuss what needs to be done. Through these new communication channels, information can be easily passed among a group, and resources such as research documents and drafts of works in progress can be distributed instantly.

Increased Sharing of Knowledge: In the traditional classroom, the instructor is the primary source of information. In distance learning, using tools such as a discussion group, students have a greater opportunity to share their knowledge and experience, allowing the members of the group to learn from each other. In addition, access to the Internet allows students to access the experience and knowledge of others outside their immediate classroom setting.

Immediate Access to Updated Material: Any material or announcements that have been changed can be distributed instantly, reducing distribution costs and providing students with access to the most current information.

Developing Needed Technology Skills: Students are learning technology skills that they can apply later in their work setting.

Some important factors should be considered when deciding whether a distance education model is right for you. It has been shown that students can learn course content by distance methods as well as or better than in the traditional classroom setting. Less information is available on socialization issues related to the nurse generalist, specialist, or practitioner roles. Socialization involves internalizing attitudes, values, and norms. The role modeling, mentoring, and collegial friendships may or may not be as adaptable to distance methods. Careful selection of clinical settings for experience, on-site preceptors, requirements for certain on-campus experiences, and group attendance of students and faculty members at regional or national meetings are some methods used to assist socialization.

Distance learning will not suffice for the "college experience" of joining sororities and fraternities and of participating in athletic and social activities that many young undergraduate students desire. On the other hand, for the adult learner with job and family responsibilities, the distance education methodologies can provide the opportunity to participate in educational experiences that might otherwise have been beyond consideration.

When selecting your educational program, you should clearly define your goals for your educational experiences. If you want to have clinical experience in a particular setting, to be a research or teaching assistant to a certain person, or to be mentored by a selected expert, then your choice would be an on-site educational environment in a particular setting. However, if you want a degree from a particular institution but do not want to move or travel there, explore the distance learning opportunities offered. You need to remember that it is not an either-or proposition. You may be able to combine traditional classroom-based courses with distance learning for selected courses to optimize your overall educational program.

Distance learning is used by more and more educational institutions to provide both degree and continuing education. Many schools collaborate to offer students a selection of courses taught by different colleges and universities. A recent collaborative effort is the Western Governors University, a virtual university that is a partnership involving eighteen states and approximately 100 participating colleges and universities.

As noted above, the world is changing and so is the way we deliver nursing education. Distance education has opened a world of opportunities to students and faculty members. Students now have the ability to further their education by removing many of the time and access barriers they previously faced. Faculty members are presented with new and exciting challenges as they begin to use innovative technologies in their course delivery. With careful consideration and planning, the outcome will enhance the overall learning experience of both learner and teacher.

THE INTERNATIONAL NURSING STUDENT

For many international students completing baccalaureate, master's, or doctoral nursing programs, their choice of learning institutions is obvious. U.S. and Canadian colleges and universities are thought to offer the finest programs of nursing education available anywhere in the world. U.S. and Canadian nursing programs are renowned for their breadth and flexibility, for the excellence of their basic curriculum structure, and for their commitment to extensive on-site clinical training. Nursing study in the United States and Canada also affords students the opportunity for hands-on learning and practice in the world's most technologically advanced health-care systems. For many international nursing students, and especially for students from countries that are medically underserved, these features make U.S. and Canadian nursing programs unsurpassed.

Applying to Nursing School

The application process for international students often involves the completion of two separate written applications. Many colleges screen international candidates with a brief preliminary application requesting basic biographical and educational information. This document helps the admission officer determine whether the student has the minimum credentials for admission before requiring him or her to begin the lengthy process of completing and submitting final application forms.

Final applications to U.S. and Canadian colleges and universities vary widely in length and complexity, just as specific admission requirements vary from institution to institution. However, international nursing students must typically have a satisfactory scholastic record and demonstrated proficiency in English. To be admitted to any postsecondary institution in the United States or Canada, you must have satisfactorily completed a minimum of twelve years of elementary and secondary education. The customary cycle for this education includes a six-year elementary program, a three-year intermediate program, and a three-year postsecondary program, generally referred to as high school in the United States. In addition, nursing school programs generally require successful completion of several years of high school-level mathematics and science.

The documentation of satisfactory completion of secondary schooling (and university education, in the case of graduate-level applicants) is achieved through submission of school reports, transcripts, and teacher recommendations. Because academic records and systems of evaluation differ widely from one educational system to the next, request that your school include a guide to grading standards. If you have received your secondary education at a school in which English is not the language of instruction, be certain to include official translations of all documents.

International students who have completed some university-level course work in their native country may be eligible to receive credit for equivalent courses at the U.S. or Canadian institution in which they enroll. Under special circumstances, practical nursing experience may also qualify for university credit. Policies regarding the transfer of or qualification for credits based on education or nursing experience outside the United States (or Canada for Canadian schools) vary widely, so be certain to inquire about these policies at the universities or colleges that interest you.

Language skills are a key to scholastic success. "The ability to speak, write, and understand English is an important determinant of success," says Joann Weiss, former Director of the Nursing and Latin American Studies dual-degree programs at the University of New Mexico in Albuquerque. Her advice for potential international applicants is simple: "Develop a true command of written and spoken English." English proficiency for students who have not received formal education in English-speaking schools is usually demonstrated via the Test of English as a Foreign Language (TOEFL); minimum test scores of 550 to 580 are commonly required. This policy, as well as the level of proficiency required, varies from school to school, so be sure to investigate each college's policies.

In addition, most universities offer some form of English language instruction for international students, often under the rubric ESL (English as a second language). Students who require additional language study to meet admission requirements or students who wish to deepen their skills in written or verbal English should inquire about ESL program availability.

Many colleges and universities also require that all undergraduate applicants take a standardized test—either the SAT and three SAT Subject Tests or the ACT. Like their U.S. and Canadian counterparts, international applicants to graduate-level nursing programs are required by most institutions to take the standardized Graduate Record Examinations (GRE).

Applicants should also be aware that financial assistance for international students is usually quite limited. To spare international students economic hardship during their schooling in the United States or Canada, many colleges and universities require them to demonstrate the availability of sufficient financial resources for tuition and minimum living expenses and supplies. As with so many admission requirements, policies regarding financial aid vary considerably; find out early what the policies are at the colleges that interest you.

Attending School in the United States or Canada

Once you are accepted by the college or university of your choice, take full advantage of the academic and personal advising systems offered to international students. Most institutions of higher education in the United States and Canada maintain an international student advisory office staffed with trained counselors. In addition to general academic counseling and planning, an international adviser can assist in a broad range of matters ranging from immigration and visa concerns to employment opportunities and health-care issues.

With few exceptions, all university students also obtain specialized academic counseling from an assigned faculty adviser. Faculty advisers monitor academic performance and progress and try to ensure that students meet the institutional requirements for their degree. Faculty advisers are excellent sources of information regarding course selection, and some advisers offer tutorials or special language or educational support to international students.

Although all university students face academic challenges, international students often find life outside the classroom equally demanding. Suddenly introduced into a new culture where the way of life may be dramatically different from that of their native country, international students often face a variety of social, domestic, medical, religious, or emotional concerns. Questions about social conventions, meal preparation, or other personal concerns can often be addressed by your international or faculty adviser.

Lorraine Rudowski, Assistant Professor and Coordinator of the International Health Program at the College of Health and Human Services at George Mason University in Fairfax, Virginia, emphasizes the benefits of a strong relationship with your advisers: "My job as an adviser is to provide comprehensive support to my students—from academic counseling and opportunities for language development to emotional support and guidance to attending parties or other informal social events to ease the sense of social and personal isolation often experienced by foreign students."

Dr. Rudowski says that international students would do well to find a sponsor or confidant within the university who understands the conventions of the student's native country. "A culturally sensitive sponsor is better equipped to understand the unique needs of each international student and is much more likely to help students obtain the assistance they need, whether we're talking about religious issues, help with study methods or social skills, or simply knowing how to deal with such everyday chores as cooking and cleaning. All of these matters can be sources of deep concern to international students."

Yet for all the academic, social, and personal challenges facing international nursing students, there is good news. Deans of nursing, professors, and advisers typically praise the motivation and determination of their international students, and international nursing students often boast matriculation rates that match or exceed those of their U.S. and Canadian counterparts.

For more information about the rules and regulations governing international students' entrance to U.S. schools, log on to educationUSA, part of the U.S. Department of State's Web site, at http:// educationusa.state.gov.

SPECIALTY NURSING ORGANIZATIONS

Academy of Medical-Surgical Nurses
East Holly Avenue
Box 56
Pitman, NJ 08071-0056
866-877-AMSN (2676) (toll-free)
E-mail: amsn@ajj.com
www.amsn.org

Air & Surface Transport Nurses Association
7995 East Prentice Avenue
Suite 100
Greenwood Village, CO 80111
800-897-NFNA (6362) (toll-free)
Fax: 303-770-1614
E-mail: astna@gwami.com
www.astna.org

American Academy of Ambulatory Care Nursing
East Holly Avenue
Box 56
Pitman, NJ 08071-0056
800-262-6877 (toll-free)
E-mail: aaacn@ajj.com
www.aaacn.org

American Association of Critical-Care Nurses
101 Columbia
Aliso Viejo, CA 92656-4109
949-362-2000
800-899-AACN (2226) (toll-free)
E-mail: info@aacn.org
www.aacn.org

American Association of Diabetes Educators
200 West Madison Street
Suite 800
Chicago, IL 60606
800-338-3633 (toll-free)
Fax: 312-424-2427
E-mail: education@aadenet.org
www.aadenet.org

American Association of Legal Nurse Consultants
330 N. Wabash Avenue
Chicago, IL 60611
877-402-2562 (toll-free)
Fax: 312-673-6655
E-mail: info@aalnc.org
www.aalnc.org

American Association of Neuroscience Nurses
4700 West Lake Avenue
Glenview, IL 60025
847-375-4733
888-557-2266 (toll-free in the U.S. only)
Fax: 847-375-6430
E-mail: info@aann.org
www.aann.org

American Association of Nurse Anesthetists
222 South Prospect Avenue
Park Ridge, IL 60068-4037
847-692-7050
Fax: 847-692-6968
E-mail: info@aana.com
www.aana.com

The American Association of Nurse Attorneys
3416 Primm Lane
Birmingham, AL 35216
205-824-7615
877-538-2262 (toll-free)
Fax: 205-823-2760
E-mail: taana@primemanagement.net

American Association of Occupational Health Nurses, Inc.
7794 Grow Drive
Pensacola, FL 32514
850-474-6963
800-241-8014 (toll-free)
Fax: 850-484-8762
E-mail: aaohn@dancyamc.com
www.aaohn.org

American College of Nurse-Midwives
8403 Colesville Road
Suite 1550
Silver Spring, MD 20910
240-485-1800
Fax: 240-485-1818
www.midwife.org

American College of Nurse Practitioners
225 Reinekers Lane
Suite 525
Alexandria, VA 22314
703-740-2529
Fax: 703-740-2533
E-mail: acnp@acnpweb.org
www.acnpweb.org

American Holistic Nurses Association
100 SE 9th Street
Suite 3A
Topeka, KS 66612-1213
785-234-1712
800-278-2462 (toll-free)
Fax: 785-234-1713
E-mail: info@ahna.org
www.ahna.org

American Nephrology Nurses' Association
East Holly Avenue
Box 56
Pitman, NJ 08071-0056
856-256-2320
888-600-2662 (toll-free)
Fax: 856-589-7463
E-mail: anna@ajj.com
www.annanurse.org

American Psychiatric Nurses Association
3141 Fairview Park Drive
Suite 625
Falls Church, VA 22042
855-863-APNA (2762)
571-533-1919
www.apna.org

American Public Health Association
800 I Street, NW
Washington, DC 20001-3710
202-777-APHA
Fax: 202-777-2534
E-mail: comments@apha.org
www.apha.org

American Society for Pain Management Nursing
P.O. Box 15473
Lenexa, KS 66285-5473
888-34ASPMN (toll-free)
913-895-4606
Fax: 913-895-4652
E-mail: aspmn@goamp.com
www.aspmn.org

American Society of Ophthalmic Registered Nurses
P.O. Box 193030
San Francisco, CA 94119-3030
415-561-8513
Fax: 415-561-8531
E-mail: asorn@aao.org
http://www.asorn.org/

American Society of PeriAnesthesia Nurses
90 Frontage Road
Cherry Hill, NJ 08034-1424
877-737-9696 (toll-free)
Fax: 856-616-9601
E-mail: aspan@aspan.org
www.aspan.org

American Society of Plastic Surgical Nurses
500 Cummings Center
Suite 4550
Beverly, MA 01915
877-337-9315 (toll-free)
Fax: 978-524-8890
www.aspsn.org

Association for Death Education and Counseling
111 Deer Lake Road
Suite 100
Deerfield, IL 60015
847-509-0403
Fax: 847-480-9282
E-mail: info@adec.org
www.adec.org

Association for Professionals in Infection Control and Epidemiology, Inc.
1275 K Street, NW
Suite 1000
Washington, DC 20005-4006
202-789-1890
Fax: 202-789-1899
E-mail: info@apic.org
www.apic.org

Association for Radiologic & Imaging Nursing (ARIN)
7794 Grow Drive
Pensacola, FL 32514
866-486-2762 (toll-free)
850-474-7292
Fax: 850-484-8762
E-mail: arin@dancyamc.com
www.arinursing.org

Association of Nurses in AIDS Care
3538 Ridgewood Road
Akron, OH 44333-3122
800-260-6780 (toll-free)
330-670-0101
Fax: 330-670-0109
E-mail: anac@anacnet.org
www.anacnet.org

Association of Pediatric Hematology/Oncology Nurses
4700 West Lake Avenue
Glenview, IL 60025-1485
847-375-4724
Fax: 847-375-6478
E-mail: info@aphon.org
www.aphon.org

Association of Perioperative Registered Nurses
2170 South Parker Road
Suite 400
Denver, CO 80231
800-755-2676 (toll-free)
303-755-6300
Fax: 800-847-0045 (toll-free)
E-mail: custsvc@aorn.org
www.aorn.org

Association of Rehabilitation Nurses
4700 West Lake Avenue
Glenview, IL 60025
800-229-7530 (toll-free)
E-mail: info@rehabnurse.org
www.rehabnurse.org

Association of Women's Health, Obstetric and Neonatal Nurses
2000 L Street, NW
Suite 740
Washington, DC 20036
202-261-2400
800-673-8499 (toll-free in the U.S.)
800-245-0231 (toll-free in Canada)
Fax: 202-728-0575
E-mail: customerservice@awhonn.org
www.awhonn.org

Dermatology Nurses' Association
15000 Commerce Parkway
Suite C
Mount Laurel, NJ 08054
800-454-4362 (toll-free)
Fax: 856-439-0525
E-mail: dna@dnanurse.org
www.dnanurse.org

Developmental Disabilities Nurses Association
P.O. Box 536489
Orlando, FL 32853-6489
800-888-6733 (toll-free)
407-835-0642
Fax: 407-426-7440
www.ddna.org

Emergency Nurses Association
915 Lee Street
Des Plaines, IL 60016-6569
800-900-9659 (toll-free)
Fax: 847-460-4001
E-mail: enainfo@ena.org
www.ena.org

Hospice and Palliative Nurses Association
One Penn Center West
Suite 229
Pittsburgh, PA 15276-0100
412-787-9301
Fax: 412-787-9305
E-mail: hpna@hpna.org
www.hpna.org

Infusion Nurses Society
315 Norwood Park South
Norwood, MA 02062
781-440-9408
Fax: 781-440-9409
E-mail: ins@ins1.org
www.ins1.org

International Nurses Society on Addictions
P.O. Box 14846
Lenexa, KS 66285-4846
877-6-INTNSA (646-8672) (toll-free)
Fax: 913-895-4652
E-mail: intnsa@intnsa.org
www.intnsa.org

National Association for Home Care & Hospice
228 Seventh Street, SE
Washington, DC 20003
202-547-7424
Fax: 202-547-3540
E-mail: exec@nahc.org
www.nahc.org

National Association of Clinical Nurse Specialists
100 North 20th Street
4th Floor
Philadelphia, PA 19103
215-320-3881
Fax: 215-564-2175
E-mail: info@nacns.org
www.nacns.org

National Association of Directors of Nursing Administration/Long Term Care
11353 Reed Hartman Highway
Suite 210
Cincinnati, OH 45241
800-222-0539 (toll-free)
513-791-3679
Fax: 513-791-3699
www.nadona.org

National Association of Neonatal Nurses
4700 West Lake Avenue
Glenview, IL 60025
847-375-3660
800-451-3795 (toll-free)
Fax: 866-927-5321
E-mail: info@nann.org
www.nann.org

National Association of Nurse Practitioners in Women's Health
505 C Street, NE
Washington, DC 20002
202-543-9693, Ext. 1
E-mail: info@npwh.org
www.npwh.org

National Association of Orthopaedic Nurses
401 North Michigan Avenue
Suite 2200
Chicago, IL 60611
800-289-NAON (6266) (toll-free)
Fax: 312-673-6941
E-mail: naon@smithbucklin.com
www.orthonurse.org

National Association of Pediatric Nurse Practitioners
5 Hanover Square
Suite 1401
New York, NY 10004
917-746-8300
Fax: 212-785-1713
E-mail: info@napnap.org
www.napnap.org

National Association of School Nurses
8484 Georgia Avenue
Suite 420
Silver Spring, MD 20910
240-821-1130
E-mail: nasn@nasn.org
www.nasn.org

National Gerontological Nursing Association
3493 Lansdowne Drive
Suite 2
Lexington, KY 40517
800-723-0560 (toll-free)
859-977-7453
Fax: 859-271-0607
E-mail: info@ngna.org
www.ngna.org

National Organization of Nurse Practitioner Faculties
900 19th Street, NW
Suite 200B
Washington, DC 20006
202-289-8044
Fax: 202-384-1444
E-mail: nonpf@nonpf.org
www.nonpf.com

Oncology Nursing Society
125 Enterprise Drive
Pittsburgh, PA 15275
866-257-4ONS (4667) (toll-free)
412-859-6100
Fax: 877-369-5497 (toll-free)
E-mail: customer.service@ons.org
www.ons.org

Preventive Cardiovascular Nurses Association
613 Williamson Street
Suite 200
Madison, WI 53703
608-250-2440
E-mail: info@pcna.net
www.pcna.net

Respiratory Nursing Society
Tracy S. Estes
3816 Hawthorne Avenue
Richmond, VA 23222
E-mail: tsestes@southuniversity.edu
www.respiratorynursingsociety.org

Society for Vascular Nursing
100 Cummings Center
Suite 124A
Beverly, MA 01915
888-536-4SVN (4786) (toll-free)
978-927-7800
Fax: 978-927-7872
www.svnnet.org

Society of Gastroenterology Nurses and Associates, Inc.
330 N. Wabash Avenue
Suite 2000
Chicago, IL 60611-7621
800-245-7462 (toll-free)
312-321-5165 (in Illinois)
Fax: 312-673-6694
E-mail: sgna@smithbucklin.com
www.sgna.org

Society of Otorhinolaryngology and Head-Neck Nurses
207 Downing Street
New Smyrna Beach, FL 32168
386-428-1695
Fax: 386-423-7566
E-mail: info@sohnnurse.com
www.sohnnurse.com

Society of Urologic Nurses and Associates
East Holly Avenue
Box 56
Pitman, NJ 08071-0056
888-827-7862 (toll-free)
E-mail: suna@ajj.com
www.suna.org

Wound, Ostomy and Continence Nurses Society
15000 Commerce Parkway
Suite C
Mt. Laurel, NJ 08054
888-224-WOCN (9626) (toll-free)
Fax: 856-439-0525
E-mail: wocn_info@wocn.org
www.wocn.org

PAYING FOR YOUR NURSING EDUCATION

Whether you are considering a baccalaureate degree in nursing or have completed your undergraduate education and are planning to attend graduate school, finding a way to pay for that education is essential.

The cost to attend college is considerable and is increasing each year at a rate faster than most other products and services. In fact, the cost of a nursing education at a public four-year college can be more than $14,000 per year, including tuition, fees, books, room and board, transportation, and miscellaneous expenses. The cost at a private college or university, at either the graduate or undergraduate level, can be more than $30,000 per year.

This is where financial aid comes in. Financial aid is money made available by the government and other sources to help students who otherwise would be unable to attend college. More than $143 billion in aid is provided to students each year (College Board, *Trends in Student Aid 2008*). Most college students in this country receive some form of aid, and all prospective students should investigate what may be available. Most of this aid is given to students because neither they nor their families have sufficient personal resources to pay for college. This type of aid is referred to as need-based aid. Recipients of need-based aid include traditional students just out of high school or college and older, nontraditional students who are returning to college or graduate school.

There is also merit-based aid, which is awarded to students who display a particular ability. Merit scholarships are based primarily on academic merit, but may include other special talents. Many colleges and graduate schools offer merit-based aid in addition to need-based aid to their students.

Types and Sources of Financial Aid

There are four types of aid:

1. Scholarships
2. Grants
3. Loans
4. Student employment (including fellowships and assistantships)

Scholarships and grants are outright gifts and do not have to be repaid. Loans are borrowed money that must be repaid with interest, usually after graduation. Student employment provides jobs during the academic year for which students are paid. For graduate students, student employment may include fellowships and assistantships in which students work, receive free or reduced tuition, and may be paid a stipend for living expenses.

Most of the aid available to students is need-based and comes from the federal government through nine financial aid programs. Four of these programs are grant-based and are only available to undergraduate students:

1. Federal Pell Grants
2. Academic Competitive Grants
3. SMART Grants
4. Federal Supplemental Educational Opportunity Grants

Four are loan programs:

1. Federal Perkins Loan
2. Federal Stafford Student/Direct Loans (subsidized and unsubsidized)
3. Federal Graduate PLUS loans
4. Federal PLUS Loans

The final program is a student employment program called the Federal Work-Study Program, which is also awarded to undergraduate and graduate students based on financial need.

The federal government also offers a number of programs especially for nursing students. For example, the U.S. Department of Health and Human Services offers Nursing Student Scholarships, Nursing Student Loans, the Nursing Education Loan Repayment Program, and the Scholarship for Disadvantaged Students (SDS) program. Some of these programs require that the student work in a designated nursing shortage area for a period of time. These programs are administered by the nursing school's financial aid office. For more information, log on to http://bhpr.hrsa.gov/dsa.

The second-largest source of aid is from the colleges and universities themselves. Almost all colleges have aid programs from institutional resources, most of which are grants, scholarships, and fellowships. These can be either need-or merit-based.

A third source of aid is from state governments. Nearly every state provides aid for students attending college in their home state, although most only have programs for undergraduates. Most state aid programs are scholarships and grants, but many states now have low-interest loan and work-study programs. Most state grants and scholarships are not "portable," meaning that they cannot be used outside of your home state of residence.

A fourth source of aid is from private sources such as corporations, hospitals, civic associations, unions, fraternal organizations, foundations, and religious groups that give scholarships, grants, and fellowships to students. Most of these are not based on need, although the amount of the scholarship may vary depending upon financial need. The compe-

Federal Financial Aid Programs

Program	Who Benefits?	Maximum/Year
Federal Pell Grants	Undergraduate students	$5550
Federal Supplemental Educational Opportunity Grants (FSEOG)	Undergraduate students	$4000
Academic Competitivess Grants	Undergraduate students who are eligible for Federal Pell Grants	$750 (first-year students) $1300 (second-year students)
SMART Grants	Undergraduate students who are eligible for Federal Pell Grants	$4000 (third- and fourth-year students)
Federal Perkins Loans	Undergraduate students	$5500
	Graduate students	$8000
Federal Direct Loans (subsidized)	Undergraduate students	$3500 (first-year students) $4500 (second-year students) $5500 (third-year students and above)
	Graduate students*	$8500
Federal Direct Loans (unsubsidized)	Dependent undergraduate students	$2000
	Independent undergraduate students	$6000 (first- and second-year students) $7000 (third-year students and above)
	Graduate students	$12,000
Federal PLUS Loans	Dependent undergraduate students	Up to cost of attendance (less other financial aid received)
Federal Graduate PLUS loans	Graduate and professional students	Up to cost of attendance (less other financial aid received)

*Only eligible if period(s) of enrollment began prior to 7/1/2012.

The unsubsidized Federal Direct Loan amounts provided are in addition to the subsidized Federal Direct Loan amounts.

tition for these scholarships can be formidable, but the rewards are well worth the process. Many companies also offer tuition reimbursement to employees and their dependents. Check with the personnel or human resources department at your or your parents' place of employment for benefit and eligibility information.

Eligibility for Financial Aid

Since most of the financial aid that college students receive is need-based, colleges employ a process called "need analysis" to determine student awards. For most applicants, the student and parents (if the student is a dependent) fill out one form on which family income, assets, and household information are reported. This form is the Free Application for Federal Student Aid (FAFSA). The end result of this need analysis is the student's "Expected Family Contribution," or EFC, representing the amount a family should be able to contribute toward education expenses.

Dependent or Independent

The basic principle of financial aid is that the primary responsibility for paying college expenses resides with the family. In determining your EFC, you will first need to know who makes up your "family." That will tell you whose income is counted when the need analysis is done.

Graduate Students: By definition, all graduate nursing students are considered independent for federal aid purposes. Therefore, only your income and assets (and your spouse's if you are married) count in determining your expected family contribution.

Undergraduate Students: If you are financially dependent upon your parents, their income and assets, as well as yours, are counted toward the family contribution. If you are financially independent of your parents, only your income (and your spouse's if you are married) counts in the calculation.

According to the U.S. Department of Education, in order to be considered independent for financial aid for 2013–14, you must meet any ONE of the following:

- You were born before January 1, 1987.

- You are or will be enrolled in a master's or doctoral program (beyond a bachelor's degree) during the 2013–14 school year.

- You are married on the day you apply (even if you are separated but not divorced).

- You have children who receive more than half their support from you.

- You have dependents (other than your children or spouse) who live with you and who receive more than half of their support from you and will continue to receive more than half their support from you through June 30, 2013.

- Both your parents are deceased, or you are an orphan or ward of the court (or were a ward of the court until age 18).

- You are engaged in active duty in the U.S. Armed Forces or are a National Guard or Reserves enlistee and are called to active duty for purposes other than training.

- You are a veteran of the U.S. Armed Forces. ("Veteran" includes students who attended a U.S. service academy and who were released under a condition other than dishonorable. Contact your financial aid office for more information.)

- You were verified on or after the start of the award year for which the FAFSA is filed, as either an unaccompanied youth who is homeless or at risk of being homeless and self-supporting.

If you meet any one of these conditions, you are considered independent and only your income and assets (and your spouse's if you are married) count toward your family contribution. Remember, if you are attending school as a graduate student, you are automatically independent for federal aid consideration.

If there are extraordinary circumstances, the financial aid administrator at the college you will be attending has the authority to make a change to your dependency status. You will need to provide extensive documentation of your family situation.

Determining Cost and Need

Now that you know approximately how much you and your family will be expected to contribute toward your college expenses, you can subtract the EFC from the total cost of attending a college or graduate school to determine the amount of need-based financial aid for which you will be eligible. The average cost listed assumes that you will be attending nursing school full-time. If you will be attending part-time, you should adjust costs accordingly. For a more accurate estimate of the cost of attendance at a particular college, check the financial aid information usually available on the college's Web site or in its publications.

Applying for Financial Aid

After you have subtracted your EFC from the cost of your education and determined your financial need, you will have a

better understanding of how much assistance you will need. Even if you do not demonstrate financial need, you are still encouraged to file the FAFSA, as you may be eligible for assistance that is not based on need. The process for applying for aid can be confusing if you are not familiar with completing these types of applications. If you need assistance, you should contact the financial aid office for help.

Undergraduate and graduate students applying for aid must fill out the FAFSA. This application is available in high school guidance offices, college financial aid offices, state education department offices, and many local libraries. You are strongly encouraged to file the FAFSA online at www.fafsa.ed.gov. If you file online, you will need to have a Personal Identification Number (PIN). The PIN can easily be obtained at www.pin.ed.gov. Dependent students will need a PIN for themselves and one parent. When you file online, your application is processed more rapidly, and you are far less likely to make major errors. The FAFSA, whether you file a paper application or online, becomes available in November or December, almost a year before the fall term in which you will enroll, but you cannot complete it until after January 1.

If you file a paper application, you and your parents (if appropriate) must sign your completed FAFSA and mail it to a processing center in the envelope provided. Do not send any additional materials, but do make copies of everything you filled out.

The processing center enters the data into a computer that runs the federal methodology of need analysis to calculate your EFC. This center then distributes the information to the schools and agencies you listed on the FAFSA. The actual determination of need and the awarding of aid are handled by each college financial aid office.

It is generally recommended that you complete the FAFSA as soon as possible after January 1. You should check with each college to which you are applying to determine its filing deadline. It is important to meet all college deadlines for financial aid, since there is a limited amount of funds available. However, students who procrastinate can still file for federal aid any time during the year.

What Happens After You Submit the FAFSA?

Two to four weeks after you send in your completed FAFSA, you will receive a Student Aid Report (SAR) that shows the information you reported and your official EFC. This is an opportunity for you to make corrections or to have the information sent to any new school you are considering that you did not list on the original FAFSA. The SAR contains instructions on how to make corrections or to designate additional schools. If you provided an e-mail address on the FAFSA, this information will be sent to this address rather than through conventional mail.

At the same time that you receive the SAR, the college(s) you specified also receive the information. The financial aid office at the school may request additional information from you or may ask you to provide documentation verifying the information you reported on the FAFSA. For example, they may ask you for a copy of your (and your parents') income tax return or official forms verifying any untaxed income you or your parents received (e.g., Social Security, disability, or welfare benefits).

Once the financial aid office is satisfied that the information is correct, you will receive a financial aid offer. Many colleges like to make this offer in the spring prior to the fall enrollment so that students have ample opportunity to make their plans. However, some colleges will wait until summer to notify you.

Other Applications

The FAFSA is the required form for applying for federal and most state financial aid programs. Most schools also use the FASFA to determine eligibility for institutional aid; however, some colleges and graduate schools require additional information to determine eligibility for institutional aid. Nearly 500 colleges and universities, plus more than 200 private scholarship programs, employ a form called the Financial Aid PRO-FILEt from the College Scholarship Service (CSS). While the form is similar to the FAFSA, several additional questions must be answered for colleges that award their own funds. You begin the process in October or November by completing a PROFILE Registration form on which you designate the schools to which you are applying. A few weeks later, you will receive a customized, individualized application that you complete and send back to CSS, which, in turn, forwards your application information to the schools you selected. There is a fee charged for each school listed on the application.

Financial Aid Offer

If you qualify for need-based aid, a college will typically offer a combination of different types of assistance— scholarship, grant, loan, and work-study—to meet this need. An offer of aid usually is made after you have been admitted to the college or program. You may accept all or part of the financial aid package. If you will be enrolling part-time (fewer than 12 credits per term), be sure to contact the financial aid office in advance since this may have impact on your overall aid eligibility.

If you are awarded Federal Work-Study Program aid, the amount you are awarded represents your earnings limit for the academic year under the program. In general, schools assume you will earn this money on an hourly basis, so it cannot be used to pay your term bill charges. On most campuses there are many jobs available for students. Not all of these are limited to students in the Federal Work-Study Program. Check with your placement office or financial aid office for more information.

Keep in mind that the student budget used to establish eligibility for financial aid is based on averages. It may not reflect your actual expenses. Student budgets usually reflect most expenses for categories of students (for example, single students living in their parents' home, campus-provided housing, or living in an apartment or house near campus, etc.). But if you have unusual expenses that are not included, you should consult with your school's financial aid office regarding a budget adjustment.

If Your Family or Job Situation Changes

Because a family contribution is based on the previous year's income, many nursing students find they do not qualify for need-based aid (or not enough to pay their full expenses). This is particularly true of older students who were working full-time last year but are no longer doing so or who will not work during the academic year. If this is your situation, you should speak to a counselor in the financial aid office about making an adjustment in your family contribution need analysis. Financial aid administrators may make changes to any of the elements that go into the need analysis if there are conditions that merit a change. Contact the financial aid office for more information.

Don't Qualify for Need-Based Aid?

If you don't qualify for need-based aid but feel you do not have the resources necessary to pay for college or graduate school, you still have several options available.

First, there is a student loan program for which need is not a consideration. This is the Federal Direct Loan (unsubsidized) program. There are also non-need-based loan programs for parents of dependent students or for graduate or professional students called the Federal PLUS Loans and the Direct PLUS Loan program. If you or your parents are interested in borrowing through one of these programs, you should check with the financial aid office for more information. There are also numerous private or alternative loan sources available. For many students, borrowing to pay for a nursing education can be an excellent investment in one's future. At the same time, be sure that you do not overburden yourself when it comes to paying back the loans. Before you accept a federal student loan, the financial aid office will schedule a counseling session to make certain that you know the terms of the loan and that you understand the ramifications of borrowing. If you can do without, it is often suggested that you postpone student loans until they are absolutely necessary.

For graduate nursing students, Federal PLUS Loans are now available to graduate and professional students. Students who are looking into alternative loan programs should be sure to compare any terms and conditions with this federal program. Students should borrow through the Federal Graduate PLUS loans (or other alternative loan) program only after they have used the Federal Stafford Student Loan or Direct Loan program. You can borrow Federal Graduate PLUS loans and alternative loan funds up to the cost of attendance less any other financial aid received.

A second option if you do not qualify for need-based aid is to search for scholarships. Be wary of scholarship search companies that promise to find you scholarships but require you to pay a fee. There are many resources that provide lists of scholarships, including the annually published *Peterson's Scholarships, Grants & Prizes* and *How to Get Money for College,* which are available in libraries, counselors' offices, and bookstores. Non-need scholarships require application forms and are extremely competitive; only a handful of students from thousands of applicants receive awards.

Another option is to work more hours at an existing job or to find a paying position if you do not already have one. The student employment or placement office at your college should be able to help you find a job, either on or off campus. Many colleges have vacancies remaining after they have placed Federal Work-Study Program eligible students in their jobs.

You should always contact the financial aid office at the school you plan to attend for advice concerning sources of college-based and private aid.

Employer-Paid Financial Aid

Robert Atwater is a certified personnel consultant and certified medical staff recruiter and founder of Atwater Consulting in Lilburn, Georgia, a consulting firm for the employment and recruitment of physician assistants, nurse practitioners, certified nurse midwives, nurses, and nursing managers.

Health-care administrators, Atwater says, have coined a phrase to characterize their efforts to meet the growing demand for nurses with better skills and training: "Grow your own."

"Constant training through the course of a nursing career is the only way to keep pace with the technological and medical advances, but it can be a financial burden on the nurse," Atwater says.

That is why many employers now give qualified employees a benefits package that includes a continuing education allowance.

For the employer, this type of benefits package can help to recruit candidates willing to further their careers through education. Administrators feel it is the best way to build a staff of nurses with up-to-date certifications in all areas.

In a constantly expanding field, nurses should be required to continue and update their education. The nurses get a paid education, can keep their job, and work flexible hours while they are going to school. Inquiries about these allowances should be made during an interview with the company's human resources department. Additional information can be obtained from the nursing school, local hospitals in the area, or from other health-care professionals. There are many attractive options available because of the nationwide shortage of qualified nurses. Check with a number of potential employers before agreeing to any long-term contract.

SOURCES OF FINANCIAL AID FOR NURSING STUDENTS

The largest proportion of financial aid for college expenses comes from the federal government and is given on the basis of financial need. Beyond this federal need-based aid—which should always be the primary source of financial aid that a prospective student investigates and which is given regardless of one's field of study—a sizable amount of scholarship assistance specifically meant to help students in nursing programs is also available from government agencies, associations, civic or fraternal organizations, and corporations. These sources of aid can be particularly attractive for students who may not be eligible for need-based aid. The following list presents some of the major sources of financial aid specifically for nursing students. Not listed are scholarships that are specific to individual colleges and universities or are limited to residents of a particular place or to individuals who have relatively unusual qualifications. Students seeking financial aid should investigate all appropriate possibilities, including sources not listed here. You can find this information in libraries, bookstores, and guidance offices guides, including two of Peterson's annually updated publications: *Peterson's How to Get Money for College: Financing Your Future Beyond Federal Aid,* for information about undergraduate awards given by the federal government, state governments, and specific colleges, and *Peterson's Scholarships, Grants & Prizes,* for information about awards from private sources.

Air Force Institute of Technology
Award Name: Air Force Active Duty Health Professions Loan Repayment Program
Program Description: Program provides up to $40,000 (2009) to repay qualified educational loans in exchange for active duty service in the U.S. armed forces.
Application Contact:
Air Force Institute of Technology
AFIT/ENEM
Attn: Ms. Patricia Faustman
2950 Hobson Way
Wright Patterson AFB, OH 45433-7765
800-543-3490, Ext. 3015 (toll-free)
E-mail: enem.adhplrp@afit.edu
www.afit.edu/adhplrp

Alaska Native Tribal Health Consortium
Award Name: ANTHC Scholarship Program
Program Description: Provides undergraduate and graduate scholarships for Alaska Native/American Indian students pursuing an education in the health-care field. Must be a full-time student, a permanent Alaska resident, and be enrolled in or descended from a federally recognized tribe.

Application Contact:
Courtney Bridges, Trainer
Education, Development & Training
Alaska Native Tribal Health Consortium
3900 Ambassador Drive
Suite 101
Anchorage, Alaska 99508
907-729-1301
E-mail: cbridges@anthc.org
www.anthc.org

American Association of Colleges of Nursing (AACN)
Award Name: AfterCollege/AACN Scholarship Fund
Program Description: This scholarship program supports students who are seeking a baccalaureate, master's, or doctoral degree in nursing. Special consideration is given to students enrolled in a master's or doctoral program with the goal of pursuing a nursing faculty career, completing an RN to baccalaureate program (B.S.N.), or enrolled in an accelerated baccalaureate or master's degree nursing program.
Application Contact:
American Association of Colleges of Nursing
One Dupont Circle, NW
Suite 530
Washington, DC 20036
202-463-6930
Fax: 202-785-8320
E-mail: scholarship@aacn.nche.edu
http://bit.ly/aftercollege_AACN

American Association of Critical-Care Nurses
Award Name: AACN Educational Advancement Scholarships
Program Description: Nonrenewable scholarships for AACN members who are RNs currently enrolled in undergraduate or graduate NLNAC-accredited programs. The undergraduate award is for use in the junior or senior year. Minimum 3.0 GPA.
Application Contact:
American Association of Critical-Care Nurses
Scholarships
101 Columbia
Aliso Viejo, CA 92656-4109
800-899-2226 (toll-free)
E-mail: scholarships@aacn.org
www.aacn.nche.edu/education/financialaid.htm

American Cancer Society
Award Name: Scholarships in Cancer Nursing
Program Description: Renewable awards for graduate students in nursing pursuing advanced preparation in cancer nursing: research, education, administration, or clinical practice. Must be U.S. citizen.

Application Contact:
American Cancer Society
Extramural Grants Program
250 Williams Street, NW
Atlanta, GA 30303-1002
800-ACS-2345 (toll-free)
Fax: 404-417-5974
E-mail: grants@cancer.org
www.cancer.org

American Holistic Nurses' Association (AHNA)

Award Name: Charlotte McGuire Scholarship Program
Program Description: Open to any licensed nurse or nursing student pursuing holistic education. Experience in holistic health care or alternative health practices is preferred. Must be an AHNA member with a minimum 3.0 GPA.
Application Contact:
Charlotte McGuire Scholarships
American Holistic Nurses' Association
100 SE 9th Street
Suite 3A
Topeka, KS 66612
800-278-2462 Ext. 10 (toll-free)
E-mail: info@ahna.org
www.ahna.org/AboutUs/DonateSponsor/
CharlotteMcGuireScholarships/tabid/2139/Default.aspx

American Indian Graduate Center (AIGC)

Award Name: AIGC Fellowships
Program Description: Graduate fellowships available for American Indian and Alaska Native students from federally recognized U.S. tribes. Applicants must be pursuing a postbaccalaureate graduate or professional degree as a full-time student at an accredited institution in the U.S., demonstrate financial need, and be enrolled in a federally recognized American Indian tribe or Alaska Native group or provide documentation of Indian descent.
Application Contact:
American Indian Graduate Center Fellowships
American Indian Graduate Center
3701 San Mateo, NE
Suite 200
Albuquerque, NM 87110
800-628-1920 (toll-free)
505-881-4584
E-mail: web@aigcs.org
www.aigc.com

Association of Perioperative Registered Nurses (AORN)

Award Name: AORN Foundation Scholarships
Program Description: Applicant must be an active RN and a member of AORN for twelve consecutive months prior to application. Reapplication for each period is required. For baccalaureate, master's of nursing, or doctoral degree at an accredited institution. Minimum 3.0 GPA required.
Application Contact:
AORN Foundation Scholarship Program
2170 South Parker Road
Suite 400

Denver, CO 80231-5711
800-755-2676 (toll-free)
E-mail: foundation@aorn.org
www.aorn.org/

Bethesda Lutheran Communities

Award Name: Nursing Scholastic Achievement Scholarship
Program Description: Award for college nursing students with a minimum 3.0 GPA who are Lutheran and have completed their sophomore year of a four-year nursing program or one year of a two-year program. Must be interested in working with people with developmental disabilities.
Application Contact:
Bethesda Lutheran Communities
Executive Assistant for Mission Advancement
600 Hoffmann Drive
Watertown, WI 53094
800-383-8743, Ext. 4410 (toll-free)
E-mail: bethesda.institute@mailblc.org
http://bethesdalutherancommunities.org/scholarships

Foundation of the National Student Nurses' Association, Inc.

Award Names: Scholarship Program
Program Description: One-time awards available to nursing students in various educational situations: enrolled in programs leading to an RN license, RNs enrolled in programs leading to a bachelor's or master's degree in nursing, enrolled in a state approved school in a specialty area of nursing, and minority students enrolled in nursing or prenursing programs. High school students are not eligible. Funds for graduate study are available only for a first degree in nursing. Based on financial need, academic ability, and health-related nursing and community activities. Application fee of $10. Send self-addressed stamped envelope with two stamps along with application request.
Application Contact:
Scholarship Chairperson
Foundation of the National Student Nurses' Association, Inc.
45 Main Street
Suite 606
Brooklyn, NY 11201
718-210-0705
E-mail: nsna@nsna.org
www.nsna.org/FoundationScholarships.aspx

Heart and Stroke Foundation of Canada

Award Name: Nursing Research Fellowships
Program Description: In-training awards for study in an area of cardiovascular or cerebrovascular nursing. Award is directed toward preparing nurses who have completed their doctoral degree and who intend to undertake independent research programs. For master's degree candidates, the programs must include a thesis or project requirement.
Application Contact:
Heart and Stroke Foundation of Canada
222 Queen Street, Suite 1402
Ottawa, Ontario K1P-5V9
Canada

613-569-4361, Ext. 275

E-mail: research@hsf.ca

www.hsf.ca/

International Order of the King's Daughters and Sons, Inc.

Award Name: International Order of King's Daughters and Sons Health Careers Scholarships

Program Description: For study in the health fields. B.A./B.S. students are eligible in junior year. Application must be for at least third year of college. RN students must have completed first year of schooling. Send #10 self-addressed stamped envelope for application and information.

Application Contact: Director

Health Careers Scholarship Department

P.O. Box 1040

Chautauqua, NY 14722

716-357-4951

E-mail: iokds5@windstream.net

www.iokds.org/scholarship.html

March of Dimes

Award Name: Graduate Scholarships

Program Description: Scholarships for registered nurses enrolled in graduate programs in maternal-child nursing. Must be a member of the Association of Women's Health, Obstetric and Neonatal Nurses; the American College of Nurse-Midwives; or the National Association of Neonatal Nurses (NANN).

Application Contact: Education Services

March of Dimes

1275 Mamaroneck Avenue

White Plains, NY 10605

914-997-4609

E-mail: mlavan@marchofdimes.com

www.marchofdimes.com/professionals/grants.html

National Association of Hispanic Nurses (NAHN)

Award Name: National Scholarship Awards

Program Description: One-time award to an outstanding Hispanic nursing student. Must have at least a 3.0 GPA and be a member of NAHN. Based on academic merit, potential contribution to nursing, and financial need.

Application Contact:

National Association of Hispanic Nurses

Awards/Scholarship Committee

1455 Pennsylvania Avenue

Suite 400

Washington, DC 20004

202-387-2477

E-mail: info@thehispanicnurses.org

www.thehispanicnurses.org

National Black Nurses Association, Inc. (NBNA)

Award Names: NBNA Scholarships

Program Description: Scholarships available to nursing students who are members of NBNA and are enrolled in an accredited school of nursing. Must demonstrate involvement in African-American community and present letter of recommendation from local chapter of NBNA.

Application Contact:

National Black Nurses Association, Inc.

Scholarship Committee

8630 Fenton Street, Suite 330

Silver Spring, MD 20910

301-589-3200

E-mail: contact@nbna.org

www.nbna.org/

National Student Nurses' Association (NSNA)

Award Name: Educational Advancement Scholarships

Program Description: Scholarships are awarded based on academic achievement and demonstrated commitment to nursing through involvement in student organizations and school and community activities related to health care.

Application Contact:

National Student Nurses' Association Foundation

45 Main Street

Suite 606

Brooklyn, NY 11201

718-210-0705

E-mail: nsna@nsna.org

www.nsna.org

Nurses' Educational Funds, Inc.

Award Name: Nurses' Educational Fund Scholarships

Program Description: Awards for full-time students at master's level, full-time or part-time at doctoral level, or RNs who are U.S. citizens and members of a national professional nursing association. Application fee: $10.

Application Contact:

Nurses' Educational Funds, Inc.

304 Park Avenue South

11th Floor

New York, NY 10010

212-590-2443

E-mail: info@n-e-f.org

www.n-e-f.org

Oncology Nursing Society

Award Name: Scholarships

Program Description: ONF offers nearly a dozen one-time scholarships and awards at all levels of study, with various requirements and purposes, to nursing students who are interested in pursuing oncology nursing. Contact the foundation for details about appropriate awards. Application fee: $5.

Application Contact:

Oncology Nursing Society

Development Coordinator

125 Enterprise Drive

Pittsburgh, PA 15275-1214

866-257-4667 (toll-free)

E-mail: awards@ons.org

www.ons.org/awards

United States Air Force Reserve Officer Training Corps

Award Name: Air Force ROTC Nursing Scholarships

Program Description: One- to four-year programs available to students of nursing and high school seniors. Nursing graduates agree to accept a commission in the Air Force Nurse Corps and serve four years on active duty after successfully completing their licensing examination. Must have at least a 2.5 GPA for one- and four-year scholarships or at least a 2.65 GPA for two- and three-year scholarships. Two exam failures result in a four-year assignment as an Air Force line officer.

Application Contact:
Air Force ROTC
551 East Maxwell Boulevard
Maxwell AFB, AL 36112
866-423-7682 (toll-free)
www.afrotc.com/scholarships

United States Army Reserve Officers' Training Corps

Award Name: Army ROTC Nursing Scholarships

Program Description: Two- to four-year programs available to students of nursing and high school seniors. Nursing graduates agree to accept a commission in the Army Nurse Corps and serve in the military for a period of eight years. This may be fulfilled by serving on active duty for two to four years, followed by service in the Army National Guard or the United States Army Reserve or in the Inactive Ready Reserve for the remainder of the eight-year obligation.

Application Contact:
Army ROTC Cadet Command
Army ROTC Scholarship
Fort Monroe, VA 23651-1052
800-USA-ROTC (toll-free)
www.goarmy.com/rotc/scholarships.html

United States Department of Health and Human Services, Health Resources and Services Administration

Award Names: NURSE Corps Scholarship Program

Program Description: Awards for U.S. citizens enrolled or accepted for enrollment as a full- or part-time student in an accredited school of nursing in a professional registered nurse program (baccalaureate, graduate, associate degree, or diploma)

Application Contact:
Division of Nursing
U.S. Dept. of Health and Human Services
5600 Fishers Lane, Room 8-37
Parklawn Building
Rockville, MD 20857
800-221-9393 (toll-free)
GetHelp@hrsa.gov
www.hrsa.gov/loanscholarships/scholarships/Nursing

HOW TO USE THIS GUIDE

The following includes an overview of the various components of *Peterson's Nursing Programs 2014*, along with background information on the criteria used for including institutions and nursing programs in the guide, and explanatory material to help users interpret details presented within the guide.

Profiles of Nursing Programs

The **Profiles of Nursing Programs** section contains detailed profiles of schools that responded to our online survey and the nursing programs they offer. This section is organized geographically; U.S. schools are listed alphabetically by state or territory, followed by Canadian schools listed alphabetically by province.

The profiles contain basic information about the colleges and universities, along with details specific to the nursing school or department, the nursing student body, and the nursing programs offered.

Schools that are members of a consortium appear with an abbreviated profile. The abbreviated profile lists only the school heading and the specific college or university information, followed by a reference line that refers readers to the consortium profile, which contains detailed program information.

An outline of the profile follows. The items of information found under each section heading are defined and displayed. Any item discussed below that is omitted from an individual profile either does not apply to that particular college or university or is one for which no information was supplied. Each profile begins with a heading with the name of the institution (the college or university), the nursing college or unit, the location of the nursing facilities, the school's Web address, and the institution's founding date, specifically the year in which it was chartered or the year when instruction actually began, whichever date is earlier. In most cases, the location is identical to the main campus of the institution. However, in a few instances, the nursing facilities are not located in the same city or state as the main campus of the college or university.

Basic information about the college follows:

Nursing Program Faculty: The total number of full-time and part-time faculty members, followed by, if provided, the percentage of faculty members holding doctoral degrees.

Baccalaureate Enrollment: The total number of matriculated full-time and part-time baccalaureate program students as of fall 2012 is given. This snapshot of the nursing student body indicates the total number of matriculated students, both full-time and part-time, in the baccalaureate-level nursing program; the school's estimate of the percentage of nursing students in each of the following categories is provided, if applicable: Women, Men, Minority, International, and Part-time.

Graduate Enrollment: The total number of matriculated full-time and part-time students in graduate programs in fall 2012 and the percentages of **Women, Men, Minority, International,** and **Part-time** students are given.

Distance Learning Courses: This section appears if distance learning courses are available.

Nursing Student Activities: This section lists organizations open only to nursing students, including nursing clubs, Sigma Theta Tau (the international honor society for nursing), recruiter clubs, and Student Nurses' Association.

Nursing Student Resources: This section lists special learning resources available for nursing students within the nursing school's (or unit's) facilities.

Library Facilities: Figures are provided for the total number of bound volumes held by the college or university, the number of those volumes in health-related subjects, and the number in nursing and the number of periodical subscriptions held and the number of those in health-related subjects.

BACCALAUREATE PROGRAMS

Degree: Baccalaureate degree or degrees awarded are specified.

Available Programs: If, in addition to a generic baccalaureate program in nursing, a school has other baccalaureate nursing programs (e.g., accelerated programs or programs for RNs, LPNs, or college graduates with non-nursing degrees) they are specified here.

Site Options: Locations other than the nursing program's main campus at which baccalaureate programs may be taken are listed. Off-campus classes generally are held in health-care facilities or other educational facilities that are part of or affiliated with the college or nursing school.

Study Options: Lists full-time and part-time options.

Online Degree Options: This section appears if online baccalaureate degrees are available. It also specifies if the distance learning options are only available online.

Program Entrance Requirements: Lists special requirements typically required to enter a program of nursing leading to a baccalaureate degree, including completion of a specific program of prerequisite courses, sometimes called prenursing courses. These are specific course credits that must be earned by students who wish to enter the generic baccalaureate program. Students entering into other tracks may be required to prove that they have completed analogous courses. Often the minimum GPA requirement for prerequisite courses differs from that expected for general college courses. Other requirements are generally self-explanatory. This paragraph also indicates if transfer students are accepted into the program. Special tracks will require appropriate proof of experience, diplomas, or other credentials. Finally, application deadlines and fees are given.

Advanced Placement: This entry indicates that program credits may be granted on the basis of examinations or evaluations of earned credits at other facilities by the program's faculty and administrators.

Expenses: In this section, figures are provided for tuition, mandatory and other fees, and room and board, as well as an estimate of costs for books and supplies, based on the 2012–13 academic year. If a school did not return a survey, expenses for the 2010–11 or 2011–12 academic year are listed. Unless otherwise indicated, tuition is for one full academic year. If applicable, distinct tuition figures are given for state residents and nonresidents. Part-time tuition is expressed in terms of the per-unit rate (per credit, per semester hour, etc.) specified by the institution. The tuition structure at some institutions is very complex, with different rates for freshmen and sophomores than for juniors and seniors or with part-time tuition prorated on a sliding scale according to the number of credit hours taken. Mandatory fees include such items as activity fees, health insurance, and malpractice insurance.

Financial Aid: This section combines data from our online nursing survey with data received on available financial aid programs. It provides information on college-administered aid for baccalaureate-level students, including the percentage of undergraduate nursing students receiving financial aid, all types of aid offered, and application deadlines. Financial aid programs are organized into these categories: gift aid (need-based), awards based on a student's formally designated inability to pay some or all of the cost of education; gift aid (non-need-based), scholarships given on the basis of a student's special achievements, abilities, or personal characteristics; loans, subsidized low-interest student loans that can be need-based or not; and work-study, a need-based program of part-time work offered to help pay educational expenditures. The application deadline is the deadline by which application forms and need calculations, such as the FAFSA, must be submitted to the institution in order to qualify for need-based and institutional aid.

Contact: This section lists the name, title, mailing address, telephone number, and, if available, fax number and e-mail address of the person to contact for admission information about the baccalaureate program.

GRADUATE PROGRAMS

The first three paragraphs provide information that is common to the college's graduate programs in nursing.

Expenses: In this section, figures are provided for tuition, room and board, and required fees based on the 2012–13 academic year. If a school did not return a survey, expenses for the 2010–11 or 2011–12 academic year are listed. Unless otherwise indicated, tuition is for one full academic year. If applicable, distinct tuition figures are given for state residents and nonresidents. Part-time tuition is expressed in terms of the per-

unit rate (per credit, per semester hour, etc.) specified by the institution.

Financial Aid: This section combines data from our online nursing survey with data received on available financial aid programs. It provides information on college-administered aid including the percentage of graduate nursing students receiving financial aid, all types of aid offered, and application deadlines. The major kinds of aid available are listed, including traineeships, low-interest student loans, fellowships, research assistantships, teaching assistantships, and full and partial tuition waivers. If aid is available to part-time students, this is indicated. The application deadline is the deadline by which application forms must be submitted to the college's financial aid office.

Contact: Lists the name, title, mailing address, telephone number, and, if available, fax number and e-mail address of the person to contact for admission information about graduate programs.

MASTER'S DEGREE PROGRAM

Degree(s): Master's degree or degrees awarded are specified. Joint degrees specify which two degrees are given, e.g., M.S.N./Ed. D., M.S.N./M.B.A., M.S./M.H.A., M.S.N./M.P.H., in programs that combine a master's degree (or doctorate) in nursing with a master's degree in another discipline, such as business administration, hospital administration, or public health.

Available Programs: If a college has special tracks that give credit, accelerated programs, or advanced courses designed for students with previous nursing experience or higher education credentials that enable students to complete programs in less time than regularly required, these are specified here in three categories:

① For RNs—programs that admit registered nurses with associate degrees or diplomas in nursing and award a master's degree. These include RN-to-master's programs that combine the baccalaureate and master's degrees into one program for nurses who are graduates of associate or hospital diploma programs and programs that admit registered nurses with non-nursing baccalaureate degrees.

② For LPNs—programs that admit licensed practical nurses and award a master's degree.

③ For College Graduates with Non-Nursing Degrees— programs that admit students with baccalaureate or master's degrees in areas other than nursing and award a master's degree in nursing.

Concentrations Available: Specific areas of study and concentrations offered by the school are listed. Areas of specialization in case management, health-care administration, legal nurse consultant, nurse anesthesia, nurse-midwifery, nursing administration, nursing education, and nursing informatics are noted. Clinical nurse specialist and nurse practitioner programs and areas of specialization within them are noted.

Site Options: Locations other than the nursing program's main campus at which the master's degree programs are offered are listed. Off-campus classes generally are held in health-care facilities or other educational facilities that are part of or affiliated with the nursing school.

Study Options: Lists full-time and part-time options.

Online Degree Options: This section appears if online master's degrees are available. It also specifies if the distance learning options are only available online.

Program Entrance Requirements: Lists generally self-explanatory requirements.

Advanced Placement: Indicates that program credits may be granted on the basis of examinations or evaluations of earned credits at other facilities by the program's faculty and administrators.

Degree Requirements: Indicates the number of master's program credit hours required to earn the master's degree and the need for a thesis or qualifying score on a comprehensive examination.

POST-MASTER'S PROGRAM

Areas of Study: Listed here are the specific areas of clinical nurse specialist programs, nurse practitioner programs, and other specializations offered as postmaster's programs.

DOCTORAL DEGREE PROGRAM

Degree: Doctoral degree awarded is specified.

Areas of Study: Lists specific areas of study and concentration offered by the school.

Program Entrance Requirements: Lists generally self-explanatory requirements.

Degree Requirements: Indicates the number of program credit hours required to earn the doctorate and the need for a dissertation, oral examination, written examination, or residency.

POSTDOCTORAL PROGRAM

Areas of Study: Lists areas of study currently reported. These may change, dependent upon the individuals in the program.

Postdoctoral Program Contact: Lists the name, title, mailing address, telephone number, and, if available, fax number and e-mail address of the person to contact for information about postdoctoral programs.

CONTINUING EDUCATION PROGRAM

Contact: The appearance of this heading indicates that the nursing school has a program of continuing education. If provided, the name, title, mailing address, telephone number, fax number, and e-mail address of the person to contact regarding the program are given.

Display Ads

Display ads, which appear near some of the institutions' profiles, have been provided by those colleges or universities that wished to pay for and supplement the profile data with information about their institutions or nursing programs.

Two-Page Descriptions

The **Two-Page Descriptions** section is an open forum for nursing schools to communicate their particular message to prospective students. The absence of any college or university from this section does not constitute an editorial decision on the part of Peterson's Publishing. Those who have submitted and paid for these inclusions are responsible for the accuracy of the content. Statements regarding a school's objectives and accomplishments represent its own beliefs and are not the opinions of the editors. The **Two-Page Descriptions** are arranged alphabetically by the official institution name.

Indexes

Indexes at the back of the book provide references to profiles by baccalaureate, master's, doctoral, postdoctoral, online, and continuing education programs offered; for master's-level programs, by area of study or concentration; and by institution name.

Abbreviations Used in This Guide

AACN	American Association of Colleges of Nursing
AACSB	AACSB International—The Association to Advance Collegiate Schools of Business
AAHC	Association of Academic Health Centers
AAS	Associate in Applied Science
ABSN	Accelerated Bachelor of Science in Nursing
ACT	American College Testing, Inc.
ACT ASSET	American College Testing Assessment of Skills for Successful Entry and Transfer
ACT COMP	American College Testing College Outcomes Measures Program
ACT PEP	American College Testing Proficiency Examination Program
AD	Associate Degree
ADN	Associate Degree in Nursing
AHNP	Adult Health Nurse Practitioner
ALE	American Language Exam
AMEDD	Army Medical Department
ANA	American Nurses Association
ANP	Adult Nurse Practitioner
APN	Advanced Practice Nurse
ARNP	Advanced Registered Nurse Practitioner
AS	Associate of Science
ASN	Associate of Science in Nursing
BA	Bachelor of Arts
BAA	Bachelor of Applied Arts
BN	Bachelor of Nursing
BNSc	Bachelor of Nursing Science

BRN	Baccalaureate for the Registered Nurse	ICEOP	Illinois Consortium for Educational Opportunities Program
BS	Bachelor of Science	ICU	intensive care unit
BScMH	Bachelor of Science in Mental Health	ISP	Internet service provider
BScN	Bachelor of Science in Nursing	ITV	interactive television
BSEd	Bachelor of Science in Education	LD	Licensed Dietician
BSN	Bachelor of Science in Nursing	LPN	Licensed Practical Nurse
CAI	computer-assisted instruction	LVN	Licensed Vocational Nurse
CAUSN	Canadian Association of University Schools of Nursing	MA	Master of Arts
		MAEd	Master of Arts in Education
CCNE	Commission on Collegiate Nursing Education	MAT	Miller Analogies Test
CCRN	Critical-Care Registered Nurse	MBA	Master of Business Administration
CFNP	Certified Family Nurse Practitioner	MCSc	Master of Clinical Science
CGFNS	Commission on Graduates of Foreign Nursing Schools	MDiv	Master of Divinity
		MEd	Master of Education
CINAHL	Cumulative Index to Nursing and Allied Health Literature	MEDLINE	MEDLARS On-Line
		MELAB	Michigan English Language Assessment Battery
CLAST	College-Level Academic Skills Test	MHA	Master of Hospital Administration
CLEP	College-Level Examination Program		Master of Health Administration
CNA	Certified Nurse Assistant, Certified Nursing Assistant, Certified Nurses' Aide	MHD	Master of Human Development
		MHSA	Master of Health Services Administration
CNAT	Canadian Nurses Association Testing	MN	Master of Nursing
CNL	Clinical Nurse Leader	MNSc	Master of Nursing Science
CNM	Certified Nurse-Midwife	MOM	Master of Organizational Management
CNS	Clinical Nurse Specialist	MPA	Master of Public Affairs
CODEC	coder/decoder	MPH	Master of Public Health
CPR	cardiopulmonary resuscitation	MPS	Master of Public Service
CRNA	Certified Registered Nurse Anesthetist	MS	Master of Science
CS	Certified Specialist	MSBA	Master of Science in Business Administration
CSS	College Scholarship Service	M Sc	Master of Science
DAP	Doctor of Anesthesia Practice	MSc(A)	Master of Science (Applied)
DNP	Doctor of Nursing Practice	MScN	Master of Science in Nursing
DNS	Doctor of Nursing Science	MTS	Master of Theological Studies
DNSc	Doctor of Nursing Science	MSEd	Master of Science in Education
DOE	U.S. Department of Education	MSN	Master of Science in Nursing
DrPH	Doctor of Public Health	MSOB	Master of Science in Organizational Behavior
DSN	Doctor of Science in Nursing	NCAA	National Collegiate Athletic Association
EdD	Doctor of Education	NCLEX-RN	National Council Licensure Examination for Registered Nurses
EFC	expected family contribution		
ERIC	Educational Resources Information Center	ND	Doctor of Nursing
ESL	English as a second language	NLN	National League for Nursing
ETN	Enterostomal Nurse	NNP	Neonatal Nurse Practitioner
FAAN	Fellow in the American Academy of Nursing	NP	Nurse Practitioner
FAF	Financial Aid Form	NSNA	National Student Nurses' Association
FAFSA	Free Application for Federal Student Aid	OB	Organizational Behavior
FC	family contribution	OB/GYN	obstetrics/gynecology
FNP	Family Nurse Practitioner	OCLC	Online Computer Library Center
FSEOG	Federal Supplemental Educational Opportunity Grants	OM	Organizational Management
		PEP	Proficiency Examination Program
GED	General Educational Development test	PhD	Doctor of Philosophy
GMAT	Graduate Management Admission Test	PHEAA	Pennsylvania Higher Education Assistance Agency
GPA	grade point average		
GPO	Government Printing Office	PHS	Public Health Service
GRE	Graduate Record Examinations	PLUS	Parents' Loan for Undergraduate Students
Gyn	gynecology		
HIV	human immunodeficiency virus	PNNP	Perinatal Nurse Practitioner
HMO	health maintenance organization	PNP	Pediatric Nurse Practitioner

PSAT	Preliminary SAT
RD	Registered Dietician
RN	Registered Nurse
RN, C	Registered Nurse, Certified
RN, CAN	Registered Nurse, Certified in Nursing Administration
RN, CNAA	Registered Nurse, Certified in Nursing Administration, Advanced
RN, CS	Registered Nurse, Certified Specialist
ROTC	Reserve Officers' Training Corps
RPN	Registered Psychiatric Nurse
SAR	Student Aid Report
SAT	SAT and SAT Subject Tests
SLS	Supplemental Loans to Students
SNA	Student Nurses' Association
SNAP	Student Nurses Acting for Progress
SNO	Student Nurses Organization
SUNY	State University of New York
TAP	Tuition Assistance Program
TB	tuberculosis
TOEFL	Test of English as a Foreign Language
TSE	Test of Spoken English
TWE	Test of Written English
USIS	United States Information Service
WHNP	Women's Health Nurse Practitioner

Data Collection Procedures

The data contained in the preponderant number of nursing college profiles, as well as in the indexes to them, were collected through *Peterson's Survey of Nursing Programs* during winter 2012–13. Questionnaires were posted online for more than 800 colleges and universities with baccalaureate and graduate programs in nursing. With minor exceptions, data for those colleges or schools of nursing that responded to the questionnaires were submitted by officials at the schools themselves. All usable information received in time for publication has been included. The omission of a particular item from a profile means that it is either not applicable to that institution or was not available or usable. In the handful of instances in which no information regarding an eligible nursing program was submitted and research of reliable secondary sources was unable to elicit the desired information, the name, location, and some general information regarding the nursing program appear in the profile section to indicate the existence of the program. Because of the extensive system of checks performed on the data collected by Peterson's, we believe that the information presented in this guide is accurate. Nonetheless, errors and omissions are possible in a data collection and processing endeavor of this scope. Also, facts and figures, such as tuition and fees, can suddenly change. Therefore, students should check with a specific college or university at the time of application to verify all pertinent information.

Criteria for Inclusion in This Book

Peterson's Nursing Programs 2014 covers accredited institutions in the United States, U.S. territories, and Canada that grant baccalaureate and graduate degrees. The institutions that sponsor the nursing programs must be accredited by accrediting agencies approved by the U.S. Department of Education (USDE) or the Council for Higher Education Accreditation (CHEA) or be candidates for accreditation with an agency recognized by the USDE for its preaccreditation category. Canadian schools may be provincially chartered instead of accredited.

Baccalaureate-level and master's-level nursing programs represented by a profile within the guide are accredited by the National League for Nursing Accrediting Commission (NLNAC) or the Commission on Collegiate Nursing Education (CCNE). Canadian nursing schools are members of the Canadian Association of University Schools of Nursing (CAUSN).

Doctoral, postdoctoral, continuing education, and other nursing programs included in the profiles are offered by nursing schools or departments affiliated with colleges or universities that meet the criteria outlined above.

NOTICE: Certain portions of or information contained in this book have been submitted and paid for by the educational institution identified, and such institutions take full responsibility for the accuracy, timeliness, completeness and functionality of such contents. Such portions or information include (i) each display ad in the "Profiles of Nursing Programs" section from pages 81 through 472 that comprises a one-half page of information covering a single educational institution, and (ii) each two-page in-depth description in the "Two-Page Descriptions" section from Pages 474 through 513.

QUICK REFERENCE CHART

	Baccalaureate	Masters	Accelerated	Joint Degree	Post-Masters	Doctoral	Postdoctoral	Continuing Education
United States								
Alabama								
Auburn University	•	•						•
Auburn University Montgomery	•	•						
Jacksonville State University	•	•						•
Oakwood University	•							
Samford University	•	•	B	•		•		•
Spring Hill College	•	•	M					
Stillman College	•							
Troy University	•	•				•	•	
Tuskegee University	•							
The University of Alabama	•	•				•	•	
The University of Alabama at Birmingham	•	•	M	•	•	•	•	
The University of Alabama in Huntsville	•	•			•	•		•
University of Mobile	•	•						•
University of North Alabama	•	•						•
University of South Alabama	•	•	B,M			•		
Alaska								
University of Alaska Anchorage	•	•						
Arizona								
Arizona State University at the Downtown Phoenix Campus	•	•	B	•	•	•		•
Chamberlain College of Nursing	•	•	B					
Grand Canyon University	•	•		•	•			•
Northern Arizona University	•	•	B		•	•		
The University of Arizona	•	•	M		•	•		
University of Phoenix–Online Campus	•	•	B		•			
University of Phoenix–Phoenix Main Campus	•	•	B	•	•			•
University of Phoenix–Southern Arizona Campus	•	•	B		•			
Arkansas								
Arkansas State University	•	•	B		•			
Arkansas Tech University	•	•						
Harding University	•							•
Henderson State University	•							
Southern Arkansas University–Magnolia	•							
University of Arkansas	•	•						•
University of Arkansas at Little Rock	•							
University of Arkansas at Monticello	•							
University of Arkansas at Pine Bluff	•							
University of Arkansas for Medical Sciences	•	•	B			•	•	•
University of Arkansas–Fort Smith	•							
University of Central Arkansas	•	•				•		

B = Baccalaureate; M = Masters

	Baccalaureate	Masters	Accelerated	Joint Degree	Post-Masters	Doctoral	Postdoctoral	Continuing Education
California								
American University of Health Sciences	•		B					
Azusa Pacific University	•	•	B,M		•	•		•
Biola University	•							
Brandman University	•	•				•		•
California Baptist University	•	•	M					
California State University, Bakersfield	•							•
California State University Channel Islands	•							
California State University, Chico	•	•						•
California State University, Dominguez Hills	•	•			•			
California State University, East Bay	•							
California State University, Fresno	•	•	M		•	•		•
California State University, Fullerton	•	•				•		
California State University, Long Beach	•	•	B,M		•			
California State University, Los Angeles	•	•	M		•			
California State University, Northridge	•		B					
California State University, Sacramento	•	•						
California State University, San Bernardino	•	•						
California State University, San Marcos	•		B					
California State University, Stanislaus	•							
Charles Drew University of Medicine and Science		•	M					
Concordia University	•		B					
Dominican University of California	•	•						•
Fresno Pacific University	•							
Holy Names University	•	•		•	•			
Loma Linda University	•	•	B		•	•		
Mount St. Mary's College	•	•	B					
National University	•	•			•	•		
Pacific Union College	•							•
Point Loma Nazarene University	•	•			•			•
Samuel Merritt University	•	•	B		•	•		
San Diego State University	•	•			•			•
San Francisco State University	•	•	B,M		•			•
San Jose State University	•	•						
Sonoma State University	•							
University of California, Davis		•				•	•	
University of California, Irvine	•	•			•			
University of California, Los Angeles	•	•		•	•	•	•	
University of California, San Francisco		•			•	•	•	
University of Phoenix–Bay Area Campus	•	•	B	•				
University of Phoenix–Central Valley Campus	•							
University of Phoenix–Sacramento Valley Campus	•	•	B,M		•			•
University of Phoenix–San Diego Campus	•	•	B					
University of Phoenix–Southern California Campus	•	•	B	•	•			•

B = Baccalaureate; M = Masters

	Baccalaureate	Masters	Accelerated	Joint Degree	Post-Masters	Doctoral	Postdoctoral	Continuing Education
University of San Diego		•	M			•		
University of San Francisco	•	•	M		•	•		
Vanguard University of Southern California	•							
West Coast University	•		B					
Western University of Health Sciences		•	M		•	•		
Colorado								
Adams State University	•							
American Sentinel University	•	•						
Aspen University		•						
Colorado Christian University	•							
Colorado Mesa University	•							
Colorado State University–Pueblo	•	•	B		•			
Colorado Technical University Online	•							
Denver College of Nursing	•		B					
Metropolitan State University of Denver	•		B					
Platt College	•		B					
Regis University	•	•	B					
University of Colorado at Colorado Springs	•	•	B		•	•		•
University of Colorado Denver	•	•	B		•	•	•	•
University of Northern Colorado	•	•	B		•	•		
University of Phoenix–Denver Campus	•	•	B					
University of Phoenix–Southern Colorado Campus								
Connecticut								
Central Connecticut State University	•							
Fairfield University	•	•	B		•	•		•
Quinnipiac University	•	•	B		•	•		•
Sacred Heart University	•	•			•	•		
Southern Connecticut State University	•	•	B		•	•		
University of Connecticut	•	•	B	•	•	•		•
University of Hartford	•	•		•	•			
University of Saint Joseph	•	•			•			
Western Connecticut State University	•	•						
Yale University		•		•	•	•	•	
Delaware								
Delaware State University	•	•						
University of Delaware	•	•	B		•	•		•
Wesley College	•	•	M		•			•
Wilmington University	•	•	B,M	•	•			
District of Columbia								
The Catholic University of America	•	•	B	•	•	•		
Georgetown University	•	•	B		•			
The George Washington University	•	•	B		•	•		
Howard University	•	•			•			

B = Baccalaureate; M = Masters

	Baccalaureate	Masters	Accelerated	Joint Degree	Post-Masters	Doctoral	Postdoctoral	Continuing Education
Trinity Washington University	•							
University of the District of Columbia	•							
Florida								
Adventist University of Health Sciences	•							
Barry University	•	•	B	•	•	•		
Bethune-Cookman University	•							
Broward College	•							
Edison State College	•							
Florida Agricultural and Mechanical University	•	•			•	•		•
Florida Atlantic University	•	•	B		•	•		•
Florida Gulf Coast University	•	•			•			•
Florida International University	•	•	B,M		•	•		
Florida Southern College	•	•	B	•	•			
Florida State College at Jacksonville	•							
Florida State University	•	•	B		•	•		
Indian River State College	•							
Jacksonville University	•	•	B	•	•			
Kaplan University Online	•	•						
Keiser University	•	•						
Keiser University	•	•						
Keiser University	•	•						
Keiser University	•	•						
Keiser University	•	•						
Keiser University	•	•						
Keiser University	•	•						
Keiser University	•	•						
Keiser University	•	•						
Keiser University	•	•						
Keiser University	•	•						
Keiser University	•	•						
Keiser University	•	•						
Miami Dade College	•							
Northwest Florida State College	•		B					
Nova Southeastern University	•	•						
Palm Beach Atlantic University	•							
Remington College of Nursing	•		B					
St. Petersburg College	•							•
South University	•	•						
South University	•	•						
State College of Florida Manatee-Sarasota	•							
University of Central Florida	•	•	B		•	•		
University of Florida	•	•	B	•	•	•		
University of Miami	•	•	B		•	•		•
University of North Florida	•	•	B		•			
University of Phoenix–Central Florida Campus	•	•	B					

B = Baccalaureate; M = Masters

	Baccalaureate	Masters	Accelerated	Joint Degree	Post-Masters	Doctoral	Postdoctoral	Continuing Education
University of Phoenix–North Florida Campus	•	•	B					
University of Phoenix–South Florida Campus	•	•		•				
University of Phoenix–West Florida Campus	•		B					
University of South Florida	•	•	B	•		•		•
The University of Tampa	•	•			•			•
University of West Florida	•	•						
Georgia								
Albany State University	•	•	B,M		•			
Armstrong Atlantic State University	•	•		•	•			
Augusta State University	•							
Brenau University	•	•	M		•	•		
Clayton State University	•	•						
College of Coastal Georgia	•		B					
Columbus State University	•							
Emory University	•	•	B	•	•	•		
Georgia College & State University	•	•			•	•		
Georgia Regents University	•	•	M		•	•		
Georgia Southern University	•	•						
Georgia Southwestern State University	•							
Georgia State University	•	•	B		•	•		
Gordon State College	•							
Kennesaw State University	•	•	B					•
LaGrange College	•							
Macon State College	•							
Mercer University Georgia Baptist College of Nursing	•	•			•	•		
Piedmont College	•							
Shorter University	•							
Thomas University	•	•	B,M	•	•			
University of North Georgia	•	•			•			
University of Phoenix–Atlanta Campus								
University of West Georgia	•	•	B,M		•	•		
Valdosta State University	•	•						•
Guam								
University of Guam	•							
Hawaii								
Chaminade University of Honolulu	•							
Hawai`i Pacific University	•	•		•	•			
University of Hawaii at Hilo	•							
University of Hawaii at Manoa	•	•	M	•	•	•		
University of Phoenix–Hawaii Campus	•	•	B					
Idaho								
Boise State University	•	•	B					
Brigham Young University–Idaho	•							

B = Baccalaureate; M = Masters

	Baccalaureate	Masters	Accelerated	Joint Degree	Post-Masters	Doctoral	Postdoctoral	Continuing Education
Idaho State University	•	•	B,M		•			
Lewis-Clark State College	•							
Northwest Nazarene University	•	•						
Illinois								
Aurora University		•						
Benedictine University	•	•	B,M					
Blessing–Rieman College of Nursing	•	•	B					
Bradley University	•	•	B					
Chicago State University	•							
DePaul University		•			•			
Eastern Illinois University								
Elmhurst College	•	•		•				
Governors State University	•	•			•			
Illinois State University	•	•	B		•	•		
Illinois Wesleyan University	•							
Lakeview College of Nursing	•		B					
Lewis University	•	•	B,M	•	•			•
Loyola University Chicago	•	•	B	•	•	•		
MacMurray College	•							
McKendree University	•	•			•			
Methodist College	•		B					
Millikin University	•	•	M					
Northern Illinois University	•	•			•	•		
North Park University	•	•			•	•		
Olivet Nazarene University	•	•	B					•
Resurrection University	•	•	B,M		•			
Rockford College	•							
Rush University		•			•	•		•
Saint Anthony College of Nursing	•	•			•			
Saint Francis Medical Center College of Nursing	•	•	M		•	•		
St. John's College	•							
Saint Xavier University	•	•		•	•			•
Southern Illinois University Edwardsville	•	•	B		•	•		•
Trinity Christian College	•							
Trinity College of Nursing and Health Sciences	•		B					
University of Illinois at Chicago	•	•		•	•	•	•	•
University of St. Francis	•	•	B		•	•		
Western Illinois University	•							
Indiana								
Anderson University	•	•		•	•			
Ball State University	•	•	B		•	•		
Bethel College	•	•			•			
Goshen College	•	•						
Huntington University	•							

B = Baccalaureate; M = Masters

	Baccalaureate	Masters	Accelerated	Joint Degree	Post-Masters	Doctoral	Postdoctoral	Continuing Education
Indiana State University	•	•	B		•	•		•
Indiana University Bloomington	•							
Indiana University East	•							
Indiana University Kokomo	•		B					•
Indiana University Northwest	•							
Indiana University–Purdue University Fort Wayne	•	•			•			
Indiana University–Purdue University Indianapolis	•	•	B	•	•	•	•	•
Indiana University South Bend	•	•	B					
Indiana University Southeast	•							
Indiana Wesleyan University	•	•	B		•			
Marian University	•		B					•
Purdue University	•	•	B		•	•		
Purdue University Calumet	•	•	B		•			
Purdue University North Central	•		B					
Saint Joseph's College	•		B					
Saint Mary's College	•		B					
University of Evansville	•							
University of Indianapolis	•	•	B,M	•	•	•		
University of Saint Francis	•	•			•			
University of Southern Indiana	•	•			•	•		•
Valparaiso University	•	•	B	•	•			•
Vincennes University	•							
Iowa								
Allen College	•	•	B		•	•		•
Briar Cliff University	•	•						•
Clarke University	•	•			•			•
Coe College	•							
Dordt College	•							
Grand View University	•	•						•
Iowa Wesleyan College	•							
Luther College	•							•
Mercy College of Health Sciences	•							
Morningside College	•							
Mount Mercy University	•	•	B					•
Northwestern College	•							
St. Ambrose University	•	•						•
University of Dubuque	•							
The University of Iowa	•	•	M	•	•	•	•	•
Upper Iowa University	•							
Kansas								
Baker University	•							
Benedictine College	•							
Bethel College	•							
Emporia State University	•							
Fort Hays State University	•	•			•			

B = Baccalaureate; M = Masters

	Baccalaureate	Masters	Accelerated	Joint Degree	Post-Masters	Doctoral	Postdoctoral	Continuing Education
Kansas Wesleyan University	•							
MidAmerica Nazarene University	•	•	B,M					
Newman University	•							
Pittsburg State University	•	•			•			•
Southwestern College	•		B					
Tabor College	•		B					
The University of Kansas	•	•		•	•	•	•	•
University of Saint Mary	•							
Washburn University	•	•			•			•
Wichita State University	•		B			•		
Kentucky								
Bellarmine University	•	•	B	•	•	•		•
Berea College	•							
Eastern Kentucky University	•	•	B					
Frontier Nursing University		•	M			•		
Kentucky Christian University	•							•
Kentucky State University	•							
Midway College	•		B					•
Morehead State University	•							
Murray State University	•	•			•			•
Northern Kentucky University	•	•	B		•	•		•
Spalding University	•	•	B,M		•			•
Thomas More College	•							
University of Kentucky	•	•			•	•		•
University of Louisville	•	•	B		•	•		•
Western Kentucky University	•	•	M			•		•
Louisiana								
Dillard University	•							•
Grambling State University	•	•			•			
Louisiana College	•							
Louisiana State University at Alexandria	•							
Louisiana State University Health Sciences Center	•	•	B			•		•
Loyola University New Orleans	•	•			•			
McNeese State University	•	•			•			
Nicholls State University	•							•
Northwestern State University of Louisiana	•	•			•			•
Our Lady of Holy Cross College	•							
Our Lady of the Lake College	•	•	B					•
Southeastern Louisiana University	•	•	B		•	•		
Southern University and Agricultural and Mechanical College	•	•			•	•		
University of Louisiana at Lafayette	•	•	B		•			•
University of Louisiana at Monroe								•
University of Phoenix–Louisiana Campus	•		B					

B = Baccalaureate; M = Masters

	Baccalaureate	Masters	Accelerated	Joint Degree	Post-Masters	Doctoral	Postdoctoral	Continuing Education
Maine								
Husson University	•	•			•			
Saint Joseph's College of Maine	•	•						•
University of Maine	•	•						
University of Maine at Fort Kent	•		B					
University of New England	•		B					•
University of Southern Maine	•	•	B	•	•			•
Maryland								
Bowie State University	•	•	B					
Coppin State University	•	•	B		•			
Frostburg State University	•							
The Johns Hopkins University	•	•	B	•	•	•	•	•
Notre Dame of Maryland University	•		B					
Salisbury University	•	•	B		•	•		
Stevenson University	•	•	B,M					
Towson University	•	•				•		
University of Maryland, Baltimore	•	•	M	•	•	•		•
Washington Adventist University	•		B					
Massachusetts								
American International College	•	•						
Anna Maria College	•							•
Boston College	•	•	M	•	•	•		•
Curry College	•	•	B					
Elms College	•	•						
Emmanuel College	•	•						
Endicott College	•	•						•
Fitchburg State University	•	•	B		•			
Framingham State University	•	•						•
Massachusetts College of Pharmacy and Health Sciences	•		B					
MGH Institute of Health Professions	•		B		•	•		
Northeastern University	•	•				•		•
Regis College	•	•	B,M		•	•		
Salem State University	•	•	B,M	•				
Simmons College	•	•	B,M		•	•		
University of Massachusetts Amherst	•	•	B			•		•
University of Massachusetts Boston	•	•	B		•	•	•	
University of Massachusetts Dartmouth	•	•			•	•		
University of Massachusetts Lowell	•	•	M		•	•		
University of Massachusetts Worcester		•	M		•	•		
Worcester State University	•	•				•		•
Michigan								
Andrews University	•	•						
Calvin College	•							
Davenport University	•							

B = Baccalaureate; M = Masters

	Baccalaureate	Masters	Accelerated	Joint Degree	Post-Masters	Doctoral	Postdoctoral	Continuing Education
Davenport University	•							
Eastern Michigan University	•	•						
Ferris State University	•	•	B,M	•				
Finlandia University	•							
Grand Valley State University	•	•				•		•
Hope College	•							
Lake Superior State University	•							
Madonna University	•	•		•	•	•		•
Michigan State University	•	•	B		•	•		•
Northern Michigan University	•	•	B		•			•
Oakland University	•	•			•			•
The Robert B. Miller College	•							
Rochester College	•							
Saginaw Valley State University	•	•	B,M		•	•		•
Siena Heights University	•							
Spring Arbor University	•	•		•				
University of Detroit Mercy	•	•	B,M	•				
University of Michigan	•	•	B,M	•	•	•	•	
University of Michigan–Flint	•	•	B,M		•			
University of Phoenix–Metro Detroit Campus	•	•	B					
University of Phoenix–West Michigan Campus								
Wayne State University	•	•	B		•	•	•	•
Western Michigan University	•	•						•
Minnesota								
Augsburg College	•	•						
Bemidji State University	•							•
Bethel University	•	•						
Capella University	•	•	M			•		
College of Saint Benedict	•							
The College of St. Scholastica	•	•	B		•	•		
Concordia College	•	•	B					
Crown College	•							
Globe University–Woodbury	•							
Gustavus Adolphus College	•							
Herzing University	•							
Metropolitan State University	•	•			•			
Minnesota Intercollegiate Nursing Consortium	•							
Minnesota State University Mankato	•	•	B,M		•	•		•
Minnesota State University Moorhead	•	•						
St. Catherine University	•	•			•	•		
St. Cloud State University	•							
Saint Mary's University of Minnesota	•							
St. Olaf College	•							
University of Minnesota, Twin Cities Campus	•					•		•

B = Baccalaureate; M = Masters

	Baccalaureate	Masters	Accelerated	Joint Degree	Post-Masters	Doctoral	Postdoctoral	Continuing Education
Walden University	•	•			•	•		
Winona State University	•	•			•	•		
Mississippi								
Alcorn State University	•	•			•			
Delta State University	•	•			•			
Mississippi College	•							
Mississippi University for Women	•	•			•			
University of Mississippi Medical Center	•	•	B,M		•	•		•
University of Southern Mississippi	•	•			•	•		
William Carey University	•	•				•		
Missouri								
Avila University	•							
Central Methodist University	•	•						
Chamberlain College of Nursing	•		B					
College of the Ozarks	•							
Cox College	•	•	B					•
Goldfarb School of Nursing at Barnes-Jewish College	•	•	B		•	•		
Graceland University	•	•	B		•	•		
Lincoln University	•							
Maryville University of Saint Louis	•	•	B,M			•		
Missouri Southern State University	•	•						
Missouri State University	•	•	B,M		•	•		•
Missouri Western State University	•	•						•
Research College of Nursing	•	•	B		•			
Saint Louis University	•	•	B,M	•	•	•		
Saint Luke's College of Health Sciences	•							
Southeast Missouri State University	•	•	B		•			
Southwest Baptist University	•	•						
Truman State University	•	•						
University of Central Missouri	•	•						
University of Missouri	•	•	B	•	•	•		•
University of Missouri–Kansas City	•	•	B		•	•		
University of Missouri–St. Louis	•	•	B		•	•		
Webster University	•	•						
William Jewell College	•		B					
Montana								
Carroll College	•							
Montana State University	•	•	B		•	•		
Montana State University–Northern	•							
Salish Kootenai College	•							
University of Great Falls	•							
Nebraska								
BryanLGH College of Health Sciences	•	•						

B = Baccalaureate; M = Masters

	Baccalaureate	Masters	Accelerated	Joint Degree	Post-Masters	Doctoral	Postdoctoral	Continuing Education
Clarkson College	•	•	B		•			•
College of Saint Mary	•							
Creighton University	•	•	B		•	•		
Midland University	•							
Nebraska Methodist College	•	•	B		•			•
Nebraska Wesleyan University	•	•	B,M		•			
Union College	•							
University of Nebraska Medical Center	•	•	B		•	•	•	•
Nevada								
Great Basin College	•							
Nevada State College at Henderson	•		B					
Roseman University of Health Sciences	•		B					
Touro University	•	•				•		
University of Nevada, Las Vegas	•	•	B		•	•		•
University of Nevada, Reno	•	•	B	•	•	•		
New Hampshire								
Colby-Sawyer College	•							
Franklin Pierce University	•	•						
Rivier University	•	•			•			
Saint Anselm College	•							•
University of New Hampshire	•	•			•			
New Jersey								
Bloomfield College	•							
Caldwell College	•							
The College of New Jersey	•	•			•			
College of Saint Elizabeth	•		B					•
Fairleigh Dickinson University, Metropolitan Campus	•	•	B,M		•	•		•
Felician College	•	•	B,M	•	•			
Kean University	•	•	M	•				
Monmouth University	•	•			•			•
New Jersey City University	•		B					
Ramapo College of New Jersey	•	•			•			•
The Richard Stockton College of New Jersey	•	•						
Rowan University	•							
Rutgers School of Nursing–Camden	•		B					•
Rutgers, The State University of New Jersey, College of Nursing	•	•	B	•	•	•		•
Saint Peter's University	•	•			•			
Seton Hall University	•	•	B,M	•	•	•		
Thomas Edison State College	•	•						
University of Medicine and Dentistry of New Jersey	•	•	B	•	•	•		•
William Paterson University of New Jersey	•	•	B		•	•		
New Mexico								
Eastern New Mexico University	•							

B = Baccalaureate; M = Masters

	Baccalaureate	Masters	Accelerated	Joint Degree	Post-Masters	Doctoral	Postdoctoral	Continuing Education
New Mexico Highlands University	•							
New Mexico State University	•	•				•		•
Northern New Mexico College	•							
University of New Mexico	•	•	B	•	•	•		
University of Phoenix–New Mexico Campus	•	•	B					
Western New Mexico University	•							
New York								
Adelphi University	•	•	B	•	•	•		•
Binghamton University, State University of New York	•	•	B		•	•		•
The College at Brockport, State University of New York	•							
College of Mount Saint Vincent	•	•						
The College of New Rochelle	•	•	B		•			
College of Staten Island of the City University of New York	•	•			•			
Columbia University	•	•	B,M	•	•	•	•	•
Concordia College–New York	•		B					
Daemen College	•	•	B,M		•	•		
Dominican College	•	•	B					
D'Youville College	•	•			•			
Elmira College	•							•
Excelsior College	•	•			•			
Farmingdale State College	•							
Hartwick College	•		B					
Hunter College of the City University of New York	•	•	B	•	•	•		•
Keuka College	•		B					
Lehman College of the City University of New York	•	•	B		•	•		•
Le Moyne College	•	•			•			
Long Island University–Brooklyn Campus	•	•	B		•			
Long Island University–C. W. Post Campus	•	•						
Medgar Evers College of the City University of New York	•		B					
Mercy College	•	•	B,M		•			
Molloy College	•	•	B		•	•		•
Mount Saint Mary College	•	•	B		•			
Nazareth College of Rochester	•							
New York City College of Technology of the City University of New York	•							
New York Institute of Technology	•							
New York University	•	•	B	•	•	•		•
Niagara University	•							
Pace University	•	•	B		•	•		
Roberts Wesleyan College	•	•			•			
The Sage Colleges	•	•	B,M	•	•	•		•
St. Francis College	•							
St. John Fisher College	•	•	B		•	•		
St. Joseph's College, New York	•	•						
State University of New York at Plattsburgh	•							
State University of New York College of Technology at Delhi	•							

B = Baccalaureate; M = Masters

	Baccalaureate	Masters	Accelerated	Joint Degree	Post-Masters	Doctoral	Postdoctoral	Continuing Education
State University of New York Downstate Medical Center	•	•	B	•	•			•
State University of New York Empire State College	•							
State University of New York Institute of Technology	•	•	B,M		•			•
State University of New York Upstate Medical University	•	•	M		•			•
Stony Brook University, State University of New York	•	•	B		•	•		•
University at Buffalo, the State University of New York	•		B			•		
University of Rochester	•	•	B,M	•	•	•	•	•
Utica College	•		B					
Wagner College	•	•				•		
York College of the City University of New York	•							
North Carolina								
Appalachian State University	•							
Barton College	•							
Cabarrus College of Health Sciences	•							
Duke University	•	•	B	•	•	•		
East Carolina University	•	•	M		•	•		
Fayetteville State University	•							
Gardner-Webb University	•	•		•		•		
Lees-McRae College	•							
Lenoir-Rhyne University	•							
North Carolina Agricultural and Technical State University	•		B					
North Carolina Central University	•							
Queens University of Charlotte	•	•	B	•				•
The University of North Carolina at Chapel Hill	•	•	B		•	•	•	•
The University of North Carolina at Charlotte	•	•			•			
The University of North Carolina at Greensboro	•	•		•	•	•		
The University of North Carolina at Pembroke	•							
The University of North Carolina Wilmington	•	•			•			
Western Carolina University	•	•	B		•			
Winston-Salem State University	•	•	B					•
North Dakota								
Dickinson State University	•							
Jamestown College	•							
Minot State University	•							
North Dakota State University	•	•				•		
Sanford College of Nursing	•							
University of Mary	•	•						
University of North Dakota	•	•	B		•	•		
Ohio								
Ashland University	•		B					
Capital University	•	•	B	•	•			
Case Western Reserve University	•	•	M	•	•	•	•	•
Cedarville University	•	•						
Chamberlain College of Nursing	•	•	B					

B = Baccalaureate; M = Masters

	Baccalaureate	Masters	Accelerated	Joint Degree	Post-Masters	Doctoral	Postdoctoral	Continuing Education
Cleveland State University	•	•	B	•	•	•		•
College of Mount St. Joseph	•	•	B,M					
Defiance College	•							
Franciscan University of Steubenville	•	•						
Hiram College	•							
Kent State University	•	•	B,M	•	•	•		•
Kettering College	•							
Lourdes University	•	•						
Malone University	•	•						
Mercy College of Ohio	•							
Miami University	•							
Miami University Hamilton	•							
Mount Carmel College of Nursing	•	•	B		•			
Mount Vernon Nazarene University	•							
Muskingum University	•							
Notre Dame College	•							
Ohio Northern University	•							
The Ohio State University	•	•	M	•	•	•		•
Ohio University	•	•						
Otterbein University	•	•	B		•			•
Shawnee State University	•							•
The University of Akron	•	•	B		•	•		•
University of Cincinnati	•	•	B,M	•	•	•		•
University of Phoenix–Cleveland Campus	•	•	B					
University of Rio Grande	•							
The University of Toledo	•	•			•	•		•
Urbana University	•	•						•
Ursuline College	•	•	B,M		•	•		
Walsh University	•	•	B,M			•		
Wright State University	•	•	B	•	•	•		•
Xavier University	•	•	M	•				
Youngstown State University	•	•						
Oklahoma								
Bacone College	•		B					
East Central University	•							
Langston University	•							
Northeastern State University	•	•	B					
Northwestern Oklahoma State University	•		B					
Oklahoma Baptist University	•	•						
Oklahoma Christian University	•							
Oklahoma City University	•	•	B,M	•	•	•		•
Oklahoma Panhandle State University	•							
Oklahoma Wesleyan University	•		B					
Oral Roberts University	•							
Rogers State University	•							

B = Baccalaureate; M = Masters

	Baccalaureate	Masters	Accelerated	Joint Degree	Post-Masters	Doctoral	Postdoctoral	Continuing Education
Southern Nazarene University	•	•	M					
Southwestern Oklahoma State University	•							
University of Central Oklahoma	•							
University of Oklahoma Health Sciences Center	•	•	B		•	•		•
University of Phoenix–Oklahoma City Campus								
University of Phoenix–Tulsa Campus								
University of Tulsa	•							
Oregon								
George Fox University	•							
Linfield College	•		B					•
Oregon Health & Science University	•	•	B,M	•	•	•	•	•
University of Portland	•	•				•		
Pennsylvania								
Alvernia University	•							•
Bloomsburg University of Pennsylvania	•	•			•	•		•
California University of Pennsylvania	•							
Carlow University	•	•	B,M		•			•
Cedar Crest College	•	•						
Chatham University	•	•					•	
Clarion University of Pennsylvania	•	•				•		
DeSales University	•	•	B,M	•	•			•
Drexel University	•	•	B		•	•		•
Duquesne University	•	•	B		•	•		•
Eastern University	•		B					
East Stroudsburg University of Pennsylvania	•							
Edinboro University of Pennsylvania	•		B					
Gannon University	•	•	M		•	•		
Gwynedd-Mercy College	•	•	B		•			
Holy Family University	•	•	B		•			
Immaculata University	•	•	B					•
Indiana University of Pennsylvania	•	•				•		
Lancaster General College of Nursing & Health Sciences	•							
La Roche College	•	•	B					•
La Salle University	•	•		•	•			•
Mansfield University of Pennsylvania	•	•						
Marywood University	•	•		•				•
Messiah College	•							
Millersville University of Pennsylvania	•	•				•		
Misericordia University	•	•	B			•		
Moravian College	•	•						
Mount Aloysius College	•		B					•
Neumann University	•	•	B		•			
Penn State University Park	•	•		•	•	•	•	•
Pennsylvania College of Technology	•							

B = Baccalaureate; M = Masters

	Baccalaureate	Masters	Accelerated	Joint Degree	Post-Masters	Doctoral	Postdoctoral	Continuing Education
Robert Morris University	•	•				•		
Saint Francis University	•							
Slippery Rock University of Pennsylvania								
Temple University	•	•			•	•		•
Thomas Jefferson University	•	•	B,M		•	•		•
University of Pennsylvania	•	•	B,M	•	•	•	•	•
University of Pittsburgh	•	•	B		•	•	•	•
University of Pittsburgh at Bradford	•							
The University of Scranton	•	•	M		•			
Villanova University	•	•	B		•	•		
Waynesburg University	•	•	B,M	•		•		
West Chester University of Pennsylvania	•	•	B					
Widener University	•	•		•	•	•		•
Wilkes University	•	•	B,M		•			•
York College of Pennsylvania	•	•			•	•		
Puerto Rico								
Inter American University of Puerto Rico, Aguadilla Campus	•							
Inter American University of Puerto Rico, Arecibo Campus	•							
Inter American University of Puerto Rico, Metropolitan Campus	•		B					
Pontifical Catholic University of Puerto Rico	•							
Universidad Adventista de las Antillas	•							•
Universidad del Turabo	•							
Universidad Metropolitana	•							
University of Puerto Rico at Arecibo	•							
University of Puerto Rico at Humacao	•							
University of Puerto Rico, Mayagüez Campus	•							•
University of Puerto Rico, Medical Sciences Campus	•	•						•
University of the Sacred Heart	•	•						
Rhode Island								
Rhode Island College	•	•						
Salve Regina University	•							•
University of Rhode Island	•	•			•	•		
South Carolina								
Charleston Southern University	•	•						
Clemson University	•	•	B		•			
Coastal Carolina University	•							
Francis Marion University	•							
Lander University	•		B					
Medical University of South Carolina	•	•	B			•	•	
Newberry College	•							
South Carolina State University	•							
University of South Carolina	•	•			•	•		•
University of South Carolina Aiken	•							

B = Baccalaureate; M = Masters

	Baccalaureate	Masters	Accelerated	Joint Degree	Post-Masters	Doctoral	Postdoctoral	Continuing Education
University of South Carolina Beaufort	•							
University of South Carolina Upstate	•							
South Dakota								
Augustana College	•							
Mount Marty College	•		B					
National American University	•							
Presentation College	•							
South Dakota State University	•	•	B			•	•	•
University of Sioux Falls	•		B					
Tennessee								
Aquinas College	•	•	B			•		
Austin Peay State University	•	•				•		
Baptist College of Health Sciences	•							
Belmont University	•	•	B			•		
Bethel University								
Carson-Newman University	•	•	B,M			•		
Cumberland University	•		B					
East Tennessee State University	•	•	B			•	•	•
King College	•	•	B,M	•				
Lincoln Memorial University	•	•	B			•		
Lipscomb University	•							
Martin Methodist College	•							
Middle Tennessee State University	•	•	M			•		
Milligan College	•							
South College	•							
Southern Adventist University	•	•	M	•			•	•
Tennessee State University	•	•				•		•
Tennessee Technological University	•	•						
Tennessee Wesleyan College	•							
Union University	•	•	B			•		•
University of Memphis	•	•	B,M			•		
The University of Tennessee	•	•	B,M			•	•	•
The University of Tennessee at Chattanooga	•	•				•	•	
The University of Tennessee at Martin	•							
The University of Tennessee Health Science Center		•	M			•	•	
Vanderbilt University		•		•	•	•	•	
Texas								
Angelo State University	•	•						
Baylor University	•	•	B			•	•	
East Texas Baptist University	•							
Houston Baptist University	•							
Lamar University	•	•		•	•			•
Lubbock Christian University	•							
Midwestern State University	•	•				•		•

B = Baccalaureate; M = Masters

	Baccalaureate	Masters	Accelerated	Joint Degree	Post-Masters	Doctoral	Postdoctoral	Continuing Education
Patty Hanks Shelton School of Nursing	•	•			•			•
Prairie View A&M University	•	•			•			
Southwestern Adventist University	•							
Stephen F. Austin State University	•							
Tarleton State University	•							•
Texas A&M Health Science Center	•		B					
Texas A&M International University	•	•						
Texas A&M University–Corpus Christi	•	•	B		•			•
Texas A&M University–Texarkana	•	•						
Texas Christian University	•	•	B		•	•		•
Texas State University–San Marcos	•							
Texas Tech University Health Sciences Center	•	•	B		•	•		
Texas Woman's University	•	•			•	•		
University of Houston–Victoria	•	•	B					
University of Mary Hardin-Baylor	•	•			•			
The University of Texas at Arlington	•	•	B	•	•	•		•
The University of Texas at Austin	•	•		•	•	•		
The University of Texas at Brownsville	•	•						•
The University of Texas at El Paso	•	•	B					
The University of Texas at Tyler	•	•	B,M	•	•	•		
The University of Texas Health Science Center at Houston	•	•	B	•	•	•		•
The University of Texas Health Science Center at San Antonio	•	•	B		•	•		•
The University of Texas Medical Branch	•	•	B		•	•		
The University of Texas–Pan American	•	•			•			
University of the Incarnate Word	•	•	M		•	•		
Wayland Baptist University	•							
West Texas A&M University	•	•			•			
Utah								
Brigham Young University	•	•			•			
Dixie State College of Utah	•							
Southern Utah University	•							
University of Phoenix–Utah Campus								
University of Utah	•	•	B		•	•	•	
Utah Valley University	•							
Weber State University	•	•						
Western Governors University	•	•	B,M					
Westminster College	•	•			•			
Vermont								
Norwich University	•							
Southern Vermont College	•							
University of Vermont	•	•			•			
Virgin Islands								
University of the Virgin Islands	•							

B = Baccalaureate; M = Masters

	Baccalaureate	Masters	Accelerated	Joint Degree	Post-Masters	Doctoral	Postdoctoral	Continuing Education
Virginia								
Bon Secours Memorial College of Nursing	•							
Eastern Mennonite University	•	•						
ECPI College of Technology	•							
George Mason University	•	•	B		•	•		•
Hampton University	•	•	B			•		
James Madison University	•	•			•	•		
Jefferson College of Health Sciences	•	•						•
Liberty University	•	•						
Lynchburg College	•	•	B	•				
Marymount University	•	•	B		•	•		
Norfolk State University	•		B					
Old Dominion University	•	•	B		•	•		•
Radford University	•	•			•	•		
Sentara College of Health Sciences	•							
Shenandoah University	•	•	B	•	•	•		•
University of Virginia	•	•		•	•	•	•	
The University of Virginia's College at Wise	•							
Virginia Commonwealth University	•	•	B		•	•	•	
Washington								
Gonzaga University	•	•	M		•			
Northwest University	•							
Olympic College	•							
Pacific Lutheran University	•	•	M	•				•
Seattle Pacific University	•	•			•			
Seattle University	•	•	M		•	•		
University of Washington	•	•	B	•	•	•	•	•
Walla Walla University	•							
Washington State University College of Nursing	•	•	M		•	•		•
West Virginia								
Alderson-Broaddus College	•							
Bluefield State College	•							
Fairmont State University	•		B					•
Marshall University	•	•	B		•			
Shepherd University	•							•
University of Charleston	•							
West Liberty University	•		B					
West Virginia University	•	•	B,M		•	•		•
West Virginia Wesleyan College	•	•						
Wheeling Jesuit University	•	•	B		•			

B = Baccalaureate; M = Masters

	Baccalaureate	Masters	Accelerated	Joint Degree	Post-Masters	Doctoral	Postdoctoral	Continuing Education
Wisconsin								
Alverno College	•	•						•
Bellin College	•	•	B					
Cardinal Stritch University	•	•	M					
Carroll University	•							
Columbia College of Nursing/Mount Mary College Nursing Program	•							
Concordia University Wisconsin	•	•			•	•		
Edgewood College	•	•	B	•				
Herzing University Online	•							
Maranatha Baptist Bible College	•							
Marian University	•	•			•			
Marquette University	•	•			•	•		
Milwaukee School of Engineering	•							
Silver Lake College of the Holy Family	•							
University of Phoenix–Milwaukee Campus	•	•				•		
University of Wisconsin–Eau Claire	•	•	B		•	•		•
University of Wisconsin–Green Bay	•							
University of Wisconsin–Madison	•					•	•	•
University of Wisconsin–Milwaukee	•	•				•		
University of Wisconsin–Oshkosh	•	•	B,M		•	•		
Viterbo University	•	•				•		•
Wisconsin Lutheran College	•							
Wyoming								
University of Wyoming	•	•	B		•	•		

Canada

Alberta

Athabasca University	•	•		•	•			
University of Alberta	•	•	B		•	•		
University of Calgary	•	•	B		•	•		
University of Lethbridge	•	•	B					

British Columbia

British Columbia Institute of Technology	•							•
Kwantlen Polytechnic University	•		B					
Thompson Rivers University	•							•
Trinity Western University	•	•						
The University of British Columbia	•	•	B			•	•	
University of Northern British Columbia	•	•					•	
University of Victoria	•	•				•		
Vancouver Island University	•							•

B = Baccalaureate; M = Masters

	Baccalaureate	Masters	Accelerated	Joint Degree	Post-Masters	Doctoral	Postdoctoral	Continuing Education
Manitoba								
Brandon University	•							
University of Manitoba	•	•				•		•
New Brunswick								
Université de Moncton	•	•						•
University of New Brunswick Fredericton	•	•	B					•
Newfoundland and Labrador								
Memorial University of Newfoundland	•	•	B		•			
Nova Scotia								
St. Francis Xavier University	•		B					•
Ontario								
Brock University	•							
Lakehead University	•		B					
Laurentian University	•	•	B					•
McMaster University	•	•		•		•		
Nipissing University	•							
Queen's University at Kingston	•	•	B			•		
Ryerson University	•	•						•
Trent University	•		B					
University of Ottawa	•	•				•	•	
University of Toronto	•	•	B		•	•	•	•
The University of Western Ontario	•	•	B			•	•	
University of Windsor	•	•				•		•
York University	•							•
Prince Edward Island								
University of Prince Edward Island	•							
Quebec								
McGill University	•	•	B			•	•	
Université de Montréal	•	•			•	•	•	•
Université de Sherbrooke	•	•				•	•	
Université du Québec à Chicoutimi	•	•	B,M	•				
Université du Québec à Rimouski	•	•						•
Université du Québec à Trois-Rivières	•	•						
Université du Québec en Abitibi-Témiscamingue	•							
Université du Québec en Outaouais	•	•						
Université Laval	•	•	B,M		•	•	•	•
Saskatchewan								
University of Saskatchewan	•	•	B		•	•		•

B = Baccalaureate; M = Masters

PROFILES OF NURSING PROGRAMS

ALABAMA

Auburn University

School of Nursing
Auburn University, Alabama

http://www.auburn.edu/academic/nursing/
Founded in 1856
DEGREES • BSN • MSN
Nursing Program Faculty 15
Baccalaureate Enrollment 237 **Women** 90% **Men** 10% **Minority** 3%
Graduate Enrollment 55 **Women** 96% **Men** 4% **Minority** 7% **Part-time** 20%
Nursing Student Activities Nursing Honor Society, Sigma Theta Tau, Student Nurses' Association, nursing club.
Nursing Student Resources Academic advising; academic or career counseling; assistance for students with disabilities; bookstore; campus computer network; career placement assistance; computer lab; computer-assisted instruction; e-mail services; employment services for current students; interactive nursing skills videos; Internet; library services; nursing audiovisuals; placement services for program completers; remedial services; resume preparation assistance; skills, simulation, or other laboratory; tutoring.
Library Facilities 3.5 million volumes; 256,354 periodical subscriptions.

BACCALAUREATE PROGRAMS

Degree BSN
Available Programs Generic Baccalaureate.
Study Options Full-time.
Program Entrance Requirements Minimum overall college GPA of 2.5, transcript of college record, CPR certification, health exam, health insurance, immunizations, interview, minimum GPA in nursing prerequisites of 2.5, professional liability insurance/malpractice insurance, prerequisite course work. Transfer students are accepted. *Application deadline:* 2/1 (fall), 5/1 (spring).
Expenses (2012–13) *Tuition, state resident:* full-time $9446. *Tuition, nonresident:* full-time $25,190. *Room and board:* $10,606 per academic year.
Financial Aid 85% of baccalaureate students in nursing programs received some form of financial aid in 2011–12.
Contact Pam Hennessey, Academic Advisor, School of Nursing, Auburn University, 118 Miller Hall, Auburn University, AL 36849. *Telephone:* 334-844-5665. *Fax:* 334-844-4177. *E-mail:* hennepp@auburn.edu.

GRADUATE PROGRAMS

Expenses (2012–13) *Tuition, state resident:* full-time $9440. *Tuition, nonresident:* full-time $25,172. *Room and board:* $10,606 per academic year.
Contact Dr. Barbara Wilder, Director, MSN Program, School of Nursing, Auburn University, 118 Miller Hall, Auburn University, AL 36849. *Telephone:* 334-844-5665. *E-mail:* wildebf@auburn.edu.

MASTER'S DEGREE PROGRAM

Degree MSN
Available Programs Master's.
Concentrations Available Nursing education. *Clinical nurse specialist programs in:* adult health, gerontology, pediatric.
Study Options Full-time and part-time.
Program Entrance Requirements Minimum overall college GPA of 3.0, transcript of college record, nursing research course, statistics course.
Degree Requirements 51 total credit hours, thesis or project.

CONTINUING EDUCATION PROGRAM

Contact Dr. Stuart Pope, Outreach Coordinator, School of Nursing, Auburn University, Miller Hall, Auburn University, AL 36849-5505. *Telephone:* 334-844-5665. *Fax:* 334-844-4177.

Auburn University Montgomery

School of Nursing
Montgomery, Alabama

http://www.aum.edu/nursing
Founded in 1967
DEGREES • BSN • MSN
Nursing Program Faculty 20 (70% with doctorates).
Baccalaureate Enrollment 650 **Women** 80% **Men** 20% **Minority** 33% **International** 1% **Part-time** 20%
Graduate Enrollment 30
Nursing Student Activities Nursing Honor Society, Sigma Theta Tau, Student Nurses' Association.
Nursing Student Resources Academic advising; academic or career counseling; assistance for students with disabilities; bookstore; campus computer network; career placement assistance; computer lab; computer-assisted instruction; daycare for children of students; e-mail services; housing assistance; interactive nursing skills videos; Internet; learning resource lab; library services; nursing audiovisuals; remedial services; resume preparation assistance; skills, simulation, or other laboratory; tutoring.
Library Facilities 9,568 volumes in nursing; 273 periodical subscriptions health-care related.

BACCALAUREATE PROGRAMS

Degree BSN
Available Programs Generic Baccalaureate; RN Baccalaureate.
Study Options Full-time.
Program Entrance Requirements Transcript of college record, CPR certification, health exam, high school transcript, immunizations, interview, minimum GPA in nursing prerequisites of 2.5, professional liability insurance/malpractice insurance, prerequisite course work. Transfer students are accepted. *Application deadline:* 2/1 (fall), 5/1 (spring).
Contact *Telephone:* 334-244-3431. *Fax:* 334-244-3243.

GRADUATE PROGRAMS

Contact *Telephone:* 334-844-5613. *Fax:* 334-844-4177.

MASTER'S DEGREE PROGRAM

Degree MSN
Available Programs Master's.
Concentrations Available Nursing education. *Clinical nurse specialist programs in:* adult health, gerontology, pediatric. *Nurse practitioner programs in:* primary care.
Study Options Full-time and part-time.
Program Entrance Requirements Clinical experience, minimum overall college GPA of 3.0, written essay, 3 letters of recommendation, resume, statistics course.
Advanced Placement Credit given for nursing courses completed elsewhere dependent upon specific evaluations.
Degree Requirements 42 total credit hours, thesis or project, comprehensive exam.

Jacksonville State University
College of Nursing and Health Sciences
Jacksonville, Alabama

http://www.jsu.edu/nursing/index.html
Founded in 1883
DEGREES • BSN • MSN
Nursing Program Faculty 35 (34% with doctorates).
Baccalaureate Enrollment 569 **Women** 86% **Men** 14% **Minority** 30%
International 3% **Part-time** 22%
Graduate Enrollment 64 **Women** 92% **Men** 8% **Minority** 25% **International** 3% **Part-time** 86%
Distance Learning Courses Available.
Nursing Student Activities Sigma Theta Tau, Student Nurses' Association.
Nursing Student Resources Academic advising; academic or career counseling; campus computer network; computer lab; computer-assisted instruction; e-mail services; Internet; learning resource lab; nursing audiovisuals; remedial services; skills, simulation, or other laboratory; tutoring.
Library Facilities 685,991 volumes (23,465 in health, 1,768 in nursing); 14,376 periodical subscriptions (1,443 health-care related).

BACCALAUREATE PROGRAMS

Degree BSN
Available Programs Generic Baccalaureate; RN Baccalaureate.
Study Options Full-time and part-time.
Online Degree Options Yes.
Program Entrance Requirements Transcript of college record, CPR certification, health exam, health insurance, high school transcript, immunizations, minimum GPA in nursing prerequisites, professional liability insurance/malpractice insurance, prerequisite course work. Transfer students are accepted. *Application deadline:* 6/1 (fall), 10/1 (spring).
Expenses (2012–13) *Tuition, area resident:* full-time $6360; part-time $265 per credit hour. *Tuition, state resident:* full-time $7848; part-time $327 per credit hour. *Tuition, nonresident:* full-time $12,720; part-time $530 per credit hour. *International tuition:* $12,720 full-time. *Room and board:* $6562; room only: $3812 per academic year.
Financial Aid 70% of baccalaureate students in nursing programs received some form of financial aid in 2011–12.
Contact Mr. David Hofland, Student Services Coordinator, College of Nursing and Health Sciences, Jacksonville State University, 700 Pelham Road North, Jacksonville, AL 36265-1602. *Telephone:* 256-782-5276. *Fax:* 256-782-5406. *E-mail:* hofland@jsu.edu.

GRADUATE PROGRAMS

Expenses (2012–13) *Tuition, state resident:* full-time $7902; part-time $439 per credit hour. *Tuition, nonresident:* full-time $7902; part-time $439 per credit hour. *International tuition:* $7902 full-time. *Room and board:* $6562; room only: $3812 per academic year.
Financial Aid 60% of graduate students in nursing programs received some form of financial aid in 2011–12.
Contact Dr. Rebecca D. Peinhardt, Director, Graduate Studies, College of Nursing and Health Sciences, Jacksonville State University, 700 Pelham Road North, Jacksonville, AL 36265-1602. *Telephone:* 256-782-5960. *Fax:* 256-782-5406. *E-mail:* rpeinhardt@jsu.edu.

MASTER'S DEGREE PROGRAM
Degree MSN
Available Programs Master's.
Concentrations Available *Clinical nurse specialist programs in:* community health.
Study Options Full-time and part-time.
Online Degree Options Yes (online only).
Program Entrance Requirements Minimum overall college GPA of 3.0, transcript of college record, written essay, interview, 3 letters of recommendation, nursing research course, physical assessment course, statistics course. *Application deadline:* Applications may be processed on a rolling basis for some programs.
Advanced Placement Credit given for nursing courses completed elsewhere dependent upon specific evaluations.
Degree Requirements 36 total credit hours, thesis or project, comprehensive exam.

CONTINUING EDUCATION PROGRAM

Contact Mr. David Hofland, Student Services Coordinator, College of Nursing and Health Sciences, Jacksonville State University, 700 Pelham

Road North, Jacksonville, AL 36265-1602. *Telephone:* 256-782-5276. *Fax:* 256-782-5406. *E-mail:* hofland@jsu.edu.

Oakwood University
Department of Nursing
Huntsville, Alabama

http://www.oakwood.edu/academics/academic-departments/nursing
Founded in 1896
DEGREE • BS
Nursing Program Faculty 10 (33% with doctorates).
Baccalaureate Enrollment 94 **Women** 90% **Men** 10% **Minority** 99% **International** 5%
Nursing Student Activities Nursing club.
Nursing Student Resources Academic advising; academic or career counseling; assistance for students with disabilities; bookstore; campus computer network; career placement assistance; computer lab; computer-assisted instruction; e-mail services; employment services for current students; externships; interactive nursing skills videos; Internet; learning resource lab; library services; nursing audiovisuals; paid internships; placement services for program completers; remedial services; resume preparation assistance; skills, simulation, or other laboratory; tutoring; unpaid internships.
Library Facilities 133,106 volumes (5,147 in health, 3,474 in nursing); 726 periodical subscriptions (47 health-care related).

BACCALAUREATE PROGRAMS

Degree BS
Available Programs Generic Baccalaureate; RN Baccalaureate.
Study Options Full-time and part-time.
Program Entrance Requirements Minimum overall college GPA of 3.0, transcript of college record, CPR certification, written essay, health exam, health insurance, high school transcript, immunizations, interview, 3 letters of recommendation, minimum high school GPA of 3.0, minimum GPA in nursing prerequisites of 3.0, prerequisite course work. Transfer students are accepted. *Application deadline:* 1/16 (fall), 1/15 (winter).
Expenses (2012–13) *Tuition:* full-time $24,264; part-time $563 per contact hour. *International tuition:* $24,264 full-time. *Room and board:* $11,414; room only: $6614 per academic year. *Required fees:* full-time $792; part-time $792 per term.
Financial Aid 95% of baccalaureate students in nursing programs received some form of financial aid in 2011–12.
Contact Mrs. Denise Finley, Secretary, Department of Nursing, Oakwood University, 7000 Adventist Boulevard, Huntsville, AL 35896. *Telephone:* 256-726-7287. *Fax:* 256-726-8338. *E-mail:* dfinley@oakwood.edu.

Samford University
Ida V. Moffett School of Nursing
Birmingham, Alabama

http://www.samford.edu/nursing/
Founded in 1841
DEGREES • BSN • DNP • MSN • MSN/MBA
Nursing Program Faculty 39 (49% with doctorates).
Baccalaureate Enrollment 427 **Women** 90% **Men** 10% **Minority** 12% **International** 1% **Part-time** 7%
Graduate Enrollment 301 **Women** 68% **Men** 32% **Minority** 22% **Part-time** 10%
Distance Learning Courses Available.
Nursing Student Activities Nursing Honor Society, Sigma Theta Tau, Student Nurses' Association, nursing club.
Nursing Student Resources Academic advising; academic or career counseling; assistance for students with disabilities; bookstore; campus computer network; career placement assistance; computer lab; computer-assisted instruction; e-mail services; employment services for current students; externships; housing assistance; interactive nursing skills videos; Internet; learning resource lab; library services; nursing audiovisuals; paid internships; placement services for program completers; resume preparation assistance; skills, simulation, or other laboratory; tutoring; unpaid internships.

Library Facilities 737,129 volumes (7,973 in health, 896 in nursing); 4,014 periodical subscriptions health-care related.

BACCALAUREATE PROGRAMS

Degree BSN
Available Programs Accelerated Baccalaureate for Second Degree; Baccalaureate for Second Degree; Generic Baccalaureate.
Site Options Birmingham, AL.
Study Options Full-time and part-time.
Program Entrance Requirements Minimum overall college GPA of 2.7, transcript of college record, CPR certification, written essay, health exam, health insurance, high school biology, high school chemistry, 2 years high school math, 2 years high school science, high school transcript, immunizations, minimum high school GPA of 3.0, minimum GPA in nursing prerequisites of 2.0, professional liability insurance/malpractice insurance, prerequisite course work. Transfer students are accepted. *Application deadline:* 5/1 (fall). Applications may be processed on a rolling basis for some programs. *Application fee:* $45.
Expenses (2012–13) *Tuition:* full-time $24,570; part-time $821 per credit. *International tuition:* $24,570 full-time. *Room and board:* $8250; room only: $4250 per academic year. *Required fees:* full-time $800.
Financial Aid 83% of baccalaureate students in nursing programs received some form of financial aid in 2011–12.
Contact Mrs. Janice G. Paine, Director, Undergraduate Student Services, Ida V. Moffett School of Nursing, Samford University, 800 Lakeshore Drive, Birmingham, AL 35229. *Telephone:* 205-726-2872 Ext. 2746. *Fax:* 205-726-4269. *E-mail:* jgpaine@samford.edu.

GRADUATE PROGRAMS

Expenses (2012–13) *Tuition:* full-time $17,625; part-time $705 per credit. *International tuition:* $17,625 full-time. *Room and board:* $9500 per academic year. *Required fees:* full-time $680.
Financial Aid 90% of graduate students in nursing programs received some form of financial aid in 2011–12. Institutionally sponsored loans, scholarships, and traineeships available. *Financial aid application deadline:* 3/1.
Contact Dr. Marian W. Carter, Director, Graduate Student Services, Ida V. Moffett School of Nursing, Samford University, 800 Lakeshore Drive, Birmingham, AL 35229. *Telephone:* 205-726-2047. *Fax:* 205-726-4179. *E-mail:* mwcarter@samford.edu.

MASTER'S DEGREE PROGRAM

Degrees MSN; MSN/MBA
Available Programs Master's; RN to Master's.
Concentrations Available Nurse anesthesia; nursing administration; nursing education. *Nurse practitioner programs in:* family health.
Site Options Birmingham, AL.
Study Options Full-time and part-time.
Online Degree Options Yes.
Program Entrance Requirements Clinical experience, computer literacy, minimum overall college GPA of 3.0, transcript of college record, CPR certification, immunizations, interview, 3 letters of recommendation, nursing research course, physical assessment course, professional liability insurance/malpractice insurance, prerequisite course work, MAT; GRE (for nurse anesthesia). *Application deadline:* 6/1 (fall), 9/1 (spring). *Application fee:* $65.
Degree Requirements 38 total credit hours, thesis or project.

DOCTORAL DEGREE PROGRAM

Degree DNP
Available Programs Doctorate.
Areas of Study Advanced practice nursing, nursing administration.
Site Options Birmingham, AL.
Online Degree Options Yes (online only).
Program Entrance Requirements Clinical experience, minimum overall college GPA of 3.5, interview by faculty committee, interview, 3 letters of recommendation, MSN or equivalent, vita, writing sample. *Application deadline:* 9/1 (spring), 2/1 (summer). *Application fee:* $65.
Degree Requirements 38 total credit hours, oral exam.

CONTINUING EDUCATION PROGRAM

Contact Mrs. Suzanne Scharf, Coordinator, Ida V. Moffett School of Nursing, Samford University, 800 Lakeshore Drive, Birmingham, AL 35229. *Telephone:* 205-726-2045. *Fax:* 205-726-2219. *E-mail:* shscharf@samford.edu.

Spring Hill College
Division of Nursing
Mobile, Alabama

http://www.shc.edu/
Founded in 1830
DEGREES • BSN • MSN
Nursing Program Faculty 8 (84% with doctorates).
Baccalaureate Enrollment 124 Women 86% Men 14% Minority 12%
Graduate Enrollment 62 Women 95% Men 5% Minority 45% Part-time 40%
Distance Learning Courses Available.
Nursing Student Activities Nursing Honor Society, Sigma Theta Tau, Student Nurses' Association.
Nursing Student Resources Academic advising; academic or career counseling; assistance for students with disabilities; bookstore; campus computer network; career placement assistance; computer lab; computer-assisted instruction; e-mail services; employment services for current students; externships; interactive nursing skills videos; Internet; learning resource lab; library services; nursing audiovisuals; placement services for program completers; resume preparation assistance; skills, simulation, or other laboratory; tutoring; unpaid internships.
Library Facilities 330 volumes in health, 300 volumes in nursing; 58 periodical subscriptions health-care related.

BACCALAUREATE PROGRAMS

Degree BSN
Available Programs Baccalaureate for Second Degree; Generic Baccalaureate.
Study Options Full-time.
Program Entrance Requirements Minimum overall college GPA of 2.75, transcript of college record, CPR certification, written essay, health exam, health insurance, high school transcript, immunizations, 1 letter of recommendation, minimum GPA in nursing prerequisites of 2.75, prerequisite course work. Transfer students are accepted. *Application deadline:* 3/1 (spring).
Advanced Placement Credit by examination available.
Contact *Telephone:* 334-380-4492. *Fax:* 334-380-4495.

GRADUATE PROGRAMS

Contact *Telephone:* 251-380-3067. *Fax:* 251-460-2190.

MASTER'S DEGREE PROGRAM

Degree MSN
Available Programs Accelerated AD/RN to Master's; Master's; RN to Master's.
Concentrations Available Clinical nurse leader.
Study Options Full-time and part-time.
Online Degree Options Yes (online only).
Program Entrance Requirements Clinical experience, minimum overall college GPA of 3.0, transcript of college record, immunizations, professional liability insurance/malpractice insurance, prerequisite course work, resume, statistics course. *Application deadline:* Applications may be processed on a rolling basis for some programs.
Advanced Placement Credit by examination available. Credit given for nursing courses completed elsewhere dependent upon specific evaluations.
Degree Requirements 36 total credit hours, thesis or project.

Stillman College
Nursing Major
Tuscaloosa, Alabama

Founded in 1876
DEGREE • BSN
Library Facilities 116,945 volumes; 31,867 periodical subscriptions.

BACCALAUREATE PROGRAMS

Degree BSN
Available Programs RN Baccalaureate.
Contact *Telephone:* 205-349-4240. *Fax:* 205-366-8996.

Troy University
School of Nursing
Troy, Alabama

http://www.troy.edu
Founded in 1887
DEGREES • BSN • DNP • MSN
Nursing Program Faculty 39 (49% with doctorates).
Baccalaureate Enrollment 800 **Women** 88% **Men** 12% **Minority** 35%
International 4% **Part-time** 10%
Graduate Enrollment 200 **Women** 97% **Men** 3% **Minority** 23% **Part-time** 29%
Distance Learning Courses Available.
Nursing Student Activities Sigma Theta Tau, Student Nurses' Association.
Nursing Student Resources Academic advising; academic or career counseling; assistance for students with disabilities; bookstore; campus computer network; career placement assistance; computer lab; computer-assisted instruction; e-mail services; employment services for current students; externships; housing assistance; interactive nursing skills videos; Internet; learning resource lab; library services; nursing audiovisuals; placement services for program completers; resume preparation assistance; skills, simulation, or other laboratory; tutoring; unpaid internships.
Library Facilities 580,895 volumes (45,006 in health, 3,843 in nursing); 30,072 periodical subscriptions (703 health-care related).

BACCALAUREATE PROGRAMS
Degree BSN
Available Programs Generic Baccalaureate; RN Baccalaureate.
Site Options Montgomery, AL; Phenix City, AL; Dothan, AL.
Study Options Full-time.
Program Entrance Requirements Minimum overall college GPA of 2.5, transcript of college record, CPR certification, health exam, health insurance, immunizations, professional liability insurance/malpractice insurance, prerequisite course work. Transfer students are accepted. *Application deadline:* 3/15 (fall), 9/15 (spring). *Application fee:* $20.
Advanced Placement Credit by examination available. Credit given for nursing courses completed elsewhere dependent upon specific evaluations.
Contact *Telephone:* 334-670-3428. *Fax:* 334-670-3744.

GRADUATE PROGRAMS
Contact *Telephone:* 334-834-2320. *Fax:* 334-241-8627.

MASTER'S DEGREE PROGRAM
Degree MSN
Available Programs Master's.
Concentrations Available Nursing administration; nursing education; nursing informatics. *Clinical nurse specialist programs in:* adult health, maternity-newborn. *Nurse practitioner programs in:* family health.
Site Options Montgomery, AL; Phenix City, AL.
Study Options Full-time and part-time.
Online Degree Options Yes.
Program Entrance Requirements Minimum overall college GPA of 3.0, transcript of college record, CPR certification, immunizations, 3 letters of recommendation, physical assessment course, professional liability insurance/malpractice insurance. *Application deadline:* Applications may be processed on a rolling basis for some programs. *Application fee:* $20.
Advanced Placement Credit given for nursing courses completed elsewhere dependent upon specific evaluations.
Degree Requirements 39 total credit hours, thesis or project, comprehensive exam.

POST-MASTER'S PROGRAM
Areas of Study *Nurse practitioner programs in:* family health.

DOCTORAL DEGREE PROGRAM
Degree DNP
Available Programs Doctorate; Post-Baccalaureate Doctorate.
Areas of Study Advanced practice nursing.
Site Options Montgomery, AL; Phenix City, AL.
Online Degree Options Yes (online only).
Program Entrance Requirements Clinical experience, minimum overall college GPA of 3.0, interview by faculty committee, 2 letters of recommendation, MSN or equivalent, vita, writing sample. *Application deadline:* 2/1 (fall). *Application fee:* $75.
Degree Requirements 74 total credit hours, oral exam, residency.

Tuskegee University
Program in Nursing
Tuskegee, Alabama

http://www.tuskegee.edu/home.aspx
Founded in 1881
DEGREE • BSN
Nursing Program Faculty 7 (43% with doctorates).
Baccalaureate Enrollment 145 **Women** 99% **Men** 1% **Minority** 100%
Nursing Student Activities Nursing Honor Society, Student Nurses' Association, nursing club.
Nursing Student Resources Academic advising; academic or career counseling; assistance for students with disabilities; bookstore; campus computer network; career placement assistance; computer lab; computer-assisted instruction; e-mail services; interactive nursing skills videos; Internet; learning resource lab; library services; nursing audiovisuals; placement services for program completers; remedial services; resume preparation assistance; skills, simulation, or other laboratory; tutoring; unpaid internships.
Library Facilities 623,824 volumes (4,500 in health, 600 in nursing); 81,157 periodical subscriptions (250 health-care related).

BACCALAUREATE PROGRAMS
Degree BSN
Available Programs ADN to Baccalaureate; Generic Baccalaureate; RN Baccalaureate.
Study Options Full-time and part-time.
Program Entrance Requirements Minimum overall college GPA of 3.0, transcript of college record, CPR certification, written essay, health exam, health insurance, high school biology, high school chemistry, 2 years high school math, 1 year of high school science, high school transcript, immunizations, interview, minimum high school GPA of 3.0, minimum GPA in nursing prerequisites of 3.0, professional liability insurance/malpractice insurance, prerequisite course work. Transfer students are accepted. *Application deadline:* 5/30 (fall), 11/30 (spring), 4/30 (summer). Applications may be processed on a rolling basis for some programs. *Application fee:* $35.
Advanced Placement Credit given for nursing courses completed elsewhere dependent upon specific evaluations.
Expenses (2011–12) *Tuition:* full-time $17,070; part-time $945 per credit hour. *International tuition:* $17,070 full-time. *Room and board:* $7380; room only: $4845 per academic year. *Required fees:* full-time $850; part-time $850 per term.
Financial Aid 85% of baccalaureate students in nursing programs received some form of financial aid in 2010–11.
Contact Dr. Doris S. Holeman, Associate Dean and Director, Program in Nursing, Tuskegee University, 209 Basil O'Connor Hall, Tuskegee, AL 36083. *Telephone:* 334-727-8382. *Fax:* 334-727-5461. *E-mail:* dholeman@tuskegee.edu.

The University of Alabama
Capstone College of Nursing
Tuscaloosa, Alabama

http://nursing.ua.edu/
Founded in 1831
DEGREES • BSN • DNP • MSN • MSN/ED D • MSN/MA
Nursing Program Faculty 57 (51% with doctorates).
Baccalaureate Enrollment 1,567 **Women** 90% **Men** 10% **Minority** 19% **International** .13% **Part-time** 12%
Graduate Enrollment 383 **Women** 89% **Men** 11% **Minority** 32% **Part-time** 79%
Distance Learning Courses Available.
Nursing Student Activities Sigma Theta Tau, Student Nurses' Association.
Nursing Student Resources Academic advising; academic or career counseling; assistance for students with disabilities; bookstore; campus computer network; career placement assistance; computer lab; computer-assisted instruction; e-mail services; interactive nursing skills videos;

Internet; learning resource lab; library services; paid internships; placement services for program completers; skills, simulation, or other laboratory; tutoring; unpaid internships.

Library Facilities 3.6 million volumes (21,000 in health, 400 in nursing); 101,538 periodical subscriptions (1,500 health-care related).

BACCALAUREATE PROGRAMS

Degree BSN

Available Programs Baccalaureate for Second Degree; Generic Baccalaureate; RN Baccalaureate.

Study Options Full-time.

Program Entrance Requirements Minimum overall college GPA of 3.0, transcript of college record, CPR certification, health exam, health insurance, 4 years high school math, 4 years high school science, high school transcript, immunizations, minimum high school GPA of 2.5, minimum GPA in nursing prerequisites of 3.0, professional liability insurance/malpractice insurance, prerequisite course work. Transfer students are accepted. *Application deadline:* 6/1 (fall), 3/1 (summer). *Application fee:* $25.

Expenses (2012–13) *Tuition, state resident:* full-time $9200; part-time $695 per credit hour. *Tuition, nonresident:* full-time $22,950; part-time $1260 per credit hour. *Room and board:* $11,850; room only: $8800 per academic year. *Required fees:* full-time $1350.

Financial Aid 75% of baccalaureate students in nursing programs received some form of financial aid in 2011–12.

Contact Ms. Rebekah Welch, Director of Nursing Student Services, Capstone College of Nursing, The University of Alabama, Box 870358, Tuscaloosa, AL 35487-0358. *Telephone:* 205-348-6639. *Fax:* 205-348-5559. *E-mail:* rebekah.welch@ua.edu.

GRADUATE PROGRAMS

Expenses (2012–13) *Tuition, state resident:* part-time $330 per credit hour. *Tuition, nonresident:* full-time $5940; part-time $330 per credit hour. *Required fees:* full-time $246.

Financial Aid 49% of graduate students in nursing programs received some form of financial aid in 2011–12.

Contact Dr. Marsha Howell Adams, Interim Assistant Dean, Graduate Program, Capstone College of Nursing, The University of Alabama, Box 870358, Tuscaloosa, AL 35487-0358. *Telephone:* 205-348-1044. *Fax:* 205-348-5559. *E-mail:* madams@ua.edu.

MASTER'S DEGREE PROGRAM

Degrees MSN; MSN/Ed D; MSN/MA

Available Programs Master's; RN to Master's.

Concentrations Available Clinical nurse leader; nurse case management; nursing administration; nursing education. *Nurse practitioner programs in:* family health, psychiatric/mental health.

Study Options Full-time and part-time.

Online Degree Options Yes (online only).

Program Entrance Requirements Minimum overall college GPA of 3.0, transcript of college record, written essay. *Application deadline:* 7/1 (fall), 11/1 (spring), 4/1 (summer). Applications may be processed on a rolling basis for some programs. *Application fee:* $25.

Degree Requirements 36 total credit hours, thesis or project.

POST-MASTER'S PROGRAM

Areas of Study Clinical nurse leader; nurse case management.

DOCTORAL DEGREE PROGRAM

Degree DNP

Available Programs Doctorate.

Areas of Study Advanced practice nursing, nursing administration.

Online Degree Options Yes (online only).

Program Entrance Requirements Minimum overall college GPA of 3.0, interview, 2 letters of recommendation, MSN or equivalent, writing sample. *Application deadline:* 7/1 (fall). Applications may be processed on a rolling basis for some programs. *Application fee:* $25.

Degree Requirements 34 total credit hours, residency.

The University of Alabama at Birmingham
School of Nursing
Birmingham, Alabama

http://www.uab.edu/son/
Founded in 1969
DEGREES • BSN • DNP • MSN • MSN/MPH • PHD
Nursing Program Faculty 108 (67% with doctorates).
Baccalaureate Enrollment 498 **Women** 83% **Men** 17% **Minority** 32% **International** 4% **Part-time** 41%
Graduate Enrollment 1,563 **Women** 89% **Men** 11% **Minority** 23% **International** 2% **Part-time** 67%
Distance Learning Courses Available.
Nursing Student Activities Sigma Theta Tau, Student Nurses' Association, nursing club.
Nursing Student Resources Academic advising; academic or career counseling; assistance for students with disabilities; bookstore; campus computer network; career placement assistance; computer lab; computer-assisted instruction; e-mail services; housing assistance; interactive nursing skills videos; Internet; learning resource lab; library services; nursing audiovisuals; paid internships; placement services for program completers; resume preparation assistance; skills, simulation, or other laboratory; tutoring.
Library Facilities 1.4 million volumes (318,000 in health, 6,862 in nursing); 36,371 periodical subscriptions (2,566 health-care related).

BACCALAUREATE PROGRAMS

Degree BSN

Available Programs Baccalaureate for Second Degree; Generic Baccalaureate; RN Baccalaureate.

Study Options Full-time.

Program Entrance Requirements Minimum overall college GPA of 2.75, transcript of college record, CPR certification, written essay, health exam, health insurance, high school biology, high school transcript, immunizations, minimum high school GPA of 2.0, minimum GPA in nursing prerequisites of 2.75, prerequisite course work. Transfer students are accepted. *Application deadline:* 4/12 (fall), 9/7 (spring).

Expenses (2012–13) *Tuition, state resident:* full-time $8658; part-time $3792 per semester. *Tuition, nonresident:* full-time $19,786; part-time $9342 per semester. *International tuition:* $19,786 full-time. *Room and board:* $9294; room only: $5400 per academic year. *Required fees:* full-time $1130; part-time $340 per term.

Financial Aid 84% of baccalaureate students in nursing programs received some form of financial aid in 2011–12. *Gift aid (need-based):* Federal Pell, FSEOG, state, private, college/university gift aid from institutional funds, United Negro College Fund. *Loans:* Federal Direct (Subsidized and Unsubsidized Stafford PLUS), Perkins, state, college/university. *Work-study:* Federal Work-Study. *Financial aid application deadline (priority):* 3/1.

Contact Mr. Peter Tofani, Assistant Dean for Student Affairs, School of Nursing, The University of Alabama at Birmingham, NB 1003, 1720 2nd Avenue South, Birmingham, AL 35294-1210. *Telephone:* 205-975-7529. *Fax:* 205-934-5490. *E-mail:* tofanip@uab.edu.

GRADUATE PROGRAMS

Expenses (2012–13) *Tuition, state resident:* full-time $8343; part-time $2781 per semester. *Tuition, nonresident:* full-time $18,819; part-time $6273 per semester. *International tuition:* $18,819 full-time. *Room and board:* $9294; room only: $5400 per academic year. *Required fees:* full-time $1710; part-time $770 per term.

Financial Aid 66% of graduate students in nursing programs received some form of financial aid in 2011–12. Fellowships, research assistantships, teaching assistantships, Federal Work-Study available. Aid available to part-time students.

Contact Mr. Peter Tofani, Assistant Dean for Student Affairs, School of Nursing, The University of Alabama at Birmingham, NB 1003, 1720 2nd Avenue South, Birmingham, AL 35294-1210. *Telephone:* 205-975-7529. *Fax:* 205-934-5490. *E-mail:* tofanip@uab.edu.

MASTER'S DEGREE PROGRAM

Degrees MSN; MSN/MPH

Available Programs Accelerated AD/RN to Master's; Accelerated Master's for Non-Nursing College Graduates; Master's.

Concentrations Available Clinical nurse leader; health-care administration; nurse anesthesia; nursing administration; nursing education;

nursing informatics. *Nurse practitioner programs in:* acute care, adult health, family health, gerontology, neonatal health, occupational health, pediatric, primary care, psychiatric/mental health, women's health.
Study Options Full-time and part-time.
Program Entrance Requirements Clinical experience, computer literacy, minimum overall college GPA of 3.0, transcript of college record, CPR certification, written essay, immunizations, 3 letters of recommendation, prerequisite course work, resume, statistics course, GRE General Test. *Application deadline:* 3/16 (fall), 9/7 (spring). *Application fee:* $45.
Advanced Placement Credit given for nursing courses completed elsewhere dependent upon specific evaluations.
Degree Requirements 30 total credit hours, comprehensive exam.

POST-MASTER'S PROGRAM
Areas of Study *Nurse practitioner programs in:* acute care, adult health, family health, gerontology, neonatal health, pediatric, psychiatric/mental health.

DOCTORAL DEGREE PROGRAM
Degree DNP
Available Programs Doctorate.
Areas of Study Advanced practice nursing, health-care systems, nursing administration.
Program Entrance Requirements Minimum overall college GPA of 3.0, clinical experience, 3 letters of recommendation, statistics course, vita, writing sample. *Application deadline:* 1/18 (fall). *Application fee:* $45.
Degree Requirements 66 total credit hours, dissertation, residency, written exam.
Degree PhD
Available Programs Doctorate; Post-Baccalaureate Doctorate.
Areas of Study Nursing research, nursing science.
Program Entrance Requirements Clinical experience, minimum overall college GPA of 3.0, interview by faculty committee, interview, 3 letters of recommendation, scholarly papers, statistics course, vita, writing sample, GRE General Test. *Application deadline:* 1/18 (fall). *Application fee:* $45.
Degree Requirements 66 total credit hours, dissertation, oral exam, written exam, residency.

POSTDOCTORAL PROGRAM
Areas of Study Nursing research, outcomes.
Postdoctoral Program Contact Dr. Patricia Patrician, Donna Brown Banton Endowed Professorship and Associate Professor, School of Nursing, The University of Alabama at Birmingham, 1720 2nd Avenue South, Birmingham, AL 35294-1210. *Telephone:* 205-996-5211. *Fax:* 205-934-5490. *E-mail:* ppatrici@uab.edu.

The University of Alabama in Huntsville
College of Nursing
Huntsville, Alabama

http://onlinenurse.nb.uah.edu/
Founded in 1950
DEGREES • BSN • DNP • MSN
Nursing Program Faculty 46 (30% with doctorates).
Baccalaureate Enrollment 662 **Women** 90% **Men** 10% **Minority** 14% **International** 1% **Part-time** 22%
Graduate Enrollment 106 **Women** 92% **Men** 8% **Minority** 15% **International** 1% **Part-time** 65%
Distance Learning Courses Available.
Nursing Student Activities Sigma Theta Tau, Student Nurses' Association.
Nursing Student Resources Academic advising; academic or career counseling; assistance for students with disabilities; bookstore; campus computer network; career placement assistance; computer lab; computer-assisted instruction; e-mail services; employment services for current students; housing assistance; interactive nursing skills videos; Internet; learning resource lab; library services; nursing audiovisuals; placement services for program completers; remedial services; resume preparation assistance; skills, simulation, or other laboratory; tutoring.
Library Facilities 302,503 volumes (13,004 in health, 3,480 in nursing); 628 periodical subscriptions (3,200 health-care related).

BACCALAUREATE PROGRAMS
Degree BSN
Available Programs Baccalaureate for Second Degree; Generic Baccalaureate; RN Baccalaureate.
Study Options Full-time and part-time.
Program Entrance Requirements Minimum overall college GPA of 2.0, transcript of college record, CPR certification, health exam, health insurance, immunizations, minimum GPA in nursing prerequisites of 2.0, professional liability insurance/malpractice insurance, prerequisite course work. Transfer students are accepted. *Application deadline:* 3/1 (fall), 9/1 (spring).
Advanced Placement Credit by examination available. Credit given for nursing courses completed elsewhere dependent upon specific evaluations.
Contact *Telephone:* 256-824-6742. *Fax:* 256-824-2850.

GRADUATE PROGRAMS
Contact *Telephone:* 256-824-6742. *Fax:* 256-824-6026.

MASTER'S DEGREE PROGRAM
Degree MSN
Available Programs Master's; RN to Master's.
Concentrations Available Clinical nurse leader; health-care administration. *Clinical nurse specialist programs in:* adult health. *Nurse practitioner programs in:* acute care, family health.
Study Options Full-time and part-time.
Online Degree Options Yes.
Program Entrance Requirements Minimum overall college GPA of 3.0, transcript of college record, CPR certification, immunizations, 3 letters of recommendation, professional liability insurance/malpractice insurance, statistics course, MAT or GRE. *Application deadline:* 4/15 (fall).
Advanced Placement Credit given for nursing courses completed elsewhere dependent upon specific evaluations.
Degree Requirements 42 total credit hours, thesis or project, comprehensive exam.

POST-MASTER'S PROGRAM
Areas of Study Nursing education. *Nurse practitioner programs in:* family health.

DOCTORAL DEGREE PROGRAM
Degree DNP
Available Programs Doctorate.
Areas of Study Advanced practice nursing, nursing administration.
Online Degree Options Yes (online only).
Program Entrance Requirements interview by faculty committee, letters of recommendation, MSN or equivalent, vita, writing sample. *Application deadline:* 4/15 (fall). *Application fee:* $40.
Degree Requirements 34 total credit hours, oral exam, written exam.

CONTINUING EDUCATION PROGRAM
Contact *Telephone:* 256-824-2456. *Fax:* 256-824-6026.

University of Mobile
School of Nursing
Mobile, Alabama

http://www.umobile.edu/
Founded in 1961
DEGREES • BSN • MSN
Nursing Program Faculty 14 (22% with doctorates).
Baccalaureate Enrollment 105 **Women** 93% **Men** 7% **Minority** 34%
Graduate Enrollment 19 **Women** 90% **Men** 10% **Minority** 54% **Part-time** 21%
Nursing Student Activities Sigma Theta Tau, Student Nurses' Association.
Nursing Student Resources Academic advising; academic or career counseling; assistance for students with disabilities; bookstore; campus computer network; career placement assistance; computer lab; computer-assisted instruction; e-mail services; employment services for current students; interactive nursing skills videos; Internet; learning resource lab; library services; nursing audiovisuals; remedial services; resume preparation assistance; skills, simulation, or other laboratory; tutoring; unpaid internships.

Library Facilities 107,379 volumes (10,000 in health, 6,500 in nursing); 239 periodical subscriptions (4,373 health-care related).

BACCALAUREATE PROGRAMS

Degree BSN
Available Programs ADN to Baccalaureate; Generic Baccalaureate; RN Baccalaureate.
Study Options Full-time.
Program Entrance Requirements Minimum overall college GPA of 2.75, transcript of college record, CPR certification, health exam, health insurance, high school transcript, immunizations, minimum GPA in nursing prerequisites of 2.75, prerequisite course work. Transfer students are accepted. *Application deadline:* 3/1 (fall).
Advanced Placement Credit given for nursing courses completed elsewhere dependent upon specific evaluations.
Expenses (2012–13) *Tuition:* full-time $17,110; part-time $609 per credit hour. *International tuition:* $17,110 full-time. *Room and board:* $8650; room only: $5100 per academic year. *Required fees:* full-time $570; part-time $346 per term.
Financial Aid 96% of baccalaureate students in nursing programs received some form of financial aid in 2011–12.
Contact Mrs. Mattie Easter, Assistant Professor, School of Nursing, University of Mobile, 5735 College Parkway, Mobile, AL 36613-2842. *Telephone:* 251-442-2337. *Fax:* 251-442-2520. *E-mail:* measter@mail.umobile.edu.

GRADUATE PROGRAMS

Expenses (2012–13) *Tuition:* full-time $8604; part-time $478 per credit hour. *International tuition:* $8604 full-time. *Required fees:* full-time $146; part-time $73 per term.
Financial Aid 50% of graduate students in nursing programs received some form of financial aid in 2011–12.
Contact Dr. Janith C. Wood, Department Chair, School of Nursing, University of Mobile, 5735 College Parkway, Mobile, AL 36613-2842. *Telephone:* 251-442-2446. *Fax:* 251-442-2520. *E-mail:* jwood@mail.umobile.edu.

MASTER'S DEGREE PROGRAM

Degree MSN
Available Programs Master's.
Concentrations Available Nursing administration; nursing education.
Study Options Full-time and part-time.
Program Entrance Requirements Minimum overall college GPA of 3.0, transcript of college record, CPR certification, immunizations, 3 letters of recommendation, statistics course. *Application deadline:* Applications may be processed on a rolling basis for some programs. *Application fee:* $40.
Advanced Placement Credit given for nursing courses completed elsewhere dependent upon specific evaluations.
Degree Requirements 39 total credit hours, thesis or project, comprehensive exam.

CONTINUING EDUCATION PROGRAM

Contact Dr. Janith C. Wood, Dean, School of Nursing, School of Nursing, University of Mobile, 5735 College Parkway, Mobile, AL 36613. *Telephone:* 251-442-2446. *Fax:* 251-442-2520. *E-mail:* Jwood@mail.umobile.edu.

University of North Alabama
College of Nursing and Allied Health
Florence, Alabama

http://www.una.edu/nursing/
Founded in 1830
DEGREES • BSN • MSN
Nursing Program Faculty 37 (22% with doctorates).
Baccalaureate Enrollment 390 **Women** 87% **Men** 13% **Minority** 20.5% **International** 1% **Part-time** 31%
Graduate Enrollment 36 **Women** 97% **Men** 3% **Minority** 17% **Part-time** 25%
Distance Learning Courses Available.
Nursing Student Activities Sigma Theta Tau, Student Nurses' Association.
Nursing Student Resources Academic advising; academic or career counseling; assistance for students with disabilities; bookstore; campus

computer network; career placement assistance; computer lab; e-mail services; employment services for current students; housing assistance; interactive nursing skills videos; Internet; learning resource lab; library services; nursing audiovisuals; remedial services; resume preparation assistance; skills, simulation, or other laboratory; tutoring.
Library Facilities 409,163 volumes; 19,633 periodical subscriptions.

BACCALAUREATE PROGRAMS

Degree BSN
Available Programs Generic Baccalaureate; RN Baccalaureate.
Study Options Full-time and part-time.
Online Degree Options Yes (online only).
Program Entrance Requirements Transcript of college record, CPR certification, health exam, health insurance, high school transcript, immunizations, minimum GPA in nursing prerequisites of 2.5, professional liability insurance/malpractice insurance, prerequisite course work. Transfer students are accepted.
Contact *Telephone:* 256-765-4984. *Fax:* 256-765-4935.

GRADUATE PROGRAMS

Contact *Telephone:* 256-765-4931. *Fax:* 256-765-4701.

MASTER'S DEGREE PROGRAM

Degree MSN
Available Programs Master's.
Concentrations Available Nursing administration; nursing education.
Study Options Full-time and part-time.
Online Degree Options Yes (online only).
Program Entrance Requirements Clinical experience, minimum overall college GPA of 3.0, transcript of college record, written essay, 3 letters of recommendation, professional liability insurance/malpractice insurance.
Degree Requirements 42 total credit hours, thesis or project.

CONTINUING EDUCATION PROGRAM

Contact *Telephone:* 256-765-4787. *Fax:* 256-765-4872.

University of South Alabama
College of Nursing
Mobile, Alabama

http://www.southalabama.edu/nursing/
Founded in 1963
DEGREES • BSN • MSN
Nursing Program Faculty 57 (30% with doctorates).
Baccalaureate Enrollment 316 **Women** 82% **Men** 18% **Minority** 24% **International** 3% **Part-time** 11%
Graduate Enrollment 368 **Women** 86% **Men** 14% **Minority** 19% **Part-time** 22%
Nursing Student Activities Sigma Theta Tau, Student Nurses' Association.
Nursing Student Resources Academic advising; academic or career counseling; assistance for students with disabilities; bookstore; campus computer network; career placement assistance; computer lab; learning resource lab; library services; nursing audiovisuals; resume preparation assistance.
Library Facilities 854,298 volumes (2,406 in health, 2,300 in nursing); 985 periodical subscriptions (299 health-care related).

BACCALAUREATE PROGRAMS

Degree BSN
Available Programs ADN to Baccalaureate; Accelerated Baccalaureate; Generic Baccalaureate; RN Baccalaureate.
Site Options Fairhope, AL.
Study Options Full-time and part-time.
Program Entrance Requirements Minimum overall college GPA of 2.5, transcript of college record, CPR certification, health exam, health insurance, immunizations, minimum GPA in nursing prerequisites of 2.5, professional liability insurance/malpractice insurance, prerequisite course work. Transfer students are accepted.
Advanced Placement Credit given for nursing courses completed elsewhere dependent upon specific evaluations.
Contact *Telephone:* 251-434-3410. *Fax:* 251-434-3413.

GRADUATE PROGRAMS

Contact *Telephone:* 251-434-3410. *Fax:* 251-434-3413.

MASTER'S DEGREE PROGRAM
Degree MSN
Available Programs Accelerated Master's; Master's; Master's for Nurses with Non-Nursing Degrees.
Concentrations Available Nursing administration; nursing education. *Clinical nurse specialist programs in:* acute care, community health, family health, gerontology, maternity-newborn, pediatric, psychiatric/mental health, women's health. *Nurse practitioner programs in:* acute care, family health, gerontology, neonatal health, pediatric, psychiatric/mental health, women's health.
Study Options Full-time and part-time.
Program Entrance Requirements Computer literacy, minimum overall college GPA of 3.0, transcript of college record, immunizations, nursing research course, physical assessment course, resume.
Advanced Placement Credit given for nursing courses completed elsewhere dependent upon specific evaluations.
Degree Requirements 30 total credit hours, thesis or project.

POST-MASTER'S PROGRAM
Areas of Study Nursing administration; nursing education. *Clinical nurse specialist programs in:* acute care, community health, family health, gerontology, maternity-newborn, pediatric, psychiatric/mental health, women's health. *Nurse practitioner programs in:* acute care, family health, gerontology, neonatal health, pediatric, psychiatric/mental health, women's health.

ALASKA

University of Alaska Anchorage
School of Nursing
Anchorage, Alaska

http://www.uaa.alaska.edu/schoolofnursing/
Founded in 1954
DEGREES • BS • MS
Nursing Program Faculty 26 (42% with doctorates).
Baccalaureate Enrollment 224 **Women** 80% **Men** 20% **Minority** 31% **International** 3% **Part-time** 18%
Graduate Enrollment 60 **Women** 94% **Men** 6% **Minority** 9% **Part-time** 12%
Nursing Student Activities Sigma Theta Tau, Student Nurses' Association.
Nursing Student Resources Academic advising; academic or career counseling; assistance for students with disabilities; bookstore; campus computer network; career placement assistance; computer lab; computer-assisted instruction; daycare for children of students; e-mail services; interactive nursing skills videos; Internet; learning resource lab; library services; nursing audiovisuals; placement services for program completers; remedial services; resume preparation assistance; skills, simulation, or other laboratory; tutoring.
Library Facilities 23,000 volumes in health, 150 volumes in nursing; 780 periodical subscriptions health-care related.

BACCALAUREATE PROGRAMS

Degree BS
Available Programs Generic Baccalaureate; RN Baccalaureate.
Study Options Full-time and part-time.
Program Entrance Requirements Minimum overall college GPA of 2.7, transcript of college record, CPR certification, written essay, immunizations, 3 letters of recommendation, minimum GPA in nursing prerequisites of 2.7, professional liability insurance/malpractice insurance, prerequisite course work. Transfer students are accepted.
Advanced Placement Credit given for nursing courses completed elsewhere dependent upon specific evaluations.
Contact *Telephone:* 907-786-4550. *Fax:* 907-786-4558.

GRADUATE PROGRAMS

Contact *Telephone:* 907-786-4570. *Fax:* 907-786-4559.

MASTER'S DEGREE PROGRAM
Degree MS
Available Programs Master's.
Concentrations Available Health-care administration; nursing education. *Clinical nurse specialist programs in:* community health, psychiatric/mental health. *Nurse practitioner programs in:* family health, psychiatric/mental health.
Study Options Full-time and part-time.
Program Entrance Requirements Clinical experience, minimum overall college GPA of 3.0, transcript of college record, written essay, 3 letters of recommendation, nursing research course, prerequisite course work, statistics course, GRE or MAT.
Advanced Placement Credit given for nursing courses completed elsewhere dependent upon specific evaluations.
Degree Requirements 50 total credit hours, thesis or project.

ARIZONA

Arizona State University at the Downtown Phoenix Campus
College of Nursing
Phoenix, Arizona

http://campus.asu.edu/downtown/
Founded in 2006
DEGREES • BSN • DNP • MS • MS/MPH
Nursing Program Faculty 119 (44% with doctorates).
Baccalaureate Enrollment 1,085 **Women** 88% **Men** 12% **Minority** 31% **International** 1% **Part-time** 18%
Graduate Enrollment 363 **Women** 91% **Men** 9% **Minority** 7% **Part-time** 46%
Distance Learning Courses Available.
Nursing Student Activities Nursing Honor Society, Sigma Theta Tau, Student Nurses' Association, nursing club.
Nursing Student Resources Academic advising; academic or career counseling; assistance for students with disabilities; bookstore; campus computer network; career placement assistance; computer lab; computer-assisted instruction; daycare for children of students; e-mail services; employment services for current students; housing assistance; interactive nursing skills videos; Internet; learning resource lab; library services; nursing audiovisuals; paid internships; placement services for program completers; remedial services; resume preparation assistance; skills, simulation, or other laboratory; tutoring; unpaid internships.
Library Facilities 77,814 volumes in health, 7,501 volumes in nursing; 755 periodical subscriptions health-care related.

BACCALAUREATE PROGRAMS

Degree BSN
Available Programs Accelerated Baccalaureate for Second Degree; Accelerated RN Baccalaureate; Baccalaureate for Second Degree; Generic Baccalaureate; RN Baccalaureate.
Site Options Phoenix, AZ; Scottsdale, AZ.
Study Options Full-time.
Online Degree Options Yes.
Program Entrance Requirements Minimum overall college GPA of 3.50, transcript of college record, CPR certification, health exam, health insurance, high school biology, high school chemistry, high school foreign language, 4 years high school math, 3 years high school science, high school transcript, immunizations, minimum high school GPA of 3.5, minimum high school rank 25%, minimum GPA in nursing prerequisites of 3.75, professional liability insurance/malpractice insurance, prerequisite course work. *Application deadline:* 5/1 (fall), 9/1 (spring), 2/1 (summer). *Application fee:* $65.
Expenses (2012–13) *Tuition, state resident:* full-time $11,722; part-time $955 per credit hour. *Tuition, nonresident:* full-time $24,975; part-time $1233 per credit hour. *International tuition:* $25,000 full-time. *Room and board:* $9100; room only: $6000 per academic year.
Financial Aid 70% of baccalaureate students in nursing programs received some form of financial aid in 2011–12.
Contact Sara Sullivan, Senior Student Support Specialist, College of Nursing, Arizona State University at the Downtown Phoenix Campus, 502 East Monroe Street, Suite C 250, Phoenix, AZ 85004-4431.

Telephone: 602-496-0887. *Fax:* 602-496-0705. *E-mail:* sara.sullivan@asu.edu.

GRADUATE PROGRAMS

Expenses (2012–13) *Tuition, state resident:* full-time $14,515; part-time $1154 per credit hour. *Tuition, nonresident:* full-time $22,928; part-time $1463 per credit hour. *International tuition:* $23,000 full-time. *Room and board:* $9100; room only: $6000 per academic year.

Financial Aid 75% of graduate students in nursing programs received some form of financial aid in 2011–12.

Contact Ms. Eula Bradley, Manager, Graduate Student Success, College of Nursing, Arizona State University at the Downtown Phoenix Campus, 550 North 3rd Street, Phoenix, AZ 85004. *Telephone:* 602-496-0703. *E-mail:* eula.bradley@asu.edu.

MASTER'S DEGREE PROGRAM

Degrees MS; MS/MPH

Available Programs Master's.

Concentrations Available *Clinical nurse specialist programs in:* acute care, adult health, community health, pediatric, psychiatric/mental health. *Nurse practitioner programs in:* acute care, adult health, family health, neonatal health, pediatric, psychiatric/mental health, women's health.

Site Options Phoenix, AZ.

Study Options Full-time and part-time.

Program Entrance Requirements Clinical experience, minimum overall college GPA of 3.0, transcript of college record, immunizations, interview, 3 letters of recommendation, physical assessment course, prerequisite course work, resume, statistics course, GRE.

Advanced Placement Credit given for nursing courses completed elsewhere dependent upon specific evaluations.

Degree Requirements 40 total credit hours, thesis or project.

POST-MASTER'S PROGRAM

Areas of Study *Clinical nurse specialist programs in:* acute care, adult health, community health, pediatric, psychiatric/mental health. *Nurse practitioner programs in:* acute care, adult health, family health, neonatal health, pediatric, psychiatric/mental health, women's health.

DOCTORAL DEGREE PROGRAM

Degree DNP

Available Programs Doctorate.

Areas of Study Advanced practice nursing.

Site Options Phoenix, AZ.

CONTINUING EDUCATION PROGRAM

Contact Amy Fitzgerald, RN, Assistant Director, College of Nursing, Arizona State University at the Downtown Phoenix Campus, 550 North 3rd Street, Phoenix, AZ 85004. *Telephone:* 602-496-2175. *E-mail:* Amy.Fitzgerald@asu.edu.

Chamberlain College of Nursing

Chamberlain College of Nursing
Phoenix, Arizona

DEGREES • BSN • MSN

Distance Learning Courses Available.

BACCALAUREATE PROGRAMS

Degree BSN

Available Programs Accelerated Baccalaureate; Accelerated Baccalaureate for Second Degree; RN Baccalaureate.

Contact *Telephone:* 888-556-8226.

GRADUATE PROGRAMS

Contact *Telephone:* 888-556-8226.

MASTER'S DEGREE PROGRAM

Degree MSN

Available Programs Master's.

Grand Canyon University

College of Nursing and Health Sciences
Phoenix, Arizona

Founded in 1949

DEGREES • BSN • MS • MSN/MBA

Nursing Program Faculty 122 (3% with doctorates).

Baccalaureate Enrollment 1,067 **Women** 90% **Men** 10% **International** .01% **Part-time** 58%

Graduate Enrollment 297 **Women** 93% **Men** 7% **Part-time** 89%

Distance Learning Courses Available.

Nursing Student Activities Sigma Theta Tau, Student Nurses' Association.

Nursing Student Resources Academic advising; academic or career counseling; assistance for students with disabilities; bookstore; campus computer network; career placement assistance; computer lab; computer-assisted instruction; e-mail services; employment services for current students; housing assistance; Internet; learning resource lab; library services; nursing audiovisuals; other; paid internships; remedial services; resume preparation assistance; skills, simulation, or other laboratory; tutoring; unpaid internships.

Library Facilities 158,587 volumes (9,663 in health); 57,802 periodical subscriptions (177 health-care related).

BACCALAUREATE PROGRAMS

Degree BSN

Available Programs ADN to Baccalaureate; RN Baccalaureate.

Site Options Phoenix, AZ; Tucson, AZ; Albuquerque, NM.

Study Options Full-time.

Online Degree Options Yes.

Program Entrance Requirements Minimum overall college GPA of 3.0, transcript of college record, CPR certification, health exam, health insurance, high school transcript, immunizations, minimum GPA in nursing prerequisites of 3.0, prerequisite course work. Transfer students are accepted. *Application deadline:* 5/15 (fall), 9/15 (spring), 1/15 (summer).

Advanced Placement Credit by examination available. Credit given for nursing courses completed elsewhere dependent upon specific evaluations.

Contact *Telephone:* 602-639-6429.

GRADUATE PROGRAMS

Contact *Telephone:* 602-639-7982.

MASTER'S DEGREE PROGRAM

Degrees MS; MSN/MBA

Available Programs Master's.

Concentrations Available Nursing administration; nursing education. *Clinical nurse specialist programs in:* adult health. *Nurse practitioner programs in:* acute care, family health.

Site Options Phoenix, AZ; Tucson, AZ.

Study Options Full-time and part-time.

Online Degree Options Yes.

Program Entrance Requirements Clinical experience, computer literacy, minimum overall college GPA of 3.0, transcript of college record, CPR certification, written essay, immunizations, interview, nursing research course, physical assessment course, professional liability insurance/malpractice insurance, prerequisite course work, resume, statistics course. *Application deadline:* Applications may be processed on a rolling basis for some programs.

Advanced Placement Credit given for nursing courses completed elsewhere dependent upon specific evaluations.

Degree Requirements 52 total credit hours, thesis or project.

POST-MASTER'S PROGRAM

Areas of Study Nursing education. *Clinical nurse specialist programs in:* adult health. *Nurse practitioner programs in:* acute care, family health.

CONTINUING EDUCATION PROGRAM

Contact *Telephone:* 602-639-7982. *Fax:* 602-639-7982.

Northern Arizona University
School of Nursing
Flagstaff, Arizona

http://nau.edu/chhs/nursing/
Founded in 1899

DEGREES • BSN • DNP • MS

Nursing Program Faculty 60 (30% with doctorates).
Baccalaureate Enrollment 875 **Women** 88% **Men** 12% **Minority** 20% **International** 1% **Part-time** 50%
Graduate Enrollment 120 **Women** 96% **Men** 4% **Minority** 20% **Part-time** 65%
Distance Learning Courses Available.
Nursing Student Activities Sigma Theta Tau, Student Nurses' Association.
Nursing Student Resources Academic advising; academic or career counseling; assistance for students with disabilities; bookstore; campus computer network; computer lab; computer-assisted instruction; e-mail services; interactive nursing skills videos; Internet; learning resource lab; library services; nursing audiovisuals; remedial services; skills, simulation, or other laboratory; tutoring.
Library Facilities 892,809 volumes; 59,863 periodical subscriptions.

BACCALAUREATE PROGRAMS

Degree BSN
Available Programs ADN to Baccalaureate; Accelerated Baccalaureate for Second Degree; Generic Baccalaureate; RN Baccalaureate.
Site Options St. Michaels/Window Rock, AZ; Yuma, AZ; Tucson, AZ.
Study Options Full-time.
Online Degree Options Yes.
Program Entrance Requirements Transcript of college record, CPR certification, health exam, health insurance, high school transcript, immunizations, 2 letters of recommendation, minimum GPA in nursing prerequisites of 2.75, professional liability insurance/malpractice insurance, prerequisite course work. Transfer students are accepted. *Application deadline:* 3/15 (fall), 10/15 (spring).
Advanced Placement Credit given for nursing courses completed elsewhere dependent upon specific evaluations.
Financial Aid 75% of baccalaureate students in nursing programs received some form of financial aid in 2011–12. *Gift aid (need-based):* Federal Pell, FSEOG, state, private, college/university gift aid from institutional funds, Federal Nursing, TEACH Grants, tribal grants, LEAP Grants. *Loans:* Federal Nursing Student Loans, Federal Direct (Subsidized and Unsubsidized Stafford PLUS), Perkins, state, college/university. *Work-study:* Federal Work-Study, part-time campus jobs. *Financial aid application deadline (priority):* 2/14.
Contact Mr. Gregg Schneider, Senior Academic Advisor, School of Nursing, Northern Arizona University, Box 15035, Flagstaff, AZ 86011. *Telephone:* 928-523-6717. *Fax:* 928-523-7171. *E-mail:* gregg.schneider@nau.edu.

GRADUATE PROGRAMS

Financial Aid 75% of graduate students in nursing programs received some form of financial aid in 2011–12. Career-related internships or fieldwork, Federal Work-Study, scholarships, traineeships, tuition waivers, and unspecified assistantships available.
Contact Dr. Barbara Tomlinson, Graduate Program Coordinator, School of Nursing, Northern Arizona University, Box 15035, Flagstaff, AZ 86011. *Telephone:* 928-523-3536. *Fax:* 928-523-7171. *E-mail:* barbara.tomlinson@nau.edu.

MASTER'S DEGREE PROGRAM

Degree MS
Available Programs Master's.
Concentrations Available *Nurse practitioner programs in:* family health.
Site Options St. Michaels/Window Rock, AZ; Yuma, AZ; Tucson, AZ.
Study Options Full-time and part-time.
Online Degree Options Yes (online only).
Program Entrance Requirements Clinical experience, computer literacy, minimum overall college GPA of 3.0, transcript of college record, CPR certification, written essay, immunizations, 3 letters of recommendation, nursing research course, physical assessment course, professional liability insurance/malpractice insurance, prerequisite course work, resume, statistics course, GRE General Test or minimum GPA of 3.0. *Application deadline:* 10/15 (fall), 1/15 (spring), 7/15 (summer).

Advanced Placement Credit given for nursing courses completed elsewhere dependent upon specific evaluations.
Degree Requirements 40 total credit hours, thesis or project.

POST-MASTER'S PROGRAM
Areas of Study *Nurse practitioner programs in:* family health.

DOCTORAL DEGREE PROGRAM
Degree DNP
Available Programs Doctorate.
Areas of Study Clinical practice, family health.
Site Options St. Michaels/Window Rock, AZ; Yuma, AZ; Tucson, AZ.
Online Degree Options Yes (online only).
Program Entrance Requirements Clinical experience, minimum overall college GPA of 3.0, interview by faculty committee, 3 letters of recommendation, MSN or equivalent, statistics course, vita. *Application deadline:* Applications may be processed on a rolling basis for some programs.
Degree Requirements 31 total credit hours, dissertation.

The University of Arizona
College of Nursing
Tucson, Arizona

http://www.nursing.arizona.edu/
Founded in 1885

DEGREES • BSN • MSN • PHD

Nursing Program Faculty 75 (57% with doctorates).
Baccalaureate Enrollment 214 **Women** 90.2% **Men** 9.8% **Minority** 32.7% **International** .01%
Graduate Enrollment 363 **Women** 93.5% **Men** 6.5% **Minority** 37.7% **International** .01% **Part-time** 14%
Distance Learning Courses Available.
Nursing Student Activities Nursing Honor Society, Sigma Theta Tau, Student Nurses' Association, nursing club.
Nursing Student Resources Academic advising; academic or career counseling; assistance for students with disabilities; bookstore; campus computer network; career placement assistance; computer lab; computer-assisted instruction; e-mail services; externships; housing assistance; interactive nursing skills videos; Internet; learning resource lab; library services; nursing audiovisuals; other; placement services for program completers; remedial services; resume preparation assistance; skills, simulation, or other laboratory; tutoring.
Library Facilities 112,500 volumes in health, 5,400 volumes in nursing; 10,785 periodical subscriptions health-care related.

BACCALAUREATE PROGRAMS

Degree BSN
Available Programs Generic Baccalaureate.
Study Options Full-time.
Program Entrance Requirements Minimum overall college GPA of 3.0, transcript of college record, CPR certification, written essay, health insurance, high school transcript, immunizations, interview, minimum GPA in nursing prerequisites of 3.0, prerequisite course work. Transfer students are accepted. *Application deadline:* 2/1 (fall), 9/1 (spring).
Advanced Placement Credit given for nursing courses completed elsewhere dependent upon specific evaluations.
Expenses (2012–13) *Tuition, state resident:* full-time $12,048; part-time $820 per credit hour. *Tuition, nonresident:* full-time $28,244; part-time $1224 per credit hour. *International tuition:* $28,244 full-time. *Required fees:* full-time $930; part-time $86 per credit.
Financial Aid 82% of baccalaureate students in nursing programs received some form of financial aid in 2011–12. *Gift aid (need-based):* Federal Pell, FSEOG, state, private, college/university gift aid from institutional funds, Federal Nursing. *Loans:* Federal Nursing Student Loans, Federal Direct (Subsidized and Unsubsidized Stafford PLUS), Perkins, college/university. *Work-study:* Federal Work-Study, part-time campus jobs. *Financial aid application deadline:* Continuous.
Contact Mr. Thomas M. Dickson, Director for Student Affairs, College of Nursing, The University of Arizona, 1305 North Martin, PO Box 210203, Tucson, AZ 85721-0203. *Telephone:* 520-626-3808. *Fax:* 520-626-6424. *E-mail:* tdickson@nursing.arizona.edu.

GRADUATE PROGRAMS

Expenses (2012–13) *Tuition, state resident:* full-time $10,200; part-time $729 per credit hour. *Tuition, nonresident:* full-time $25,616; part-time

$1423 per credit hour. *International tuition:* $25,616 full-time. *Required fees:* full-time $5200; part-time $351 per credit.
Financial Aid 72% of graduate students in nursing programs received some form of financial aid in 2011–12. 4 research assistantships with full tuition reimbursements available (averaging $18,220 per year), 3 teaching assistantships (averaging $18,327 per year) were awarded; career-related internships or fieldwork, institutionally sponsored loans, scholarships, traineeships, tuition waivers (full), and unspecified assistantships also available. *Financial aid application deadline:* 6/1.
Contact Graduate Support Services, Senior, College of Nursing, The University of Arizona, 1305 North Martin, PO Box 210203, Tucson, AZ 85721-0203. *Telephone:* 520-626-3808. *Fax:* 520-626-6424. *E-mail:* advanced@nursing.arizona.edu.

MASTER'S DEGREE PROGRAM
Degree MSN
Available Programs Accelerated Master's; Accelerated Master's for Non-Nursing College Graduates; RN to Master's.
Study Options Full-time.
Online Degree Options Yes.
Program Entrance Requirements Minimum overall college GPA of 3.0, transcript of college record, CPR certification, written essay, immunizations, interview, prerequisite course work, statistics course. *Application deadline:* 1/15 (fall). *Application fee:* $75.
Advanced Placement Credit given for nursing courses completed elsewhere dependent upon specific evaluations.
Degree Requirements 56 total credit hours, thesis or project, comprehensive exam.

POST-MASTER'S PROGRAM
Areas of Study *Nurse practitioner programs in:* acute care, adult health, family health, gerontology, pediatric, psychiatric/mental health.

DOCTORAL DEGREE PROGRAM
Degree PhD
Available Programs Doctorate; Post-Baccalaureate Doctorate.
Areas of Study Addiction/substance abuse, advanced practice nursing, aging, bio-behavioral research, biology of health and illness, clinical practice, community health, faculty preparation, family health, gerontology, health policy, health promotion/disease prevention, illness and transition, individualized study, information systems, neuro-behavior, nursing research, nursing science, oncology.
Online Degree Options Yes (online only).
Program Entrance Requirements Minimum overall college GPA of 3.0, interview by faculty committee, interview, 3 letters of recommendation, statistics course, vita. *Application deadline:* 12/15 (fall). *Application fee:* $75.
Degree Requirements 64 total credit hours, dissertation, oral exam, written exam, residency.

POSTDOCTORAL PROGRAM
Postdoctoral Program Contact Ms. Vickie Radoye, Assistant Dean for Student Affairs, College of Nursing, The University of Arizona, 1305 North Martin, PO Box 210203, Tucson, AZ 85721-0203. *Telephone:* 520-626-3808. *Fax:* 520-626-6424. *E-mail:* vradoye@nursing.arizona.edu.

University of Phoenix–Online Campus
Online Campus
Phoenix, Arizona

http://www.uopxonline.com/
Founded in 1989
DEGREES • BSN • MSN • MSN/MBA • MSN/MHA • PHD
Nursing Program Faculty 444 (29% with doctorates).
Baccalaureate Enrollment 5,644 **Women** 92.2% **Men** 7.8% **Minority** 18.1%
Graduate Enrollment 5,878 **Women** 92.5% **Men** 7.5% **Minority** 23%
Distance Learning Courses Available.
Nursing Student Activities Sigma Theta Tau.
Nursing Student Resources Academic advising; academic or career counseling; assistance for students with disabilities; bookstore; campus computer network; computer lab; computer-assisted instruction; e-mail services; interactive nursing skills videos; Internet; learning resource lab; library services; nursing audiovisuals; remedial services; skills, simulation, or other laboratory; tutoring.
Library Facilities 16,781 periodical subscriptions (1,300 health-care related).

BACCALAUREATE PROGRAMS
Degree BSN
Available Programs Accelerated Baccalaureate.
Study Options Full-time.
Online Degree Options Yes.
Program Entrance Requirements Transcript of college record, CPR certification, immunizations, 1 letter of recommendation, RN licensure. Transfer students are accepted. *Application deadline:* Applications may be processed on a rolling basis for some programs.
Advanced Placement Credit by examination available. Credit given for nursing courses completed elsewhere dependent upon specific evaluations.
Contact *Telephone:* 602-387-7000.

GRADUATE PROGRAMS
Contact *Telephone:* 602-387-7000.

MASTER'S DEGREE PROGRAM
Degrees MSN; MSN/MBA; MSN/MHA
Available Programs Master's; Master's for Nurses with Non-Nursing Degrees.
Concentrations Available Health-care administration; nursing administration; nursing education. *Nurse practitioner programs in:* family health.
Study Options Full-time.
Online Degree Options Yes.
Program Entrance Requirements Clinical experience, computer literacy, minimum overall college GPA of 3.0, transcript of college record, CPR certification. *Application deadline:* Applications may be processed on a rolling basis for some programs.
Advanced Placement Credit given for nursing courses completed elsewhere dependent upon specific evaluations.
Degree Requirements 39 total credit hours, thesis or project.

POST-MASTER'S PROGRAM
Areas of Study *Nurse practitioner programs in:* family health.

DOCTORAL DEGREE PROGRAM
Degree PhD
Available Programs Doctorate.
Areas of Study Nursing administration, nursing education.
Online Degree Options Yes (online only).
Program Entrance Requirements Minimum overall college GPA of 3.0, MSN or equivalent. *Application deadline:* Applications may be processed on a rolling basis for some programs. *Application fee:* $45.
Degree Requirements 62 total credit hours, dissertation, residency.

CONTINUING EDUCATION PROGRAM
Contact *Telephone:* 602-387-7000.

University of Phoenix–Phoenix Main Campus
College of Nursing
Tempe, Arizona

Founded in 1976
DEGREES • BSN • MSN • MSN/MBA • MSN/MHA
Nursing Program Faculty 38 (32% with doctorates).
Baccalaureate Enrollment 239 **Women** 89.5% **Men** 10.5% **Minority** 23.4%
Graduate Enrollment 148 **Women** 91.9% **Men** 8.1% **Minority** 14.86%
Nursing Student Activities Sigma Theta Tau.
Nursing Student Resources Academic advising; academic or career counseling; assistance for students with disabilities; bookstore; campus computer network; computer lab; computer-assisted instruction; interactive nursing skills videos; Internet; learning resource lab; library services; nursing audiovisuals; skills, simulation, or other laboratory; tutoring.
Library Facilities 16,781 periodical subscriptions (1,300 health-care related).

BACCALAUREATE PROGRAMS

Degree BSN
Available Programs Accelerated Baccalaureate; LPN to Baccalaureate.
Site Options Scottsdale, AZ; Mesa, AZ; Chandler, AZ.
Study Options Full-time.
Online Degree Options Yes.
Program Entrance Requirements Transcript of college record, CPR certification, immunizations, 1 letter of recommendation, RN licensure. Transfer students are accepted. *Application deadline:* Applications may be processed on a rolling basis for some programs.
Advanced Placement Credit by examination available. Credit given for nursing courses completed elsewhere dependent upon specific evaluations.
Contact *Telephone:* 480-804-7600.

GRADUATE PROGRAMS

Contact *Telephone:* 480-804-7600.

MASTER'S DEGREE PROGRAM

Degrees MSN; MSN/MBA; MSN/MHA
Available Programs Master's.
Concentrations Available Health-care administration; nursing administration; nursing education. *Nurse practitioner programs in:* family health.
Site Options Scottsdale, AZ; Mesa, AZ; Chandler, AZ.
Study Options Full-time.
Online Degree Options Yes.
Program Entrance Requirements Clinical experience, computer literacy, minimum overall college GPA of 2.5, transcript of college record. *Application deadline:* Applications may be processed on a rolling basis for some programs. *Application fee:* $45.
Advanced Placement Credit given for nursing courses completed elsewhere dependent upon specific evaluations.
Degree Requirements 39 total credit hours, thesis or project.

POST-MASTER'S PROGRAM

Areas of Study *Nurse practitioner programs in:* family health.

CONTINUING EDUCATION PROGRAM

Contact *Telephone:* 480-557-2279. *Fax:* 480-557-2338.

University of Phoenix–Southern Arizona Campus

College of Social Sciences
Tucson, Arizona

Founded in 1979
DEGREES · BSN · MSN
Nursing Program Faculty 19 (32% with doctorates).
Baccalaureate Enrollment 67 **Women** 85.1% **Men** 14.9% **Minority** 33.8%
Graduate Enrollment 97 **Women** 80.4% **Men** 19.6% **Minority** 18.56%
Nursing Student Activities Sigma Theta Tau.
Nursing Student Resources Academic advising; academic or career counseling; assistance for students with disabilities; bookstore; campus computer network; computer lab; computer-assisted instruction; e-mail services; interactive nursing skills videos; Internet; learning resource lab; library services; nursing audiovisuals; remedial services; skills, simulation, or other laboratory; tutoring.
Library Facilities 16,781 periodical subscriptions (1,300 health-care related).

BACCALAUREATE PROGRAMS

Degree BSN
Available Programs Accelerated Baccalaureate; LPN to Baccalaureate.
Site Options Sierra Vista, AZ; Yuma, AZ; Nogales, AZ.
Study Options Full-time.
Online Degree Options Yes.
Program Entrance Requirements Transcript of college record, CPR certification, immunizations, 1 letter of recommendation, RN licensure. Transfer students are accepted. *Application deadline:* Applications may be processed on a rolling basis for some programs.
Advanced Placement Credit by examination available. Credit given for nursing courses completed elsewhere dependent upon specific evaluations.

Contact *Telephone:* 520-881-6512.

GRADUATE PROGRAMS

Contact *Telephone:* 520-881-6512.

MASTER'S DEGREE PROGRAM

Degree MSN
Available Programs Master's.
Concentrations Available Health-care administration; nursing administration; nursing education. *Nurse practitioner programs in:* family health.
Site Options Sierra Vista, AZ; Yuma, AZ; Nogales, AZ.
Study Options Full-time.
Online Degree Options Yes.
Program Entrance Requirements Clinical experience, computer literacy, minimum overall college GPA of 2.5, transcript of college record. *Application deadline:* Applications may be processed on a rolling basis for some programs. *Application fee:* $45.
Advanced Placement Credit given for nursing courses completed elsewhere dependent upon specific evaluations.
Degree Requirements 39 total credit hours, thesis or project.

POST-MASTER'S PROGRAM

Areas of Study *Nurse practitioner programs in:* family health.

CONTINUING EDUCATION PROGRAM

Contact *Telephone:* 520-881-6512.

ARKANSAS

Arkansas State University
Department of Nursing
Jonesboro, State University, Arkansas

http://www.astate.edu/
Founded in 1909
DEGREES · BSN · MSN
Nursing Program Faculty 91 (17% with doctorates).
Baccalaureate Enrollment 305 **Women** 83% **Men** 17% **Minority** 14% **International** 1% **Part-time** 35%
Graduate Enrollment 206 **Women** 48% **Men** 52% **Minority** 18% **Part-time** 50%
Distance Learning Courses Available.
Nursing Student Activities Sigma Theta Tau, Student Nurses' Association.
Nursing Student Resources Academic advising; academic or career counseling; assistance for students with disabilities; bookstore; campus computer network; computer lab; computer-assisted instruction; daycare for children of students; e-mail services; housing assistance; Internet; learning resource lab; library services; nursing audiovisuals; resume preparation assistance; skills, simulation, or other laboratory; tutoring.
Library Facilities 643,148 volumes; 33,458 periodical subscriptions.

BACCALAUREATE PROGRAMS

Degree BSN
Available Programs Accelerated Baccalaureate for Second Degree; Generic Baccalaureate; LPN to Baccalaureate; RN Baccalaureate.
Site Options Mountain Home, AR; West Memphis, AR; Beebe, AR.
Study Options Full-time.
Online Degree Options Yes.
Program Entrance Requirements Minimum overall college GPA of 2.8, transcript of college record, CPR certification, written essay, immunizations, 3 letters of recommendation, professional liability insurance/malpractice insurance, prerequisite course work. Transfer students are accepted. *Application deadline:* 6/15 (fall).
Advanced Placement Credit by examination available. Credit given for nursing courses completed elsewhere dependent upon specific evaluations.
Expenses (2012–13) *Tuition, state resident:* full-time $5792; part-time $181 per credit hour. *Tuition, nonresident:* full-time $11,584; part-time $362 per credit hour. *International tuition:* $11,584 full-time. *Room and board:* $3195; room only: $1850 per academic year.

Contact Jenafer Wray, Nursing Advisor, Department of Nursing, Arkansas State University, PO Box 910, State University, AR 72467. *Telephone:* 870-972-3074. *Fax:* 870-972-2954. *E-mail:* jwray@astate.edu.

GRADUATE PROGRAMS

Expenses (2012–13) *Tuition, state resident:* full-time $4140; part-time $230 per credit hour. *Tuition, nonresident:* full-time $8280; part-time $460 per credit hour. *International tuition:* $8280 full-time. *Room and board:* $3830; room only: $2630 per academic year. *Required fees:* full-time $1924.
Contact Dr. Angela Schmidt, MSN Program Director, Department of Nursing, Arkansas State University, PO Box 910, MSN Program, State University, AR 72467. *Telephone:* 870-972-3701. *Fax:* 870-972-2954. *E-mail:* aschmidt@astate.edu.

MASTER'S DEGREE PROGRAM
Degree MSN
Available Programs Master's.
Concentrations Available Nurse anesthesia; nursing administration; nursing education. *Clinical nurse specialist programs in:* adult health. *Nurse practitioner programs in:* primary care.
Study Options Full-time and part-time.
Program Entrance Requirements Clinical experience, minimum overall college GPA of 2.75, transcript of college record, CPR certification, written essay, immunizations, physical assessment course, professional liability insurance/malpractice insurance, statistics course. *Application deadline:* 4/15 (fall), 10/15 (spring). *Application fee:* $30.
Degree Requirements 45 total credit hours, thesis or project, comprehensive exam.

POST-MASTER'S PROGRAM
Areas of Study Nursing education. *Nurse practitioner programs in:* primary care.

Arkansas Tech University
Program in Nursing
Russellville, Arkansas

http://nursing.atu.edu/
Founded in 1909
DEGREES • BSN • MSN
Nursing Program Faculty 27 (20% with doctorates).
Baccalaureate Enrollment 248 **Women** 87% **Men** 13% **Minority** 11% **International** 4% **Part-time** 14%
Graduate Enrollment 23 **Women** 87% **Men** 13% **Part-time** 50%
Distance Learning Courses Available.
Nursing Student Activities Nursing Honor Society, Sigma Theta Tau, Student Nurses' Association.
Nursing Student Resources Academic advising; academic or career counseling; assistance for students with disabilities; bookstore; campus computer network; career placement assistance; computer lab; computer-assisted instruction; e-mail services; employment services for current students; housing assistance; interactive nursing skills videos; Internet; learning resource lab; library services; nursing audiovisuals; other; paid internships; placement services for program completers; remedial services; resume preparation assistance; skills, simulation, or other laboratory; tutoring.
Library Facilities 285,591 volumes (16,900 in health, 2,100 in nursing); 774 periodical subscriptions (130 health-care related).

BACCALAUREATE PROGRAMS
Degree BSN
Available Programs ADN to Baccalaureate; Baccalaureate for Second Degree; Generic Baccalaureate; LPN to Baccalaureate; RN Baccalaureate.
Site Options Russellville, AR.
Study Options Full-time and part-time.
Online Degree Options Yes.
Program Entrance Requirements Transcript of college record, CPR certification, health exam, immunizations, minimum GPA in nursing prerequisites of 3.0, professional liability insurance/malpractice insurance, prerequisite course work. Transfer students are accepted. *Application deadline:* 3/1 (fall), 10/1 (spring).

Advanced Placement Credit by examination available. Credit given for nursing courses completed elsewhere dependent upon specific evaluations.
Expenses (2012–13) *Tuition, state resident:* full-time $5610; part-time $187 per credit hour. *Tuition, nonresident:* full-time $11,220; part-time $374 per credit hour. *International tuition:* $11,400 full-time. *Room and board:* $6000; room only: $3600 per academic year. *Required fees:* full-time $918; part-time $50 per credit; part-time $318 per term.
Financial Aid 80% of baccalaureate students in nursing programs received some form of financial aid in 2011–12. *Gift aid (need-based):* Federal Pell, FSEOG, state, private. *Loans:* Federal Direct (Subsidized and Unsubsidized Stafford PLUS), Perkins.*Work-study:* Federal Work-Study, part-time campus jobs.*Financial aid application deadline (priority):* 4/15.
Contact Dr. Rebecca F. Burris, Professor and Department Chair, Program in Nursing, Arkansas Tech University, 402 West O Street, Russellville, AR 72801. *Telephone:* 479-968-0383. *Fax:* 479-968-0219. *E-mail:* rburris@atu.edu.

GRADUATE PROGRAMS
Expenses (2012–13) *Tuition, state resident:* full-time $5160; part-time $215 per credit hour. *Tuition, nonresident:* full-time $10,320; part-time $430 per credit hour. *International tuition:* $10,350 full-time. *Required fees:* full-time $780; part-time $50 per credit; part-time $318 per term.
Financial Aid 75% of graduate students in nursing programs received some form of financial aid in 2011–12.
Contact Dr. Mary Gunter, Dean of Graduate College, Program in Nursing, Arkansas Tech University, Tomlinson Graduate College, Russellville, AR 72801. *Telephone:* 479-968-0398. *E-mail:* mgunter@atu.edu.

MASTER'S DEGREE PROGRAM
Degree MSN
Available Programs Master's; Master's for Nurses with Non-Nursing Degrees; RN to Master's.
Concentrations Available Nursing administration.
Site Options Russellville, AR.
Study Options Full-time and part-time.
Program Entrance Requirements Clinical experience, computer literacy, minimum overall college GPA of 3.0, transcript of college record, statistics course. *Application deadline:* 5/1 (fall). Applications may be processed on a rolling basis for some programs. *Application fee:* $25.
Advanced Placement Credit given for nursing courses completed elsewhere dependent upon specific evaluations.
Degree Requirements 39 total credit hours, thesis or project.

Harding University
College of Nursing
Searcy, Arkansas

http://www.harding.edu/nursing
Founded in 1924
DEGREE • BSN
Nursing Program Faculty 19 (25% with doctorates).
Baccalaureate Enrollment 102 **Women** 83% **Men** 17% **Minority** 1% **International** 1% **Part-time** 20%
Nursing Student Activities Nursing Honor Society, Sigma Theta Tau, Student Nurses' Association.
Nursing Student Resources Academic advising; academic or career counseling; assistance for students with disabilities; bookstore; campus computer network; career placement assistance; computer lab; computer-assisted instruction; e-mail services; employment services for current students; externships; housing assistance; interactive nursing skills videos; Internet; learning resource lab; library services; nursing audiovisuals; placement services for program completers; remedial services; resume preparation assistance; skills, simulation, or other laboratory; tutoring.
Library Facilities 237,077 volumes (5,000 in health, 1,729 in nursing); 41,954 periodical subscriptions (120 health-care related).

BACCALAUREATE PROGRAMS
Degree BSN
Available Programs ADN to Baccalaureate; Generic Baccalaureate; LPN to Baccalaureate; LPN to RN Baccalaureate; RN Baccalaureate.
Site Options Searcy, AR.
Study Options Full-time and part-time.

Program Entrance Requirements Minimum overall college GPA of 2.0, transcript of college record, CPR certification, health exam, high school transcript, immunizations, 3 letters of recommendation, minimum GPA in nursing prerequisites of 2.5, prerequisite course work. Transfer students are accepted. *Application deadline:* 3/1 (fall), 10/1 (spring).

Advanced Placement Credit by examination available. Credit given for nursing courses completed elsewhere dependent upon specific evaluations.

Expenses (2012–13) *Tuition:* full-time $6930; part-time $462 per credit hour. *International tuition:* $6930 full-time. *Room and board:* $6192; room only: $3094 per academic year.

Financial Aid 95% of baccalaureate students in nursing programs received some form of financial aid in 2011–12. *Gift aid (need-based):* Federal Pell, FSEOG, state, private, college/university gift aid from institutional funds. *Loans:* Federal Nursing Student Loans, Federal Direct (Subsidized and Unsubsidized Stafford PLUS), Perkins, state, college/university.*Work-study:* Federal Work-Study, part-time campus jobs.*Financial aid application deadline (priority):* 4/15.

Contact Ms. Jeanne L. Castleberry, Assistant to the Dean, College of Nursing, Harding University, Box 12265, 914 East Market Avenue, Searcy, AR 72149-2265. *Telephone:* 501-279-4682. *Fax:* 501-305-8902. *E-mail:* nursing@harding.edu.

CONTINUING EDUCATION PROGRAM

Contact Dr. Cathleen M. Shultz, Dean and Professor, College of Nursing, Harding University, Carr College of Nursing, Box 12265, Searcy, AR 72149-2265. *Telephone:* 501-279-4476. *Fax:* 501-279-4669. *E-mail:* nursing@harding.edu.

Henderson State University

Department of Nursing
Arkadelphia, Arkansas

http://www.hsu.edu/nursing/
Founded in 1890

DEGREE • BSN

Nursing Program Faculty 7 (29% with doctorates).

Baccalaureate Enrollment 50 **Women** 64% **Men** 36% **Minority** 35% **International** 2%

Distance Learning Courses Available.

Nursing Student Activities Student Nurses' Association, nursing club.

Nursing Student Resources Academic advising; academic or career counseling; assistance for students with disabilities; bookstore; campus computer network; career placement assistance; computer lab; computer-assisted instruction; e-mail services; interactive nursing skills videos; Internet; learning resource lab; library services; nursing audiovisuals; remedial services; resume preparation assistance; skills, simulation, or other laboratory; tutoring.

Library Facilities 26.9 million volumes (1,000 in health, 200 in nursing); 277 periodical subscriptions (40 health-care related).

BACCALAUREATE PROGRAMS

Degree BSN

Available Programs ADN to Baccalaureate; Generic Baccalaureate; LPN to Baccalaureate.

Study Options Full-time.

Program Entrance Requirements Minimum overall college GPA of 2.5, transcript of college record, CPR certification, immunizations, minimum GPA in nursing prerequisites of 2.50, prerequisite course work. Transfer students are accepted. *Application deadline:* 2/15 (fall). *Application fee:* $57.

Advanced Placement Credit given for nursing courses completed elsewhere dependent upon specific evaluations.

Contact *Telephone:* 870-230-5508. *Fax:* 870-230-5390.

Southern Arkansas University–Magnolia

Department of Nursing
Magnolia, Arkansas

http://web.saumag.edu/science/departments/nursing/
Founded in 1909

DEGREE • BSN

Nursing Program Faculty 13 (23% with doctorates).

Baccalaureate Enrollment 51 **Women** 90% **Men** 10% **Minority** 15% **Part-time** 58%

Distance Learning Courses Available.

Nursing Student Activities Student Nurses' Association.

Nursing Student Resources Academic advising; academic or career counseling; assistance for students with disabilities; bookstore; campus computer network; career placement assistance; computer lab; computer-assisted instruction; e-mail services; employment services for current students; housing assistance; interactive nursing skills videos; Internet; learning resource lab; library services; nursing audiovisuals; remedial services; resume preparation assistance; skills, simulation, or other laboratory; tutoring.

Library Facilities 165,894 volumes (800 in health, 200 in nursing); 1,855 periodical subscriptions (2,000 health-care related).

BACCALAUREATE PROGRAMS

Degree BSN

Available Programs ADN to Baccalaureate; Generic Baccalaureate; RN Baccalaureate.

Study Options Full-time.

Online Degree Options Yes.

Program Entrance Requirements Minimum overall college GPA of 2.5, transcript of college record, CPR certification, high school chemistry, immunizations, minimum GPA in nursing prerequisites of 2.5, prerequisite course work. Transfer students are accepted. *Application deadline:* 2/28 (fall). Applications may be processed on a rolling basis for some programs.

Advanced Placement Credit given for nursing courses completed elsewhere dependent upon specific evaluations.

Contact *Telephone:* 870-235-4331. *Fax:* 870-235-5058.

University of Arkansas
Eleanor Mann School of Nursing
Fayetteville, Arkansas

http://nurs.uark.edu/
Founded in 1871

DEGREES • BSN • MSN

Nursing Program Faculty 25 (26% with doctorates).

Baccalaureate Enrollment 220 **Women** 95% **Men** 5% **Minority** 7% **Graduate Enrollment** 20

Nursing Student Activities Sigma Theta Tau, Student Nurses' Association.

Nursing Student Resources Academic advising; academic or career counseling; assistance for students with disabilities; bookstore; campus computer network; career placement assistance; computer lab; computer-assisted instruction; e-mail services; employment services for current students; housing assistance; interactive nursing skills videos; Internet; learning resource lab; library services; nursing audiovisuals; other; placement services for program completers; remedial services; resume preparation assistance; skills, simulation, or other laboratory; tutoring.

Library Facilities 1.9 million volumes (60,000 in health, 20,000 in nursing); 27,518 periodical subscriptions (130,000 health-care related).

BACCALAUREATE PROGRAMS

Degree BSN

Available Programs Generic Baccalaureate; LPN to Baccalaureate; LPN to RN Baccalaureate; RN Baccalaureate.

Study Options Full-time and part-time.

Program Entrance Requirements Minimum overall college GPA of 2.75, transcript of college record, CPR certification, health insurance, immunizations, minimum GPA in nursing prerequisites of 2.75, professional liability insurance/malpractice insurance, prerequisite course work. Transfer students are accepted.

Advanced Placement Credit by examination available. Credit given for nursing courses completed elsewhere dependent upon specific evaluations.
Contact *Telephone:* 479-575-3907. *Fax:* 479-575-3218.

GRADUATE PROGRAMS

Contact *Telephone:* 479-575-3907. *Fax:* 479-575-3218.

MASTER'S DEGREE PROGRAM
Degree MSN
Available Programs Master's.
Concentrations Available Nursing education. *Clinical nurse specialist programs in:* acute care, medical-surgical.
Study Options Full-time and part-time.
Online Degree Options Yes.
Program Entrance Requirements Computer literacy, minimum overall college GPA of 3.0, transcript of college record, CPR certification, immunizations, nursing research course, physical assessment course, statistics course.
Degree Requirements 42 total credit hours, thesis or project, comprehensive exam.

CONTINUING EDUCATION PROGRAM

Contact *Telephone:* 479-575-3907. *Fax:* 479-575-3218.

University of Arkansas at Little Rock
BSN Programs
Little Rock, Arkansas

Founded in 1927
DEGREE • BSN

BACCALAUREATE PROGRAMS

Degree BSN
Available Programs RN Baccalaureate.
Contact *Telephone:* 501-569-8081.

University of Arkansas at Monticello
School of Nursing
Monticello, Arkansas

http://www.uamont.edu/Nursing/
Founded in 1909
DEGREE • BSN
Nursing Program Faculty 10
Baccalaureate Enrollment 30 **Women** 87% **Men** 13% **Minority** 23%
Distance Learning Courses Available.
Nursing Student Activities Sigma Theta Tau, Student Nurses' Association.
Nursing Student Resources Academic advising; academic or career counseling; assistance for students with disabilities; bookstore; campus computer network; computer lab; computer-assisted instruction; e-mail services; interactive nursing skills videos; Internet; learning resource lab; library services; nursing audiovisuals; resume preparation assistance; skills, simulation, or other laboratory; tutoring.
Library Facilities 241,822 volumes (3,888 in health, 539 in nursing); 956 periodical subscriptions (5,015 health-care related).

BACCALAUREATE PROGRAMS

Degree BSN
Available Programs ADN to Baccalaureate; Generic Baccalaureate; LPN to Baccalaureate; RN Baccalaureate.
Study Options Full-time.
Program Entrance Requirements Minimum overall college GPA, transcript of college record, immunizations, minimum GPA in nursing prerequisites of 2.5, prerequisite course work. Transfer students are accepted. *Application deadline:* 3/1 (spring).

Advanced Placement Credit by examination available. Credit given for nursing courses completed elsewhere dependent upon specific evaluations.
Financial Aid 83% of baccalaureate students in nursing programs received some form of financial aid in 2011–12.
Contact Dr. Laura K. Evans, Dean, School of Nursing, University of Arkansas at Monticello, 124 University Place, PO Box 3606, Monticello, AR 71656. *Telephone:* 870-460-1069. *Fax:* 870-460-1969. *E-mail:* evansl@uamont.edu.

University of Arkansas at Pine Bluff
Department of Nursing
Pine Bluff, Arkansas

http://www.uapb.edu/
Founded in 1873
DEGREE • BSN
Nursing Program Faculty 5 (40% with doctorates).
Baccalaureate Enrollment 20 **Women** 95% **Men** 5% **Minority** 100% **International** 20%
Nursing Student Activities Student Nurses' Association.
Nursing Student Resources Academic advising; academic or career counseling; assistance for students with disabilities; bookstore; campus computer network; career placement assistance; computer lab; computer-assisted instruction; e-mail services; housing assistance; interactive nursing skills videos; Internet; learning resource lab; library services; nursing audiovisuals; remedial services; resume preparation assistance; skills, simulation, or other laboratory; tutoring.
Library Facilities 187,582 volumes (2,600 in health, 1,550 in nursing); 3,041 periodical subscriptions (60 health-care related).

BACCALAUREATE PROGRAMS

Degree BSN
Available Programs Generic Baccalaureate.
Study Options Full-time and part-time.
Program Entrance Requirements Minimum overall college GPA of 2.5, transcript of college record, CPR certification, written essay, health exam, immunizations, 3 letters of recommendation, minimum GPA in nursing prerequisites of 2.5, professional liability insurance/malpractice insurance, prerequisite course work. Transfer students are accepted.
Advanced Placement Credit by examination available. Credit given for nursing courses completed elsewhere dependent upon specific evaluations.
Contact *Telephone:* 870-575-8220. *Fax:* 870-575-8229.

University of Arkansas for Medical Sciences
College of Nursing
Little Rock, Arkansas

http://www.nursing.uams.edu/
Founded in 1879
DEGREES • BSN • DNP • MN SC • PHD
Nursing Program Faculty 85 (38% with doctorates).
Baccalaureate Enrollment 384 **Women** 83.07% **Men** 16.93% **Minority** 13.02%
Graduate Enrollment 262 **Women** 85.5% **Men** 14.5% **Minority** 15.27%
Distance Learning Courses Available.
Nursing Student Activities Nursing Honor Society, Sigma Theta Tau, Student Nurses' Association.
Nursing Student Resources Academic advising; academic or career counseling; assistance for students with disabilities; bookstore; campus computer network; computer lab; computer-assisted instruction; e-mail services; externships; interactive nursing skills videos; Internet; learning resource lab; library services; nursing audiovisuals; remedial services; skills, simulation, or other laboratory; tutoring.
Library Facilities 183,975 volumes (183,975 in health); 1,567 periodical subscriptions (1,567 health-care related).

BACCALAUREATE PROGRAMS

Degree BSN

Available Programs ADN to Baccalaureate; Accelerated RN Baccalaureate; Baccalaureate for Second Degree; Generic Baccalaureate; LPN to Baccalaureate; RN Baccalaureate.

Site Options Fayetteville, AR; El Dorado, AR; Texarkana, AR; Helena, AR; Jonesboro, AR; Hope, AR.

Study Options Full-time.

Online Degree Options Yes.

Program Entrance Requirements Minimum overall college GPA of 2.5, transcript of college record, CPR certification, health insurance, immunizations, interview, minimum high school GPA of 2.5, minimum GPA in nursing prerequisites of 2.5, prerequisite course work. Transfer students are accepted. *Application deadline:* 2/1 (summer). *Application fee:* $60.

Advanced Placement Credit by examination available. Credit given for nursing courses completed elsewhere dependent upon specific evaluations.

Expenses (2012–13) *Tuition, state resident:* full-time $2844; part-time $237 per credit hour. *Tuition, nonresident:* full-time $7080; part-time $590 per credit hour. *International tuition:* $7080 full-time.

Financial Aid 90% of baccalaureate students in nursing programs received some form of financial aid in 2011–12.

Contact Dr. Donna Middaugh, Associate Dean for Academic Programs, College of Nursing, University of Arkansas for Medical Sciences, 4301 West Markham, #529, Little Rock, AR 72205-7199. *Telephone:* 501-686-5374. *Fax:* 501-686-8350. *E-mail:* middaughdonnaj@uams.edu.

GRADUATE PROGRAMS

Expenses (2012–13) *Tuition, state resident:* full-time $3078; part-time $342 per credit hour. *Tuition, nonresident:* full-time $7080; part-time $590 per credit hour. *International tuition:* $7080 full-time.

Financial Aid 90% of graduate students in nursing programs received some form of financial aid in 2011–12. Career-related internships or fieldwork and traineeships available. Aid available to part-time students.

Contact Dr. Donna Middaugh, Associate Dean for Academic Programs, College of Nursing, University of Arkansas for Medical Sciences, 4301 West Markham, #529, Little Rock, AR 72205-7199. *Telephone:* 501-686-8349. *Fax:* 501-686-8350. *E-mail:* middaughdonnaj@uams.edu.

MASTER'S DEGREE PROGRAM

Degree MN Sc

Available Programs Master's; Master's for Nurses with Non-Nursing Degrees; RN to Master's.

Concentrations Available Nursing administration; nursing education. *Clinical nurse specialist programs in:* acute care, adult health, pediatric. *Nurse practitioner programs in:* acute care, family health, pediatric, psychiatric/mental health.

Site Options Fayetteville, AR; El Dorado, AR; Texarkana, AR; Helena, AR; Jonesboro, AR.

Study Options Full-time and part-time.

Program Entrance Requirements Clinical experience, minimum overall college GPA of 2.85, transcript of college record, CPR certification, immunizations, physical assessment course, professional liability insurance/malpractice insurance, statistics course. *Application deadline:* 4/1 (fall), 9/1 (spring). *Application fee:* $60.

Advanced Placement Credit given for nursing courses completed elsewhere dependent upon specific evaluations.

Degree Requirements 39 total credit hours, thesis or project, comprehensive exam.

DOCTORAL DEGREE PROGRAM

Degree DNP

Available Programs Doctorate.

Areas of Study Clinical practice.

Program Entrance Requirements Minimum overall college GPA of 3.4, clinical experience, interview, interview by faculty committee, 3 letters of recommendation, MSN or equivalent, statistics course. *Application deadline:* 3/1 (spring). *Application fee:* $60.

Degree Requirements 29 total credit hours, oral exam, written exam.

Contact Dr. Matthew V. Hadley, RN, DNP, University of Arkansas for Medical Sciences, 4301 West Markham, #529, Little Rock, AR 72205-7199. *Telephone:* 501-686-5374. *Fax:* 501-686-8350. *E-mail:* hadleymatthewv@uams.edu.

DOCTORAL DEGREE PROGRAM

Degree PhD

Available Programs Doctorate; Post-Baccalaureate Doctorate.

Areas of Study Advanced practice nursing, clinical practice, gerontology, health-care systems, nursing administration, nursing education, nursing research, nursing science, oncology.

Program Entrance Requirements Minimum overall college GPA of 3.65, interview by faculty committee, interview, 4 letters of recommendation, MSN or equivalent, scholarly papers, statistics course, writing sample, GRE. *Application deadline:* 3/1 (spring). *Application fee:* $60.

Degree Requirements 60 total credit hours, dissertation, oral exam, written exam.

POSTDOCTORAL PROGRAM

Areas of Study Aging, cancer care, gerontology, nursing research, nursing science.

Postdoctoral Program Contact Dr. Jean McSweeney, Postdoctoral Contact, College of Nursing, University of Arkansas for Medical Sciences, 4301 West Markham, #529, Little Rock, AR 72205-7199. *Telephone:* 501-686-5374. *Fax:* 501-686-8350. *E-mail:* mcsweeneyjeanc@uams.edu.

CONTINUING EDUCATION PROGRAM

Contact Dr. Lorraine Frazier, Dean and Professor, College of Nursing, University of Arkansas for Medical Sciences, 4301 West Markham, #529, Little Rock, AR 72205-7199. *Telephone:* 501-686-5374. *Fax:* 501-686-8350. *E-mail:* lfrazier@uams.edu.

University of Arkansas–Fort Smith

Carol McKelvey Moore School of Nursing
Fort Smith, Arkansas

Founded in 1928

DEGREE • BSN

Nursing Program Faculty 18

Baccalaureate Enrollment 20 **Women** 60% **Men** 40% **Minority** 5%

Distance Learning Courses Available.

Nursing Student Activities Student Nurses' Association.

Nursing Student Resources Academic advising; academic or career counseling; assistance for students with disabilities; bookstore; campus computer network; career placement assistance; computer lab; computer-assisted instruction; e-mail services; housing assistance; interactive nursing skills videos; Internet; learning resource lab; library services; nursing audiovisuals; remedial services; resume preparation assistance; skills, simulation, or other laboratory; tutoring.

Library Facilities 86,725 volumes (2,231 in health, 1,183 in nursing); 3,230 periodical subscriptions (5,350 health-care related).

BACCALAUREATE PROGRAMS

Degree BSN

Available Programs ADN to Baccalaureate; Generic Baccalaureate.

Study Options Full-time.

Online Degree Options Yes (online only).

Program Entrance Requirements Minimum overall college GPA of 2.5, transcript of college record, CPR certification, health exam, health insurance, immunizations, interview, minimum GPA in nursing prerequisites of 2.5, prerequisite course work. Transfer students are accepted.

Advanced Placement Credit given for nursing courses completed elsewhere dependent upon specific evaluations.

Contact *Telephone:* 479-788-7840. *Fax:* 479-788-7869.

University of Central Arkansas

Department of Nursing
Conway, Arkansas

http://www.uca.edu/nursing/

Founded in 1907

DEGREES • BSN • MSN

Nursing Program Faculty 32 (28% with doctorates).

Baccalaureate Enrollment 245 **Women** 84.9% **Men** 15.1% **Minority** 12.65% **International** 2.04% **Part-time** 23.67%

Graduate Enrollment 136 **Women** 95.59% **Men** 4.41% **Minority** 11.76% **International** .74% **Part-time** 95.59%

Distance Learning Courses Available.

Nursing Student Activities Sigma Theta Tau, Student Nurses' Association.
Nursing Student Resources Academic advising; academic or career counseling; assistance for students with disabilities; bookstore; campus computer network; career placement assistance; computer lab; computer-assisted instruction; e-mail services; employment services for current students; externships; housing assistance; interactive nursing skills videos; Internet; learning resource lab; library services; nursing audiovisuals; paid internships; placement services for program completers; remedial services; resume preparation assistance; skills, simulation, or other laboratory; tutoring; unpaid internships.
Library Facilities 600,084 volumes; 804 periodical subscriptions.

BACCALAUREATE PROGRAMS

Degree BSN
Available Programs ADN to Baccalaureate; Generic Baccalaureate; LPN to Baccalaureate; LPN to RN Baccalaureate; RN Baccalaureate.
Study Options Full-time and part-time.
Program Entrance Requirements Minimum overall college GPA of 2.5, transcript of college record, health exam, health insurance, immunizations, minimum GPA in nursing prerequisites, prerequisite course work. Transfer students are accepted. *Application deadline:* 3/1 (fall). *Application fee:* $50.
Advanced Placement Credit given for nursing courses completed elsewhere dependent upon specific evaluations.
Contact *Telephone:* 501-450-5526. *Fax:* 501-450-5560.

GRADUATE PROGRAMS

Contact *Telephone:* 501-450-5532. *Fax:* 501-450-5560.

MASTER'S DEGREE PROGRAM
Degree MSN
Available Programs Master's; RN to Master's.
Concentrations Available Nursing education. *Clinical nurse specialist programs in:* medical-surgical. *Nurse practitioner programs in:* adult health, family health.
Site Options Russelville, AR; Pine Bluff, AR; Fort Smith, AR.
Study Options Full-time and part-time.
Online Degree Options Yes (online only).
Program Entrance Requirements Clinical experience, minimum overall college GPA of 2.7, transcript of college record, CPR certification, immunizations, professional liability insurance/malpractice insurance, prerequisite course work, resume, statistics course, GRE General Test. *Application deadline:* 4/1 (fall), 8/1 (spring). *Application fee:* $50.
Degree Requirements 39 total credit hours, comprehensive exam.

POST-MASTER'S PROGRAM
Areas of Study Nursing education. *Clinical nurse specialist programs in:* medical-surgical. *Nurse practitioner programs in:* adult health, family health.

CALIFORNIA

American University of Health Sciences
School of Nursing
Signal Hill, California

DEGREE • BSN

BACCALAUREATE PROGRAMS

Degree BSN
Available Programs Accelerated Baccalaureate; Generic Baccalaureate.
Program Entrance Requirements Minimum overall college GPA of 2.5, written essay, interview, 2 letters of recommendation, prerequisite course work.
Contact School of Nursing, School of Nursing, American University of Health Sciences, 1600 East Hill Street, Building #1, Signal Hill, CA 90755. *Telephone:* 562-988-2278. *E-mail:* bsninfo@auhs.edu.

Azusa Pacific University
School of Nursing
Azusa, California

http://www.apu.edu/nursing/
Founded in 1899
DEGREES • BSN • MSN • PHD
Nursing Program Faculty 77 (22% with doctorates).
Baccalaureate Enrollment 236 **Women** 90% **Men** 10% **Minority** 44% **International** 11% **Part-time** 2%
Graduate Enrollment 110 **Women** 89% **Men** 11% **Minority** 37%
Nursing Student Activities Sigma Theta Tau, Student Nurses' Association, nursing club.
Nursing Student Resources Academic advising; academic or career counseling; bookstore; campus computer network; career placement assistance; computer lab; computer-assisted instruction; e-mail services; employment services for current students; housing assistance; interactive nursing skills videos; Internet; learning resource lab; library services; nursing audiovisuals; remedial services; resume preparation assistance; skills, simulation, or other laboratory; tutoring.
Library Facilities 14,206 volumes in health, 4,712 volumes in nursing; 432 periodical subscriptions health-care related.

BACCALAUREATE PROGRAMS

Degree BSN
Available Programs ADN to Baccalaureate; Accelerated Baccalaureate; Accelerated RN Baccalaureate; Generic Baccalaureate.
Study Options Full-time and part-time.
Program Entrance Requirements Minimum overall college GPA of 3.0, transcript of college record, CPR certification, written essay, health exam, high school biology, high school chemistry, 2 years high school math, high school transcript, immunizations, 3 letters of recommendation, minimum high school GPA of 3.0, minimum GPA in nursing prerequisites of 3.0. Transfer students are accepted.
Advanced Placement Credit by examination available. Credit given for nursing courses completed elsewhere dependent upon specific evaluations.
Contact *Telephone:* 626-815-6000 Ext. 5501. *Fax:* 626-815-5414.

GRADUATE PROGRAMS

Contact *Telephone:* 626-815-5386. *Fax:* 626-815-5414.

MASTER'S DEGREE PROGRAM
Degree MSN
Available Programs Accelerated Master's for Non-Nursing College Graduates; Accelerated Master's for Nurses with Non-Nursing Degrees; Master's.
Concentrations Available Nursing administration; nursing education. *Clinical nurse specialist programs in:* adult health, medical-surgical, parent-child, pediatric, school health. *Nurse practitioner programs in:* adult health, family health, pediatric, primary care.
Study Options Full-time and part-time.
Program Entrance Requirements Clinical experience, computer literacy, minimum overall college GPA of 3.0, transcript of college record, CPR certification, written essay, immunizations, 3 letters of recommendation, nursing research course, physical assessment course, professional liability insurance/malpractice insurance, prerequisite course work, resume, statistics course.
Advanced Placement Credit by examination available. Credit given for nursing courses completed elsewhere dependent upon specific evaluations.
Degree Requirements 42 total credit hours, thesis or project, comprehensive exam.

POST-MASTER'S PROGRAM
Areas of Study Nursing administration; nursing education. *Clinical nurse specialist programs in:* adult health, medical-surgical, parent-child, pediatric, school health. *Nurse practitioner programs in:* adult health, family health, pediatric, primary care.

DOCTORAL DEGREE PROGRAM
Degree PhD
Available Programs Doctorate.
Areas of Study Community health, family health, nursing education.
Program Entrance Requirements Clinical experience, minimum overall college GPA of 3.5, interview by faculty committee, interview, 3

letters of recommendation, MSN or equivalent, scholarly papers, statistics course, vita, writing sample.
Degree Requirements 64 total credit hours, dissertation, oral exam, written exam.

CONTINUING EDUCATION PROGRAM

Contact *Telephone:* 626-815-5385. *Fax:* 626-815-5414.

Biola University
Department of Nursing
La Mirada, California

http://www.biola.edu/
Founded in 1908
DEGREE • BSN
Nursing Program Faculty 18 (39% with doctorates).
Baccalaureate Enrollment 115 **Women** 90% **Men** 10% **Minority** 38% **International** 1% **Part-time** 1%
Nursing Student Activities Student Nurses' Association.
Nursing Student Resources Academic advising; academic or career counseling; assistance for students with disabilities; bookstore; campus computer network; career placement assistance; computer lab; computer-assisted instruction; e-mail services; employment services for current students; housing assistance; Internet; learning resource lab; library services; nursing audiovisuals; placement services for program completers; remedial services; resume preparation assistance; skills, simulation, or other laboratory; tutoring.
Library Facilities 545,611 volumes (20,000 in health, 10,000 in nursing); 994 periodical subscriptions (750 health-care related).

BACCALAUREATE PROGRAMS

Degree BSN
Available Programs ADN to Baccalaureate; Generic Baccalaureate; LPN to Baccalaureate; RN Baccalaureate.
Study Options Full-time.
Program Entrance Requirements Minimum overall college GPA of 3.0, transcript of college record, written essay, high school chemistry, 2 years high school math, high school transcript, interview, 2 letters of recommendation, minimum high school GPA of 3.5, minimum GPA in nursing prerequisites of 3.0, prerequisite course work. Transfer students are accepted. *Application deadline:* 1/15 (fall). *Application fee:* $50.
Advanced Placement Credit given for nursing courses completed elsewhere dependent upon specific evaluations.
Expenses (2012–13) *Tuition:* full-time $31,004; part-time $1292 per unit. *International tuition:* $31,004 full-time. *Room and board:* $9316; room only: $5076 per academic year. *Required fees:* full-time $600; part-time $300 per term.
Financial Aid 95% of baccalaureate students in nursing programs received some form of financial aid in 2011–12.
Contact Ms. Shannon Gramatky, Nursing Department Advisor, Department of Nursing, Biola University, 13800 Biola Avenue, La Mirada, CA 90639. *Telephone:* 562-903-4850. *Fax:* 562-903-4803. *E-mail:* shannon.gramatky@biola.edu.

Brandman University
School of Nursing and Health Professions
Irvine, California

Founded in 2009
DEGREES • BSN • DNP • MS

BACCALAUREATE PROGRAMS

Degree BSN
Available Programs RN Baccalaureate.
Program Entrance Requirements Minimum overall college GPA of 2.0, transcript of college record, prerequisite course work. *Application deadline:* 8/1 (fall), 12/1 (winter).
Contact Nursing Representative, School of Nursing and Health Professions, Brandman University, 16355 Laguna Canyon Road, Irvine, CA 92618. *Telephone:* 800-581-4100. *Fax:* 949-754-1335. *E-mail:* nursing@brandman.edu.

GRADUATE PROGRAMS

Contact Nursing Representative, School of Nursing and Health Professions, Brandman University, 16355 Laguna Canyon Road, Irvine, CA 92618. *Telephone:* 800-581-4100. *Fax:* 949-754-1335. *E-mail:* nursing@brandman.edu.

MASTER'S DEGREE PROGRAM

Degree MS
Available Programs Master's.
Concentrations Available Nursing administration.
Online Degree Options Yes.
Program Entrance Requirements Transcript of college record, 3 letters of recommendation, resume. *Application deadline:* 8/1 (fall), 12/1 (winter).

DOCTORAL DEGREE PROGRAM

Degree DNP
Available Programs Doctorate; Post-Baccalaureate Doctorate.
Areas of Study Family health, gerontology, maternity-newborn.
Program Entrance Requirements 3 letters of recommendation. *Application deadline:* 12/1 (winter).

CONTINUING EDUCATION PROGRAM

Contact Nursing Representative, School of Nursing and Health Professions, Brandman University, 16355 Laguna Canyon Road, Irvine, CA 92618. *Telephone:* 800-581-4100. *Fax:* 949-754-1335. *E-mail:* nursing@brandman.edu.

California Baptist University
School of Nursing
Riverside, California

http://www.calbaptist.edu/nursing
Founded in 1950
DEGREES • BSN • MSN
Nursing Program Faculty 26 (4% with doctorates).
Baccalaureate Enrollment 180 **Women** 87.78% **Men** 12.22% **Minority** 33.89% **International** 1.67%
Graduate Enrollment 16 **Women** 87.5% **Men** 12.5% **Minority** 56.25%
Nursing Student Activities Student Nurses' Association.
Nursing Student Resources Academic advising; academic or career counseling; bookstore; campus computer network; career placement assistance; computer lab; e-mail services; employment services for current students; interactive nursing skills videos; Internet; learning resource lab; library services; nursing audiovisuals; resume preparation assistance; skills, simulation, or other laboratory; tutoring.
Library Facilities 219,033 volumes (335 in health, 236 in nursing); 32,656 periodical subscriptions (286 health-care related).

BACCALAUREATE PROGRAMS

Degree BSN
Available Programs ADN to Baccalaureate; Generic Baccalaureate; RN Baccalaureate.
Site Options Corona, CA; San Bernardino, CA; Fullerton, CA.
Study Options Full-time.
Program Entrance Requirements Minimum overall college GPA of 2.7, transcript of college record, CPR certification, written essay, health exam, health insurance, immunizations, 2 letters of recommendation, minimum GPA in nursing prerequisites of 2.7, professional liability insurance/malpractice insurance, prerequisite course work. Transfer students are accepted. *Application deadline:* 3/11 (fall), 8/31 (spring). *Application fee:* $50.
Contact *Telephone:* 951-343-4336.

GRADUATE PROGRAMS

Contact *Telephone:* 951-343-4336. *Fax:* 951-343-4703.

MASTER'S DEGREE PROGRAM

Degree MSN
Available Programs Accelerated Master's for Non-Nursing College Graduates; Master's.
Concentrations Available Clinical nurse leader; nursing education. *Clinical nurse specialist programs in:* adult health.
Study Options Part-time.

Program Entrance Requirements Computer literacy, minimum overall college GPA of 3.25, transcript of college record, CPR certification, written essay, immunizations, interview, 3 letters of recommendation, professional liability insurance/malpractice insurance, prerequisite course work, resume, statistics course. *Application deadline:* Applications may be processed on a rolling basis for some programs. *Application fee:* $45.
Degree Requirements 42 total credit hours, thesis or project, comprehensive exam.

California State University, Bakersfield
Program in Nursing
Bakersfield, California

http://www.csub.edu/nursing
Founded in 1970
DEGREE • BSN
Nursing Program Faculty 24 (15% with doctorates).
Baccalaureate Enrollment 208 **Women** 86% **Men** 14% **Minority** 60% **International** 4% **Part-time** 6%
Distance Learning Courses Available.
Nursing Student Activities Nursing Honor Society, Sigma Theta Tau, Student Nurses' Association, nursing club.
Nursing Student Resources Academic advising; academic or career counseling; assistance for students with disabilities; bookstore; campus computer network; career placement assistance; computer lab; computer-assisted instruction; daycare for children of students; e-mail services; employment services for current students; externships; housing assistance; interactive nursing skills videos; Internet; learning resource lab; library services; nursing audiovisuals; paid internships; placement services for program completers; remedial services; resume preparation assistance; skills, simulation, or other laboratory; tutoring; unpaid internships.
Library Facilities 20,000 volumes in health, 1,850 volumes in nursing; 255 periodical subscriptions health-care related.

BACCALAUREATE PROGRAMS

Degree BSN
Available Programs ADN to Baccalaureate; Generic Baccalaureate.
Site Options Visalia, CA; Lancaster, CA.
Study Options Full-time.
Program Entrance Requirements Minimum overall college GPA of 2.0, transcript of college record, CPR certification, health exam, health insurance, high school transcript, immunizations, interview, minimum GPA in nursing prerequisites of 2.8, professional liability insurance/malpractice insurance, prerequisite course work. Transfer students are accepted. *Application deadline:* 4/30 (fall), 12/31 (spring). *Application fee:* $25.
Advanced Placement Credit by examination available. Credit given for nursing courses completed elsewhere dependent upon specific evaluations.
Contact *Telephone:* 661-654-2508. *Fax:* 661-654-6347.

CONTINUING EDUCATION PROGRAM

Contact *Telephone:* 661-654-2446. *Fax:* 661-664-2447.

California State University Channel Islands
Nursing Program
Camarillo, California

Founded in 2002
DEGREE • BSN
Nursing Program Faculty 13 (20% with doctorates).
Baccalaureate Enrollment 120
Nursing Student Activities Student Nurses' Association.
Nursing Student Resources Academic advising; academic or career counseling; assistance for students with disabilities; bookstore; campus computer network; career placement assistance; computer lab; e-mail services; housing assistance; interactive nursing skills videos; Internet;

learning resource lab; library services; nursing audiovisuals; remedial services; skills, simulation, or other laboratory; tutoring.

BACCALAUREATE PROGRAMS

Degree BSN
Available Programs Generic Baccalaureate; RN Baccalaureate.
Contact *Telephone:* 805-437-3307.

California State University, Chico
School of Nursing
Chico, California

http://www.csuchico.edu/nurs/
Founded in 1887
DEGREES • BSN • MSN
Nursing Program Faculty 35 (25% with doctorates).
Baccalaureate Enrollment 230 **Women** 90% **Men** 10% **Minority** 35% **Part-time** 13%
Graduate Enrollment 20 **Women** 88% **Men** 12% **Minority** 29% **Part-time** 100%
Distance Learning Courses Available.
Nursing Student Activities Sigma Theta Tau, Student Nurses' Association, nursing club.
Nursing Student Resources Academic advising; academic or career counseling; assistance for students with disabilities; bookstore; campus computer network; career placement assistance; computer lab; computer-assisted instruction; daycare for children of students; e-mail services; employment services for current students; externships; housing assistance; interactive nursing skills videos; Internet; learning resource lab; library services; nursing audiovisuals; paid internships; placement services for program completers; remedial services; resume preparation assistance; skills, simulation, or other laboratory; tutoring; unpaid internships.
Library Facilities 942,304 volumes (17,727 in health, 1,467 in nursing); 22,000 periodical subscriptions (133 health-care related).

BACCALAUREATE PROGRAMS

Degree BSN
Available Programs ADN to Baccalaureate; Baccalaureate for Second Degree; Generic Baccalaureate; LPN to RN Baccalaureate; RN Baccalaureate.
Study Options Full-time.
Program Entrance Requirements Minimum overall college GPA of 3.0, transcript of college record, CPR certification, health insurance, immunizations, minimum GPA in nursing prerequisites of 3.0, prerequisite course work. Transfer students are accepted. *Application deadline:* 3/1 (fall), 11/1 (spring).
Advanced Placement Credit by examination available. Credit given for nursing courses completed elsewhere dependent upon specific evaluations.
Expenses (2012–13) *Tuition, state resident:* full-time $5970; part-time $3462 per semester. *Tuition, nonresident:* full-time $13,393; part-time $4697 per semester. *Room and board:* $11,208; room only: $6800 per academic year. *Required fees:* full-time $1468; part-time $122 per credit; part-time $734 per term.
Financial Aid 75% of baccalaureate students in nursing programs received some form of financial aid in 2011–12.
Contact Dr. Carol L. Huston, Director, School of Nursing, California State University, Chico, Holt Hall 369, Chico, CA 95929-0200. *Telephone:* 530-898-5891. *Fax:* 530-898-4363. *E-mail:* chuston@csuchico.edu.

GRADUATE PROGRAMS

Expenses (2012–13) *Tuition, state resident:* full-time $7052; part-time $2867 per semester. *Tuition, nonresident:* full-time $17,752; part-time $5099 per semester. *Room and board:* $11,208; room only: $6800 per academic year. *Required fees:* full-time $3336; part-time $278 per credit; part-time $1668 per term.
Financial Aid 25% of graduate students in nursing programs received some form of financial aid in 2011–12. Career-related internships or fieldwork and scholarships available. *Financial aid application deadline:* 3/1.
Contact Irene Morgan, Graduate Coordinator, School of Nursing, California State University, Chico, 400 West 1st Street, Chico, CA

95929-0200. *Telephone:* 530-898-5891. *Fax:* 530-898-6709. *E-mail:* imorgan@csuchico.edu.

MASTER'S DEGREE PROGRAM
Degree MSN
Available Programs Master's.
Concentrations Available Nursing education.
Study Options Part-time.
Online Degree Options Yes (online only).
Program Entrance Requirements Clinical experience, minimum overall college GPA of 3.0, transcript of college record, CPR certification, written essay, immunizations, prerequisite course work, statistics course, GRE. *Application deadline:* 3/1 (fall), 3/1 (spring).
Advanced Placement Credit given for nursing courses completed elsewhere dependent upon specific evaluations.
Degree Requirements 30 total credit hours, thesis or project.

CONTINUING EDUCATION PROGRAM

Contact Dr. Carol L. Huston, Director, School of Nursing, School of Nursing, California State University, Chico, Holt Hall 369, Chico, CA 95929-0200. *Telephone:* 530-898-5891. *Fax:* 530-898-6709. *E-mail:* chuston@csuchico.edu.

California State University, Dominguez Hills
Program in Nursing
Carson, California

http://www.csudh.edu/cps/son
Founded in 1960
DEGREES • BSN • MSN
Nursing Program Faculty 79 (34% with doctorates).
Baccalaureate Enrollment 725 **Women** 91% **Men** 9% **Minority** 37% **Part-time** 81%
Graduate Enrollment 456 **Women** 91% **Men** 9% **Minority** 28% **Part-time** 95%
Distance Learning Courses Available.
Nursing Student Activities Nursing Honor Society, Sigma Theta Tau, nursing club.
Nursing Student Resources Academic advising; academic or career counseling; assistance for students with disabilities; bookstore; campus computer network; career placement assistance; computer lab; computer-assisted instruction; daycare for children of students; e-mail services; housing assistance; interactive nursing skills videos; Internet; learning resource lab; library services; nursing audiovisuals; remedial services; skills, simulation, or other laboratory; tutoring.
Library Facilities 451,000 volumes (10,000 in nursing); 11,344 periodical subscriptions (215 health-care related).

BACCALAUREATE PROGRAMS

Degree BSN
Available Programs Baccalaureate for Second Degree; RN Baccalaureate.
Site Options Ventura, CA; Santa Monica, CA; Whittier, CA.
Online Degree Options Yes.
Program Entrance Requirements Minimum overall college GPA of 2.0, transcript of college record, minimum GPA in nursing prerequisites of 2.0, prerequisite course work, RN licensure. Transfer students are accepted. *Application fee:* $55.
Expenses (2011–12) *Tuition, area resident:* full-time $6100; part-time $1901 per semester.
Financial Aid 58% of baccalaureate students in nursing programs received some form of financial aid in 2010–11.
Contact Dr. Kathleen T. Chai, BSN Coordinator, Program in Nursing, California State University, Dominguez Hills, 1000 East Victoria Street, WH 335, Carson, CA 90747. *Telephone:* 310-243-2005. *Fax:* 310-516-3542. *E-mail:* kchai@csudh.edu.

GRADUATE PROGRAMS

Expenses (2011–12) *Tuition, area resident:* full-time $7366; part-time $2267 per semester.
Financial Aid 59% of graduate students in nursing programs received some form of financial aid in 2010–11.
Contact Dr. Cynthia Johnson, MSN Coordinator, Program in Nursing, California State University, Dominguez Hills, 1000 East Victoria Street,

WH A320, Carson, CA 90747. *Telephone:* 310-243-2522. *Fax:* 310-516-3542. *E-mail:* cjohnson@csudh.edu.

MASTER'S DEGREE PROGRAM
Degree MSN
Available Programs Master's; Master's for Non-Nursing College Graduates; Master's for Nurses with Non-Nursing Degrees.
Concentrations Available Clinical nurse leader; nursing administration; nursing education. *Clinical nurse specialist programs in:* gerontology, parent-child. *Nurse practitioner programs in:* family health.
Site Options Whittier, CA.
Study Options Full-time and part-time.
Online Degree Options Yes (online only).
Program Entrance Requirements Minimum overall college GPA of 3.0, transcript of college record, written essay, nursing research course, physical assessment course, prerequisite course work, resume, statistics course. *Application deadline:* 4/1 (fall), 11/1 (spring). Applications may be processed on a rolling basis for some programs. *Application fee:* $55.
Advanced Placement Credit given for nursing courses completed elsewhere dependent upon specific evaluations.
Degree Requirements 45 total credit hours, comprehensive exam.

POST-MASTER'S PROGRAM
Areas of Study Nursing administration; nursing education. *Clinical nurse specialist programs in:* gerontology, parent-child. *Nurse practitioner programs in:* family health.

California State University, East Bay
Department of Nursing and Health Sciences
Hayward, California

http://www20.csueastbay.edu/csci/departments/nursing/
Founded in 1957
DEGREE • BS
Nursing Program Faculty 53 (23% with doctorates).
Baccalaureate Enrollment 494 **Women** 80% **Men** 20% **Minority** 40% **International** 5% **Part-time** 10%
Distance Learning Courses Available.
Nursing Student Activities Sigma Theta Tau, Student Nurses' Association.
Nursing Student Resources Academic advising; academic or career counseling; assistance for students with disabilities; bookstore; campus computer network; career placement assistance; computer lab; computer-assisted instruction; e-mail services; employment services for current students; externships; interactive nursing skills videos; Internet; learning resource lab; library services; nursing audiovisuals; other; paid internships; placement services for program completers; remedial services; resume preparation assistance; skills, simulation, or other laboratory; tutoring; unpaid internships.

BACCALAUREATE PROGRAMS

Degree BS
Available Programs ADN to Baccalaureate; Generic Baccalaureate.
Site Options Concord, CA.
Study Options Full-time.
Program Entrance Requirements Transcript of college record, CPR certification, health exam, health insurance, immunizations, minimum GPA in nursing prerequisites of 3.0, prerequisite course work. Transfer students are accepted. *Application deadline:* 11/30 (fall).
Advanced Placement Credit given for nursing courses completed elsewhere dependent upon specific evaluations.
Expenses (2012–13) *Tuition, state resident:* full-time $6500. *Tuition, nonresident:* full-time $15,500. *International tuition:* $15,500 full-time.
Financial Aid *Gift aid (need-based):* Federal Pell, FSEOG, state, private, college/university gift aid from institutional funds. *Loans:* Federal Direct (Subsidized and Unsubsidized Stafford PLUS), Perkins, college/university.*Work-study:* Federal Work-Study.*Financial aid application deadline (priority):* 3/2.
Contact Lara Dungan, Admissions Coordinator/Advisor, Department of Nursing and Health Sciences, California State University, East Bay, 25800 Carlos Bee Boulevard, Hayward, CA 94542. *Telephone:* 510-885-3481. *Fax:* 510-885-2156. *E-mail:* lara.dungan@csueastbay.edu.

California State University, Fresno

Department of Nursing
Fresno, California

http://www.csufresno.edu/chhs/depts_programs/nursing/
Founded in 1911
DEGREES • BSN • DNP • MSN
Nursing Program Faculty 54 (30% with doctorates).
Baccalaureate Enrollment 450 **Women** 80% **Men** 20% **Minority** 49%
Part-time 5%
Graduate Enrollment 125 **Women** 86% **Men** 14% **Minority** 53%
International 4% **Part-time** 36%
Distance Learning Courses Available.
Nursing Student Activities Sigma Theta Tau, Student Nurses' Association.
Nursing Student Resources Academic advising; academic or career counseling; assistance for students with disabilities; bookstore; campus computer network; career placement assistance; computer lab; computer-assisted instruction; daycare for children of students; e-mail services; externships; housing assistance; interactive nursing skills videos; Internet; learning resource lab; library services; nursing audiovisuals; paid internships; placement services for program completers; remedial services; skills, simulation, or other laboratory; tutoring.
Library Facilities 28,197 volumes in health, 1,287 volumes in nursing; 1,700 periodical subscriptions health-care related.

BACCALAUREATE PROGRAMS

Degree BSN
Available Programs ADN to Baccalaureate; Generic Baccalaureate.
Study Options Full-time.
Program Entrance Requirements Transcript of college record, CPR certification, health exam, immunizations, minimum GPA in nursing prerequisites of 3.0, professional liability insurance/malpractice insurance, prerequisite course work. Transfer students are accepted. *Application deadline:* 3/31 (fall), 8/31 (spring).
Advanced Placement Credit by examination available. Credit given for nursing courses completed elsewhere dependent upon specific evaluations.
Expenses (2011–12) *Tuition, state resident:* full-time $5970; part-time $1731 per semester. *Room and board:* $8000 per academic year. *Required fees:* full-time $397.
Financial Aid 65% of baccalaureate students in nursing programs received some form of financial aid in 2010–11. *Gift aid (need-based):* Federal Pell, FSEOG, state, private, college/university gift aid from institutional funds. *Loans:* Federal Nursing Student Loans, Perkins, college/university, alternative loans. *Work-study:* Federal Work-Study. *Financial aid application deadline (priority):* 3/2.
Contact Dr. Mary Barakzai, Co-Chair, Department of Nursing, California State University, Fresno, 2345 East San Ramon Avenue, MH25, Fresno, CA 93740-8031. *Telephone:* 559-278-2429. *Fax:* 559-278-6360. *E-mail:* maryb@csufresno.edu.

GRADUATE PROGRAMS

Financial Aid 30% of graduate students in nursing programs received some form of financial aid in 2010–11. 2 teaching assistantships were awarded; career-related internships or fieldwork, Federal Work-Study, scholarships, and traineeships also available. Aid available to part-time students. *Financial aid application deadline:* 3/1.
Contact Dr. Ndidi Griffin, Graduate Coordinator, Department of Nursing, California State University, Fresno, 2345 East San Ramon Avenue, MH25, Fresno, CA 93740-8031. *Telephone:* 559-278-6697. *Fax:* 559-278-6360. *E-mail:* ndidig@csufresno.edu.

MASTER'S DEGREE PROGRAM

Degree MSN
Available Programs Accelerated Master's; Master's; Master's for Nurses with Non-Nursing Degrees.
Concentrations Available Nursing education. *Clinical nurse specialist programs in:* adult health, gerontology, pediatric. *Nurse practitioner programs in:* family health, pediatric.
Study Options Full-time and part-time.
Program Entrance Requirements Computer literacy, minimum overall college GPA of 3.0, transcript of college record, CPR certification, written essay, 3 letters of recommendation, nursing research course, physical assessment course, professional liability insurance/malpractice insurance, prerequisite course work, resume, statistics course, GRE General Test. *Application deadline:* 4/1 (fall).
Advanced Placement Credit given for nursing courses completed elsewhere dependent upon specific evaluations.
Degree Requirements 38 total credit hours, thesis or project, comprehensive exam.

POST-MASTER'S PROGRAM

Areas of Study *Nurse practitioner programs in:* family health, pediatric, psychiatric/mental health.

DOCTORAL DEGREE PROGRAM

Degree DNP
Available Programs Doctorate.
Online Degree Options Yes (online only).
Program Entrance Requirements Clinical experience, minimum overall college GPA of 3.0, interview by faculty committee, 3 letters of recommendation, MSN or equivalent, vita, writing sample. *Application deadline:* 1/31 (fall).
Degree Requirements 37 total credit hours, oral exam.

CONTINUING EDUCATION PROGRAM

Contact Dr. Lynnette Zelezny, Associate Vice President, Department of Nursing, California State University, Fresno, 5005 North Maple Avenue, ED76, Fresno, CA 93740-0076. *Telephone:* 559-278-2691. *Fax:* 559-278-0333. *E-mail:* lynnette@csufresno.edu.

California State University, Fullerton

Department of Nursing
Fullerton, California

http://nursing.fullerton.edu/
Founded in 1957
DEGREES • BSN • DNP • MSN
Nursing Program Faculty 71 (28% with doctorates).
Baccalaureate Enrollment 464 **Women** 83.2% **Men** 16.8% **Minority** 60.8% **International** 4.3% **Part-time** 69%
Graduate Enrollment 372 **Women** 84.9% **Men** 15.1% **Minority** 44.9% **International** 1.1% **Part-time** 46.5%
Distance Learning Courses Available.
Nursing Student Activities Nursing Honor Society, Sigma Theta Tau, Student Nurses' Association.
Nursing Student Resources Academic advising; academic or career counseling; assistance for students with disabilities; bookstore; campus computer network; computer lab; computer-assisted instruction; daycare for children of students; e-mail services; housing assistance; Internet; learning resource lab; library services; resume preparation assistance; skills, simulation, or other laboratory; tutoring.
Library Facilities 1.3 million volumes (17,340 in health, 837 in nursing); 55,756 periodical subscriptions (8,145 health-care related).

BACCALAUREATE PROGRAMS

Degree BSN
Available Programs ADN to Baccalaureate; Baccalaureate for Second Degree; Generic Baccalaureate; LPN to Baccalaureate; RN Baccalaureate.
Site Options Los Angeles, CA; Riverside, CA; Mission Viejo, CA.
Study Options Full-time.
Program Entrance Requirements Minimum overall college GPA, transcript of college record, minimum GPA in nursing prerequisites, prerequisite course work. *Application deadline:* 2/15 (fall).
Advanced Placement Credit given for nursing courses completed elsewhere dependent upon specific evaluations.
Expenses (2012–13) *Tuition, state resident:* full-time $3313.
Financial Aid 50% of baccalaureate students in nursing programs received some form of financial aid in 2011–12.
Contact Nursing Advisor, Department of Nursing, California State University, Fullerton, EC-182, PO Box 6868, Fullerton, CA 92834-6868. *Telephone:* 657-278-3217. *Fax:* 657-278-2096. *E-mail:* nursingadvising@fullerton.edu.

GRADUATE PROGRAMS

Expenses (2012–13) *Tuition, state resident:* full-time $4006; part-time $2461 per semester.

Financial Aid 44% of graduate students in nursing programs received some form of financial aid in 2011–12.
Contact Ms. Mary Lehn-Mooney, Advisor, Department of Nursing, California State University, Fullerton, EC 190, 800 North State College Boulevard, Fullerton, CA 92834-6868. *Telephone:* 714-278-3217. *Fax:* 714-278-2096. *E-mail:* mlehn-mooney@fullerton.edu.

MASTER'S DEGREE PROGRAM
Degree MSN
Available Programs Master's; Master's for Non-Nursing College Graduates.
Concentrations Available Nurse anesthesia; nurse-midwifery; nursing administration; nursing education. *Clinical nurse specialist programs in:* school health. *Nurse practitioner programs in:* women's health.
Study Options Full-time and part-time.
Online Degree Options Yes.
Program Entrance Requirements Clinical experience, minimum overall college GPA of 3.0, transcript of college record, CPR certification, written essay, immunizations, interview, 3 letters of recommendation, nursing research course, professional liability insurance/malpractice insurance, prerequisite course work, statistics course. *Application deadline:* 11/30 (fall). Applications may be processed on a rolling basis for some programs. *Application fee:* $55.
Advanced Placement Credit given for nursing courses completed elsewhere dependent upon specific evaluations.
Degree Requirements 71 total credit hours, thesis or project, comprehensive exam.

DOCTORAL DEGREE PROGRAM
Degree DNP
Available Programs Doctorate; Doctorate for Nurses with Non-Nursing Degrees; Post-Baccalaureate Doctorate.
Areas of Study Advanced practice nursing, clinical practice, community health, critical care, family health, nursing administration, nursing education, nursing research, nursing science, women's health.
Program Entrance Requirements Clinical experience, minimum overall college GPA of 3.5, interview, 3 letters of recommendation, MSN or equivalent, statistics course, writing sample. *Application deadline:* 12/15 (fall). *Application fee:* $55.
Degree Requirements 36 total credit hours, dissertation, written exam.

California State University, Long Beach
School of Nursing
Long Beach, California

http://www.csulb.edu/colleges/chhs/departments/nursing/
Founded in 1949
DEGREES • BSN • MSN • MSN/MHA
Nursing Program Faculty 76 (40% with doctorates).
Baccalaureate Enrollment 539 **Women** 79.2% **Men** 20.8% **Minority** 73.6% **International** .01% **Part-time** 10%
Graduate Enrollment 484 **Women** 86.4% **Men** 13.6% **Minority** 71.7% **International** .02% **Part-time** 50%
Nursing Student Activities Nursing Honor Society, Sigma Theta Tau, Student Nurses' Association.
Nursing Student Resources Academic advising; academic or career counseling; assistance for students with disabilities; bookstore; e-mail services; interactive nursing skills videos; Internet; learning resource lab; library services; nursing audiovisuals; remedial services; resume preparation assistance; skills, simulation, or other laboratory; tutoring; unpaid internships.
Library Facilities 2 million volumes; 21,002 periodical subscriptions.

BACCALAUREATE PROGRAMS
Degree BSN
Available Programs ADN to Baccalaureate; Accelerated Baccalaureate; Baccalaureate for Second Degree; Generic Baccalaureate; LPN to Baccalaureate.
Site Options Huntington Beach, CA.
Study Options Full-time.
Program Entrance Requirements Transcript of college record, CPR certification, health exam, health insurance, immunizations, interview, minimum GPA in nursing prerequisites of 3.0, professional liability insurance/malpractice insurance, prerequisite course work. Transfer stu-

dents are accepted. *Application deadline:* 2/15 (fall), 9/15 (spring). *Application fee:* $55.
Advanced Placement Credit given for nursing courses completed elsewhere dependent upon specific evaluations.
Expenses (2012–13) *Tuition, state resident:* full-time $6700; part-time $4230 per semester. *Tuition, nonresident:* full-time $15,666; part-time $8694 per semester. *International tuition:* $15,666 full-time. *Room and board:* $11,000; room only: $8200 per academic year. *Required fees:* full-time $3000; part-time $300 per credit; part-time $1500 per term.
Financial Aid 75% of baccalaureate students in nursing programs received some form of financial aid in 2011–12. *Gift aid (need-based):* Federal Pell, FSEOG, state, private, college/university gift aid from institutional funds. *Loans:* Federal Direct (Subsidized and Unsubsidized Stafford PLUS), Perkins. *Work-study:* Federal Work-Study. *Financial aid application deadline (priority):* 3/2.
Contact Dr. Beth R. Keely, Assistant Director, Undergraduate Nursing Programs, School of Nursing, California State University, Long Beach, 1250 Bellflower Boulevard, Long Beach, CA 90840. *Telephone:* 562-985-4478. *Fax:* 562-985-2382. *E-mail:* bkeely@csulb.edu.

GRADUATE PROGRAMS
Expenses (2012–13) *Tuition, state resident:* full-time $8124; part-time $5034 per semester. *Tuition, nonresident:* full-time $12,588; part-time $9498 per semester. *International tuition:* $12,588 full-time. *Room and board:* $10,658; room only: $8208 per academic year. *Required fees:* full-time $3000; part-time $372 per credit; part-time $1500 per term.
Financial Aid 25% of graduate students in nursing programs received some form of financial aid in 2011–12. Federal Work-Study, institutionally sponsored loans, and scholarships available. *Financial aid application deadline:* 3/2.
Contact Alison Kliachko-Trafas, Administrative Assistant, School of Nursing, California State University, Long Beach, 1250 Bellflower Boulevard, Long Beach, CA 90840. *Telephone:* 562-985-4473. *Fax:* 562-985-2382. *E-mail:* akliachk@csulb.edu.

MASTER'S DEGREE PROGRAM
Degrees MSN; MSN/MHA
Available Programs Accelerated Master's; Master's; Master's for Non-Nursing College Graduates.
Concentrations Available Health-care administration; nursing administration; nursing education. *Clinical nurse specialist programs in:* adult health. *Nurse practitioner programs in:* adult health, family health, gerontology, pediatric, psychiatric/mental health, women's health.
Site Options Long Beach, CA; Huntington Beach, CA.
Study Options Full-time and part-time.
Program Entrance Requirements Clinical experience, minimum overall college GPA of 2.75, transcript of college record, written essay, 3 letters of recommendation, physical assessment course, prerequisite course work, resume, statistics course. *Application deadline:* 3/15 (fall), 10/15 (spring). *Application fee:* $55.
Advanced Placement Credit given for nursing courses completed elsewhere dependent upon specific evaluations.
Degree Requirements 37 total credit hours, thesis or project, comprehensive exam.

POST-MASTER'S PROGRAM
Areas of Study Nursing administration. *Clinical nurse specialist programs in:* adult health. *Nurse practitioner programs in:* adult health, family health, gerontology, pediatric, psychiatric/mental health, women's health.

California State University, Los Angeles
School of Nursing
Los Angeles, California

http://www.calstatela.edu/dept/nursing/
Founded in 1947
DEGREES • BSN • MSN
Nursing Program Faculty 31 (39% with doctorates).
Baccalaureate Enrollment 300
Graduate Enrollment 100
Nursing Student Resources Academic advising.
Library Facilities 2.1 million volumes; 648 periodical subscriptions.

BACCALAUREATE PROGRAMS

Degree BSN
Available Programs Generic Baccalaureate; LPN to RN Baccalaureate; RN Baccalaureate.
Study Options Full-time.
Program Entrance Requirements Minimum overall college GPA of 2.75, CPR certification, health exam, health insurance, high school biology, immunizations, minimum GPA in nursing prerequisites of 2.75, professional liability insurance/malpractice insurance, prerequisite course work. Transfer students are accepted. *Application deadline:* 12/1 (fall).
Advanced Placement Credit given for nursing courses completed elsewhere dependent upon specific evaluations.
Contact *Telephone:* 323-343-4700. *Fax:* 323-343-6454.

GRADUATE PROGRAMS

Contact *Telephone:* 323-343-4700. *Fax:* 323-343-6454.

MASTER'S DEGREE PROGRAM
Degree MSN
Available Programs Accelerated Master's for Nurses with Non-Nursing Degrees; Accelerated RN to Master's; Master's; Master's for Non-Nursing College Graduates.
Concentrations Available Nursing administration; nursing education. *Clinical nurse specialist programs in:* psychiatric/mental health. *Nurse practitioner programs in:* acute care, adult health, family health, pediatric, primary care, psychiatric/mental health.
Study Options Full-time and part-time.
Program Entrance Requirements Clinical experience, minimum overall college GPA of 3.0, transcript of college record, written essay, immunizations, letters of recommendation, nursing research course, physical assessment course, professional liability insurance/malpractice insurance, resume, statistics course. *Application deadline:* 11/15 (fall), 5/15 (spring).
Advanced Placement Credit given for nursing courses completed elsewhere dependent upon specific evaluations.
Degree Requirements 45 total credit hours, comprehensive exam.

POST-MASTER'S PROGRAM
Areas of Study *Nurse practitioner programs in:* acute care, adult health, family health, pediatric, primary care.

California State University, Northridge
Nursing Program
Northridge, California

http://www.csun.edu/~nursing/
Founded in 1958
DEGREE • BSN
Nursing Program Faculty 18 (3.6% with doctorates).
Baccalaureate Enrollment 140 **Women** 92% **Men** 8% **Minority** 60% **International** 12% **Part-time** 66%
Nursing Student Activities Sigma Theta Tau, Student Nurses' Association.
Nursing Student Resources Academic advising; academic or career counseling; assistance for students with disabilities; bookstore; campus computer network; career placement assistance; computer lab; computer-assisted instruction; daycare for children of students; e-mail services; housing assistance; interactive nursing skills videos; Internet; learning resource lab; library services; nursing audiovisuals; remedial services; resume preparation assistance; skills, simulation, or other laboratory; tutoring.
Library Facilities 1.4 million volumes (61,848 in health, 1,401 in nursing); 1,063 periodical subscriptions (303 health-care related).

BACCALAUREATE PROGRAMS

Degree BSN
Available Programs ADN to Baccalaureate; Accelerated Baccalaureate.
Site Options Panorama City, CA; Ventura , CA; Antelope Valley, CA.
Study Options Full-time and part-time.
Program Entrance Requirements Minimum overall college GPA of 3.0, transcript of college record, CPR certification, written essay, health exam, health insurance, immunizations, interview, 3 letters of recommendation, minimum GPA in nursing prerequisites of 3.0, professional lia-

bility insurance/malpractice insurance, prerequisite course work, RN licensure. Transfer students are accepted. *Application deadline:* 11/30 (fall), 11/30 (summer). *Application fee:* $55.
Advanced Placement Credit by examination available. Credit given for nursing courses completed elsewhere dependent upon specific evaluations.
Expenses (2012–13) *Tuition, state resident:* full-time $7002; part-time $4494 per semester. *Tuition, nonresident:* full-time $11,466; part-time $6726 per semester. *International tuition:* $11,466 full-time. *Room and board:* $11,511; room only: $6771 per academic year. *Required fees:* full-time $1032; part-time $516 per term.
Financial Aid 90% of baccalaureate students in nursing programs received some form of financial aid in 2011–12.
Contact Department of Nursing, Nursing Program, California State University, Northridge, 18111 Nordhoff Street, Northridge, CA 91330-8285. *Telephone:* 818-677-3101. *Fax:* 818-677-2045. *E-mail:* absn@csun.edu.

California State University, Sacramento
School of Nursing
Sacramento, California

http://www.hhs.csus.edu/nrs
Founded in 1947
DEGREES • BSN • MS
Nursing Program Faculty 64 (50% with doctorates).
Baccalaureate Enrollment 286 **Women** 89% **Men** 11%
Graduate Enrollment 180 **Women** 95% **Men** 5% **Part-time** 100%
Distance Learning Courses Available.
Nursing Student Activities Sigma Theta Tau, Student Nurses' Association.
Nursing Student Resources Academic advising; academic or career counseling; assistance for students with disabilities; bookstore; campus computer network; computer lab; computer-assisted instruction; daycare for children of students; e-mail services; externships; housing assistance; interactive nursing skills videos; Internet; learning resource lab; library services; nursing audiovisuals; paid internships; placement services for program completers; remedial services; resume preparation assistance; skills, simulation, or other laboratory; tutoring.
Library Facilities 33,000 volumes in health; 327 periodical subscriptions health-care related.

BACCALAUREATE PROGRAMS

Degree BSN
Available Programs ADN to Baccalaureate; Baccalaureate for Second Degree; Generic Baccalaureate; LPN to RN Baccalaureate.
Study Options Full-time.
Program Entrance Requirements Transcript of college record, CPR certification, health exam, health insurance, high school biology, high school math, immunizations, minimum GPA in nursing prerequisites of 3.3, professional liability insurance/malpractice insurance, prerequisite course work. Transfer students are accepted. *Application deadline:* 3/1 (fall), 10/1 (spring).
Advanced Placement Credit by examination available. Credit given for nursing courses completed elsewhere dependent upon specific evaluations.
Contact *Telephone:* 916-278-6525.

GRADUATE PROGRAMS

Contact *Fax:* 916-278-6311.

MASTER'S DEGREE PROGRAM
Degree MS
Available Programs Master's.
Concentrations Available Nursing administration; nursing education. *Nurse practitioner programs in:* family health, primary care.
Study Options Part-time.
Program Entrance Requirements Clinical experience, computer literacy, minimum overall college GPA of 3.0, transcript of college record, CPR certification, immunizations, nursing research course, professional liability insurance/malpractice insurance, prerequisite course work, statistics course, GRE. *Application deadline:* 11/30 (fall).

Advanced Placement Credit given for nursing courses completed elsewhere dependent upon specific evaluations.

Degree Requirements 33 total credit hours, comprehensive exam.

California State University, San Bernardino

Department of Nursing
San Bernardino, California

http://nursing.csusb.edu/
Founded in 1965

DEGREES • BSN • MSN

Nursing Program Faculty 42 (19% with doctorates).

Baccalaureate Enrollment 457 **Women** 81% **Men** 19% **Minority** 59%

Graduate Enrollment 19 **Women** 89% **Men** 11% **Minority** 47%

Distance Learning Courses Available.

Nursing Student Activities Sigma Theta Tau, Student Nurses' Association.

Nursing Student Resources Academic advising; academic or career counseling; assistance for students with disabilities; bookstore; campus computer network; computer lab; computer-assisted instruction; daycare for children of students; e-mail services; Internet; learning resource lab; library services; nursing audiovisuals; remedial services; skills, simulation, or other laboratory.

Library Facilities 731,259 volumes (1,500 in health, 1,000 in nursing); 2,028 periodical subscriptions (5,000 health-care related).

BACCALAUREATE PROGRAMS

Degree BSN

Available Programs Generic Baccalaureate; LPN to Baccalaureate; RN Baccalaureate.

Site Options Palm Desert, CA.

Study Options Full-time.

Program Entrance Requirements Minimum overall college GPA of 2.5, transcript of college record, 3 letters of recommendation, minimum GPA in nursing prerequisites of 2.5, prerequisite course work. Transfer students are accepted. *Application deadline:* 3/1 (fall), 10/1 (winter).

Advanced Placement Credit given for nursing courses completed elsewhere dependent upon specific evaluations.

Contact *Telephone:* 909-537-5381.

GRADUATE PROGRAMS

Contact *Telephone:* 909-537-7241.

MASTER'S DEGREE PROGRAM

Degree MSN

Available Programs Master's.

Concentrations Available Nursing administration; nursing education. *Clinical nurse specialist programs in:* community health.

Study Options Full-time and part-time.

Program Entrance Requirements Clinical experience, minimum overall college GPA of 3.0, transcript of college record, letters of recommendation, prerequisite course work, resume, statistics course. *Application deadline:* 6/10 (fall).

Advanced Placement Credit given for nursing courses completed elsewhere dependent upon specific evaluations.

Degree Requirements 65 total credit hours, thesis or project, comprehensive exam.

California State University, San Marcos

School of Nursing
San Marcos, California

Founded in 1990

DEGREE • BSN

Nursing Student Activities Student Nurses' Association.

Library Facilities 401,041 volumes; 41,825 periodical subscriptions.

BACCALAUREATE PROGRAMS

Degree BSN

Available Programs Accelerated Baccalaureate; Generic Baccalaureate.

Contact *Telephone:* 706-750-7550. *Fax:* 706-750-3646.

California State University, Stanislaus

Department of Nursing
Turlock, California

http://www.csustan.edu/academics/CHHS/Nursing.html
Founded in 1957

DEGREE • BSN

Nursing Program Faculty 17 (24% with doctorates).

Baccalaureate Enrollment 164 **Women** 88% **Men** 12% **Minority** 42% **Part-time** 30%

Nursing Student Activities Sigma Theta Tau, Student Nurses' Association.

Nursing Student Resources Academic advising; academic or career counseling; assistance for students with disabilities; bookstore; campus computer network; career placement assistance; computer lab; computer-assisted instruction; daycare for children of students; e-mail services; employment services for current students; externships; interactive nursing skills videos; Internet; learning resource lab; library services; nursing audiovisuals; resume preparation assistance; skills, simulation, or other laboratory; tutoring.

Library Facilities 498,803 volumes (12,642 in health, 1,338 in nursing); 59,768 periodical subscriptions (93 health-care related).

BACCALAUREATE PROGRAMS

Degree BSN

Available Programs ADN to Baccalaureate; Generic Baccalaureate; LPN to Baccalaureate.

Study Options Full-time.

Program Entrance Requirements Minimum overall college GPA of 3.0, transcript of college record, CPR certification, health exam, immunizations, minimum GPA in nursing prerequisites of 3.0, professional liability insurance/malpractice insurance, prerequisite course work. Transfer students are accepted.

Advanced Placement Credit given for nursing courses completed elsewhere dependent upon specific evaluations.

Contact *Telephone:* 209-667-3141. *Fax:* 209-667-3690.

Charles Drew University of Medicine and Science

School of Nursing
Los Angeles, California

Founded in 1966

DEGREE • MSN

Library Facilities 84,336 volumes; 36,693 periodical subscriptions.

GRADUATE PROGRAMS

Contact School of Nursing, School of Nursing, Charles Drew University of Medicine and Science, 1731 East 120th Street, Los Angeles, CA 90059. *Telephone:* 323-568-3301. *E-mail:* mmdson@cdrewu.edu.

MASTER'S DEGREE PROGRAM

Degree MSN

Available Programs Accelerated Master's for Nurses with Non-Nursing Degrees; Master's.

Program Entrance Requirements Minimum overall college GPA of 3.0, written essay, 3 letters of recommendation, resume. *Application fee:* $100.

Concordia University
Bachelor of Science in Nursing Program
Irvine, California

Founded in 1972

DEGREE • BSN

Library Facilities 79,909 volumes; 24,600 periodical subscriptions.

BACCALAUREATE PROGRAMS

Degree BSN

Available Programs Accelerated Baccalaureate for Second Degree; RN Baccalaureate.

Program Entrance Requirements Transcript of college record, prerequisite course work, RN licensure.

Contact *Telephone:* 949-854-8002 Ext. 1144.

Dominican University of California
Program in Nursing
San Rafael, California

http://www.dominican.edu/
Founded in 1890

DEGREES • BSN • MSN

Nursing Program Faculty 53 (23% with doctorates).

Baccalaureate Enrollment 497 **Women** 88% **Men** 12% **Minority** 55% **International** 1% **Part-time** 17%

Graduate Enrollment 30 **Women** 87% **Men** 13% **Minority** 23% **Part-time** 50%

Nursing Student Activities Sigma Theta Tau, Student Nurses' Association, nursing club.

Nursing Student Resources Academic advising; academic or career counseling; assistance for students with disabilities; bookstore; campus computer network; career placement assistance; computer lab; computer-assisted instruction; e-mail services; employment services for current students; housing assistance; interactive nursing skills videos; Internet; learning resource lab; library services; nursing audiovisuals; remedial services; resume preparation assistance; skills, simulation, or other laboratory; tutoring; unpaid internships.

Library Facilities 114,625 volumes (1,200 in health, 1,000 in nursing); 93,144 periodical subscriptions (1,300 health-care related).

BACCALAUREATE PROGRAMS

Degree BSN

Available Programs Baccalaureate for Second Degree; Generic Baccalaureate; RN Baccalaureate.

Study Options Full-time and part-time.

Program Entrance Requirements Minimum overall college GPA of 3.0, transcript of college record, CPR certification, written essay, health exam, health insurance, high school biology, high school chemistry, 2 years high school math, high school transcript, immunizations, 1 letter of recommendation, minimum high school GPA of 3.0, minimum GPA in nursing prerequisites of 3.0, prerequisite course work. Transfer students are accepted. *Application deadline:* 2/1 (fall), 9/1 (spring). Applications may be processed on a rolling basis for some programs. *Application fee:* $40.

Advanced Placement Credit given for nursing courses completed elsewhere dependent upon specific evaluations.

Expenses (2011–12) *Tuition:* full-time $36,900; part-time $1560 per credit hour. *International tuition:* $36,900 full-time. *Room and board:* $13,900; room only: $8400 per academic year. *Required fees:* full-time $450; part-time $450 per term.

Financial Aid 95% of baccalaureate students in nursing programs received some form of financial aid in 2010–11.

Contact Rebecca Finn Kenney, Assistant Vice President of Undergraduate Admissions, Program in Nursing, Dominican University of California, 50 Acacia Avenue, San Rafael, CA 94901-2298. *Telephone:* 415-485-3204. *Fax:* 415-485-3214. *E-mail:* rebecca.finnkenney@dominican.edu.

GRADUATE PROGRAMS

Expenses (2011–12) *Tuition:* full-time $16,380; part-time $910 per credit. *International tuition:* $16,380 full-time. *Required fees:* full-time $300; part-time $300 per term.

Financial Aid 61% of graduate students in nursing programs received some form of financial aid in 2010–11. Scholarships available. Aid available to part-time students. *Financial aid application deadline:* 3/2.

Contact Mr. Larry Schwartz, Director of Graduate and Pathways Admissions, Program in Nursing, Dominican University of California, 50 Acacia Avenue, San Rafael, CA 94901-2298. *Telephone:* 415-458-3748. *E-mail:* larry.schwartz@dominican.edu.

MASTER'S DEGREE PROGRAM

Degree MSN

Available Programs Master's; Master's for Nurses with Non-Nursing Degrees; RN to Master's.

Concentrations Available Clinical nurse leader.

Study Options Full-time and part-time.

Program Entrance Requirements Clinical experience, minimum overall college GPA of 3.0, transcript of college record, CPR certification, written essay, interview, 2 letters of recommendation, nursing research course, prerequisite course work, resume, statistics course. *Application deadline:* 6/15 (fall), 11/15 (spring). Applications may be processed on a rolling basis for some programs. *Application fee:* $40.

Advanced Placement Credit given for nursing courses completed elsewhere dependent upon specific evaluations.

Degree Requirements 32 total credit hours, thesis or project.

CONTINUING EDUCATION PROGRAM

Contact Mr. Larry Schwartz, Director of Graduate and Pathways Admissions, Program in Nursing, Dominican University of California, 50 Acacia Avenue, San Rafael, CA 94901. *Telephone:* 415-458-3748. *E-mail:* larry.schwartz@dominican.edu.

Fresno Pacific University
RN to BSN Program
Fresno, California

Founded in 1944

DEGREE • BSN

Library Facilities 196,000 volumes; 16,000 periodical subscriptions.

BACCALAUREATE PROGRAMS

Degree BSN

Available Programs RN Baccalaureate.

Contact *Telephone:* 559-453-2000.

Holy Names University
Department of Nursing
Oakland, California

http://www.hnu.edu/
Founded in 1868

DEGREES • BSN • MSN • MSN/MBA

Nursing Program Faculty 44 (8% with doctorates).

Baccalaureate Enrollment 68 **Women** 90% **Men** 10% **Minority** 52% **International** 1% **Part-time** 100%

Graduate Enrollment 70 **Women** 85% **Men** 15% **Minority** 60% **International** 2% **Part-time** 10%

Distance Learning Courses Available.

Nursing Student Activities Nursing Honor Society, Sigma Theta Tau, nursing club.

Nursing Student Resources Academic advising; academic or career counseling; assistance for students with disabilities; bookstore; campus computer network; career placement assistance; computer lab; computer-assisted instruction; e-mail services; employment services for current students; externships; housing assistance; interactive nursing skills videos; Internet; learning resource lab; library services; nursing audiovisuals; placement services for program completers; remedial services; resume preparation assistance; skills, simulation, or other laboratory; tutoring.

Library Facilities 86,954 volumes (500 in health, 200 in nursing); 27,803 periodical subscriptions (200 health-care related).

BACCALAUREATE PROGRAMS

Degree BSN
Available Programs LPN to RN Baccalaureate; RN Baccalaureate.
Site Options Stanford, CA.
Study Options Full-time and part-time.
Program Entrance Requirements Minimum overall college GPA of 2.75, transcript of college record, written essay, prerequisite course work, RN licensure. Transfer students are accepted. *Application deadline:* Applications may be processed on a rolling basis for some programs. *Application fee:* $50.
Advanced Placement Credit given for nursing courses completed elsewhere dependent upon specific evaluations.
Financial Aid 95% of baccalaureate students in nursing programs received some form of financial aid in 2011–12.
Contact Ms. Nancy Flinn, Admission Counselor, Department of Nursing, Holy Names University, 3500 Mountain Boulevard, Oakland, CA 94619-1699. *Telephone:* 510-436-1325. *Fax:* 510-436-1376. *E-mail:* flinn@hnu.edu.

GRADUATE PROGRAMS

Financial Aid 95% of graduate students in nursing programs received some form of financial aid in 2011–12. Scholarships available. Aid available to part-time students. *Financial aid application deadline:* 3/2.
Contact Ms. Lisa Marie Gibson, Admission Counselor, Department of Nursing, Holy Names University, 3500 Mountain Boulevard, Oakland, CA 94619-1699. *Telephone:* 510-436-1317. *Fax:* 510-436-1376. *E-mail:* lgibson@hnu.edu.

MASTER'S DEGREE PROGRAM

Degrees MSN; MSN/MBA
Available Programs Master's; Master's for Nurses with Non-Nursing Degrees.
Concentrations Available Nursing administration; nursing education. *Nurse practitioner programs in:* family health.
Site Options Arroyo Grande.
Study Options Full-time and part-time.
Program Entrance Requirements Minimum overall college GPA of 2.8, transcript of college record, written essay, 2 letters of recommendation, resume. *Application deadline:* Applications may be processed on a rolling basis for some programs. *Application fee:* $65.
Degree Requirements 45 total credit hours, thesis or project.

POST-MASTER'S PROGRAM

Areas of Study Nursing administration; nursing education. *Nurse practitioner programs in:* family health.

Loma Linda University

School of Nursing
Loma Linda, California

http://www.llu.edu/nursing
Founded in 1905
DEGREES • BS • MS • PHD
Nursing Program Faculty 47 (55% with doctorates).
Baccalaureate Enrollment 496 **Women** 81% **Men** 19% **Minority** 62% **International** 19% **Part-time** 22%
Graduate Enrollment 191 **Women** 98% **Men** 2% **Minority** 40% **International** 8% **Part-time** 73%
Nursing Student Activities Nursing Honor Society, Sigma Theta Tau, Student Nurses' Association, nursing club.
Nursing Student Resources Academic advising; academic or career counseling; assistance for students with disabilities; bookstore; campus computer network; computer lab; computer-assisted instruction; e-mail services; employment services for current students; externships; housing assistance; interactive nursing skills videos; Internet; learning resource lab; library services; nursing audiovisuals; paid internships; remedial services; resume preparation assistance; skills, simulation, or other laboratory; tutoring.
Library Facilities 338,418 volumes (73,702 in health, 4,965 in nursing); 1,671 periodical subscriptions (6,516 health-care related).

BACCALAUREATE PROGRAMS

Degree BS

Available Programs ADN to Baccalaureate; Accelerated Baccalaureate for Second Degree; Accelerated RN Baccalaureate; Baccalaureate for Second Degree; Generic Baccalaureate; LPN to Baccalaureate; RN Baccalaureate.
Study Options Full-time and part-time.
Program Entrance Requirements Minimum overall college GPA of 3.0, transcript of college record, CPR certification, written essay, health exam, high school transcript, immunizations, interview, 3 letters of recommendation, minimum GPA in nursing prerequisites of 3.0, prerequisite course work. Transfer students are accepted. *Application deadline:* 3/31 (fall), 8/15 (winter), 11/1 (spring). Applications may be processed on a rolling basis for some programs. *Application fee:* $120.
Advanced Placement Credit by examination available. Credit given for nursing courses completed elsewhere dependent upon specific evaluations.
Expenses (2012–13) *Tuition:* full-time $27,600; part-time $575 per quarter hour. *International tuition:* $27,600 full-time. *Room and board:* room only: $2640 per academic year. *Required fees:* full-time $3650; part-time $1200 per term.
Financial Aid 95% of baccalaureate students in nursing programs received some form of financial aid in 2011–12.
Contact Mrs. Heather Krause, Director of Admissions, Marketing, and Recruitment, School of Nursing, Loma Linda University, 11262 Campus Street, Loma Linda, CA 92350. *Telephone:* 909-558-4923. *Fax:* 909-558-0175. *E-mail:* hkrause@llu.edu.

GRADUATE PROGRAMS

Expenses (2012–13) *Tuition:* part-time $690 per quarter hour. *Room and board:* room only: $2640 per academic year. *Required fees:* part-time $702 per term.
Financial Aid 26% of graduate students in nursing programs received some form of financial aid in 2011–12.
Contact Mrs. Michelle Mohr, Assistant Director of Admissions, Marketing, and Recruitment, School of Nursing, Loma Linda University, 11262 Campus Street, Loma Linda, CA 92350. *Telephone:* 909-558-1000 Ext. 83113. *Fax:* 909-558-4134. *E-mail:* graduatenursing@llu.edu.

MASTER'S DEGREE PROGRAM

Degree MS
Available Programs Master's; RN to Master's.
Concentrations Available Health-care administration; nurse anesthesia; nursing administration; nursing education. *Clinical nurse specialist programs in:* adult health, family health, maternity-newborn, medical-surgical, parent-child, pediatric, perinatal. *Nurse practitioner programs in:* adult health, family health, pediatric, primary care, psychiatric/mental health.
Study Options Full-time and part-time.
Program Entrance Requirements Clinical experience, minimum overall college GPA of 3.0, transcript of college record, written essay, immunizations, interview, 3 letters of recommendation, nursing research course, prerequisite course work, statistics course. *Application fee:* $60.
Advanced Placement Credit given for nursing courses completed elsewhere dependent upon specific evaluations.
Degree Requirements Comprehensive exam.

POST-MASTER'S PROGRAM

Areas of Study *Clinical nurse specialist programs in:* adult health, family health, maternity-newborn, medical-surgical, parent-child, pediatric, perinatal. *Nurse practitioner programs in:* adult health, family health, pediatric, primary care, psychiatric/mental health.

DOCTORAL DEGREE PROGRAM

Degree PhD
Available Programs Doctorate.
Areas of Study Ethics, faculty preparation, gerontology, health policy, health promotion/disease prevention, human health and illness, nursing education, nursing research.
Program Entrance Requirements Clinical experience, minimum overall college GPA of 3.5, interview by faculty committee, interview, 3 letters of recommendation, MSN or equivalent, scholarly papers, statistics course, vita, writing sample. *Application deadline:* 3/1 (summer). *Application fee:* $60.
Degree Requirements 90 total credit hours, dissertation, oral exam, written exam, residency.

Mount St. Mary's College
Department of Nursing
Los Angeles, California

http://www.msmc.la.edu/index.asp
Founded in 1925
DEGREES • BSN • BSC PN • MSN
Nursing Program Faculty 112 (10% with doctorates).
Baccalaureate Enrollment 326 **Women** 87% **Men** 13% **Minority** 80%
Graduate Enrollment 51 **Women** 91% **Men** 9% **Minority** 54%
Distance Learning Courses Available.
Nursing Student Activities Nursing Honor Society, Student Nurses' Association, nursing club.
Nursing Student Resources Academic advising; academic or career counseling; assistance for students with disabilities; bookstore; campus computer network; career placement assistance; computer lab; computer-assisted instruction; daycare for children of students; e-mail services; employment services for current students; housing assistance; interactive nursing skills videos; Internet; learning resource lab; library services; nursing audiovisuals; remedial services; resume preparation assistance; skills, simulation, or other laboratory; tutoring.
Library Facilities 150,000 volumes (4,000 in health, 1,000 in nursing); 29 periodical subscriptions (150 health-care related).

BACCALAUREATE PROGRAMS

Degrees BSN; BSc PN
Available Programs ADN to Baccalaureate; Accelerated Baccalaureate; Generic Baccalaureate.
Study Options Full-time.
Program Entrance Requirements Minimum overall college GPA of 2.7, transcript of college record, CPR certification, written essay, health exam, high school chemistry, high school transcript, immunizations, 1 letter of recommendation, minimum GPA in nursing prerequisites of 2.5, professional liability insurance/malpractice insurance, prerequisite course work. Transfer students are accepted. *Application deadline:* 2/1 (fall). *Application fee:* $20.
Advanced Placement Credit by examination available. Credit given for nursing courses completed elsewhere dependent upon specific evaluations.
Contact *Telephone:* 310-954-4279. *Fax:* 310-954-4229.

GRADUATE PROGRAMS

Contact *Telephone:* 213-477-2980. *Fax:* 213-477-2639.

MASTER'S DEGREE PROGRAM
Degree MSN
Available Programs Master's; RN to Master's.
Concentrations Available Nursing administration; nursing education. *Clinical nurse specialist programs in:* adult health, community health.
Study Options Full-time and part-time.
Program Entrance Requirements Minimum overall college GPA of 3.0, transcript of college record, CPR certification, written essay, immunizations, interview, professional liability insurance/malpractice insurance, statistics course. *Application deadline:* Applications may be processed on a rolling basis for some programs. *Application fee:* $50.
Advanced Placement Credit given for nursing courses completed elsewhere dependent upon specific evaluations.
Degree Requirements 39 total credit hours, thesis or project.

National University
Department of Nursing
La Jolla, California

http://www.nu.edu
Founded in 1971
DEGREES • BSN • DNP • MSN
Nursing Program Faculty 26 (69% with doctorates).
Baccalaureate Enrollment 620 **Women** 88% **Men** 12% **Minority** 60%
Distance Learning Courses Available.

Nursing Student Activities Nursing Honor Society, Student Nurses' Association.
Nursing Student Resources Academic advising; academic or career counseling; assistance for students with disabilities; bookstore; campus computer network; computer lab; Internet; library services; nursing audiovisuals; other; remedial services; resume preparation assistance; skills, simulation, or other laboratory; tutoring.
Library Facilities 303,000 volumes (14,446 in health, 1,167 in nursing); 22,700 periodical subscriptions (2,047 health-care related).

BACCALAUREATE PROGRAMS

Degree BSN
Available Programs ADN to Baccalaureate; Baccalaureate for Second Degree; Generic Baccalaureate; LPN to Baccalaureate; RN Baccalaureate.
Site Options Los Angeles, CA; Fresno, CA.
Study Options Full-time.
Program Entrance Requirements Minimum overall college GPA of 2.75, transcript of college record, CPR certification, written essay, health exam, health insurance, immunizations, minimum GPA in nursing prerequisites of 2.75, professional liability insurance/malpractice insurance, prerequisite course work. Transfer students are accepted. *Application deadline:* Applications may be processed on a rolling basis for some programs.
Advanced Placement Credit given for nursing courses completed elsewhere dependent upon specific evaluations.
Expenses (2012–13) *Tuition:* full-time $30,000.
Financial Aid 89% of baccalaureate students in nursing programs received some form of financial aid in 2011–12.
Contact Mr. Joel Sedano, Admissions Advisor, Department of Nursing, National University, 11255 North Torrey Pines Road, La Jolla, CA 92037. *Telephone:* 800-628-8648 Ext. 8211. *Fax:* 858-642-8709. *E-mail:* jsedano@nu.edu.

GRADUATE PROGRAMS

Expenses (2012–13) *Tuition:* full-time $30,000; part-time $5000 per term.
Financial Aid Institutionally sponsored loans, scholarships, and tuition waivers (full and partial) available.
Contact Dr. Mary L. McHugh, Professor and Chair, Department of Nursing, National University, 3678 Aero Court, San Diego, CA 92123. *Telephone:* 858-309-3519. *Fax:* 858-309-3480. *E-mail:* mmchugh@nu.edu.

MASTER'S DEGREE PROGRAM
Degree MSN
Available Programs Master's.
Concentrations Available Nurse anesthesia; nursing administration; nursing informatics. *Clinical nurse specialist programs in:* forensic nursing.
Study Options Part-time.
Online Degree Options Yes (online only).
Program Entrance Requirements Minimum overall college GPA of 3.0, transcript of college record, nursing research course, professional liability insurance/malpractice insurance, statistics course. *Application deadline:* Applications may be processed on a rolling basis for some programs. *Application fee:* $65.
Advanced Placement Credit given for nursing courses completed elsewhere dependent upon specific evaluations.
Degree Requirements 36 total credit hours, thesis or project.

POST-MASTER'S PROGRAM
Areas of Study Nursing administration; nursing informatics.

DOCTORAL DEGREE PROGRAM
Degree DNP
Available Programs Doctorate.
Areas of Study Information systems, nursing administration.
Online Degree Options Yes (online only).
Program Entrance Requirements Minimum overall college GPA of 3.0, interview by faculty committee, 3 letters of recommendation, MSN or equivalent, statistics course, vita, writing sample. *Application deadline:* Applications may be processed on a rolling basis for some programs. *Application fee:* $65.

Pacific Union College
Department of Nursing
Angwin, California

http://www.puc.edu
Founded in 1882
DEGREE • BSN
Nursing Program Faculty 16 (14% with doctorates).
Baccalaureate Enrollment 56 **Women** 77% **Men** 23% **Minority** 39% **Part-time** 59%
Nursing Student Activities Student Nurses' Association.
Nursing Student Resources Academic advising; academic or career counseling; assistance for students with disabilities; bookstore; campus computer network; career placement assistance; computer lab; daycare for children of students; e-mail services; employment services for current students; externships; housing assistance; Internet; learning resource lab; library services; nursing audiovisuals; skills, simulation, or other laboratory; tutoring.
Library Facilities 185,668 volumes (125 in health, 75 in nursing); 36,988 periodical subscriptions (109 health-care related).

BACCALAUREATE PROGRAMS

Degree BSN
Available Programs ADN to Baccalaureate.
Site Options Napa, CA.
Study Options Full-time and part-time.
Program Entrance Requirements Transcript of college record, CPR certification, health exam, health insurance, immunizations, interview, 2 letters of recommendation, minimum GPA in nursing prerequisites of 2.0, professional liability insurance/malpractice insurance, prerequisite course work, RN licensure. Transfer students are accepted.
Advanced Placement Credit given for nursing courses completed elsewhere dependent upon specific evaluations.
Contact *Telephone:* 707-965-7618. *Fax:* 707-965-6499.

CONTINUING EDUCATION PROGRAM

Contact *Telephone:* 707-965-7262. *Fax:* 707-965-6499.

Point Loma Nazarene University
School of Nursing
San Diego, California

http://www.pointloma.edu/experience/academics/schools-departments/school-nursing
Founded in 1902
DEGREES • BSN • MSN
Nursing Program Faculty 28 (40% with doctorates).
Baccalaureate Enrollment 170 **Women** 90% **Men** 10% **Minority** 23% **International** 1% **Part-time** 2%
Graduate Enrollment 43 **Women** 92% **Men** 8% **Minority** 45% **Part-time** 5%
Nursing Student Activities Sigma Theta Tau, Student Nurses' Association.
Nursing Student Resources Academic advising; academic or career counseling; bookstore; campus computer network; computer lab; computer-assisted instruction; daycare for children of students; e-mail services; employment services for current students; externships; housing assistance; interactive nursing skills videos; Internet; learning resource lab; library services; nursing audiovisuals; paid internships; resume preparation assistance; skills, simulation, or other laboratory; tutoring; unpaid internships.
Library Facilities 177,189 volumes; 439 periodical subscriptions.

BACCALAUREATE PROGRAMS

Degree BSN
Available Programs ADN to Baccalaureate; Generic Baccalaureate; LPN to RN Baccalaureate; RN Baccalaureate.
Site Options San Diego, CA.
Study Options Full-time.
Program Entrance Requirements Minimum overall college GPA of 2.7, transcript of college record, CPR certification, written essay, health exam, health insurance, 2 years high school math, immunizations, 1 letter

of recommendation, minimum GPA in nursing prerequisites of 2.7, prerequisite course work. Transfer students are accepted. *Application deadline:* 2/1 (fall), 2/1 (winter).
Advanced Placement Credit by examination available. Credit given for nursing courses completed elsewhere dependent upon specific evaluations.
Contact *Telephone:* 619-849-7055. *Fax:* 619-849-2672.

GRADUATE PROGRAMS

Contact *Telephone:* 619-849-2863. *Fax:* 619-849-2672.

MASTER'S DEGREE PROGRAM
Degree MSN
Available Programs Master's; RN to Master's.
Concentrations Available Nursing education. *Clinical nurse specialist programs in:* family health, gerontology, medical-surgical, psychiatric/mental health.
Site Options San Diego, CA.
Study Options Full-time and part-time.
Program Entrance Requirements Clinical experience, computer literacy, minimum overall college GPA of 3.0, transcript of college record, CPR certification, written essay, immunizations, interview, 3 letters of recommendation, professional liability insurance/malpractice insurance, resume. *Application deadline:* 8/1 (fall), 12/1 (winter), 8/1 (summer). *Application fee:* $40.
Degree Requirements 43 total credit hours, thesis or project.

POST-MASTER'S PROGRAM
Areas of Study Nursing education. *Clinical nurse specialist programs in:* family health, gerontology, medical-surgical, psychiatric/mental health.

CONTINUING EDUCATION PROGRAM

Contact *Telephone:* 619-849-7055. *Fax:* 619-849-2672.

Samuel Merritt University
School of Nursing
Oakland, California

http://www.samuelmerritt.edu/nursing
Founded in 1909
DEGREES • BSN • DNP • MSN
Nursing Program Faculty 179 (27% with doctorates).
Baccalaureate Enrollment 513 **Women** 83% **Men** 17% **Minority** 57% **Part-time** 2%
Graduate Enrollment 404 **Women** 82% **Men** 18% **Minority** 51% **Part-time** 51%
Distance Learning Courses Available.
Nursing Student Activities Sigma Theta Tau, Student Nurses' Association.
Nursing Student Resources Academic advising; academic or career counseling; assistance for students with disabilities; bookstore; campus computer network; computer lab; computer-assisted instruction; e-mail services; housing assistance; interactive nursing skills videos; Internet; learning resource lab; library services; nursing audiovisuals; remedial services; skills, simulation, or other laboratory; tutoring; unpaid internships.
Library Facilities 34,729 volumes (14,115 in health, 10,073 in nursing); 9,188 periodical subscriptions (18,123 health-care related).

BACCALAUREATE PROGRAMS

Degree BSN
Available Programs Accelerated Baccalaureate; Generic Baccalaureate.
Site Options San Mateo, CA; Sacramento, CA; San Francisco, CA.
Study Options Full-time and part-time.
Program Entrance Requirements Minimum overall college GPA of 3.0, transcript of college record, CPR certification, written essay, health exam, immunizations, 1 letter of recommendation, minimum GPA in nursing prerequisites of 3.0, prerequisite course work. Transfer students are accepted. *Application deadline:* 3/1 (fall), 9/1 (spring). *Application fee:* $50.
Advanced Placement Credit by examination available. Credit given for nursing courses completed elsewhere dependent upon specific evaluations.

Expenses (2012–13) *Tuition:* full-time $39,456; part-time $1663 per credit hour. *International tuition:* $39,456 full-time. *Required fees:* full-time $1385.
Financial Aid 75% of baccalaureate students in nursing programs received some form of financial aid in 2011–12.
Contact Ms. Anne E. Seed, Director of Admissions, School of Nursing, Samuel Merritt University, 3100 Telegraph Avenue, Office of Admissions, Oakland, CA 94609. *Telephone:* 510-869-6610. *Fax:* 510-869-6525. *E-mail:* admission@samuelmerritt.edu.

GRADUATE PROGRAMS

Expenses (2012–13) *Tuition:* full-time $38,247; part-time $1118 per credit hour. *Required fees:* full-time $572.
Financial Aid 84% of graduate students in nursing programs received some form of financial aid in 2011–12. Career-related internships or fieldwork, Federal Work-Study, scholarships, and traineeships available. Aid available to part-time students. *Financial aid application deadline:* 3/2.
Contact Ms. Anne E. Seed, Director of Admissions, School of Nursing, Samuel Merritt University, 3100 Telegraph Avenue, Office of Admissions, Oakland, CA 94609. *Telephone:* 510-869-6610. *Fax:* 510-869-6525. *E-mail:* aseed@samuelmerritt.edu.

MASTER'S DEGREE PROGRAM
Degree MSN
Available Programs Master's; Master's for Non-Nursing College Graduates; Master's for Nurses with Non-Nursing Degrees.
Concentrations Available Nurse anesthesia; nurse case management. *Nurse practitioner programs in:* family health.
Site Options Sacramento, CA.
Study Options Full-time and part-time.
Program Entrance Requirements Computer literacy, minimum overall college GPA of 3.0, transcript of college record, CPR certification, written essay, immunizations, interview, 2 letters of recommendation, prerequisite course work, statistics course. *Application deadline:* 1/15 (fall), 7/1 (spring). *Application fee:* $50.
Advanced Placement Credit by examination available. Credit given for nursing courses completed elsewhere dependent upon specific evaluations.
Degree Requirements 49 total credit hours, thesis or project, comprehensive exam.

POST-MASTER'S PROGRAM
Areas of Study Nurse anesthesia; nurse case management. *Nurse practitioner programs in:* family health.

DOCTORAL DEGREE PROGRAM
Degree DNP
Available Programs Doctorate.
Online Degree Options Yes (online only).
Program Entrance Requirements Minimum overall college GPA of 3.0, MSN or equivalent, statistics course. *Application deadline:* 8/1 (spring). *Application fee:* $50.
Degree Requirements 36 total credit hours.

San Diego State University
School of Nursing
San Diego, California

http://nursing.sdsu.edu/
Founded in 1897
DEGREES • BSN • MSN
Nursing Program Faculty 65 (30% with doctorates).
Baccalaureate Enrollment 419 **Women** 85% **Men** 15% **Minority** 50% **International** 1% **Part-time** 2%
Graduate Enrollment 96 **Women** 95% **Men** 5% **Minority** 10% **Part-time** 77%
Distance Learning Courses Available.
Nursing Student Activities Sigma Theta Tau, Student Nurses' Association.
Nursing Student Resources Academic advising; academic or career counseling; assistance for students with disabilities; bookstore; campus computer network; career placement assistance; computer lab; daycare for children of students; e-mail services; housing assistance; Internet; learning resource lab; library services; nursing audiovisuals; paid internships; placement services for program completers; remedial services;

resume preparation assistance; skills, simulation, or other laboratory; unpaid internships.
Library Facilities 1.3 million volumes (36,000 in health, 14,000 in nursing); 8,245 periodical subscriptions (335 health-care related).

BACCALAUREATE PROGRAMS

Degree BSN
Available Programs ADN to Baccalaureate; Generic Baccalaureate; RN Baccalaureate.
Study Options Full-time and part-time.
Program Entrance Requirements Minimum overall college GPA of 2.8, transcript of college record, high school transcript, minimum GPA in nursing prerequisites of 2.8, prerequisite course work. Transfer students are accepted. *Application deadline:* 11/30 (fall). Applications may be processed on a rolling basis for some programs.
Advanced Placement Credit by examination available. Credit given for nursing courses completed elsewhere dependent upon specific evaluations.
Expenses (2011–12) *Tuition, state resident:* full-time $5472. *Tuition, nonresident:* full-time $14,400. *International tuition:* $15,100 full-time. *Room and board:* $11,549; room only: $7304 per academic year. *Required fees:* full-time $1106; part-time $553 per term.
Financial Aid 75% of baccalaureate students in nursing programs received some form of financial aid in 2010–11. *Gift aid (need-based):* Federal Pell, FSEOG, state, private, college/university gift aid from institutional funds, Federal Nursing. *Loans:* Federal Direct (Subsidized and Unsubsidized Stafford PLUS), Perkins, college/university. *Work-study:* Federal Work-Study. *Financial aid application deadline:* 3/2.
Contact Nursing Contact, School of Nursing, San Diego State University, 5500 Campanile Drive, San Diego, CA 92182-4158. *Telephone:* 619-594-2540. *Fax:* 619-594-2765. *E-mail:* nursing@mail.sdsu.edu.

GRADUATE PROGRAMS

Expenses (2011–12) *Tuition, state resident:* full-time $6348. *Tuition, nonresident:* full-time $13,044. *International tuition:* $13,744 full-time. *Room and board:* $11,549; room only: $7304 per academic year. *Required fees:* full-time $1106; part-time $1106 per term.
Financial Aid 90% of graduate students in nursing programs received some form of financial aid in 2010–11. Career-related internships or fieldwork, scholarships, traineeships, and unspecified assistantships available.
Contact Dr. Beverly Carlson, Graduate Adviser, School of Nursing, San Diego State University, 5500 Campanile Drive, San Diego, CA 92182-4158. *Telephone:* 619-594-2766. *Fax:* 619-594-2765. *E-mail:* bcarlson@mail.sdsu.edu.

MASTER'S DEGREE PROGRAM
Degree MSN
Available Programs Master's.
Concentrations Available Nurse-midwifery; nursing administration; nursing education. *Clinical nurse specialist programs in:* adult health, community health, critical care, gerontology, maternity-newborn, school health, women's health. *Nurse practitioner programs in:* acute care, adult health, gerontology, women's health.
Study Options Full-time and part-time.
Program Entrance Requirements Clinical experience, minimum overall college GPA of 3.0, transcript of college record, written essay, 3 letters of recommendation, nursing research course, physical assessment course, professional liability insurance/malpractice insurance, resume, statistics course, GRE General Test. *Application deadline:* 2/1 (fall), 2/1 (spring). Applications may be processed on a rolling basis for some programs.
Advanced Placement Credit by examination available. Credit given for nursing courses completed elsewhere dependent upon specific evaluations.
Degree Requirements 39 total credit hours, thesis or project, comprehensive exam.

POST-MASTER'S PROGRAM
Areas of Study Nurse-midwifery.

CONTINUING EDUCATION PROGRAM

Contact Dr. Beverly Carlson, Graduate Advisor, School of Nursing, San Diego State University, 5500 Campanile Drive, San Diego, CA 92182-4158. *Telephone:* 619-594-2766. *Fax:* 619-594-2765. *E-mail:* bcarlson@mail.sdsu.edu.

San Francisco State University
School of Nursing
San Francisco, California

http://www.nursing.sfsu.edu/
Founded in 1899
DEGREES • BSN • MSN
Nursing Program Faculty 40 (50% with doctorates).
Baccalaureate Enrollment 250 **Women** 88% **Men** 12% **Minority** 53% **International** 2% **Part-time** 5%
Graduate Enrollment 180 **Women** 80% **Men** 20% **Minority** 80% **International** 10% **Part-time** 20%
Nursing Student Activities Sigma Theta Tau, Student Nurses' Association.
Nursing Student Resources Academic advising; academic or career counseling; assistance for students with disabilities; bookstore; campus computer network; career placement assistance; computer lab; computer-assisted instruction; daycare for children of students; e-mail services; employment services for current students; externships; housing assistance; interactive nursing skills videos; Internet; learning resource lab; library services; nursing audiovisuals; other; placement services for program completers; remedial services; resume preparation assistance; skills, simulation, or other laboratory; tutoring.
Library Facilities 921,744 volumes (11,000 in health; 1,500 in nursing); 73,735 periodical subscriptions (200 health-care related).

BACCALAUREATE PROGRAMS

Degree BSN
Available Programs ADN to Baccalaureate; Accelerated LPN to Baccalaureate; Generic Baccalaureate; RN Baccalaureate.
Study Options Full-time.
Program Entrance Requirements Minimum overall college GPA of 2.5, transcript of college record, CPR certification, health exam, health insurance, immunizations, minimum GPA in nursing prerequisites of 2.5, professional liability insurance/malpractice insurance, prerequisite course work. Transfer students are accepted.
Advanced Placement Credit by examination available. Credit given for nursing courses completed elsewhere dependent upon specific evaluations.
Contact *Telephone:* 415-338-2315 Ext. 1. *Fax:* 415-338-0555.

GRADUATE PROGRAMS

Contact *Telephone:* 415-338-1802. *Fax:* 415-338-0555.

MASTER'S DEGREE PROGRAM
Degree MSN
Available Programs Accelerated Master's for Non-Nursing College Graduates; Accelerated Master's for Nurses with Non-Nursing Degrees; Master's; Master's for Non-Nursing College Graduates; Master's for Nurses with Non-Nursing Degrees.
Concentrations Available Nurse case management; nursing administration. *Clinical nurse specialist programs in:* adult health, perinatal, public health. *Nurse practitioner programs in:* family health.
Study Options Full-time and part-time.
Program Entrance Requirements Minimum overall college GPA of 3.0, transcript of college record, CPR certification, written essay, immunizations, 3 letters of recommendation, nursing research course, professional liability insurance/malpractice insurance, resume, statistics course.
Advanced Placement Credit by examination available. Credit given for nursing courses completed elsewhere dependent upon specific evaluations.
Degree Requirements 36 total credit hours, thesis or project.

POST-MASTER'S PROGRAM
Areas of Study Nursing administration. *Nurse practitioner programs in:* family health.

CONTINUING EDUCATION PROGRAM

Contact *Telephone:* 415-405-3660. *Fax:* 415-338-0555.

San Jose State University
The Valley Foundation School of Nursing
San Jose, California

Founded in 1857
DEGREES • BS • MS
Nursing Program Faculty 55 (52% with doctorates).
Baccalaureate Enrollment 550 **Women** 92% **Men** 8% **Minority** 76% **Part-time** 20%
Graduate Enrollment 101 **Women** 92% **Men** 8% **Minority** 46% **Part-time** 83%
Nursing Student Activities Sigma Theta Tau, Student Nurses' Association, nursing club.
Nursing Student Resources Academic advising; academic or career counseling; assistance for students with disabilities; bookstore; career placement assistance; computer lab; computer-assisted instruction; housing assistance; interactive nursing skills videos; Internet; learning resource lab; library services; nursing audiovisuals; skills, simulation, or other laboratory; tutoring.
Library Facilities 280 volumes in health, 250 volumes in nursing; 80 periodical subscriptions health-care related.

BACCALAUREATE PROGRAMS

Degree BS
Available Programs Generic Baccalaureate; RPN to Baccalaureate.
Site Options Salinas, CA; Gilroy, CA.
Study Options Full-time and part-time.
Program Entrance Requirements Transcript of college record, health insurance, 3 years high school math, minimum high school GPA of 2.0, minimum GPA in nursing prerequisites of 2.0, professional liability insurance/malpractice insurance, prerequisite course work. Transfer students are accepted.
Advanced Placement Credit by examination available. Credit given for nursing courses completed elsewhere dependent upon specific evaluations.
Contact *Telephone:* 408-924-3131. *Fax:* 408-924-3135.

GRADUATE PROGRAMS

Contact *Telephone:* 408-924-3144. *Fax:* 408-924-3135.

MASTER'S DEGREE PROGRAM
Degree MS
Available Programs Master's.
Concentrations Available Nursing administration; nursing education. *Clinical nurse specialist programs in:* gerontology, school health. *Nurse practitioner programs in:* family health.
Study Options Full-time and part-time.
Program Entrance Requirements Minimum overall college GPA of 3.0, transcript of college record, CPR certification, written essay, immunizations, 3 letters of recommendation, nursing research course, physical assessment course, professional liability insurance/malpractice insurance, resume, statistics course.
Degree Requirements 36 total credit hours, thesis or project.

Sonoma State University
Department of Nursing
Rohnert Park, California

http://www.sonoma.edu/nursing
Founded in 1960
DEGREE • BSN
Library Facilities 584,247 volumes; 141,421 periodical subscriptions.

BACCALAUREATE PROGRAMS

Degree BSN
Available Programs Generic Baccalaureate.
Study Options Full-time.
Program Entrance Requirements Written essay, health exam, high school biology, high school chemistry, high school foreign language, 3 years high school math, 2 years high school science, high school transcript, immunizations, minimum high school GPA of 3.5. Transfer students are accepted. *Application deadline:* 2/28 (fall).
Contact Nursing Department, Department of Nursing, Sonoma State University, 1801 East Cotati Avenue, Rohnert Park, CA 94928.

Telephone: 707-664-2465. *Fax:* 707-664-2653. *E-mail:* nursing@sonoma.edu.

University of California, Davis
The Betty Irene Moore School of Nursing
Davis, California

http://www.ucdmc.ucdavis.edu/nursing/
Founded in 1905
DEGREES • MS • PHD
Nursing Program Faculty 17 (100% with doctorates).
Graduate Enrollment 73 **Women** 85% **Men** 15% **Minority** 27% **International** 3%
Distance Learning Courses Available.
Nursing Student Activities Sigma Theta Tau.
Nursing Student Resources Academic advising; academic or career counseling; assistance for students with disabilities; bookstore; campus computer network; career placement assistance; computer lab; computer-assisted instruction; e-mail services; employment services for current students; Internet; learning resource lab; library services; remedial services; resume preparation assistance; skills, simulation, or other laboratory; tutoring.
Library Facilities 371,673 volumes in health, 5,492 volumes in nursing; 97,413 periodical subscriptions (1,076 health-care related).

GRADUATE PROGRAMS

Contact Anna Libonati, Student Affairs Officer, The Betty Irene Moore School of Nursing, University of California, Davis, School of Nursing, 4610 X Street, Sacramento, CA 95817. *Telephone:* 916-734-2145. *E-mail:* BettyIreneMooreSON@ucdmc.ucdavis.edu.

MASTER'S DEGREE PROGRAM
Degree MS
Available Programs Master's.
Concentrations Available *Nurse practitioner programs in:* family health.
Study Options Full-time.
Program Entrance Requirements Minimum overall college GPA of 3.0, transcript of college record, written essay, immunizations, 3 letters of recommendation. *Application deadline:* 1/15 (fall). *Application fee:* $80.
Degree Requirements 31 total credit hours, thesis or project.

DOCTORAL DEGREE PROGRAM
Degree PhD
Available Programs Doctorate; Post-Baccalaureate Doctorate.
Areas of Study Health policy, individualized study, nursing research, nursing science.
Program Entrance Requirements Minimum overall college GPA of 3.0, interview by faculty committee, interview, 3 letters of recommendation, MSN or equivalent. *Application deadline:* 1/15 (fall). *Application fee:* $80.
Degree Requirements 43 total credit hours, dissertation.

POSTDOCTORAL PROGRAM
Areas of Study Individualized study, nursing research, nursing science.
Postdoctoral Program Contact Lisa Reevesman, Academic Personnel Coordinator, The Betty Irene Moore School of Nursing, University of California, Davis, School of Nursing, 4610 X Street, Sacramento, CA 95817. *Telephone:* 916-734-4737. *E-mail:* lisa.reevesman@ucdmc.ucdavis.edu.

University of California, Irvine
Program in Nursing Science
Irvine, California

http://www.nursing.uci.edu/
Founded in 1965
DEGREES • BS • MS
Nursing Program Faculty 36 (27% with doctorates).
Baccalaureate Enrollment 162 **Women** 89% **Men** 11% **Minority** 72%
Graduate Enrollment 26 **Women** 88% **Men** 12% **Minority** 54% **Part-time** 35%
Nursing Student Activities Student Nurses' Association.

Nursing Student Resources Academic advising; academic or career counseling; assistance for students with disabilities; bookstore; campus computer network; computer lab; computer-assisted instruction; daycare for children of students; e-mail services; employment services for current students; housing assistance; interactive nursing skills videos; Internet; learning resource lab; library services; nursing audiovisuals; skills, simulation, or other laboratory; tutoring.
Library Facilities 3.4 million volumes (365,965 in health, 6,047 in nursing); 85,870 periodical subscriptions.

BACCALAUREATE PROGRAMS

Degree BS
Available Programs Generic Baccalaureate.
Study Options Full-time.
Program Entrance Requirements Written essay, high school biology, high school chemistry, 2 years high school science, 3 letters of recommendation. Transfer students are accepted. *Application deadline:* 11/30 (fall). *Application fee:* $60.
Contact *Telephone:* 949-824-3580. *Fax:* 949-824-0470.

GRADUATE PROGRAMS

Contact *Telephone:* 949-824-3580. *Fax:* 949-824-0470.

MASTER'S DEGREE PROGRAM
Degree MS
Available Programs Master's.
Concentrations Available *Nurse practitioner programs in:* adult health, family health, gerontology.
Study Options Full-time and part-time.
Program Entrance Requirements Clinical experience, transcript of college record, 3 letters of recommendation, statistics course. *Application deadline:* 3/1 (winter). *Application fee:* $70.
Degree Requirements 72 total credit hours, comprehensive exam.

POST-MASTER'S PROGRAM
Areas of Study *Nurse practitioner programs in:* adult health, family health, gerontology.

University of California, Los Angeles
School of Nursing
Los Angeles, California

http://nursing.ucla.edu
Founded in 1919
DEGREES • BS • MSN • MSN/MBA • PHD
Nursing Program Faculty 87 (54% with doctorates).
Baccalaureate Enrollment 212 **Women** 87% **Men** 13% **Minority** 69%
Graduate Enrollment 391 **Women** 90% **Men** 10% **Minority** 51% **International** 3%
Nursing Student Activities Nursing Honor Society, Sigma Theta Tau, Student Nurses' Association, nursing club.
Nursing Student Resources Academic advising; academic or career counseling; assistance for students with disabilities; bookstore; campus computer network; computer lab; daycare for children of students; e-mail services; housing assistance; Internet; library services; nursing audiovisuals; skills, simulation, or other laboratory.
Library Facilities 9 million volumes (760,000 in health, 8,000 in nursing); 38,975 periodical subscriptions (600,000 health-care related).

BACCALAUREATE PROGRAMS

Degree BS
Available Programs Generic Baccalaureate.
Study Options Full-time.
Program Entrance Requirements Transcript of college record, written essay, high school transcript, 2 letters of recommendation, minimum high school GPA, prerequisite course work. Transfer students are accepted. *Application deadline:* 11/30 (fall). *Application fee:* $60.
Expenses (2012–13) *Tuition, state resident:* full-time $14,010. *Tuition, nonresident:* full-time $36,888. *International tuition:* $36,888 full-time. *Room and board:* $13,892; room only: $10,148 per academic year.
Financial Aid 76% of baccalaureate students in nursing programs received some form of financial aid in 2011–12. *Gift aid (need-based):* Federal Pell, FSEOG, state, private, college/university gift aid from institutional funds, United Negro College Fund, Federal Nursing. *Loans:*

Federal Nursing Student Loans, Federal Direct (Subsidized and Unsubsidized Stafford PLUS), Perkins, state, college/university.*Work-study:* Federal Work-Study, part-time campus jobs.*Financial aid application deadline (priority):* 3/2.

Contact Ms. Rhonda Flenoy-Younger, Director of Recruitment, Outreach, and Admissions, School of Nursing, University of California, Los Angeles, Box 951702, Los Angeles, CA 90095-1702. *Telephone:* 310-825-9193. *Fax:* 310-206-7433. *E-mail:* rflenoy@sonnet.ucla.edu.

GRADUATE PROGRAMS

Expenses (2012–13) *Tuition, state resident:* full-time $22,549. *Tuition, nonresident:* full-time $34,794. *International tuition:* $34,794 full-time.

Financial Aid 89% of graduate students in nursing programs received some form of financial aid in 2011–12. 254 fellowships with full and partial tuition reimbursements available, 10 research assistantships with full and partial tuition reimbursements available, 43 teaching assistantships with full and partial tuition reimbursements available were awarded; Federal Work-Study, institutionally sponsored loans, scholarships, tuition waivers (full and partial), and unspecified assistantships also available. *Financial aid application deadline:* 3/1.

Contact Ms. Rhonda Flenoy-Younger, Director of Recruitment, Outreach, and Admissions, School of Nursing, University of California, Los Angeles, Box 951702, Los Angeles, CA 90095-1702. *Telephone:* 310-825-9193. *Fax:* 310-267-0330. *E-mail:* rflenoy@sonnet.ucla.edu.

MASTER'S DEGREE PROGRAM
Degrees MSN; MSN/MBA

Available Programs Master's; Master's for Non-Nursing College Graduates.

Concentrations Available Clinical nurse leader; nursing administration. *Clinical nurse specialist programs in:* acute care, oncology, pediatric. *Nurse practitioner programs in:* acute care, adult health, family health, gerontology, occupational health, oncology, pediatric.

Study Options Full-time.

Program Entrance Requirements Minimum overall college GPA of 3.0, transcript of college record, written essay, 3 letters of recommendation, nursing research course, physical assessment course, prerequisite course work, statistics course. *Application deadline:* 12/1 (fall). *Application fee:* $80.

Degree Requirements 72 total credit hours, comprehensive exam.

POST-MASTER'S PROGRAM
Areas of Study Nursing administration. *Clinical nurse specialist programs in:* acute care, oncology, pediatric. *Nurse practitioner programs in:* acute care, adult health, family health, gerontology, oncology, pediatric.

DOCTORAL DEGREE PROGRAM
Degree PhD

Available Programs Doctorate; Post-Baccalaureate Doctorate.

Areas of Study Addiction/substance abuse, advanced practice nursing, aging, bio-behavioral research, biology of health and illness, clinical practice, community health, critical care, family health, gerontology, health policy, health promotion/disease prevention, health-care systems, human health and illness, illness and transition, neuro-behavior, nursing administration, nursing research, nursing science, oncology, women's health.

Program Entrance Requirements Minimum overall college GPA of 3.5, interview, 3 letters of recommendation, scholarly papers, statistics course, vita, writing sample, GRE General Test. *Application deadline:* 12/1 (fall). *Application fee:* $80.

Degree Requirements 127 total credit hours, dissertation, oral exam, written exam, residency.

POSTDOCTORAL PROGRAM
Areas of Study Addiction/substance abuse, adolescent health, aging, cancer care, gerontology, health promotion/disease prevention, nursing research, vulnerable population, women's health.

Postdoctoral Program Contact Dr. Sally Maliski, Associate Dean for Academic Affairs, School of Nursing, University of California, Los Angeles, Box 951702, Los Angeles, CA 90095-1702. *Telephone:* 310-206-2825. *Fax:* 310-206-7433. *E-mail:* smaliski@sonnet.ucla.edu.

CONTINUING EDUCATION PROGRAM
Contact Ms. Salpy Akaragian, Education Specialist, School of Nursing, University of California, Los Angeles, Box 951701, Los Angeles, CA 90095-1701. *Telephone:* 310-206-9581. *E-mail:* nssa@mednet.ucla.edu.

University of California, San Francisco
School of Nursing
San Francisco, California

http://www.nurseweb.ucsf.edu/
Founded in 1864

DEGREES • MS • PHD
Nursing Program Faculty 151 (72% with doctorates).
Graduate Enrollment 721 **Women** 87% **Men** 13% **Minority** 30% **International** 10% **Part-time** 1%
Distance Learning Courses Available.
Nursing Student Activities Nursing Honor Society, Sigma Theta Tau, Student Nurses' Association, nursing club.
Nursing Student Resources Academic advising; academic or career counseling; assistance for students with disabilities; bookstore; campus computer network; career placement assistance; computer lab; computer-assisted instruction; daycare for children of students; e-mail services; employment services for current students; housing assistance; interactive nursing skills videos; Internet; learning resource lab; library services; nursing audiovisuals; other; paid internships; placement services for program completers; remedial services; resume preparation assistance; skills, simulation, or other laboratory; tutoring; unpaid internships.
Library Facilities 856,169 volumes in health, 131,046 volumes in nursing; 3,270 periodical subscriptions health-care related.

GRADUATE PROGRAMS
Contact *Telephone:* 415-476-1435. *Fax:* 415-476-9707.

MASTER'S DEGREE PROGRAM
Degree MS

Available Programs Master's; Master's for Non-Nursing College Graduates; Master's for Nurses with Non-Nursing Degrees.

Concentrations Available Nurse-midwifery; nursing administration. *Clinical nurse specialist programs in:* cardiovascular, community health, critical care, gerontology, occupational health, oncology, pediatric, perinatal, psychiatric/mental health. *Nurse practitioner programs in:* acute care, adult health, family health, gerontology, neonatal health, occupational health, pediatric, psychiatric/mental health.

Study Options Full-time.

Program Entrance Requirements Clinical experience, computer literacy, minimum overall college GPA of 3.0, transcript of college record, written essay, immunizations, 4 letters of recommendation, statistics course, GRE General Test. *Application deadline:* 2/1 (fall). *Application fee:* $60.

Advanced Placement Credit given for nursing courses completed elsewhere dependent upon specific evaluations.

Degree Requirements 44 total credit hours, comprehensive exam.

POST-MASTER'S PROGRAM
Areas of Study *Clinical nurse specialist programs in:* cardiovascular, community health, critical care, gerontology, occupational health, oncology, pediatric, perinatal, psychiatric/mental health. *Nurse practitioner programs in:* acute care, adult health, family health, gerontology, neonatal health, occupational health, pediatric, psychiatric/mental health.

DOCTORAL DEGREE PROGRAM
Degree PhD

Available Programs Doctorate; Post-Baccalaureate Doctorate.

Areas of Study Addiction/substance abuse, aging, bio-behavioral research, biology of health and illness, community health, critical care, ethics, family health, gerontology, health policy, health promotion/disease prevention, health-care systems, human health and illness, illness and transition, individualized study, information systems, maternity-newborn, nursing administration, nursing policy, nursing research, nursing science, oncology, urban health, women's health.

Program Entrance Requirements Minimum overall college GPA of 3.0, 4 letters of recommendation, statistics course, writing sample, GRE General Test. *Application deadline:* 12/15 (fall). *Application fee:* $60.

Degree Requirements Dissertation, oral exam, written exam, residency.

POSTDOCTORAL PROGRAM
Areas of Study Individualized study.
Postdoctoral Program Contact *Telephone:* 415-476-1435. *Fax:* 415-476-9707.

University of Phoenix–Bay Area Campus

College of Nursing
San Jose, California

DEGREES • BSN • MSN • MSN/MBA • MSN/MHA

Nursing Program Faculty 12 (58% with doctorates).
Baccalaureate Enrollment 39 **Women** 92.3% **Men** 7.7% **Minority** 35.9%
Graduate Enrollment 22 **Women** 86.4% **Men** 13.6% **Minority** 40.91%
Nursing Student Activities Sigma Theta Tau.
Nursing Student Resources Academic advising; academic or career counseling; assistance for students with disabilities; bookstore; campus computer network; computer lab; computer-assisted instruction; e-mail services; interactive nursing skills videos; Internet; learning resource lab; library services; nursing audiovisuals; remedial services; skills, simulation, or other laboratory; tutoring.
Library Facilities 16,781 periodical subscriptions (1,300 health-care related).

BACCALAUREATE PROGRAMS

Degree BSN
Available Programs Accelerated Baccalaureate.
Site Options Oakland, CA; San Francisco, CA; Novato, CA.
Study Options Full-time.
Program Entrance Requirements Transcript of college record, CPR certification, immunizations, 1 letter of recommendation, RN licensure. Transfer students are accepted. *Application deadline:* Applications may be processed on a rolling basis for some programs.
Advanced Placement Credit by examination available. Credit given for nursing courses completed elsewhere dependent upon specific evaluations.
Contact *Telephone:* 877-416-4100.

GRADUATE PROGRAMS

Contact *Telephone:* 877-416-4100.

MASTER'S DEGREE PROGRAM

Degrees MSN; MSN/MBA; MSN/MHA
Available Programs Master's.
Concentrations Available Health-care administration; nursing administration; nursing education.
Site Options Oakland, CA; San Francisco, CA; Novato, CA.
Study Options Full-time.
Program Entrance Requirements Clinical experience, computer literacy, minimum overall college GPA of 2.5, transcript of college record. *Application deadline:* Applications may be processed on a rolling basis for some programs. *Application fee:* $45.
Advanced Placement Credit given for nursing courses completed elsewhere dependent upon specific evaluations.
Degree Requirements 39 total credit hours, thesis or project.

University of Phoenix–Central Valley Campus

College of Health and Human Services
Fresno, California

Founded in 2004
DEGREE • BSN
Nursing Program Faculty 8 (13% with doctorates).
Baccalaureate Enrollment 53 **Women** 94.3% **Men** 5.7% **Minority** 30.2%
Nursing Student Activities Sigma Theta Tau.
Nursing Student Resources Academic advising; academic or career counseling; bookstore; campus computer network; computer lab; computer-assisted instruction; e-mail services; interactive nursing skills videos; Internet; learning resource lab; library services; nursing audiovisuals; remedial services; skills, simulation, or other laboratory; tutoring.
Library Facilities 1,300 periodical subscriptions health-care related.

BACCALAUREATE PROGRAMS

Degree BSN
Available Programs RN Baccalaureate.
Site Options Fresno, CA; Visalia, CA; Bakersfield, CA.
Study Options Full-time.
Program Entrance Requirements Transcript of college record, CPR certification, immunizations, 1 letter of recommendation, RN licensure. Transfer students are accepted.
Advanced Placement Credit by examination available. Credit given for nursing courses completed elsewhere dependent upon specific evaluations.
Contact *Telephone:* 661-663-0300. *Fax:* 661-633-2711.

University of Phoenix–Sacramento Valley Campus

College of Nursing
Sacramento, California

Founded in 1993
DEGREES • BSN • MSN • MSN/MHA
Nursing Program Faculty 29 (28% with doctorates).
Baccalaureate Enrollment 250 **Women** 88.8% **Men** 11.2% **Minority** 32%
Graduate Enrollment 53 **Women** 90.6% **Men** 9.4% **Minority** 15.09%
Nursing Student Activities Sigma Theta Tau.
Nursing Student Resources Academic advising; academic or career counseling; assistance for students with disabilities; bookstore; campus computer network; computer lab; computer-assisted instruction; e-mail services; interactive nursing skills videos; Internet; learning resource lab; library services; nursing audiovisuals; skills, simulation, or other laboratory; tutoring.
Library Facilities 16,781 periodical subscriptions (1,300 health-care related).

BACCALAUREATE PROGRAMS

Degree BSN
Available Programs Accelerated Baccalaureate; LPN to Baccalaureate.
Site Options Lathrop, CA; Modesto, CA; Fairfield, CA.
Study Options Full-time.
Online Degree Options Yes.
Program Entrance Requirements Transcript of college record, CPR certification, immunizations, 1 letter of recommendation, RN licensure. Transfer students are accepted. *Application deadline:* Applications may be processed on a rolling basis for some programs.
Advanced Placement Credit by examination available. Credit given for nursing courses completed elsewhere dependent upon specific evaluations.
Contact *Telephone:* 800-266-2107.

GRADUATE PROGRAMS

Contact *Telephone:* 800-266-2107.

MASTER'S DEGREE PROGRAM

Degrees MSN; MSN/MHA
Available Programs Accelerated Master's.
Concentrations Available Health-care administration; nursing administration; nursing education. *Nurse practitioner programs in:* family health.
Site Options Lathrop, CA; Modesto, CA; Fairfield, CA.
Study Options Full-time and part-time.
Program Entrance Requirements Clinical experience, computer literacy, minimum overall college GPA of 2.5, transcript of college record. *Application deadline:* Applications may be processed on a rolling basis for some programs. *Application fee:* $45.
Advanced Placement Credit given for nursing courses completed elsewhere dependent upon specific evaluations.
Degree Requirements 39 total credit hours, thesis or project.

POST-MASTER'S PROGRAM

Areas of Study *Nurse practitioner programs in:* family health.

CONTINUING EDUCATION PROGRAM

Contact *Telephone:* 800-266-2107.

University of Phoenix–San Diego Campus

College of Nursing
San Diego, California

Founded in 1988

DEGREES • BSN • MSN • MSN/ED D
Nursing Program Faculty 30 (37% with doctorates).
Baccalaureate Enrollment 103 **Women** 81.6% **Men** 18.4% **Minority** 29.1%
Graduate Enrollment 46 **Women** 89.1% **Men** 10.9% **Minority** 58.7%
Nursing Student Activities Sigma Theta Tau.
Nursing Student Resources Academic advising; academic or career counseling; assistance for students with disabilities; bookstore; campus computer network; computer lab; computer-assisted instruction; e-mail services; interactive nursing skills videos; Internet; learning resource lab; library services; nursing audiovisuals; skills, simulation, or other laboratory; tutoring.
Library Facilities 16,781 periodical subscriptions (1,300 health-care related).

BACCALAUREATE PROGRAMS

Degree BSN
Available Programs Accelerated Baccalaureate.
Site Options Chula Vista, CA; Imperial, CA; Palm Desert, CA.
Study Options Full-time.
Program Entrance Requirements Transcript of college record, CPR certification, immunizations, 1 letter of recommendation, RN licensure. Transfer students are accepted. *Application deadline:* Applications may be processed on a rolling basis for some programs.
Advanced Placement Credit by examination available. Credit given for nursing courses completed elsewhere dependent upon specific evaluations.
Contact *Telephone:* 888-867-4636.

GRADUATE PROGRAMS

Contact *Telephone:* 888-867-4636.

MASTER'S DEGREE PROGRAM
Degrees MSN; MSN/Ed D
Available Programs Master's.
Concentrations Available Health-care administration; nursing administration; nursing education.
Site Options Chula Vista, CA; Imperial, CA; Palm Desert, CA.
Study Options Full-time.
Program Entrance Requirements Clinical experience, computer literacy, minimum overall college GPA of 2.5, transcript of college record. *Application deadline:* Applications may be processed on a rolling basis for some programs. *Application fee:* $45.
Advanced Placement Credit given for nursing courses completed elsewhere dependent upon specific evaluations.
Degree Requirements 39 total credit hours, thesis or project.

University of Phoenix–Southern California Campus

College of Nursing
Costa Mesa, California

Founded in 1980

DEGREES • BSN • MSN • MSN/MBA • MSN/MHA
Nursing Program Faculty 109 (23% with doctorates).
Baccalaureate Enrollment 563 **Women** 89.2% **Men** 10.8% **Minority** 36.8%
Graduate Enrollment 379 **Women** 90.2% **Men** 9.8% **Minority** 40.9%
Nursing Student Activities Sigma Theta Tau.
Nursing Student Resources Academic advising; academic or career counseling; assistance for students with disabilities; bookstore; campus computer network; computer lab; computer-assisted instruction; e-mail services; interactive nursing skills videos; Internet; learning resource lab; library services; nursing audiovisuals; remedial services; skills, simulation, or other laboratory; tutoring.

Library Facilities 16,781 periodical subscriptions (1,300 health-care related).

BACCALAUREATE PROGRAMS

Degree BSN
Available Programs Accelerated Baccalaureate.
Site Options Diamond Bar, CA; La Marada, CA; Lancaster, CA.
Study Options Full-time.
Program Entrance Requirements Transcript of college record, CPR certification, immunizations, 1 letter of recommendation, RN licensure. Transfer students are accepted. *Application deadline:* Applications may be processed on a rolling basis for some programs.
Advanced Placement Credit by examination available. Credit given for nursing courses completed elsewhere dependent upon specific evaluations.
Contact *Telephone:* 800-697-8223.

GRADUATE PROGRAMS

Contact *Telephone:* 800-697-8223.

MASTER'S DEGREE PROGRAM
Degrees MSN; MSN/MBA; MSN/MHA
Available Programs Master's.
Concentrations Available Health-care administration; nursing administration; nursing education. *Nurse practitioner programs in:* family health.
Site Options Diamond Bar, CA; La Marada, CA; Lancaster, CA.
Study Options Full-time.
Program Entrance Requirements Clinical experience, computer literacy, minimum overall college GPA of 2.5, transcript of college record, 1 letter of recommendation. *Application deadline:* Applications may be processed on a rolling basis for some programs. *Application fee:* $45.
Advanced Placement Credit given for nursing courses completed elsewhere dependent upon specific evaluations.
Degree Requirements 39 total credit hours, thesis or project.

POST-MASTER'S PROGRAM
Areas of Study *Nurse practitioner programs in:* family health.

CONTINUING EDUCATION PROGRAM

Contact *Telephone:* 714-338-1720.

University of San Diego

Hahn School of Nursing and Health Science
San Diego, California

http://www.sandiego.edu/nursing
Founded in 1949

DEGREES • DNP • MSN • PHD
Nursing Program Faculty 44 (75% with doctorates).
Graduate Enrollment 355 **Women** 85% **Men** 15% **Minority** 39% **International** 1% **Part-time** 35%
Nursing Student Activities Nursing Honor Society, Sigma Theta Tau, Student Nurses' Association.
Nursing Student Resources Academic advising; academic or career counseling; assistance for students with disabilities; bookstore; campus computer network; career placement assistance; computer lab; computer-assisted instruction; daycare for children of students; e-mail services; employment services for current students; externships; interactive nursing skills videos; Internet; learning resource lab; library services; nursing audiovisuals; resume preparation assistance; skills, simulation, or other laboratory; tutoring.
Library Facilities 1 million volumes (47,500 in health, 24,600 in nursing); 38,810 periodical subscriptions (2,200 health-care related).

GRADUATE PROGRAMS

Expenses (2012–13) *Tuition:* full-time $30,840; part-time $1285 per credit hour. *Required fees:* full-time $650; part-time $125 per credit.
Financial Aid 90% of graduate students in nursing programs received some form of financial aid in 2011–12. Scholarships and traineeships available. Aid available to part-time students. *Financial aid application deadline:* 4/1.
Contact Ms. Cathleen Mumper, Director of Student Services and Admissions Officer, Hahn School of Nursing and Health Science, University of San Diego, 5998 Alcala Park, San Diego, CA 92110-2492.

Telephone: 619-260-4548. *Fax:* 619-260-6814. *E-mail:* cmm@sandiego.edu.

MASTER'S DEGREE PROGRAM

Degree MSN

Available Programs Accelerated Master's for Non-Nursing College Graduates; Master's; Master's for Nurses with Non-Nursing Degrees.

Concentrations Available Clinical nurse leader; nursing administration; nursing education; nursing informatics. *Clinical nurse specialist programs in:* acute care, adult health, critical care, medical-surgical, palliative care. *Nurse practitioner programs in:* adult health, family health, pediatric, primary care, psychiatric/mental health.

Study Options Full-time and part-time.

Program Entrance Requirements Clinical experience, computer literacy, minimum overall college GPA of 3.0, transcript of college record, CPR certification, written essay, immunizations, interview, 3 letters of recommendation, prerequisite course work, resume, statistics course, GRE General Test (entry-level nursing). *Application deadline:* 3/1 (fall), 11/1 (spring). *Application fee:* $45.

Advanced Placement Credit by examination available. Credit given for nursing courses completed elsewhere dependent upon specific evaluations.

DOCTORAL DEGREE PROGRAM

Degree DNP

Available Programs Doctorate, Post-Baccalaureate Doctorate.

Areas of Study Addiction/substance abuse, advanced practice nursing, aging, bio-behavioral research, biology of health and illness, clinical practice, community health, ethics, faculty preparation, family health, gerontology, health policy, health promotion/disease prevention, health-care systems, human health and illness, illness and transition, information systems, maternity-newborn, nursing education, women's health.

Program Entrance Requirements Minimum overall college GPA of 3.5, clinical experience, interview, 3 letters of recommendation, MSN or equivalent, vita, writing sample. *Application deadline:* 3/1 (fall).

Degree Requirements Residency.

DOCTORAL DEGREE PROGRAM

Degree PhD

Available Programs Doctorate; Post-Baccalaureate Doctorate.

Areas of Study Addiction/substance abuse, advanced practice nursing, aging, bio-behavioral research, clinical practice, community health, critical care, ethics, faculty preparation, family health, gerontology, health policy, health promotion/disease prevention, health-care systems, human health and illness, illness and transition, individualized study, information systems, maternity-newborn, nurse case management, nursing administration, nursing education, nursing policy, nursing research, nursing science, oncology, urban health, women's health.

Program Entrance Requirements Clinical experience, minimum overall college GPA of 3.5, interview by faculty committee, interview, 3 letters of recommendation, MSN or equivalent, statistics course, vita, writing sample. *Application deadline:* 2/1 (fall). *Application fee:* $45.

Degree Requirements 48 total credit hours, dissertation, residency.

See display below and full description on page 508.

University of San Francisco
School of Nursing and Health Professions
San Francisco, California

http://www.usfca.edu/nursing/
Founded in 1855

DEGREES • BSN • DNP • MSN

Nursing Program Faculty 112 (75% with doctorates).

Baccalaureate Enrollment 756 **Women** 86% **Men** 14% **Minority** 57% **International** 1% **Part-time** 1%

Graduate Enrollment 378 **Women** 84% **Men** 16% **Minority** 40% **Part-time** 5%

Distance Learning Courses Available.

Nursing Student Activities Nursing Honor Society, Sigma Theta Tau, Student Nurses' Association, nursing club.

Nursing Student Resources Academic advising; academic or career counseling; assistance for students with disabilities; bookstore; campus computer network; career placement assistance; computer lab; computer-assisted instruction; e-mail services; employment services for current students; housing assistance; interactive nursing skills videos; Internet; learning resource lab; library services; nursing audiovisuals; remedial services; resume preparation assistance; skills, simulation, or other laboratory; tutoring; unpaid internships.

Library Facilities 1.1 million volumes; 5,560 periodical subscriptions (200 health-care related).

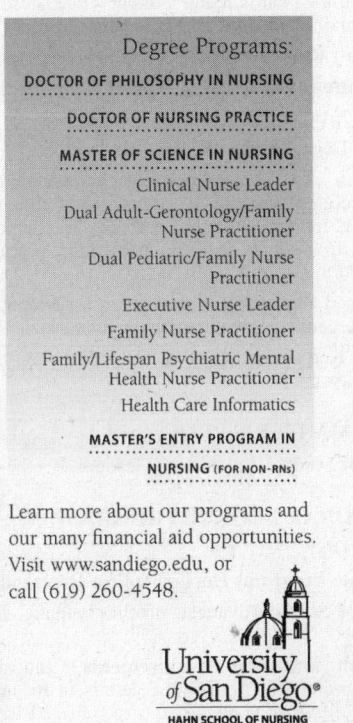

BACCALAUREATE PROGRAMS

Degree BSN

Available Programs Generic Baccalaureate.

Study Options Full-time.

Online Degree Options Yes.

Program Entrance Requirements Minimum overall college GPA of 3.0, transcript of college record, written essay, health insurance, high school biology, high school chemistry, 3 years high school math, 2 years high school science, high school transcript, immunizations, 2 letters of recommendation, minimum high school GPA of 3.9, prerequisite course work. Transfer students are accepted. *Application deadline:* 1/15 (fall), 12/15 (winter). *Application fee:* $55.

Advanced Placement Credit given for nursing courses completed elsewhere dependent upon specific evaluations.

Expenses (2011–12) *Tuition:* full-time $38,490. *Room and board:* $14,700; room only: $10,550 per academic year. *Required fees:* full-time $1574.

Financial Aid 95% of baccalaureate students in nursing programs received some form of financial aid in 2010–11.

Contact Office of Undergraduate Admissions, School of Nursing and Health Professions, University of San Francisco, 2130 Fulton Street, San Francisco, CA 94117. *Telephone:* 800-422-6563. *Fax:* 415-422-6877. *E-mail:* admission@usfca.edu.

GRADUATE PROGRAMS

Expenses (2011–12) *Tuition:* part-time $1130 per unit. *Required fees:* full-time $150.

Financial Aid 75% of graduate students in nursing programs received some form of financial aid in 2010–11. Institutionally sponsored loans available. *Financial aid application deadline:* 3/2.

Contact Mr. Robert Horgan, Recruiter, School of Nursing and Health Professions, University of San Francisco, 2130 Fulton Street, Cowell Hall, San Francisco, CA 94117-1080. *Telephone:* 415-422-6681. *Fax:* 415-422-6877. *E-mail:* rjhorgan@usfca.edu.

MASTER'S DEGREE PROGRAM

Degree MSN

Available Programs Accelerated AD/RN to Master's; Accelerated Master's for Non-Nursing College Graduates; Master's for Nurses with Non-Nursing Degrees; RN to Master's.

Concentrations Available Clinical nurse leader.

Site Options San Jose, CA; San Ramon, CA; Santa Rosa, CA.

Study Options Full-time.

Online Degree Options Yes.

Program Entrance Requirements Clinical experience, minimum overall college GPA of 3.5, transcript of college record, written essay, 2 letters of recommendation, prerequisite course work, resume, statistics course. *Application deadline:* 6/15 (fall), 10/15 (spring), 2/15 (summer). *Application fee:* $55.

Advanced Placement Credit given for nursing courses completed elsewhere dependent upon specific evaluations.

Degree Requirements 40 total credit hours, thesis or project, comprehensive exam.

POST-MASTER'S PROGRAM

Areas of Study Clinical nurse leader.

DOCTORAL DEGREE PROGRAM

Degree DNP

Available Programs Doctorate; Post-Baccalaureate Doctorate.

Areas of Study Advanced practice nursing, family health, health-care systems.

Program Entrance Requirements Clinical experience, minimum overall college GPA of 3.0, 3 letters of recommendation, vita, writing sample. *Application deadline:* 6/15 (fall), 10/15 (spring). *Application fee:* $55.

Degree Requirements Dissertation, oral exam, residency.

Vanguard University of Southern California
Nursing Program
Costa Mesa, California

Founded in 1920

DEGREE • BSN

Baccalaureate Enrollment 75

Library Facilities 164,333 volumes; 17,342 periodical subscriptions.

BACCALAUREATE PROGRAMS

Degree BSN

Available Programs RN Baccalaureate.

Contact *Telephone:* 714-668-6130 Ext. 3902. *Fax:* 714-668-6194.

West Coast University
Nursing Programs
North Hollywood, California

Founded in 1909

DEGREE • BSN

BACCALAUREATE PROGRAMS

Degree BSN

Available Programs Accelerated RN Baccalaureate; RN Baccalaureate.

Contact *Telephone:* 866-508-2684.

Western University of Health Sciences
College of Graduate Nursing
Pomona, California

http://www.westernu.edu/nursing-visitor

Founded in 1975

DEGREES • DNP • MSN

Nursing Program Faculty 25 (65% with doctorates).

Graduate Enrollment 285 **Women** 85% **Men** 15% **Minority** 54% **International** 1% **Part-time** 5%

Distance Learning Courses Available.

Nursing Student Activities Nursing Honor Society, Sigma Theta Tau, Student Nurses' Association, nursing club.

Nursing Student Resources Academic advising; academic or career counseling; assistance for students with disabilities; bookstore; campus computer network; career placement assistance; computer lab; computer-assisted instruction; e-mail services; interactive nursing skills videos; Internet; learning resource lab; library services; nursing audiovisuals; other; remedial services; resume preparation assistance; skills, simulation, or other laboratory; tutoring.

Library Facilities 17,171 volumes in health, 322 volumes in nursing; 5,000 periodical subscriptions health-care related.

GRADUATE PROGRAMS

Contact *Telephone:* 909-469-5255. *Fax:* 909-469-5521.

MASTER'S DEGREE PROGRAM

Degree MSN

Available Programs Accelerated AD/RN to Master's; Accelerated Master's; Accelerated Master's for Non-Nursing College Graduates; Master's.

Concentrations Available Clinical nurse leader; nursing administration. *Nurse practitioner programs in:* family health.

Study Options Full-time and part-time.

Online Degree Options Yes (online only).

Program Entrance Requirements Computer literacy, minimum overall college GPA of 3.0, transcript of college record, CPR certification, written essay, immunizations, interview, 3 letters of recommendation, prerequisite course work, resume, statistics course. *Application deadline:* 3/1 (fall). Applications may be processed on a rolling basis for some programs. *Application fee:* $60.

Advanced Placement Credit given for nursing courses completed elsewhere dependent upon specific evaluations.

Degree Requirements 50 total credit hours, thesis or project.

POST-MASTER'S PROGRAM

Areas of Study *Nurse practitioner programs in:* family health.

DOCTORAL DEGREE PROGRAM

Degree DNP

Available Programs Doctorate.

Online Degree Options Yes (online only).

Program Entrance Requirements Minimum overall college GPA of 3.0, 3 letters of recommendation, MSN or equivalent, scholarly papers, statistics course, vita, writing sample. *Application deadline:* 3/1 (fall). Applications may be processed on a rolling basis for some programs. *Application fee:* $60.

Degree Requirements 30 total credit hours, dissertation.

COLORADO

Adams State University

Nursing Program
Alamosa, Colorado

Founded in 1921

DEGREE • BSN

Nursing Program Faculty 10 (10% with doctorates).

Baccalaureate Enrollment 67 **Women** 89% **Men** 11% **Minority** 48% **International** 1% **Part-time** 39%

Nursing Student Activities Nursing Honor Society, Sigma Theta Tau, Student Nurses' Association.

Nursing Student Resources Academic advising; academic or career counseling; assistance for students with disabilities; bookstore; campus computer network; computer lab; computer-assisted instruction; daycare for children of students; e-mail services; employment services for current students; housing assistance; interactive nursing skills videos; Internet; learning resource lab; library services; nursing audiovisuals; remedial services; resume preparation assistance; skills, simulation, or other laboratory; tutoring; unpaid internships.

Library Facilities 565 volumes in health, 565 volumes in nursing; 200 periodical subscriptions health-care related.

BACCALAUREATE PROGRAMS

Degree BSN

Available Programs Generic Baccalaureate; RN Baccalaureate.

Site Options Salida, CO; Trinidad, CO.

Study Options Full-time.

Program Entrance Requirements Minimum overall college GPA of 3.0, transcript of college record, written essay, immunizations, interview, 2 letters of recommendation, minimum GPA in nursing prerequisites of 3.0, prerequisite course work. Transfer students are accepted. *Application deadline:* 8/1 (fall).

Advanced Placement Credit by examination available. Credit given for nursing courses completed elsewhere dependent upon specific evaluations.

Contact *Telephone:* 719-587-8134. *Fax:* 719-587-7522.

American Sentinel University

RN to Bachelor of Science Nursing
Aurora, Colorado

Founded in 1988

DEGREES • BSN • MSN

Distance Learning Courses Available.

BACCALAUREATE PROGRAMS

Degree BSN

Available Programs RN Baccalaureate.

Program Entrance Requirements Transcript of college record, RN licensure.

Contact *Telephone:* 866-922-5690.

GRADUATE PROGRAMS

Contact *Telephone:* 866-922-5690.

MASTER'S DEGREE PROGRAM

Degree MSN

Available Programs Master's.

Concentrations Available Nurse case management; nursing administration; nursing education; nursing informatics.

Program Entrance Requirements Transcript of college record.

Degree Requirements 36 total credit hours.

Aspen University

Graduate School of Health Professions and Studies
Denver, Colorado

http://www.aspen.edu
Founded in 1987

DEGREE • MSN

Nursing Program Faculty 4 (100% with doctorates).

Graduate Enrollment 206

Distance Learning Courses Available.

Nursing Student Resources Academic advising; computer-assisted instruction.

GRADUATE PROGRAMS

Contact Enrollment Office, Graduate School of Health Professions and Studies, Aspen University, 720 South Colorado Boulevard, Suite 1150N, Denver, CO 80246. *Telephone:* 800-373-7814. *E-mail:* enrollment@aspen.edu.

MASTER'S DEGREE PROGRAM

Degree MSN

Available Programs Master's; RN to Master's.

Concentrations Available Nursing administration; nursing education.

Study Options Full-time and part-time.

Online Degree Options Yes (online only).

Program Entrance Requirements Clinical experience, minimum overall college GPA of 3.0, transcript of college record, written essay, resume. *Application deadline:* Applications may be processed on a rolling basis for some programs.

Advanced Placement Credit given for nursing courses completed elsewhere dependent upon specific evaluations.

Degree Requirements 36 total credit hours, thesis or project, comprehensive exam.

Colorado Christian University

Nursing Programs
Lakewood, Colorado

Founded in 1914

DEGREE • BSN

BACCALAUREATE PROGRAMS

Degree BSN

Available Programs Generic Baccalaureate; RN Baccalaureate.

Online Degree Options Yes.

Contact College of Adult and Graduate Studies, Nursing Programs, Colorado Christian University, 8787 West Alameda Avenue, Lakewood, CO 80226. *Telephone:* 303-963-3311. *E-mail:* agsadmission@ccu.edu.

Colorado Mesa University

Department of Nursing and Radiologic Sciences
Grand Junction, Colorado

http://www.coloradomesa.edu/healthsciences/index.html
Founded in 1925
DEGREE • BSN
Nursing Program Faculty 40 (7% with doctorates).
Baccalaureate Enrollment 190 **Women** 88% **Men** 12% **Minority** 11%
International 4% **Part-time** 8%
Distance Learning Courses Available.
Nursing Student Activities Sigma Theta Tau, Student Nurses' Association.
Nursing Student Resources Academic advising; academic or career counseling; assistance for students with disabilities; bookstore; campus computer network; career placement assistance; computer lab; computer-assisted instruction; daycare for children of students; e-mail services; employment services for current students; housing assistance; interactive nursing skills videos; Internet; learning resource lab; library services; nursing audiovisuals; placement services for program completers; resume preparation assistance; skills, simulation, or other laboratory; tutoring; unpaid internships.
Library Facilities 545,373 volumes (7,500 in health, 6,576 in nursing); 76,724 periodical subscriptions (100 health-care related).

BACCALAUREATE PROGRAMS

Degree BSN
Available Programs ADN to Baccalaureate; Generic Baccalaureate; LPN to Baccalaureate; LPN to RN Baccalaureate; RN Baccalaureate.
Study Options Full-time and part-time.
Online Degree Options Yes.
Program Entrance Requirements Minimum overall college GPA of 2.0, transcript of college record, CPR certification, health exam, immunizations, minimum GPA in nursing prerequisites of 2.0, professional liability insurance/malpractice insurance, prerequisite course work. Transfer students are accepted. *Application deadline:* 3/1 (fall), 10/1 (spring).
Advanced Placement Credit by examination available. Credit given for nursing courses completed elsewhere dependent upon specific evaluations.
Contact *Telephone:* 970-248-1840. *Fax:* 970-248-1133.

Colorado State University–Pueblo

Department of Nursing
Pueblo, Colorado

Founded in 1933
DEGREES • BSN • MS
Nursing Program Faculty 30 (10% with doctorates).
Baccalaureate Enrollment 134 **Women** 90% **Men** 10% **Minority** 42%
International 1% **Part-time** 2%
Graduate Enrollment 26 **Women** 73% **Men** 27% **Minority** 50% **Part-time** 92%
Nursing Student Activities Sigma Theta Tau, Student Nurses' Association.
Nursing Student Resources Academic advising; academic or career counseling; assistance for students with disabilities; bookstore; campus computer network; computer lab; computer-assisted instruction; daycare for children of students; e-mail services; employment services for current students; housing assistance; Internet; learning resource lab; library services; nursing audiovisuals; remedial services; resume preparation assistance; skills, simulation, or other laboratory; tutoring.
Library Facilities 274,890 volumes (2,891 in health, 1,168 in nursing); 14,672 periodical subscriptions (101 health-care related).

BACCALAUREATE PROGRAMS

Degree BSN
Available Programs ADN to Baccalaureate; Accelerated Baccalaureate for Second Degree; Accelerated RN Baccalaureate; Baccalaureate for Second Degree; Generic Baccalaureate; LPN to Baccalaureate; LPN to RN Baccalaureate; RN Baccalaureate.
Study Options Full-time.

Program Entrance Requirements Minimum overall college GPA of 2.75, transcript of college record, CPR certification, health exam, immunizations, minimum GPA in nursing prerequisites of 2.75, professional liability insurance/malpractice insurance, prerequisite course work. Transfer students are accepted. *Application deadline:* 5/25 (fall), 10/1 (summer). *Application fee:* $25.
Advanced Placement Credit by examination available. Credit given for nursing courses completed elsewhere dependent upon specific evaluations.
Contact *Telephone:* 719-549-2422. *Fax:* 719-549-2113.

GRADUATE PROGRAMS

Contact *Telephone:* 719-549-2502. *Fax:* 719-549-2949.

MASTER'S DEGREE PROGRAM

Degree MS
Available Programs Master's.
Concentrations Available Nursing education. *Clinical nurse specialist programs in:* acute care, psychiatric/mental health. *Nurse practitioner programs in:* acute care, family health, pediatric.
Study Options Full-time and part-time.
Program Entrance Requirements Clinical experience, computer literacy, minimum overall college GPA of 3.0, transcript of college record, CPR certification, written essay, immunizations, 3 letters of recommendation, nursing research course, professional liability insurance/malpractice insurance, prerequisite course work, resume, statistics course. *Application deadline:* 5/25 (fall). *Application fee:* $35.
Advanced Placement Credit given for nursing courses completed elsewhere dependent upon specific evaluations.
Degree Requirements 46 total credit hours, thesis or project, comprehensive exam.

POST-MASTER'S PROGRAM

Areas of Study Nursing education. *Clinical nurse specialist programs in:* acute care, psychiatric/mental health. *Nurse practitioner programs in:* acute care, family health, pediatric.

Colorado Technical University Online

Nursing Program
Colorado Springs, Colorado

DEGREE • BSN

BACCALAUREATE PROGRAMS

Degree BSN
Available Programs RN Baccalaureate.
Online Degree Options Yes.
Contact Admissions, Nursing Program, Colorado Technical University Online, 4435 North Chestnut Street, Suite E, Colorado Springs, CO 80907. *Telephone:* 800-416-8904. *E-mail:* enroll@ctuonline.edu.

Denver College of Nursing

Denver College of Nursing
Denver, Colorado

DEGREE • BSN
Nursing Program Faculty 78 (7% with doctorates).
Baccalaureate Enrollment 270 **Women** 80% **Men** 20% **Minority** 15%
Distance Learning Courses Available.
Nursing Student Activities Student Nurses' Association.
Nursing Student Resources Academic advising; academic or career counseling; assistance for students with disabilities; bookstore; campus computer network; career placement assistance; computer lab; computer-assisted instruction; e-mail services; employment services for current students; externships; interactive nursing skills videos; Internet; learning resource lab; library services; nursing audiovisuals; placement services for program completers; remedial services; resume preparation assistance; skills, simulation, or other laboratory; tutoring; unpaid internships.
Library Facilities 1,000 volumes in health, 1,000 volumes in nursing; 26,000 periodical subscriptions health-care related.

BACCALAUREATE PROGRAMS

Degree BSN

Available Programs ADN to Baccalaureate; Accelerated Baccalaureate; Accelerated Baccalaureate for Second Degree; Generic Baccalaureate; LPN to RN Baccalaureate; RN Baccalaureate.

Site Options Denver, CO.

Study Options Full-time.

Program Entrance Requirements Transcript of college record, written essay, health exam, health insurance, immunizations, interview, 3 letters of recommendation, minimum high school GPA of 2.0, minimum GPA in nursing prerequisites of 2.0. Transfer students are accepted. *Application deadline:* Applications may be processed on a rolling basis for some programs. *Application fee:* $50.

Advanced Placement Credit given for nursing courses completed elsewhere dependent upon specific evaluations.

Expenses (2011–12) *Tuition, state resident:* full-time $6220; part-time $430 per credit hour. *Tuition, nonresident:* full-time $6220; part-time $430 per credit hour. *International tuition:* $6220 full-time.

Financial Aid 60% of baccalaureate students in nursing programs received some form of financial aid in 2010–11.

Contact Mr. Jeff Johnson, Director of Admissions, Denver College of Nursing, 1401 Nineteenth Street, Denver, CO 80202. *Telephone:* 303-292-0015 Ext. 3611. *Fax:* 720-974-0290. *E-mail:* j.johnson@denverschoolofnursing.edu.

Metropolitan State University of Denver

Department of Health Professions
Denver, Colorado

http://www.mscd.edu/
Founded in 1963

DEGREE • BSN

Nursing Program Faculty 19 (10% with doctorates).

Baccalaureate Enrollment 124 **Women** 89% **Men** 11% **Minority** 17% **International** 2% **Part-time** 63%

Distance Learning Courses Available.

Nursing Student Activities Nursing club.

Nursing Student Resources Academic advising; academic or career counseling; assistance for students with disabilities; bookstore; campus computer network; computer lab; computer-assisted instruction; daycare for children of students; e-mail services; interactive nursing skills videos; Internet; library services; nursing audiovisuals; remedial services; resume preparation assistance; skills, simulation, or other laboratory.

Library Facilities 607,971 volumes (21,503 in health); 2,380 periodical subscriptions (204 health-care related).

BACCALAUREATE PROGRAMS

Degree BSN

Available Programs ADN to Baccalaureate; Accelerated Baccalaureate for Second Degree.

Study Options Full-time and part-time.

Program Entrance Requirements Transcript of college record, CPR certification, written essay, immunizations, minimum GPA in nursing prerequisites of 2.5, professional liability insurance/malpractice insurance, prerequisite course work, RN licensure. Transfer students are accepted. *Application deadline:* 4/15 (spring). *Application fee:* $25.

Advanced Placement Credit given for nursing courses completed elsewhere dependent upon specific evaluations.

Expenses (2012–13) *Tuition, area resident:* full-time $2152; part-time $1076 per semester. *Tuition, nonresident:* full-time $7993; part-time $3996 per semester. *Required fees:* full-time $1037; part-time $518 per term.

Financial Aid 35% of baccalaureate students in nursing programs received some form of financial aid in 2011–12.

Contact M. Linda Stroup, Associate Chair of the Nursing Department. *Telephone:* 303-556-4391. *Fax:* 303-556-5165. *E-mail:* lstroup@msudenver.edu.

Platt College

School of Nursing
Aurora, Colorado

http://www.plattcolorado.edu/
Founded in 1986

DEGREE • BSN

Nursing Program Faculty 8 (2% with doctorates).

Baccalaureate Enrollment 134 **Women** 90% **Men** 10% **Minority** 2.5%

Nursing Student Activities Student Nurses' Association.

Nursing Student Resources Academic advising; academic or career counseling; assistance for students with disabilities; campus computer network; career placement assistance; housing assistance; Internet; learning resource lab; library services; nursing audiovisuals; resume preparation assistance; skills, simulation, or other laboratory; tutoring; unpaid internships.

Library Facilities 1,000 volumes in health, 888 volumes in nursing; 12 periodical subscriptions health-care related.

BACCALAUREATE PROGRAMS

Degree BSN

Available Programs Accelerated Baccalaureate.

Study Options Full-time.

Program Entrance Requirements Transcript of college record, CPR certification, written essay, health exam, health insurance, high school transcript, interview, letters of recommendation, minimum GPA in nursing prerequisites. Transfer students are accepted. *Application deadline:* 7/15 (fall), 11/15 (winter), 2/15 (spring), 5/15 (summer). Applications may be processed on a rolling basis for some programs. *Application fee:* $50.

Advanced Placement Credit by examination available. Credit given for nursing courses completed elsewhere dependent upon specific evaluations.

Contact *Telephone:* 303-369-5151.

Regis University

School of Nursing
Denver, Colorado

Founded in 1877

DEGREES • BSN • MS

Nursing Program Faculty 18 (55% with doctorates).

Distance Learning Courses Available.

Nursing Student Activities Nursing Honor Society, Sigma Theta Tau, Student Nurses' Association.

Nursing Student Resources Academic advising; academic or career counseling; assistance for students with disabilities; bookstore; campus computer network; computer lab; computer-assisted instruction; e-mail services; interactive nursing skills videos; Internet; learning resource lab; library services; nursing audiovisuals; resume preparation assistance; skills, simulation, or other laboratory; tutoring; unpaid internships.

Library Facilities 618,544 volumes; 35,000 periodical subscriptions.

BACCALAUREATE PROGRAMS

Degree BSN

Available Programs Accelerated Baccalaureate; Generic Baccalaureate; RN Baccalaureate.

Site Options Cheyenne, WY.

Study Options Full-time.

Program Entrance Requirements Minimum overall college GPA of 2.5, transcript of college record, written essay, 2 letters of recommendation, prerequisite course work. Transfer students are accepted.

Advanced Placement Credit by examination available.

Contact *Telephone:* 303-964-5178. *Fax:* 303-964-5400.

GRADUATE PROGRAMS

Contact *Telephone:* 303-458-3534. *Fax:* 303-964-5400.

MASTER'S DEGREE PROGRAM
Degree MS

Available Programs Master's; RN to Master's.

Concentrations Available Health-care administration; nursing administration; nursing education. *Nurse practitioner programs in:* family health, neonatal health.

Study Options Full-time and part-time.
Online Degree Options Yes.
Program Entrance Requirements Minimum overall college GPA of 2.75, transcript of college record, written essay, 3 letters of recommendation, prerequisite course work, statistics course.
Advanced Placement Credit by examination available.
Degree Requirements 42 total credit hours, thesis or project.

University of Colorado at Colorado Springs

Beth-El College of Nursing and Health Sciences
Colorado Springs, Colorado

http://www.uccs.edu/~bethel/
Founded in 1965
DEGREES • BSN • DNP • MSN
Nursing Program Faculty 43 (32% with doctorates).
Baccalaureate Enrollment 332 **Women** 92% **Men** 8% **Minority** 6.5% **Part-time** 5%
Graduate Enrollment 155 **Women** 94% **Men** 6% **Minority** 8% **Part-time** 38%
Distance Learning Courses Available.
Nursing Student Activities Nursing Honor Society, Sigma Theta Tau, Student Nurses' Association, nursing club.
Nursing Student Resources Academic advising; academic or career counseling; assistance for students with disabilities; bookstore; campus computer network; career placement assistance; computer lab; computer-assisted instruction; daycare for children of students; e-mail services; employment services for current students; externships; housing assistance; interactive nursing skills videos; Internet; learning resource lab; library services; nursing audiovisuals; resume preparation assistance; skills, simulation, or other laboratory; tutoring; unpaid internships.
Library Facilities 408,018 volumes (10,454 in health, 1,040 in nursing); 4,807 periodical subscriptions (331 health-care related).

BACCALAUREATE PROGRAMS

Degree BSN
Available Programs Accelerated Baccalaureate for Second Degree; Generic Baccalaureate; RN Baccalaureate.
Study Options Full-time.
Online Degree Options Yes.
Program Entrance Requirements Minimum overall college GPA of 3.3, transcript of college record, CPR certification, health insurance, high school biology, high school chemistry, high school foreign language, 3 years high school math, 1 year of high school science, high school transcript, immunizations, minimum high school GPA of 3.3, minimum GPA in nursing prerequisites of 3.0. Transfer students are accepted. *Application deadline:* Applications may be processed on a rolling basis for some programs. *Application fee:* $50.
Advanced Placement Credit given for nursing courses completed elsewhere dependent upon specific evaluations.
Contact *Telephone:* 719-255-3867. *Fax:* 719-255-3645.

GRADUATE PROGRAMS

Contact *Telephone:* 719-255-4424. *Fax:* 719-255-4496.

MASTER'S DEGREE PROGRAM
Degree MSN
Available Programs Master's.
Concentrations Available *Clinical nurse specialist programs in:* adult health. *Nurse practitioner programs in:* adult health, family health.
Study Options Full-time and part-time.
Online Degree Options Yes (online only).
Program Entrance Requirements Clinical experience, computer literacy, minimum overall college GPA of 3.0, transcript of college record, CPR certification, immunizations, 4 letters of recommendation, nursing research course, physical assessment course, professional liability insurance/malpractice insurance, prerequisite course work, resume, statistics course. *Application deadline:* 7/1 (fall), 11/1 (spring). *Application fee:* $60.
Advanced Placement Credit given for nursing courses completed elsewhere dependent upon specific evaluations.
Degree Requirements 47 total credit hours, thesis or project, comprehensive exam.

POST-MASTER'S PROGRAM
Areas of Study Nursing education. *Clinical nurse specialist programs in:* adult health. *Nurse practitioner programs in:* adult health, family health.

DOCTORAL DEGREE PROGRAM
Degree DNP
Available Programs Doctorate.
Areas of Study Forensic nursing, gerontology, individualized study.
Online Degree Options Yes (online only).
Program Entrance Requirements Clinical experience, minimum overall college GPA of 3.3, interview, 3 letters of recommendation, MSN or equivalent, statistics course, vita. *Application deadline:* 3/1 (summer). *Application fee:* $60.
Degree Requirements 36 total credit hours, written exam, residency.

CONTINUING EDUCATION PROGRAM

Contact *Telephone:* 719-255-4651. *Fax:* 719-255-4284.

University of Colorado Denver

College of Nursing
Aurora, Colorado

http://www.nursing.ucdenver.edu/
Founded in 1912
DEGREES • BS • DNP • MS • PHD
Nursing Program Faculty 87 (57% with doctorates).
Baccalaureate Enrollment 487 **Women** 86.25% **Men** 13.75% **Minority** 21.97% **International** .41% **Part-time** 13.9%
Graduate Enrollment 466 **Women** 92.92% **Men** 7.08% **Minority** 13.73% **International** 1.07% **Part-time** 30.9%
Distance Learning Courses Available.
Nursing Student Activities Nursing Honor Society, Sigma Theta Tau, Student Nurses' Association, nursing club.
Nursing Student Resources Academic advising; academic or career counseling; assistance for students with disabilities; bookstore; campus computer network; computer lab; computer-assisted instruction; e-mail services; housing assistance; interactive nursing skills videos; Internet; learning resource lab; library services; nursing audiovisuals; resume preparation assistance; skills, simulation, or other laboratory; tutoring.
Library Facilities 107,073 volumes in health, 4,552 volumes in nursing; 8,948 periodical subscriptions health-care related.

BACCALAUREATE PROGRAMS

Degree BS
Available Programs Accelerated Baccalaureate; Generic Baccalaureate; RN Baccalaureate.
Study Options Full-time and part-time.
Online Degree Options Yes.
Program Entrance Requirements Minimum overall college GPA of 3.0, transcript of college record, CPR certification, written essay, health exam, health insurance, immunizations, interview, minimum GPA in nursing prerequisites of 2.0, professional liability insurance/malpractice insurance, prerequisite course work. Transfer students are accepted. *Application deadline:* 6/15 (spring), 10/15 (summer). *Application fee:* $65.
Expenses (2012–13) *Tuition, state resident:* part-time $340 per credit hour. *Tuition, nonresident:* part-time $819 per credit hour.
Contact Pre-Admissions Advising, College of Nursing, University of Colorado Denver, 13120 East 19th Avenue, Campus Box C288-6, Aurora, CO 80045. *Telephone:* 303-724-1812. *Fax:* 303-724-1710. *E-mail:* nursing.admissions@ucdenver.edu.

GRADUATE PROGRAMS

Expenses (2012–13) *Tuition, state resident:* part-time $490 per credit hour. *Tuition, nonresident:* part-time $990 per credit hour.
Financial Aid Fellowships, research assistantships, teaching assistantships, Federal Work-Study, scholarships, and unspecified assistantships available.
Contact Pre-Admissions Advising, College of Nursing, University of Colorado Denver, 13120 East 19th Avenue, Box C288-6, Aurora, CO 80045. *Telephone:* 303-724-1812. *Fax:* 303-724-1710. *E-mail:* nursing.admissions@ucdenver.edu.

MASTER'S DEGREE PROGRAM
Degree MS
Available Programs Master's.
Concentrations Available Nurse-midwifery; nursing administration; nursing informatics. *Clinical nurse specialist programs in:* adult health. *Nurse practitioner programs in:* adult health, family health, pediatric, psychiatric/mental health, women's health.
Study Options Full-time and part-time.
Online Degree Options Yes.
Program Entrance Requirements Computer literacy, minimum overall college GPA of 3.0, transcript of college record, written essay, immunizations, 4 letters of recommendation, nursing research course, prerequisite course work, resume, statistics course, GRE if cumulative undergraduate GPA is less than 3.0. *Application deadline:* 7/1 (fall), 2/1 (spring). *Application fee:* $50.
Degree Requirements 30 total credit hours, thesis or project, comprehensive exam.

POST-MASTER'S PROGRAM
Areas of Study Nurse-midwifery; nursing administration; nursing informatics. *Clinical nurse specialist programs in:* adult health. *Nurse practitioner programs in:* adult health, family health, pediatric, psychiatric/mental health, women's health.

DOCTORAL DEGREE PROGRAM
Degree DNP
Available Programs Doctorate.
Areas of Study Advanced practice nursing, clinical nurse specialist--general, nurse anesthesia, nurse-midwifery.
Online Degree Options Yes (online only).
Program Entrance Requirements Minimum overall college GPA of 3.0, essay, interview, letters of recommendation, MSN or equivalent, vita. *Application deadline:* 2/1 (fall), 7/1 (spring). *Application fee:* $65.
Degree Requirements 41 total credit hours, Capstone project.

DOCTORAL DEGREE PROGRAM
Degree PhD
Available Programs Doctorate.
Areas of Study Bio-behavioral research, health-care systems.
Program Entrance Requirements Minimum overall college GPA of 3.0, interview by faculty committee, interview, 4 letters of recommendation, MSN or equivalent, statistics course, vita, writing sample, GRE. *Application deadline:* 3/1 (fall). *Application fee:* $50.
Degree Requirements 72 total credit hours, dissertation, oral exam, written exam.

POSTDOCTORAL PROGRAM
Postdoctoral Program Contact Pre-Admissions Advising, College of Nursing, University of Colorado Denver, 13120 East 19th Avenue, Campus Box C288-6, Aurora, CO 80045. *Telephone:* 303-724-1812. *Fax:* 303-724-1710. *E-mail:* nursing.admissions@ucdenver.edu.

CONTINUING EDUCATION PROGRAM
Contact Office of Lifelong Learning, College of Nursing, University of Colorado Denver, 13120 East 19th Avenue, Box C288-8, Aurora, CO 80045. *Telephone:* 303-724-1372. *E-mail:* professional.development@ucdenver.edu.

University of Northern Colorado
School of Nursing
Greeley, Colorado

http://www.unco.edu/nursing
Founded in 1890
DEGREES • BS • MS • PHD
Nursing Program Faculty 52 (60% with doctorates).
Baccalaureate Enrollment 216 **Women** 94% **Men** 6% **Minority** 18%
Graduate Enrollment 57 **Women** 98% **Men** 2% **Minority** 10% **Part-time** 60%
Distance Learning Courses Available.
Nursing Student Activities Sigma Theta Tau, Student Nurses' Association.
Nursing Student Resources Academic advising; academic or career counseling; assistance for students with disabilities; bookstore; campus computer network; career placement assistance; computer lab; computer-assisted instruction; e-mail services; employment services for current students; housing assistance; interactive nursing skills videos; Internet; learning resource lab; library services; nursing audiovisuals; paid internships; placement services for program completers; resume preparation assistance; skills, simulation, or other laboratory; tutoring.
Library Facilities 1.1 million volumes (43,602 in health, 25,700 in nursing); 40,304 periodical subscriptions (140 health-care related).

BACCALAUREATE PROGRAMS
Degree BS
Available Programs Accelerated Baccalaureate; Generic Baccalaureate; RN Baccalaureate.
Site Options Greeley, CO.
Study Options Full-time.
Program Entrance Requirements Minimum overall college GPA of 3.0, transcript of college record, CPR certification, health exam, immunizations, 2 letters of recommendation, minimum GPA in nursing prerequisites of 3.0, professional liability insurance/malpractice insurance, prerequisite course work. Transfer students are accepted.
Advanced Placement Credit given for nursing courses completed elsewhere dependent upon specific evaluations.
Contact *Telephone:* 970-351-2293. *Fax:* 970-351-1707.

GRADUATE PROGRAMS
Contact *Telephone:* 970-351-2293. *Fax:* 970-351-1707.

MASTER'S DEGREE PROGRAM
Degree MS
Available Programs Master's.
Concentrations Available Nursing education. *Clinical nurse specialist programs in:* family health. *Nurse practitioner programs in:* family health.
Site Options Greeley, CO.
Study Options Full-time and part-time.
Online Degree Options Yes (online only).
Program Entrance Requirements Clinical experience, minimum overall college GPA of 3.0, transcript of college record, CPR certification, immunizations, 2 letters of recommendation, GRE General Test.
Advanced Placement Credit given for nursing courses completed elsewhere dependent upon specific evaluations.
Degree Requirements 45 total credit hours, thesis or project, comprehensive exam.

POST-MASTER'S PROGRAM
Areas of Study Nursing education. *Nurse practitioner programs in:* family health.

DOCTORAL DEGREE PROGRAM
Degree PhD
Available Programs Doctorate.
Areas of Study Nursing education.
Site Options Greeley, CO.
Online Degree Options Yes (online only).
Program Entrance Requirements Clinical experience, minimum overall college GPA of 3.0, 2 letters of recommendation, MSN or equivalent, vita, writing sample, GRE General Test.
Degree Requirements 60 total credit hours, dissertation.

University of Phoenix–Denver Campus
College of Nursing
Lone Tree, Colorado

DEGREES • BSN • MSN • MSN/ED D • MSN/MHA
Nursing Program Faculty 19 (5% with doctorates).
Baccalaureate Enrollment 330 **Women** 86.7% **Men** 13.3% **Minority** 23.3%
Graduate Enrollment 19 **Women** 78.9% **Men** 21.1% **Minority** 21.05%
Nursing Student Activities Sigma Theta Tau.
Nursing Student Resources Academic advising; academic or career counseling; assistance for students with disabilities; bookstore; campus computer network; computer lab; computer-assisted instruction; e-mail services; interactive nursing skills videos; Internet; learning resource lab; library services; nursing audiovisuals; remedial services; skills, simulation, or other laboratory; tutoring.

Library Facilities 16,781 periodical subscriptions (1,300 health-care related).

BACCALAUREATE PROGRAMS

Degree BSN
Available Programs Accelerated Baccalaureate; LPN to Baccalaureate.
Site Options Westminister, CO; Aurora, CO; Ft. Collins, CO.
Study Options Full-time.
Program Entrance Requirements Transcript of college record, CPR certification, immunizations, 1 letter of recommendation, RN licensure. Transfer students are accepted. *Application deadline:* Applications may be processed on a rolling basis for some programs.
Advanced Placement Credit by examination available. Credit given for nursing courses completed elsewhere dependent upon specific evaluations.
Contact *Telephone:* 303-694-9093.

GRADUATE PROGRAMS

Contact *Telephone:* 303-694-9003.

MASTER'S DEGREE PROGRAM

Degrees MSN; MSN/Ed D; MSN/MHA
Available Programs Master's.
Concentrations Available Nursing administration; nursing education.
Site Options Westminister, CO; Aurora, CO.
Study Options Full-time.
Program Entrance Requirements Clinical experience, computer literacy, minimum overall college GPA of 2.5, transcript of college record. *Application deadline:* Applications may be processed on a rolling basis for some programs. *Application fee:* $45.
Advanced Placement Credit given for nursing courses completed elsewhere dependent upon specific evaluations.
Degree Requirements 39 total credit hours, thesis or project.

University of Phoenix–Southern Colorado Campus
College of Nursing
Colorado Springs, Colorado

Founded in 1999
Nursing Program Faculty 2
Nursing Student Activities Sigma Theta Tau.
Nursing Student Resources Academic advising; academic or career counseling; assistance for students with disabilities; bookstore; campus computer network; computer lab; computer-assisted instruction; e-mail services; interactive nursing skills videos; Internet; learning resource lab; library services; nursing audiovisuals; remedial services; skills, simulation, or other laboratory; tutoring.
Library Facilities 16,781 periodical subscriptions (1,300 health-care related).

CONNECTICUT

Central Connecticut State University
Department of Nursing
New Britain, Connecticut

Founded in 1849
DEGREE • BSN
Nursing Program Faculty 4 (100% with doctorates).
Nursing Student Activities Sigma Theta Tau, nursing club.
Nursing Student Resources Academic advising; academic or career counseling; assistance for students with disabilities; bookstore; campus computer network; career placement assistance; computer lab; computer-assisted instruction; e-mail services; employment services for current students; externships; Internet; learning resource lab; library services;

nursing audiovisuals; resume preparation assistance; skills, simulation, or other laboratory; tutoring.
Library Facilities 734,780 volumes; 55,879 periodical subscriptions.

BACCALAUREATE PROGRAMS

Degree BSN
Available Programs Generic Baccalaureate; RN Baccalaureate.
Site Options New Britain, CT.
Study Options Full-time and part-time.
Program Entrance Requirements Minimum overall college GPA of 2.7, CPR certification, health exam, high school transcript, immunizations, minimum GPA in nursing prerequisites of 2.7, prerequisite course work. Transfer students are accepted.
Advanced Placement Credit given for nursing courses completed elsewhere dependent upon specific evaluations.
Contact *Telephone:* 860-832-2147. *Fax:* 860-832-2188.

Fairfield University
School of Nursing
Fairfield, Connecticut

http://www.fairfield.edu/son/
Founded in 1942
DEGREES • BS • DNP • MSN
Nursing Program Faculty 61 (75% with doctorates).
Baccalaureate Enrollment 393 **Women** 96% **Men** 4% **Minority** 8% **Part-time** 19%
Graduate Enrollment 152 **Women** 86% **Men** 14% **Minority** 3% **International** 1% **Part-time** 86%
Nursing Student Activities Nursing Honor Society, Sigma Theta Tau, Student Nurses' Association.
Nursing Student Resources Academic advising; academic or career counseling; assistance for students with disabilities; bookstore; campus computer network; career placement assistance; computer lab; computer-assisted instruction; daycare for children of students; e-mail services; housing assistance; interactive nursing skills videos; Internet; learning resource lab; library services; nursing audiovisuals; placement services for program completers; resume preparation assistance; skills, simulation, or other laboratory; tutoring; unpaid internships.
Library Facilities 371,131 volumes (6,659 in health, 4,935 in nursing); 53,130 periodical subscriptions (4,874 health-care related).

BACCALAUREATE PROGRAMS

Degree BS
Available Programs Accelerated Baccalaureate for Second Degree; Generic Baccalaureate; RN Baccalaureate.
Study Options Full-time.
Program Entrance Requirements Written essay, health exam, health insurance, high school biology, high school chemistry, high school foreign language, 3 years high school math, 3 years high school science, high school transcript, immunizations, 1 letter of recommendation, minimum high school GPA of 3.0. *Application deadline:* 1/15 (fall). *Application fee:* $60.
Advanced Placement Credit given for nursing courses completed elsewhere dependent upon specific evaluations.
Expenses (2012–13) *Tuition:* full-time $41,090; part-time $650 per credit hour. *Room and board:* $12,550 per academic year. *Required fees:* full-time $1200; part-time $15 per credit; part-time $600 per term.
Financial Aid 70% of baccalaureate students in nursing programs received some form of financial aid in 2011–12. *Gift aid (need-based):* Federal Pell, FSEOG, state, private, college/university gift aid from institutional funds, Federal Nursing. *Loans:* Federal Nursing Student Loans, Federal Direct (Subsidized and Unsubsidized Stafford PLUS), Perkins, alternative loans. *Work-study:* Federal Work-Study. *Financial aid application deadline:* 2/15.
Contact Ms. Karen Pellegrino, Dean of Enrollment, School of Nursing, Fairfield University, 1073 North Benson Road, Kelley Center, Fairfield, CT 06824-5195. *Telephone:* 203-254-4100. *Fax:* 203-254-4199. *E-mail:* admis@fairfield.edu.

GRADUATE PROGRAMS

Expenses (2012–13) *Tuition:* part-time $660 per hour. *Required fees:* part-time $30 per term.

Financial Aid 34% of graduate students in nursing programs received some form of financial aid in 2011–12. Unspecified assistantships available.

Contact Ms. Marianne Gumpper, Director of Graduate and Continuing Studies Admission, School of Nursing, Fairfield University, 1073 North Benson Road, Kelley Center, Fairfield, CT 06824-5195. *Telephone:* 203-254-4184. *Fax:* 203-254-4073. *E-mail:* gradadmis@fairfield.edu.

MASTER'S DEGREE PROGRAM
Degree MSN
Available Programs Master's; Master's for Nurses with Non-Nursing Degrees.
Concentrations Available Clinical nurse leader; health-care administration; nurse anesthesia. *Nurse practitioner programs in:* family health, psychiatric/mental health.
Study Options Full-time and part-time.
Program Entrance Requirements Computer literacy, minimum overall college GPA of 3.0, transcript of college record, written essay, immunizations, interview, 2 letters of recommendation, resume, statistics course. *Application deadline:* Applications may be processed on a rolling basis for some programs. *Application fee:* $60.
Advanced Placement Credit given for nursing courses completed elsewhere dependent upon specific evaluations.
Degree Requirements 38 total credit hours.

POST-MASTER'S PROGRAM
Areas of Study *Nurse practitioner programs in:* family health, psychiatric/mental health.

DOCTORAL DEGREE PROGRAM
Degree DNP
Available Programs Doctorate; Post-Baccalaureate Doctorate.
Areas of Study Advanced practice nursing.
Program Entrance Requirements Clinical experience, minimum overall college GPA of 3.2, interview by faculty committee, interview, 2 letters of recommendation, vita, writing sample, GRE (nurse anesthesia applicants only). *Application deadline:* Applications may be processed on a rolling basis for some programs. *Application fee:* $60.
Degree Requirements 38 total credit hours, oral exam, residency.

CONTINUING EDUCATION PROGRAM
Contact Carole A. Pomarico, Adult Program Director, School of Nursing, Fairfield University, 1073 North Benson Road, Fairfield, CT 06824. *Telephone:* 203-254-4000 Ext. 2711. *Fax:* 203-254-4126. *E-mail:* capomarico@fairfield.edu.

Quinnipiac University
School of Nursing
Hamden, Connecticut

http://www.quinnipiac.edu/nursing
Founded in 1929
DEGREES • BSN • DNP • MSN
Nursing Program Faculty 78 (90% with doctorates).
Baccalaureate Enrollment 540 **Women** 97% **Men** 3% **Minority** 7% **International** 2%
Graduate Enrollment 98 **Women** 98% **Men** 2% **Minority** 6% **International** 1% **Part-time** 60%
Nursing Student Activities Sigma Theta Tau, Student Nurses' Association.
Nursing Student Resources Academic advising; academic or career counseling; bookstore; campus computer network; career placement assistance; computer lab; computer-assisted instruction; e-mail services; employment services for current students; externships; housing assistance; interactive nursing skills videos; Internet; learning resource lab; library services; nursing audiovisuals; paid internships; placement services for program completers; resume preparation assistance; skills, simulation, or other laboratory; tutoring; unpaid internships.
Library Facilities 311,000 volumes (1,700 in nursing); 44,700 periodical subscriptions.

BACCALAUREATE PROGRAMS
Degree BSN
Available Programs Accelerated Baccalaureate for Second Degree; Generic Baccalaureate.
Site Options North Haven, CT.

Study Options Full-time.
Program Entrance Requirements Minimum overall college GPA of 3.0, transcript of college record, written essay, health exam, high school biology, high school chemistry, 4 years high school math, 4 years high school science, high school transcript, immunizations, 1 letter of recommendation, minimum high school GPA of 3.0, minimum high school rank 35%, minimum GPA in nursing prerequisites of 3.0. Transfer students are accepted. *Application deadline:* 11/15 (fall), 12/1 (spring). Applications may be processed on a rolling basis for some programs. *Application fee:* $45.
Advanced Placement Credit given for nursing courses completed elsewhere dependent upon specific evaluations.
Expenses (2012–13) *Tuition:* full-time $36,510; part-time $875 per credit. *International tuition:* $36,510 full-time. *Room and board:* $13,800 per academic year. *Required fees:* full-time $1490; part-time $37 per credit; part-time $407 per term.
Financial Aid 80% of baccalaureate students in nursing programs received some form of financial aid in 2011–12. *Gift aid (need-based):* Federal Pell, FSEOG, state, private, college/university gift aid from institutional funds. *Loans:* Federal Direct (Subsidized and Unsubsidized Stafford PLUS), Perkins. *Work-study:* Federal Work-Study, part-time campus jobs. *Financial aid application deadline (priority):* 3/1.
Contact Ms. Carla Knowlton, Director of Undergraduate Admissions, School of Nursing, Quinnipiac University, 275 Mount Carmel Avenue, Hamden, CT 06518. *Telephone:* 203-582-8600. *Fax:* 203-582-8906. *E-mail:* admissions@quinnipiac.edu.

GRADUATE PROGRAMS

Expenses (2012–13) *Tuition:* full-time $24,570; part-time $895 per credit. *International tuition:* $24,570 full-time. *Required fees:* part-time $37 per credit; part-time $333 per term.
Financial Aid 30% of graduate students in nursing programs received some form of financial aid in 2011–12.
Contact Kristin Parent, Associate Director of Graduate Admissions, School of Nursing, Quinnipiac University, 275 Mount Carmel Avenue, Hamden, CT 06518. *Telephone:* 203-582-8672. *Fax:* 203-582-3443. *E-mail:* graduate@quinnipiac.edu.

MASTER'S DEGREE PROGRAM
Degree MSN
Available Programs Master's.
Concentrations Available *Nurse practitioner programs in:* adult health, family health.
Site Options North Haven, CT.
Study Options Full-time and part-time.
Program Entrance Requirements Clinical experience, minimum overall college GPA of 3.0, transcript of college record, written essay, 2 letters of recommendation. *Application deadline:* 5/15 (fall), 12/15 (spring). Applications may be processed on a rolling basis for some programs. *Application fee:* $45.
Degree Requirements 43 total credit hours.

POST-MASTER'S PROGRAM
Areas of Study *Nurse practitioner programs in:* adult health, family health.

DOCTORAL DEGREE PROGRAM
Degree DNP
Available Programs Doctorate; Post-Baccalaureate Doctorate.
Areas of Study Advanced practice nursing.
Site Options North Haven, CT.
Program Entrance Requirements Minimum overall college GPA of 3.0, interview, 2 letters of recommendation, vita, writing sample. *Application deadline:* 6/1 (fall). Applications may be processed on a rolling basis for some programs. *Application fee:* $45.
Degree Requirements 75 total credit hours, residency.

CONTINUING EDUCATION PROGRAM
Contact Ms. Mary Wargo, Director of Transfer and Part-Time Admissions, School of Nursing, Quinnipiac University, 275 Mount Carmel Avenue, Hamden, CT 06518. *Telephone:* 203-582-8612. *Fax:* 203-582-8906. *E-mail:* mary.wargo@quinnipiac.edu.

See display on next page and full description on page 498.

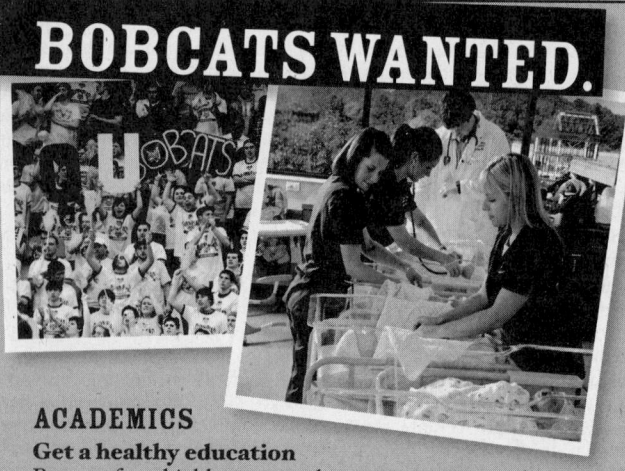
Sacred Heart University
Program in Nursing
Fairfield, Connecticut

http://www.sacredheart.edu/nursing.cfm
Founded in 1963
DEGREES • BSN • DNP • MSN
Nursing Program Faculty 77
Baccalaureate Enrollment 410 **Women** 94% **Men** 6% **Minority** 8% **Part-time** 30%
Graduate Enrollment 767 **Women** 75% **Men** 25% **Minority** 10% **International** .01% **Part-time** 100%
Distance Learning Courses Available.
Nursing Student Activities Nursing Honor Society, Sigma Theta Tau, Student Nurses' Association.
Nursing Student Resources Academic advising; academic or career counseling; assistance for students with disabilities; bookstore; campus computer network; career placement assistance; computer lab; computer-assisted instruction; e-mail services; employment services for current students; externships; housing assistance; interactive nursing skills videos; Internet; learning resource lab; library services; nursing audiovisuals; paid internships; placement services for program completers; remedial services; resume preparation assistance; skills, simulation, or other laboratory; tutoring; unpaid internships.
Library Facilities 139,720 volumes (5,000 in health, 649 in nursing); 2,199 periodical subscriptions (328 health-care related).

BACCALAUREATE PROGRAMS

Degree BSN
Available Programs Generic Baccalaureate; RN Baccalaureate.
Study Options Full-time.
Program Entrance Requirements Minimum overall college GPA of 2.8, transcript of college record, written essay, high school biology, high school chemistry, 3 years high school math, 3 years high school science, high school transcript, interview, 1 letter of recommendation, minimum high school GPA of 3.3, minimum GPA in nursing prerequisites of 3.0. Transfer students are accepted. *Application deadline:* Applications may be processed on a rolling basis for some programs. *Application fee:* $70.
Advanced Placement Credit given for nursing courses completed elsewhere dependent on specific evaluations.
Expenses (2012–13) *Tuition:* full-time $33,780; part-time $515 per credit. *International tuition:* $33,780 full-time. *Room and board:* $13,230; room only: $9380 per academic year. *Required fees:* full-time $1990.
Financial Aid 78% of baccalaureate students in nursing programs received some form of financial aid in 2011–12.
Contact Ms. Cori Nevers, Executive Director of International Admissions/Director of Admissions for the College of Health Professions, Program in Nursing, Sacred Heart University, 5151 Park Avenue, Fairfield, CT 06825-1000. *Telephone:* 203-767-0386. *E-mail:* NeversC@sacredheart.edu.

GRADUATE PROGRAMS

Expenses (2012–13) *Tuition:* part-time $580 per credit.
Financial Aid 38% of graduate students in nursing programs received some form of financial aid in 2011–12.
Contact Ms. Kathy Dilks, Associate Dean of Graduate Admissions, Program in Nursing, Sacred Heart University, 5151 Park Avenue, Fairfield, CT 06825-1000. *Telephone:* 203-396-8259. *E-mail:* dilksk@sacredheart.edu.

MASTER'S DEGREE PROGRAM

Degree MSN
Available Programs Master's; RN to Master's.
Concentrations Available Clinical nurse leader; nursing administration; nursing education. *Nurse practitioner programs in:* family health.
Study Options Full-time and part-time.
Online Degree Options Yes.
Program Entrance Requirements Clinical experience, minimum overall college GPA of 3.0, transcript of college record, written essay, interview, 2 letters of recommendation, prerequisite course work, statistics course. *Application deadline:* 2/15 (fall). Applications may be processed on a rolling basis for some programs. *Application fee:* $60.
Advanced Placement Credit given for nursing courses completed elsewhere dependent upon specific evaluations.
Degree Requirements 38 total credit hours, thesis or project.

POST-MASTER'S PROGRAM
Areas of Study *Nurse practitioner programs in:* family health.

DOCTORAL DEGREE PROGRAM
Degree DNP
Available Programs Doctorate.
Areas of Study Clinical practice, nursing administration.
Program Entrance Requirements Minimum overall college GPA of 3.2, interview by faculty committee, 2 letters of recommendation, MSN or equivalent, scholarly papers, statistics course, writing sample. *Application deadline:* 4/1 (fall). *Application fee:* $60.
Degree Requirements 39 total credit hours, dissertation.

Southern Connecticut State University
Department of Nursing
New Haven, Connecticut

http://www.southernct.edu/nursing/
Founded in 1893
DEGREES • BS • EDD • MSN
Nursing Program Faculty 45 (65% with doctorates).
Baccalaureate Enrollment 220 **Women** 85% **Men** 15% **Minority** 20% **Part-time** 5%
Graduate Enrollment 40 **Women** 97% **Men** 3% **Part-time** 97%
Distance Learning Courses Available.
Nursing Student Activities Nursing Honor Society, Sigma Theta Tau, Student Nurses' Association.
Nursing Student Resources Academic advising; academic or career counseling; assistance for students with disabilities; bookstore; campus computer network; career placement assistance; computer lab; daycare for children of students; e-mail services; employment services for current students; housing assistance; Internet; learning resource lab; library services; nursing audiovisuals; resume preparation assistance; skills, simulation, or other laboratory; tutoring.
Library Facilities 486,663 volumes (35,540 in health, 2,279 in nursing); 4,165 periodical subscriptions (318 health-care related).

BACCALAUREATE PROGRAMS
Degree BS
Available Programs ADN to Baccalaureate; Accelerated Baccalaureate; Generic Baccalaureate; RN Baccalaureate.
Study Options Full-time and part-time.
Program Entrance Requirements Minimum overall college GPA of 2.8, transcript of college record, CPR certification, health exam, high school transcript, immunizations, minimum GPA in nursing prerequisites, prerequisite course work. Transfer students are accepted. *Application deadline:* 2/1 (spring).
Advanced Placement Credit given for nursing courses completed elsewhere dependent upon specific evaluations.
Expenses (2011–12). *Tuition, state resident:* full-time $4124. *Tuition, nonresident:* full-time $13,346. *International tuition:* $13,346 full-time. *Room and board:* $10,200; room only: $5600 per academic year. *Required fees:* part-time $245 per credit; part-time $55 per term.
Financial Aid *Gift aid (need-based):* Federal Pell, FSEOG, state, private, college/university gift aid from institutional funds. *Loans:* Federal Direct (Subsidized and Unsubsidized Stafford PLUS).*Work-study:* Federal Work-Study, part-time campus jobs.*Financial aid application deadline:* 3/9(priority: 3/5).
Contact Dr. Karen Barnett, Coordinator, BSN Program in Nursing, Department of Nursing, Southern Connecticut State University, 501 Crescent Street, New Haven, CT 06515-1355. *Telephone:* 203-392-6475. *Fax:* 203-392-6493. *E-mail:* barnettk3@southernct.edu.

GRADUATE PROGRAMS
Expenses (2011–12) *Tuition, state resident:* full-time $5000; part-time $285 per credit. *Tuition, nonresident:* full-time $15,200; part-time $291 per credit. *International tuition:* $15,200 full-time. *Required fees:* full-time $4000; part-time $238 per credit; part-time $55 per term.
Contact Dr. Leslie Neal Boylan, Coordinator, Graduate Programs in Nursing, Department of Nursing, Southern Connecticut State University, 501 Crescent Street, New Haven, CT 06515. *Telephone:* 203-392-6480. *Fax:* 203-392-6493. *E-mail:* nealboylanl1@southernct.edu.

MASTER'S DEGREE PROGRAM
Degree MSN
Available Programs Master's; RN to Master's.
Concentrations Available Clinical nurse leader; nursing education. *Nurse practitioner programs in:* family health.
Study Options Full-time and part-time.
Program Entrance Requirements Clinical experience, minimum overall college GPA of 3.0, transcript of college record, CPR certification, immunizations, interview, 2 letters of recommendation, nursing research course, physical assessment course, professional liability insurance/malpractice insurance, prerequisite course work, resume, statistics course, GRE, MAT. *Application deadline:* 10/1 (fall), 3/1 (spring). Applications may be processed on a rolling basis for some programs.
Advanced Placement Credit given for nursing courses completed elsewhere dependent upon specific evaluations.
Degree Requirements 42 total credit hours, thesis or project.

POST-MASTER'S PROGRAM
Areas of Study Nursing education. *Nurse practitioner programs in:* family health.

DOCTORAL DEGREE PROGRAM
Degree EdD
Available Programs Doctorate.
Areas of Study Nursing education.
Online Degree Options Yes (online only).
Program Entrance Requirements Minimum overall college GPA of 3.0, interview, 2 letters of recommendation, MSN or equivalent, vita, writing sample. *Application deadline:* 3/1 (spring).
Degree Requirements 51 total credit hours, dissertation, written exam, residency.

University of Connecticut
School of Nursing
Storrs, Connecticut

http://www.nursing.uconn.edu/
Founded in 1881
DEGREES • BS • DNP • MS • MS/MBA • PHD
Nursing Program Faculty 64 (49% with doctorates).
Baccalaureate Enrollment 549 **Women** 87% **Men** 13% **Minority** 22%
Graduate Enrollment 169 **Women** 91% **Men** 9% **Part-time** 60%
Distance Learning Courses Available.
Nursing Student Activities Sigma Theta Tau, Student Nurses' Association, nursing club.
Nursing Student Resources Academic advising; academic or career counseling; assistance for students with disabilities; bookstore; campus computer network; career placement assistance; computer lab; e-mail services; housing assistance; interactive nursing skills videos; Internet; learning resource lab; library services; nursing audiovisuals; remedial services; resume preparation assistance; skills, simulation, or other laboratory; tutoring; unpaid internships.
Library Facilities 3 million volumes (7,648 in health, 359 in nursing); 17,378 periodical subscriptions (7,287 health-care related).

BACCALAUREATE PROGRAMS
Degree BS
Available Programs Accelerated Baccalaureate for Second Degree; Generic Baccalaureate.
Site Options Waterbury, CT; Groton, CT; Stamford, CT.
Study Options Full-time and part-time.
Program Entrance Requirements Minimum overall college GPA of 3.3, transcript of college record, written essay, health exam, health insurance, high school chemistry, high school foreign language, 3 years high school math, 2 years high school science, high school transcript, immunizations, minimum high school GPA of 3.0, minimum GPA in nursing prerequisites of 3.0, prerequisite course work. Transfer students are accepted. *Application deadline:* 1/15 (fall). *Application fee:* $70.
Advanced Placement Credit by examination available. Credit given for nursing courses completed elsewhere dependent upon specific evaluations.
Expenses (2012–13) *Tuition, state resident:* full-time $8712; part-time $363 per credit. *Tuition, nonresident:* full-time $26,544; part-time $1106 per credit. *International tuition:* $26,544 full-time. *Room and board:* $11,380; room only: $6096 per academic year. *Required fees:* full-time $2650.

Financial Aid 77% of baccalaureate students in nursing programs received some form of financial aid in 2011–12. *Gift aid (need-based):* Federal Pell, FSEOG, state, private, college/university gift aid from institutional funds. *Loans:* Federal Nursing Student Loans, Federal Direct (Subsidized and Unsubsidized Stafford PLUS), Perkins, state. *Work-study:* Federal Work-Study, part-time campus jobs. *Financial aid application deadline (priority):* 3/1.

Contact Ms. Dorine Nagy, Admissions Coordinator, School of Nursing, University of Connecticut, 231 Glenbrook Road, Unit 2026, Storrs, CT 06269-4026. *Telephone:* 860-486-1937. *Fax:* 860-486-0906. *E-mail:* Dorine.Nagy@uconn.edu.

GRADUATE PROGRAMS

Expenses (2012–13) *Tuition, state resident:* full-time $10,782; part-time $599 per credit. *Tuition, nonresident:* full-time $27,990; part-time $1555 per credit. *Room and board:* $12,534; room only: $7250 per academic year. *Required fees:* full-time $2084; part-time $940 per term.

Financial Aid 24% of graduate students in nursing programs received some form of financial aid in 2011–12. 9 research assistantships with full tuition reimbursements available, 12 teaching assistantships with full tuition reimbursements available were awarded; fellowships, Federal Work-Study, scholarships, and unspecified assistantships also available. *Financial aid application deadline:* 2/1.

Contact Ms. Dorine Nagy, Graduate Program Contact, School of Nursing, University of Connecticut, 231 Glenbrook Road, Unit 4026, Storrs, CT 06269-4026. *Telephone:* 860-486-1937. *Fax:* 860-486-0906. *E-mail:* Dorine.Nagy@uconn.edu.

MASTER'S DEGREE PROGRAM

Degrees MS; MS/MBA

Available Programs Master's; RN to Master's.

Concentrations Available Clinical nurse leader. *Clinical nurse specialist programs in:* acute care, maternity-newborn. *Nurse practitioner programs in:* acute care, family health, neonatal health, primary care.

Study Options Full-time and part-time.

Program Entrance Requirements Clinical experience, computer literacy, minimum overall college GPA of 3.0, transcript of college record, CPR certification, immunizations, interview, 3 letters of recommendation, nursing research course, physical assessment course, professional liability insurance/malpractice insurance, resume, statistics course. *Application deadline:* 5/1 (fall). Applications may be processed on a rolling basis for some programs. *Application fee:* $75.

Advanced Placement Credit given for nursing courses completed elsewhere dependent upon specific evaluations.

Degree Requirements 24 total credit hours, comprehensive exam.

POST-MASTER'S PROGRAM

Areas of Study *Clinical nurse specialist programs in:* maternity-newborn. *Nurse practitioner programs in:* acute care, family health, neonatal health, primary care.

DOCTORAL DEGREE PROGRAM

Degree DNP

Available Programs Doctorate, Post-Baccalaureate Doctorate.

Areas of Study Clinical practice, nursing research, nursing science.

Program Entrance Requirements Minimum overall college GPA of 3.25, clinical experience, interview by faculty committee, 3 letters of recommendation, MSN or equivalent, scholarly papers, statistics course, vita. *Application deadline:* 2/1 (fall). *Application fee:* $75.

Degree Requirements 59 total credit hours.

DOCTORAL DEGREE PROGRAM

Degree PhD

Available Programs Doctorate; Post-Baccalaureate Doctorate.

Areas of Study Nursing research, nursing science.

Program Entrance Requirements Minimum overall college GPA of 3.25, interview by faculty committee, interview, 3 letters of recommendation, MSN or equivalent, statistics course, vita, writing sample. *Application deadline:* 2/1 (fall). *Application fee:* $75.

Degree Requirements 59 total credit hours, dissertation, oral exam, written exam.

CONTINUING EDUCATION PROGRAM

Contact Ms. Elise Bennett, School of Nursing, University of Connecticut, School of Nursing, 231 Glenbrook Road, U-4026, Storrs, CT 06269-4026. *Telephone:* 860-486-8321. *Fax:* 860-486-0001. *E-mail:* Elise.Bennett@uconn.edu.

University of Hartford
College of Education, Nursing, and Health Professions
West Hartford, Connecticut

http://www.hartford.edu/enhp
Founded in 1877

DEGREES • BSN • MSN • MSN/MSOB

Nursing Program Faculty 5 (80% with doctorates).

Baccalaureate Enrollment 77 **Women** 91% **Men** 9% **Minority** 55% **Part-time** 100%

Graduate Enrollment 145 **Women** 94% **Men** 6% **Minority** 15% **International** 1% **Part-time** 100%

Distance Learning Courses Available.

Nursing Student Activities Sigma Theta Tau.

Nursing Student Resources Academic advising; academic or career counseling; assistance for students with disabilities; bookstore; computer lab; e-mail services; Internet; library services; resume preparation assistance; tutoring.

Library Facilities 586,150 volumes; 37,393 periodical subscriptions.

BACCALAUREATE PROGRAMS

Degree BSN

Available Programs ADN to Baccalaureate; RN Baccalaureate.

Study Options Part-time.

Program Entrance Requirements Transcript of college record, professional liability insurance/malpractice insurance, prerequisite course work, RN licensure. Transfer students are accepted. *Application deadline:* Applications may be processed on a rolling basis for some programs. *Application fee:* $45.

Advanced Placement Credit by examination available. Credit given for nursing courses completed elsewhere dependent upon specific evaluations.

Expenses (2012–13) *Tuition:* part-time $460 per credit. *Required fees:* part-time $30 per term.

Financial Aid 50% of baccalaureate students in nursing programs received some form of financial aid in 2011–12.

Contact Dr. Peter Kennedy, Chair, Department of Health Sciences and Nursing, College of Education, Nursing, and Health Professions, University of Hartford, 200 Bloomfield Avenue, West Hartford, CT 06117-1599. *Telephone:* 860-879-4823. *Fax:* 860-768-5043. *E-mail:* pkennedy@hartford.edu.

GRADUATE PROGRAMS

Expenses (2012–13) *Tuition:* part-time $480 per credit. *Required fees:* part-time $30 per term.

Financial Aid 50% of graduate students in nursing programs received some form of financial aid in 2011–12. 4 research assistantships (averaging $4,500 per year) were awarded; teaching assistantships, institutionally sponsored loans and unspecified assistantships also available. *Financial aid application deadline:* 6/1.

Contact Ms. Susan Diehl, Associate Professor of Nursing, College of Education, Nursing, and Health Professions, University of Hartford, 200 Bloomfield Avenue, West Hartford, CT 06117-1599. *Telephone:* 860-768-4214. *Fax:* 860-768-5346. *E-mail:* diehl@hartford.edu.

MASTER'S DEGREE PROGRAM

Degrees MSN; MSN/MSOB

Available Programs Master's; Master's for Nurses with Non-Nursing Degrees.

Concentrations Available Nursing administration; nursing education. *Clinical nurse specialist programs in:* public health.

Study Options Part-time.

Program Entrance Requirements Clinical experience, minimum overall college GPA of 3.0, transcript of college record, written essay, immunizations, 2 letters of recommendation, nursing research course, physical assessment course, professional liability insurance/malpractice insurance, resume. *Application deadline:* 4/15 (fall), 11/15 (spring). *Application fee:* $45.

Advanced Placement Credit given for nursing courses completed elsewhere dependent upon specific evaluations.

Degree Requirements 34 total credit hours, thesis or project.

POST-MASTER'S PROGRAM

Areas of Study Nursing education.

CONTINUING EDUCATION PROGRAM

Contact Dr. Susan H. Diehl, Associate Professor, Department of Health Sciences and Nursing, College of Education, Nursing, and Health Professions, University of Hartford, 200 Bloomfield Avenue, West Hartford, CT 06117-1599. *Telephone:* 860-768-4214. *Fax:* 860-768-5346. *E-mail:* diehl@hartford.edu.

University of Saint Joseph
Department of Nursing
West Hartford, Connecticut

http://www.usj.edu/
Founded in 1932

DEGREES • BS • MS
Nursing Program Faculty 23 (44% with doctorates).
Baccalaureate Enrollment 250 **Women** 100% **Minority** 21% **International** 4% **Part-time** 38%
Graduate Enrollment 120 **Women** 92% **Men** 8% **Minority** 35% **International** 1% **Part-time** 66%
Distance Learning Courses Available.
Nursing Student Activities Sigma Theta Tau, Student Nurses' Association, nursing club.
Nursing Student Resources Academic advising; academic or career counseling; assistance for students with disabilities; bookstore; campus computer network; career placement assistance; computer lab; computer-assisted instruction; daycare for children of students; e-mail services; employment services for current students; externships; housing assistance; interactive nursing skills videos; Internet; learning resource lab; library services; nursing audiovisuals; paid internships; placement services for program completers; remedial services; resume preparation assistance; skills, simulation, or other laboratory; tutoring; unpaid internships.
Library Facilities 7,058 volumes in health, 1,949 volumes in nursing; 1,495 periodical subscriptions health-care related.

BACCALAUREATE PROGRAMS

Degree BS
Available Programs Baccalaureate for Second Degree; Generic Baccalaureate; RN Baccalaureate.
Site Options Middletown, CT.
Study Options Full-time.
Program Entrance Requirements Minimum overall college GPA of 2.8, transcript of college record, CPR certification, written essay, health exam, health insurance, high school biology, high school chemistry, high school transcript, immunizations, minimum high school GPA, minimum GPA in nursing prerequisites of 2.8, prerequisite course work. Transfer students are accepted. *Application deadline:* 4/1 (fall), 12/1 (spring). Applications may be processed on a rolling basis for some programs. *Application fee:* $50.
Advanced Placement Credit given for nursing courses completed elsewhere dependent upon specific evaluations.
Financial Aid 85% of baccalaureate students in nursing programs received some form of financial aid in 2010–11. *Gift aid (need-based):* Federal Pell, FSEOG, state, private, college/university gift aid from institutional funds. *Loans:* Federal Direct (Subsidized and Unsubsidized Stafford PLUS), Perkins, state, private loans.*Work-study:* part-time campus jobs.*Financial aid application deadline (priority):* 2/15.
Contact Dr. Kim Joerg, Undergraduate Program Director, Department of Nursing, University of Saint Joseph, 1678 Asylum Avenue, West Hartford, CT 06117-2700. *Telephone:* 860-231-5304. *E-mail:* kjoerg@sjc.edu.

GRADUATE PROGRAMS

Expenses (2011–12) *Required fees:* part-time $650 per credit.
Financial Aid 75% of graduate students in nursing programs received some form of financial aid in 2010–11.
Contact Dr. Pamela Aselton, Graduate Program Director, Department of Nursing, University of Saint Joseph, 1678 Asylum Avenue, West Hartford, CT 06117-2700. *Telephone:* 860-231-5352. *Fax:* 860-231-8396. *E-mail:* paselton@sjc.edu.

MASTER'S DEGREE PROGRAM

Degree MS
Available Programs Master's; Master's for Nurses with Non-Nursing Degrees.

Concentrations Available Nursing education. *Nurse practitioner programs in:* family health, psychiatric/mental health.
Site Options Middletown, CT.
Study Options Full-time and part-time.
Program Entrance Requirements Clinical experience, minimum overall college GPA of 3.0, transcript of college record, CPR certification, written essay, immunizations, interview, 2 letters of recommendation, professional liability insurance/malpractice insurance, resume. *Application deadline:* Applications may be processed on a rolling basis for some programs. *Application fee:* $50.
Advanced Placement Credit given for nursing courses completed elsewhere dependent upon specific evaluations.
Degree Requirements 44 total credit hours, comprehensive exam.

POST-MASTER'S PROGRAM

Areas of Study *Nurse practitioner programs in:* psychiatric/mental health.

Western Connecticut State University
Department of Nursing
Danbury, Connecticut

http://www.wcsu.edu/
Founded in 1903

DEGREES • BS • MS
Nursing Program Faculty 18 (50% with doctorates).
Baccalaureate Enrollment 160 **Women** 95% **Men** 5% **Minority** 20%
Graduate Enrollment 35 **Women** 100% **Minority** 2% **Part-time** 100%
Distance Learning Courses Available.
Nursing Student Activities Sigma Theta Tau, Student Nurses' Association.
Nursing Student Resources Academic advising; academic or career counseling; assistance for students with disabilities; bookstore; campus computer network; career placement assistance; computer lab; computer-assisted instruction; daycare for children of students; e-mail services; employment services for current students; externships; housing assistance; interactive nursing skills videos; Internet; learning resource lab; library services; nursing audiovisuals; paid internships; remedial services; resume preparation assistance; skills, simulation, or other laboratory; tutoring.

BACCALAUREATE PROGRAMS

Degree BS
Available Programs Generic Baccalaureate; RN Baccalaureate.
Site Options Waterbury, CT.
Study Options Full-time.
Program Entrance Requirements Minimum overall college GPA of 2.5, transcript of college record, CPR certification, health exam, health insurance, high school biology, high school chemistry, high school foreign language, 3 years high school math, 2 years high school science, high school transcript, immunizations, minimum GPA in nursing prerequisites of 2.5, prerequisite course work. Transfer students are accepted. *Application deadline:* Applications may be processed on a rolling basis for some programs. *Application fee:* $60.
Advanced Placement Credit by examination available. Credit given for nursing courses completed elsewhere dependent upon specific evaluations.
Contact *Telephone:* 203-837-8556. *Fax:* 203-837-8550.

GRADUATE PROGRAMS

Contact *Telephone:* 203-837-8556. *Fax:* 203-837-8550.

MASTER'S DEGREE PROGRAM

Degree MS
Available Programs Master's.
Concentrations Available *Clinical nurse specialist programs in:* adult health. *Nurse practitioner programs in:* adult health.
Study Options Part-time.
Program Entrance Requirements Clinical experience, computer literacy, minimum overall college GPA of 3.0, transcript of college record, CPR certification, immunizations, interview, 2 letters of recommendation, nursing research course, physical assessment course, professional liability insurance/malpractice insurance, prerequisite course work,

resume, statistics course. *Application deadline:* Applications may be processed on a rolling basis for some programs. *Application fee:* $60.

Advanced Placement Credit by examination available. Credit given for nursing courses completed elsewhere dependent upon specific evaluations.

Degree Requirements 36 total credit hours, thesis or project.

POST-MASTER'S PROGRAM

Areas of Study *Clinical nurse specialist programs in:* adult health. *Nurse practitioner programs in:* adult health.

Yale University
School of Nursing
New Haven, Connecticut

http://www.nursing.yale.edu/
Founded in 1701

DEGREES • DNP • MSN • MSN/MDIV • MSN/MPH • PHD

Nursing Program Faculty 42 (70% with doctorates).
Graduate Enrollment 349 **Women** 89% **Men** 11% **Minority** 24%
International 5% **Part-time** 19%
Distance Learning Courses Available.
Nursing Student Activities Nursing Honor Society, Sigma Theta Tau.
Nursing Student Resources Academic advising; academic or career counseling; assistance for students with disabilities; bookstore; campus computer network; career placement assistance; computer lab; computer-assisted instruction; daycare for children of students; e-mail services; employment services for current students; housing assistance; interactive nursing skills videos; Internet; learning resource lab; library services; nursing audiovisuals; placement services for program completers; remedial services; resume preparation assistance; skills, simulation, or other laboratory; tutoring; unpaid internships.
Library Facilities 400,000 volumes in health; 2,900 periodical subscriptions health-care related.

GRADUATE PROGRAMS

Financial Aid 90% of graduate students in nursing programs received some form of financial aid in 2011–12. 239 fellowships (averaging $5,905 per year), 13 research assistantships with tuition reimbursements available (averaging $28,450 per year) were awarded; Federal Work-Study, scholarships, and traineeships also available. Aid available to part-time students. *Financial aid application deadline:* 2/1.
Contact Ms. Melissa Pucci, Director of Admissions, School of Nursing, Yale University, PO Box 9740, New Haven, CT 06536-0740. *Telephone:* 203-737-1793. *Fax:* 203-737-5409. *E-mail:* melissa.pucci@yale.edu.

MASTER'S DEGREE PROGRAM

Degrees MSN; MSN/MDIV; MSN/MPH
Available Programs Master's; Master's for Non-Nursing College Graduates; Master's for Nurses with Non-Nursing Degrees.
Concentrations Available Nurse-midwifery; nursing administration. *Nurse practitioner programs in:* acute care, family health, pediatric, psychiatric/mental health.
Study Options Full-time.
Online Degree Options Yes.
Program Entrance Requirements Minimum overall college GPA of 3.0, transcript of college record, CPR certification, written essay, immunizations, interview, 3 letters of recommendation, resume, GRE General Test. *Application deadline:* 11/1 (fall). *Application fee:* $100.
Advanced Placement Credit by examination available. Credit given for nursing courses completed elsewhere dependent upon specific evaluations.
Degree Requirements 40 total credit hours.

POST-MASTER'S PROGRAM

Areas of Study *Nurse practitioner programs in:* acute care, family health, pediatric, psychiatric/mental health.

DOCTORAL DEGREE PROGRAM

Degree DNP
Available Programs Doctorate.
Areas of Study Health policy, health-care systems, nursing administration, nursing policy.
Online Degree Options Yes (online only).

Program Entrance Requirements Clinical experience, minimum overall college GPA of 3.0, interview by faculty committee, interview, 3 letters of recommendation, MSN or equivalent, vita, GRE General Test. *Application deadline:* 3/1 (fall). *Application fee:* $100.
Degree Requirements 40 total credit hours.

DOCTORAL DEGREE PROGRAM

Degree PhD
Available Programs Doctorate.
Areas of Study Aging, critical care, family health, gerontology, health policy, health promotion/disease prevention, health-care systems, human health and illness, maternity-newborn, neuro-behavior, nursing policy, nursing research, oncology.
Program Entrance Requirements Minimum overall college GPA of 3.0, clinical experience, interview, interview by faculty committee, 3 letters of recommendation, MSN or equivalent, statistics course, vita, writing sample. *Application deadline:* 1/2 (fall). *Application fee:* $100.
Degree Requirements 60 total credit hours, dissertation, oral exam, written exam.

POSTDOCTORAL PROGRAM

Areas of Study Adolescent health, chronic illness.
Postdoctoral Program Contact Ms. Sarah Zaino, Assistant Director, Research Activities, School of Nursing, Yale University, PO Box 9740, New Haven, CT 06536-0740. *Telephone:* 203-737-2420. *Fax:* 203-737-4480. *E-mail:* sarah.zaino@yale.edu.

DELAWARE

Delaware State University
Department of Nursing
Dover, Delaware

http://www.desu.edu/department-nursing
Founded in 1891

DEGREES • BSN • MS

Nursing Program Faculty 11
Baccalaureate Enrollment 72 **Women** 93% **Men** 7%
Nursing Student Activities Sigma Theta Tau, Student Nurses' Association.
Nursing Student Resources Academic advising; assistance for students with disabilities; bookstore; campus computer network; computer lab; daycare for children of students; e-mail services; interactive nursing skills videos; library services; nursing audiovisuals; skills, simulation, or other laboratory.
Library Facilities 190,613 volumes; 74,881 periodical subscriptions.

BACCALAUREATE PROGRAMS

Degree BSN
Available Programs Generic Baccalaureate; LPN to Baccalaureate; RN Baccalaureate.
Study Options Full-time and part-time.
Program Entrance Requirements CPR certification, health exam, high school biology, high school chemistry, high school transcript, immunizations, minimum high school GPA of 2.0, professional liability insurance/malpractice insurance, prerequisite course work. Transfer students are accepted. *Application deadline:* 2/25 (winter).
Expenses (2011–12) *Tuition, state resident:* full-time $7056; part-time $260 per credit hour. *Tuition, nonresident:* full-time $15,052; part-time $593 per credit hour. *International tuition:* $15,052 full-time. *Room and board:* $10,620; room only: $7168 per academic year. *Required fees:* full-time $200; part-time $100 per term.
Financial Aid 75% of baccalaureate students in nursing programs received some form of financial aid in 2010–11. *Gift aid (need-based):* Federal Pell, FSEOG, state, Federal Nursing. *Loans:* Federal Nursing Student Loans, Perkins. *Work-study:* Federal Work-Study, part-time campus jobs.
Contact Dr. Bernardine Lacey, Interim Chairperson, Department of Nursing, Delaware State University, 1200 North DuPont Highway, Dover, DE 19901-2277. *Telephone:* 302-857-6700. *E-mail:* blacey@desu.edu.

GRADUATE PROGRAMS

Expenses (2011–12) *Tuition, state resident:* full-time $3591; part-time $399 per credit hour. *Tuition, nonresident:* full-time $7920; part-time $880 per credit hour. *Room and board:* $10,740; room only: $7168 per academic year. *Required fees:* full-time $230; part-time $115 per term.
Financial Aid 100% of graduate students in nursing programs received some form of financial aid in 2010–11.
Contact Dr. Bernardine Lacey, Interim Chairperson, Department of Nursing, Delaware State University, 1200 DuPont Highway, Dover, DE 19901. *Telephone:* 302-857-6700. *E-mail:* blacey@desu.edu.

MASTER'S DEGREE PROGRAM

Degree MS
Available Programs Master's.
Concentrations Available Nursing education. *Clinical nurse specialist programs in:* public health.
Study Options Full-time.
Program Entrance Requirements Clinical experience, minimum overall college GPA of 3.0, transcript of college record, CPR certification, written essay, immunizations, 3 letters of recommendation, professional liability insurance/malpractice insurance, resume. *Application deadline:* 2/1 (winter). *Application fee:* $35.
Advanced Placement Credit given for nursing courses completed elsewhere dependent upon specific evaluations.
Degree Requirements 39 total credit hours, thesis or project.

University of Delaware
School of Nursing
Newark, Delaware

http://www.udel.edu/nursing/
Founded in 1743
DEGREES • BSN • MSN • PHD
Nursing Program Faculty 37 (70% with doctorates).
Baccalaureate Enrollment 579 **Women** 93% **Men** 7% **Minority** 23% **International** 1% **Part-time** 21%
Graduate Enrollment 180 **Women** 90% **Men** 10% **Minority** 26% **Part-time** 74%
Distance Learning Courses Available.
Nursing Student Activities Sigma Theta Tau, Student Nurses' Association.
Nursing Student Resources Academic advising; academic or career counseling; assistance for students with disabilities; bookstore; campus computer network; career placement assistance; computer lab; computer-assisted instruction; e-mail services; employment services for current students; externships; housing assistance; interactive nursing skills videos; Internet; learning resource lab; library services; nursing audiovisuals; paid internships; resume preparation assistance; skills, simulation, or other laboratory; tutoring.
Library Facilities 2.8 million volumes (2.7 million in health, 40,000 in nursing); 42,000 periodical subscriptions (240 health-care related).

BACCALAUREATE PROGRAMS

Degree BSN
Available Programs Accelerated Baccalaureate for Second Degree; Generic Baccalaureate; RN Baccalaureate.
Study Options Full-time.
Online Degree Options Yes.
Program Entrance Requirements Written essay, high school biology, high school chemistry, high school foreign language, 3 years high school math, 4 years high school science, high school transcript, 1 letter of recommendation, minimum high school GPA of 3.0. *Application deadline:* 1/15 (fall). *Application fee:* $75.
Advanced Placement Credit given for nursing courses completed elsewhere dependent upon specific evaluations.
Expenses (2012–13) *Tuition, state resident:* full-time $10,150; part-time $423 per credit. *Tuition, nonresident:* full-time $27,240; part-time $1135 per credit. *Room and board:* $10,758; room only: $6516 per academic year. *Required fees:* full-time $1652; part-time $160 per term.
Financial Aid 71% of baccalaureate students in nursing programs received some form of financial aid in 2011–12. *Gift aid (need-based):* Federal Pell, FSEOG, state, private, college/university gift aid from institutional funds. *Loans:* Federal Nursing Student Loans, Federal Direct (Subsidized and Unsubsidized Stafford PLUS), Perkins.*Work-study:* Federal Work-Study, part-time campus jobs.*Financial aid application deadline:* 3/15(priority: 2/1).

Contact Ms. Anne DeCaire, Nursing Recruiter, School of Nursing, University of Delaware, 385 McDowell Hall, Newark, DE 19716. *Telephone:* 302-831-0442. *Fax:* 302-831-2382. *E-mail:* aderb@udel.edu.

GRADUATE PROGRAMS

Expenses (2012–13) *Tuition, state resident:* full-time $12,258; part-time $681 per credit. *Tuition, nonresident:* full-time $12,258; part-time $681 per credit. *Required fees:* part-time $60 per term.
Financial Aid 90% of graduate students in nursing programs received some form of financial aid in 2011–12. Research assistantships with tuition reimbursements available (averaging $15,000 per year); scholarships, traineeships, tuition waivers (full), and unspecified assistantships also available. Aid available to part-time students.. *Financial aid application deadline:* 7/1.
Contact Ms. Joanne Marra, Office Coordinator, School of Nursing, University of Delaware, 349 McDowell Hall, Newark, DE 19716. *Telephone:* 302-831-8386. *Fax:* 302-831-2382. *E-mail:* udgradnursing@udel.edu.

MASTER'S DEGREE PROGRAM

Degree MSN
Available Programs Master's; RN to Master's.
Concentrations Available Health-care administration. *Clinical nurse specialist programs in:* adult health, pediatric. *Nurse practitioner programs in:* adult health, family health.
Study Options Full-time and part-time.
Online Degree Options Yes.
Program Entrance Requirements Clinical experience, minimum overall college GPA of 3.0, transcript of college record, CPR certification, written essay, immunizations, interview, 3 letters of recommendation, resume. *Application deadline:* 3/1 (fall), 10/1 (spring). *Application fee:* $75.
Advanced Placement Credit given for nursing courses completed elsewhere dependent upon specific evaluations.
Degree Requirements 46 total credit hours.

POST-MASTER'S PROGRAM

Areas of Study Health-care administration. *Clinical nurse specialist programs in:* adult health, pediatric. *Nurse practitioner programs in:* adult health, family health.

DOCTORAL DEGREE PROGRAM

Degree PhD
Available Programs Doctorate.
Areas of Study Advanced practice nursing, aging, bio-behavioral research, community health, faculty preparation, gerontology, health policy, health promotion/disease prevention, illness and transition, individualized study, nursing education, nursing research, nursing science, oncology.
Program Entrance Requirements Clinical experience, minimum overall college GPA of 3.5, interview by faculty committee, 3 letters of recommendation, MSN or equivalent, statistics course, vita, writing sample. *Application deadline:* 2/1 (fall). *Application fee:* $75.
Degree Requirements 50 total credit hours, dissertation, oral exam, written exam, residency.

CONTINUING EDUCATION PROGRAM

Contact Dr. Dayle Thorpe, Division of Professional and Continuing Studies, School of Nursing, University of Delaware, 201 Clayton Hall, Newark, DE 19716. *Telephone:* 302-831-7600. *Fax:* 302-831-0701. *E-mail:* continuing-ed@udel.edu.

Wesley College
Nursing Program
Dover, Delaware

http://www.wesley.edu/
Founded in 1873
DEGREES • BSN • MSN
Nursing Program Faculty 12 (80% with doctorates).
Baccalaureate Enrollment 210 **Women** 85% **Men** 15% **Minority** 35% **International** 1% **Part-time** 2%
Graduate Enrollment 87 **Women** 90% **Men** 10% **Minority** 25% **Part-time** 10%
Distance Learning Courses Available.

Nursing Student Activities Sigma Theta Tau, Student Nurses' Association.

Nursing Student Resources Academic advising; academic or career counseling; assistance for students with disabilities; bookstore; campus computer network; career placement assistance; computer lab; computer-assisted instruction; e-mail services; employment services for current students; externships; housing assistance; interactive nursing skills videos; Internet; learning resource lab; library services; nursing audiovisuals; placement services for program completers; remedial services; resume preparation assistance; skills, simulation, or other laboratory; tutoring; unpaid internships.

Library Facilities 104,636 volumes (15,000 in health, 1,500 in nursing); 252 periodical subscriptions (40 health-care related).

BACCALAUREATE PROGRAMS

Degree BSN

Available Programs Generic Baccalaureate; International Nurse to Baccalaureate; LPN to Baccalaureate.

Study Options Full-time and part-time.

Program Entrance Requirements Minimum overall college GPA of 2.75, transcript of college record, CPR certification, written essay, health exam, health insurance, high school biology, high school chemistry, 2 years high school math, 2 years high school science, high school transcript, immunizations, minimum high school GPA of 2.75, minimum GPA in nursing prerequisites of 2.5, professional liability insurance/malpractice insurance. Transfer students are accepted. *Application deadline:* Applications may be processed on a rolling basis for some programs. *Application fee:* $25.

Advanced Placement Credit by examination available. Credit given for nursing courses completed elsewhere dependent upon specific evaluations.

Expenses (2011–12) *Tuition:* full-time $19,700; part-time $835 per credit. *International tuition:* $19,700 full-time. *Room and board:* $9500; room only: $4750 per academic year. *Required fees:* full-time $150; part-time $50 per term.

Financial Aid 90% of baccalaureate students in nursing programs received some form of financial aid in 2010–11. *Gift aid (need-based):* Federal Pell, FSEOG, state, private, college/university gift aid from institutional funds. *Loans:* Federal Direct (Subsidized and Unsubsidized Stafford PLUS), Perkins, state, college/university. *Work-study:* Federal Work-Study, part-time campus jobs. *Financial aid application deadline (priority):* 4/15.

Contact Dr. Karen Panunto, Program Director, Nursing Program, Wesley College, 120 North State Street, Dulany Hall, Dover, DE 19901. *Telephone:* 302-736-2511. *Fax:* 302-736-2548. *E-mail:* panuntka@wesley.edu.

GRADUATE PROGRAMS

Expenses (2011–12) *Tuition:* part-time $475 per credit. *International tuition:* $475 full-time. *Required fees:* full-time $150.

Financial Aid 100% of graduate students in nursing programs received some form of financial aid in 2010–11. Traineeships available.

Contact Dr. Lucille C. Gambardella, Chairperson, Nursing Program, Wesley College, 120 North State Street, Dover, DE 19901. *Telephone:* 302-736-2512. *Fax:* 302-736-2548. *E-mail:* gambarlu@wesley.edu.

MASTER'S DEGREE PROGRAM

Degree MSN

Available Programs Accelerated AD/RN to Master's; Accelerated RN to Master's; Master's; RN to Master's.

Concentrations Available *Clinical nurse specialist programs in:* community health, women's health. *Nurse practitioner programs in:* women's health.

Site Options New Castle, DE.

Study Options Full-time and part-time.

Program Entrance Requirements Clinical experience, computer literacy, minimum overall college GPA of 3.0, transcript of college record, interview, 2 letters of recommendation, professional liability insurance/malpractice insurance, resume, statistics course, GRE or MAT. *Application deadline:* Applications may be processed on a rolling basis for some programs. *Application fee:* $35.

Advanced Placement Credit by examination available. Credit given for nursing courses completed elsewhere dependent upon specific evaluations.

Degree Requirements 39 total credit hours, thesis or project.

POST-MASTER'S PROGRAM

Areas of Study Nursing education. *Clinical nurse specialist programs in:* women's health.

CONTINUING EDUCATION PROGRAM

Contact Dr. Lucille C. Gambardella, Chair, Department of Nursing/Director, Graduate Programs, Nursing Program, Wesley College, 120 North State Street, Dover, DE 19901. *Telephone:* 302-736-2512. *Fax:* 302-736-2548. *E-mail:* gambarlu@wesley.edu.

Wilmington University
College of Health Professions
New Castle, Delaware

http://www.wilmu.edu/health/index.aspx
Founded in 1967

DEGREES • BSN • MSN • MSN/MBA • MSN/MS

Nursing Program Faculty 13 (50% with doctorates).

Baccalaureate Enrollment 620 **Women** 95% **Men** 5% **Minority** 8% **Part-time** 88%

Graduate Enrollment 253 **Women** 97% **Men** 3% **Minority** 11% **Part-time** 50%

Distance Learning Courses Available.

Nursing Student Activities Sigma Theta Tau.

Nursing Student Resources Academic advising; academic or career counseling; assistance for students with disabilities; bookstore; campus computer network; career placement assistance; computer lab; computer-assisted instruction; e-mail services; employment services for current students; housing assistance; interactive nursing skills videos; learning resource lab; library services; nursing audiovisuals; remedial services; resume preparation assistance; skills, simulation, or other laboratory; tutoring.

Library Facilities 98,713 volumes (6,000 in health, 3,500 in nursing); 425 periodical subscriptions (60 health-care related).

BACCALAUREATE PROGRAMS

Degree BSN

Available Programs Accelerated RN Baccalaureate; International Nurse to Baccalaureate; RN Baccalaureate.

Site Options Georgetown, DE; New Castle, DE; Dover, DE.

Online Degree Options Yes.

Program Entrance Requirements Transfer students are accepted. *Application deadline:* 8/31 (fall), 1/1 (spring), 5/1 (summer). Applications may be processed on a rolling basis for some programs. *Application fee:* $35.

Expenses (2011–12) *Tuition:* part-time $314 per credit.

Financial Aid 60% of baccalaureate students in nursing programs received some form of financial aid in 2010–11.

Contact Ms. Denise Westbrook, BSN Program Chair, College of Health Professions, Wilmington University, 320 North DuPont Highway, New Castle, DE 19720. *Telephone:* 302-356-6915. *Fax:* 302-322-7081. *E-mail:* denise.z.westbrook@wilmu.edu.

GRADUATE PROGRAMS

Expenses (2011–12) *Tuition:* part-time $404 per credit. *Required fees:* part-time $100 per term.

Financial Aid 65% of graduate students in nursing programs received some form of financial aid in 2010–11. Fellowships with tuition reimbursements available, traineeships available.

Contact Ms. Misty Williams, Admissions Associate, College of Health Professions, Wilmington University, Wilson Graduate Center, 31 Read's Way, New Castle, DE 19720. *Telephone:* 302-295-1121. *E-mail:* misty.b.williams@wilmu.edu.

MASTER'S DEGREE PROGRAM

Degrees MSN; MSN/MBA; MSN/MS

Available Programs Accelerated AD/RN to Master's; Accelerated Master's for Nurses with Non-Nursing Degrees; Master's.

Concentrations Available Legal nurse consultant; nursing administration; nursing education. *Nurse practitioner programs in:* adult health, family health, gerontology.

Site Options Georgetown, DE; New Castle, DE.

Study Options Full-time and part-time.

Online Degree Options Yes.

Program Entrance Requirements Minimum overall college GPA of 3.0, transcript of college record, prerequisite course work. *Application deadline:* Applications may be processed on a rolling basis for some programs. *Application fee:* $35.

Advanced Placement Credit given for nursing courses completed elsewhere dependent upon specific evaluations.
Degree Requirements 36 total credit hours, thesis or project.

POST-MASTER'S PROGRAM

Areas of Study Legal nurse consultant; nursing administration; nursing education. *Nurse practitioner programs in:* adult health, family health, gerontology.

DISTRICT OF COLUMBIA

The Catholic University of America
School of Nursing
Washington, District of Columbia

http://nursing.cua.edu/
Founded in 1887
DEGREES • BSN • MA/MSM • MSN • PHD
Nursing Program Faculty 47 (43% with doctorates).
Baccalaureate Enrollment 286 **Women** 94% **Men** 6% **Minority** 16% **International** 1% **Part-time** 1%
Graduate Enrollment 102 **Women** 96% **Men** 4% **Minority** 35% **International** 1% **Part-time** 69%
Distance Learning Courses Available.
Nursing Student Activities Nursing Honor Society, Sigma Theta Tau, Student Nurses' Association, nursing club.
Nursing Student Resources Academic advising; academic or career counseling; assistance for students with disabilities; bookstore; campus computer network; career placement assistance; computer lab; computer-assisted instruction; e-mail services; interactive nursing skills videos; Internet; learning resource lab; library services; nursing audiovisuals; remedial services; resume preparation assistance; skills, simulation, or other laboratory; tutoring.
Library Facilities 1.6 million volumes (39,000 in health, 17,500 in nursing); 10,665 periodical subscriptions (250 health-care related).

BACCALAUREATE PROGRAMS

Degree BSN
Available Programs Accelerated Baccalaureate; Accelerated Baccalaureate for Second Degree; Generic Baccalaureate.
Study Options Full-time and part-time.
Program Entrance Requirements Minimum overall college GPA of 3.0, transcript of college record, written essay, health exam, health insurance, high school chemistry, 3 years high school math, high school transcript, immunizations, 1 letter of recommendation, minimum high school GPA of 3.0, minimum GPA in nursing prerequisites of 2.75, prerequisite course work. *Application deadline:* 7/15 (fall), 11/15 (spring), 2/28 (summer). *Application fee:* $55.
Expenses (2011–12) *Tuition:* full-time $35,260; part-time $1380 per credit hour. *International tuition:* $35,260 full-time. *Room and board:* room only: $8676 per academic year. *Required fees:* full-time $200; part-time $50 per term.
Financial Aid 50% of baccalaureate students in nursing programs received some form of financial aid in 2010–11.
Contact Ms. Lynn Doyle, Administrative Assistant, School of Nursing, The Catholic University of America, 124 Gowan Hall, 620 Michigan Avenue NE, Washington, DC 20064. *Telephone:* 202-319-6457. *Fax:* 202-319-6485. *E-mail:* doyle@cua.edu.

GRADUATE PROGRAMS

Expenses (2011–12) *Tuition:* full-time $35,260; part-time $1380 per credit hour. *International tuition:* $35,260 full-time. *Required fees:* full-time $80.
Financial Aid 80% of graduate students in nursing programs received some form of financial aid in 2010–11. Fellowships, research assistantships, teaching assistantships, Federal Work-Study, scholarships, tuition waivers (full and partial), and unspecified assistantships available. *Financial aid application deadline:* 2/1.
Contact Jacqueline Tintle, Administrative Assistant, School of Nursing, The Catholic University of America, 118 Gowan Hall, Washington, DC

20064. *Telephone:* 202-319-5403. *Fax:* 202-319-5403. *E-mail:* tintlej@cua.edu.

MASTER'S DEGREE PROGRAM

Degrees MA/MSM; MSN
Available Programs Master's.
Concentrations Available *Clinical nurse specialist programs in:* adult health, community health. *Nurse practitioner programs in:* acute care, adult health, family health, pediatric.
Site Options Washington, DC.
Study Options Full-time and part-time.
Program Entrance Requirements Clinical experience, minimum overall college GPA of 3.0, transcript of college record, written essay, immunizations, 3 letters of recommendation, professional liability insurance/malpractice insurance, prerequisite course work, statistics course, GRE General Test. *Application deadline:* 8/1 (fall), 12/1 (spring). Applications may be processed on a rolling basis for some programs. *Application fee:* $55.
Advanced Placement Credit given for nursing courses completed elsewhere dependent upon specific evaluations.
Degree Requirements 44 total credit hours, comprehensive exam.

POST-MASTER'S PROGRAM

Areas of Study *Clinical nurse specialist programs in:* adult health, community health. *Nurse practitioner programs in:* acute care, adult health, family health, pediatric.

DOCTORAL DEGREE PROGRAM

Degree PhD
Available Programs Doctorate; Post-Baccalaureate Doctorate.
Areas of Study Advanced practice nursing, clinical practice, community health, ethics, gerontology, human health and illness, nursing research, nursing science, women's health.
Online Degree Options Yes.
Program Entrance Requirements Clinical experience, minimum overall college GPA of 3.5, interview by faculty committee, interview, 3 letters of recommendation, MSN or equivalent, scholarly papers, statistics course, writing sample, GRE General Test. *Application deadline:* 8/1 (fall), 12/1 (spring). Applications may be processed on a rolling basis for some programs. *Application fee:* $55.
Degree Requirements 70 total credit hours, dissertation, oral exam, written exam, residency.

Georgetown University
School of Nursing and Health Studies
Washington, District of Columbia

http://nhs.georgetown.edu/
Founded in 1789
DEGREES • BSN • MS
Nursing Program Faculty 77 (35% with doctorates).
Baccalaureate Enrollment 480 **Women** 85% **Men** 15% **Minority** 26% **International** 1% **Part-time** 2%
Graduate Enrollment 235 **Women** 73% **Men** 27% **Minority** 24% **International** 1% **Part-time** 20%
Nursing Student Activities Nursing Honor Society, Sigma Theta Tau, Student Nurses' Association.
Nursing Student Resources Academic advising; academic or career counseling; assistance for students with disabilities; bookstore; campus computer network; career placement assistance; computer lab; computer-assisted instruction; e-mail services; employment services for current students; housing assistance; interactive nursing skills videos; Internet; learning resource lab; library services; nursing audiovisuals; placement services for program completers; resume preparation assistance; skills, simulation, or other laboratory; tutoring; unpaid internships.
Library Facilities 36,000 volumes in health, 20,000 volumes in nursing; 92 periodical subscriptions health-care related.

BACCALAUREATE PROGRAMS

Degree BSN
Available Programs Accelerated Baccalaureate for Second Degree; Generic Baccalaureate.
Study Options Full-time.
Program Entrance Requirements CPR certification, written essay, health exam, health insurance, 3 years high school math, 4 years high school science, high school transcript, immunizations, interview, 2 letters

of recommendation. Transfer students are accepted. *Application deadline:* 1/10 (fall). *Application fee:* $65.
Contact *Telephone:* 202-687-3600.

GRADUATE PROGRAMS

Contact *Telephone:* 202-687-5568.

MASTER'S DEGREE PROGRAM
Degree MS
Available Programs Master's; Master's for Non-Nursing College Graduates.
Concentrations Available Health-care administration; nurse anesthesia; nurse-midwifery; nursing education. *Clinical nurse specialist programs in:* acute care, critical care. *Nurse practitioner programs in:* acute care, family health, women's health.
Study Options Full-time and part-time.
Program Entrance Requirements Clinical experience, minimum overall college GPA of 3.0, transcript of college record, CPR certification, written essay, immunizations, interview, 3 letters of recommendation, resume, statistics course, GRE General Test or MAT. *Application deadline:* 1/15 (fall). Applications may be processed on a rolling basis for some programs. *Application fee:* $75.
Advanced Placement Credit given for nursing courses completed elsewhere dependent upon specific evaluations.
Degree Requirements 40 total credit hours, thesis or project.

POST-MASTER'S PROGRAM
Areas of Study Nurse-midwifery; nursing education. *Clinical nurse specialist programs in:* acute care, critical care. *Nurse practitioner programs in:* acute care, family health, women's health.

The George Washington University
School of Nursing
Washington, District of Columbia

Founded in 1821
DEGREES • BSN • DNP • MSN
Distance Learning Courses Available.
Nursing Student Activities Sigma Theta Tau.
Nursing Student Resources Academic advising; academic or career counseling; bookstore; campus computer network; computer lab; computer-assisted instruction; e-mail services; interactive nursing skills videos; Internet; learning resource lab; library services; nursing audiovisuals; skills, simulation, or other laboratory.

BACCALAUREATE PROGRAMS

Degree BSN
Available Programs Accelerated Baccalaureate for Second Degree.
Study Options Full-time.
Program Entrance Requirements Minimum overall college GPA of 2.8, transcript of college record, CPR certification, written essay, health exam, health insurance, immunizations, 2 letters of recommendation, minimum GPA in nursing prerequisites of 3.0, prerequisite course work. *Application deadline:* 6/15 (fall). *Application fee:* $60.
Contact *Telephone:* 202-994-7901. *Fax:* 202-994-2777.

GRADUATE PROGRAMS

Contact *Telephone:* 202-994-7901. *Fax:* 202-994-2777.

MASTER'S DEGREE PROGRAM
Degree MSN
Available Programs Master's.
Concentrations Available Clinical nurse leader; health-care administration; nursing administration. *Nurse practitioner programs in:* adult health, family health.

POST-MASTER'S PROGRAM
Areas of Study *Nurse practitioner programs in:* adult health, family health.

DOCTORAL DEGREE PROGRAM
Degree DNP
Available Programs Doctorate.

Howard University
Division of Nursing
Washington, District of Columbia

http://www.cpnahs.howard.edu
Founded in 1867
DEGREES • BSN • MSN
Nursing Program Faculty 26 (54% with doctorates).
Baccalaureate Enrollment 262 **Women** 92% **Men** 8% **Minority** 99.3%
International 3% **Part-time** 34%
Graduate Enrollment 43 **Women** 86% **Men** 14% **Minority** 100%
International 7% **Part-time** 52%
Distance Learning Courses Available.
Nursing Student Activities Nursing Honor Society, Sigma Theta Tau, Student Nurses' Association, nursing club.
Nursing Student Resources Academic advising; academic or career counseling; assistance for students with disabilities; bookstore; campus computer network; career placement assistance; computer lab; computer-assisted instruction; e-mail services; externships; housing assistance; interactive nursing skills videos; Internet; learning resource lab; library services; nursing audiovisuals; paid internships; placement services for program completers; remedial services; resume preparation assistance; skills, simulation, or other laboratory; tutoring.
Library Facilities 2.5 million volumes (219,448 in health, 4,500 in nursing); 26,382 periodical subscriptions (5,247 health-care related).

BACCALAUREATE PROGRAMS

Degree BSN
Available Programs Generic Baccalaureate; LPN to Baccalaureate; RN Baccalaureate.
Study Options Full-time and part-time.
Online Degree Options Yes (online only).
Program Entrance Requirements Minimum overall college GPA of 2.8, transcript of college record, written essay, health exam, high school biology, high school chemistry, high school foreign language, 3 years high school math, 2 years high school science, high school transcript, immunizations, 2 letters of recommendation, minimum high school GPA of 2.5, minimum high school rank 50%, minimum GPA in nursing prerequisites of 2.5, prerequisite course work. Transfer students are accepted. *Application deadline:* 2/15 (fall), 11/1 (spring), 4/1 (summer). *Application fee:* $45.
Expenses (2012–13) *Tuition:* full-time $21,450; part-time $895 per credit hour. *International tuition:* $21,450 full-time. *Room and board:* $11,000; room only: $8000 per academic year. *Required fees:* full-time $1633; part-time $817 per term.
Financial Aid 92% of baccalaureate students in nursing programs received some form of financial aid in 2011–12. *Gift aid (need-based):* Federal Pell, FSEOG, state, private, college/university gift aid from institutional funds, Federal Nursing. *Loans:* Federal Nursing Student Loans, Federal Direct (Subsidized and Unsubsidized Stafford PLUS), Perkins, state, college/university.*Work-study:* Federal Work-Study, part-time campus jobs.*Financial aid application deadline:* 8/15(priority: 2/1).
Contact Miss Melissa L. Weir, Interim Chairperson, Undergraduate Program, Division of Nursing, Howard University, 516 Bryant Street NW, Annex 1, Washington, DC 20059. *Telephone:* 202-806-7854. *Fax:* 202-806-5085. *E-mail:* melissa.weir@howard.edu.

GRADUATE PROGRAMS

Expenses (2012–13) *Tuition:* full-time $29,090; part-time $1615 per credit hour. *International tuition:* $29,090 full-time. *Room and board:* $13,274; room only: $9320 per academic year. *Required fees:* full-time $2321; part-time $1160 per term.
Financial Aid 16% of graduate students in nursing programs received some form of financial aid in 2011–12. Teaching assistantships (averaging $16,000 per year); career-related internships or fieldwork, institutionally sponsored loans, and scholarships also available. *Financial aid application deadline:* 4/1.
Contact Dr. Tammi L. Damas, Chairperson, Graduate Program, Division of Nursing, Howard University, 516 Bryant Street NW, Annex 1, Washington, DC 20059. *Telephone:* 202-806-7460. *Fax:* 202-806-5085. *E-mail:* Tammi.damas@howard.edu.

MASTER'S DEGREE PROGRAM
Degree MSN
Available Programs Master's.
Concentrations Available Nursing education. *Nurse practitioner programs in:* family health.

Study Options Full-time and part-time.

Online Degree Options Yes (online only).

Program Entrance Requirements Clinical experience, minimum overall college GPA of 3.0, transcript of college record, written essay, immunizations, interview, 3 letters of recommendation, resume, statistics course. *Application deadline:* Applications may be processed on a rolling basis for some programs. *Application fee:* $45.

Advanced Placement Credit given for nursing courses completed elsewhere dependent upon specific evaluations.

Degree Requirements 46 total credit hours, thesis or project, comprehensive exam.

POST-MASTER'S PROGRAM

Areas of Study Nursing education. *Nurse practitioner programs in:* family health.

Trinity Washington University
Nursing Program
Washington, District of Columbia

Founded in 1897

DEGREE • BSN

Nursing Program Faculty 9 (4% with doctorates).

Baccalaureate Enrollment 80

Nursing Student Activities Sigma Theta Tau, Student Nurses' Association.

Nursing Student Resources Academic advising; academic or career counseling; assistance for students with disabilities; bookstore; campus computer network; career placement assistance; computer lab; computer-assisted instruction; e-mail services; employment services for current students; housing assistance; Internet; learning resource lab; library services; nursing audiovisuals; paid internships; remedial services; resume preparation assistance; skills, simulation, or other laboratory; tutoring; unpaid internships.

Library Facilities 207,000 volumes (1,200 in health, 200 in nursing); 498 periodical subscriptions (40 health-care related).

BACCALAUREATE PROGRAMS

Degree BSN

Available Programs Generic Baccalaureate; RN Baccalaureate.

Study Options Full-time and part-time.

Program Entrance Requirements Transcript of college record, CPR certification, written essay, health exam, health insurance, high school transcript, immunizations, interview, 1 letter of recommendation, minimum GPA in nursing prerequisites of 2.0, professional liability insurance/malpractice insurance, prerequisite course work, RN licensure. Transfer students are accepted. *Application deadline:* Applications may be processed on a rolling basis for some programs.

Advanced Placement Credit by examination available. Credit given for nursing courses completed elsewhere dependent upon specific evaluations.

Contact *Telephone:* 202-884-9245. *Fax:* 202-884-9308.

University of the District of Columbia
Nursing Education Program
Washington, District of Columbia

Founded in 1976

DEGREE • BSN

Nursing Program Faculty 6 (3% with doctorates).

Baccalaureate Enrollment 40 **Women** 97% **Men** 3% **Minority** 98% **International** 50% **Part-time** 50%

Nursing Student Activities Student Nurses' Association.

Nursing Student Resources Academic advising; academic or career counseling; assistance for students with disabilities; bookstore; campus computer network; career placement assistance; computer lab; computer-

assisted instruction; daycare for children of students; e-mail services; employment services for current students; Internet; learning resource lab; library services; nursing audiovisuals; remedial services; resume preparation assistance; skills, simulation, or other laboratory; tutoring.

Library Facilities 554,412 volumes (500 in health, 250 in nursing); 647 periodical subscriptions (75 health-care related).

BACCALAUREATE PROGRAMS

Degree BSN

Available Programs RN Baccalaureate.

Site Options Washington, DC.

Study Options Full-time and part-time.

Program Entrance Requirements Minimum overall college GPA of 2.7, transcript of college record, CPR certification, written essay, health exam, health insurance, immunizations, 2 letters of recommendation, minimum GPA in nursing prerequisites of 2.7, professional liability insurance/malpractice insurance, prerequisite course work, RN licensure. Transfer students are accepted. *Application deadline:* 6/15 (fall), 11/15 (spring), 4/15 (summer).

Advanced Placement Credit by examination available. Credit given for nursing courses completed elsewhere dependent upon specific evaluations.

Contact *Telephone:* 202-274-5916. *Fax:* 202-274-5952.

FLORIDA

Adventist University of Health Sciences
Department of Nursing
Orlando, Florida

Founded in 1913

DEGREE • BSN

Nursing Program Faculty 21 (23% with doctorates).

Baccalaureate Enrollment 562

Distance Learning Courses Available.

Nursing Student Activities Nursing Honor Society, Student Nurses' Association.

Nursing Student Resources Academic advising; academic or career counseling; bookstore; campus computer network; computer lab; computer-assisted instruction; e-mail services; interactive nursing skills videos; Internet; learning resource lab; library services; nursing audiovisuals; skills, simulation, or other laboratory; tutoring.

Library Facilities 74,581 volumes; 158 periodical subscriptions.

BACCALAUREATE PROGRAMS

Degree BSN

Available Programs Generic Baccalaureate; RN Baccalaureate.

Study Options Full-time and part-time.

Online Degree Options Yes (online only).

Program Entrance Requirements Minimum overall college GPA of 3.0, transcript of college record, CPR certification, written essay, health exam, high school transcript, immunizations, 2 letters of recommendation, minimum high school GPA of 3.0, prerequisite course work, RN licensure. Transfer students are accepted. *Application deadline:* 4/15 (fall).

Advanced Placement Credit by examination available. Credit given for nursing courses completed elsewhere dependent upon specific evaluations.

Expenses (2011–12) *Tuition:* part-time $315 per credit hour. *Room and board:* room only: $3500 per academic year. *Required fees:* part-time $290 per term.

Contact Dr. Lorraine Brown, Department of Nursing, Department of Nursing, Adventist University of Health Sciences, 671 Winyah Drive, Orlando, FL 32803. *Telephone:* 407-303-5762. *Fax:* 407-303-1872.

Barry University
Division of Nursing
Miami Shores, Florida

http://www.barry.edu/nursing
Founded in 1940

DEGREES • BSN • MSN • MSN/MBA • PHD
Nursing Program Faculty 30 (50% with doctorates).
Baccalaureate Enrollment 431 **Women** 87% **Men** 13% **Minority** 51% **International** 2% **Part-time** 20%
Graduate Enrollment 161 **Women** 93% **Men** 7% **Minority** 51% **International** 1% **Part-time** 99%
Nursing Student Activities Sigma Theta Tau, Student Nurses' Association.
Nursing Student Resources Academic advising; academic or career counseling; assistance for students with disabilities; bookstore; campus computer network; career placement assistance; computer lab; computer-assisted instruction; e-mail services; employment services for current students; housing assistance; interactive nursing skills videos; Internet; learning resource lab; library services; nursing audiovisuals; paid internships; remedial services; resume preparation assistance; skills, simulation, or other laboratory; tutoring.
Library Facilities 316,517 volumes (15,000 in health, 8,500 in nursing); 2,880 periodical subscriptions (400 health-care related).

BACCALAUREATE PROGRAMS

Degree BSN
Available Programs ADN to Baccalaureate; Accelerated Baccalaureate; Accelerated Baccalaureate for Second Degree; Baccalaureate for Second Degree; Generic Baccalaureate; LPN to Baccalaureate; LPN to RN Baccalaureate; RN Baccalaureate.
Site Options Kendall, FL.
Study Options Full-time and part-time.
Program Entrance Requirements Minimum overall college GPA of 3.0, transcript of college record, CPR certification, health exam, health insurance, high school biology, high school chemistry, high school math, high school science, high school transcript, immunizations, 2 letters of recommendation, minimum high school GPA of 3.0, minimum GPA in nursing prerequisites of 3.0, professional liability insurance/malpractice insurance. Transfer students are accepted. *Application deadline:* Applications may be processed on a rolling basis for some programs. *Application fee:* $30.
Advanced Placement Credit given for nursing courses completed elsewhere dependent upon specific evaluations.
Expenses (2012–13) *Tuition:* full-time $28,160; part-time $845 per credit.
Financial Aid 90% of baccalaureate students in nursing programs received some form of financial aid in 2011–12. *Gift aid (need-based):* Federal Pell, FSEOG, state, private, college/university gift aid from institutional funds, Federal Nursing. *Loans:* Federal Nursing Student Loans, Perkins, college/university, alternative loans. *Work-study:* Federal Work-Study, part-time campus jobs. *Financial aid application deadline:* Continuous.
Contact Ms. Rosanne Sonshine, Recruiter and Clinical Coordinator, Division of Nursing, Barry University, 11300 NE Second Avenue, Miami Shores, FL 33161-6695. *Telephone:* 305-899-3813. *Fax:* 305-899-3831. *E-mail:* rsonshine@mail.barry.edu.

GRADUATE PROGRAMS

Expenses (2012–13) *Tuition:* part-time $935 per credit.
Financial Aid 90% of graduate students in nursing programs received some form of financial aid in 2011–12. 3 research assistantships (averaging $5,000 per year), 3 teaching assistantships (averaging $5,000 per year) were awarded; scholarships and tuition waivers (full) also available. *Financial aid application deadline:* 5/1.
Contact Ms. Kelley Eddington, Operations Manager, Division of Nursing, Barry University, 11300 NE Second Avenue, Miami Shores, FL 33161-6695. *Telephone:* 305-899-3814. *Fax:* 305-899-3831. *E-mail:* keddington@mail.barry.edu.

MASTER'S DEGREE PROGRAM
Degrees MSN; MSN/MBA
Available Programs Master's.
Concentrations Available Nursing administration; nursing education. *Nurse practitioner programs in:* acute care, family health.
Site Options Kendall, FL.
Study Options Part-time.

Program Entrance Requirements Clinical experience, computer literacy, minimum overall college GPA of 3.0, transcript of college record, written essay, 2 letters of recommendation, nursing research course, professional liability insurance/malpractice insurance, statistics course, GRE General Test or MAT. *Application deadline:* Applications may be processed on a rolling basis for some programs.
Advanced Placement Credit given for nursing courses completed elsewhere dependent upon specific evaluations.
Degree Requirements 45 total credit hours.

POST-MASTER'S PROGRAM
Areas of Study Nursing administration; nursing education. *Nurse practitioner programs in:* acute care, family health.

DOCTORAL DEGREE PROGRAM
Degree PhD
Available Programs Doctorate.
Areas of Study Nursing research, nursing science.
Site Options Orlando, FL; Kendall, FL; Palm Beach, FL.
Program Entrance Requirements Clinical experience, minimum overall college GPA of 3.0, interview, 2 letters of recommendation, MSN or equivalent, statistics course, writing sample, GRE General Test or MAT. *Application deadline:* Applications may be processed on a rolling basis for some programs.
Degree Requirements 45 total credit hours, dissertation, written exam, residency.

Bethune-Cookman University
School of Nursing
Daytona Beach, Florida

http://www.cookman.edu/academics/schools/sn/index.html
Founded in 1904

DEGREE • BSN
Nursing Program Faculty 11 (2% with doctorates).
Baccalaureate Enrollment 137 **Women** 93% **Men** 7% **Minority** 95% **International** 2%
Nursing Student Activities Nursing Honor Society, Student Nurses' Association.
Nursing Student Resources Academic advising; bookstore; campus computer network; computer lab; computer-assisted instruction; e-mail services; interactive nursing skills videos; Internet; learning resource lab; library services; nursing audiovisuals; resume preparation assistance; skills, simulation, or other laboratory; tutoring; unpaid internships.
Library Facilities 145,033 volumes; 128 periodical subscriptions.

BACCALAUREATE PROGRAMS

Degree BSN
Available Programs Generic Baccalaureate; RN Baccalaureate.
Study Options Full-time.
Program Entrance Requirements Minimum overall college GPA of 2.8, transcript of college record, CPR certification, written essay, health exam, high school transcript, immunizations, interview, 2 letters of recommendation, minimum GPA in nursing prerequisites of 2.8, prerequisite course work. Transfer students are accepted.
Advanced Placement Credit by examination available. Credit given for nursing courses completed elsewhere dependent upon specific evaluations.
Contact *Telephone:* 386-481-2000.

Broward College
Nursing Program
Fort Lauderdale, Florida

Founded in 1960
DEGREE • BSN

BACCALAUREATE PROGRAMS

Degree BSN
Available Programs RN Baccalaureate.
Program Entrance Requirements Minimum overall college GPA of 2.5, RN licensure.

Contact RN-BSN Program Office, Nursing Program, Broward College, Building 9, Room 200, 3501 Davie Road, Davie, FL 33314. *Telephone:* 954-201-4880. *E-mail:* bsn@broward.edu.

Edison State College
Bachelor of Science in Nursing Program
Fort Myers, Florida

Founded in 1962
DEGREE • BSN
Library Facilities 181,085 volumes.

BACCALAUREATE PROGRAMS

Degree BSN
Available Programs RN Baccalaureate.
Program Entrance Requirements Minimum overall college GPA of 2.0, transcript of college record, prerequisite course work, RN licensure. *Application deadline:* 8/1 (fall), 12/1 (spring), 4/1 (summer).
Contact Admissions Office, Bachelor of Science in Nursing Program, Edison State College, 8099 College Parkway, Fort Myers, FL 33919. *Telephone:* 800-749-2322. *E-mail:* admissions@edison.edu.

Florida Agricultural and Mechanical University
School of Nursing
Tallahassee, Florida

http://www.famu.edu/index.cfm?a=nursing
Founded in 1887
DEGREES • BSN • MSN • PHD
Nursing Program Faculty 28 (18% with doctorates).
Baccalaureate Enrollment 161 **Women** 90% **Men** 10% **Minority** 98%
Graduate Enrollment 17 **Women** 83% **Men** 17% **Minority** 76% **Part-time** 12%
Nursing Student Activities Sigma Theta Tau, Student Nurses' Association.
Nursing Student Resources Academic advising; academic or career counseling; bookstore; campus computer network; career placement assistance; computer lab; computer-assisted instruction; daycare for children of students; e-mail services; employment services for current students; externships; interactive nursing skills videos; Internet; library services; nursing audiovisuals; placement services for program completers; remedial services; resume preparation assistance; skills, simulation, or other laboratory; tutoring.
Library Facilities 1 million volumes (5,000 in health, 4,091 in nursing); 105,200 periodical subscriptions (385 health-care related).

BACCALAUREATE PROGRAMS

Degree BSN
Available Programs Generic Baccalaureate.
Study Options Part-time.
Program Entrance Requirements CPR certification, health exam, immunizations, 3 letters of recommendation, minimum high school GPA of 2.5, prerequisite course work. Transfer students are accepted.
Contact *Telephone:* 850-599-3458. *Fax:* 850-599-3508.

GRADUATE PROGRAMS

Contact *Telephone:* 850-599-3017. *Fax:* 850-599-3508.

MASTER'S DEGREE PROGRAM

Degree MSN
Available Programs Master's.
Concentrations Available *Nurse practitioner programs in:* adult health, gerontology, women's health.
Study Options Full-time and part-time.
Program Entrance Requirements Clinical experience, minimum overall college GPA of 3.0, CPR certification, immunizations, interview, nursing research course, physical assessment course, professional liability insurance/malpractice insurance, statistics course.
Degree Requirements 42 total credit hours, thesis or project.

POST-MASTER'S PROGRAM

Areas of Study *Nurse practitioner programs in:* adult health, gerontology, women's health.

DOCTORAL DEGREE PROGRAM

Degree PhD
Program Entrance Requirements Minimum overall college GPA of 3.5, 3 letters of recommendation, MSN or equivalent.
Degree Requirements 90 total credit hours, dissertation, oral exam, written exam.

CONTINUING EDUCATION PROGRAM

Contact *Telephone:* 850-599-3017. *Fax:* 850-599-3508.

Florida Atlantic University
Christine E. Lynn College of Nursing
Boca Raton, Florida

http://nursing.fau.edu/
Founded in 1961
DEGREES • BSN • DNP • MS
Nursing Program Faculty 57 (75% with doctorates).
Baccalaureate Enrollment 518 **Women** 90% **Men** 10% **Minority** 35% **International** 2% **Part-time** 72%
Graduate Enrollment 395 **Women** 92% **Men** 8% **Minority** 48% **International** 5% **Part-time** 92%
Distance Learning Courses Available.
Nursing Student Activities Sigma Theta Tau, Student Nurses' Association.
Nursing Student Resources Academic advising; academic or career counseling; assistance for students with disabilities; bookstore; campus computer network; computer lab; computer-assisted instruction; e-mail services; housing assistance; interactive nursing skills videos; Internet; learning resource lab; library services; nursing audiovisuals; remedial services; skills, simulation, or other laboratory; tutoring.
Library Facilities 1.3 million volumes (28,670 in health, 5,749 in nursing); 12,811 periodical subscriptions (903 health-care related).

BACCALAUREATE PROGRAMS

Degree BSN
Available Programs Accelerated Baccalaureate for Second Degree; Generic Baccalaureate; RN Baccalaureate.
Site Options Davie, FL; Port St. Lucie, FL.
Study Options Full-time.
Online Degree Options Yes (online only).
Program Entrance Requirements Minimum overall college GPA of 3.0, transcript of college record, CPR certification, health exam, health insurance, high school transcript, immunizations, minimum GPA in nursing prerequisites of 2.0, prerequisite course work. Transfer students are accepted. *Application deadline:* 11/30 (fall). *Application fee:* $30.
Advanced Placement Credit by examination available. Credit given for nursing courses completed elsewhere dependent upon specific evaluations.
Expenses (2011–12) *Tuition, state resident:* full-time $5372; part-time $177 per credit hour. *Tuition, nonresident:* full-time $19,715; part-time $657 per credit hour. *International tuition:* $19,715 full-time. *Room and board:* $10,940 per academic year. *Required fees:* full-time $135.
Financial Aid 75% of baccalaureate students in nursing programs received some form of financial aid in 2010–11. *Gift aid (need-based):* Federal Pell, FSEOG, state, private, college/university gift aid from institutional funds, Federal Nursing. *Loans:* Perkins, college/university. *Work-study:* Federal Work-Study, part-time campus jobs. *Financial aid application deadline (priority):* 3/1.
Contact Dr. Sharon Lee Dormire, Assistant Dean of Undergraduate Programs, Christine E. Lynn College of Nursing, Florida Atlantic University, 777 Glades Road, Boca Raton, FL 33431. *Telephone:* 561-297-2535. *Fax:* 561-297-3652. *E-mail:* sdormire@fau.edu.

GRADUATE PROGRAMS

Expenses (2011–12) *Tuition, area resident:* part-time $343 per credit. *Tuition, nonresident:* part-time $997 per credit. *International tuition:* $997 full-time.
Financial Aid 15% of graduate students in nursing programs received some form of financial aid in 2010–11. Research assistantships with partial tuition reimbursements available, teaching assistantships with

partial tuition reimbursements available, career-related internships or fieldwork, Federal Work-Study, institutionally sponsored loans, scholarships, and traineeships available. Aid available to part-time students.
Contact Dr. Shirley Gordon, Masters Program Director, Christine E. Lynn College of Nursing, Florida Atlantic University, 777 Glades Road, Boca Raton, FL 33431. *Telephone:* 561-297-3389. *Fax:* 561-297-3652. *E-mail:* sgordon@fau.edu.

MASTER'S DEGREE PROGRAM

Degree MS
Available Programs Master's; Master's for Nurses with Non-Nursing Degrees; RN to Master's.
Concentrations Available Clinical nurse leader; nursing administration; nursing education. *Nurse practitioner programs in:* adult health, family health, gerontology.
Site Options Davie, FL; Port St. Lucie, FL.
Study Options Full-time and part-time.
Online Degree Options Yes.
Program Entrance Requirements Minimum overall college GPA of 3.0, transcript of college record, CPR certification, written essay, immunizations, interview, 2 letters of recommendation, nursing research course, physical assessment course, professional liability insurance/malpractice insurance, prerequisite course work, resume, statistics course, GRE General Test. *Application deadline:* 6/1 (fall), 10/1 (spring), 2/1 (summer). *Application fee:* $30.
Advanced Placement Credit given for nursing courses completed elsewhere dependent upon specific evaluations.
Degree Requirements 30 total credit hours.

POST-MASTER'S PROGRAM

Areas of Study Clinical nurse leader; nursing administration; nursing education. *Nurse practitioner programs in:* adult health, family health, gerontology.

DOCTORAL DEGREE PROGRAM

Degree DNP
Available Programs Doctorate; Post-Baccalaureate Doctorate.
Areas of Study Aging, bio-behavioral research, gerontology, health-care systems, human health and illness, individualized study, nursing administration, nursing education, nursing research, nursing science.
Program Entrance Requirements Minimum overall college GPA of 3.5, interview by faculty committee, interview, 3 letters of recommendation, MSN or equivalent, scholarly papers, statistics course, vita, writing sample, GRE General Test. *Application deadline:* 2/28 (fall), 10/15 (spring). *Application fee:* $30.
Degree Requirements 63 total credit hours, written exam, residency.

CONTINUING EDUCATION PROGRAM

Contact Dr. Beth King, Director, Christine E. Lynn College of Nursing, Florida Atlantic University, 777 Glades Road, Boca Raton, FL 33431. *Telephone:* 561-297-3249. *Fax:* 561-297-3652. *E-mail:* bking@fau.edu.

Florida Gulf Coast University
School of Nursing
Fort Myers, Florida

http://www.fgcu.edu/chp/nursing/
Founded in 1991
DEGREES • BSN • MSN
Nursing Program Faculty 17 (57% with doctorates).
Baccalaureate Enrollment 141 **Women** 89% **Men** 11% **Minority** 20.5% **Part-time** 15%
Graduate Enrollment 75 **Women** 88% **Men** 12% **Minority** 12% **Part-time** 10%
Nursing Student Activities Sigma Theta Tau, Student Nurses' Association.
Nursing Student Resources Academic advising; academic or career counseling; assistance for students with disabilities; bookstore; campus computer network; career placement assistance; computer lab; computer-assisted instruction; e-mail services; employment services for current students; Internet; learning resource lab; library services; nursing audiovisuals; skills, simulation, or other laboratory; tutoring.
Library Facilities 410,417 volumes (13,943 in health, 6,742 in nursing); 94,274 periodical subscriptions (471 health-care related).

BACCALAUREATE PROGRAMS

Degree BSN
Available Programs Generic Baccalaureate.
Study Options Full-time.
Program Entrance Requirements Minimum overall college GPA of 3.0, transcript of college record, CPR certification, health insurance, high school foreign language, immunizations, professional liability insurance/malpractice insurance, prerequisite course work. Transfer students are accepted. *Application deadline:* 2/1 (fall), 5/15 (spring).
Advanced Placement Credit given for nursing courses completed elsewhere dependent upon specific evaluations.
Contact Ms. Kim Hobart, School of Nursing Office Manager, School of Nursing, Florida Gulf Coast University, 10501 FGCU Boulevard South, Fort Myers, FL 33965-6565. *Telephone:* 239-590-7454. *Fax:* 239-590-7474. *E-mail:* khobart@fgcu.edu.

GRADUATE PROGRAMS

Financial Aid 45% of graduate students in nursing programs received some form of financial aid in 2010–11.
Contact Ms. Brenda Bartlett, MSN Program Assistant, School of Nursing, Florida Gulf Coast University, 10501 FGCU Boulevard South, Fort Myers, FL 33965-6565. *Telephone:* 239-590-7505. *Fax:* 239-590-7474. *E-mail:* bbartlett@fgcu.edu.

MASTER'S DEGREE PROGRAM

Degree MSN
Available Programs Master's.
Concentrations Available Nurse anesthesia. *Nurse practitioner programs in:* acute care, adult health, family health.
Study Options Full-time and part-time.
Program Entrance Requirements Clinical experience, minimum overall college GPA of 3.0, transcript of college record, interview, physical assessment course, resume, statistics course.
Advanced Placement Credit given for nursing courses completed elsewhere dependent upon specific evaluations.

POST-MASTER'S PROGRAM

Areas of Study *Nurse practitioner programs in:* acute care, family health.

CONTINUING EDUCATION PROGRAM

Contact Dr. Anne Nolan, Associate Professor, School of Nursing, Florida Gulf Coast University, 10501 FGCU Boulevard South, Fort Myers, FL 33931. *Telephone:* 239-590-7513. *Fax:* 239-590-7474. *E-mail:* anolan@fgcu.edu.

Florida International University
Graduate Nursing Programs
Miami, Florida

http://www.fiu.edu/
Founded in 1965
DEGREES • BSN • MSN • PHD
Nursing Program Faculty 77 (29% with doctorates).
Baccalaureate Enrollment 474 **Women** 73% **Men** 27% **Minority** 88% **International** 1% **Part-time** 25%
Graduate Enrollment 395 **Women** 82% **Men** 18% **Minority** 74% **International** 1% **Part-time** 60%
Distance Learning Courses Available.
Nursing Student Activities Sigma Theta Tau, Student Nurses' Association.
Nursing Student Resources Academic advising; academic or career counseling; assistance for students with disabilities; bookstore; campus computer network; career placement assistance; computer lab; computer-assisted instruction; daycare for children of students; e-mail services; externships; housing assistance; interactive nursing skills videos; Internet; learning resource lab; library services; nursing audiovisuals; paid internships; remedial services; resume preparation assistance; skills, simulation, or other laboratory; tutoring.
Library Facilities 2.2 million volumes (25,000 in health, 3,300 in nursing); 61,891 periodical subscriptions (1,500 health-care related).

BACCALAUREATE PROGRAMS

Degree BSN

Available Programs Accelerated Baccalaureate for Second Degree; Generic Baccalaureate; RN Baccalaureate.
Site Options St. Petersburg, FL; North Miami, FL.
Study Options Full-time.
Online Degree Options Yes.
Program Entrance Requirements Minimum overall college GPA of 3.0, transcript of college record, CPR certification, written essay, health exam, health insurance, high school foreign language, high school transcript, immunizations, minimum GPA in nursing prerequisites of 3.0, prerequisite course work. Transfer students are accepted. *Application deadline:* 5/15 (fall), 2/15 (summer). *Application fee:* $30.
Advanced Placement Credit by examination available. Credit given for nursing courses completed elsewhere dependent upon specific evaluations.
Contact *Telephone:* 305-348-7717. *Fax:* 305-348-7764.

GRADUATE PROGRAMS

Contact *Telephone:* 305-348-7717. *Fax:* 305-348-7764.

MASTER'S DEGREE PROGRAM
Degree MSN
Available Programs Accelerated AD/RN to Master's; Master's; Master's for Nurses with Non-Nursing Degrees.
Concentrations Available Nurse anesthesia; nursing administration; nursing education. *Nurse practitioner programs in:* adult health, family health, pediatric.
Study Options Full-time and part-time.
Program Entrance Requirements Clinical experience, computer literacy, minimum overall college GPA of 3.0, transcript of college record, CPR certification, written essay, immunizations, interview, 3 letters of recommendation, nursing research course, physical assessment course, professional liability insurance/malpractice insurance, prerequisite course work, resume, statistics course. *Application deadline:* 6/1 (fall), 10/1 (spring), 3/1 (summer). *Application fee:* $30.
Advanced Placement Credit given for nursing courses completed elsewhere dependent upon specific evaluations.
Degree Requirements 43 total credit hours.

POST-MASTER'S PROGRAM
Areas of Study Nursing administration; nursing education. *Nurse practitioner programs in:* adult health, family health, pediatric.

DOCTORAL DEGREE PROGRAM
Degree PhD
Available Programs Doctorate.
Areas of Study Faculty preparation, health policy, health-care systems, individualized study, nursing administration, nursing education, nursing policy, nursing research, nursing science.
Program Entrance Requirements Clinical experience, minimum overall college GPA of 3.0, interview by faculty committee, 3 letters of recommendation, MSN or equivalent, statistics course, writing sample, GRE. *Application deadline:* Applications may be processed on a rolling basis for some programs. *Application fee:* $30.
Degree Requirements 84 total credit hours, dissertation, oral exam, written exam.

Florida Southern College
School of Nursing & Health Sciences
Lakeland, Florida

http://www.flsouthern.edu/KCMS/Nursing-Health-Sciences.aspx
Founded in 1885
DEGREES • BSN • MSN • MSN/MBA
Nursing Program Faculty 12 (75% with doctorates).
Baccalaureate Enrollment 149
Graduate Enrollment 89
Nursing Student Activities Nursing Honor Society, Sigma Theta Tau, Student Nurses' Association.
Nursing Student Resources Academic advising; academic or career counseling; assistance for students with disabilities; bookstore; campus computer network; career placement assistance; computer lab; computer-assisted instruction; e-mail services; externships; interactive nursing skills videos; Internet; learning resource lab; library services; nursing audiovisuals; paid internships; placement services for program com-

pleters; remedial services; resume preparation assistance; skills, simulation, or other laboratory; tutoring.
Library Facilities 166,053 volumes (4,000 in health, 3,500 in nursing); 43,570 periodical subscriptions (40 health-care related).

BACCALAUREATE PROGRAMS

Degree BSN
Available Programs Accelerated Baccalaureate; Accelerated Baccalaureate for Second Degree; Baccalaureate for Second Degree; Generic Baccalaureate; RN Baccalaureate.
Study Options Full-time.
Program Entrance Requirements Minimum overall college GPA of 3.2, transcript of college record, CPR certification, written essay, health exam, health insurance, immunizations, minimum high school GPA of 3.2, minimum GPA in nursing prerequisites of 3.0, prerequisite course work. Transfer students are accepted. *Application deadline:* 5/1 (fall). Applications may be processed on a rolling basis for some programs.
Advanced Placement Credit by examination available. Credit given for nursing courses completed elsewhere dependent upon specific evaluations.
Expenses (2012–13) *Tuition:* full-time $26,600; part-time $750 per credit hour. *Room and board:* $9100 per academic year.
Contact Dr. John Welton, Dean, School of Nursing & Health Sciences, Florida Southern College, 111 Lake Hollingsworth Drive, Lakeland, FL 33801. *Telephone:* 863-680-3951. *Fax:* 863-680-3860. *E-mail:* jwelton@flsouthern.edu.

GRADUATE PROGRAMS

Expenses (2012–13) *Tuition:* part-time $460 per credit hour.
Contact Dr. Beverley Brown, Graduate Program Director, School of Nursing & Health Sciences, Florida Southern College, 111 Lake Hollingsworth Drive, Lakeland, FL 33801. *Telephone:* 863-680-3951. *Fax:* 863-680-3860. *E-mail:* bbrown@flsouthern.edu.

MASTER'S DEGREE PROGRAM
Degrees MSN; MSN/MBA
Available Programs Master's; Master's for Nurses with Non-Nursing Degrees.
Concentrations Available Nursing administration; nursing education. *Clinical nurse specialist programs in:* adult health, gerontology. *Nurse practitioner programs in:* adult health, primary care.
Study Options Full-time and part-time.
Program Entrance Requirements Clinical experience, computer literacy, minimum overall college GPA of 3.0, transcript of college record, CPR certification, written essay, immunizations, 3 letters of recommendation, nursing research course, physical assessment course, professional liability insurance/malpractice insurance, prerequisite course work, resume, statistics course. *Application deadline:* 6/1 (fall), 11/1 (spring). *Application fee:* $30.
Advanced Placement Credit given for nursing courses completed elsewhere dependent upon specific evaluations.
Degree Requirements 42 total credit hours, thesis or project.

POST-MASTER'S PROGRAM
Areas of Study Nursing administration; nursing education. *Clinical nurse specialist programs in:* adult health, gerontology. *Nurse practitioner programs in:* adult health, primary care.

Florida State College at Jacksonville
Nursing Department
Jacksonville, Florida

Founded in 1963
DEGREE • BSN
Nursing Program Faculty 2 (100% with doctorates).
Baccalaureate Enrollment 59 **Women** 99% **Men** 1% **Minority** 42%
Distance Learning Courses Available.
Nursing Student Activities Student Nurses' Association.
Nursing Student Resources Academic advising; academic or career counseling; assistance for students with disabilities; bookstore; campus computer network; career placement assistance; computer lab; computer-assisted instruction; daycare for children of students; e-mail services; employment services for current students; interactive nursing skills videos; Internet; learning resource lab; library services; nursing audiovi-

suals; resume preparation assistance; skills, simulation, or other laboratory; tutoring.

Library Facilities 211,361 volumes (50,000 in health, 5,000 in nursing); 3,299 periodical subscriptions (148 health-care related).

BACCALAUREATE PROGRAMS

Degree BSN

Available Programs RN Baccalaureate.

Program Entrance Requirements Transcript of college record, CPR certification, written essay, health exam, high school foreign language, high school transcript, immunizations, 1 letter of recommendation, minimum GPA in nursing prerequisites of 2.0, professional liability insurance/malpractice insurance, prerequisite course work, RN licensure. Transfer students are accepted. *Application deadline:* 6/1 (fall), 10/1 (winter). *Application fee:* $25.

Expenses (2012–13) *Tuition, state resident:* full-time $115. *Tuition, nonresident:* full-time $601. *International tuition:* $601 full-time.

Financial Aid 32% of baccalaureate students in nursing programs received some form of financial aid in 2011–12. *Loans:* college/university. *Work-study:* Federal Work-Study.

Contact Dr. Mary Kathleen Ebener, Associate Dean of Nursing for BSN Program, Nursing Department, Florida State College at Jacksonville, North Campus, 4501 Capper Road, Jacksonville, FL 32218. *Telephone:* 904-713-6015. *Fax:* 904-713-4850. *E-mail:* mebener@fscj.edu.

Florida State University

College of Nursing
Tallahassee, Florida

http://nursing.fsu.edu/
Founded in 1851

DEGREES • BSN • DNP • MSN

Nursing Program Faculty 29 (62% with doctorates).

Baccalaureate Enrollment 226 **Women** 89% **Men** 11% **Minority** 29% **International** 1% **Part-time** 10%

Graduate Enrollment 81 **Women** 98% **Men** 2% **Minority** 5% **Part-time** 55%

Distance Learning Courses Available.

Nursing Student Activities Sigma Theta Tau, Student Nurses' Association.

Nursing Student Resources Academic advising; academic or career counseling; assistance for students with disabilities; campus computer network; computer lab; e-mail services; interactive nursing skills videos; Internet; learning resource lab; nursing audiovisuals; skills, simulation, or other laboratory; unpaid internships.

Library Facilities 3 million volumes; 78,300 periodical subscriptions.

BACCALAUREATE PROGRAMS

Degree BSN

Available Programs Accelerated Baccalaureate; Generic Baccalaureate.

Study Options Full-time.

Program Entrance Requirements Minimum overall college GPA of 3.0, transcript of college record, CPR certification, health exam, health insurance, high school biology, high school chemistry, high school foreign language, 3 years high school math, immunizations, minimum high school GPA of 3.7, minimum GPA in nursing prerequisites of 3.0, professional liability insurance/malpractice insurance, prerequisite course work. Transfer students are accepted. *Application deadline:* 2/1 (fall). *Application fee:* $20.

Advanced Placement Credit given for nursing courses completed elsewhere dependent upon specific evaluations.

Expenses (2012–13) *Tuition, state resident:* full-time $6403; part-time $103 per credit hour. *Tuition, nonresident:* full-time $21,569; part-time $481 per credit hour. *International tuition:* $21,569 full-time. *Room and board:* $9818; room only: $5820 per academic year. *Required fees:* full-time $318; part-time $73 per credit; part-time $109 per term.

Financial Aid 96% of baccalaureate students in nursing programs received some form of financial aid in 2011–12.

Contact Mr. Carlos Urrutia, Director of Student Services, College of Nursing, Florida State University, 98 Varsity Way, 103 SCN, Tallahassee, FL 32306-4310. *Telephone:* 850-644-5638. *Fax:* 850-645-7249. *E-mail:* currutia@fsu.edu.

GRADUATE PROGRAMS

Expenses (2012–13) *Tuition, state resident:* full-time $12,105; part-time $481 per credit hour. *Tuition, nonresident:* full-time $18,040; part-time $601 per credit hour. *International tuition:* $18,040 full-time. *Required fees:* full-time $145.

Financial Aid 91% of graduate students in nursing programs received some form of financial aid in 2011–12. Fellowships with partial tuition reimbursements available (averaging $6,300 per year), research assistantships with partial tuition reimbursements available (averaging $3,000 per year), 3 teaching assistantships with partial tuition reimbursements available (averaging $3,000 per year) were awarded; career-related internships or fieldwork, Federal Work-Study, institutionally sponsored loans, scholarships, traineeships, and tuition waivers (partial) also available. *Financial aid application deadline:* 4/15.

Contact Mr. Carlos Urrutia, Director of Student Services, College of Nursing, Florida State University, 98 Varsity Way, 103 SCN, Tallahassee, FL 32306-4310. *Telephone:* 850-644-5638. *Fax:* 850-645-7249. *E-mail:* currutiaa@fsu.edu.

MASTER'S DEGREE PROGRAM

Degree MSN

Available Programs Master's.

Concentrations Available Nursing administration; nursing education.

Study Options Full-time and part-time.

Online Degree Options Yes (online only).

Program Entrance Requirements Minimum overall college GPA of 3.0, transcript of college record, CPR certification, immunizations, interview, 2 letters of recommendation, resume, GRE General Test, MAT. *Application deadline:* 7/1 (fall). *Application fee:* CAN$20.

Advanced Placement Credit given for nursing courses completed elsewhere dependent upon specific evaluations.

Degree Requirements 38 total credit hours.

POST-MASTER'S PROGRAM

Areas of Study Nursing administration; nursing education.

DOCTORAL DEGREE PROGRAM

Degree DNP

Available Programs Doctorate; Post-Baccalaureate Doctorate.

Areas of Study Family health, health-care systems.

Site Options Panama City, FL; Sarasota, FL.

Program Entrance Requirements Minimum overall college GPA of 3.0, interview, 2 letters of recommendation, GRE General Test, MAT. *Application deadline:* 4/15 (fall).

Degree Requirements 90 total credit hours, residency.

Indian River State College

Bachelor of Science in Nursing Program
Fort Pierce, Florida

Founded in 1960

DEGREE • BSN

Library Facilities 112,032 volumes; 200 periodical subscriptions.

BACCALAUREATE PROGRAMS

Degree BSN

Available Programs RN Baccalaureate.

Contact *Telephone:* 772-462-7415.

Jacksonville University

School of Nursing
Jacksonville, Florida

http://www.jacksonvilleu.com/?loc=logo
Founded in 1934

DEGREES • BSN • MSN • MSN/MBA

Nursing Program Faculty 31 (52% with doctorates).

Baccalaureate Enrollment 700 **Women** 90% **Men** 10% **Minority** 40% **International** .5% **Part-time** 15%

Graduate Enrollment 90 **Women** 87% **Men** 13% **Minority** 37%

Distance Learning Courses Available.

Nursing Student Activities Nursing Honor Society, Sigma Theta Tau, Student Nurses' Association, nursing club.

Nursing Student Resources Academic advising; academic or career counseling; assistance for students with disabilities; bookstore; campus computer network; career placement assistance; computer lab; computer-assisted instruction; e-mail services; employment services for current students; externships; interactive nursing skills videos; Internet; learning resource lab; library services; nursing audiovisuals; placement services for program completers; remedial services; resume preparation assistance; skills, simulation, or other laboratory; tutoring; unpaid internships.

BACCALAUREATE PROGRAMS

Degree BSN
Available Programs ADN to Baccalaureate; Accelerated Baccalaureate; Accelerated Baccalaureate for Second Degree; Baccalaureate for Second Degree; Generic Baccalaureate.
Site Options Jacksonville, FL.
Study Options Full-time.
Online Degree Options Yes.
Program Entrance Requirements Minimum overall college GPA of 2.5, transcript of college record, CPR certification, written essay, health exam, health insurance, immunizations, interview, 3 letters of recommendation, minimum GPA in nursing prerequisites of 2.0, prerequisite course work. Transfer students are accepted. *Application deadline:* 4/1 (fall), 12/1 (summer). *Application fee:* $15.
Advanced Placement Credit given for nursing courses completed elsewhere dependent upon specific evaluations.
Contact *Telephone:* 904-256-7286. *Fax:* 904-256-7287.

GRADUATE PROGRAMS

Contact *Telephone:* 904-256-7034. *Fax:* 904-256-7287.

MASTER'S DEGREE PROGRAM

Degrees MSN; MSN/MBA
Available Programs Master's.
Concentrations Available Nursing administration; nursing education. *Nurse practitioner programs in:* family health.
Site Options Jacksonville, FL.
Study Options Full-time and part-time.
Online Degree Options Yes.
Program Entrance Requirements Clinical experience, minimum overall college GPA of 3.0, transcript of college record, CPR certification, written essay, immunizations, interview, 3 letters of recommendation, prerequisite course work, resume. *Application deadline:* 4/30 (fall). Applications may be processed on a rolling basis for some programs. *Application fee:* $30.
Advanced Placement Credit given for nursing courses completed elsewhere dependent upon specific evaluations.
Degree Requirements 46 total credit hours, thesis or project, comprehensive exam.

POST-MASTER'S PROGRAM

Areas of Study *Nurse practitioner programs in:* family health.

Kaplan University Online
The School of Nursing Online
Fort Lauderdale, Florida

DEGREES • BSN • MSN

BACCALAUREATE PROGRAMS

Degree BSN
Available Programs Generic Baccalaureate.
Contact *Telephone:* 866-527-5268.

GRADUATE PROGRAMS

Contact *Telephone:* 866-527-5268.

MASTER'S DEGREE PROGRAM

Degree MSN
Available Programs Master's; RN to Master's.
Concentrations Available Health-care administration; nursing education; nursing informatics. *Nurse practitioner programs in:* adult health, family health.

Keiser University
Nursing Programs
Fort Lauderdale, Florida

Founded in 1977
DEGREES • BSN • MSN

BACCALAUREATE PROGRAMS

Degree BSN
Available Programs RN Baccalaureate.
Contact Fort Lauderdale campus, Nursing Programs, Keiser University, 1500 Northwest 49th Street, Fort Lauderdale, FL 33309. *Telephone:* 954-776-4456. *Fax:* 954-771-4894.

GRADUATE PROGRAMS

Contact Fort Lauderdale campus, Nursing Programs, Keiser University, 1500 Northwest 49th Street, Fort Lauderdale, FL 33309. *Telephone:* 954-776-4456. *Fax:* 954-771-4894.

MASTER'S DEGREE PROGRAM

Degree MSN
Available Programs Master's.
Program Entrance Requirements Minimum overall college GPA of 2.7.
Degree Requirements 33 total credit hours.

Keiser University
Nursing Programs
Fort Myers, Florida

DEGREES • BSN • MSN

BACCALAUREATE PROGRAMS

Degree BSN
Available Programs RN Baccalaureate.
Contact Ft. Myers campus, Nursing Programs, Keiser University, 9100 Forum Corporate Parkway, Ft. Myers, FL 33905. *Telephone:* 239-277-1336. *Fax:* 239-277-1259.

GRADUATE PROGRAMS

Contact Ft. Myers campus, Nursing Programs, Keiser University, 9100 Forum Corporate Parkway, Ft. Myers, FL 33905. *Telephone:* 239-277-1336. *Fax:* 239-277-1259.

MASTER'S DEGREE PROGRAM

Degree MSN
Available Programs Master's.
Program Entrance Requirements Minimum overall college GPA of 2.7.
Degree Requirements 33 total credit hours.

Keiser University
Nursing Programs
Jacksonville, Florida

DEGREES • BSN • MSN

BACCALAUREATE PROGRAMS

Degree BSN
Available Programs RN Baccalaureate.
Contact Jacksonville campus, Nursing Programs, Keiser University, 6430 Southpoint Parkway, Jacksonville, FL 32216. *Telephone:* 904-296-3440. *Fax:* 904-296-3407.

GRADUATE PROGRAMS

Contact Jacksonville campus, Nursing Programs, Keiser University, 6430 Southpoint Parkway, Jacksonville, FL 32216. *Telephone:* 904-296-3440. *Fax:* 904-296-3407.

MASTER'S DEGREE PROGRAM
Degree MSN
Available Programs Master's.
Program Entrance Requirements Minimum overall college GPA of 2.7.
Degree Requirements 33 total credit hours.

Keiser University
Nursing Programs
Lakeland, Florida

DEGREES • BSN • MSN

BACCALAUREATE PROGRAMS

Degree BSN
Available Programs RN Baccalaureate.
Contact Lakeland campus, Nursing Programs, Keiser University, 2400 Interstate Drive, Lakeland, FL 33805. *Telephone:* 863-682-6020. *Fax:* 863-688-6196.

GRADUATE PROGRAMS

Contact Lakeland campus, Nursing Programs, Keiser University, 2400 Interstate Drive, Lakeland, FL 33805. *Telephone:* 863-682-6020. *Fax:* 863-688-6196.

MASTER'S DEGREE PROGRAM

Degree MSN
Available Programs Master's.
Program Entrance Requirements Minimum overall college GPA of 2.7.
Degree Requirements 33 total credit hours.

Keiser University
Nursing Programs
Melbourne, Florida

Founded in 1989
DEGREES • BSN • MSN

BACCALAUREATE PROGRAMS

Degree BSN
Available Programs RN Baccalaureate.
Contact Melbourne campus, Nursing Programs, Keiser University, 900 South Babcock Street, Melbourne, FL 32901. *Telephone:* 321-409-4800. *Fax:* 321-725-3766.

GRADUATE PROGRAMS

Contact Melbourne campus, Nursing Programs, Keiser University, 900 South Babcock Street, Melbourne, FL 32901. *Telephone:* 321-409-4800. *Fax:* 321-725-3766.

MASTER'S DEGREE PROGRAM

Degree MSN
Available Programs Master's.
Program Entrance Requirements Minimum overall college GPA of 2.7.
Degree Requirements 33 total credit hours.

Keiser University
Nursing Programs
Miami, Florida

DEGREES • BSN • MSN

BACCALAUREATE PROGRAMS

Degree BSN

Available Programs RN Baccalaureate.
Contact Miami campus, Nursing Programs, Keiser University, 2101 NW 117th Avenue, Miami, FL 33172. *Telephone:* 305-596-2226. *Fax:* 305-596-7077.

GRADUATE PROGRAMS

Contact Miami campus, Nursing Programs, Keiser University, 2101 NW 117th Avenue, Miami, FL 33172. *Telephone:* 305-596-2226. *Fax:* 305-596-7077.

MASTER'S DEGREE PROGRAM

Degree MSN
Available Programs Master's.
Program Entrance Requirements Minimum overall college GPA of 2.7.
Degree Requirements 33 total credit hours.

Keiser University
Nursing Programs
Orlando, Florida

DEGREES • BSN • MSN

BACCALAUREATE PROGRAMS

Degree BSN
Available Programs RN Baccalaureate.
Contact Orlando campus, Nursing Programs, Keiser University, 5600 Lake Underhill Road, Orlando, FL 32807. *Telephone:* 407-273-5800. *Fax:* 407-381-1233.

GRADUATE PROGRAMS

Contact Orland campus, Nursing Programs, Keiser University, 5600 Lake Underhill Road, Orlando, FL 32807. *Telephone:* 407-273-5800. *Fax:* 407-381-1233.

MASTER'S DEGREE PROGRAM

Degree MSN
Available Programs Master's.
Program Entrance Requirements Minimum overall college GPA of 2.7.
Degree Requirements 33 total credit hours.

Keiser University
Nursing Program
Pembroke Pines, Florida

Founded in 1998
DEGREES • BSN • MSN

BACCALAUREATE PROGRAMS

Degree BSN
Available Programs RN Baccalaureate.
Contact Pembroke Pines campus, Nursing Program, Keiser University, 1640 SW 145th Avenue, Pembroke Pines, FL 33027. *Telephone:* 954-431-4300. *Fax:* 954-431-2929.

GRADUATE PROGRAMS

Contact Pembroke Pines campus, Nursing Program, Keiser University, 1640 SW 145th Avenue, Pembroke Pines, FL 33027. *Telephone:* 954-431-4300. *Fax:* 954-431-2929.

MASTER'S DEGREE PROGRAM

Degree MSN
Available Programs Master's.
Program Entrance Requirements Minimum overall college GPA of 2.7.
Degree Requirements 33 total credit hours.

Keiser University
Nursing Programs
Port St. Lucie, Florida

Founded in 1999
DEGREES • BSN • MSN

BACCALAUREATE PROGRAMS

Degree BSN
Available Programs RN Baccalaureate.
Contact Port St. Lucie campus, Nursing Programs, Keiser University, 10330 South U.S. 1, Port St. Lucie, FL 34952. *Telephone:* 772-398-9990. *Fax:* 772-335-9619.

GRADUATE PROGRAMS

Contact Port St. Lucie campus, Nursing Programs, Keiser University, 10330 South U.S. 1, Port St. Lucie, FL 34952. *Telephone:* 772-398-9990. *Fax:* 772-335-9619.

MASTER'S DEGREE PROGRAM
Degree MSN
Available Programs Master's.
Program Entrance Requirements Minimum overall college GPA of 2.7.
Degree Requirements 33 total credit hours.

Keiser University
Nursing Programs
Sarasota, Florida

Founded in 1995
DEGREES • BSN • MSN

BACCALAUREATE PROGRAMS

Degree BSN
Available Programs RN Baccalaureate.
Contact Sarasota campus, Nursing Programs, Keiser University, 6151 Lake Osprey Drive, Sarasota, FL 34240. *Telephone:* 941-907-3900. *Fax:* 941-907-2016.

GRADUATE PROGRAMS

Contact Sarasota campus, Nursing Programs, Keiser University, 6151 Lake Osprey Drive, Sarasota, FL 34240. *Telephone:* 941-907-3900. *Fax:* 941-907-2016.

MASTER'S DEGREE PROGRAM
Degree MSN
Available Programs Master's.
Program Entrance Requirements Minimum overall college GPA of 2.7.
Degree Requirements 33 total credit hours.

Keiser University
Nursing Programs
Tallahassee, Florida

Founded in 1992
DEGREES • BSN • MSN

BACCALAUREATE PROGRAMS

Degree BSN
Available Programs RN Baccalaureate.
Contact Tallahassee campus, Nursing Programs, Keiser University, 1700 Halstead Boulevard, Building 2, Tallahassee, FL 32309. *Telephone:* 850-906-9494. *Fax:* 850-906-9497.

GRADUATE PROGRAMS

Contact Tallahassee campus, Nursing Programs, Keiser University, 1700 Halstead Boulevard, Building 2, Tallahassee, FL 32309. *Telephone:* 850-906-9494. *Fax:* 850-906-9497.

MASTER'S DEGREE PROGRAM
Degree MSN
Available Programs Master's.
Program Entrance Requirements Minimum overall college GPA of 2.7.
Degree Requirements 33 total credit hours.

Keiser University
Nursing Programs
Tampa, Florida

DEGREES • BSN • MSN

BACCALAUREATE PROGRAMS

Degree BSN
Available Programs RN Baccalaureate.
Contact Tampa campus, Nursing Programs, Keiser University, 5002 West Waters Avenue, Tampa, FL 33634. *Telephone:* 813-885-4900. *Fax:* 813-885-4911.

GRADUATE PROGRAMS

Contact Tampa campus, Nursing Programs, Keiser University, 5002 West Waters Avenue, Tampa, FL 33634. *Telephone:* 813-885-4900. *Fax:* 813-885-4911.

MASTER'S DEGREE PROGRAM
Degree MSN
Available Programs Master's.
Program Entrance Requirements Minimum overall college GPA of 2.7.
Degree Requirements 33 total credit hours.

Keiser University
Nursing Programs
West Palm Beach, Florida

Founded in 1988
DEGREES • BSN • MSN

BACCALAUREATE PROGRAMS

Degree BSN
Available Programs RN Baccalaureate.
Contact West Palm Beach campus, Nursing Programs, Keiser University, 2085 Vista Parkway, West Palm Beach, FL 33411. *Telephone:* 561-471-6000. *Fax:* 561-471-7849.

GRADUATE PROGRAMS

Contact West Palm Beach campus, Nursing Programs, Keiser University, 2085 Vista Parkway, West Palm Beach, FL 33411. *Telephone:* 561-471-6000. *Fax:* 561-471-7849.

MASTER'S DEGREE PROGRAM
Degree MSN
Available Programs Master's.
Program Entrance Requirements Minimum overall college GPA of 2.7.
Degree Requirements 33 total credit hours.

Miami Dade College
School of Nursing
Miami, Florida

Founded in 1960
DEGREE • BSN
Nursing Program Faculty 14 (73% with doctorates).
Baccalaureate Enrollment 578 **Women** 88% **Men** 12% **Minority** 94% **International** 3% **Part-time** 92%
Distance Learning Courses Available.
Nursing Student Activities Nursing Honor Society, Student Nurses' Association.

Nursing Student Resources Academic advising; academic or career counseling; assistance for students with disabilities; bookstore; campus computer network; computer lab; computer-assisted instruction; e-mail services; interactive nursing skills videos; Internet; learning resource lab; library services; nursing audiovisuals; remedial services; resume preparation assistance; skills, simulation, or other laboratory; tutoring.
Library Facilities 365,224 volumes (14,000 in health, 3,580 in nursing); 14,090 periodical subscriptions health-care related.

BACCALAUREATE PROGRAMS

Degree BSN
Available Programs RN Baccalaureate.
Site Options Miami, FL.
Program Entrance Requirements CPR certification, health exam, immunizations, minimum GPA in nursing prerequisites of 2.5, prerequisite course work, RN licensure. Transfer students are accepted. Application deadline: 5/1 (fall), 9/1 (spring). Application fee: $200.
Expenses (2012–13) Tuition, state resident: full-time $3304; part-time $92 per credit hour. Tuition, nonresident: full-time $16,156; part-time $449 per credit hour. International tuition: $16,156 full-time. Required fees: full-time $1157; part-time $32 per credit; part-time $385 per term.
Financial Aid 63% of baccalaureate students in nursing programs received some form of financial aid in 2011–12. Gift aid (need-based): Federal Pell, FSEOG, state, private, college/university gift aid from institutional funds. Loans: Perkins.Work-study: Federal Work-Study, part-time campus jobs.Financial aid application deadline (priority): 2/15.
Contact Amy Pettigrew, Dean, Benjamn Len School of Nursing, School of Nursing, Miami Dade College, 950 NW 20th Street, Miami, FL 33127. Telephone: 305-237-4039. E-mail: apettigr@mdc.edu.

Northwest Florida State College
RN to BSN Degree Program
Niceville, Florida

http://www.nwfsc.edu/RNtoBSN/
Founded in 1963
DEGREE • BSN
Nursing Program Faculty 3 (2% with doctorates).
Baccalaureate Enrollment 89
Distance Learning Courses Available.
Nursing Student Activities Student Nurses' Association, nursing club.
Nursing Student Resources Academic advising; academic or career counseling; assistance for students with disabilities; bookstore; campus computer network; career placement assistance; computer lab; computer-assisted instruction; daycare for children of students; employment services for current students; interactive nursing skills videos; Internet; learning resource lab; library services; nursing audiovisuals; placement services for program completers; remedial services; resume preparation assistance; skills, simulation, or other laboratory; tutoring; unpaid internships.
Library Facilities 106,383 volumes (1,880 in health, 1,048 in nursing); 399 periodical subscriptions (70 health-care related).

BACCALAUREATE PROGRAMS

Degree BSN
Available Programs ADN to Baccalaureate; Accelerated RN Baccalaureate; RN Baccalaureate.
Study Options Full-time and part-time.
Program Entrance Requirements Transcript of college record, CPR certification, health exam, immunizations, minimum GPA in nursing prerequisites of 2.75, RN licensure. Transfer students are accepted. Application deadline: 7/1 (fall), 11/30 (spring), 3/15 (summer). Applications may be processed on a rolling basis for some programs.
Advanced Placement Credit given for nursing courses completed elsewhere dependent upon specific evaluations.
Expenses (2012–13) Tuition, state resident: full-time $2846; part-time $119 per credit hour. Tuition, nonresident: full-time $107,763; part-time $449 per credit hour.
Contact Dr. Beth C. Norton, Division Director, Allied Health and BSN Programs, RN to BSN Degree Program, Northwest Florida State College, 100 College Boulevard, Niceville, FL 32578. Telephone: 850-729-6473. Fax: 850-729-6484. E-mail: nortonb@nwfsc.edu.

Nova Southeastern University
College of Health Care Sciences
Fort Lauderdale, Florida

http://www.nova.edu/nursing
Founded in 1964
DEGREES • BSN • MSN
Distance Learning Courses Available.
Nursing Student Activities Sigma Theta Tau, Student Nurses' Association.
Nursing Student Resources Academic advising; academic or career counseling; assistance for students with disabilities; bookstore; campus computer network; career placement assistance; computer lab; computer-assisted instruction; e-mail services; employment services for current students; housing assistance; interactive nursing skills videos; Internet; learning resource lab; library services; placement services for program completers; resume preparation assistance; skills, simulation, or other laboratory; tutoring.
Library Facilities 1 million volumes; 197,340 periodical subscriptions.

BACCALAUREATE PROGRAMS

Degree BSN
Available Programs Generic Baccalaureate; RN Baccalaureate.
Site Options Fort Myers, FL; Kendall, FL.
Study Options Full-time.
Online Degree Options Yes.
Program Entrance Requirements Minimum overall college GPA of 3.0, transcript of college record, health insurance, immunizations, interview, minimum GPA in nursing prerequisites of 2.75, prerequisite course work. Application deadline: 4/1 (fall), 10/1 (winter). Application fee: $50.
Expenses (2012–13) Tuition: full-time $23,450. International tuition: $24,500 full-time. Room and board: $7530 per academic year. Required fees: full-time $1045.
Contact Dr. Mary Botter, Associate Dean (Entry Level Nursing), College of Health Care Sciences, Nova Southeastern University, 3200 South University Drive, Fort Lauderdale, FL 33328. Telephone: 800-338-4723. Fax: 954-262-8000 Ext. 7184. E-mail: aalvarez1@nova.edu.

GRADUATE PROGRAMS

Expenses (2012–13) Tuition: part-time $550 per credit. International tuition: $550 full-time. Room and board: $14,050 per academic year. Required fees: full-time $1045; part-time $300 per term.
Financial Aid 1 fellowship (averaging $10,000 per year), 4 teaching assistantships (averaging $10,200 per year) were awarded; institutionally sponsored loans and unspecified assistantships also available.
Contact Dr. Diane Whitehead, Associate Dean, College of Health Care Sciences, Nova Southeastern University, 3200 South University Drive, Fort Lauderdale, FL 33328. Telephone: 954-262-1101. Fax: 877-640-0218. E-mail: keatta@nova.edu.

MASTER'S DEGREE PROGRAM
Degree MSN
Available Programs Master's; RN to Master's.
Concentrations Available Nursing administration; nursing education; nursing informatics.
Study Options Full-time and part-time.
Online Degree Options Yes (online only).
Program Entrance Requirements Minimum overall college GPA of 3.0, transcript of college record, written essay, immunizations, 2 letters of recommendation, statistics course, GRE General Test. Application deadline: 8/1 (fall), 12/1 (winter). Application fee: $50.
Degree Requirements 36 total credit hours, thesis or project.

Palm Beach Atlantic University
School of Nursing
West Palm Beach, Florida

Founded in 1968
DEGREE • BSN
Nursing Student Activities Student Nurses' Association.
Library Facilities 220,428 volumes; 66,424 periodical subscriptions.

BACCALAUREATE PROGRAMS

Degree BSN
Available Programs RN Baccalaureate.
Program Entrance Requirements RN licensure.
Contact *Telephone:* 561-803-2825. *Fax:* 561-803-2828.

Remington College of Nursing
Remington College of Nursing
Lake Mary, Florida

DEGREE • BSN

Nursing Program Faculty 23 (8% with doctorates).
Baccalaureate Enrollment 77 **Women** 86% **Men** 14% **Minority** 49%
International 4% **Part-time** 1%
Distance Learning Courses Available.
Nursing Student Activities Student Nurses' Association.
Nursing Student Resources Academic advising; academic or career counseling; assistance for students with disabilities; campus computer network; career placement assistance; computer-assisted instruction; e-mail services; interactive nursing skills videos; Internet; learning resource lab; library services; nursing audiovisuals; other; remedial services; resume preparation assistance; skills, simulation, or other laboratory; tutoring.
Library Facilities 990 volumes in health, 880 volumes in nursing; 905 periodical subscriptions health-care related.

BACCALAUREATE PROGRAMS

Degree BSN
Available Programs Accelerated Baccalaureate for Second Degree.
Study Options Full-time.
Program Entrance Requirements Minimum overall college GPA of 2.5, transcript of college record, CPR certification, written essay, health exam, health insurance, immunizations, interview, 2 letters of recommendation, prerequisite course work. *Application deadline:* 12/1 (winter), 4/1 (summer). Applications may be processed on a rolling basis for some programs. *Application fee:* $50.
Advanced Placement Credit given for nursing courses completed elsewhere dependent upon specific evaluations.
Expenses (2011–12) *Tuition, state resident:* full-time $36,000; part-time $480 per credit hour. *Tuition, nonresident:* full-time $36,000; part-time $480 per credit hour.
Financial Aid 38% of baccalaureate students in nursing programs received some form of financial aid in 2010–11.
Contact Pamela Milkowski, Admissions Coordinator, Remington College of Nursing, 660 Century Point, Suite 1050, Lake Mary, FL 32746. *Telephone:* 800-294-4434. *E-mail:* nursing.info@ remingtoncollege.edu.

St. Petersburg College
Department of Nursing
St. Petersburg, Florida

http://www.spcollege.edu/
Founded in 1927
DEGREE • BSN

Nursing Program Faculty 27 (56% with doctorates).
Baccalaureate Enrollment 688 **Women** 85% **Men** 15% **Minority** 28%
International 1%
Distance Learning Courses Available.
Nursing Student Activities Sigma Theta Tau, Student Nurses' Association.
Nursing Student Resources Academic advising; academic or career counseling; assistance for students with disabilities; bookstore; campus computer network; computer lab; computer-assisted instruction; e-mail services; employment services for current students; interactive nursing skills videos; Internet; learning resource lab; library services; nursing audiovisuals; placement services for program completers; remedial services; resume preparation assistance; skills, simulation, or other laboratory; tutoring; unpaid internships.
Library Facilities 241,761 volumes (1,390 in health, 484 in nursing); 1,987 periodical subscriptions (77 health-care related).

BACCALAUREATE PROGRAMS

Degree BSN
Available Programs ADN to Baccalaureate; RN Baccalaureate.
Site Options Pinellas Park, FL.
Online Degree Options Yes.
Program Entrance Requirements Minimum overall college GPA of 2.0, transcript of college record, high school transcript, prerequisite course work, RN licensure. Transfer students are accepted. *Application deadline:* 7/13 (fall), 11/9 (spring). *Application fee:* $40.
Expenses (2012–13) *Tuition, state resident:* full-time $5879; part-time $117 per credit hour. *Tuition, nonresident:* full-time $18,002; part-time $420 per credit hour. *Required fees:* full-time $3000; part-time $1000 per term.
Financial Aid 45% of baccalaureate students in nursing programs received some form of financial aid in 2011–12. *Gift aid (need-based):* Federal Pell, FSEOG, state, private, college/university gift aid from institutional funds. *Loans:* college/university. *Work-study:* Federal Work-Study. *Financial aid application deadline (priority):* 4/15.
Contact Dr. Susan Anita Baker, Dean, Department of Nursing, St. Petersburg College, PO Box 13489, St. Petersburg, FL 33733. *Telephone:* 727-341-3640. *Fax:* 727-341-3646. *E-mail:* baker.susan@spcollege.edu.

CONTINUING EDUCATION PROGRAM

Contact Denise Kerwin, Program Director, Department of Nursing, St. Petersburg College, PO Box 13489, St. Petersburg, FL 33733. *Telephone:* 727-341-3374. *Fax:* 727-341-4197. *E-mail:* kerwin.denise@ spcollege.edu.

South University
Nursing Program
Royal Palm Beach, Florida

http://www.southuniversity.edu/nursing-and-health-professions-programs-125.aspx
Founded in 1899
DEGREES • BSN • MSN

Nursing Program Faculty 89 (50% with doctorates).
Baccalaureate Enrollment 1,150 **Women** 93% **Men** 7% **Minority** 40%
Graduate Enrollment 212 **Women** 93% **Men** 7% **Minority** 40%
Distance Learning Courses Available.
Nursing Student Activities Nursing Honor Society, Student Nurses' Association.
Nursing Student Resources Academic advising; academic or career counseling; assistance for students with disabilities; bookstore; campus computer network; career placement assistance; computer lab; computer-assisted instruction; e-mail services; externships; interactive nursing skills videos; Internet; learning resource lab; library services; nursing audiovisuals; placement services for program completers; remedial services; resume preparation assistance; skills, simulation, or other laboratory; tutoring.
Library Facilities 6,000 volumes in health, 2,000 volumes in nursing; 50 periodical subscriptions health-care related.

BACCALAUREATE PROGRAMS

Degree BSN
Available Programs Generic Baccalaureate; RN Baccalaureate.
Site Options Tampa, FL; West Palm Beach, FL; Columbia, SC.
Study Options Full-time.
Online Degree Options Yes.
Program Entrance Requirements Minimum overall college GPA of 2.5, transcript of college record, health exam, high school transcript, immunizations, minimum GPA in nursing prerequisites of 2.5, prerequisite course work. Transfer students are accepted.
Contact *Telephone:* 800-688-0932.

GRADUATE PROGRAMS

Contact *Telephone:* 888-444-3404.

MASTER'S DEGREE PROGRAM
Degree MSN
Available Programs Master's; RN to Master's.
Concentrations Available Nursing education.
Site Options West Palm Beach, FL.
Study Options Full-time and part-time.
Online Degree Options Yes.

Program Entrance Requirements Minimum overall college GPA of 2.7, transcript of college record, written essay, 3 letters of recommendation, nursing research course, prerequisite course work, resume, statistics course. *Application deadline:* Applications may be processed on a rolling basis for some programs.
Advanced Placement Credit given for nursing courses completed elsewhere dependent upon specific evaluations.
Degree Requirements 48 total credit hours, thesis or project.

South University
College of Nursing
Tampa, Florida

DEGREES • BSN • MS

BACCALAUREATE PROGRAMS

Degree BSN
Available Programs RN Baccalaureate.
Online Degree Options Yes.
Program Entrance Requirements Minimum overall college GPA of 2.5, RN licensure.
Contact *Telephone:* 800-846-1472. *Fax:* 813-393-3814.

GRADUATE PROGRAMS

Contact *Telephone:* 800-846-1472. *Fax:* 813-393-3814.

MASTER'S DEGREE PROGRAM

Degree MS
Available Programs Master's.
Program Entrance Requirements 3 Letters of recommendation, resume.

State College of Florida Manatee-Sarasota
Nursing Degree Program
Bradenton, Florida

Founded in 1957
DEGREE • BSN
Library Facilities 65,386 volumes; 378 periodical subscriptions.

BACCALAUREATE PROGRAMS

Degree BSN
Available Programs RN Baccalaureate.
Program Entrance Requirements Prerequisite course work, RN licensure. *Application deadline:* 3/1 (summer).
Contact Admissions, Nursing Degree Program; State College of Florida Manatee-Sarasota, 5840 26th Street West, Bradenton, FL 34206. *Telephone:* 941-752-5050. *Fax:* 941-727-6380. *E-mail:* admissions@scf.edu.

University of Central Florida
College of Nursing
Orlando, Florida

http://www.nursing.ucf.edu/
Founded in 1963
DEGREES • BSN • MSN • PHD
Nursing Program Faculty 56 (43% with doctorates).
Baccalaureate Enrollment 379 **Women** 91% **Men** 9% **Minority** 25% **Part-time** 32%
Graduate Enrollment 136 **Women** 87% **Men** 13% **Minority** 10% **Part-time** 75%
Nursing Student Activities Sigma Theta Tau, Student Nurses' Association.
Nursing Student Resources Academic advising; academic or career counseling; assistance for students with disabilities; bookstore; campus computer network; computer lab; computer-assisted instruction; daycare for children of students; e-mail services; employment services for current

students; externships; housing assistance; interactive nursing skills videos; Internet; learning resource lab; library services; nursing audiovisuals; skills, simulation, or other laboratory; tutoring.
Library Facilities 2.4 million volumes (38,944 in health, 2,848 in nursing); 43,333 periodical subscriptions (360 health-care related).

BACCALAUREATE PROGRAMS

Degree BSN
Available Programs Accelerated Baccalaureate for Second Degree; Generic Baccalaureate; RN Baccalaureate.
Study Options Full-time and part-time.
Program Entrance Requirements Minimum overall college GPA of 2.5, transcript of college record, CPR certification, health exam, health insurance, high school foreign language, high school math, high school transcript, immunizations, minimum high school GPA of 2.5, prerequisite course work. Transfer students are accepted.
Advanced Placement Credit given for nursing courses completed elsewhere dependent upon specific evaluations.
Contact *Telephone:* 407-823-2744. *Fax:* 407-823-5675.

GRADUATE PROGRAMS

Contact *Telephone:* 407-823-2744. *Fax:* 407-823-5675.

MASTER'S DEGREE PROGRAM

Degree MSN
Available Programs Master's; RN to Master's.
Concentrations Available Nurse case management; nursing administration; nursing education. *Clinical nurse specialist programs in:* acute care, critical care. *Nurse practitioner programs in:* adult health, family health, pediatric.
Study Options Full-time and part-time.
Program Entrance Requirements Clinical experience, minimum overall college GPA of 3.0, transcript of college record, CPR certification, written essay, immunizations, 3 letters of recommendation, physical assessment course, resume, statistics course.
Advanced Placement Credit given for nursing courses completed elsewhere dependent upon specific evaluations.
Degree Requirements 47 total credit hours, thesis or project.

POST-MASTER'S PROGRAM

Areas of Study *Nurse practitioner programs in:* adult health, family health, pediatric.

DOCTORAL DEGREE PROGRAM

Degree PhD
Available Programs Doctorate.
Areas of Study Health policy, health-care systems, individualized study, information systems, nursing research.
Program Entrance Requirements Minimum overall college GPA of 3.5, interview by faculty committee, 3 letters of recommendation, MSN or equivalent, statistics course, vita.
Degree Requirements 57 total credit hours, dissertation.

University of Florida
College of Nursing
Gainesville, Florida

http://www.nursing.ufl.edu/
Founded in 1853
DEGREES • BSN • MSN • MSN/PHD • PHD
Nursing Program Faculty 62 (50% with doctorates).
Baccalaureate Enrollment 374 **Women** 94% **Men** 6% **Minority** 23% **International** 1%
Graduate Enrollment 364 **Women** 97% **Men** 3% **Minority** 17% **International** 1% **Part-time** 56%
Distance Learning Courses Available.
Nursing Student Activities Nursing Honor Society, Sigma Theta Tau, Student Nurses' Association.
Nursing Student Resources Academic advising; academic or career counseling; assistance for students with disabilities; bookstore; campus computer network; career placement assistance; computer lab; computer-assisted instruction; daycare for children of students; e-mail services; employment services for current students; housing assistance; interactive nursing skills videos; Internet; learning resource lab; library services; nursing audiovisuals; placement services for program completers;

remedial services; resume preparation assistance; skills, simulation, or other laboratory; tutoring.

Library Facilities 5.8 million volumes (260,000 in health, 3,000 in nursing); 132,028 periodical subscriptions (200 health-care related).

BACCALAUREATE PROGRAMS

Degree BSN

Available Programs Accelerated Baccalaureate for Second Degree; Generic Baccalaureate.

Study Options Full-time.

Program Entrance Requirements Minimum overall college GPA of 2.8, transcript of college record, CPR certification, written essay, health exam, health insurance, high school biology, high school chemistry, high school foreign language, high school transcript, immunizations, 2 letters of recommendation, minimum GPA in nursing prerequisites of 2.8, prerequisite course work. Transfer students are accepted. *Application deadline:* 3/15 (fall), 1/15 (summer). *Application fee:* $30.

Advanced Placement Credit by examination available. Credit given for nursing courses completed elsewhere dependent upon specific evaluations.

Contact *Telephone:* 352-273-6383. *Fax:* 352-273-6440.

GRADUATE PROGRAMS

Contact *Telephone:* 352-273-6331. *Fax:* 352-273-6440.

MASTER'S DEGREE PROGRAM

Degrees MSN; MSN/PhD

Available Programs Master's.

Concentrations Available Clinical nurse leader; nurse-midwifery. *Clinical nurse specialist programs in:* psychiatric/mental health, public health. *Nurse practitioner programs in:* acute care, adult health, family health, neonatal health, pediatric, psychiatric/mental health.

Site Options Jacksonville, FL.

Study Options Full-time and part-time.

Online Degree Options Yes.

Program Entrance Requirements Minimum overall college GPA of 3.0, transcript of college record, CPR certification, written essay, immunizations, 2 letters of recommendation, resume, GRE General Test. *Application deadline:* 3/15 (fall). Applications may be processed on a rolling basis for some programs. *Application fee:* $30.

Advanced Placement Credit given for nursing courses completed elsewhere dependent upon specific evaluations.

Degree Requirements 46 total credit hours, comprehensive exam.

POST-MASTER'S PROGRAM

Areas of Study Clinical nurse leader; nurse-midwifery. *Clinical nurse specialist programs in:* psychiatric/mental health, public health. *Nurse practitioner programs in:* acute care, adult health, family health, neonatal health, pediatric, psychiatric/mental health.

DOCTORAL DEGREE PROGRAM

Degree PhD

Available Programs Doctorate; Post-Baccalaureate Doctorate.

Areas of Study Aging, bio-behavioral research, health policy, nursing policy, nursing science, oncology, women's health.

Site Options Jacksonville, FL.

Online Degree Options Yes.

Program Entrance Requirements Minimum overall college GPA of 3.5, 3 letters of recommendation, MSN or equivalent, vita, writing sample, GRE General Test. *Application deadline:* 3/15 (fall). Applications may be processed on a rolling basis for some programs. *Application fee:* $30.

Degree Requirements 62 total credit hours, dissertation.

University of Miami
School of Nursing and Health Studies
Coral Gables, Florida

http://www.miami.edu/sonhs
Founded in 1925
DEGREES • BSN • MSN • PHD
Nursing Program Faculty 75 (26% with doctorates).
Baccalaureate Enrollment 324 **Women** 86.73% **Men** 13.27% **Minority** 64.2% **International** 1.23% **Part-time** 3.4%
Graduate Enrollment 270 **Women** 74.44% **Men** 25.56% **Minority** 68.52% **International** 4.07% **Part-time** 33.33%

Distance Learning Courses Available.

Nursing Student Activities Nursing Honor Society, Sigma Theta Tau, Student Nurses' Association.

Nursing Student Resources Academic advising; academic or career counseling; assistance for students with disabilities; bookstore; campus computer network; career placement assistance; computer lab; computer-assisted instruction; e-mail services; employment services for current students; externships; housing assistance; interactive nursing skills videos; Internet; learning resource lab; library services; nursing audiovisuals; placement services for program completers; remedial services; resume preparation assistance; skills, simulation, or other laboratory; tutoring; unpaid internships.

Library Facilities 54,924 volumes in health, 1,892 volumes in nursing; 8,441 periodical subscriptions health-care related.

BACCALAUREATE PROGRAMS

Degree BSN

Available Programs Accelerated Baccalaureate for Second Degree; Baccalaureate for Second Degree; Generic Baccalaureate; RN Baccalaureate.

Study Options Full-time.

Program Entrance Requirements Minimum overall college GPA of 3.5, transcript of college record, CPR certification, written essay, health exam, health insurance, immunizations, 2 letters of recommendation, minimum high school GPA of 4.0, minimum GPA in nursing prerequisites of 3.3, professional liability insurance/malpractice insurance, prerequisite course work. Transfer students are accepted. *Application deadline:* 3/1 (fall), 10/15 (spring), 3/1 (summer). Applications may be processed on a rolling basis for some programs. *Application fee:* $70.

Expenses (2012–13) *Tuition:* full-time $39,980; part-time $1660 per credit. *International tuition:* $39,980 full-time. *Room and board:* $11,882; room only: $6914 per academic year. *Required fees:* full-time $1040; part-time $510 per term.

Financial Aid 90% of baccalaureate students in nursing programs received some form of financial aid in 2011–12. *Gift aid (need-based):* Federal Pell, FSEOG, state, private, college/university gift aid from institutional funds, Federal Nursing, Academic Competitiveness Grants, National SMART Grants. *Loans:* Federal Nursing Student Loans, Federal Direct (Subsidized and Unsubsidized Stafford PLUS), Perkins, college/university, private loans. *Work-study:* Federal Work-Study, part-time campus jobs. *Financial aid application deadline (priority):* 2/1.

Contact Ms. Deborah Paris, Associate Dean for Student Services, School of Nursing and Health Studies, University of Miami, PO Box 248153-3850, Coral Gables, FL 33124-3850. *Telephone:* 305-284-4099. *Fax:* 305-284-5686. *E-mail:* dparis@miami.edu.

GRADUATE PROGRAMS

Expenses (2012–13) *Tuition:* part-time $1660 per credit. *Room and board:* $11,882; room only: $6914 per academic year. *Required fees:* part-time $260 per term.

Financial Aid 90% of graduate students in nursing programs received some form of financial aid in 2011–12. 1 fellowship (averaging $36,000 per year), 6 research assistantships with tuition reimbursements available (averaging $36,000 per year), 4 teaching assistantships with tuition reimbursements available (averaging $36,000 per year) were awarded; Federal Work-Study, institutionally sponsored loans, scholarships, and unspecified assistantships also available. Aid available to part-time students. *Financial aid application deadline:* 3/1.

Contact Ms. Deborah Paris, Associate Dean for Student Services, School of Nursing and Health Studies, University of Miami, PO Box 248153, M. Christine Schwartz Center, Coral Gables, FL 33124-3850. *Telephone:* 305-284-4099. *Fax:* 305-284-5686. *E-mail:* dparis@miami.edu.

MASTER'S DEGREE PROGRAM

Degree MSN

Available Programs Master's.

Concentrations Available Nurse anesthesia; nurse-midwifery; nursing education. *Nurse practitioner programs in:* acute care, adult health, family health.

Study Options Full-time and part-time.

Program Entrance Requirements Clinical experience, minimum overall college GPA of 3.0, transcript of college record, CPR certification, written essay, immunizations, interview, 3 letters of recommendation, professional liability insurance/malpractice insurance, resume, statistics course, GRE General Test. *Application deadline:* 4/1 (fall), 10/15 (spring). Applications may be processed on a rolling basis for some programs. *Application fee:* $65.

Degree Requirements 30 total credit hours, comprehensive exam.

POST-MASTER'S PROGRAM

Areas of Study Nurse-midwifery. *Nurse practitioner programs in:* acute care, adult health, family health.

DOCTORAL DEGREE PROGRAM

Degree PhD

Available Programs Doctorate; Post-Baccalaureate Doctorate.

Areas of Study Addiction/substance abuse, bio-behavioral research, biology of health and illness, clinical practice, family health, health policy, health promotion/disease prevention, maternity-newborn, nursing policy, nursing research, nursing science.

Program Entrance Requirements Minimum overall college GPA of 3.0, interview, 3 letters of recommendation, MSN or equivalent, statistics course, vita, writing sample, GRE General Test. *Application deadline:* 6/1 (fall), 3/1 (summer). Applications may be processed on a rolling basis for some programs. *Application fee:* $65.

Degree Requirements 40 total credit hours, dissertation, oral exam, written exam, residency.

CONTINUING EDUCATION PROGRAM

Contact Ms. Deborah Paris, Assistant Dean, School of Nursing and Health Studies, University of Miami, PO Box 248153, M. Christine Schwartz Center, Room 152, Coral Gables, FL 33124-3850. *Telephone:* 305-284-4325. *Fax:* 305-284-4827. *E-mail:* dparis@miami.edu.

University of North Florida

School of Nursing
Jacksonville, Florida

http://www.unf.edu/brooks/nursing/
Founded in 1965

DEGREES • BSN • MSN

Nursing Program Faculty 19 (50% with doctorates).

Baccalaureate Enrollment 279 **Women** 85% **Men** 15% **Minority** 20% **International** 1% **Part-time** 27%

Graduate Enrollment 35 **Women** 86% **Men** 14% **Minority** 6% **Part-time** 70%

Nursing Student Activities Sigma Theta Tau, Student Nurses' Association.

Nursing Student Resources Academic advising; academic or career counseling; assistance for students with disabilities; bookstore; campus computer network; career placement assistance; computer lab; computer-assisted instruction; e-mail services; interactive nursing skills videos; Internet; learning resource lab; library services; nursing audiovisuals; resume preparation assistance; skills, simulation, or other laboratory.

Library Facilities 840,423 volumes (30,466 in health, 3,000 in nursing); 2,800 periodical subscriptions (200 health-care related).

BACCALAUREATE PROGRAMS

Degree BSN

Available Programs Accelerated Baccalaureate for Second Degree; Generic Baccalaureate; RN Baccalaureate.

Study Options Full-time.

Program Entrance Requirements Minimum overall college GPA of 2.7, CPR certification, written essay, health exam, immunizations, interview, minimum high school GPA, minimum GPA in nursing prerequisites of 3.0, professional liability insurance/malpractice insurance, prerequisite course work. Transfer students are accepted.

Advanced Placement Credit given for nursing courses completed elsewhere dependent upon specific evaluations.

Contact *Telephone:* 904-620-2418.

GRADUATE PROGRAMS

Contact *Telephone:* 904-620-2684. *Fax:* 904-620-2848.

MASTER'S DEGREE PROGRAM

Degree MSN

Available Programs Master's; RN to Master's.

Concentrations Available *Clinical nurse specialist programs in:* adult health, cardiovascular, community health, critical care, gerontology,

maternity-newborn, medical-surgical, pediatric, psychiatric/mental health, women's health. *Nurse practitioner programs in:* family health, primary care.

Study Options Full-time and part-time.

Program Entrance Requirements Clinical experience, computer literacy, minimum overall college GPA of 3.0, transcript of college record, CPR certification, written essay, immunizations, 2 letters of recommendation, nursing research course, physical assessment course, professional liability insurance/malpractice insurance, resume, statistics course.

Advanced Placement Credit given for nursing courses completed elsewhere dependent upon specific evaluations.

Degree Requirements 43 total credit hours, thesis or project.

POST-MASTER'S PROGRAM

Areas of Study *Nurse practitioner programs in:* family health, primary care.

University of Phoenix–Central Florida Campus

College of Nursing
Maitland, Florida

Founded in 1996

DEGREES • BSN • MSN • MSN/ED D

Nursing Program Faculty 10 (60% with doctorates).

Baccalaureate Enrollment 35 **Women** 88.6% **Men** 11.4% **Minority** 45.7%

Graduate Enrollment 18 **Women** 94.4% **Men** 5.6% **Minority** 50%

Nursing Student Activities Sigma Theta Tau.

Nursing Student Resources Academic advising; academic or career counseling; assistance for students with disabilities; bookstore; campus computer network; computer lab; computer-assisted instruction; e-mail services; interactive nursing skills videos; Internet; learning resource lab; library services; nursing audiovisuals; remedial services; skills, simulation, or other laboratory; tutoring.

Library Facilities 16,781 periodical subscriptions (1,300 health-care related).

BACCALAUREATE PROGRAMS

Degree BSN

Available Programs Accelerated Baccalaureate.

Site Options Orlando, FL; Daytona Beach, FL.

Study Options Full-time.

Program Entrance Requirements Transcript of college record, CPR certification, immunizations, 1 letter of recommendation, RN licensure. Transfer students are accepted. *Application deadline:* Applications may be processed on a rolling basis for some programs.

Advanced Placement Credit by examination available. Credit given for nursing courses completed elsewhere dependent upon specific evaluations.

Contact *Telephone:* 407-667-0555.

GRADUATE PROGRAMS

Contact *Telephone:* 407-667-0555.

MASTER'S DEGREE PROGRAM

Degrees MSN; MSN/Ed D

Available Programs Master's.

Concentrations Available Nursing administration; nursing education.

Site Options Orlando, FL; Daytona Beach, FL.

Study Options Full-time.

Program Entrance Requirements Clinical experience, computer literacy, minimum overall college GPA of 2.5, transcript of college record. *Application deadline:* Applications may be processed on a rolling basis for some programs. *Application fee:* $45.

Advanced Placement Credit given for nursing courses completed elsewhere dependent upon specific evaluations.

Degree Requirements 39 total credit hours, thesis or project.

University of Phoenix–North Florida Campus
College of Nursing
Jacksonville, Florida

Founded in 1976
DEGREES • BSN • MSN • MSN/ED D • MSN/MHA
Nursing Program Faculty 7 (29% with doctorates).
Baccalaureate Enrollment 13 **Women** 92.3% **Men** 7.7% **Minority** 38.5%
Graduate Enrollment 10 **Women** 100% **Minority** 20%
Nursing Student Activities Sigma Theta Tau.
Nursing Student Resources Academic advising; academic or career counseling; assistance for students with disabilities; bookstore; campus computer network; computer lab; computer-assisted instruction; e-mail services; interactive nursing skills videos; Internet; learning resource lab; library services; nursing audiovisuals; remedial services; skills, simulation, or other laboratory; tutoring.
Library Facilities 1,300 periodical subscriptions health-care related.

BACCALAUREATE PROGRAMS

Degree BSN
Available Programs Accelerated Baccalaureate.
Site Options Orange Park, FL.
Study Options Full-time.
Program Entrance Requirements Transcript of college record, CPR certification, immunizations, 1 letter of recommendation, RN licensure. Transfer students are accepted. *Application deadline:* Applications may be processed on a rolling basis for some programs.
Advanced Placement Credit by examination available. Credit given for nursing courses completed elsewhere dependent upon specific evaluations.
Contact *Telephone:* 904-636-6645.

GRADUATE PROGRAMS

Contact *Telephone:* 904-636-6645.

MASTER'S DEGREE PROGRAM
Degrees MSN; MSN/Ed D; MSN/MHA
Available Programs Master's.
Concentrations Available Health-care administration; nursing administration; nursing education.
Site Options Orange Park, FL.
Study Options Full-time.
Program Entrance Requirements Clinical experience, computer literacy, minimum overall college GPA of 2.5, transcript of college record. *Application deadline:* Applications may be processed on a rolling basis for some programs. *Application fee:* $45.
Advanced Placement Credit given for nursing courses completed elsewhere dependent upon specific evaluations.
Degree Requirements 39 total credit hours, thesis or project.

University of Phoenix–South Florida Campus
College of Nursing
Fort Lauderdale, Florida

DEGREES • BSN • MSN • MSN/MBA • MSN/MHA
Nursing Program Faculty 24 (21% with doctorates).
Baccalaureate Enrollment 135 **Women** 96.3% **Men** 3.7% **Minority** 38.5%
Graduate Enrollment 102 **Women** 91.2% **Men** 8.8% **Minority** 41.18%
Nursing Student Activities Sigma Theta Tau.
Nursing Student Resources Academic advising; academic or career counseling; assistance for students with disabilities; bookstore; campus computer network; computer lab; computer-assisted instruction; e-mail services; interactive nursing skills videos; Internet; learning resource lab; library services; nursing audiovisuals; skills, simulation, or other laboratory; tutoring.

Library Facilities 16,781 periodical subscriptions (1,300 health-care related).

BACCALAUREATE PROGRAMS

Degree BSN
Available Programs RN Baccalaureate.
Site Options Palm Beach Gardens, FL; Ft. Lauderdale, FL; Miramar, FL.
Study Options Full-time.
Online Degree Options Yes.
Program Entrance Requirements Transcript of college record, CPR certification, immunizations, 1 letter of recommendation, RN licensure. Transfer students are accepted. *Application deadline:* Applications may be processed on a rolling basis for some programs.
Advanced Placement Credit by examination available. Credit given for nursing courses completed elsewhere dependent upon specific evaluations.
Contact *Telephone:* 954-382-5303.

GRADUATE PROGRAMS

Contact *Telephone:* 954-382-5303.

MASTER'S DEGREE PROGRAM
Degrees MSN; MSN/MBA; MSN/MHA
Available Programs Master's.
Concentrations Available Health-care administration; nursing administration; nursing education.
Site Options Palm Beach Gardens, FL; Ft. Lauderdale, FL; Miramar, FL.
Study Options Full-time.
Online Degree Options Yes.
Program Entrance Requirements Clinical experience, computer literacy, minimum overall college GPA of 2.5, transcript of college record. *Application deadline:* Applications may be processed on a rolling basis for some programs. *Application fee:* $45.
Advanced Placement Credit given for nursing courses completed elsewhere dependent upon specific evaluations.
Degree Requirements 39 total credit hours, thesis or project.

University of Phoenix–West Florida Campus
College of Nursing
Temple Terrace, Florida

DEGREE • BSN
Nursing Program Faculty 5 (60% with doctorates).
Baccalaureate Enrollment 8 **Women** 87.5% **Men** 12.5% **Minority** 12.5%
Nursing Student Activities Sigma Theta Tau.
Nursing Student Resources Academic advising; academic or career counseling; assistance for students with disabilities; bookstore; campus computer network; computer lab; computer-assisted instruction; e-mail services; interactive nursing skills videos; Internet; learning resource lab; library services; nursing audiovisuals; remedial services; skills, simulation, or other laboratory; tutoring.
Library Facilities 16,781 periodical subscriptions (1,300 health-care related).

BACCALAUREATE PROGRAMS

Degree BSN
Available Programs Accelerated Baccalaureate.
Site Options Tampa, FL; Clearwater, FL; Sarasota, FL.
Study Options Full-time.
Online Degree Options Yes.
Program Entrance Requirements Transcript of college record, CPR certification, immunizations, 1 letter of recommendation, RN licensure. Transfer students are accepted. *Application deadline:* Applications may be processed on a rolling basis for some programs.
Advanced Placement Credit by examination available. Credit given for nursing courses completed elsewhere dependent upon specific evaluations.
Contact *Telephone:* 813-626-7911.

University of South Florida
College of Nursing
Tampa, Florida

http://hsc.usf.edu/nursing
Founded in 1956
DEGREES • BS • MS • MS/MPH • PHD
Nursing Program Faculty 77 (48% with doctorates).
Baccalaureate Enrollment 702 **Women** 81% **Men** 19% **Minority** 32% **International** 2% **Part-time** 38%
Graduate Enrollment 684 **Women** 86% **Men** 14% **Minority** 21% **International** 1% **Part-time** 85%
Distance Learning Courses Available.
Nursing Student Activities Nursing Honor Society, Sigma Theta Tau, Student Nurses' Association.
Nursing Student Resources Academic advising; academic or career counseling; assistance for students with disabilities; bookstore; campus computer network; career placement assistance; computer lab; computer-assisted instruction; daycare for children of students; e-mail services; employment services for current students; housing assistance; interactive nursing skills videos; Internet; learning resource lab; library services; nursing audiovisuals; remedial services; resume preparation assistance; skills, simulation, or other laboratory; tutoring.
Library Facilities 2.6 million volumes (106,028 in health, 4,000 in nursing); 82,706 periodical subscriptions (1,750 health-care related).

BACCALAUREATE PROGRAMS

Degree BS
Available Programs ADN to Baccalaureate; Accelerated Baccalaureate for Second Degree; Generic Baccalaureate.
Study Options Full-time.
Online Degree Options Yes.
Program Entrance Requirements Minimum overall college GPA of 3.2, transcript of college record, CPR certification, written essay, health insurance, immunizations, prerequisite course work. Transfer students are accepted. *Application deadline:* 6/15 (fall), 3/15 (summer). *Application fee:* $30.
Expenses (2012–13) *Tuition, state resident:* full-time $9391; part-time $209 per credit hour. *Tuition, nonresident:* full-time $24,274; part-time $539 per credit hour. *International tuition:* $24,274 full-time. *Room and board:* $12,574; room only: $7324 per academic year. *Required fees:* full-time $2795; part-time $62 per credit; part-time $932 per term.
Financial Aid 60% of baccalaureate students in nursing programs received some form of financial aid in 2011–12.
Contact Ms. Joylynn Grier, Coordinator, Undergraduate Admissions, College of Nursing, University of South Florida, 12901 Bruce B. Downs Boulevard, MDC Box 22, Tampa, FL 33612-4766. *Telephone:* 813-974-2191. *Fax:* 813-974-3118. *E-mail:* nurstudent@health.usf.edu.

GRADUATE PROGRAMS

Expenses (2012–13) *Tuition, state resident:* full-time $14,971; part-time $416 per credit hour. *Tuition, nonresident:* full-time $30,142; part-time $837 per credit hour. *International tuition:* $30,142 full-time. *Room and board:* $12,574; room only: $7324 per academic year. *Required fees:* full-time $2161; part-time $72 per credit; part-time $720 per term.
Financial Aid 30% of graduate students in nursing programs received some form of financial aid in 2011–12. 7 research assistantships with tuition reimbursements available (averaging $18,935 per year), 29 teaching assistantships with tuition reimbursements available (averaging $30,814 per year) were awarded; tuition waivers (partial) and unspecified assistantships also available. *Financial aid application deadline:* 2/1.
Contact Ms. Zuzanna Moore, Admissions Recruiter Advisor, College of Nursing, University of South Florida, 12901 Bruce B. Downs Boulevard, MDC Box 22, Tampa, FL 33612-4766. *Telephone:* 813-974-2952. *Fax:* 813-974-5418. *E-mail:* nurstudent@health.usf.edu.

MASTER'S DEGREE PROGRAM

Degrees MS; MS/MPH
Available Programs Master's; Master's for Nurses with Non-Nursing Degrees; RN to Master's.
Concentrations Available Clinical nurse leader; nurse anesthesia; nursing education. *Nurse practitioner programs in:* acute care, adult health, family health, gerontology, occupational health, oncology, pediatric.
Study Options Full-time and part-time.
Program Entrance Requirements Computer literacy, minimum overall college GPA of 3.0, transcript of college record, CPR certification, immu-

nizations, interview, 3 letters of recommendation, resume, GRE General Test. *Application deadline:* 2/15 (fall), 10/15 (spring). *Application fee:* $30.
Advanced Placement Credit given for nursing courses completed elsewhere dependent upon specific evaluations.
Degree Requirements 45 total credit hours, thesis or project, comprehensive exam.

DOCTORAL DEGREE PROGRAM

Degree PhD
Available Programs Doctorate.
Areas of Study Bio-behavioral research, clinical practice, critical care, ethics, faculty preparation, family health, gerontology, health promotion/disease prevention, human health and illness, illness and transition, maternity-newborn, nursing education, nursing research, nursing science, oncology, women's health.
Program Entrance Requirements Minimum overall college GPA of 3.0, interview by faculty committee, interview, 3 letters of recommendation, MSN or equivalent, vita, writing sample, GRE General Test. *Application deadline:* 2/1 (fall). *Application fee:* $30.
Degree Requirements 63 total credit hours, dissertation.

CONTINUING EDUCATION PROGRAM

Contact Dr. Deborah Sutherland, Senior Vice President, College of Nursing, University of South Florida, 124 South Franklin Street, Tampa, FL 33602. *Telephone:* 813-224-7840.

The University of Tampa
Department of Nursing
Tampa, Florida

http://www.ut.edu/nursing
Founded in 1931
DEGREES • BSN • MSN
Nursing Program Faculty 25 (45% with doctorates).
Baccalaureate Enrollment 95 **Women** 80% **Men** 20% **Minority** 24% **International** 5% **Part-time** 5%
Graduate Enrollment 177 **Women** 95% **Men** 5% **Minority** 25% **Part-time** 66%
Nursing Student Activities Sigma Theta Tau, Student Nurses' Association.
Nursing Student Resources Academic advising; academic or career counseling; assistance for students with disabilities; bookstore; campus computer network; career placement assistance; computer lab; computer-assisted instruction; e-mail services; employment services for current students; externships; housing assistance; interactive nursing skills videos; Internet; learning resource lab; library services; nursing audiovisuals; paid internships; placement services for program completers; remedial services; resume preparation assistance; skills, simulation, or other laboratory; tutoring; unpaid internships.
Library Facilities 291,457 volumes (252,147 in health, 3,000 in nursing); 51,978 periodical subscriptions (10,854 health-care related).

BACCALAUREATE PROGRAMS

Degree BSN
Available Programs ADN to Baccalaureate; Generic Baccalaureate; RN Baccalaureate.
Study Options Full-time.
Program Entrance Requirements Minimum overall college GPA of 3.25, transcript of college record, CPR certification, written essay, health exam, health insurance, high school transcript, immunizations, 1 letter of recommendation, minimum GPA in nursing prerequisites, professional liability insurance/malpractice insurance, prerequisite course work. Transfer students are accepted. *Application deadline:* 10/15 (spring).
Expenses (2011–12) *Tuition:* full-time $22,834; part-time $486 per credit. *International tuition:* $22,834 full-time. *Room and board:* $8830; room only: $4700 per academic year. *Required fees:* full-time $1142; part-time $354 per term.
Financial Aid 85% of baccalaureate students in nursing programs received some form of financial aid in 2010–11. *Gift aid (need-based):* Federal Pell, FSEOG, state, private, college/university gift aid from institutional funds. *Loans:* Federal Direct (Subsidized and Unsubsidized Stafford PLUS), Perkins, college/university. *Work-study:* Federal Work-Study, part-time campus jobs. *Financial aid application deadline:* Continuous.

Contact Admissions Office, Department of Nursing, The University of Tampa, 401 West Kennedy Boulevard, Box F, Tampa, FL 33606. *Telephone:* 813-253-6211. *Fax:* 813-258-7398. *E-mail:* admissions@ut.edu.

GRADUATE PROGRAMS

Expenses (2011–12) *Tuition:* part-time $520 per credit. *Room and board:* $8830; room only: $4700 per academic year.
Financial Aid 80% of graduate students in nursing programs received some form of financial aid in 2010–11.
Contact Graduate Studies Office, Department of Nursing, The University of Tampa, 401 West Kennedy Boulevard, Tampa, FL 33606. *Telephone:* 813-258-7409. *Fax:* 813-259-5403. *E-mail:* utgrad@ut.edu.

MASTER'S DEGREE PROGRAM

Degree MSN
Available Programs Master's; RN to Master's.
Concentrations Available *Nurse practitioner programs in;* adult health, family health.
Study Options Full-time and part-time.
Program Entrance Requirements Computer literacy, minimum overall college GPA of 3.0, transcript of college record, CPR certification, written essay, immunizations, interview, 2 letters of recommendation, physical assessment course, professional liability insurance/malpractice insurance, prerequisite course work, resume, statistics course. *Application deadline:* Applications may be processed on a rolling basis for some programs.
Advanced Placement Credit given for nursing courses completed elsewhere dependent upon specific evaluations.
Degree Requirements 48 total credit hours, comprehensive exam.

POST-MASTER'S PROGRAM

Areas of Study *Nurse practitioner programs in:* adult health, family health.

CONTINUING EDUCATION PROGRAM

Contact Dr. Kim Curry, Assistant Professor/Associate Director, Department of Nursing, The University of Tampa, 401 West Kennedy Boulevard, Box 10-F, Tampa, FL 33606-1490. *Telephone:* 813-257-3633. *Fax:* 813-258-7214. *E-mail:* kcurry@ut.edu.

University of West Florida
Department of Nursing
Pensacola, Florida

http://uwf.edu/nursing
Founded in 1963
DEGREES • BSN • MSN
Nursing Program Faculty 13 (23% with doctorates).
Baccalaureate Enrollment 133 **Women** 89% **Men** 11% **Minority** 14% **International** 3% **Part-time** 47%
Graduate Enrollment 8 **Women** 87% **Men** 13% **Minority** 13% **Part-time** 13%
Distance Learning Courses Available.
Nursing Student Activities Sigma Theta Tau, Student Nurses' Association.
Nursing Student Resources Academic advising; academic or career counseling; assistance for students with disabilities; bookstore; campus computer network; career placement assistance; computer lab; computer-assisted instruction; daycare for children of students; e-mail services; employment services for current students; housing assistance; interactive nursing skills videos; Internet; learning resource lab; library services; nursing audiovisuals; remedial services; resume preparation assistance; skills, simulation, or other laboratory; tutoring; unpaid internships.
Library Facilities 503,353 volumes (3,500 in health, 1,950 in nursing); 4,466 periodical subscriptions (54 health-care related).

BACCALAUREATE PROGRAMS

Degree BSN
Available Programs ADN to Baccalaureate; Generic Baccalaureate; RN Baccalaureate.
Study Options Full-time.
Program Entrance Requirements Minimum overall college GPA of 3.0, transcript of college record, CPR certification, health exam, health insurance, immunizations, professional liability insurance/malpractice

insurance, prerequisite course work. Transfer students are accepted. *Application deadline:* 3/1 (fall).
Advanced Placement Credit by examination available. Credit given for nursing courses completed elsewhere dependent upon specific evaluations.
Expenses (2011–12) *Tuition, state resident:* full-time $4702. *Tuition, nonresident:* full-time $15,866. *Room and board:* $8094 per academic year.
Financial Aid 70% of baccalaureate students in nursing programs received some form of financial aid in 2010–11. *Gift aid (need-based):* Federal Pell, FSEOG, state, private, college/university gift aid from institutional funds. *Loans:* Federal Direct (Subsidized and Unsubsidized Stafford PLUS), Perkins, college/university.*Work-study:* Federal Work-Study, part-time campus jobs.*Financial aid application deadline:* Continuous.
Contact Ms. Carol K. Hatcher, Nursing Advisor, Department of Nursing, University of West Florida, 11000 University Parkway, Pensacola, FL 32514. *Telephone:* 850-473-7757. *Fax:* 850-473-7769. *E-mail:* chatcher@uwf.edu.

GRADUATE PROGRAMS

Expenses (2011–12) *Tuition, state resident:* full-time $6032; part-time $314 per credit hour. *Tuition, nonresident:* full-time $19,224; part-time $973 per credit hour. *Room and board:* $8094 per academic year.
Contact Dr. Angela Blackburn, Assistant Professor, Department of Nursing, University of West Florida, 11000 University Parkway, Building 37, Pensacola, FL 32514. *Telephone:* 850-473-7760. *Fax:* 850-473-7769. *E-mail:* ablackburn@uwf.edu.

MASTER'S DEGREE PROGRAM

Degree MSN
Available Programs Master's.
Concentrations Available Nursing administration; nursing education.
Study Options Full-time and part-time.
Online Degree Options Yes (online only).
Program Entrance Requirements Clinical experience, computer literacy, minimum overall college GPA of 3.0, transcript of college record, CPR certification, immunizations, 3 letters of recommendation, professional liability insurance/malpractice insurance, resume. *Application deadline:* 6/1 (fall), 10/1 (spring), 3/1 (summer). Applications may be processed on a rolling basis for some programs.
Advanced Placement Credit given for nursing courses completed elsewhere dependent upon specific evaluations.
Degree Requirements 39 total credit hours, thesis or project.

GEORGIA

Albany State University
College of Sciences and Health Professions
Albany, Georgia

http://www.asurams.edu/
Founded in 1903
DEGREES • BSN • MSN
Nursing Program Faculty 22 (41% with doctorates).
Baccalaureate Enrollment 206 **Women** 93% **Men** 7% **Minority** 96% **International** 1% **Part-time** 26%
Graduate Enrollment 101 **Women** 90% **Men** 10% **Minority** 49% **International** 3% **Part-time** 40%
Distance Learning Courses Available.
Nursing Student Activities Nursing Honor Society, Student Nurses' Association, nursing club.
Nursing Student Resources Academic advising; academic or career counseling; assistance for students with disabilities; bookstore; campus computer network; career placement assistance; computer lab; computer-assisted instruction; e-mail services; interactive nursing skills videos; Internet; learning resource lab; library services; nursing audiovisuals; paid internships; placement services for program completers; remedial services; resume preparation assistance; skills, simulation, or other laboratory; tutoring; unpaid internships.
Library Facilities 201,063 volumes (15,075 in health, 7,032 in nursing); 327 periodical subscriptions (75 health-care related).

BACCALAUREATE PROGRAMS

Degree BSN

Available Programs ADN to Baccalaureate; Accelerated Baccalaureate for Second Degree; Generic Baccalaureate.

Study Options Full-time.

Online Degree Options Yes.

Program Entrance Requirements Minimum overall college GPA of 2.75, transcript of college record, CPR certification, health exam, health insurance, high school biology, high school foreign language, 4 years high school math, 3 years high school science, high school transcript, immunizations, minimum GPA in nursing prerequisites of 2.75, professional liability insurance/malpractice insurance, prerequisite course work. Transfer students are accepted. *Application deadline:* 7/1 (fall), 11/1 (spring), 4/1 (summer). Applications may be processed on a rolling basis for some programs. *Application fee:* $20.

Advanced Placement Credit given for nursing courses completed elsewhere dependent upon specific evaluations.

Expenses (2012–13) *Tuition, state resident:* full-time $5912; part-time $529 per credit. *Tuition, nonresident:* full-time $17,816; part-time $926 per credit. *Room and board:* $5672; room only: $2724 per academic year. *Required fees:* full-time $300.

Financial Aid 92% of baccalaureate students in nursing programs received some form of financial aid in 2011–12. *Gift aid (need-based):* Federal Pell, FSEOG, state, private, college/university gift aid from institutional funds, Federal Nursing, Thurgood Marshall Scholarship Fund. *Loans:* Federal Nursing Student Loans, Federal Direct (Subsidized and Unsubsidized Stafford PLUS), Perkins, state.*Work-study:* Federal Work-Study, part-time campus jobs.*Financial aid application deadline:* 6/1(priority: 4/15).

Contact Dr. Cathy H. Williams, Chair, Department of Nursing, College of Sciences and Health Professions, Albany State University, 504 College Drive, Albany, GA 31705. *Telephone:* 229-430-4728. *Fax:* 229-434-7118. *E-mail:* cathy.williams@asurams.edu.

GRADUATE PROGRAMS

Expenses (2012–13) *Tuition, state resident:* full-time $5796; part-time $563 per credit. *Tuition, nonresident:* full-time $18,978; part-time $1112 per credit. *Room and board:* $5672; room only: $2724 per academic year.

Financial Aid 70% of graduate students in nursing programs received some form of financial aid in 2011–12. Scholarships and traineeships available. *Financial aid application deadline:* 4/15.

Contact Dr. Cathy H. Williams, Chair, Department of Nursing, College of Sciences and Health Professions, Albany State University, 504 College Drive, Albany, GA 31705. *Telephone:* 229-430-4728. *Fax:* 229-434-7118. *E-mail:* cathy.williams@asurams.edu.

MASTER'S DEGREE PROGRAM

Degree MSN

Available Programs Accelerated AD/RN to Master's; Accelerated Master's; Master's; RN to Master's.

Concentrations Available Nursing education. *Nurse practitioner programs in:* family health.

Study Options Full-time and part-time.

Online Degree Options Yes (online only).

Program Entrance Requirements Clinical experience, computer literacy, minimum overall college GPA of 3.0, transcript of college record, CPR certification, immunizations, 2 letters of recommendation, nursing research course, physical assessment course, professional liability insurance/malpractice insurance, prerequisite course work, resume, statistics course, GRE or MAT. *Application deadline:* 7/1 (fall), 11/1 (spring), 4/1 (summer). Applications may be processed on a rolling basis for some programs. *Application fee:* $20.

Advanced Placement Credit given for nursing courses completed elsewhere dependent upon specific evaluations.

Degree Requirements 36 total credit hours, thesis or project, comprehensive exam.

POST-MASTER'S PROGRAM

Areas of Study Nursing education. *Nurse practitioner programs in:* family health.

Armstrong Atlantic State University
Program in Nursing
Savannah, Georgia

http://armstrong.edu/Health_professions/nursing/
Founded in 1935
DEGREES • BSN • MS/MHSA • MSN
Nursing Program Faculty 53 (19% with doctorates).
Baccalaureate Enrollment 350 **Women** 85% **Men** 15% **Minority** 35% **International** 2% **Part-time** 10%
Graduate Enrollment 45 **Women** 89% **Men** 11% **Minority** 33% **Part-time** 75%
Distance Learning Courses Available.
Nursing Student Activities Nursing Honor Society, Sigma Theta Tau, Student Nurses' Association.
Nursing Student Resources Academic advising; academic or career counseling; assistance for students with disabilities; bookstore; campus computer network; career placement assistance; computer lab; computer-assisted instruction; e-mail services; employment services for current students; externships; housing assistance; interactive nursing skills videos; Internet; learning resource lab; library services; nursing audiovisuals; placement services for program completers; remedial services; resume preparation assistance; skills, simulation, or other laboratory; tutoring.
Library Facilities 214,900 volumes (8,500 in nursing); 496 periodical subscriptions (200 health-care related).

BACCALAUREATE PROGRAMS

Degree BSN

Available Programs ADN to Baccalaureate; Baccalaureate for Second Degree; Generic Baccalaureate; LPN to Baccalaureate; RN Baccalaureate.

Study Options Full-time and part-time.

Program Entrance Requirements Minimum overall college GPA of 3.0, transcript of college record, CPR certification, health exam, health insurance, immunizations, minimum GPA in nursing prerequisites of 3.0, professional liability insurance/malpractice insurance, prerequisite course work. Transfer students are accepted. *Application deadline:* 2/28 (fall), 10/15 (spring). *Application fee:* $250.

Advanced Placement Credit by examination available. Credit given for nursing courses completed elsewhere dependent upon specific evaluations.

Financial Aid 90% of baccalaureate students in nursing programs received some form of financial aid in 2011–12.

Contact Ms. Kristy Gose, Administrative Assistant, Program in Nursing, Armstrong Atlantic State University, 11935 Abercorn Street, Savannah, GA 31419-1997. *Telephone:* 912-344-2575. *Fax:* 912-344-3481. *E-mail:* kristy.gose@armstrong.edu.

GRADUATE PROGRAMS

Financial Aid 85% of graduate students in nursing programs received some form of financial aid in 2011–12. Research assistantships with full tuition reimbursements available (averaging $5,000 per year); Federal Work-Study, scholarships, and unspecified assistantships also available. Aid available to part-time students.

Contact Dr. Anita Nivens, Graduate Program Coordinator, Program in Nursing, Armstrong Atlantic State University, 11935 Abercorn Street, Savannah, GA 31419-1997. *Telephone:* 912-344-2724. *Fax:* 912-344-3481. *E-mail:* anita.nivens@armstrong.edu.

MASTER'S DEGREE PROGRAM

Degrees MS/MHSA; MSN
Available Programs Master's; RN to Master's.
Concentrations Available *Clinical nurse specialist programs in:* acute care, adult health. *Nurse practitioner programs in:* acute care, adult health.
Study Options Full-time and part-time.
Program Entrance Requirements Clinical experience, minimum overall college GPA of 3.0, transcript of college record, CPR certification, written essay, immunizations, interview, 3 letters of recommendation, nursing research course, physical assessment course, professional liability insurance/malpractice insurance, prerequisite course work, statistics course, GRE General Test or MAT. *Application deadline:* 5/15 (fall), 11/15 (spring).

Advanced Placement Credit by examination available. Credit given for nursing courses completed elsewhere dependent upon specific evaluations.

Degree Requirements 36 total credit hours, thesis or project.

POST-MASTER'S PROGRAM

Areas of Study *Clinical nurse specialist programs in:* acute care, adult health. *Nurse practitioner programs in:* acute care, adult health.

Augusta State University

Department of Nursing
Augusta, Georgia

Founded in 1925

DEGREE • BSN

BACCALAUREATE PROGRAMS

Degree BSN
Available Programs Generic Baccalaureate; LPN to Baccalaureate; RN Baccalaureate.
Contact *Telephone:* 706-737-1725. *Fax:* 706-737-1726.

Brenau University

College of Health and Science
Gainesville, Georgia

Founded in 1878

DEGREES • BSN • DNP • MSN

Nursing Program Faculty 15 (65% with doctorates).
Baccalaureate Enrollment 300 Women 95% Men 5% Minority 40% International 10% Part-time 50%
Graduate Enrollment 100 Women 95% Men 5% Minority 40% Part-time 100%
Distance Learning Courses Available.
Nursing Student Activities Sigma Theta Tau, Student Nurses' Association.
Nursing Student Resources Academic advising; academic or career counseling; assistance for students with disabilities; bookstore; campus computer network; career placement assistance; computer lab; computer-assisted instruction; e-mail services; housing assistance; interactive nursing skills videos; Internet; learning resource lab; library services; nursing audiovisuals; remedial services; skills, simulation, or other laboratory; tutoring.
Library Facilities 86,590 volumes (6,000 in health, 5,000 in nursing); 20,128 periodical subscriptions (500 health-care related).

BACCALAUREATE PROGRAMS

Degree BSN
Available Programs ADN to Baccalaureate; Generic Baccalaureate; RN Baccalaureate.
Study Options Full-time and part-time.
Online Degree Options Yes.
Program Entrance Requirements Minimum overall college GPA of 2.75, transcript of college record, high school biology, high school chemistry, high school foreign language, 2 years high school math, 1 year of high school science, high school transcript, minimum high school GPA of 2.75, minimum GPA in nursing prerequisites of 2.5. Transfer students are accepted. *Application deadline:* 7/15 (spring), 11/15 (summer). *Application fee:* $35.
Advanced Placement Credit by examination available. Credit given for nursing courses completed elsewhere dependent upon specific evaluations.
Financial Aid 75% of baccalaureate students in nursing programs received some form of financial aid in 2010–11.
Contact Ms. Christina White, Undergraduate Admissions Coordinator for Women's College, College of Health and Science, Brenau University, 500 Washington Street SE, Gainesville, GA 30501. *Telephone:* 770-534-6100. *Fax:* 770-538-4306. *E-mail:* cwhite@brenau.edu.

GRADUATE PROGRAMS

Financial Aid 90% of graduate students in nursing programs received some form of financial aid in 2010–11. Scholarships and traineeships

available. Aid available to part-time students. *Financial aid application deadline:* 7/15.
Contact Dr. Cathy Dyches, Coordinator of Graduate Nursing Programs, College of Health and Science, Brenau University, 500 Washington Street SE, Gainesville, GA 30501. *Telephone:* 770-534-6125. *Fax:* 770-534-4666. *E-mail:* cdyches@brenau.edu.

MASTER'S DEGREE PROGRAM

Degree MSN
Available Programs Accelerated AD/RN to Master's; Accelerated RN to Master's; Master's; RN to Master's.
Concentrations Available Clinical nurse leader; nursing education. *Nurse practitioner programs in:* family health.
Site Options Atlanta, GA.
Study Options Part-time.
Program Entrance Requirements Clinical experience, minimum overall college GPA of 3.0, transcript of college record, CPR certification, written essay, immunizations, 2 letters of recommendation, nursing research course, physical assessment course, prerequisite course work, statistics course, GRE General Test or MAT (for some programs). *Application deadline:* Applications may be processed on a rolling basis for some programs.
Degree Requirements Thesis or project.

POST-MASTER'S PROGRAM

Areas of Study *Nurse practitioner programs in:* family health.

DOCTORAL DEGREE PROGRAM

Degree DNP
Available Programs Doctorate.
Site Options Atlanta, GA.
Program Entrance Requirements Clinical experience, minimum overall college GPA of 3.0, letters of recommendation, MSN or equivalent, statistics course, vita, writing sample.

Clayton State University

Department of Nursing
Morrow, Georgia

http://nursing.clayton.edu/default.htm
Founded in 1969

DEGREES • BSN • MSN

Nursing Program Faculty 42 (35% with doctorates).
Baccalaureate Enrollment 258 Women 85.7% Men 14.3% Minority 69% International 14.3% Part-time 38%
Graduate Enrollment 25 Women 96% Men 4% Minority 76% International 4% Part-time 64%
Distance Learning Courses Available.
Nursing Student Activities Nursing Honor Society, Sigma Theta Tau, Student Nurses' Association.
Nursing Student Resources Academic advising; academic or career counseling; assistance for students with disabilities; bookstore; campus computer network; career placement assistance; computer lab; computer-assisted instruction; e-mail services; employment services for current students; externships; housing assistance; interactive nursing skills videos; Internet; learning resource lab; library services; nursing audiovisuals; paid internships; placement services for program completers; remedial services; resume preparation assistance; skills, simulation, or other laboratory; tutoring.
Library Facilities 148,798 volumes (3,450 in health, 1,800 in nursing); 618 periodical subscriptions (151 health-care related).

BACCALAUREATE PROGRAMS

Degree BSN
Available Programs Generic Baccalaureate; RN Baccalaureate.
Study Options Full-time.
Online Degree Options Yes.
Program Entrance Requirements Minimum overall college GPA of 2.5, transcript of college record, CPR certification, health exam, health insurance, immunizations, interview, minimum GPA in nursing prerequisites of 2.5, professional liability insurance/malpractice insurance, prerequisite course work. Transfer students are accepted. *Application deadline:* 2/15 (fall), 9/15 (spring). *Application fee:* $25.
Expenses (2012–13) *Tuition, state resident:* full-time $3610; part-time $150 per credit hour. *Tuition, nonresident:* full-time $13,113; part-time $547 per credit hour. *International tuition:* $13,113 full-time. *Room and*

board: $8862; room only: $5574 per academic year. *Required fees:* full-time $1404.
Financial Aid 61% of baccalaureate students in nursing programs received some form of financial aid in 2011–12.
Contact Dr. Sue E. Odom, Director of the Undergraduate Nursing Program, Department of Nursing, Clayton State University, 2000 Clayton State Boulevard, Morrow, GA 30260. *Telephone:* 678-466-4959. *Fax:* 678-466-4999. *E-mail:* sueodom@clayton.edu.

GRADUATE PROGRAMS

Expenses (2012–13) *Tuition, state resident:* part-time $385 per credit hour. *Tuition, nonresident:* part-time $385 per credit hour. *Room and board:* $8862; room only: $5574 per academic year.
Financial Aid 3.8% of graduate students in nursing programs received some form of financial aid in 2011–12.
Contact Dr. Betty Lane, Director of the MSN Program, Department of Nursing, Clayton State University, 2000 Clayton State Boulevard, Morrow, GA 30260. *Telephone:* 678-466-4953. *Fax:* 678-466-4999. *E-mail:* bettylane@clayton.edu.

MASTER'S DEGREE PROGRAM

Degree MSN
Available Programs Master's; RN to Master's.
Concentrations Available Nursing administration; nursing education.
Study Options Full-time and part-time.
Online Degree Options Yes (online only).
Program Entrance Requirements Computer literacy, minimum overall college GPA of 3.0, transcript of college record, CPR certification, written essay, immunizations, interview, 3 letters of recommendation, professional liability insurance/malpractice insurance. *Application deadline:* 7/1 (fall), 11/1 (spring), 3/1 (summer). Applications may be processed on a rolling basis for some programs. *Application fee:* $25.
Advanced Placement Credit given for nursing courses completed elsewhere dependent upon specific evaluations.
Degree Requirements 36 total credit hours, thesis or project.

College of Coastal Georgia
Department of Nursing and Health Sciences
Brunswick, Georgia

http://www.ccga.edu/Academics/SchoolNursing/
Founded in 1961
DEGREE • BS
Nursing Program Faculty 16 (31% with doctorates).
Baccalaureate Enrollment 146 **Women** 85% **Men** 15% **Minority** 20% **Part-time** 5%
Distance Learning Courses Available.
Nursing Student Activities Student Nurses' Association.
Nursing Student Resources Academic advising; academic or career counseling; assistance for students with disabilities; bookstore; campus computer network; career placement assistance; computer lab; computer-assisted instruction; e-mail services; employment services for current students; externships; housing assistance; interactive nursing skills videos; Internet; learning resource lab; library services; nursing audiovisuals; placement services for program completers; remedial services; resume preparation assistance; skills, simulation, or other laboratory; tutoring; unpaid internships.
Library Facilities 15.3 million volumes (1,730 in health, 282 in nursing); 362 periodical subscriptions (48 health-care related).

BACCALAUREATE PROGRAMS

Degree BS
Available Programs Accelerated Baccalaureate; Generic Baccalaureate; RN Baccalaureate.
Study Options Full-time.
Online Degree Options Yes.
Program Entrance Requirements Minimum overall college GPA of 2.8, transcript of college record, CPR certification, health exam, health insurance, immunizations, minimum GPA in nursing prerequisites of 2.8, professional liability insurance/malpractice insurance, prerequisite course work. Transfer students are accepted. *Application deadline:* 1/15 (fall), 9/15 (spring).
Expenses (2012–13) *Tuition, state resident:* full-time $2846; part-time $95 per credit hour. *Tuition, nonresident:* full-time $10,514; part-time $350 per credit hour. *Room and board:* $12,168; room only: $9168 per academic year. *Required fees:* full-time $1260.

Financial Aid 98% of baccalaureate students in nursing programs received some form of financial aid in 2011–12. *Gift aid (need-based):* Federal Pell, FSEOG, state, private, college/university gift aid from institutional funds. *Work-study:* Federal Work-Study. *Financial aid application deadline (priority):* 7/1.
Contact Dr. Patricia Kraft, Southeast Georgia Health System Distinguished Dean of Nursing and Health Sciences, Department of Nursing and Health Sciences, College of Coastal Georgia, One College Drive, Brunswick, GA 31520. *Telephone:* 912-279-5860. *Fax:* 912-279-5912. *E-mail:* pkraft@ccga.edu.

Columbus State University
Nursing Program
Columbus, Georgia

http://nursing.ColumbusState.edu/
Founded in 1958
DEGREE • BSN
Nursing Program Faculty 31 (12% with doctorates).
Baccalaureate Enrollment 187 **Women** 91% **Men** 9% **Minority** 42% **International** 6% **Part-time** 3%
Distance Learning Courses Available.
Nursing Student Activities Sigma Theta Tau, Student Nurses' Association.
Nursing Student Resources Academic advising; academic or career counseling; assistance for students with disabilities; bookstore; campus computer network; career placement assistance; computer lab; computer-assisted instruction; e-mail services; housing assistance; interactive nursing skills videos; Internet; learning resource lab; library services; nursing audiovisuals; remedial services; resume preparation assistance; skills, simulation, or other laboratory; tutoring.
Library Facilities 376,614 volumes (284 in health, 260 in nursing); 1,392 periodical subscriptions (81 health-care related).

BACCALAUREATE PROGRAMS

Degree BSN
Available Programs Generic Baccalaureate; RN Baccalaureate.
Study Options Full-time.
Online Degree Options Yes.
Program Entrance Requirements Minimum overall college GPA of 2.75, transcript of college record, CPR certification, health exam, health insurance, immunizations, 3 letters of recommendation, minimum GPA in nursing prerequisites of 2.75, professional liability insurance/malpractice insurance, prerequisite course work. *Application deadline:* 2/28 (fall).
Advanced Placement Credit given for nursing courses completed elsewhere dependent upon specific evaluations.
Contact *Telephone:* 706-568-5050. *Fax:* 706-569-3101.

Emory University
Nell Hodgson Woodruff School of Nursing
Atlanta, Georgia

http://www.nursing.emory.edu/
Founded in 1836
DEGREES • BSN • MSN • MSN/MPH • PHD
Nursing Program Faculty 102 (55% with doctorates).
Baccalaureate Enrollment 264 **Women** 89% **Men** 11% **Minority** 41% **International** 2%
Graduate Enrollment 190 **Women** 92% **Men** 8% **Minority** 24% **International** 1% **Part-time** 20%
Nursing Student Activities Sigma Theta Tau, Student Nurses' Association.
Nursing Student Resources Academic advising; academic or career counseling; assistance for students with disabilities; bookstore; campus computer network; career placement assistance; computer lab; computer-assisted instruction; daycare for children of students; e-mail services; employment services for current students; externships; housing assistance; interactive nursing skills videos; Internet; learning resource lab; library services; nursing audiovisuals; other; resume preparation assistance; skills, simulation, or other laboratory; tutoring; unpaid internships.
Library Facilities 3.7 million volumes (250,000 in health); 99,168 periodical subscriptions (1,800 health-care related).

BACCALAUREATE PROGRAMS

Degree BSN

Available Programs Accelerated Baccalaureate; Accelerated Baccalaureate for Second Degree; Baccalaureate for Second Degree; Generic Baccalaureate.

Study Options Full-time.

Program Entrance Requirements Minimum overall college GPA of 3.0, transcript of college record, written essay, 3 letters of recommendation, minimum GPA in nursing prerequisites of 3.0, prerequisite course work. Transfer students are accepted. *Application deadline:* 1/15 (fall), 12/1 (summer). *Application fee:* $50.

Advanced Placement Credit given for nursing courses completed elsewhere dependent upon specific evaluations.

Expenses (2012–13) *Tuition:* full-time $37,600; part-time $1567 per credit hour. *International tuition:* $37,600 full-time. *Room and board:* $12,000; room only: $7200 per academic year. *Required fees:* full-time $580.

Financial Aid 92% of baccalaureate students in nursing programs received some form of financial aid in 2011–12. *Gift aid (need-based):* Federal Pell, FSEOG, private, college/university gift aid from institutional funds. *Loans:* Federal Nursing Student Loans, Federal Direct (Subsidized and Unsubsidized Stafford PLUS), Perkins, college/university.*Work-study:* Federal Work-Study, part-time campus jobs.*Financial aid application deadline:* 3/1(priority: 2/15).

Contact Mrs. Katie Kennedy, Office of Enrollment and Student Affairs, Nell Hodgson Woodruff School of Nursing, Emory University, 1520 Clifton Road NE, Atlanta, GA 30322. *Telephone:* 404-727-7980. *Fax:* 404-727-8509. *E-mail:* admit@nursing.emory.edu.

GRADUATE PROGRAMS

Expenses (2012–13) *Tuition:* full-time $56,400; part-time $1567 per credit hour. *International tuition:* $56,400 full-time. *Required fees:* full-time $771.

Financial Aid 88% of graduate students in nursing programs received some form of financial aid in 2011–12. 14 fellowships (averaging $28,000 per year) were awarded; career-related internships or fieldwork, Federal Work-Study, institutionally sponsored loans, and scholarships also available. Aid available to part-time students. *Financial aid application deadline:* 3/1.

Contact Mrs. Katie Kennedy, Office of Enrollment and Student Affairs, Nell Hodgson Woodruff School of Nursing, Emory University, 1520 Clifton Road NE, Atlanta, GA 30322. *Telephone:* 404-727-7980. *Fax:* 404-727-8509. *E-mail:* admit@nursing.emory.edu.

MASTER'S DEGREE PROGRAM

Degrees MSN; MSN/MPH

Available Programs Master's; RN to Master's.

Concentrations Available Nurse-midwifery. *Clinical nurse specialist programs in:* public health. *Nurse practitioner programs in:* acute care, adult health, family health, gerontology, pediatric, primary care, women's health.

Study Options Full-time and part-time.

Program Entrance Requirements Clinical experience, minimum overall college GPA of 3.0, transcript of college record, written essay, interview, 3 letters of recommendation, physical assessment course, prerequisite course work, resume, statistics course, GRE General Test or MAT. *Application deadline:* 1/15 (fall), 10/1 (spring), 1/15 (summer). Applications may be processed on a rolling basis for some programs. *Application fee:* $50.

Advanced Placement Credit given for nursing courses completed elsewhere dependent upon specific evaluations.

Degree Requirements 41 total credit hours.

POST-MASTER'S PROGRAM

Areas of Study Nurse-midwifery. *Clinical nurse specialist programs in:* public health. *Nurse practitioner programs in:* acute care, adult health, family health, gerontology, pediatric, primary care, women's health.

DOCTORAL DEGREE PROGRAM

Degree PhD

Available Programs Doctorate; Post-Baccalaureate Doctorate.

Areas of Study Aging, biology of health and illness, ethics, faculty preparation, gerontology, health policy, human health and illness, illness and transition, individualized study, neuro-behavior, nursing policy, nursing research, nursing science, women's health.

Program Entrance Requirements Minimum overall college GPA of 3.0, interview by faculty committee, 3 letters of recommendation, MSN or equivalent, statistics course, vita, writing sample. *Application*

deadline: 1/3 (fall). Applications may be processed on a rolling basis for some programs.

Degree Requirements 50 total credit hours, dissertation, oral exam, written exam, residency.

POSTDOCTORAL PROGRAM

Postdoctoral Program Contact Ms. Teresa Fosque, Senior Business Manager, Nell Hodgson Woodruff School of Nursing, Emory University, 1520 Clifton Road NE, Atlanta, GA 30322. *E-mail:* tfosque@emory.edu.

Georgia College & State University
College of Health Sciences
Milledgeville, Georgia

http://www.gcsu.edu/nursing
Founded in 1889

DEGREES • BSN • DNP • MSN

Nursing Program Faculty 22 (50% with doctorates).

Baccalaureate Enrollment 267 **Women** 85% **Men** 15% **Minority** 12% **International** 1% **Part-time** 30%

Graduate Enrollment 80 **Women** 80% **Men** 20% **Minority** 16% **International** 1% **Part-time** 20%

Distance Learning Courses Available.

Nursing Student Activities Sigma Theta Tau, Student Nurses' Association.

Nursing Student Resources Academic advising; academic or career counseling; assistance for students with disabilities; bookstore; campus computer network; career placement assistance; computer lab; computer-assisted instruction; e-mail services; employment services for current students; housing assistance; interactive nursing skills videos; Internet; learning resource lab; library services; nursing audiovisuals; remedial services; resume preparation assistance; skills, simulation, or other laboratory; tutoring; unpaid internships.

Library Facilities 207,038 volumes (3,095 in health, 1,465 in nursing); 55,550 periodical subscriptions (315 health-care related).

BACCALAUREATE PROGRAMS

Degree BSN

Available Programs Generic Baccalaureate; RN Baccalaureate.

Study Options Full-time.

Program Entrance Requirements Minimum overall college GPA of 2.75, transcript of college record, CPR certification, health exam, health insurance, high school foreign language, 4 years high school math, 4 years high school science, high school transcript, immunizations, minimum high school GPA of 2.5, minimum GPA in nursing prerequisites of 2.75, professional liability insurance/malpractice insurance, prerequisite course work. Transfer students are accepted. *Application deadline:* 2/1 (fall), 7/15 (spring). *Application fee:* $10.

Advanced Placement Credit by examination available. Credit given for nursing courses completed elsewhere dependent upon specific evaluations.

Expenses (2012–13) *Tuition, state resident:* full-time $8618. *Tuition, nonresident:* full-time $26,082. *Required fees:* full-time $1350.

Financial Aid 94% of baccalaureate students in nursing programs received some form of financial aid in 2011–12. *Gift aid (need-based):* Federal Pell, FSEOG, state, college/university gift aid from institutional funds. *Loans:* Federal Direct PLUS), Perkins, state, college/university.*Work-study:* Federal Work-Study.*Financial aid application deadline (priority):* 3/1.

Contact Ms. Tamette Farrington, Pre-Nursing Advisor, College of Health Sciences, Georgia College & State University, Campus Box 115, Milledgeville, GA 31061. *Telephone:* 478-445-2634. *E-mail:* tamette.farrington@gcsu.edu.

GRADUATE PROGRAMS

Expenses (2012–13) *Tuition, state resident:* full-time $7546. *Tuition, nonresident:* full-time $20,560. *Room and board:* $9970 per academic year. *Required fees:* full-time $1350.

Financial Aid 51% of graduate students in nursing programs received some form of financial aid in 2011–12. 28 research assistantships with tuition reimbursements available were awarded; career-related internships or fieldwork and unspecified assistantships also available. Aid available to part-time students.

Contact Dr. Debby MacMilllan, Assistant Director, Graduate Programs, College of Health Sciences, Georgia College & State University, Macon Graduate Center, 433 Cherry Street, Macon, GA 31204. *Telephone:* 478-752-1074. *E-mail:* debby.macmillan@gcsu.edu.

MASTER'S DEGREE PROGRAM
Degree MSN
Available Programs Master's.
Concentrations Available *Nurse practitioner programs in:* family health.
Site Options Macon, GA.
Study Options Full-time and part-time.
Online Degree Options Yes (online only).
Program Entrance Requirements Clinical experience, computer literacy, minimum overall college GPA of 2.75, transcript of college record, CPR certification, immunizations, interview, nursing research course, physical assessment course, professional liability insurance/malpractice insurance, statistics course, GRE, GMAT or MAT. *Application deadline:* 1/10 (summer).
Advanced Placement Credit given for nursing courses completed elsewhere dependent upon specific evaluations.
Degree Requirements 36 total credit hours, thesis or project, comprehensive exam.

POST-MASTER'S PROGRAM
Areas of Study *Nurse practitioner programs in:* family health.

DOCTORAL DEGREE PROGRAM
Degree DNP
Available Programs Doctorate.
Site Options Macon, GA.
Online Degree Options Yes (online only).
Program Entrance Requirements Clinical experience, minimum overall college GPA of 3.2, interview by faculty committee, 2 letters of recommendation, MSN or equivalent, statistics course, vita, writing sample. *Application deadline:* 1/16 (spring). *Application fee:* $10.
Degree Requirements 37 total credit hours.

Georgia Regents University
School of Nursing
Augusta, Georgia

http://www.georgiahealth.edu/nursing
Founded in 1828
DEGREES • BSN • DNP • MSN • PHD
Nursing Program Faculty 61 (47% with doctorates).
Baccalaureate Enrollment 162
Graduate Enrollment 396
Distance Learning Courses Available.
Nursing Student Activities Nursing Honor Society, Sigma Theta Tau, Student Nurses' Association, nursing club.
Nursing Student Resources Academic advising; academic or career counseling; assistance for students with disabilities; bookstore; campus computer network; career placement assistance; computer lab; computer-assisted instruction; daycare for children of students; e-mail services; employment services for current students; externships; housing assistance; interactive nursing skills videos; Internet; learning resource lab; library services; nursing audiovisuals; paid internships; remedial services; skills, simulation, or other laboratory; tutoring.
Library Facilities 166,744 volumes (178,650 in health, 14,650 in nursing); 4,674 periodical subscriptions (1,307 health-care related).

BACCALAUREATE PROGRAMS
Degree BSN
Available Programs Generic Baccalaureate.
Site Options Athens, GA.
Study Options Full-time.
Program Entrance Requirements Minimum overall college GPA of 2.8, transcript of college record, CPR certification, written essay, health insurance, immunizations, 2 letters of recommendation, prerequisite course work. Transfer students are accepted. *Application deadline:* 2/15 (fall). *Application fee:* $50.
Contact Office of Academic Admissions, School of Nursing, Georgia Regents University, AA-170 Kelly Building, Augusta, GA 30912. *Telephone:* 706-721-2725. *Fax:* 706-721-0186. *E-mail:* admissions@georgiahealth.edu.

GRADUATE PROGRAMS
Contact Director, Academic Admissions, School of Nursing, Georgia Regents University, AA-170 Kelly Building, Augusta, GA 30912. *Telephone:* 706-721-2725. *Fax:* 706-721-0186. *E-mail:* admissions@georgiahealth.edu.

MASTER'S DEGREE PROGRAM
Degree MSN
Available Programs Accelerated Master's for Non-Nursing College Graduates; Master's.
Concentrations Available Clinical nurse leader; nurse anesthesia. *Nurse practitioner programs in:* family health, pediatric.
Site Options Columbus, GA; Athens, GA.
Study Options Full-time and part-time.
Online Degree Options Yes.
Program Entrance Requirements Clinical experience, computer literacy, minimum overall college GPA of 3.0, transcript of college record, CPR certification, written essay, immunizations, interview, 3 letters of recommendation, professional liability insurance/malpractice insurance, prerequisite course work, resume, statistics course. *Application fee:* $50.
Degree Requirements Thesis or project.

POST-MASTER'S PROGRAM
Areas of Study *Nurse practitioner programs in:* family health, pediatric, psychiatric/mental health.

DOCTORAL DEGREE PROGRAM
Degree DNP
Available Programs Doctorate, Post-Baccalaureate Doctorate.
Areas of Study Advanced practice nursing.
Online Degree Options Yes.
Program Entrance Requirements Minimum overall college GPA of 3.3, clinical experience, interview, interview by faculty committee, 3 letters of recommendation, statistics course, vita, writing sample. *Application deadline:* 2/1 (fall). *Application fee:* $50.
Degree Requirements Capstone project.

DOCTORAL DEGREE PROGRAM
Degree PhD
Available Programs Doctorate; Post-Baccalaureate Doctorate.
Areas of Study Bio-behavioral research, nursing research.
Site Options Columbus, GA; Athens, GA.
Program Entrance Requirements Clinical experience, minimum overall college GPA of 3.2, interview by faculty committee, interview, 3 letters of recommendation, MSN or equivalent, scholarly papers, statistics course, vita, writing sample. *Application fee:* $50.
Degree Requirements Dissertation, oral exam, written exam.

Georgia Southern University
School of Nursing
Statesboro, Georgia

http://chhs.georgiasouthern.edu/nursing/
Founded in 1906
DEGREES • BSN • DNP • MSN
Nursing Program Faculty 36 (18% with doctorates).
Baccalaureate Enrollment 267 **Women** 86.5% **Men** 13.5% **Minority** 15.3% **International** .4% **Part-time** 24.7%
Graduate Enrollment 66 **Women** 94% **Men** 6% **Minority** 27% **Part-time** 1.5%
Distance Learning Courses Available.
Nursing Student Activities Sigma Theta Tau, Student Nurses' Association.
Nursing Student Resources Academic advising; academic or career counseling; assistance for students with disabilities; bookstore; campus computer network; career placement assistance; computer lab; computer-assisted instruction; daycare for children of students; e-mail services; employment services for current students; housing assistance; interactive nursing skills videos; Internet; learning resource lab; library services; nursing audiovisuals; placement services for program completers; resume preparation assistance; skills, simulation, or other laboratory; tutoring.
Library Facilities 620,975 volumes (25,000 in health, 12,000 in nursing); 40,936 periodical subscriptions (20,000 health-care related).

BACCALAUREATE PROGRAMS
Degree BSN

Available Programs ADN to Baccalaureate; Generic Baccalaureate; LPN to RN Baccalaureate.

Study Options Full-time.

Online Degree Options Yes.

Program Entrance Requirements Minimum overall college GPA of 3.0, transcript of college record, CPR certification, written essay, health exam, health insurance, high school biology, high school chemistry, high school foreign language, 2 years high school math, 4 years high school science, high school transcript, immunizations, minimum GPA in nursing prerequisites of 3.0, professional liability insurance/malpractice insurance, prerequisite course work. Transfer students are accepted. *Application deadline:* 2/4 (fall), 8/5 (spring).

Advanced Placement Credit by examination available. Credit given for nursing courses completed elsewhere dependent upon specific evaluations.

Expenses (2012–13) *Tuition, state resident:* full-time $2246; part-time $162 per credit hour. *Tuition, nonresident:* full-time $8564; part-time $571 per credit hour. *Room and board:* $4010; room only: $2810 per academic year. *Required fees:* full-time $950.

Financial Aid 94% of baccalaureate students in nursing programs received some form of financial aid in 2011–12.

Contact Dr. Melissa Garno, BSN Program Director, School of Nursing, Georgia Southern University, PO Box 8158, Statesboro, GA 30460-8158. *Telephone:* 912-478-5454. *Fax:* 912-478-1159. *E-mail:* mel@georgiasouthern.edu.

GRADUATE PROGRAMS

Expenses (2012–13) *Tuition, state resident:* full-time $3150; part-time $263 per credit hour. *Tuition, nonresident:* full-time $12,587; part-time $1049 per credit hour. *Room and board:* $4010; room only: $2810 per academic year. *Required fees:* full-time $936.

Financial Aid 39% of graduate students in nursing programs received some form of financial aid in 2011–12. Research assistantships with partial tuition reimbursements available (averaging $7,200 per year), teaching assistantships with partial tuition reimbursements available (averaging $7,200 per year) were awarded; career-related internships or fieldwork, Federal Work-Study, scholarships, traineeships, tuition waivers (partial), and unspecified assistantships also available. Aid available to part-time students. *Financial aid application deadline:* 4/15.

Contact Dr. Deborah Allen, Director, Graduate Program, School of Nursing, Georgia Southern University, PO Box 8158, Statesboro, GA 30460-8158. *Telephone:* 912-478-0017. *Fax:* 912-478-1679. *E-mail:* debbieallen@georgiasouthern.edu.

MASTER'S DEGREE PROGRAM

Degree MSN

Available Programs Master's; RN to Master's.

Concentrations Available *Clinical nurse specialist programs in:* community health. *Nurse practitioner programs in:* family health.

Study Options Full-time and part-time.

Program Entrance Requirements Clinical experience, computer literacy, minimum overall college GPA of 3.0, transcript of college record, CPR certification, immunizations, interview, 3 letters of recommendation, professional liability insurance/malpractice insurance, prerequisite course work, statistics course, GRE General Test or MAT. *Application deadline:* 3/15 (fall).

Advanced Placement Credit given for nursing courses completed elsewhere dependent upon specific evaluations.

Degree Requirements 48 total credit hours, comprehensive exam.

POST-MASTER'S PROGRAM

Areas of Study *Clinical nurse specialist programs in:* community health. *Nurse practitioner programs in:* family health.

DOCTORAL DEGREE PROGRAM

Degree DNP

Available Programs Doctorate.

Areas of Study Nursing science.

Online Degree Options Yes (online only).

Program Entrance Requirements Minimum overall college GPA of 3.0, interview by faculty committee, 3 letters of recommendation, MSN or equivalent, vita, writing sample, GRE, MAT. *Application deadline:* 3/1 (fall).

Degree Requirements 40 total credit hours, oral exam, written exam.

Georgia Southwestern State University
School of Nursing
Americus, Georgia

http://www.gsw.edu/
Founded in 1906

DEGREES • BSN • MSN

Nursing Program Faculty 15 (33% with doctorates).

Baccalaureate Enrollment 331 **Women** 87% **Men** 13% **Minority** 33% **International** 8% **Part-time** 35%

Graduate Enrollment 10

Distance Learning Courses Available.

Nursing Student Activities Sigma Theta Tau, Student Nurses' Association.

Nursing Student Resources Academic advising; academic or career counseling; assistance for students with disabilities; bookstore; campus computer network; career placement assistance; computer lab; computer-assisted instruction; e-mail services; employment services for current students; interactive nursing skills videos; Internet; learning resource lab; library services; nursing audiovisuals; placement services for program completers; remedial services; resume preparation assistance; skills, simulation, or other laboratory; tutoring.

Library Facilities 627 volumes in health, 528 volumes in nursing; 141 periodical subscriptions health-care related.

BACCALAUREATE PROGRAMS

Degree BSN

Available Programs Baccalaureate for Second Degree; Generic Baccalaureate; LPN to RN Baccalaureate; RN Baccalaureate.

Study Options Full-time.

Online Degree Options Yes.

Program Entrance Requirements Minimum overall college GPA of 2.8, transcript of college record, CPR certification, written essay, health exam, health insurance, high school foreign language, 4 years high school math, 4 years high school science, high school transcript, immunizations, 2 letters of recommendation, minimum high school GPA of 2.8, minimum GPA in nursing prerequisites of 2.8, professional liability insurance/malpractice insurance, prerequisite course work, RN licensure. Transfer students are accepted. *Application deadline:* 2/15 (fall), 8/15 (spring).

Expenses (2012–13) *Tuition, state resident:* full-time $2256; part-time $150 per credit hour. *Tuition, nonresident:* full-time $8208; part-time $547 per credit hour. *International tuition:* $8208 full-time. *Room and board:* $2769; room only: $1390 per academic year. *Required fees:* full-time $634; part-time $292 per term.

Financial Aid 91% of baccalaureate students in nursing programs received some form of financial aid in 2011–12.

Contact Dr. Sandra Daniel, Dean and Professor, School of Nursing, Georgia Southwestern State University, 800 Georgia Southwestern State University Drive, Americus, GA 31709. *Telephone:* 229-931-2280. *Fax:* 229-931-2288. *E-mail:* sandra.daniel@gsw.edu.

GRADUATE PROGRAMS

Expenses (2012–13) *Tuition, state resident:* part-time $385 per credit hour. *Room and board:* $3304; room only: $1925 per academic year.

Contact Dr. Sandra Daniel, Dean, School of Nursing, Georgia Southwestern State University, 800 GSW State University Drive, Americus, GA 31709. *Telephone:* 912-931-2275. *Fax:* 912-931-2288. *E-mail:* Sandra.Daniel@gsw.edu.

MASTER'S DEGREE PROGRAM

Degree MSN

Available Programs Master's; RN to Master's.

Concentrations Available Nursing administration; nursing education.

Study Options Full-time and part-time.

Online Degree Options Yes (online only).

Program Entrance Requirements Clinical experience, computer literacy, minimum overall college GPA of 3.0, transcript of college record, CPR certification, written essay, immunizations, interview, 3 letters of recommendation, nursing research course, physical assessment course, professional liability insurance/malpractice insurance, prerequisite course work, resume, statistics course. *Application deadline:* Applications may be processed on a rolling basis for some programs. *Application fee:* $25.

Degree Requirements 36 total credit hours, thesis or project, comprehensive exam.

Georgia State University

Byrdine F. Lewis School of Nursing and Health Professions
Atlanta, Georgia

http://nursing.gsu.edu
Founded in 1913

DEGREES • BS • MSN • PHD

Nursing Program Faculty 60 (40% with doctorates).

Baccalaureate Enrollment 297 **Women** 86% **Men** 14% **Minority** 35% **International** 5% **Part-time** 5%

Graduate Enrollment 300 **Women** 90% **Men** 10% **Minority** 31% **International** 2% **Part-time** 90%

Distance Learning Courses Available.

Nursing Student Activities Sigma Theta Tau, Student Nurses' Association.

Nursing Student Resources Academic advising; academic or career counseling; assistance for students with disabilities; bookstore; campus computer network; career placement assistance; computer lab; computer-assisted instruction; e-mail services; interactive nursing skills videos; Internet; learning resource lab; library services; nursing audiovisuals; remedial services; resume preparation assistance; skills, simulation, or other laboratory; tutoring.

Library Facilities 1.7 million volumes (52,835 in health, 20,856 in nursing); 18,492 periodical subscriptions (725 health-care related).

BACCALAUREATE PROGRAMS

Degree BS

Available Programs Accelerated RN Baccalaureate; Generic Baccalaureate.

Study Options Full-time and part-time.

Program Entrance Requirements Minimum overall college GPA of 3.5, transcript of college record, CPR certification, written essay, health exam, immunizations, 2 letters of recommendation, minimum GPA in nursing prerequisites of 3.0, professional liability insurance/malpractice insurance, prerequisite course work. Transfer students are accepted. *Application deadline:* 3/1 (fall), 10/1 (spring).

Advanced Placement Credit given for nursing courses completed elsewhere dependent upon specific evaluations.

Expenses (2012–13) *Tuition, state resident:* full-time $7034; part-time $251 per credit hour. *Tuition, nonresident:* full-time $24,030; part-time $858 per credit hour. *International tuition:* $24,030 full-time. *Room and board:* $11,046; room only: $5661 per academic year. *Required fees:* full-time $1064; part-time $312 per credit; part-time $642 per term.

Financial Aid 90% of baccalaureate students in nursing programs received some form of financial aid in 2011–12. *Gift aid (need-based):* Federal Pell, FSEOG, state, private, college/university gift aid from institutional funds. *Loans:* Federal Direct (Subsidized and Unsubsidized Stafford PLUS), Perkins, state.*Work-study:* Federal Work-Study.*Financial aid application deadline:* 11/1(priority: 4/1).

Contact Ms. Denisa Hightower, Admissions Counselor, Byrdine F. Lewis School of Nursing and Health Professions, Georgia State University, College of Health and Human Sciences, Office of Academic Assistance, Atlanta, GA 30303-3083. *Telephone:* 404-413-1000. *Fax:* 404-413-1001. *E-mail:* dhightower@gsu.edu.

GRADUATE PROGRAMS

Expenses (2012–13) *Tuition, state resident:* full-time $9234; part-time $342 per credit hour. *Tuition, nonresident:* full-time $32,562; part-time $1206 per credit hour. *International tuition:* $32,562 full-time. *Required fees:* full-time $1064; part-time $312 per credit; part-time $642 per term.

Financial Aid 50% of graduate students in nursing programs received some form of financial aid in 2011–12. Fellowships with full tuition reimbursements available, research assistantships with full and partial tuition reimbursements available, teaching assistantships, Federal Work-Study, institutionally sponsored loans, scholarships, traineeships, tuition waivers (partial), and unspecified assistantships available. Aid available to part-time students. *Financial aid application deadline:* 4/1.

Contact Ms. Barbara Smith, Admissions Counselor, Byrdine F. Lewis School of Nursing and Health Professions, Georgia State University, College of Health and Human Sciences, PO Box 3995, Atlanta, GA 30302-3995. *Telephone:* 404-413-1007. *Fax:* 404-413-1001. *E-mail:* alhbbs@langate.gsu.edu.

MASTER'S DEGREE PROGRAM

Degree MSN

Available Programs Master's; RN to Master's.

Concentrations Available Nursing administration; nursing informatics. *Clinical nurse specialist programs in:* adult health, pediatric, perinatal, psychiatric/mental health, women's health. *Nurse practitioner programs in:* adult health, family health, pediatric, psychiatric/mental health, women's health.

Site Options Alpharetta, GA.

Study Options Full-time and part-time.

Program Entrance Requirements Clinical experience, computer literacy, minimum overall college GPA of 3.0, transcript of college record, CPR certification, written essay, interview, 2 letters of recommendation, professional liability insurance/malpractice insurance, MAT (preferred) or GRE. *Application deadline:* 3/1 (fall), 10/15 (spring), 3/1 (summer). *Application fee:* $50.

Advanced Placement Credit given for nursing courses completed elsewhere dependent upon specific evaluations.

Degree Requirements 48 total credit hours.

POST-MASTER'S PROGRAM

Areas of Study *Clinical nurse specialist programs in:* adult health, pediatric, perinatal, psychiatric/mental health, women's health. *Nurse practitioner. programs in:* adult health, family health, pediatric, psychiatric/mental health, women's health.

DOCTORAL DEGREE PROGRAM

Degree PhD

Available Programs Doctorate; Post-Baccalaureate Doctorate.

Areas of Study Bio-behavioral research, health promotion/disease prevention, individualized study, nursing research, nursing science.

Site Options Alpharetta, GA.

Program Entrance Requirements Minimum overall college GPA of 3.0, interview by faculty committee, interview, 3 letters of recommendation, MSN or equivalent, statistics course, vita, GRE General Test. *Application deadline:* 3/1 (fall). *Application fee:* $50.

Degree Requirements 60 total credit hours, dissertation, written exam, residency.

Gordon State College

Division of Nursing and Health Sciences
Barnesville, Georgia

http://www.gdn.edu/
Founded in 1852

DEGREE • BSN

Nursing Program Faculty 2 (50% with doctorates).

Baccalaureate Enrollment 26

Nursing Student Activities Student Nurses' Association.

Nursing Student Resources Academic advising; academic or career counseling; assistance for students with disabilities; bookstore; campus computer network; computer lab; computer-assisted instruction; e-mail services; employment services for current students; externships; interactive nursing skills videos; Internet; learning resource lab; library services; nursing audiovisuals; remedial services; skills, simulation, or other laboratory; tutoring.

Library Facilities 15 volumes in nursing.

BACCALAUREATE PROGRAMS

Degree BSN

Available Programs RN Baccalaureate.

Program Entrance Requirements Transcript of college record.

Contact *Telephone:* 678-359-5085. *Fax:* 678-359-5064.

Kennesaw State University
School of Nursing
Kennesaw, Georgia

http://www.kennesaw.edu/
Founded in 1963
DEGREES • BSN • MSN
Distance Learning Courses Available.
Nursing Student Activities Sigma Theta Tau, Student Nurses' Association.
Nursing Student Resources Academic advising; academic or career counseling; assistance for students with disabilities; bookstore; campus computer network; career placement assistance; computer lab; computer-assisted instruction; e-mail services; employment services for current students; externships; housing assistance; interactive nursing skills videos; Internet; learning resource lab; library services; nursing audiovisuals; paid internships; placement services for program completers; remedial services; resume preparation assistance; skills, simulation, or other laboratory; tutoring.
Library Facilities 585,200 volumes (20,000 in health, 10,000 in nursing); 50,000 periodical subscriptions (503 health-care related).

BACCALAUREATE PROGRAMS

Degree BSN
Available Programs ADN to Baccalaureate; Accelerated Baccalaureate; Accelerated Baccalaureate for Second Degree; Baccalaureate for Second Degree; Generic Baccalaureate; RN Baccalaureate.
Site Options Rome, GA; Jasper, GA.
Study Options Full-time and part-time.
Program Entrance Requirements Minimum overall college GPA of 2.7, transcript of college record, CPR certification, health exam, health insurance, 2 years high school math, 2 years high school science, high school transcript, immunizations, interview, 1 letter of recommendation, minimum high school GPA of 2.5, minimum GPA in nursing prerequisites of 2.7, professional liability insurance/malpractice insurance, prerequisite course work. Transfer students are accepted.
Advanced Placement Credit by examination available. Credit given for nursing courses completed elsewhere dependent upon specific evaluations.
Contact *Telephone:* 770-499-3211. *Fax:* 770-423-6627.

GRADUATE PROGRAMS

Contact *Telephone:* 770-423-6061. *Fax:* 770-423-6627.

MASTER'S DEGREE PROGRAM
Degree MSN
Available Programs Master's.
Concentrations Available *Clinical nurse specialist programs in:* adult health. *Nurse practitioner programs in:* adult health, family health, primary care.
Study Options Full-time.
Program Entrance Requirements Clinical experience, minimum overall college GPA of 3.0, transcript of college record, CPR certification, written essay, immunizations, 2 letters of recommendation, nursing research course, physical assessment course, professional liability insurance/malpractice insurance, prerequisite course work, resume.
Advanced Placement Credit given for nursing courses completed elsewhere dependent upon specific evaluations.
Degree Requirements 40 total credit hours, thesis or project.

CONTINUING EDUCATION PROGRAM

Contact *Telephone:* 770-423-6064. *Fax:* 770-423-6627.

LaGrange College
Department of Nursing
LaGrange, Georgia

http://www.lagrange.edu/
Founded in 1831
DEGREE • BSN
Nursing Program Faculty 6 (20% with doctorates).

Baccalaureate Enrollment 80 **Women** 85% **Men** 15% **Minority** 20%
Nursing Student Activities Nursing Honor Society, Student Nurses' Association.
Nursing Student Resources Academic advising; academic or career counseling; assistance for students with disabilities; bookstore; campus computer network; career placement assistance; computer lab; computer-assisted instruction; e-mail services; employment services for current students; externships; interactive nursing skills videos; Internet; learning resource lab; library services; nursing audiovisuals; paid internships; placement services for program completers; remedial services; resume preparation assistance; skills, simulation, or other laboratory; tutoring; unpaid internships.
Library Facilities 379,805 volumes (19,000 in health, 10,000 in nursing); 223 periodical subscriptions (100 health-care related).

BACCALAUREATE PROGRAMS

Degree BSN
Available Programs Generic Baccalaureate; RN Baccalaureate.
Study Options Full-time.
Program Entrance Requirements Minimum overall college GPA of 2.5, transcript of college record, CPR certification, written essay, health exam, health insurance, immunizations, interview, 2 letters of recommendation, minimum GPA in nursing prerequisites of 2.5, professional liability insurance/malpractice insurance, prerequisite course work. Transfer students are accepted. *Application deadline:* 4/15 (fall).
Advanced Placement Credit given for nursing courses completed elsewhere dependent upon specific evaluations.
Expenses (2012–13) *Tuition:* full-time $18,000. *International tuition:* $18,000 full-time. *Room and board:* $9000 per academic year. *Required fees:* full-time $800.
Financial Aid 95% of baccalaureate students in nursing programs received some form of financial aid in 2011–12. *Gift aid (need-based):* Federal Pell, FSEOG, state, private, college/university gift aid from institutional funds. *Loans:* Perkins, state. *Work-study:* Federal Work-Study, part-time campus jobs. *Financial aid application deadline (priority):* 3/1.
Contact Dr. Celia G. Hay, Chair, Department of Nursing, LaGrange College, 601 Broad Street, LaGrange, GA 30240-2999. *Telephone:* 706-880-8220. *Fax:* 706-880-8029. *E-mail:* chay@lagrange.edu.

Macon State College
School of Nursing and Health Sciences
Macon, Georgia

http://www.maconstate.edu
Founded in 1968
DEGREE • BSN
Nursing Program Faculty 30 (7% with doctorates).
Baccalaureate Enrollment 104 **Women** 88% **Men** 12% **Minority** 21% **International** 2%
Nursing Student Activities Student Nurses' Association.
Nursing Student Resources Academic advising; academic or career counseling; assistance for students with disabilities; bookstore; campus computer network; career placement assistance; computer lab; computer-assisted instruction; e-mail services; interactive nursing skills videos; Internet; learning resource lab; library services; nursing audiovisuals; remedial services; resume preparation assistance; skills, simulation, or other laboratory; tutoring.
Library Facilities 80,000 volumes (4,000 in health, 920 in nursing); 513 periodical subscriptions (90 health-care related).

BACCALAUREATE PROGRAMS

Degree BSN
Available Programs ADN to Baccalaureate; Generic Baccalaureate.
Study Options Full-time and part-time.
Program Entrance Requirements Minimum overall college GPA of 2.0, transcript of college record, CPR certification, health exam, health insurance, immunizations, minimum GPA in nursing prerequisites of 2.5, professional liability insurance/malpractice insurance, prerequisite course work. Transfer students are accepted. *Application deadline:* 2/15 (fall).
Contact *Telephone:* 478-471-2761. *Fax:* 478-471-2983.

Mercer University Georgia Baptist College of Nursing

Mercer University Georgia Baptist College of Nursing
Atlanta, Georgia

http://www.mercer.edu/nursing

DEGREES • BSN • DNP • MSN • PHD

Nursing Program Faculty 31 (58% with doctorates).

Baccalaureate Enrollment 298 **Women** 92% **Men** 8% **Minority** 38% **International** 1% **Part-time** 6%

Graduate Enrollment 95 **Women** 95% **Men** 5% **Minority** 43% **International** 2% **Part-time** 36%

Nursing Student Activities Sigma Theta Tau, Student Nurses' Association, nursing club.

Nursing Student Resources Academic advising; academic or career counseling; assistance for students with disabilities; bookstore; campus computer network; career placement assistance; computer lab; computer-assisted instruction; e-mail services; employment services for current students; housing assistance; interactive nursing skills videos; Internet; learning resource lab; library services; nursing audiovisuals; placement services for program completers; remedial services; resume preparation assistance; skills, simulation, or other laboratory; tutoring.

Library Facilities 4,072 volumes in health, 2,805 volumes in nursing; 218 periodical subscriptions health-care related.

BACCALAUREATE PROGRAMS

Degree BSN

Available Programs Generic Baccalaureate; RN Baccalaureate.

Study Options Full-time.

Program Entrance Requirements Transcript of college record, written essay, health exam, health insurance, high school biology, high school foreign language, 3 years high school math, 3 years high school science, high school transcript, immunizations, prerequisite course work. Transfer students are accepted. *Application deadline:* 5/1 (fall). Applications may be processed on a rolling basis for some programs. *Application fee:* $50.

Advanced Placement Credit by examination available. Credit given for nursing courses completed elsewhere dependent upon specific evaluations.

Expenses (2012–13) *Tuition:* full-time $21,100; part-time $875 per credit hour. *International tuition:* $21,100 full-time. *Room and board:* room only: $9660 per academic year. *Required fees:* full-time $1461; part-time $1106 per term.

Financial Aid 90% of baccalaureate students in nursing programs received some form of financial aid in 2011–12.

Contact Mrs. Lynn Vines, Director of Admissions, Mercer University Georgia Baptist College of Nursing, 3001 Mercer University Drive, Atlanta, GA 30341. *Telephone:* 678-547-6700. *Fax:* 678-547-6794. *E-mail:* vines_ml@mercer.edu.

GRADUATE PROGRAMS

Expenses (2012–13) *Tuition:* full-time $19,764; part-time $1098 per credit hour. *International tuition:* $19,764 full-time. *Room and board:* room only: $9660 per academic year. *Required fees:* full-time $1210; part-time $735 per term.

Financial Aid 90% of graduate students in nursing programs received some form of financial aid in 2011–12.

Contact Dr. Virginia Dare Domico, Associate Dean for Graduate Programs, Mercer University Georgia Baptist College of Nursing, 3001 Mercer University Drive, Atlanta, GA 30341. *Telephone:* 678-547-6741. *Fax:* 678-547-6777. *E-mail:* domico_vd@mercer.edu.

MASTER'S DEGREE PROGRAM

Degree MSN

Available Programs Master's.

Concentrations Available Nursing education. *Clinical nurse specialist programs in:* acute care, adult health, critical care, gerontology, pediatric. *Nurse practitioner programs in:* family health.

Study Options Full-time and part-time.

Program Entrance Requirements Clinical experience, computer literacy, minimum overall college GPA of 3.0, transcript of college record, CPR certification, written essay, immunizations, interview, 3 letters of recommendation, nursing research course, physical assessment course,

statistics course. *Application deadline:* 7/1 (fall), 11/1 (spring), 4/15 (summer). Applications may be processed on a rolling basis for some programs. *Application fee:* $50.

Advanced Placement Credit given for nursing courses completed elsewhere dependent upon specific evaluations.

Degree Requirements 38 total credit hours, thesis or project.

POST-MASTER'S PROGRAM

Areas of Study Nursing education.

DOCTORAL DEGREE PROGRAM

Degree DNP

Available Programs Doctorate.

Areas of Study Advanced practice nursing, nursing research.

Program Entrance Requirements Minimum overall college GPA of 3.5, clinical experience, interview, interview by faculty committee, 3 letters of recommendation, MSN or equivalent, scholarly papers, statistics course, vita, writing sample. *Application deadline:* 3/15 (fall). Applications may be processed on a rolling basis for some programs. *Application fee:* $50.

Degree Requirements 45 total credit hours, oral exam, written exam.

DOCTORAL DEGREE PROGRAM

Degree PhD

Available Programs Doctorate.

Areas of Study Clinical practice, ethics, nursing education.

Online Degree Options Yes (online only).

Program Entrance Requirements Minimum overall college GPA of 3.5, interview, 3 letters of recommendation, MSN or equivalent, scholarly papers, statistics course, vita, writing sample. *Application deadline:* 3/15 (fall). Applications may be processed on a rolling basis for some programs. *Application fee:* $50.

Degree Requirements 58 total credit hours, dissertation, oral exam, written exam.

Piedmont College

School of Nursing
Demorest, Georgia

http://www.piedmont.edu/pc/index.php/nursing-home
Founded in 1897

DEGREE • BSN

Nursing Program Faculty 8 (25% with doctorates).

Baccalaureate Enrollment 60 **Women** 99% **Men** 1% **Minority** 10% **International** 1% **Part-time** 20%

Distance Learning Courses Available.

Nursing Student Activities Nursing Honor Society, Student Nurses' Association.

Nursing Student Resources Academic advising; academic or career counseling; assistance for students with disabilities; bookstore; campus computer network; career placement assistance; computer lab; computer-assisted instruction; e-mail services; externships; housing assistance; interactive nursing skills videos; Internet; learning resource lab; library services; nursing audiovisuals; other; paid internships; resume preparation assistance; skills, simulation, or other laboratory; tutoring.

Library Facilities 311,722 volumes (3,000 in health, 500 in nursing); 290 periodical subscriptions (75 health-care related).

BACCALAUREATE PROGRAMS

Degree BSN

Available Programs Generic Baccalaureate; LPN to Baccalaureate; RN Baccalaureate.

Study Options Full-time.

Program Entrance Requirements Transcript of college record, CPR certification, health exam, health insurance, high school foreign language, 2 years high school math, 3 years high school science, high school transcript, immunizations, minimum GPA in nursing prerequisites of 3.0, professional liability insurance/malpractice insurance, prerequisite course work. Transfer students are accepted. *Application deadline:* 10/15 (fall).

Advanced Placement Credit given for nursing courses completed elsewhere dependent upon specific evaluations.

Contact *Telephone:* 706-776-0116. *Fax:* 706-778-0701.

Shorter University
School of Nursing
Rome, Georgia

http://www.shorter.edu/academics/nursing/nursing.htm
Founded in 1873
DEGREE • BSN
Nursing Program Faculty 9 (10% with doctorates).
Baccalaureate Enrollment 62 **Women** 75% **Men** 25% **Minority** 10% **International** 5%
Nursing Student Activities Nursing club.
Nursing Student Resources Academic advising; academic or career counseling; assistance for students with disabilities; bookstore; campus computer network; computer lab; e-mail services; housing assistance; interactive nursing skills videos; Internet; learning resource lab; library services; nursing audiovisuals; resume preparation assistance; skills, simulation, or other laboratory; tutoring.
Library Facilities 144,475 volumes; 8,511 periodical subscriptions.

BACCALAUREATE PROGRAMS

Degree BSN
Available Programs Generic Baccalaureate.
Site Options Rome, GA.
Study Options Full-time.
Program Entrance Requirements Minimum overall college GPA of 2.8, CPR certification, written essay, health exam, health insurance, immunizations, minimum GPA in nursing prerequisites of 2.8, professional liability insurance/malpractice insurance, prerequisite course work. Transfer students are accepted. *Application deadline:* 2/1 (fall).
Expenses (2011–12) *Tuition:* full-time $17,500. *International tuition:* $17,500 full-time. *Room and board:* $8600; room only: $4600 per academic year. *Required fees:* full-time $700.
Financial Aid 60% of baccalaureate students in nursing programs received some form of financial aid in 2010–11. *Gift aid (need-based):* Federal Pell, FSEOG, state, private, college/university gift aid from institutional funds. *Loans:* Federal Direct (Subsidized and Unsubsidized Stafford PLUS), Perkins. *Work-study:* Federal Work-Study, part-time campus jobs. *Financial aid application deadline (priority):* 4/1.
Contact April Allen, Administrative Assistant to the Dean, School of Nursing, Shorter University, 315 Shorter Avenue, Rome, GA 30165. *Telephone:* 706-233-7464. *Fax:* 706-291-4283. *E-mail:* aallen@shorter.edu.

Thomas University
Division of Nursing
Thomasville, Georgia

http://www.thomasu.edu/nursing.htm
Founded in 1950
DEGREES • BSN • MSN • MSN/MBA
Nursing Program Faculty 10 (60% with doctorates).
Baccalaureate Enrollment 88 **Women** 85% **Men** 15% **Minority** 30%
Graduate Enrollment 42 **Women** 90% **Men** 10% **Minority** 40% **Part-time** 50%
Distance Learning Courses Available.
Nursing Student Activities Nursing Honor Society, Sigma Theta Tau.
Nursing Student Resources Academic advising; academic or career counseling; assistance for students with disabilities; bookstore; campus computer network; career placement assistance; computer lab; computer-assisted instruction; e-mail services; housing assistance; interactive nursing skills videos; Internet; learning resource lab; library services; nursing audiovisuals; remedial services; resume preparation assistance; skills, simulation, or other laboratory; tutoring.
Library Facilities 41,467 volumes (1,200 in health, 400 in nursing); 451 periodical subscriptions (150 health-care related).

BACCALAUREATE PROGRAMS

Degree BSN
Available Programs ADN to Baccalaureate; Accelerated RN Baccalaureate; International Nurse to Baccalaureate; RN Baccalaureate.
Site Options Tallahassee, FL; Moultrie, GA.
Study Options Full-time and part-time.
Program Entrance Requirements Minimum overall college GPA of 2.5, transcript of college record, CPR certification, health exam, health insurance, immunizations, minimum GPA in nursing prerequisites of 2.5, professional liability insurance/malpractice insurance, prerequisite course work, RN licensure. Transfer students are accepted. *Application deadline:* 8/1 (fall), 12/1 (spring), 4/15 (summer). Applications may be processed on a rolling basis for some programs. *Application fee:* $35.
Advanced Placement Credit by examination available. Credit given for nursing courses completed elsewhere dependent upon specific evaluations.
Financial Aid 90% of baccalaureate students in nursing programs received some form of financial aid in 2011–12. *Gift aid (need-based):* Federal Pell, FSEOG, state, private, college/university gift aid from institutional funds. *Loans:* Federal Direct (Subsidized and Unsubsidized Stafford PLUS), state, alternative loans. *Work-study:* Federal Work-Study. *Financial aid application deadline (priority):* 5/1.
Contact Kerri Knight, Director of Admissions, Division of Nursing, Thomas University, 1501 Millpond Road, Thomasville, GA 31792. *Fax:* 229-226-1653. *E-mail:* kknight@thomasu.edu.

GRADUATE PROGRAMS

Financial Aid 50% of graduate students in nursing programs received some form of financial aid in 2011–12.
Contact Kerri Knight, Admissions Representative, Division of Nursing, Thomas University, 1501 Millpond Road, Thomasville, GA 31792. *Fax:* 229-226-1653. *E-mail:* kknight@thomasu.edu.

MASTER'S DEGREE PROGRAM
Degrees MSN; MSN/MBA
Available Programs Accelerated Master's; Master's; RN to Master's.
Concentrations Available Health-care administration; nursing administration; nursing education.
Study Options Full-time and part-time.
Program Entrance Requirements Computer literacy, minimum overall college GPA of 3.0, transcript of college record, CPR certification, written essay, immunizations, 3 letters of recommendation, professional liability insurance/malpractice insurance, resume, statistics course. *Application deadline:* 8/1 (fall), 12/1 (spring), 4/15 (summer). Applications may be processed on a rolling basis for some programs. *Application fee:* $50.
Advanced Placement Credit given for nursing courses completed elsewhere dependent upon specific evaluations.
Degree Requirements 36 total credit hours, thesis or project.

POST-MASTER'S PROGRAM
Areas of Study Health-care administration; nursing administration; nursing education.

University of North Georgia
Department of Nursing
Dahlonega, Georgia

http://www.northgeorgia.edu/
Founded in 1873
DEGREES • BSN • MS
Nursing Program Faculty 42 (17% with doctorates).
Baccalaureate Enrollment 70 **Women** 90% **Men** 10% **Minority** 12% **International** 4% **Part-time** 40%
Graduate Enrollment 50 **Women** 90% **Men** 10% **Minority** 10% **International** 2% **Part-time** 5%
Distance Learning Courses Available.
Nursing Student Activities Nursing Honor Society, Sigma Theta Tau, Student Nurses' Association.
Nursing Student Resources Academic advising; academic or career counseling; assistance for students with disabilities; bookstore; campus computer network; career placement assistance; computer lab; computer-assisted instruction; e-mail services; externships; interactive nursing skills videos; Internet; learning resource lab; library services; nursing audiovisuals; remedial services; resume preparation assistance; skills, simulation, or other laboratory; tutoring.
Library Facilities 228,298 volumes (6,875 in health, 619 in nursing); 13,747 periodical subscriptions (2,377 health-care related).

BACCALAUREATE PROGRAMS

Degree BSN
Available Programs ADN to Baccalaureate.
Study Options Full-time and part-time.
Online Degree Options Yes (online only).

Program Entrance Requirements Minimum overall college GPA of 2.75, transcript of college record, CPR certification, health exam, health insurance, high school biology, high school chemistry, high school foreign language, 3 years high school math, 2 years high school science, high school transcript, immunizations, 2 letters of recommendation, professional liability insurance/malpractice insurance, prerequisite course work, RN licensure. Transfer students are accepted. *Application deadline:* 2/1 (fall). *Application fee:* $25.
Contact *Telephone:* 706-864-1937. *Fax:* 706-864-1845.

GRADUATE PROGRAMS

Contact *Telephone:* 706-864-1489. *Fax:* 706-864-1845.

MASTER'S DEGREE PROGRAM
Degree MS
Available Programs Master's.
Concentrations Available Nursing education. *Nurse practitioner programs in:* family health.
Study Options Full-time and part-time.
Program Entrance Requirements Clinical experience, computer literacy, minimum overall college GPA of 2.75, transcript of college record, CPR certification, written essay, immunizations, 3 letters of recommendation, nursing research course, physical assessment course, professional liability insurance/malpractice insurance, prerequisite course work. *Application deadline:* 2/28 (spring). *Application fee:* $25.
Degree Requirements 46 total credit hours, thesis or project, comprehensive exam.

POST-MASTER'S PROGRAM
Areas of Study Nursing education. *Nurse practitioner programs in:* family health.

University of Phoenix–Atlanta Campus
College of Health and Human Services
Sandy Springs, Georgia

Nursing Student Activities Sigma Theta Tau.
Nursing Student Resources Academic advising; academic or career counseling; assistance for students with disabilities; bookstore; campus computer network; computer lab; computer-assisted instruction; e-mail services; interactive nursing skills videos; Internet; learning resource lab; library services; nursing audiovisuals; remedial services; skills, simulation, or other laboratory; tutoring.
Library Facilities 16,781 periodical subscriptions (1,300 health-care related).

University of West Georgia
School of Nursing
Carrollton, Georgia

http://www.westga.edu/~nurs/
Founded in 1933
DEGREES • BSN • EDD • MSN
Nursing Program Faculty 42 (36% with doctorates).
Baccalaureate Enrollment 351 **Women** 88% **Men** 12% **Minority** 30% **International** 1% **Part-time** 69%
Graduate Enrollment 89 **Women** 97% **Men** 3% **Minority** 42% **Part-time** 17%
Distance Learning Courses Available.
Nursing Student Activities Sigma Theta Tau, Student Nurses' Association.
Nursing Student Resources Academic advising; academic or career counseling; assistance for students with disabilities; bookstore; campus computer network; career placement assistance; computer lab; computer-assisted instruction; e-mail services; employment services for current students; externships; housing assistance; interactive nursing skills videos; Internet; learning resource lab; library services; nursing audiovisuals; remedial services; resume preparation assistance; skills, simulation, or other laboratory; tutoring.
Library Facilities 850,195 volumes (1,487 in health, 980 in nursing); 65,301 periodical subscriptions (134 health-care related).

BACCALAUREATE PROGRAMS
Degree BSN
Available Programs Accelerated RN Baccalaureate; Generic Baccalaureate.
Site Options Newnan, GA.
Study Options Full-time and part-time.
Program Entrance Requirements Minimum overall college GPA of 2.75, transcript of college record, CPR certification, written essay, health exam, health insurance, immunizations, minimum GPA in nursing prerequisites of 2.75, professional liability insurance/malpractice insurance, prerequisite course work. Transfer students are accepted. *Application deadline:* 2/1 (summer). *Application fee:* $40.
Expenses (2012–13) *Tuition, state resident:* full-time $3855; part-time $162 per credit hour. *Tuition, nonresident:* full-time $9993; part-time $571 per credit hour. *Room and board:* $4077; room only: $2386 per academic year. *Required fees:* full-time $400; part-time $200 per term.
Financial Aid 82% of baccalaureate students in nursing programs received some form of financial aid in 2011–12.
Contact Dr. Cynthia D. Epps, Associate Dean and Undergraduate Program Coordinator, School of Nursing, University of West Georgia, 1601 Maple Street, Carrollton, GA 30118. *Telephone:* 678-839-6552. *Fax:* 678-839-6553. *E-mail:* cepps@westga.edu.

GRADUATE PROGRAMS
Expenses (2012–13) *Tuition, state resident:* part-time $343 per credit hour. *Tuition, nonresident:* part-time $343 per credit hour. *Room and board:* $4077; room only: $3855 per academic year. *Required fees:* part-time $150 per term.
Financial Aid 54% of graduate students in nursing programs received some form of financial aid in 2011–12.
Contact Dr. Laurie Jowers Ware, Assistant Dean and Director of Graduate Program, School of Nursing, University of West Georgia, 1601 Maple Street, Carrollton, GA 30118. *Telephone:* 678-839-6552. *Fax:* 678-839-6553. *E-mail:* lware@westga.edu.

MASTER'S DEGREE PROGRAM
Degree MSN
Available Programs Accelerated RN to Master's; Master's.
Concentrations Available Clinical nurse leader; nursing administration; nursing education.
Study Options Full-time and part-time.
Online Degree Options Yes (online only).
Program Entrance Requirements Clinical experience, computer literacy, minimum overall college GPA of 3.0, transcript of college record, CPR certification, immunizations, 2 letters of recommendation, nursing research course, professional liability insurance/malpractice insurance, prerequisite course work, resume, statistics course. *Application deadline:* 7/1 (fall). *Application fee:* $40.
Degree Requirements 36 total credit hours, thesis or project, comprehensive exam.

POST-MASTER'S PROGRAM
Areas of Study Clinical nurse leader; nursing administration; nursing education.

DOCTORAL DEGREE PROGRAM
Degree EdD
Available Programs Doctorate.
Areas of Study Nursing education.
Online Degree Options Yes (online only).
Program Entrance Requirements Minimum overall college GPA of 3.0, 3 letters of recommendation, MSN or equivalent, statistics course, vita, writing sample. *Application deadline:* 5/1 (fall). *Application fee:* $40.
Degree Requirements 60 total credit hours, dissertation, oral exam, written exam.

Valdosta State University
College of Nursing
Valdosta, Georgia

http://www.valdosta.edu/nursing/
Founded in 1906
DEGREES • BSN • MSN
Nursing Program Faculty 23 (52% with doctorates).

Baccalaureate Enrollment 183 **Women** 87% **Men** 13% **Minority** 21% **International** 1% **Part-time** 7%
Graduate Enrollment 25 **Women** 99% **Men** 1% **Minority** 15% **International** 1% **Part-time** 49%
Nursing Student Activities Sigma Theta Tau, Student Nurses' Association.
Nursing Student Resources Academic advising; academic or career counseling; assistance for students with disabilities; bookstore; campus computer network; career placement assistance; computer lab; computer-assisted instruction; e-mail services; employment services for current students; externships; housing assistance; Internet; learning resource lab; library services; nursing audiovisuals; placement services for program completers; resume preparation assistance; skills, simulation, or other laboratory; tutoring; unpaid internships.
Library Facilities 660,108 volumes (21,688 in health); 2,598 periodical subscriptions (75 health-care related).

BACCALAUREATE PROGRAMS

Degree BSN
Available Programs Generic Baccalaureate; RN Baccalaureate.
Study Options Full-time.
Program Entrance Requirements Minimum overall college GPA of 2.8, transcript of college record, CPR certification, health exam, health insurance, immunizations, minimum GPA in nursing prerequisites of 2.8, professional liability insurance/malpractice insurance, prerequisite course work. Transfer students are accepted.
Advanced Placement Credit given for nursing courses completed elsewhere dependent upon specific evaluations.
Contact *Telephone:* 229-333-5959. *Fax:* 229-333-7300.

GRADUATE PROGRAMS

Contact *Telephone:* 229-333-5959. *Fax:* 229-333-7300.

MASTER'S DEGREE PROGRAM
Degree MSN
Available Programs Master's; RN to Master's.
Concentrations Available Nurse case management; nursing administration; nursing education. *Clinical nurse specialist programs in:* adult health, family health, psychiatric/mental health.
Study Options Full-time and part-time.
Program Entrance Requirements Minimum overall college GPA of 2.8, transcript of college record, CPR certification, immunizations, 3 letters of recommendation, physical assessment course, professional liability insurance/malpractice insurance, statistics course, GRE General Test.
Advanced Placement Credit given for nursing courses completed elsewhere dependent upon specific evaluations.
Degree Requirements 36 total credit hours, thesis or project, comprehensive exam.

CONTINUING EDUCATION PROGRAM

Contact *Telephone:* 229-333-5960.

GUAM

University of Guam
School of Nursing and Health Sciences
Mangilao, Guam

http://www.uog.edu
Founded in 1952
DEGREE • BSN
Nursing Program Faculty 10 (30% with doctorates).
Baccalaureate Enrollment 175 **Women** 97% **Men** 3% **International** 2%
Nursing Student Activities Student Nurses' Association.
Nursing Student Resources Academic advising; academic or career counseling; assistance for students with disabilities; bookstore; campus computer network; career placement assistance; computer lab; daycare for children of students; e-mail services; employment services for current students; interactive nursing skills videos; Internet; learning resource lab; library services; nursing audiovisuals; remedial services; skills, simulation, or other laboratory; tutoring.
Library Facilities 315,478 volumes (5,246 in health, 982 in nursing); 28,845 periodical subscriptions (53 health-care related).

BACCALAUREATE PROGRAMS

Degree BSN
Available Programs ADN to Baccalaureate; Generic Baccalaureate; RN Baccalaureate.
Study Options Full-time and part-time.
Program Entrance Requirements Transcript of college record, CPR certification, written essay, health exam, high school biology, high school chemistry, 1 year of high school math, 1 year of high school science, high school transcript, immunizations, interview, minimum high school GPA of 2.5, minimum GPA in nursing prerequisites of 2.7, prerequisite course work. Transfer students are accepted.
Advanced Placement Credit by examination available. Credit given for nursing courses completed elsewhere dependent upon specific evaluations.
Financial Aid 73% of baccalaureate students in nursing programs received some form of financial aid in 2010–11.
Contact Dr. Deborah Leon Guerrero, Registrar, School of Nursing and Health Sciences, University of Guam, Admissions and Records Office, UOG Station, Mangilao, GU 96923. *Telephone:* 671-735-2210. *Fax:* 671-734-4245. *E-mail:* admitme@uog9.uog.edu.

HAWAII

Chaminade University of Honolulu
Nursing Program
Honolulu, Hawaii

http://www.chaminade.edu/nursing
Founded in 1955
DEGREE • BSN
Nursing Program Faculty 7 (28% with doctorates).
Baccalaureate Enrollment 145
Nursing Student Activities Sigma Theta Tau, nursing club.
Nursing Student Resources Academic advising; academic or career counseling; assistance for students with disabilities; bookstore; campus computer network; computer lab; computer-assisted instruction; e-mail services; employment services for current students; interactive nursing skills videos; Internet; learning resource lab; library services; nursing audiovisuals; placement services for program completers; remedial services; resume preparation assistance; skills, simulation, or other laboratory; tutoring.
Library Facilities 78,000 volumes; 6,730 periodical subscriptions.

BACCALAUREATE PROGRAMS

Degree BSN
Available Programs Generic Baccalaureate.
Study Options Full-time.
Program Entrance Requirements Minimum overall college GPA of 2.75, transcript of college record, written essay, high school chemistry, 4 years high school math, high school transcript, 2 letters of recommendation, minimum high school GPA of 2.75. Transfer students are accepted. *Application deadline:* 2/1 (fall). *Application fee:* $25.
Expenses (2011–12) *Tuition:* full-time $23,660; part-time $11,830 per semester. *Room and board:* $6000; room only: $4000 per academic year. *Required fees:* full-time $400.
Contact Ashley Wiswell, Nursing Program Assistant, Nursing Program, Chaminade University of Honolulu, 3140 Waialae Ave, Henry Hall 110, Honolulu, HI 96816. *Telephone:* 808-735-4813. *E-mail:* ashley.wiswell@chaminade.edu.

Hawaii Pacific University
College of Nursing and Health Sciences
Honolulu, Hawaii

http://www.hpu.edu/
Founded in 1965

DEGREES • BSN • MSN • MSN/MBA
Nursing Program Faculty 102 (16% with doctorates).
Baccalaureate Enrollment 1,279 **Women** 82% **Men** 18% **Minority** 74% **International** 2% **Part-time** 26%
Graduate Enrollment 65 **Women** 81% **Men** 19% **Minority** 90% **International** 20% **Part-time** 22%
Distance Learning Courses Available.
Nursing Student Activities Nursing Honor Society, Sigma Theta Tau, Student Nurses' Association.
Nursing Student Resources Academic advising; academic or career counseling; assistance for students with disabilities; bookstore; campus computer network; career placement assistance; computer lab; computer-assisted instruction; e-mail services; employment services for current students; externships; housing assistance; Internet; learning resource lab; library services; paid internships; placement services for program completers; resume preparation assistance; skills, simulation, or other laboratory; tutoring.
Library Facilities 175,000 volumes (5,314 in health, 1,996 in nursing); 45,000 periodical subscriptions (7,243 health-care related).

BACCALAUREATE PROGRAMS

Degree BSN
Available Programs Generic Baccalaureate; International Nurse to Baccalaureate; LPN to Baccalaureate; RN Baccalaureate.
Site Options Kaneohe, HI; Honolulu, HI.
Study Options Full-time and part-time.
Program Entrance Requirements Minimum overall college GPA of 2.75, transcript of college record, CPR certification, health exam, health insurance, immunizations, minimum GPA in nursing prerequisites of 2.75, prerequisite course work. Transfer students are accepted. *Application deadline:* Applications may be processed on a rolling basis for some programs. *Application fee:* $50.
Advanced Placement Credit given for nursing courses completed elsewhere dependent upon specific evaluations.
Expenses (2012–13) *Tuition:* full-time $18,500; part-time $617 per credit. *International tuition:* $18,500 full-time. *Room and board:* $12,482 per academic year. *Required fees:* full-time $100.
Financial Aid 79% of baccalaureate students in nursing programs received some form of financial aid in 2011–12.
Contact Miss Sara Sato, Director of Admissions, College of Nursing and Health Sciences, Hawai`i Pacific University, 1164 Bishop Street, Honolulu, HI 96813. *Telephone:* 808-544-0238. *Fax:* 808-544-1136. *E-mail:* ssato@hpu.edu.

GRADUATE PROGRAMS

Expenses (2012–13) *Tuition:* full-time $13,590; part-time $755 per credit hour. *International tuition:* $13,590 full-time. *Required fees:* full-time $100.
Financial Aid 60% of graduate students in nursing programs received some form of financial aid in 2011–12. Career-related internships or fieldwork, Federal Work-Study, scholarships, traineeships, and tuition waivers available. *Financial aid application deadline:* 3/1.
Contact Dr. Diane Knight, Chair, Department of Graduate and Post-Baccalaureate Nursing Programs, College of Nursing and Health Sciences, Hawai`i Pacific University, 45-045 Kamehameha Highway, Kaneohe, HI 96744-5297. *Telephone:* 808-236-3552. *Fax:* 808-236-3524. *E-mail:* dknight@hpu.edu.

MASTER'S DEGREE PROGRAM

Degrees MSN; MSN/MBA
Available Programs Master's; RN to Master's.
Concentrations Available Nursing education. *Clinical nurse specialist programs in:* community health. *Nurse practitioner programs in:* family health.
Site Options Kaneohe, HI.
Study Options Full-time and part-time.
Program Entrance Requirements Clinical experience, minimum overall college GPA of 3.0, transcript of college record, written essay, 2 letters of recommendation, nursing research course, prerequisite course work, statistics course. *Application deadline:* Applications may be processed on a rolling basis for some programs. *Application fee:* $50.

Advanced Placement Credit given for nursing courses completed elsewhere dependent upon specific evaluations.
Degree Requirements 48 total credit hours, thesis or project.

POST-MASTER'S PROGRAM
Areas of Study Nursing education. *Nurse practitioner programs in:* family health.

University of Hawaii at Hilo
Department in Nursing
Hilo, Hawaii

http://www.uhh.hawaii.edu/
Founded in 1970

DEGREE • BSN
Nursing Program Faculty 10 (50% with doctorates).
Baccalaureate Enrollment 78 **Women** 83% **Men** 17% **Minority** 68% **International** 1% **Part-time** 18%
Distance Learning Courses Available.
Nursing Student Activities Nursing Honor Society, Sigma Theta Tau, Student Nurses' Association.
Nursing Student Resources Academic advising; academic or career counseling; assistance for students with disabilities; bookstore; campus computer network; career placement assistance; computer lab; computer-assisted instruction; e-mail services; employment services for current students; externships; housing assistance; interactive nursing skills videos; Internet; learning resource lab; library services; nursing audiovisuals; paid internships; remedial services; resume preparation assistance; skills, simulation, or other laboratory; tutoring.
Library Facilities 250,000 volumes (680 in health, 284 in nursing); 2,500 periodical subscriptions (15,000 health-care related).

BACCALAUREATE PROGRAMS

Degree BSN
Available Programs ADN to Baccalaureate; Generic Baccalaureate; RN Baccalaureate.
Site Options Kona, HI; Lihue, HI; Kahalui, HI.
Study Options Full-time.
Program Entrance Requirements Minimum overall college GPA of 2.7, transcript of college record, CPR certification, written essay, health exam, health insurance, high school biology, high school chemistry, high school foreign language, 1 year of high school math, 3 years high school science, high school transcript, immunizations, 2 letters of recommendation, minimum high school GPA of 3.0, minimum GPA in nursing prerequisites of 2.7, professional liability insurance/malpractice insurance, prerequisite course work. *Application deadline:* 1/15 (fall).
Expenses (2011–12) *Tuition, state resident:* full-time $7990; part-time $235 per credit hour. *Tuition, nonresident:* full-time $24,242; part-time $713 per credit hour. *Room and board:* $6460; room only: $2756 per academic year. *Required fees:* full-time $5705; part-time $84 per credit; part-time $168 per term.
Financial Aid 90% of baccalaureate students in nursing programs received some form of financial aid in 2010–11. *Gift aid (need-based):* Federal Pell, FSEOG, state, private, college/university gift aid from institutional funds. *Loans:* Federal Direct (Subsidized and Unsubsidized Stafford PLUS), Perkins, state. *Work-study:* Federal Work-Study, part-time campus jobs. *Financial aid application deadline (priority):* 3/1.
Contact Dr. Katharyn Daub, Chair and Program Director, Department in Nursing, University of Hawaii at Hilo, 200 West Kawili Street, UCB 235, Hilo, HI 96720. *Telephone:* 808-974-7760. *Fax:* 808-974-7665. *E-mail:* katharyn@hawaii.edu.

University of Hawaii at Manoa
School of Nursing and Dental Hygiene
Honolulu, Hawaii

http://www.nursing.hawaii.edu/
Founded in 1907

DEGREES • BSN • MS • MSN/MBA • PHD
Nursing Program Faculty 97 (35% with doctorates).
Baccalaureate Enrollment 336 **Women** 77% **Men** 23% **Minority** 83% **International** 3% **Part-time** 56%

Graduate Enrollment 170 **Women** 88% **Men** 12% **Minority** 60% **International** 2% **Part-time** 66%

Distance Learning Courses Available.

Nursing Student Activities Nursing Honor Society, Sigma Theta Tau, Student Nurses' Association, nursing club.

Nursing Student Resources Academic advising; academic or career counseling; assistance for students with disabilities; bookstore; computer lab; computer-assisted instruction; e-mail services; employment services for current students; housing assistance; Internet; learning resource lab; library services; nursing audiovisuals; resume preparation assistance; skills, simulation, or other laboratory.

Library Facilities 3.4 million volumes; 58,434 periodical subscriptions.

BACCALAUREATE PROGRAMS

Degree BSN

Available Programs ADN to Baccalaureate; Generic Baccalaureate; RN Baccalaureate.

Study Options Full-time and part-time.

Program Entrance Requirements Minimum overall college GPA of 2.5, transcript of college record, CPR certification, health exam, health insurance, immunizations, minimum GPA in nursing prerequisites of 2.5, prerequisite course work. Transfer students are accepted. *Application deadline:* 3/1 (fall), 10/1 (spring). *Application fee:* $50.

Advanced Placement Credit by examination available. Credit given for nursing courses completed elsewhere dependent upon specific evaluations.

Contact *Telephone:* 808-956-8939. *Fax:* 808-956-5977.

GRADUATE PROGRAMS

Contact *Telephone:* 808-956-3519. *Fax:* 808-956-5977.

MASTER'S DEGREE PROGRAM

Degrees MS; MSN/MBA

Available Programs Accelerated Master's; Master's; Master's for Non-Nursing College Graduates; RN to Master's.

Concentrations Available Nursing administration; nursing education. *Clinical nurse specialist programs in:* psychiatric/mental health. *Nurse practitioner programs in:* adult health, community health, family health, gerontology, pediatric.

Site Options Kahului, HI; Lihue, HI; Kailua Kona, HI.

Study Options Full-time and part-time.

Online Degree Options Yes.

Program Entrance Requirements Minimum overall college GPA of 3.0, transcript of college record, CPR certification, written essay, immunizations, interview, 2 letters of recommendation, resume, statistics course. *Application deadline:* 3/1 (fall). *Application fee:* $60.

Advanced Placement Credit given for nursing courses completed elsewhere dependent upon specific evaluations.

Degree Requirements 52 total credit hours.

POST-MASTER'S PROGRAM

Areas of Study Nursing administration; nursing education. *Clinical nurse specialist programs in:* psychiatric/mental health. *Nurse practitioner programs in:* adult health, community health, family health, gerontology, pediatric.

DOCTORAL DEGREE PROGRAM

Degree PhD

Available Programs Doctorate.

Areas of Study Faculty preparation, nursing education, nursing research, nursing science.

Site Options Kahului, HI; Lihue, HI; Kailua Kona, HI.

Online Degree Options Yes (online only).

Program Entrance Requirements Clinical experience, minimum overall college GPA of 3.0, interview by faculty committee, interview, 3 letters of recommendation, MSN or equivalent, scholarly papers, statistics course, vita, writing sample. *Application deadline:* 2/1 (fall).

Degree Requirements 46 total credit hours, dissertation, oral exam, residency.

University of Phoenix–Hawaii Campus

College of Nursing
Honolulu, Hawaii

DEGREES • BSN • MSN • MSN/ED D

Nursing Program Faculty 26 (15% with doctorates).

Baccalaureate Enrollment 70 **Women** 90% **Men** 10% **Minority** 40%

Graduate Enrollment 14 **Women** 71.4% **Men** 28.6% **Minority** 57.14%

Nursing Student Activities Sigma Theta Tau.

Nursing Student Resources Academic advising; academic or career counseling; assistance for students with disabilities; bookstore; campus computer network; computer lab; computer-assisted instruction; e-mail services; interactive nursing skills videos; Internet; learning resource lab; library services; nursing audiovisuals; remedial services; skills, simulation, or other laboratory; tutoring.

Library Facilities 16,781 periodical subscriptions (1,300 health-care related).

BACCALAUREATE PROGRAMS

Degree BSN

Available Programs Accelerated Baccalaureate; LPN to Baccalaureate.

Site Options Kaneohe, HI; Mililani, HI; Kapolei, HI.

Study Options Full-time.

Program Entrance Requirements Transcript of college record, CPR certification, immunizations, 1 letter of recommendation, RN licensure. Transfer students are accepted. *Application deadline:* Applications may be processed on a rolling basis for some programs.

Advanced Placement Credit by examination available. Credit given for nursing courses completed elsewhere dependent upon specific evaluations.

Contact *Telephone:* 808-536-2686.

GRADUATE PROGRAMS

Contact *Telephone:* 808-536-2686.

MASTER'S DEGREE PROGRAM

Degrees MSN; MSN/Ed D

Available Programs Master's.

Concentrations Available Health-care administration; nursing administration; nursing education. *Nurse practitioner programs in:* family health.

Site Options Kaneohe, HI; Mililani, HI; Kapolei, HI.

Study Options Full-time.

Program Entrance Requirements Clinical experience, computer literacy, minimum overall college GPA of 2.5, transcript of college record. *Application deadline:* Applications may be processed on a rolling basis for some programs. *Application fee:* $45.

Advanced Placement Credit given for nursing courses completed elsewhere dependent upon specific evaluations.

Degree Requirements 39 total credit hours, thesis or project.

IDAHO

Boise State University

Department of Nursing
Boise, Idaho

http://nursing.boisestate.edu/
Founded in 1932

DEGREES • BS • MSN • MSN/MS

Nursing Program Faculty 55 (25% with doctorates).

Baccalaureate Enrollment 540 **Women** 75% **Men** 25% **Minority** 1% **International** 1%

Graduate Enrollment 12

Distance Learning Courses Available.

Nursing Student Activities Nursing Honor Society, Sigma Theta Tau, Student Nurses' Association.

Nursing Student Resources Academic advising; academic or career counseling; assistance for students with disabilities; bookstore; campus computer network; career placement assistance; computer lab; computer-

assisted instruction; daycare for children of students; e-mail services; employment services for current students; housing assistance; interactive nursing skills videos; Internet; learning resource lab; library services; nursing audiovisuals; placement services for program completers; remedial services; resume preparation assistance; skills, simulation, or other laboratory; tutoring.
Library Facilities 838,932 volumes (27,919 in health, 2,617 in nursing); 5,575 periodical subscriptions (158 health-care related).

BACCALAUREATE PROGRAMS

Degree BS
Available Programs Accelerated RN Baccalaureate; Generic Baccalaureate; LPN to Baccalaureate; RN Baccalaureate.
Site Options Nampa, ID.
Study Options Full-time.
Online Degree Options Yes.
Program Entrance Requirements Transcript of college record, immunizations, minimum GPA in nursing prerequisites of 3.0, professional liability insurance/malpractice insurance, prerequisite course work. Transfer students are accepted. *Application deadline:* 3/1 (fall), 10/1 (spring). *Application fee:* $20.
Advanced Placement Credit by examination available. Credit given for nursing courses completed elsewhere dependent upon specific evaluations.
Contact *Telephone:* 208-426-4143. *Fax:* 208-426-1370.

GRADUATE PROGRAMS

Contact *Telephone:* 208-426-4143.

MASTER'S DEGREE PROGRAM

Degrees MSN; MSN/MS
Available Programs Master's.
Concentrations Available Clinical nurse leader; health-care administration; nurse case management; nursing administration; nursing education.
Study Options Part-time.
Program Entrance Requirements Minimum overall college GPA of 3.0, transcript of college record, CPR certification, written essay, letters of recommendation, nursing research course, professional liability insurance/malpractice insurance, prerequisite course work, resume, statistics course. *Application deadline:* 3/31 (spring).
Degree Requirements 39 total credit hours, thesis or project.

Brigham Young University–Idaho
Department of Nursing
Rexburg, Idaho

Founded in 1888
DEGREE • BSN

BACCALAUREATE PROGRAMS

Degree BSN
Available Programs RN Baccalaureate.
Program Entrance Requirements RN licensure. Transfer students are accepted. *Application deadline:* 6/1 (fall), 10/1 (winter), 2/1 (spring).
Contact *Telephone:* 208-496-4555. *Fax:* 208-496-4553.

Idaho State University
Department of Nursing
Pocatello, Idaho

http://www.isu.edu/nursing
Founded in 1901
DEGREES • BSN • MS
Nursing Program Faculty 22 (36% with doctorates).
Baccalaureate Enrollment 195 **Women** 76% **Men** 24% **Minority** 14%
Graduate Enrollment 124 **Women** 85% **Men** 15% **Minority** 6% **Part-time** 58%
Distance Learning Courses Available.
Nursing Student Activities Sigma Theta Tau, Student Nurses' Association.

Nursing Student Resources Academic advising; academic or career counseling; assistance for students with disabilities; bookstore; campus computer network; computer lab; computer-assisted instruction; daycare for children of students; e-mail services; employment services for current students; housing assistance; interactive nursing skills videos; Internet; learning resource lab; library services; nursing audiovisuals; resume preparation assistance; skills, simulation, or other laboratory; tutoring.
Library Facilities 35,948 volumes in health, 1,775 volumes in nursing; 5,312 periodical subscriptions health-care related.

BACCALAUREATE PROGRAMS

Degree BSN
Available Programs ADN to Baccalaureate; Accelerated Baccalaureate for Second Degree; Generic Baccalaureate; LPN to Baccalaureate.
Site Options Boise, ID; Idaho Falls, ID; Twin Falls, ID.
Study Options Full-time.
Program Entrance Requirements Minimum overall college GPA, transcript of college record, CPR certification, written essay, health exam, health insurance, high school transcript, immunizations, 3 letters of recommendation, minimum high school GPA of 2.0, minimum GPA in nursing prerequisites of 3.0, professional liability insurance/malpractice insurance, prerequisite course work. Transfer students are accepted. *Application deadline:* 9/15 (spring). *Application fee:* $50.
Advanced Placement Credit given for nursing courses completed elsewhere dependent upon specific evaluations.
Contact *Telephone:* 208-282-2443. *Fax:* 208-236-4476.

GRADUATE PROGRAMS

Contact *Telephone:* 208-282-2443. *Fax:* 208-282-4476.

MASTER'S DEGREE PROGRAM

Degree MS
Available Programs Accelerated AD/RN to Master's; Master's.
Concentrations Available Clinical nurse leader; nursing administration; nursing education. *Clinical nurse specialist programs in:* adult health. *Nurse practitioner programs in:* family health.
Study Options Full-time and part-time.
Online Degree Options Yes (online only).
Program Entrance Requirements Minimum overall college GPA of 3.0, transcript of college record, CPR certification, immunizations, interview, 3 letters of recommendation, professional liability insurance/malpractice insurance, prerequisite course work, statistics course, GRE General Test. *Application deadline:* 2/2 (fall). *Application fee:* $50.
Advanced Placement Credit given for nursing courses completed elsewhere dependent upon specific evaluations.
Degree Requirements 46 total credit hours, comprehensive exam.

POST-MASTER'S PROGRAM

Areas of Study Nursing administration; nursing education. *Clinical nurse specialist programs in:* adult health. *Nurse practitioner programs in:* family health.

Lewis-Clark State College
Division of Nursing and Health Sciences
Lewiston, Idaho

http://www.lcsc.edu/Nurdiv/
Founded in 1893
DEGREE • BSN
Nursing Program Faculty 32 (16% with doctorates).
Baccalaureate Enrollment 193 **Women** 83% **Men** 17% **Minority** 10% **International** 5% **Part-time** 21%
Distance Learning Courses Available.
Nursing Student Activities Student Nurses' Association.
Nursing Student Resources Academic advising; academic or career counseling; assistance for students with disabilities; bookstore; campus computer network; career placement assistance; computer lab; computer-assisted instruction; daycare for children of students; e-mail services; housing assistance; interactive nursing skills videos; Internet; learning resource lab; library services; nursing audiovisuals; remedial services; resume preparation assistance; skills, simulation, or other laboratory; tutoring; unpaid internships.
Library Facilities 19,920 volumes in health, 5,101 volumes in nursing; 12,058 periodical subscriptions health-care related.

BACCALAUREATE PROGRAMS

Degree BSN
Available Programs ADN to Baccalaureate; Generic Baccalaureate; LPN to Baccalaureate; LPN to RN Baccalaureate.
Site Options Coeur d'Alene, ID.
Study Options Full-time.
Program Entrance Requirements Minimum overall college GPA of 2.5, transcript of college record, CPR certification, health insurance, immunizations, minimum GPA in nursing prerequisites of 2.5, prerequisite course work. Transfer students are accepted. *Application deadline:* 2/15 (fall), 9/30 (spring). *Application fee:* $35.
Advanced Placement Credit given for nursing courses completed elsewhere dependent upon specific evaluations.
Expenses (2012–13) *Tuition, state resident:* full-time $2781; part-time $285 per credit. *Tuition, nonresident:* full-time $7738. *International tuition:* $7738 full-time. *Room and board:* $5950; room only: $3200 per academic year. *Required fees:* full-time $340.
Financial Aid 75% of baccalaureate students in nursing programs received some form of financial aid in 2011–12.
Contact Advising Center, Division of Nursing and Health Sciences, Lewis-Clark State College, 500 8th Avenue, Lewiston, ID 83501. *Telephone:* 208-792-2688. *Fax:* 208-792-2062. *E-mail:* nhs@lcsc.edu.

Northwest Nazarene University
School of Health and Science
Nampa, Idaho

http://www.nnu.edu/
Founded in 1913
DEGREES • BSN • MSN
Nursing Program Faculty 26 (27% with doctorates).
Baccalaureate Enrollment 120 **Women** 88% **Men** 12% **Minority** 12% **International** 3% **Part-time** 1%
Graduate Enrollment 17 **Women** 100%
Distance Learning Courses Available.
Nursing Student Activities Student Nurses' Association.
Nursing Student Resources Academic advising; academic or career counseling; assistance for students with disabilities; bookstore; campus computer network; career placement assistance; computer lab; computer-assisted instruction; e-mail services; housing assistance; interactive nursing skills videos; Internet; learning resource lab; library services; nursing audiovisuals; remedial services; resume preparation assistance; skills, simulation, or other laboratory; tutoring; unpaid internships.
Library Facilities 1,500 volumes in health, 950 volumes in nursing; 218 periodical subscriptions health-care related.

BACCALAUREATE PROGRAMS

Degree BSN
Available Programs Generic Baccalaureate.
Study Options Full-time.
Program Entrance Requirements Transcript of college record, CPR certification, health exam, health insurance, high school chemistry, immunizations, minimum GPA in nursing prerequisites of 2.75, professional liability insurance/malpractice insurance, prerequisite course work. Transfer students are accepted. *Application deadline:* 4/15 (fall).
Advanced Placement Credit given for nursing courses completed elsewhere dependent upon specific evaluations.
Expenses (2012–13) *Tuition:* full-time $24,790; part-time $1074 per credit. *Room and board:* $6400 per academic year. *Required fees:* full-time $660.
Financial Aid 90% of baccalaureate students in nursing programs received some form of financial aid in 2011–12.
Contact Dr. Barbara A. Lester, Chair, Department of Nursing, School of Health and Science, Northwest Nazarene University, 623 South University Boulevard, Nampa, ID 83686. *Telephone:* 208-467-8650. *Fax:* 208-467-8651. *E-mail:* nursing@nnu.edu.

GRADUATE PROGRAMS

Financial Aid 90% of graduate students in nursing programs received some form of financial aid in 2011–12.
Contact Mrs. Kathy L. Hanson, Program Administrator, School of Health and Science, Northwest Nazarene University, 623 South University Boulevard, Nampa, ID 83686. *Telephone:* 208-467-8642. *Fax:* 208-467-8651. *E-mail:* klhanson@nnu.edu.

MASTER'S DEGREE PROGRAM

Degree MSN
Available Programs Master's; RN to Master's.
Concentrations Available Nursing education.
Study Options Full-time.
Online Degree Options Yes (online only).
Program Entrance Requirements Computer literacy, minimum overall college GPA of 3.0, transcript of college record, nursing research course, prerequisite course work, resume, statistics course. *Application deadline:* 7/31 (fall). Applications may be processed on a rolling basis for some programs. *Application fee:* $50.
Degree Requirements 36 total credit hours, thesis or project.

ILLINOIS

Aurora University
School of Nursing
Aurora, Illinois

http://www.aurora.edu/
Founded in 1893
DEGREES • BSN • MSN
Nursing Program Faculty 23 (17% with doctorates).
Baccalaureate Enrollment 291 **Women** 92% **Men** 8% **Minority** 29% **Part-time** 41%
Graduate Enrollment 30 **Women** 93% **Men** 7% **Minority** 40% **Part-time** 93%
Distance Learning Courses Available.
Nursing Student Activities Sigma Theta Tau, Student Nurses' Association, nursing club.
Nursing Student Resources Academic advising; academic or career counseling; assistance for students with disabilities; bookstore; campus computer network; career placement assistance; computer lab; computer-assisted instruction; e-mail services; externships; interactive nursing skills videos; Internet; learning resource lab; library services; nursing audiovisuals; remedial services; resume preparation assistance; skills, simulation, or other laboratory; tutoring.
Library Facilities 95,869 volumes (4,908 in health, 620 in nursing); 30,124 periodical subscriptions (1,700 health-care related).

BACCALAUREATE PROGRAMS

Degree BSN
Available Programs Generic Baccalaureate; RN Baccalaureate.
Site Options Winfield, IL; Williams Bay, WI; Aurora, IL.
Study Options Full-time.
Online Degree Options Yes.
Program Entrance Requirements Minimum overall college GPA of 2.75, transcript of college record, CPR certification, written essay, health exam, health insurance, immunizations, interview, minimum GPA in nursing prerequisites of 2.75, prerequisite course work. Transfer students are accepted. *Application deadline:* 1/15 (fall). *Application fee:* $25.
Advanced Placement Credit given for nursing courses completed elsewhere dependent upon specific evaluations.
Expenses (2012–13) *Tuition:* full-time $19,900; part-time $590 per credit hour. *International tuition:* $19,900 full-time. *Room and board:* $8714 per academic year. *Required fees:* full-time $200.
Financial Aid 85% of baccalaureate students in nursing programs received some form of financial aid in 2011–12. *Gift aid (need-based):* Federal Pell, FSEOG, state, private, college/university gift aid from institutional funds. *Loans:* Federal Direct (Subsidized and Unsubsidized Stafford PLUS), Perkins, college/university, alternative loans. *Work-study:* Federal Work-Study, part-time campus jobs. *Financial aid application deadline (priority):* 1/1.
Contact Dr. Carmella M. Moran, Director and Associate Professor of Nursing, School of Nursing, Aurora University, 347 South Gladstone Avenue, Aurora, IL 60506-4892. *Telephone:* 630-844-5130. *Fax:* 630-844-7822. *E-mail:* cmoran@aurora.edu.

GRADUATE PROGRAMS

Expenses (2012–13) *Tuition:* part-time $640 per credit hour.
Financial Aid 75% of graduate students in nursing programs received some form of financial aid in 2011–12.

Contact Dr. Barbara Lockwood, Coordinator, MSN Program, School of Nursing, Aurora University, 347 South Gladstone Avenue, Aurora, IL 60506-4892. *Telephone:* 630-844-5139. *Fax:* 630-844-7822. *E-mail:* lockwood@aurora.edu.

MASTER'S DEGREE PROGRAM

Degree MSN
Available Programs Master's.
Concentrations Available Nursing administration; nursing education.
Site Options Aurora, IL.
Study Options Part-time.
Program Entrance Requirements Clinical experience, computer literacy, minimum overall college GPA of 3.0, transcript of college record, CPR certification, written essay, immunizations, interview, 3 letters of recommendation, nursing research course, physical assessment course, professional liability insurance/malpractice insurance, resume, statistics course. *Application deadline:* 7/15 (fall), 10/15 (spring). Applications may be processed on a rolling basis for some programs. *Application fee:* $25.
Degree Requirements 36 total credit hours, thesis or project.

Benedictine University
Department of Nursing
Lisle, Illinois

http://www.ben.edu/nursing
Founded in 1887
DEGREES • BSN • MSN
Nursing Program Faculty 30 (80% with doctorates).
Baccalaureate Enrollment 157 **Women** 95% **Men** 5% **Minority** 25% **International** 1%
Graduate Enrollment 322 **Women** 96% **Men** 4% **Minority** 37%
Distance Learning Courses Available.
Nursing Student Activities Nursing Honor Society, Sigma Theta Tau.
Nursing Student Resources Academic advising; academic or career counseling; assistance for students with disabilities; bookstore; campus computer network; career placement assistance; computer lab; computer-assisted instruction; e-mail services; interactive nursing skills videos; Internet; learning resource lab; library services; nursing audiovisuals; placement services for program completers; remedial services; resume preparation assistance; skills, simulation, or other laboratory; tutoring.
Library Facilities 267,649 volumes (1,350 in health, 850 in nursing); 24,106 periodical subscriptions (291 health-care related).

BACCALAUREATE PROGRAMS

Degree BSN
Available Programs Accelerated RN Baccalaureate.
Site Options Springfield, IL; Glen Ellyn, IL; River Grove, IL.
Study Options Full-time.
Program Entrance Requirements Minimum overall college GPA of 2.5, transcript of college record, 1 letter of recommendation, RN licensure. Transfer students are accepted. *Application deadline:* 7/1 (fall), 11/1 (winter), 2/1 (spring), 5/1 (summer). Applications may be processed on a rolling basis for some programs.
Advanced Placement Credit given for nursing courses completed elsewhere dependent upon specific evaluations.
Financial Aid 50% of baccalaureate students in nursing programs received some form of financial aid in 2010–11. *Gift aid (need-based):* Federal Pell, FSEOG, state, private, college/university gift aid from institutional funds. *Loans:* Federal Direct (Subsidized and Unsubsidized Stafford PLUS), Perkins, alternative loans. *Work-study:* Federal Work-Study, part-time campus jobs. *Financial aid application deadline:* Continuous.
Contact Crystal Pace, Office Assistant, Department of Nursing, Benedictine University, 5700 College Road, Kindlon Hall 249, Lisle, IL 60532-0900. *Telephone:* 630-829-1152. *Fax:* 630-829-1154. *E-mail:* cpace@ben.edu.

GRADUATE PROGRAMS

Financial Aid 90% of graduate students in nursing programs received some form of financial aid in 2010–11.
Contact Tracy Cole, Admissions Manager, Department of Nursing, Benedictine University, 851 Trafalgar Court, Suite 420, Matland, FL 32751. *Telephone:* 866-295-3104 Ext. 5411. *Fax:* 866-789-5608. *E-mail:* tcole@ben.edu.

MASTER'S DEGREE PROGRAM

Degree MSN
Available Programs Accelerated Master's; Master's.
Study Options Full-time and part-time.
Online Degree Options Yes (online only).
Program Entrance Requirements Minimum overall college GPA of 3.0, transcript of college record, written essay, 1 letter of recommendation, resume. *Application deadline:* Applications may be processed on a rolling basis for some programs.
Advanced Placement Credit given for nursing courses completed elsewhere dependent upon specific evaluations.
Degree Requirements 36 total credit hours, thesis or project.

Blessing–Rieman College of Nursing
Blessing–Rieman College of Nursing
Quincy, Illinois

http://www.brcn.edu/
DEGREES • BSN • MSN
Nursing Program Faculty 29 (21% with doctorates).
Baccalaureate Enrollment 300 **Women** 85% **Men** 15% **Minority** 5% **International** 1% **Part-time** 8%
Graduate Enrollment 8 **Women** 90% **Men** 10% **Minority** 2% **Part-time** 100%
Distance Learning Courses Available.
Nursing Student Activities Nursing Honor Society, Sigma Theta Tau, Student Nurses' Association.
Nursing Student Resources Academic advising; academic or career counseling; bookstore; campus computer network; computer lab; computer-assisted instruction; daycare for children of students; e-mail services; employment services for current students; externships; interactive nursing skills videos; Internet; learning resource lab; library services; nursing audiovisuals; paid internships; resume preparation assistance; skills, simulation, or other laboratory; tutoring.
Library Facilities 3,752 volumes in health, 3,752 volumes in nursing; 125 periodical subscriptions health-care related.

BACCALAUREATE PROGRAMS

Degree BSN
Available Programs ADN to Baccalaureate; Accelerated Baccalaureate for Second Degree; Generic Baccalaureate; RN Baccalaureate.
Study Options Full-time and part-time.
Online Degree Options Yes.
Program Entrance Requirements Minimum overall college GPA of 2.7, transcript of college record, CPR certification, health insurance, high school biology, high school chemistry, 2 years high school math, 2 years high school science, high school transcript, immunizations, minimum high school GPA of 3.0, minimum GPA in nursing prerequisites of 2.7, prerequisite course work. Transfer students are accepted. *Application deadline:* Applications may be processed on a rolling basis for some programs.
Advanced Placement Credit by examination available. Credit given for nursing courses completed elsewhere dependent upon specific evaluations.
Expenses (2012–13) *Tuition:* full-time $18,840; part-time $500 per credit hour. *Room and board:* room only: $2982 per academic year. *Required fees:* full-time $415.
Financial Aid 90% of baccalaureate students in nursing programs received some form of financial aid in 2011–12.
Contact Mrs. Heather Mutter, Admission Counselor, Blessing–Rieman College of Nursing, Broadway at 11th Street, PO Box 7005, Quincy, IL 62305-7005. *Telephone:* 217-228-5520 Ext. 6949. *Fax:* 217-223-4661. *E-mail:* admissions@brcn.edu.

GRADUATE PROGRAMS

Expenses (2012–13) *Tuition:* part-time $500 per credit hour.
Contact Mrs. Heather Mutter, Admissions Counselor, Blessing–Rieman College of Nursing, Broadway at 11th Street, PO Box 7005, Quincy, IL 62305-7005. *Telephone:* 217-228-5520 Ext. 6949. *Fax:* 217-223-4661. *E-mail:* admissions@brcn.edu.

MASTER'S DEGREE PROGRAM

Degree MSN
Available Programs Master's; RN to Master's.

Concentrations Available Nursing administration; nursing education.
Study Options Part-time.
Program Entrance Requirements Clinical experience, computer literacy, minimum overall college GPA of 3.0, transcript of college record, CPR certification, written essay, immunizations, letters of recommendation, nursing research course, physical assessment course, professional liability insurance/malpractice insurance, resume, statistics course. *Application deadline:* 4/15 (spring). Applications may be processed on a rolling basis for some programs.
Advanced Placement Credit given for nursing courses completed elsewhere dependent upon specific evaluations.
Degree Requirements 44 total credit hours, thesis or project.

Bradley University
Department of Nursing
Peoria, Illinois

http://www.bradley.edu/academic/departments/nursing/
Founded in 1897
DEGREES • BSN • BSC PN • MSN
Nursing Program Faculty 52 (13% with doctorates).
Baccalaureate Enrollment 334 **Women** 94% **Men** 6% **Minority** 18% **Part-time** 4%
Graduate Enrollment 38 **Women** 72% **Men** 28% **Minority** 2% **Part-time** 98%
Nursing Student Activities Sigma Theta Tau, Student Nurses' Association.
Nursing Student Resources Academic advising; academic or career counseling; assistance for students with disabilities; bookstore; campus computer network; career placement assistance; computer lab; computer-assisted instruction; e-mail services; employment services for current students; externships; housing assistance; Internet; learning resource lab; library services; nursing audiovisuals; placement services for program completers; remedial services; resume preparation assistance; skills, simulation, or other laboratory; tutoring.
Library Facilities 511,000 volumes (11,159 in health, 2,214 in nursing); 41,689 periodical subscriptions (210 health-care related).

BACCALAUREATE PROGRAMS

Degrees BSN; BSc PN
Available Programs ADN to Baccalaureate; Accelerated Baccalaureate for Second Degree; Generic Baccalaureate; LPN to Baccalaureate; RN Baccalaureate.
Study Options Full-time.
Program Entrance Requirements Written essay, high school biology, high school chemistry, 3 years high school math, 3 years high school science, high school transcript, immunizations, 1 letter of recommendation, minimum high school GPA of 3.25. Transfer students are accepted. *Application deadline:* Applications may be processed on a rolling basis for some programs.
Expenses (2011–12) *Tuition:* full-time $26,400; part-time $850 per hour. *Room and board:* $8200; room only: $4850 per academic year. *Required fees:* full-time $350.
Financial Aid 93% of baccalaureate students in nursing programs received some form of financial aid in 2010–11.
Contact Mr. Rodney San Jose, Director of Admissions, Department of Nursing, Bradley University, 1501 West Bradley Avenue, Peoria, IL 61625. *Telephone:* 309-677-1000. *Fax:* 309-677-2797. *E-mail:* admissions@bradley.edu.

GRADUATE PROGRAMS

Expenses (2011–12) *Tuition:* part-time $710 per hour. *Room and board:* $8200; room only: $4850 per academic year. *Required fees:* full-time $100.
Financial Aid 80% of graduate students in nursing programs received some form of financial aid in 2010–11. Research assistantships, scholarships, tuition waivers (partial), and unspecified assistantships available. *Financial aid application deadline:* 4/1.
Contact Dr. Peggy Flannigan, Graduate Coordinator, Department of Nursing, Bradley University, 1501 West Bradley Avenue, Peoria, IL 61625. *Telephone:* 309-677-2568. *Fax:* 309-677-2527. *E-mail:* pnflan@bradley.edu.

MASTER'S DEGREE PROGRAM
Degree MSN
Available Programs Master's; RN to Master's.

Concentrations Available Nurse anesthesia; nursing administration; nursing education.
Study Options Full-time and part-time.
Program Entrance Requirements Clinical experience, minimum overall college GPA of 3.0, transcript of college record, interview, 3 letters of recommendation, nursing research course, physical assessment course, resume, statistics course, GRE General Test or MAT. *Application deadline:* Applications may be processed on a rolling basis for some programs.
Advanced Placement Credit given for nursing courses completed elsewhere dependent upon specific evaluations.
Degree Requirements 36 total credit hours, thesis or project, comprehensive exam.

Chicago State University
Department of Nursing
Chicago, Illinois

http://www.csu.edu/
Founded in 1867
DEGREE • BSN
Nursing Program Faculty 23 (60% with doctorates).
Baccalaureate Enrollment 372 **Women** 90% **Men** 10% **Minority** 97% **International** 15% **Part-time** 24%
Nursing Student Activities Nursing Honor Society, Student Nurses' Association.
Nursing Student Resources Academic advising; academic or career counseling; assistance for students with disabilities; bookstore; campus computer network; computer lab; computer-assisted instruction; daycare for children of students; e-mail services; employment services for current students; externships; interactive nursing skills videos; Internet; learning resource lab; library services; nursing audiovisuals; remedial services; resume preparation assistance; skills, simulation, or other laboratory; tutoring; unpaid internships.
Library Facilities 426,691 volumes; 1,654 periodical subscriptions.

BACCALAUREATE PROGRAMS

Degree BSN
Available Programs Generic Baccalaureate; LPN to Baccalaureate; RN Baccalaureate.
Study Options Full-time.
Program Entrance Requirements Minimum overall college GPA of 2.5, transcript of college record, written essay, health exam, health insurance, 3 years high school math, 3 years high school science, high school transcript, immunizations, interview, 3 letters of recommendation, minimum GPA in nursing prerequisites of 2.5, professional liability insurance/malpractice insurance, prerequisite course work. Transfer students are accepted.
Advanced Placement Credit by examination available.
Contact *Telephone:* 773-995-3992. *Fax:* 773-821-2438.

DePaul University
Department of Nursing
Chicago, Illinois

http://www.depaul.edu
Founded in 1898
DEGREE • DNP • MS
Nursing Program Faculty 33 (39% with doctorates).
Graduate Enrollment 285 **Women** 85% **Men** 15% **Minority** 27% **International** 1% **Part-time** 11%
Nursing Student Activities Sigma Theta Tau, Student Nurses' Association.
Nursing Student Resources Academic advising; academic or career counseling; assistance for students with disabilities; bookstore; campus computer network; career placement assistance; computer lab; computer-assisted instruction; e-mail services; employment services for current students; housing assistance; interactive nursing skills videos; Internet; learning resource lab; library services; nursing audiovisuals; resume preparation assistance; skills, simulation, or other laboratory; tutoring.
Library Facilities 27,000 volumes in health, 5,800 volumes in nursing; 1,800 periodical subscriptions health-care related.

GRADUATE PROGRAMS

Financial Aid 82% of graduate students in nursing programs received some form of financial aid in 2011–12. 6 fellowships (averaging $1,500 per year) were awarded; traineeships also available.
Contact The Office of Graduate Admission, Department of Nursing, DePaul University, DePaul University, 2400 North Sheffield Avenue, Chicago, IL 60614. *Telephone:* 773-325-7315. *Fax:* 312-476-3244. *E-mail:* GradDePaul@depaul.edu.

MASTER'S DEGREE PROGRAM

Degree MS
Available Programs Master's; Master's for Non-Nursing College Graduates.
Concentrations Available Nurse anesthesia. *Nurse practitioner programs in:* adult health, family health.
Study Options Full-time and part-time.
Program Entrance Requirements Computer literacy, minimum overall college GPA of 3.0, transcript of college record, CPR certification, written essay, immunizations, interview, 2 letters of recommendation, professional liability insurance/malpractice insurance, prerequisite course work, resume, GRE (if bachelor's GPA less than 3.2). *Application deadline:* 1/15 (fall), 6/15 (winter). *Application fee:* $40.
Advanced Placement Credit given for nursing courses completed elsewhere dependent upon specific evaluations.
Degree Requirements 107 total credit hours, thesis or project.

POST-MASTER'S PROGRAM

Areas of Study Nurse anesthesia. *Nurse practitioner programs in:* adult health, family health.

DOCTORAL DEGREE PROGRAM

Degree DNP
Available Programs Doctorate; Post-Baccalaureate Doctorate.
Areas of Study Advanced practice nursing.
Program Entrance Requirements Clinical experience, minimum overall college GPA of 3.5, interview by faculty committee, interview, 2 letters of recommendation, vita. *Application deadline:* 3/15 (fall). *Application fee:* $40.
Degree Requirements 100 total credit hours.

Eastern Illinois University

Nursing Program
Charleston, Illinois

http://eiu.edu/nursing
Founded in 1895
DEGREE • BSN
Nursing Program Faculty 5 (100% with doctorates).
Baccalaureate Enrollment 55 **Women** 65% **Men** 35% **Minority** 45% **Part-time** 80%
Distance Learning Courses Available.
Nursing Student Resources Academic advising; academic or career counseling; assistance for students with disabilities; bookstore; campus computer network; computer lab; computer-assisted instruction; e-mail services; interactive nursing skills videos; Internet; library services; nursing audiovisuals; remedial services; resume preparation assistance; skills, simulation, or other laboratory; tutoring.
Library Facilities 1.1 million volumes (500 in nursing); 36,675 periodical subscriptions (50 health-care related).

BACCALAUREATE PROGRAMS

Degree BSN
Available Programs ADN to Baccalaureate.
Study Options Full-time and part-time.
Online Degree Options Yes (online only).
Program Entrance Requirements Minimum overall college GPA of 2.5, transcript of college record, CPR certification, written essay, health exam, health insurance, high school transcript, immunizations, 2 letters of recommendation, professional liability insurance/malpractice insurance, prerequisite course work, RN licensure. *Application deadline:* 11/15 (fall), 7/15 (summer). *Application fee:* $30.
Advanced Placement Credit given for nursing courses completed elsewhere dependent upon specific evaluations.
Expenses (2011–12) *Tuition, state resident:* part-time $233 per credit hour. *Tuition, nonresident:* part-time $473 per credit hour.

Financial Aid 50% of baccalaureate students in nursing programs received some form of financial aid in 2010–11.
Contact RN to BS in Nursing Program, Nursing Program, Eastern Illinois University, 600 Lincoln Avenue, 2230 McAfee, Charleston, IL 61920. *Telephone:* 217-581-7049. *Fax:* 217-581-7050.

Elmhurst College

Deicke Center for Nursing Education
Elmhurst, Illinois

Founded in 1871
DEGREES • BS • MS • MSN/MBA
Nursing Program Faculty 13 (55% with doctorates).
Baccalaureate Enrollment 195
Graduate Enrollment 34
Nursing Student Activities Sigma Theta Tau, Student Nurses' Association.
Nursing Student Resources Academic advising; academic or career counseling; assistance for students with disabilities; bookstore; campus computer network; career placement assistance; computer lab; daycare for children of students; e-mail services; employment services for current students; housing assistance; Internet; learning resource lab; library services; nursing audiovisuals; remedial services; resume preparation assistance; skills, simulation, or other laboratory; tutoring.
Library Facilities 230,055 volumes (6,000 in health); 1,859 periodical subscriptions (80 health-care related).

BACCALAUREATE PROGRAMS

Degree BS
Available Programs Generic Baccalaureate; RN Baccalaureate.
Study Options Full-time.
Program Entrance Requirements Minimum overall college GPA of 2.75, transcript of college record, CPR certification, written essay, health insurance, immunizations, 2 letters of recommendation, minimum GPA in nursing prerequisites of 2.75, prerequisite course work. Transfer students are accepted. *Application deadline:* 6/1 (fall).
Advanced Placement Credit given for nursing courses completed elsewhere dependent upon specific evaluations.
Contact *Telephone:* 630-617-3344. *Fax:* 630-617-3237.

GRADUATE PROGRAMS

Contact *Fax:* 630-617-3514.

MASTER'S DEGREE PROGRAM

Degrees MS; MSN/MBA
Available Programs Master's.
Concentrations Available Clinical nurse leader; nursing education.
Study Options Full-time.
Program Entrance Requirements Clinical experience, computer literacy, transcript of college record, CPR certification, written essay, immunizations, interview, 3 letters of recommendation, nursing research course, physical assessment course, prerequisite course work, resume, statistics course. *Application deadline:* Applications may be processed on a rolling basis for some programs.
Degree Requirements 33 total credit hours.

Governors State University

College of Health and Human Services
University Park, Illinois

http://www.govst.edu/chhs/dn/
Founded in 1969
DEGREES • BS • MS
Nursing Program Faculty 7 (85% with doctorates).
Baccalaureate Enrollment 31 **Women** 98% **Men** 2% **Minority** 92% **International** 1% **Part-time** 100%
Graduate Enrollment 72 **Women** 97% **Men** 3% **Minority** 89% **International** 6% **Part-time** 4%
Nursing Student Activities Sigma Theta Tau.
Nursing Student Resources Academic advising; assistance for students with disabilities; bookstore; campus computer network; computer lab; daycare for children of students; e-mail services; Internet; learning resource lab; library services; nursing audiovisuals; tutoring.

BACCALAUREATE PROGRAMS

Degree BS
Available Programs RN Baccalaureate.
Study Options Part-time.
Program Entrance Requirements Transcript of college record, CPR certification, health exam, health insurance, immunizations, minimum GPA in nursing prerequisites of 2.0, professional liability insurance/malpractice insurance, prerequisite course work, RN licensure. Transfer students are accepted.
Contact *Telephone:* 708-534-4053. *Fax:* 708-534-2197.

GRADUATE PROGRAMS

Contact *Telephone:* 708-534-4053. *Fax:* 708-534-2197.

MASTER'S DEGREE PROGRAM

Degree MS
Available Programs Master's.
Concentrations Available *Clinical nurse specialist programs in:* adult health.
Study Options Full-time and part-time.
Program Entrance Requirements Clinical experience, computer literacy, minimum overall college GPA of 3.0, transcript of college record, CPR certification, written essay, immunizations, nursing research course, physical assessment course, professional liability insurance/malpractice insurance, prerequisite course work, statistics course.
Degree Requirements 42 total credit hours, comprehensive exam.

POST-MASTER'S PROGRAM

Areas of Study Nursing education.

Illinois State University
Mennonite College of Nursing
Normal, Illinois

http://mcn.illinoisstate.edu/
Founded in 1857
DEGREES • BSN • MSN • PHD
Nursing Program Faculty 61 (30% with doctorates).
Baccalaureate Enrollment 283 **Women** 93% **Men** 7% **Minority** 14% **International** 1% **Part-time** 14%
Graduate Enrollment 101 **Women** 92% **Men** 8% **Minority** 4% **Part-time** 77%
Distance Learning Courses Available.
Nursing Student Activities Nursing Honor Society, Sigma Theta Tau, Student Nurses' Association.
Nursing Student Resources Academic advising; academic or career counseling; assistance for students with disabilities; bookstore; campus computer network; career placement assistance; computer lab; computer-assisted instruction; daycare for children of students; e-mail services; employment services for current students; interactive nursing skills videos; Internet; learning resource lab; library services; nursing audiovisuals; remedial services; resume preparation assistance; skills, simulation, or other laboratory; tutoring.
Library Facilities 1.6 million volumes (29,773 in health, 2,824 in nursing); 70,406 periodical subscriptions (420 health-care related).

BACCALAUREATE PROGRAMS

Degree BSN
Available Programs Accelerated Baccalaureate for Second Degree; Generic Baccalaureate; RN Baccalaureate.
Site Options Normal, IL.
Study Options Full-time and part-time.
Online Degree Options Yes.
Program Entrance Requirements Minimum overall college GPA of 2.5, transcript of college record, CPR certification, written essay, health exam, health insurance, immunizations, minimum GPA in nursing prerequisites of 2.0, prerequisite course work. Transfer students are accepted. *Application deadline:* 1/15 (fall), 6/15 (spring), 6/15 (summer). *Application fee:* $40.
Advanced Placement Credit given for nursing courses completed elsewhere dependent upon specific evaluations.
Expenses (2012–13) *Tuition, state resident:* full-time $12,460; part-time $335 per credit hour. *Tuition, nonresident:* full-time $19,354; part-time $578 per credit hour. *International tuition:* $19,354 full-time. *Room and*

board: $9880; room only: $5002 per academic year. *Required fees:* full-time $3240; part-time $76 per credit; part-time $376 per term.
Financial Aid 78% of baccalaureate students in nursing programs received some form of financial aid in 2011–12. *Gift aid (need-based):* Federal Pell, FSEOG, state, private, college/university gift aid from institutional funds, Federal Nursing. *Loans:* Federal Nursing Student Loans, Federal Direct (Subsidized and Unsubsidized Stafford PLUS), Perkins. *Work-study:* Federal Work-Study, part-time campus jobs. *Financial aid application deadline (priority):* 3/1.
Contact Ms. Nancy Jakubczyk, Academic Advisor, Mennonite College of Nursing, Illinois State University, Campus Box 5810, Normal, IL 61790-5810. *Telephone:* 309-438-7400. *Fax:* 309-438-7711. *E-mail:* njakubc@ilstu.edu.

GRADUATE PROGRAMS

Expenses (2012–13) *Tuition, state resident:* full-time $9240; part-time $308 per credit hour. *Tuition, nonresident:* full-time $19,170; part-time $639 per credit hour. *Required fees:* full-time $2268; part-time $76 per credit.
Financial Aid 83% of graduate students in nursing programs received some form of financial aid in 2011–12.
Contact Ms. Melissa K. Moody, Academic Advisor, Mennonite College of Nursing, Illinois State University, Campus Box 5810, Edwards Hall, 100 North University, Normal, IL 61790-5810. *Telephone:* 309-438-7035. *Fax:* 309-438-7711. *E-mail:* mkmoody@ilstu.edu.

MASTER'S DEGREE PROGRAM

Degree MSN
Available Programs Master's.
Concentrations Available Clinical nurse leader; nursing administration. *Nurse practitioner programs in:* family health.
Site Options Normal, IL.
Study Options Full-time and part-time.
Program Entrance Requirements Minimum overall college GPA of 3.0, transcript of college record, CPR certification, written essay, immunizations, interview, 3 letters of recommendation, nursing research course, physical assessment course, prerequisite course work, resume, statistics course. *Application deadline:* 2/1 (fall). *Application fee:* $40.
Advanced Placement Credit given for nursing courses completed elsewhere dependent upon specific evaluations.
Degree Requirements 44 total credit hours, comprehensive exam.

POST-MASTER'S PROGRAM

Areas of Study *Nurse practitioner programs in:* family health.

DOCTORAL DEGREE PROGRAM

Degree PhD
Available Programs Doctorate.
Areas of Study Aging.
Site Options Normal, IL.
Program Entrance Requirements Minimum overall college GPA of 3.0, interview by faculty committee, interview, 3 letters of recommendation, MSN or equivalent, statistics course, vita. *Application deadline:* 2/1 (fall). *Application fee:* $40.
Degree Requirements 66 total credit hours, dissertation, oral exam, written exam, residency.

Illinois Wesleyan University
School of Nursing
Bloomington, Illinois

http://www2.iwu.edu/nursing/
Founded in 1850
DEGREE • BSN
Nursing Program Faculty 23 (35% with doctorates).
Baccalaureate Enrollment 139 **Women** 92% **Men** 8% **Minority** 13%
Nursing Student Activities Nursing Honor Society, Sigma Theta Tau, Student Nurses' Association, nursing club.
Nursing Student Resources Academic advising; academic or career counseling; assistance for students with disabilities; bookstore; campus computer network; career placement assistance; computer lab; computer-assisted instruction; e-mail services; employment services for current students; externships; housing assistance; interactive nursing skills videos; Internet; learning resource lab; library services; nursing audiovisuals; paid internships; placement services for program completers; resume

preparation assistance; skills, simulation, or other laboratory; tutoring; unpaid internships.

Library Facilities 5,057 volumes in health, 3,250 volumes in nursing; 177 periodical subscriptions health-care related.

BACCALAUREATE PROGRAMS

Degree BSN
Available Programs Generic Baccalaureate.
Study Options Full-time and part-time.
Program Entrance Requirements Minimum overall college GPA of 3.0, transcript of college record, written essay, health exam, health insurance, high school biology, high school chemistry, 2 years high school math, 2 years high school science, high school transcript, immunizations, interview, minimum high school GPA of 3.0, minimum high school rank 25%, minimum GPA in nursing prerequisites of 3.0. Transfer students are accepted. *Application deadline:* Applications may be processed on a rolling basis for some programs.
Expenses (2012–13) *Tuition:* full-time $37,774; part-time $4722 per unit. *International tuition:* $37,774 full-time. *Room and board:* $8838; room only: $5584 per academic year. *Required fees:* full-time $180; part-time $90 per term.
Financial Aid 96% of baccalaureate students in nursing programs received some form of financial aid in 2011–12.
Contact Dr. Victoria N. Folse, Director and Associate Professor, School of Nursing, Illinois Wesleyan University, PO Box 2900, Bloomington, IL 61702-2900. *Telephone:* 309-556-3051. *Fax:* 309-556-3043. *E-mail:* vfolse@iwu.edu.

Lakeview College of Nursing

Lakeview College of Nursing
Danville, Illinois

http://www.lakeviewcol.edu/
Founded in 1987

DEGREE • BSN
Nursing Program Faculty 24 (2% with doctorates).
Baccalaureate Enrollment 284 **Women** 87% **Men** 13% **Minority** 20% **Part-time** 8%
Nursing Student Activities Nursing Honor Society, Sigma Theta Tau, Student Nurses' Association.
Nursing Student Resources Academic advising; academic or career counseling; assistance for students with disabilities; bookstore; campus computer network; career placement assistance; computer lab; Internet; library services; nursing audiovisuals; resume preparation assistance; skills, simulation, or other laboratory; tutoring.
Library Facilities 2,000 volumes in health; 41 periodical subscriptions health-care related.

BACCALAUREATE PROGRAMS

Degree BSN
Available Programs Accelerated RN Baccalaureate; Generic Baccalaureate; RN Baccalaureate.
Site Options Charleston, IL.
Study Options Full-time and part-time.
Program Entrance Requirements Minimum overall college GPA of 2.5, transcript of college record, CPR certification, written essay, health exam, immunizations, 2 letters of recommendation, prerequisite course work. Transfer students are accepted. *Application deadline:* 4/1 (fall), 10/1 (spring). *Application fee:* $100.
Advanced Placement Credit given for nursing courses completed elsewhere dependent upon specific evaluations.
Contact *Telephone:* 217-709-0931. *Fax:* 217-709-0953.

Lewis University

Program in Nursing
Romeoville, Illinois

http://www.lewisu.edu/academics/nursing/index.htm
Founded in 1932

DEGREES • BSN • MSN • MSN/MBA
Nursing Program Faculty 30 (40% with doctorates).
Baccalaureate Enrollment 630 **Women** 90% **Men** 10% **Minority** 31% **International** 9% **Part-time** 69%

Graduate Enrollment 147 **Women** 91% **Men** 9% **Minority** 16% **International** 2%
Distance Learning Courses Available.
Nursing Student Activities Sigma Theta Tau, Student Nurses' Association.
Nursing Student Resources Academic advising; academic or career counseling; assistance for students with disabilities; bookstore; campus computer network; career placement assistance; computer lab; computer-assisted instruction; e-mail services; employment services for current students; externships; interactive nursing skills videos; Internet; learning resource lab; library services; nursing audiovisuals; other; placement services for program completers; remedial services; resume preparation assistance; skills, simulation, or other laboratory; tutoring.
Library Facilities 154,602 volumes (3,100 in health, 2,038 in nursing); 44,925 periodical subscriptions (90 health-care related).

BACCALAUREATE PROGRAMS

Degree BSN
Available Programs Accelerated Baccalaureate for Second Degree; Accelerated RN Baccalaureate; Generic Baccalaureate.
Site Options Hickory Hills, IL; Shorewood, IL; Oak Brook, IL; Tinley Park, IL.
Study Options Full-time.
Program Entrance Requirements Minimum overall college GPA of 2.75, transcript of college record, CPR certification, health exam, health insurance, high school biology, high school chemistry, 3 years high school math, high school transcript, immunizations, minimum high school GPA of 2.75, minimum GPA in nursing prerequisites of 2.75, prerequisite course work. Transfer students are accepted.
Advanced Placement Credit given for nursing courses completed elsewhere dependent upon specific evaluations.
Contact *Telephone:* 815-836-5245. *Fax:* 815-838-8306.

GRADUATE PROGRAMS

Contact *Telephone:* 815-836-5878 Ext. 815. *Fax:* 815-836-5806.

MASTER'S DEGREE PROGRAM
Degrees MSN; MSN/MBA
Available Programs Accelerated Master's; Accelerated Master's for Nurses with Non-Nursing Degrees; Accelerated RN to Master's; RN to Master's.
Concentrations Available Nurse case management; nursing administration; nursing education. *Nurse practitioner programs in:* adult health.
Site Options Hickory Hills, IL; Shorewood, IL; Oak Brook, IL; Tinley Park, IL.
Study Options Full-time and part-time.
Online Degree Options Yes (online only).
Program Entrance Requirements Clinical experience, computer literacy, minimum overall college GPA of 3.0, transcript of college record, CPR certification, immunizations, interview, 2 letters of recommendation, nursing research course, physical assessment course, professional liability insurance/malpractice insurance, prerequisite course work, resume, statistics course.
Advanced Placement Credit given for nursing courses completed elsewhere dependent upon specific evaluations.
Degree Requirements 45 total credit hours, thesis or project.

POST-MASTER'S PROGRAM
Areas of Study Nursing administration; nursing education. *Nurse practitioner programs in:* adult health.

CONTINUING EDUCATION PROGRAM
Contact *Telephone:* 815-836-5889. *Fax:* 815-838-8306.

Loyola University Chicago

Marcella Niehoff School of Nursing
Maywood, Illinois

http://www.luc.edu/nursing/
Founded in 1870

DEGREES • BSN • DNP • MSN • MSN/MBA • PHD
Nursing Program Faculty 48 (82% with doctorates).
Baccalaureate Enrollment 957 **Women** 89% **Men** 11% **Minority** 30%
Graduate Enrollment 370 **Women** 92.7% **Men** 7.3% **Minority** 27.3% **Part-time** 82.9%

Distance Learning Courses Available.
Nursing Student Activities Nursing Honor Society, Sigma Theta Tau, Student Nurses' Association.
Nursing Student Resources Academic advising; academic or career counseling; assistance for students with disabilities; bookstore; campus computer network; computer lab; computer-assisted instruction; e-mail services; interactive nursing skills videos; Internet; learning resource lab; library services; nursing audiovisuals; remedial services; resume preparation assistance; skills, simulation, or other laboratory; tutoring.
Library Facilities 1.4 million volumes (51,674 in health, 4,966 in nursing); 52,370 periodical subscriptions (2,630 health-care related).

BACCALAUREATE PROGRAMS

Degree BSN
Available Programs Accelerated Baccalaureate for Second Degree; Generic Baccalaureate; RN Baccalaureate.
Site Options Maywood, IL; Chicago, IL.
Study Options Full-time.
Program Entrance Requirements Transcript of college record, CPR certification, written essay, health exam, health insurance, high school biology, high school chemistry, 2 years high school math, high school transcript, immunizations, 2 letters of recommendation, minimum high school GPA of 3.0, minimum high school rank 25%, prerequisite course work. *Application deadline:* 3/1 (fall). Applications may be processed on a rolling basis for some programs.
Expenses (2012–13) *Tuition:* full-time $34,570; part-time $750 per credit hour. *Room and board:* $12,010; room only: $7820 per academic year. *Required fees:* full-time $1130; part-time $150 per term.
Financial Aid *Gift aid (need-based):* Federal Pell, FSEOG, state, private, college/university gift aid from institutional funds. *Loans:* Federal Nursing Student Loans, Federal Direct (Subsidized and Unsubsidized Stafford PLUS), Perkins. *Work-study:* Federal Work-Study. *Financial aid application deadline:* Continuous.
Contact Mr. Mike Summers, Director, Undergraduate Student Affairs, Marcella Niehoff School of Nursing, Loyola University Chicago, 1032 West Sheridan Road, GC 360, Chicago, IL 60660. *Telephone:* 773-508-3263. *Fax:* 773-508-3241. *E-mail:* msummers@luc.edu.

GRADUATE PROGRAMS

Expenses (2012–13) *Tuition:* part-time $945 per credit hour.
Financial Aid 1 fellowship, 4 research assistantships, 1 teaching assistantship were awarded; career-related internships or fieldwork, Federal Work-Study, institutionally sponsored loans, traineeships, and unspecified assistantships also available.
Contact Ms. Amy Weatherford, Enrollment Advisor, Marcella Niehoff School of Nursing, Loyola University Chicago, 2160 South 1st Avenue, 125-4524, Maywood, IL 60153. *Telephone:* 708-216-3751. *Fax:* 708-216-9555. *E-mail:* aweatherford@luc.edu.

MASTER'S DEGREE PROGRAM

Degrees MSN; MSN/MBA
Available Programs Master's; RN to Master's.
Concentrations Available Nursing administration; nursing informatics. *Clinical nurse specialist programs in:* acute care, adult health, critical care, oncology. *Nurse practitioner programs in:* acute care, adult health, family health, primary care, women's health.
Site Options Maywood, IL; Chicago, IL.
Study Options Full-time and part-time.
Online Degree Options Yes (online only).
Program Entrance Requirements Clinical experience, minimum overall college GPA of 3.0, transcript of college record, CPR certification, written essay, immunizations, 3 letters of recommendation, physical assessment course, professional liability insurance/malpractice insurance, resume, statistics course. *Application deadline:* 7/1 (fall), 11/15 (spring), 3/15 (summer). Applications may be processed on a rolling basis for some programs.
Advanced Placement Credit given for nursing courses completed elsewhere dependent upon specific evaluations.
Degree Requirements 48 total credit hours, comprehensive exam.

POST-MASTER'S PROGRAM

Areas of Study Nursing administration; nursing informatics. *Clinical nurse specialist programs in:* acute care, adult health, critical care, oncology. *Nurse practitioner programs in:* acute care, adult health, family health, primary care, women's health.

DOCTORAL DEGREE PROGRAM

Degree DNP
Available Programs Doctorate, Post-Baccalaureate Doctorate.

Areas of Study Advanced practice nursing.
Program Entrance Requirements Minimum overall college GPA of 3.0, clinical experience, interview, interview by faculty committee, 3 letters of recommendation, MSN or equivalent, vita. *Application deadline:* 7/15 *(fall). Applications may be processed on a rolling basis for some programs.
Degree Requirements 39 total credit hours.

DOCTORAL DEGREE PROGRAM

Degree PhD
Available Programs Doctorate; Post-Baccalaureate Doctorate.
Areas of Study Nursing research, nursing science.
Site Options Maywood, IL; Chicago, IL.
Program Entrance Requirements Minimum overall college GPA of 3.0, interview by faculty committee, interview, 3 letters of recommendation, MSN or equivalent, statistics course, vita, writing sample, GRE General Test. *Application deadline:* 7/1 (fall). Applications may be processed on a rolling basis for some programs.
Degree Requirements 45 total credit hours, dissertation, oral exam, written exam.

MacMurray College
Department of Nursing
Jacksonville, Illinois

http://www.mac.edu/academics/programs/nursing.asp
Founded in 1846
DEGREE • BSN
Nursing Program Faculty 10 (20% with doctorates).
Baccalaureate Enrollment 108 **Women** 90% **Men** 10% **Minority** 8% **Part-time** 6%
Distance Learning Courses Available.
Nursing Student Activities Sigma Theta Tau, nursing club.
Nursing Student Resources Academic advising; academic or career counseling; bookstore; campus computer network; career placement assistance; computer lab; computer-assisted instruction; e-mail services; Internet; learning resource lab; library services; nursing audiovisuals; resume preparation assistance; skills, simulation, or other laboratory; tutoring.
Library Facilities 150,000 volumes (1,800 in health, 1,300 in nursing); 125 periodical subscriptions (50 health-care related).

BACCALAUREATE PROGRAMS

Degree BSN
Available Programs ADN to Baccalaureate; Generic Baccalaureate; LPN to RN Baccalaureate.
Study Options Full-time and part-time.
Program Entrance Requirements Minimum overall college GPA of 2.5, transcript of college record, CPR certification, health exam, health insurance, high school chemistry, high school transcript, immunizations, minimum high school GPA of 2.5, minimum GPA in nursing prerequisites of 2.5. Transfer students are accepted. *Application deadline:* 3/1 (fall).
Advanced Placement Credit by examination available.
Expenses (2012–13) *Tuition:* full-time $20,900; part-time $693 per credit hour. *Room and board:* $15,300 per academic year. *Required fees:* full-time $1000; part-time $50 per credit.
Financial Aid 98% of baccalaureate students in nursing programs received some form of financial aid in 2011–12.
Contact Director of Admissions, Department of Nursing, MacMurray College, 447 East College Avenue, Jacksonville, IL 62650. *Telephone:* 800-252-7485. *Fax:* 217-291-0702. *E-mail:* admissions@mac.edu.

McKendree University
Department of Nursing
Lebanon, Illinois

http://www.mckendree.edu/nursing
Founded in 1828
DEGREES • BSN • MSN
Nursing Program Faculty 21 (38% with doctorates).
Baccalaureate Enrollment 240 **Women** 92% **Men** 8% **Minority** 11% **Part-time** 83%

Graduate Enrollment 83 **Women** 94% **Men** 6% **Minority** 10% **International** 1% **Part-time** 100%
Distance Learning Courses Available.
Nursing Student Activities Nursing Honor Society.
Nursing Student Resources Academic advising; academic or career counseling; assistance for students with disabilities; bookstore; campus computer network; career placement assistance; computer lab; computer-assisted instruction; e-mail services; interactive nursing skills videos; Internet; learning resource lab; library services; nursing audiovisuals; resume preparation assistance; tutoring.
Library Facilities 110,000 volumes (4,450 in health, 2,880 in nursing); 1,231 periodical subscriptions (80 health-care related).

BACCALAUREATE PROGRAMS

Degree BSN
Available Programs ADN to Baccalaureate.
Site Options Louisville, KY; Belleville, IL; Marion, IL.
Study Options Full-time and part-time.
Online Degree Options Yes.
Program Entrance Requirements Minimum overall college GPA of 2.0, transcript of college record, CPR certification, health exam, high school transcript, immunizations, prerequisite course work, RN licensure. Transfer students are accepted. *Application deadline:* Applications may be processed on a rolling basis for some programs.
Advanced Placement Credit given for nursing courses completed elsewhere dependent upon specific evaluations.
Expenses (2012–13) *Tuition:* part-time $305 per credit hour.
Financial Aid 40% of baccalaureate students in nursing programs received some form of financial aid in 2011–12. *Gift aid (need-based):* Federal Pell, FSEOG, state, private, college/university gift aid from institutional funds. *Loans:* Federal Direct (Subsidized and Unsubsidized Stafford PLUS), Perkins. *Work-study:* Federal Work-Study, part-time campus jobs. *Financial aid application deadline (priority):* 5/31.
Contact Kim Eichelberger, Director of Nursing Admissions, Department of Nursing, McKendree University, 701 College Road, Lebanon, IL 62254. *Telephone:* 800-232-7228 Ext. 6411. *Fax:* 618-537-6259. *E-mail:* kaeichelberger@mckendree.edu.

GRADUATE PROGRAMS

Expenses (2012–13) *Tuition:* part-time $400 per credit hour.
Financial Aid 35% of graduate students in nursing programs received some form of financial aid in 2011–12.
Contact Katherine Markuson, MSN Admissions, Department of Nursing, McKendree University, 701 College Road, Lebanon, IL 62254. *Telephone:* 502-266-6696. *Fax:* 502-267-4340. *E-mail:* klmarkuson@mckendree.edu.

MASTER'S DEGREE PROGRAM

Degree MSN
Available Programs Master's; RN to Master's.
Concentrations Available Nursing administration; nursing education.
Site Options Louisville, KY; Belleville, IL; Marion, IL.
Study Options Full-time and part-time.
Online Degree Options Yes.
Program Entrance Requirements Minimum overall college GPA of 3.0, transcript of college record, CPR certification, written essay, immunizations, interview, resume. *Application deadline:* Applications may be processed on a rolling basis for some programs.
Advanced Placement Credit given for nursing courses completed elsewhere dependent upon specific evaluations.
Degree Requirements 38 total credit hours, thesis or project.

POST-MASTER'S PROGRAM

Areas of Study Nursing administration; nursing education.

Methodist College
Methodist College
Peoria, Illinois

DEGREE • BSN
Nursing Program Faculty 44 (13% with doctorates).
Baccalaureate Enrollment 522 **Women** 87% **Men** 13% **Minority** 16% **Part-time** 12%
Distance Learning Courses Available.
Nursing Student Activities Nursing Honor Society, Student Nurses' Association.

Nursing Student Resources Academic advising; academic or career counseling; assistance for students with disabilities; bookstore; campus computer network; career placement assistance; computer lab; computer-assisted instruction; daycare for children of students; e-mail services; employment services for current students; externships; housing assistance; interactive nursing skills videos; Internet; learning resource lab; library services; nursing audiovisuals; remedial services; resume preparation assistance; skills, simulation, or other laboratory; tutoring; unpaid internships.
Library Facilities 2,425 volumes in health, 1,175 volumes in nursing; 880 periodical subscriptions health-care related.

BACCALAUREATE PROGRAMS

Degree BSN
Available Programs Accelerated Baccalaureate for Second Degree; Baccalaureate for Second Degree; Generic Baccalaureate; RN Baccalaureate.
Study Options Full-time and part-time.
Online Degree Options Yes (online only).
Program Entrance Requirements Transcript of college record, CPR certification, health exam, high school transcript, immunizations, minimum high school GPA of 2.5, minimum GPA in nursing prerequisites of 3.0, professional liability insurance/malpractice insurance. Transfer students are accepted. *Application deadline:* 4/15 (fall), 9/15 (spring). *Application fee:* $35.
Advanced Placement Credit by examination available. Credit given for nursing courses completed elsewhere dependent upon specific evaluations.
Expenses (2011–12) *Tuition:* full-time $14,088; part-time $587 per credit hour. *Room and board:* $4500; room only: $4000 per academic year. *Required fees:* full-time $1130; part-time $283 per term.
Financial Aid 91% of baccalaureate students in nursing programs received some form of financial aid in 2010–11.
Contact Mary Jane Dowling, Recruitment Coordinator, Methodist College, 415 St. Mark Court, Peoria, IL 60613. *Telephone:* 309-672-5513. *Fax:* 309-671-8303. *E-mail:* mjdowling@mcon.edu.

Millikin University
School of Nursing
Decatur, Illinois

http://www.millikin.edu/Pages/default.aspx
Founded in 1901
DEGREES • BSN • MSN
Nursing Program Faculty 23 (72% with doctorates).
Baccalaureate Enrollment 255 **Women** 90% **Men** 10% **Minority** 17% **Part-time** 4%
Graduate Enrollment 63 **Women** 75% **Men** 25% **Minority** 5% **Part-time** 28%
Distance Learning Courses Available.
Nursing Student Activities Nursing Honor Society, Sigma Theta Tau, Student Nurses' Association, nursing club.
Nursing Student Resources Academic advising; academic or career counseling; assistance for students with disabilities; bookstore; campus computer network; career placement assistance; computer lab; computer-assisted instruction; e-mail services; employment services for current students; housing assistance; interactive nursing skills videos; Internet; learning resource lab; library services; nursing audiovisuals; other; placement services for program completers; remedial services; resume preparation assistance; skills, simulation, or other laboratory; tutoring; unpaid internships.
Library Facilities 218,110 volumes (10,000 in health, 6,000 in nursing); 365 periodical subscriptions (64 health-care related).

BACCALAUREATE PROGRAMS

Degree BSN
Available Programs Baccalaureate for Second Degree; Generic Baccalaureate; RN Baccalaureate.
Study Options Full-time and part-time.
Program Entrance Requirements Minimum overall college GPA of 2.5, transcript of college record, CPR certification, written essay, health exam, high school biology, high school chemistry, 2 years high school math, 2 years high school science, high school transcript, immunizations, 2 letters of recommendation, minimum high school GPA of 3.0, minimum high school rank 75%, minimum GPA in nursing prerequisites of 2.5. Transfer students are accepted. *Application deadline:* Applications may be processed on a rolling basis for some programs.

Advanced Placement Credit given for nursing courses completed elsewhere dependent upon specific evaluations.

Expenses (2012–13) *Tuition:* full-time $27,852; part-time $931 per credit hour. *International tuition:* $27,852 full-time. *Room and board:* $8857; room only: $4887 per academic year. *Required fees:* full-time $798; part-time $11 per credit.

Financial Aid 95% of baccalaureate students in nursing programs received some form of financial aid in 2011–12.

Contact Ms. Kim Wenthe, Administrative Assistant, School of Nursing, Millikin University, 1184 West Main Street, Decatur, IL 62522. *Telephone:* 217-424-6348. *Fax:* 217-420-6731. *E-mail:* kwenthe@mail.millikin.edu.

GRADUATE PROGRAMS

Expenses (2012–13) *Tuition:* part-time $700 per credit hour. *International tuition:* $700 full-time. *Room and board:* $8857; room only: $4887 per academic year.

Financial Aid 3% of graduate students in nursing programs received some form of financial aid in 2011–12.

Contact Ms. Marianne G. Taylor, Administrative Assistant II, School of Nursing, Millikin University, 1184 West Main Street, Decatur, IL 62522. *Telephone:* 800-373-7733 Ext. 5034. *Fax:* 217-424-5034. *E-mail:* mgtaylor@mail.millikin.edu.

MASTER'S DEGREE PROGRAM

Degree MSN

Available Programs Accelerated Master's for Non-Nursing College Graduates; Master's.

Concentrations Available Clinical nurse leader; nurse anesthesia; nursing education.

Study Options Full-time and part-time.

Program Entrance Requirements Clinical experience, minimum overall college GPA of 3.0, transcript of college record, CPR certification, written essay, immunizations, interview, 3 letters of recommendation, nursing research course, professional liability insurance/malpractice insurance, prerequisite course work, resume, statistics course. *Application deadline:* Applications may be processed on a rolling basis for some programs.

Advanced Placement Credit given for nursing courses completed elsewhere dependent upon specific evaluations.

Degree Requirements 37 total credit hours, thesis or project.

Northern Illinois University
School of Nursing and Health Studies
De Kalb, Illinois

http://www.nursing.niu.edu/
Founded in 1895

DEGREES • BS • MS • MSN/MPH

Nursing Program Faculty 43 (44% with doctorates).

Baccalaureate Enrollment 469 **Women** 92% **Men** 8% **Minority** 20% **Part-time** 23%

Graduate Enrollment 164 **Women** 96% **Men** 4% **Minority** 23% **Part-time** 96%

Distance Learning Courses Available.

Nursing Student Activities Nursing Honor Society, Sigma Theta Tau, Student Nurses' Association, nursing club.

Nursing Student Resources Academic advising; academic or career counseling; assistance for students with disabilities; bookstore; campus computer network; career placement assistance; computer lab; computer-assisted instruction; daycare for children of students; e-mail services; employment services for current students; externships; housing assistance; interactive nursing skills videos; Internet; learning resource lab; library services; nursing audiovisuals; paid internships; placement services for program completers; remedial services; resume preparation assistance; skills, simulation, or other laboratory; tutoring; unpaid internships.

Library Facilities 3.4 million volumes (39,869 in health, 7,600 in nursing); 43,970 periodical subscriptions (676 health-care related).

BACCALAUREATE PROGRAMS

Degree BS

Available Programs ADN to Baccalaureate; Generic Baccalaureate; RN Baccalaureate.

Site Options Rockford, IL; Palatine, IL; Aurora, IL.

Study Options Full-time and part-time.

Program Entrance Requirements Transcript of college record, CPR certification, health exam, health insurance, high school transcript, immunizations, minimum high school GPA of 3.25, minimum high school rank 50%, minimum GPA in nursing prerequisites of 2.5, professional liability insurance/malpractice insurance. Transfer students are accepted.

Advanced Placement Credit given for nursing courses completed elsewhere dependent upon specific evaluations.

Contact *Telephone:* 815-753-0665. *Fax:* 815-753-0814.

GRADUATE PROGRAMS

Contact *Telephone:* 815-753-6551. *Fax:* 815-753-0814.

MASTER'S DEGREE PROGRAM

Degrees MS; MSN/MPH

Available Programs Master's.

Concentrations Available Nursing education. *Clinical nurse specialist programs in:* adult health, community health. *Nurse practitioner programs in:* adult health, family health.

Study Options Full-time and part-time.

Program Entrance Requirements Minimum overall college GPA of 3.0, transcript of college record, CPR certification, written essay, immunizations, 2 letters of recommendation, nursing research course, physical assessment course, professional liability insurance/malpractice insurance, statistics course.

Degree Requirements 48 total credit hours.

POST-MASTER'S PROGRAM

Areas of Study Nursing education. *Nurse practitioner programs in:* family health.

North Park University
School of Nursing
Chicago, Illinois

http://www.northpark.edu/nursing/
Founded in 1891

DEGREES • BS • MS • MSN/MA • MSN/MBA • MSN/MM

Nursing Program Faculty 35 (63% with doctorates).

Baccalaureate Enrollment 278 **Women** 88.4% **Men** 11.6% **Minority** 57% **International** 4% **Part-time** 36%

Graduate Enrollment 189 **Women** 95% **Men** 5% **Minority** 76% **International** 7% **Part-time** 80%

Nursing Student Activities Sigma Theta Tau, Student Nurses' Association.

Nursing Student Resources Academic advising; academic or career counseling; assistance for students with disabilities; bookstore; campus computer network; career placement assistance; computer lab; computer-assisted instruction; e-mail services; employment services for current students; interactive nursing skills videos; Internet; learning resource lab; library services; nursing audiovisuals; remedial services; skills, simulation, or other laboratory; tutoring.

Library Facilities 260,685 volumes (3,959 in health, 1,791 in nursing); 1,178 periodical subscriptions (239 health-care related).

BACCALAUREATE PROGRAMS

Degree BS

Available Programs Generic Baccalaureate; RN Baccalaureate.

Site Options Evanston, IL; Arlington Heights, IL; Grayslake, IL.

Study Options Full-time.

Program Entrance Requirements Minimum overall college GPA of 2.75, transcript of college record, CPR certification, health exam, health insurance, immunizations, 1 letter of recommendation, minimum GPA in nursing prerequisites of 2.75, prerequisite course work. Transfer students are accepted.

Contact *Telephone:* 773-244-5516.

GRADUATE PROGRAMS

Contact *Telephone:* 773-244-5508. *Fax:* 773-279-7082.

MASTER'S DEGREE PROGRAM

Degrees MS; MSN/MA; MSN/MBA; MSN/MM

Available Programs Master's; RN to Master's.

Concentrations Available Nursing administration. *Clinical nurse specialist programs in:* community health. *Nurse practitioner programs in:* adult health, family health.
Site Options Arlington Heights, IL; Grayslake, IL.
Study Options Full-time and part-time.
Program Entrance Requirements Clinical experience, minimum overall college GPA of 3.0, transcript of college record, CPR certification, immunizations, 2 letters of recommendation, nursing research course, physical assessment course, professional liability insurance/malpractice insurance, prerequisite course work, resume, statistics course.
Degree Requirements 37 total credit hours.

POST-MASTER'S PROGRAM

Areas of Study *Nurse practitioner programs in:* adult health, family health.

Olivet Nazarene University
Division of Nursing
Bourbonnais, Illinois

http://olivet.edu/
Founded in 1907
DEGREES • BSN • MSN
Nursing Program Faculty 24 (29% with doctorates).
Baccalaureate Enrollment 382 Women 91% Men 9% Minority 24% Part-time 62%
Graduate Enrollment 290 Women 93% Men 7% Minority 53% Part-time 64%
Nursing Student Activities Sigma Theta Tau, Student Nurses' Association.
Nursing Student Resources Academic advising; academic or career counseling; assistance for students with disabilities; bookstore; campus computer network; career placement assistance; computer lab; computer-assisted instruction; e-mail services; employment services for current students; externships; housing assistance; interactive nursing skills videos; Internet; learning resource lab; library services; nursing audiovisuals; placement services for program completers; remedial services; resume preparation assistance; skills, simulation, or other laboratory; tutoring.
Library Facilities 160,039 volumes (4,249 in health, 2,067 in nursing); 925 periodical subscriptions (4,182 health-care related).

BACCALAUREATE PROGRAMS

Degree BSN.
Available Programs Accelerated Baccalaureate; Generic Baccalaureate; RN Baccalaureate.
Site Options Oak Brook, IL; Chicago, IL.
Study Options Full-time.
Program Entrance Requirements Minimum overall college GPA of 2.75, transcript of college record, CPR certification, health exam, health insurance, high school biology, high school chemistry, 2 years high school science, high school transcript, immunizations, minimum GPA in nursing prerequisites of 2.75, prerequisite course work. Transfer students are accepted. *Application deadline:* Applications may be processed on a rolling basis for some programs.
Expenses (2012–13) *Tuition:* full-time $13,375; part-time $1115 per credit hour. *Room and board:* $3200 per academic year. *Required fees:* full-time $420; part-time $420 per term.
Financial Aid 88% of baccalaureate students in nursing programs received some form of financial aid in 2011–12.
Contact Mrs. Susan Wolff, Director of Admissions, Division of Nursing, Olivet Nazarene University, One University Avenue, Bourbonnais, IL 60914-2345. *Telephone:* 815-939-5203. *Fax:* 815-935-4998. *E-mail:* swolff@olivet.edu.

GRADUATE PROGRAMS

Expenses (2012–13) *Tuition:* full-time $20,380.
Financial Aid 89% of graduate students in nursing programs received some form of financial aid in 2011–12.
Contact Dr. Patty Nielsen, Division of Nursing, Olivet Nazarene University, One University Avenue, Bourbonnais, IL 60914-2345. *Telephone:* 815-939-5062. *Fax:* 815-935-4991. *E-mail:* pnielsen@olivet.edu.

MASTER'S DEGREE PROGRAM
Degree MSN
Available Programs Master's.

Concentrations Available *Nurse practitioner programs in:* family health.
Study Options Full-time.
Program Entrance Requirements Computer literacy, minimum overall college GPA of 2.75, transcript of college record, nursing research course, statistics course. *Application deadline:* Applications may be processed on a rolling basis for some programs. *Application fee:* $50.
Degree Requirements 34 total credit hours, thesis or project.

CONTINUING EDUCATION PROGRAM

Contact Dr. Pamela Lee, Professor of Nursing, Division of Nursing, Olivet Nazarene University, One University Avenue, Bourbonnais, IL 60914. *Telephone:* 815-939-5316. *Fax:* 815-939-5383. *E-mail:* plee@olivet.edu.

Quincy University
Blessing–Rieman College of Nursing
Quincy, Illinois

http://www.quincy.edu/

See description of programs under Blessing–Rieman College of Nursing (Quincy, Illinois).

Resurrection University
Resurrection University
Oak Park, Illinois

Founded in 1982
DEGREES • BSN • MSN
Nursing Program Faculty 20 (20% with doctorates).
Baccalaureate Enrollment 237 Women 82.7% Men 17.3% Minority 64.5% Part-time 21.5%
Graduate Enrollment 20 Women 98% Men 2% Minority 52% Part-time 100%
Distance Learning Courses Available.
Nursing Student Activities Student Nurses' Association.
Nursing Student Resources Academic advising; academic or career counseling; bookstore; campus computer network; career placement assistance; computer lab; computer-assisted instruction; e-mail services; employment services for current students; externships; Internet; learning resource lab; library services; nursing audiovisuals; resume preparation assistance; skills, simulation, or other laboratory; tutoring.
Library Facilities 4,000 volumes (2,400 in health, 1,100 in nursing); 300 periodical subscriptions (300 health-care related).

BACCALAUREATE PROGRAMS

Degree BSN.
Available Programs ADN to Baccalaureate; Accelerated Baccalaureate; Accelerated Baccalaureate for Second Degree; Accelerated RN Baccalaureate; Baccalaureate for Second Degree; RN Baccalaureate.
Study Options Full-time and part-time.
Program Entrance Requirements Minimum overall college GPA of 2.75, transcript of college record, CPR certification, written essay, health exam, health insurance, immunizations, 1 letter of recommendation, minimum GPA in nursing prerequisites of 2.75, prerequisite course work. Transfer students are accepted. *Application deadline:* 2/1 (fall), 9/15 (spring), 2/1 (summer). Applications may be processed on a rolling basis for some programs. *Application fee:* $30.
Advanced Placement Credit by examination available. Credit given for nursing courses completed elsewhere dependent upon specific evaluations.
Contact *Telephone:* 708-763-6532. *Fax:* 708-763-1531.

GRADUATE PROGRAMS

Contact *Telephone:* 708-763-6532. *Fax:* 708-763-1531.

MASTER'S DEGREE PROGRAM
Degree MSN
Available Programs Accelerated Master's for Nurses with Non-Nursing Degrees; Master's; Master's for Nurses with Non-Nursing Degrees; RN to Master's.

Concentrations Available Clinical nurse leader; health-care administration; nursing administration; nursing education.
Study Options Part-time.
Program Entrance Requirements Computer literacy, minimum overall college GPA of 3.0, transcript of college record, CPR certification, written essay, immunizations, 3 letters of recommendation, resume. *Application deadline:* 7/1 (fall). Applications may be processed on a rolling basis for some programs. *Application fee:* $30.
Advanced Placement Credit given for nursing courses completed elsewhere dependent upon specific evaluations.
Degree Requirements 32 total credit hours, thesis or project.

POST-MASTER'S PROGRAM
Areas of Study Clinical nurse leader; health-care administration; nursing administration; nursing education.

Rockford College
Department of Nursing
Rockford, Illinois

http://www.rockford.edu/
Founded in 1847
DEGREE • BSN
Nursing Program Faculty 7
Baccalaureate Enrollment 101 **Women** 94% **Men** 6% **Minority** 22%
Part-time 7%
Nursing Student Activities Student Nurses' Association.
Nursing Student Resources Academic advising; academic or career counseling; assistance for students with disabilities; bookstore; campus computer network; career placement assistance; computer lab; computer-assisted instruction; e-mail services; employment services for current students; externships; housing assistance; interactive nursing skills videos; Internet; learning resource lab; library services; nursing audiovisuals; paid internships; placement services for program completers; remedial services; resume preparation assistance; skills, simulation, or other laboratory; tutoring.
Library Facilities 140,000 volumes (655 in health, 600 in nursing); 831 periodical subscriptions (55 health-care related).

BACCALAUREATE PROGRAMS
Degree BSN
Available Programs ADN to Baccalaureate; Generic Baccalaureate; RN Baccalaureate.
Study Options Full-time.
Program Entrance Requirements Minimum overall college GPA of 2.75, transcript of college record, CPR certification, health exam, health insurance, high school biology, high school chemistry, 4 years high school math, 2 years high school science, high school transcript, immunizations, minimum high school GPA of 2.75, minimum high school rank 50%, minimum GPA in nursing prerequisites of 2.75, prerequisite course work. Transfer students are accepted. *Application deadline:* 3/1 (fall), 9/1 (spring).
Advanced Placement Credit given for nursing courses completed elsewhere dependent upon specific evaluations.
Contact *Telephone:* 815-226-4050.

Rush University
College of Nursing
Chicago, Illinois

http://www.rushu.rush.edu/nursing
Founded in 1969
DEGREES • MSN • PHD
Nursing Program Faculty 90 (69% with doctorates).
Graduate Enrollment 700 **Women** 91% **Men** 9% **Minority** 16% **Part-time** 68%
Distance Learning Courses Available.
Nursing Student Activities Nursing Honor Society, Sigma Theta Tau, Student Nurses' Association.
Nursing Student Resources Academic advising; academic or career counseling; assistance for students with disabilities; bookstore; campus computer network; computer lab; computer-assisted instruction; e-mail services; employment services for current students; housing assistance; interactive nursing skills videos; Internet; learning resource lab; library services; nursing audiovisuals; remedial services; resume preparation assistance; skills, simulation, or other laboratory; tutoring; unpaid internships.
Library Facilities 120,042 volumes; 1,100 periodical subscriptions (5,228 health-care related).

GRADUATE PROGRAMS
Expenses (2011–12) *Tuition:* full-time $32,232; part-time $708 per quarter hour. *International tuition:* $32,232 full-time. *Room and board:* room only: $10,236 per academic year.
Financial Aid 88% of graduate students in nursing programs received some form of financial aid in 2010–11. Fellowships, research assistantships with partial tuition reimbursements available, teaching assistantships with partial tuition reimbursements available, Federal Work-Study, institutionally sponsored loans, scholarships, and traineeships available. Aid available to part-time students. *Financial aid application deadline:* 4/15.
Contact Dr. Lisa Rosenberg, Associate Dean for Admissions and Recruitment, College of Nursing, Rush University, 600 South Paulina Street, Armour Academic Center, Room 440, Chicago, IL 60612. *Telephone:* 312-942-7100. *Fax:* 312-942-3043. *E-mail:* rush_admissions@rush.edu.

MASTER'S DEGREE PROGRAM
Degree MSN
Available Programs Master's; Master's for Nurses with Non-Nursing Degrees.
Concentrations Available Clinical nurse leader; nurse anesthesia. *Clinical nurse specialist programs in:* adult health, community health, critical care, gerontology, pediatric, public health. *Nurse practitioner programs in:* acute care, adult health, family health, gerontology, neonatal health, pediatric, psychiatric/mental health.
Study Options Full-time and part-time.
Online Degree Options Yes.
Program Entrance Requirements Minimum overall college GPA of 3.0, transcript of college record, CPR certification, written essay, immunizations, interview, 3 letters of recommendation, resume, GRE General Test (waived if nursing GPA is greater than 3.0 or cumulative GPA is greater than 3.25). *Application deadline:* 2/1 (fall), 6/1 (winter). *Application fee:* $65.
Advanced Placement Credit given for nursing courses completed elsewhere dependent upon specific evaluations.
Degree Requirements 68 total credit hours, thesis or project.

POST-MASTER'S PROGRAM
Areas of Study *Clinical nurse specialist programs in:* adult health, community health, gerontology, pediatric, public health. *Nurse practitioner programs in:* adult health, family health, gerontology, neonatal health, pediatric, psychiatric/mental health.

DOCTORAL DEGREE PROGRAM
Degree PhD
Available Programs Doctorate; Post-Baccalaureate Doctorate.
Areas of Study Addiction/substance abuse, advanced practice nursing, aging, bio-behavioral research, biology of health and illness, clinical practice, community health, critical care, family health, gerontology, health policy, health promotion/disease prevention, health-care systems, human health and illness, illness and transition, maternity-newborn, neuro-behavior, nursing research, nursing science, oncology, urban health, women's health.
Online Degree Options Yes (online only).
Program Entrance Requirements Minimum overall college GPA of 3.0, interview by faculty committee, interview, 3 letters of recommendation, statistics course, vita, GRE General Test. *Application deadline:* 2/1 (fall). Applications may be processed on a rolling basis for some programs. *Application fee:* $65.
Degree Requirements 56 total credit hours, dissertation, residency.

POSTDOCTORAL PROGRAM
Postdoctoral Program Contact Dr. Carol Farran, PhD Program Director, College of Nursing, Rush University, 600 South Paulina Street, 1064 AR, Chicago, IL 60612. *Telephone:* 312-942-6955. *Fax:* 312-942-3043. *E-mail:* carol_j_farran@rush.edu.

CONTINUING EDUCATION PROGRAM
Contact Dr. Marilyn Wideman, Director of Faculty Practice, College of Nursing, Rush University, 600 South Paulina Street, Suite 1080, Chicago,

IL 60612-3832. *Telephone:* 312-942-7013. *Fax:* 312-942-3043. *E-mail:* marlyn_wideman@rush.edu.

Saint Anthony College of Nursing

Saint Anthony College of Nursing

Rockford, Illinois

http://www.sacn.edu/

Founded in 1915

DEGREES • BSN • MSN

Nursing Program Faculty 17 (23% with doctorates).

Baccalaureate Enrollment 178 **Women** 93% **Men** 7% **Minority** 30% **Part-time** 24%

Graduate Enrollment 25 **Women** 96% **Men** 4% **Minority** 8% **Part-time** 100%

Nursing Student Activities Nursing Honor Society, Student Nurses' Association.

Nursing Student Resources Academic advising; academic or career counseling; campus computer network; computer lab; computer-assisted instruction; e-mail services; interactive nursing skills videos; Internet; learning resource lab; library services; nursing audiovisuals; skills, simulation, or other laboratory; tutoring.

Library Facilities 1,258 volumes (1,751 in health, 1,385 in nursing); 3,136 periodical subscriptions (60 health-care related).

BACCALAUREATE PROGRAMS

Degree BSN

Available Programs Baccalaureate for Second Degree; Generic Baccalaureate; RN Baccalaureate.

Site Options Freeport, IL.

Study Options Full-time and part-time.

Program Entrance Requirements Minimum overall college GPA of 2.5, transcript of college record, CPR certification, written essay, health exam, health insurance, immunizations, interview, 3 letters of recommendation, minimum GPA in nursing prerequisites of 2.7, prerequisite course work. Transfer students are accepted. *Application deadline:* 2/15 (fall), 9/15 (spring). *Application fee:* $50.

Advanced Placement Credit by examination available. Credit given for nursing courses completed elsewhere dependent upon specific evaluations.

Contact *Telephone:* 815-227-2141. *Fax:* 815-227-2730.

GRADUATE PROGRAMS

Contact *Telephone:* 815-395-5476. *Fax:* 815-395-2275.

MASTER'S DEGREE PROGRAM

Degree MSN

Available Programs Master's.

Concentrations Available Clinical nurse leader; nursing education. *Clinical nurse specialist programs in:* adult health. *Nurse practitioner programs in:* family health.

Study Options Part-time.

Program Entrance Requirements Minimum overall college GPA of 2.7, transcript of college record, CPR certification, written essay, immunizations, interview, 3 letters of recommendation, professional liability insurance/malpractice insurance, prerequisite course work, resume, statistics course. *Application deadline:* 4/1 (fall). *Application fee:* $50.

Advanced Placement Credit given for nursing courses completed elsewhere dependent upon specific evaluations.

Degree Requirements 48 total credit hours, thesis or project.

POST-MASTER'S PROGRAM

Areas of Study Nursing education.

See display below and full description on page 502.

Saint Francis Medical Center College of Nursing
Baccalaureate Nursing Program
Peoria, Illinois

http://www.sfmccon.edu/
Founded in 1986
DEGREES • BSN • DNP • MSN
Nursing Program Faculty 52 (15% with doctorates).
Baccalaureate Enrollment 402 **Women** 89% **Men** 11% **Minority** 11% **Part-time** 27%
Graduate Enrollment 236 **Women** 94% **Men** 6% **Minority** 1% **Part-time** 93%
Distance Learning Courses Available.
Nursing Student Activities Sigma Theta Tau, Student Nurses' Association.
Nursing Student Resources Academic advising; academic or career counseling; campus computer network; computer lab; computer-assisted instruction; e-mail services; housing assistance; interactive nursing skills videos; Internet; learning resource lab; library services; nursing audiovisuals; skills, simulation, or other laboratory; tutoring.
Library Facilities 6,790 volumes (2,045 in nursing); 139 periodical subscriptions (124 health-care related).

BACCALAUREATE PROGRAMS

Degree BSN
Available Programs Generic Baccalaureate; RN Baccalaureate.
Study Options Full-time and part-time.
Program Entrance Requirements Transcript of college record, CPR certification, written essay, health exam, high school transcript, immunizations, minimum GPA in nursing prerequisites of 2.5, professional liability insurance/malpractice insurance, prerequisite course work. Transfer students are accepted. *Application deadline:* 9/15 (fall), 2/15 (spring). *Application fee:* $50.
Advanced Placement Credit given for nursing courses completed elsewhere dependent upon specific evaluations.
Expenses (2012–13) *Tuition:* full-time $15,810; part-time $510 per credit hour. *International tuition:* $15,810 full-time. *Room and board:* room only: $3000 per academic year. *Required fees:* full-time $556.
Financial Aid 89% of baccalaureate students in nursing programs received some form of financial aid in 2011–12.
Contact Ms. Janice E. Farquharson, Director of Admissions/Registrar, Baccalaureate Nursing Program, Saint Francis Medical Center College of Nursing, 511 NE Greenleaf Street, Peoria, IL 61603. *Telephone:* 309-624-8980. *Fax:* 309-624-8973. *E-mail:* janice.farquharson@osfhealthcare.org.

GRADUATE PROGRAMS

Expenses (2012–13) *Tuition:* full-time $6120; part-time $510 per credit hour. *International tuition:* $6120 full-time. *Required fees:* full-time $416.
Financial Aid 70% of graduate students in nursing programs received some form of financial aid in 2011–12.
Contact Dr. Janice F. Boundy, Associate Dean of Graduate Program, Baccalaureate Nursing Program, Saint Francis Medical Center College of Nursing, 511 NE Greenleaf Street, Peoria, IL 61603. *Telephone:* 309-655-2230. *Fax:* 309-655-3648. *E-mail:* janice.f.boundy@osfhealthcare.org.

MASTER'S DEGREE PROGRAM
Degree MSN
Available Programs Accelerated RN to Master's; Master's.
Concentrations Available Clinical nurse leader; nursing administration; nursing education. *Clinical nurse specialist programs in:* family health, medical-surgical. *Nurse practitioner programs in:* family health, neonatal health, psychiatric/mental health.
Study Options Full-time and part-time.
Online Degree Options Yes (online only).
Program Entrance Requirements Clinical experience, computer literacy, minimum overall college GPA of 2.8, transcript of college record, CPR certification, written essay, immunizations, interview, 3 letters of recommendation, nursing research course, physical assessment course, professional liability insurance/malpractice insurance, prerequisite course work, resume, statistics course. *Application deadline:* Applications may be processed on a rolling basis for some programs. *Application fee:* $50.

Advanced Placement Credit given for nursing courses completed elsewhere dependent upon specific evaluations.
Degree Requirements 45 total credit hours, thesis or project.

POST-MASTER'S PROGRAM
Areas of Study Nursing education. *Clinical nurse specialist programs in:* family health, medical-surgical.

DOCTORAL DEGREE PROGRAM
Degree DNP
Available Programs Doctorate.
Areas of Study Clinical practice.
Online Degree Options Yes (online only).
Program Entrance Requirements Clinical experience, minimum overall college GPA of 3.2, 3 letters of recommendation, scholarly papers, statistics course, vita, writing sample. *Application deadline:* Applications may be processed on a rolling basis for some programs. *Application fee:* $50.
Degree Requirements 39 total credit hours, oral exam, residency.

St. John's College
Department of Nursing
Springfield, Illinois

http://www.stjohnscollegespringfield.edu/college/Home.aspx
Founded in 1886
DEGREE • BSN
Nursing Program Faculty 15 (13% with doctorates).
Baccalaureate Enrollment 81 **Women** 93% **Men** 7% **Minority** 4% **International** 1% **Part-time** 5%
Nursing Student Activities Student Nurses' Association.
Nursing Student Resources Academic advising; computer lab; daycare for children of students; interactive nursing skills videos; Internet; library services; resume preparation assistance; skills, simulation, or other laboratory.

BACCALAUREATE PROGRAMS

Degree BSN
Available Programs Generic Baccalaureate.
Study Options Full-time and part-time.
Program Entrance Requirements Transcript of college record, CPR certification, health exam, high school transcript, immunizations, 2 letters of recommendation, minimum GPA in nursing prerequisites of 2.4, professional liability insurance/malpractice insurance, prerequisite course work. Transfer students are accepted.
Advanced Placement Credit given for nursing courses completed elsewhere dependent upon specific evaluations.
Contact *Telephone:* 217-525-5628. *Fax:* 217-757-6870.

Saint Xavier University
School of Nursing
Chicago, Illinois

http://www.sxu.edu/academics/colleges_schools/son/
Founded in 1847
DEGREES • BSN • MSN • MSN/MBA
Nursing Program Faculty 36 (53% with doctorates).
Baccalaureate Enrollment 603 **Women** 89% **Men** 11% **Minority** 36% **Part-time** 13%
Graduate Enrollment 270 **Women** 95% **Men** 5% **Minority** 30% **Part-time** 39%
Distance Learning Courses Available.
Nursing Student Activities Nursing Honor Society, Sigma Theta Tau, Student Nurses' Association.
Nursing Student Resources Academic advising; academic or career counseling; assistance for students with disabilities; bookstore; campus computer network; career placement assistance; computer lab; computer-assisted instruction; e-mail services; employment services for current students; externships; housing assistance; interactive nursing skills videos; Internet; learning resource lab; library services; nursing audiovisuals; other; placement services for program completers; remedial services; resume preparation assistance; skills, simulation, or other laboratory; tutoring; unpaid internships.

Library Facilities 179,000 volumes (4,800 in health, 3,000 in nursing); 35,000 periodical subscriptions (5,400 health-care related).

BACCALAUREATE PROGRAMS

Degree BSN
Available Programs Generic Baccalaureate; LPN to RN Baccalaureate.
Site Options Orland Park, IL; Chicago, IL.
Study Options Full-time.
Program Entrance Requirements Minimum overall college GPA of 2.75, transcript of college record, CPR certification, written essay, health exam, health insurance, high school biology, high school chemistry, high school foreign language, 3 years high school math, 4 years high school science, high school transcript, immunizations, minimum high school GPA of 2.75, minimum GPA in nursing prerequisites of 2.75, prerequisite course work. Transfer students are accepted. *Application deadline:* 5/1 (fall), 11/1 (spring). Applications may be processed on a rolling basis for some programs.
Advanced Placement Credit by examination available. Credit given for nursing courses completed elsewhere dependent upon specific evaluations.
Expenses (2012–13) *Tuition:* full-time $27,860; part-time $650 per credit hour. *International tuition:* $27,860 full-time. *Room and board:* $9490; room only: $5620 per academic year. *Required fees:* full-time $1030; part-time $470 per term.
Financial Aid 97% of baccalaureate students in nursing programs received some form of financial aid in 2011–12. *Gift aid (need-based):* Federal Pell, FSEOG, state, private, college/university gift aid from institutional funds, United Negro College Fund, Federal Nursing. *Loans:* Federal Direct (Subsidized and Unsubsidized Stafford PLUS), Perkins.*Work-study:* Federal Work-Study, part-time campus jobs.*Financial aid application deadline (priority):* 3/1.
Contact Mr. Brian Hotzfield, Director, Undergraduate Admission, School of Nursing, Saint Xavier University, 3700 West 103rd Street, Chicago, IL 60655. *Telephone:* 773-298-3050. *Fax:* 773-298-3076. *E-mail:* admission@sxu.edu.

GRADUATE PROGRAMS

Expenses (2012–13) *Tuition:* full-time $9840; part-time $820 per credit hour. *International tuition:* $9840 full-time. *Room and board:* room only: $7800 per academic year. *Required fees:* full-time $450; part-time $225 per term.
Financial Aid 74% of graduate students in nursing programs received some form of financial aid in 2011–12. Available to part-time students.
Contact Kelly Fox, Associate Director, Graduate Admission, School of Nursing, Saint Xavier University, 3700 West 103rd Street, Chicago, IL 60655. *Telephone:* 773-298-3053. *Fax:* 773-298-3951. *E-mail:* graduateadmission@sxu.edu.

MASTER'S DEGREE PROGRAM

Degrees MSN; MSN/MBA
Available Programs Master's.
Concentrations Available Clinical nurse leader; nursing administration. *Nurse practitioner programs in:* family health.
Site Options Chicago, IL.
Study Options Full-time and part-time.
Online Degree Options Yes.
Program Entrance Requirements Minimum overall college GPA of 3.0, transcript of college record, written essay, 2 letters of recommendation, prerequisite course work, GRE General Test or MAT. *Application deadline:* 4/1 (fall). Applications may be processed on a rolling basis for some programs.
Advanced Placement Credit given for nursing courses completed elsewhere dependent upon specific evaluations.
Degree Requirements 36 total credit hours, thesis or project.

POST-MASTER'S PROGRAM

Areas of Study Nursing education. *Nurse practitioner programs in:* family health.

CONTINUING EDUCATION PROGRAM

Contact Darlene O'Callaghan, Assistant Dean, Special Initiatives, School of Nursing, Saint Xavier University, 3700 West 103rd Street, Chicago, IL 60655. *Telephone:* 773-298-3742. *Fax:* 773-298-3704. *E-mail:* ocallaghan@sxu.edu.

Southern Illinois University Edwardsville

School of Nursing
Edwardsville, Illinois

http://www.siue.edu/nursing
Founded in 1957
DEGREES • BS • DNP • MS
Nursing Program Faculty 87 (38% with doctorates).
Baccalaureate Enrollment 713 Women 83% Men 17% Minority 11% International 2% Part-time 27%
Graduate Enrollment 263 Women 86% Men 14% Minority 10% International 2% Part-time 69%
Distance Learning Courses Available.
Nursing Student Activities Sigma Theta Tau, Student Nurses' Association, nursing club.
Nursing Student Resources Academic advising; academic or career counseling; assistance for students with disabilities; bookstore; campus computer network; career placement assistance; computer lab; computer-assisted instruction; daycare for children of students; e-mail services; employment services for current students; externships; housing assistance; interactive nursing skills videos; Internet; learning resource lab; library services; nursing audiovisuals; placement services for program completers; remedial services; resume preparation assistance; skills, simulation, or other laboratory; tutoring.
Library Facilities 1.4 million volumes; 26,708 periodical subscriptions.

BACCALAUREATE PROGRAMS

Degree BS
Available Programs ADN to Baccalaureate; Accelerated Baccalaureate; Generic Baccalaureate.
Site Options Carbondale, IL.
Study Options Full-time.
Program Entrance Requirements Minimum overall college GPA of 2.5, transcript of college record, minimum GPA in nursing prerequisites of 2.7, prerequisite course work. Transfer students are accepted. *Application deadline:* 3/1 (fall).
Advanced Placement Credit given for nursing courses completed elsewhere dependent upon specific evaluations.
Expenses (2012–13) *Tuition, state resident:* full-time $6948; part-time $232 per credit hour. *Tuition, nonresident:* full-time $17,370; part-time $579 per credit hour. *International tuition:* $17,370 full-time. *Room and board:* $8281; room only: $5270 per academic year. *Required fees:* full-time $3700.
Financial Aid *Gift aid (need-based):* Federal Pell, FSEOG, state, private, college/university gift aid from institutional funds, Federal Nursing. *Loans:* Federal Nursing Student Loans, Federal Direct (Subsidized and Unsubsidized Stafford PLUS), Perkins, college/university, alternative loans.*Work-study:* Federal Work-Study, part-time campus jobs.*Financial aid application deadline (priority):* 3/1.
Contact Mrs. Karen Montgomery, Coordinator, Academic Advising, School of Nursing, Southern Illinois University Edwardsville, Box 1066, Edwardsville, IL 62026-1066. *Telephone:* 618-650-3956. *Fax:* 618-650-3854. *E-mail:* kmontgo@siue.edu.

GRADUATE PROGRAMS

Expenses (2012–13) *Tuition, state resident:* full-time $4878; part-time $271 per credit hour. *Tuition, nonresident:* full-time $12,195; part-time $678 per credit hour. Missouri residents pay the in-state tuition rate of $271 per credit hour if they are taking 6 hours or less. *International tuition:* $12,195 full-time. *Room and board:* $8281; room only: $5270 per academic year. *Required fees:* full-time $1600. Nursing fees vary by graduate specialization.
Financial Aid 3 fellowships (averaging $8,370 per year), 2 research assistantships (averaging $9,927 per year), 2 teaching assistantships (averaging $9,927 per year) were awarded; institutionally sponsored loans, scholarships, and unspecified assistantships also available.
Contact Dr. Kathy Ketchum, Assistant Dean, Graduate Programs, School of Nursing, Southern Illinois University Edwardsville, Alumni Hall, Room 2107, Edwardsville, IL 62026-1066. *Telephone:* 618-650-3956. *Fax:* 618-650-3854. *E-mail:* kketchu@siue.edu.

MASTER'S DEGREE PROGRAM

Degree MS
Available Programs Master's.

Concentrations Available Health-care administration; nurse anesthesia; nursing education. *Nurse practitioner programs in:* family health.
Site Options Springfield, IL.
Study Options Full-time and part-time.
Program Entrance Requirements Clinical experience, minimum overall college GPA of 3.0, transcript of college record, written essay, interview, 3 letters of recommendation, prerequisite course work, statistics course. *Application deadline:* 3/1 (fall), 6/1 (summer).
Advanced Placement Credit given for nursing courses completed elsewhere dependent upon specific evaluations.
Degree Requirements 35 total credit hours (hours vary by specialization), thesis or project.

POST-MASTER'S PROGRAM

Areas of Study Health-care administration; nurse anesthesia; nursing education. *Nurse practitioner programs in:* family health.

DOCTORAL DEGREE PROGRAM

Degree DNP
Available Programs Doctorate.
Program Entrance Requirements Clinical experience, minimum overall college GPA of 3.0, interview by faculty committee, 3 letters of recommendation, MSN or equivalent, statistics course, vita, writing sample. *Application deadline:* 3/1 (fall).
Degree Requirements 36 total credit hours, written exam.

CONTINUING EDUCATION PROGRAM

Contact Dr. Karen Kelly, Associate Professor and Director Continuing Education, School of Nursing, Southern Illinois University Edwardsville, Box 1066, Edwardsville, IL 62026-1066. *Telephone:* 618-650-3908. *Fax:* 618-650-3854. *E-mail:* kkelly@siue.edu.

Trinity Christian College

Department of Nursing
Palos Heights, Illinois

http://tcc.trnty.edu/depts/nursing/
Founded in 1959
DEGREE • BSN
Nursing Program Faculty 8 (37% with doctorates).
Baccalaureate Enrollment 145 **Women** 94.5% **Men** 5.5% **Minority** 14% **International** 3%
Nursing Student Activities Student Nurses' Association.
Nursing Student Resources Academic advising; academic or career counseling; assistance for students with disabilities; bookstore; campus computer network; career placement assistance; computer lab; computer-assisted instruction; e-mail services; interactive nursing skills videos; Internet; learning resource lab; library services; nursing audiovisuals; resume preparation assistance; skills, simulation, or other laboratory; tutoring; unpaid internships.
Library Facilities 71,226 volumes (2,500 in health, 500 in nursing); 44,165 periodical subscriptions (100 health-care related).

BACCALAUREATE PROGRAMS

Degree BSN
Available Programs Generic Baccalaureate; RN Baccalaureate.
Study Options Full-time.
Program Entrance Requirements Minimum overall college GPA of 2.5, transcript of college record, CPR certification, health exam, health insurance, high school biology, 3 years high school math, 2 years high school science, high school transcript, immunizations, minimum high school GPA of 2.0, minimum GPA in nursing prerequisites of 2.5, prerequisite course work. Transfer students are accepted.
Advanced Placement Credit given for nursing courses completed elsewhere dependent upon specific evaluations.
Financial Aid 90% of baccalaureate students in nursing programs received some form of financial aid in 2011–12.
Contact Admissions Office, Department of Nursing, Trinity Christian College, 6601 West College Drive, Palos Heights, IL 60463. *Telephone:* 866-874-6463. *Fax:* 708-385-5665. *E-mail:* admissions@trnty.edu.

Trinity College of Nursing and Health Sciences

Trinity College of Nursing and Health Sciences
Rock Island, Illinois

http://www.trinitycollegeqc.edu/
Founded in 1994
DEGREE • BSN
Nursing Program Faculty 15 (20% with doctorates).
Baccalaureate Enrollment 76 **Women** 92% **Men** 8% **Minority** 13% **Part-time** 67%
Distance Learning Courses Available.
Nursing Student Activities Nursing Honor Society.
Nursing Student Resources Academic advising; academic or career counseling; assistance for students with disabilities; bookstore; campus computer network; career placement assistance; computer lab; computer-assisted instruction; daycare for children of students; e-mail services; interactive nursing skills videos; Internet; library services; nursing audiovisuals; placement services for program completers; remedial services; resume preparation assistance; skills, simulation, or other laboratory; tutoring.
Library Facilities 8,500 volumes (6,000 in health, 3,400 in nursing); 791 periodical subscriptions (746 health-care related).

BACCALAUREATE PROGRAMS

Degree BSN
Available Programs ADN to Baccalaureate; Accelerated Baccalaureate; Accelerated Baccalaureate for Second Degree; Generic Baccalaureate; RN Baccalaureate.
Study Options Full-time.
Program Entrance Requirements Minimum overall college GPA of 2.75, transcript of college record, prerequisite course work. Transfer students are accepted. *Application deadline:* 12/20 (fall). Applications may be processed on a rolling basis for some programs. *Application fee:* $50.
Advanced Placement Credit given for nursing courses completed elsewhere dependent upon specific evaluations.
Expenses (2011–12) *Tuition:* full-time $21,805; part-time $623 per credit hour. *Required fees:* full-time $2024; part-time $675 per term.
Financial Aid 51% of baccalaureate students in nursing programs received some form of financial aid in 2010–11.
Contact Mrs. Tracy L. Poelvoorde, Dean of Nursing and Health Sciences, Trinity College of Nursing and Health Sciences, 2122 25th Avenue, Rock Island, IL 61201. *Telephone:* 309-779-7708. *Fax:* 309-779-7798. *E-mail:* poelvoordet@ihs.org.

University of Illinois at Chicago

College of Nursing
Chicago, Illinois

http://www.uic.edu/nursing
Founded in 1946
DEGREES • BSN • MS • MS/MBA • MS/MPH • PHD
Nursing Program Faculty 200 (75% with doctorates).
Baccalaureate Enrollment 411 **Women** 84% **Men** 16% **Minority** 21% **International** 2% **Part-time** 25%
Graduate Enrollment 932 **Women** 91% **Men** 9% **Minority** 13% **International** 3% **Part-time** 62%
Distance Learning Courses Available.
Nursing Student Activities Sigma Theta Tau, Student Nurses' Association.
Nursing Student Resources Academic advising; academic or career counseling; assistance for students with disabilities; bookstore; campus computer network; computer lab; computer-assisted instruction; daycare for children of students; e-mail services; employment services for current students; externships; Internet; learning resource lab; library services; nursing audiovisuals; resume preparation assistance; skills, simulation, or other laboratory; tutoring.
Library Facilities 3.5 million volumes (500,000 in health); 65,418 periodical subscriptions (5,100 health-care related).

BACCALAUREATE PROGRAMS

Degree BSN

Available Programs ADN to Baccalaureate; Baccalaureate for Second Degree; Generic Baccalaureate; RN Baccalaureate.

Site Options Urbana, IL.

Study Options Full-time and part-time.

Online Degree Options Yes.

Program Entrance Requirements Minimum overall college GPA of 2.75, transcript of college record, written essay, immunizations, 2 letters of recommendation, minimum GPA in nursing prerequisites of 2.5, prerequisite course work. Transfer students are accepted. *Application deadline:* 1/15 (fall).

Contact Mr. Michael Behlke, Admissions Coordinator, College of Nursing, University of Illinois at Chicago, MC 802, 845 South Damen Avenue, Chicago, IL 60612. *Telephone:* 312-996-9645. *Fax:* 312-996-8066. *E-mail:* mbehlke@uic.edu.

GRADUATE PROGRAMS

Financial Aid 3 fellowships were awarded; research assistantships, teaching assistantships, career-related internships or fieldwork, Federal Work-Study, institutionally sponsored loans, scholarships, traineeships, tuition waivers (full and partial), and unspecified assistantships also available.

Contact Mr. Michael Spielman, Admissions Coordinator, College of Nursing, University of Illinois at Chicago, MC 802, 845 South Damen Avenue, Chicago, IL 60612. *Telephone:* 312-413-1550. *Fax:* 312-996-8066. *E-mail:* mspiel2@uic.edu.

MASTER'S DEGREE PROGRAM

Degrees MS; MS/MBA; MS/MPH

Available Programs Master's; Master's for Non-Nursing College Graduates; Master's for Nurses with Non-Nursing Degrees.

Concentrations Available Health-care administration; nurse-midwifery; nursing administration; nursing informatics. *Clinical nurse specialist programs in:* acute care, adult health, cardiovascular, community health, family health, gerontology, maternity-newborn, medical-surgical, occupational health, pediatric, perinatal, psychiatric/mental health, public health, school health, women's health. *Nurse practitioner programs in:* acute care, adult health, family health, gerontology, occupational health, pediatric, psychiatric/mental health, school health, women's health.

Site Options Peoria, IL; Urbana, IL; Rockford, IL.

Study Options Full-time and part-time.

Program Entrance Requirements Clinical experience, computer literacy, minimum overall college GPA of 3.0, transcript of college record, CPR certification, written essay, immunizations, interview, 3 letters of recommendation, nursing research course, physical assessment course, prerequisite course work, resume, statistics course, GRE General Test. *Application deadline:* 2/1 (fall).

Advanced Placement Credit given for nursing courses completed elsewhere dependent upon specific evaluations.

Degree Requirements Thesis or project.

POST-MASTER'S PROGRAM

Areas of Study Health-care administration; nurse-midwifery; nursing administration; nursing education; nursing informatics. *Clinical nurse specialist programs in:* acute care, adult health, cardiovascular, family health, forensic nursing, gerontology, medical-surgical, occupational health, palliative care, pediatric, psychiatric/mental health, public health, school health, women's health. *Nurse practitioner programs in:* acute care, adult health, family health, gerontology, occupational health, pediatric, psychiatric/mental health, school health, women's health.

DOCTORAL DEGREE PROGRAM

Degree PhD

Available Programs Doctorate; Post-Baccalaureate Doctorate.

Areas of Study Advanced practice nursing, aging, bio-behavioral research, clinical practice, community health, faculty preparation, family health, forensic nursing, gerontology, health policy, health-care systems, individualized study, information systems, maternity-newborn, nursing administration, nursing policy, nursing research, nursing science, women's health.

Site Options Peoria, IL; Urbana, IL; Rockford, IL.

Program Entrance Requirements Minimum overall college GPA of 3.0, interview by faculty committee, interview, 3 letters of recommendation, MSN or equivalent, statistics course, vita, writing sample, GRE General Test.

Degree Requirements 96 total credit hours, dissertation.

POSTDOCTORAL PROGRAM

Areas of Study Individualized study, information systems, nursing informatics, nursing interventions, nursing research, nursing science, vulnerable population.

Postdoctoral Program Contact Dr. Linda D. Scott, Associate Dean for Academic Affairs, College of Nursing, University of Illinois at Chicago, 845 South Damen Avenue (MS 802), Chicago, IL 60612. *Telephone:* 312-413-1505. *Fax:* 312-996-8066. *E-mail:* ldscott@uic.edu.

CONTINUING EDUCATION PROGRAM

Contact Prof. Susan M. Ohlson, Clinical Instructor, College of Nursing, University of Illinois at Chicago, 845 South Damen Avenue (MC 802), Chicago, IL 60612. *Telephone:* 312-413-2978. *E-mail:* sohlso1@uic.edu.

University of St. Francis
Leach College of Nursing
Joliet, Illinois

https://www.stfrancis.edu/academics/college-of-nursing/#.UMiqh6zbCUk

Founded in 1920

DEGREES • BSN • DNP • MSN

Nursing Program Faculty 43 (28% with doctorates).

Baccalaureate Enrollment 527 **Women** 91% **Men** 9% **Minority** 21% **International** 1% **Part-time** 27%

Graduate Enrollment 358 **Women** 91% **Men** 9% **Minority** 23% **International** 1% **Part-time** 76%

Distance Learning Courses Available.

Nursing Student Activities Sigma Theta Tau, Student Nurses' Association.

Nursing Student Resources Academic advising; academic or career counseling; assistance for students with disabilities; bookstore; campus computer network; career placement assistance; computer lab; computer-assisted instruction; e-mail services; employment services for current students; externships; housing assistance; interactive nursing skills videos; Internet; learning resource lab; library services; nursing audiovisuals; remedial services; resume preparation assistance; skills, simulation, or other laboratory; tutoring.

Library Facilities 134,800 volumes (789 in health, 661 in nursing); 15,002 periodical subscriptions (120 health-care related).

BACCALAUREATE PROGRAMS

Degree BSN

Available Programs Accelerated RN Baccalaureate; Generic Baccalaureate.

Study Options Full-time and part-time.

Online Degree Options Yes.

Program Entrance Requirements Minimum overall college GPA of 2.75, transcript of college record, health exam, high school biology, high school chemistry, 3 years high school math, 2 years high school science, high school transcript, minimum high school GPA of 2.5, minimum high school rank 50%, minimum GPA in nursing prerequisites of 2.75, prerequisite course work. Transfer students are accepted. *Application deadline:* Applications may be processed on a rolling basis for some programs.

Advanced Placement Credit by examination available. Credit given for nursing courses completed elsewhere dependent upon specific evaluations.

Expenses (2012–13) *Tuition:* full-time $26,374; part-time $795 per credit hour. *International tuition:* $26,374 full-time. *Room and board:* $8602 per academic year. *Required fees:* full-time $550.

Financial Aid 86% of baccalaureate students in nursing programs received some form of financial aid in 2011–12. *Gift aid (need-based):* Federal Pell, FSEOG, state, private, college/university gift aid from institutional funds, Federal Nursing. *Loans:* Federal Direct (Subsidized and Unsubsidized Stafford PLUS), Perkins, alternative loans. *Work-study:* Federal Work-Study, part-time campus jobs. *Financial aid application deadline (priority):* 2/15.

Contact Cynthia Cruz, Director, Undergraduate Admissions, Leach College of Nursing, University of St. Francis, 500 Wilcox Street, Joliet, IL 60435. *Telephone:* 800-735-7500. *Fax:* 815-740-5078. *E-mail:* ccruz@stfrancis.edu.

GRADUATE PROGRAMS

Expenses (2012–13) *Tuition:* part-time $679 per credit hour.

Financial Aid 65% of graduate students in nursing programs received some form of financial aid in 2011–12.
Contact Ms. Sandee Sloka, Director, Graduate/Degree Completion Admissions, Leach College of Nursing, University of St. Francis, 500 Wilcox Street, Joliet, IL 60435. *Telephone:* 800-735-7500. *Fax:* 815-740-3431. *E-mail:* ssloka@stfrancis.edu.

MASTER'S DEGREE PROGRAM
Degree MSN
Available Programs Master's; Master's for Nurses with Non-Nursing Degrees.
Concentrations Available Nursing administration; nursing education. *Nurse practitioner programs in:* family health.
Site Options Albuquerque, NM.
Study Options Part-time.
Online Degree Options Yes.
Program Entrance Requirements Clinical experience, computer literacy, minimum overall college GPA of 3.0, transcript of college record, CPR certification, written essay, immunizations, interview, 3 letters of recommendation, nursing research course, physical assessment course, professional liability insurance/malpractice insurance, prerequisite course work, resume, statistics course. *Application deadline:* Applications may be processed on a rolling basis for some programs.
Advanced Placement Credit given for nursing courses completed elsewhere dependent upon specific evaluations.
Degree Requirements 47 total credit hours, thesis or project.

POST-MASTER'S PROGRAM
Areas of Study *Nurse practitioner programs in:* family health.

DOCTORAL DEGREE PROGRAM
Degree DNP
Available Programs Doctorate.
Areas of Study Nursing education.
Online Degree Options Yes (online only).
Program Entrance Requirements Clinical experience, minimum overall college GPA of 3.0, letters of recommendation, MSN or equivalent, vita, writing sample. *Application deadline:* Applications may be processed on a rolling basis for some programs.
Degree Requirements 40 total credit hours.

Western Illinois University
School of Nursing
Macomb, Illinois

http://www.wiu.edu/nursing
Founded in 1899
DEGREE • BSN
Nursing Program Faculty 10 (30% with doctorates).
Baccalaureate Enrollment 75 Women 75% Men 25% Minority 12% International 5% Part-time 1%
Distance Learning Courses Available.
Nursing Student Activities Nursing Honor Society, Student Nurses' Association.
Nursing Student Resources Academic advising; academic or career counseling; assistance for students with disabilities; bookstore; campus computer network; career placement assistance; computer lab; computer-assisted instruction; daycare for children of students; e-mail services; housing assistance; interactive nursing skills videos; Internet; learning resource lab; library services; nursing audiovisuals; resume preparation assistance; skills, simulation, or other laboratory.
Library Facilities 998,041 volumes; 3,200 periodical subscriptions.

BACCALAUREATE PROGRAMS
Degree BSN
Available Programs Generic Baccalaureate; RN Baccalaureate.
Site Options Moline, IL.
Study Options Full-time.
Program Entrance Requirements Minimum overall college GPA of 3.0, transcript of college record, CPR certification, written essay, health exam, immunizations, 2 letters of recommendation, minimum high school GPA of 3.0, minimum GPA in nursing prerequisites of 3.0, professional liability insurance/malpractice insurance, prerequisite course work. Transfer students are accepted. *Application deadline:* 3/1 (fall).
Expenses (2012–13) *Tuition, state resident:* full-time $9082; part-time $268 per credit hour. *Tuition, nonresident:* full-time $13,622; part-time

$401 per credit hour. *Room and board:* $7786 per academic year. *Required fees:* full-time $3286; part-time $611 per term.
Financial Aid 90% of baccalaureate students in nursing programs received some form of financial aid in 2011–12. *Gift aid (need-based):* Federal Pell, FSEOG, state, private, college/university gift aid from institutional funds. *Loans:* Federal Direct (Subsidized and Unsubsidized Stafford PLUS), Perkins, college/university.*Work-study:* Federal Work-Study, part-time campus jobs.*Financial aid application deadline (priority):* 2/15.
Contact Mr. Theo E. Schultz, Academic Advisor, School of Nursing, Western Illinois University, 1 University Circle, Macomb, IL 61455. *Telephone:* 309-298-2571. *E-mail:* t-schultz@wiu.ecu.

INDIANA

Anderson University
School of Nursing
Anderson, Indiana

http://www.anderson.edu/academics/nursing
Founded in 1917
DEGREES • BSN • MSN • MSN/MBA
Nursing Program Faculty 13 (8% with doctorates).
Baccalaureate Enrollment 134 Women 94% Men 6% Minority 10%
Graduate Enrollment 50 Women 94% Men 6% Minority 28% Part-time 100%
Distance Learning Courses Available.
Nursing Student Activities Sigma Theta Tau.
Nursing Student Resources Academic advising; academic or career counseling; assistance for students with disabilities; bookstore; campus computer network; career placement assistance; computer lab; computer-assisted instruction; e-mail services; housing assistance; interactive nursing skills videos; Internet; learning resource lab; library services; nursing audiovisuals; placement services for program completers; remedial services; resume preparation assistance; skills, simulation, or other laboratory; tutoring.
Library Facilities 266,473 volumes (6,954 in health, 1,259 in nursing); 650 periodical subscriptions (818 health-care related).

BACCALAUREATE PROGRAMS
Degree BSN
Available Programs ADN to Baccalaureate; Generic Baccalaureate.
Study Options Full-time and part-time.
Program Entrance Requirements Minimum overall college GPA of 3.0, transcript of college record, CPR certification, health exam, high school biology, high school chemistry, 2 years high school math, 3 years high school science, high school transcript, immunizations, minimum high school GPA of 3.5, minimum high school rank 33%, minimum GPA in nursing prerequisites of 3.0, professional liability insurance/malpractice insurance, prerequisite course work. Transfer students are accepted. *Application deadline:* 5/31 (spring), 8/30 (summer).
Advanced Placement Credit given for nursing courses completed elsewhere dependent upon specific evaluations.
Contact Dr. Karen S. Williams, Dean, School of Nursing, School of Nursing, Anderson University, 1100 East 5th Street, Anderson, IN 46012-3495. *Telephone:* 765-641-4385. *Fax:* 765-641-3095. *E-mail:* kswilliams@anderson.edu.

GRADUATE PROGRAMS
Financial Aid 90% of graduate students in nursing programs received some form of financial aid in 2010–11.
Contact Mrs. Lynn Schmidt, Graduate Coordinator and Assistant Professor, School of Nursing, Anderson University, 1100 East 5th Street, Anderson, IN 46012-3495. *Telephone:* 765-641-4388. *Fax:* 765-641-3095. *E-mail:* lmschmidt@anderson.edu.

MASTER'S DEGREE PROGRAM
Degrees MSN; MSN/MBA
Available Programs Master's; RN to Master's.
Concentrations Available Nursing administration; nursing education.
Site Options Indianapolis, IN.
Study Options Full-time and part-time.

Program Entrance Requirements Clinical experience, minimum overall college GPA of 2.75, transcript of college record, CPR certification, written essay, immunizations, 3 letters of recommendation, professional liability insurance/malpractice insurance. *Application deadline:* Applications may be processed on a rolling basis for some programs. *Application fee:* $50.
Advanced Placement Credit given for nursing courses completed elsewhere dependent upon specific evaluations.
Degree Requirements 55 total credit hours, thesis or project.

POST-MASTER'S PROGRAM
Areas of Study Nursing administration; nursing education.

Ball State University
School of Nursing
Muncie, Indiana

http://www.bsu.edu/nursing
Founded in 1918
DEGREES • BS • DNP • MS
Nursing Program Faculty 55 (29% with doctorates).
Baccalaureate Enrollment 428 **Women** 86% **Men** 14% **Minority** 4% **International** .5% **Part-time** 6%
Graduate Enrollment 387 **Women** 92% **Men** 8% **Minority** 7% **International** 100%
Distance Learning Courses Available.
Nursing Student Activities Nursing Honor Society, Sigma Theta Tau, Student Nurses' Association.
Nursing Student Resources Academic advising; academic or career counseling; assistance for students with disabilities; bookstore; campus computer network; career placement assistance; computer lab; computer-assisted instruction; e-mail services; employment services for current students; housing assistance; interactive nursing skills videos; Internet; learning resource lab; library services; nursing audiovisuals; placement services for program completers; remedial services; resume preparation assistance; skills, simulation, or other laboratory; tutoring.
Library Facilities 1 million volumes (16,885 in health, 9,221 in nursing); 2,551 periodical subscriptions (3,713 health-care related).

BACCALAUREATE PROGRAMS
Degree BS
Available Programs Accelerated Baccalaureate for Second Degree; Baccalaureate for Second Degree; Generic Baccalaureate; LPN to Baccalaureate; RN Baccalaureate.
Study Options Full-time and part-time.
Online Degree Options Yes.
Program Entrance Requirements Minimum overall college GPA of 3.00, transcript of college record, CPR certification, health exam, immunizations, prerequisite course work. Transfer students are accepted. *Application deadline:* 8/28 (fall), 1/21 (spring).
Advanced Placement Credit given for nursing courses completed elsewhere dependent upon specific evaluations.
Contact *Telephone:* 765-285-5589. *Fax:* 765-285-2169.

GRADUATE PROGRAMS
Contact *Telephone:* 765-285-5764. *Fax:* 765-285-2169.

MASTER'S DEGREE PROGRAM
Degree MS
Available Programs Master's; RN to Master's.
Concentrations Available Nursing administration; nursing education. *Clinical nurse specialist programs in:* adult health. *Nurse practitioner programs in:* adult health, family health.
Study Options Part-time.
Online Degree Options Yes (online only).
Program Entrance Requirements Clinical experience, computer literacy, minimum overall college GPA of 2.8, transcript of college record, CPR certification, written essay, immunizations, interview, 1 letter of recommendation, nursing research course, physical assessment course, prerequisite course work, statistics course. *Application deadline:* Applications may be processed on a rolling basis for some programs. *Application fee:* $35.
Advanced Placement Credit given for nursing courses completed elsewhere dependent upon specific evaluations.

POST-MASTER'S PROGRAM
Areas of Study Nursing education. *Nurse practitioner programs in:* adult health, family health.

DOCTORAL DEGREE PROGRAM
Degree DNP
Available Programs Doctorate.
Areas of Study Advanced practice nursing.
Online Degree Options Yes (online only).
Program Entrance Requirements Clinical experience, minimum overall college GPA of 3.2, interview by faculty committee, letters of recommendation, MSN or equivalent, statistics course, writing sample. *Application deadline:* 4/5 (fall). *Application fee:* $35.
Degree Requirements 38 total credit hours, residency.

Bethel College
School of Nursing
Mishawaka, Indiana

http://www.bethelcollege.edu/
Founded in 1947
DEGREES • BSN • MSN
Nursing Program Faculty 37 (20% with doctorates).
Baccalaureate Enrollment 152 **Women** 88% **Men** 12% **Minority** 7.8% **International** 1.3% **Part-time** 34%
Graduate Enrollment 24 **Women** 96% **Men** 4% **Minority** 12.5% **Part-time** 100%
Nursing Student Activities Sigma Theta Tau, Student Nurses' Association.
Nursing Student Resources Academic advising; academic or career counseling; assistance for students with disabilities; bookstore; campus computer network; career placement assistance; computer lab; computer-assisted instruction; e-mail services; employment services for current students; housing assistance; interactive nursing skills videos; Internet; learning resource lab; library services; nursing audiovisuals; remedial services; resume preparation assistance; skills, simulation, or other laboratory; tutoring.
Library Facilities 146,059 volumes (3,000 in health, 2,050 in nursing); 2,567 periodical subscriptions (175 health-care related).

BACCALAUREATE PROGRAMS
Degree BSN
Available Programs ADN to Baccalaureate; Generic Baccalaureate; RN Baccalaureate.
Site Options Winona Lake, IN; Mishawaka, IN; St. Joseph, MI.
Study Options Full-time and part-time.
Program Entrance Requirements Minimum overall college GPA of 2.5, transcript of college record, CPR certification, written essay, health exam, health insurance, high school chemistry, high school transcript, immunizations, 1 letter of recommendation, minimum high school GPA of 2.5, minimum GPA in nursing prerequisites of 2.5, prerequisite course work. Transfer students are accepted. *Application deadline:* 8/1 (fall). Applications may be processed on a rolling basis for some programs. *Application fee:* $25.
Advanced Placement Credit by examination available. Credit given for nursing courses completed elsewhere dependent upon specific evaluations.
Expenses (2012–13) *Tuition:* full-time $23,930; part-time $600 per credit hour. *International tuition:* $23,932 full-time. *Room and board:* $3485; room only: $1700 per academic year. *Required fees:* full-time $600; part-time $300 per term.
Financial Aid 77% of baccalaureate students in nursing programs received some form of financial aid in 2011–12.
Contact Dr. Deborah R. Gillum, Dean of Nursing, School of Nursing, Bethel College, 1001 Bethel Circle, Mishawaka, IN 46545. *Telephone:* 574-807-7015. *Fax:* 574-257-2683. *E-mail:* gillumd@bethelcollege.edu.

GRADUATE PROGRAMS
Expenses (2012–13) *Tuition:* part-time $400 per credit hour.
Financial Aid 95% of graduate students in nursing programs received some form of financial aid in 2011–12.
Contact Dr. Karon Schwartz, Graduate Nursing Program Director, School of Nursing, Bethel College, 1001 Bethel Circle, Mishawaka, IN 46545. *Telephone:* 574-257-3382. *Fax:* 574-257-7616. *E-mail:* schwark@bethelcollege.edu.

MASTER'S DEGREE PROGRAM
Degree MSN
Available Programs Master's.
Concentrations Available Nursing administration; nursing education.
Site Options Mishawaka, IN.
Study Options Part-time.
Program Entrance Requirements Clinical experience, minimum overall college GPA of 3.0, transcript of college record, CPR certification, immunizations, 3 letters of recommendation, nursing research course, physical assessment course, statistics course. *Application deadline:* 8/1 (fall). Applications may be processed on a rolling basis for some programs. *Application fee:* $25.
Advanced Placement Credit given for nursing courses completed elsewhere dependent upon specific evaluations.
Degree Requirements 36 total credit hours, thesis or project.

POST-MASTER'S PROGRAM
Areas of Study Nursing administration; nursing education.

Goshen College
Department of Nursing
Goshen, Indiana

http://www.goshen.edu/
Founded in 1894
DEGREES • BSN • MSN
Nursing Program Faculty 11 (50% with doctorates).
Baccalaureate Enrollment 93 **Women** 94% **Men** 6% **Minority** 10% **International** 3%
Graduate Enrollment 39 **Women** 85% **Men** 15% **International** 3%
Nursing Student Activities Sigma Theta Tau, Student Nurses' Association.
Nursing Student Resources Academic advising; academic or career counseling; bookstore; campus computer network; career placement assistance; computer lab; e-mail services; employment services for current students; externships; library services; nursing audiovisuals; placement services for program completers; remedial services; resume preparation assistance.
Library Facilities 137,900 volumes (80 in health, 80 in nursing); 289 periodical subscriptions (68 health-care related).

BACCALAUREATE PROGRAMS
Degree BSN
Available Programs Generic Baccalaureate; RN Baccalaureate.
Site Options Elkhart, IN.
Study Options Full-time and part-time.
Program Entrance Requirements Minimum overall college GPA of 2.5, transcript of college record, CPR certification, written essay, health exam, health insurance, high school chemistry, high school foreign language, 2 years high school math, high school science, high school transcript, immunizations, 2 letters of recommendation, minimum high school GPA of 2.7, minimum high school rank 50%. Transfer students are accepted. *Application deadline:* 3/1 (spring).
Advanced Placement Credit by examination available. Credit given for nursing courses completed elsewhere dependent upon specific evaluations.
Expenses (2011–12) *Tuition:* full-time $25,700; part-time $1070 per credit hour. *International tuition:* $25,700 full-time. *Room and board:* $8650; room only: $4550 per academic year.
Financial Aid 98% of baccalaureate students in nursing programs received some form of financial aid in 2010–11.
Contact Admissions, Department of Nursing, Goshen College, 1700 South Main Street, Goshen, IN 46526. *Telephone:* 574-535-7535. *Fax:* 574-535-7609. *E-mail:* admissions@goshen.edu.

GRADUATE PROGRAMS
Expenses (2011–12) *Tuition:* part-time $550 per credit hour. *International tuition:* $550 full-time. *Room and board:* $8650; room only: $4550 per academic year.
Financial Aid 25% of graduate students in nursing programs received some form of financial aid in 2010–11.
Contact Dr. Brenda Srof, Director, Masters in Nursing, Department of Nursing, Goshen College, 1700 South Main Street, Goshen, IN 46526. *Telephone:* 574-535-7375. *Fax:* 575-535-7375. *E-mail:* brendajs@goshen.edu.

MASTER'S DEGREE PROGRAM
Degree MSN
Available Programs Master's.
Concentrations Available *Nurse practitioner programs in:* family health.
Study Options Full-time.
Program Entrance Requirements Minimum overall college GPA of 3.0, transcript of college record, CPR certification, written essay, immunizations, interview, letters of recommendation, statistics course. *Application deadline:* 3/1 (fall). *Application fee:* $50.
Degree Requirements 48 total credit hours.

Huntington University
Department of Nursing
Huntington, Indiana

http://www.huntington.edu/nursing/
Founded in 1897
DEGREE • BSN
Nursing Program Faculty 6 (17% with doctorates).
Baccalaureate Enrollment 42 **Women** 90% **Men** 10% **Minority** 15% **International** 4%
Nursing Student Activities Nursing club.
Nursing Student Resources Academic advising; academic or career counseling; assistance for students with disabilities; bookstore; campus computer network; career placement assistance; computer lab; computer-assisted instruction; daycare for children of students; e-mail services; employment services for current students; housing assistance; interactive nursing skills videos; Internet; learning resource lab; library services; nursing audiovisuals; other; remedial services; resume preparation assistance; skills, simulation, or other laboratory; tutoring; unpaid internships.
Library Facilities 165,386 volumes (1,544 in health, 100 in nursing); 48,740 periodical subscriptions (114 health-care related).

BACCALAUREATE PROGRAMS
Degree BSN
Available Programs ADN to Baccalaureate; Generic Baccalaureate; RN Baccalaureate.
Study Options Full-time.
Program Entrance Requirements Minimum overall college GPA of 2.75, transcript of college record, CPR certification, health exam, high school biology, high school chemistry, 2 years high school math, 2 years high school science, high school transcript, immunizations, interview, minimum high school GPA of 2.3, minimum high school rank 33%, minimum GPA in nursing prerequisites of 2.5, professional liability insurance/malpractice insurance, prerequisite course work. Transfer students are accepted. *Application deadline:* 3/31 (fall). *Application fee:* $20.
Expenses (2011–12) *Tuition:* full-time $22,710; part-time $680 per credit hour. *International tuition:* $22,710 full-time. *Room and board:* $7680 per academic year. *Required fees:* full-time $500.
Financial Aid 90% of baccalaureate students in nursing programs received some form of financial aid in 2010–11. *Gift aid (need-based):* Federal Pell, FSEOG, state, private, college/university gift aid from institutional funds. *Loans:* Federal Direct (Subsidized and Unsubsidized Stafford PLUS), Perkins. *Work-study:* Federal Work-Study. *Financial aid application deadline (priority):* 3/1.
Contact Dr. Margaret Winter, Director, Department of Nursing, Department of Nursing, Huntington University, 2303 College Avenue, Huntington, IN 46750. *Telephone:* 260-359-4360. *Fax:* 260-359-4133. *E-mail:* mwinter@huntington.edu.

Indiana State University
Department of Nursing
Terre Haute, Indiana

http://www.indstate.edu/nursing/
Founded in 1865
DEGREES • BS • DNP • MS
Nursing Program Faculty 68 (28% with doctorates).
Baccalaureate Enrollment 1,132 **Women** 91% **Men** 9% **Minority** 11% **International** 1% **Part-time** 21%

Graduate Enrollment 217 **Women** 92% **Men** 8% **Minority** 21% **Part-time** 92%
Distance Learning Courses Available.
Nursing Student Activities Sigma Theta Tau, Student Nurses' Association.
Nursing Student Resources Academic advising; academic or career counseling; assistance for students with disabilities; bookstore; campus computer network; career placement assistance; computer lab; computer-assisted instruction; daycare for children of students; e-mail services; employment services for current students; externships; housing assistance; interactive nursing skills videos; Internet; learning resource lab; library services; nursing audiovisuals; paid internships; placement services for program completers; remedial services; resume preparation assistance; skills, simulation, or other laboratory; tutoring; unpaid internships.
Library Facilities 51,725 volumes in health, 4,697 volumes in nursing; 3,205 periodical subscriptions health-care related.

BACCALAUREATE PROGRAMS

Degree BS
Available Programs Accelerated Baccalaureate for Second Degree; Generic Baccalaureate; LPN to Baccalaureate; RN Baccalaureate.
Study Options Full-time and part-time.
Online Degree Options Yes.
Program Entrance Requirements Minimum overall college GPA of 2.5, transcript of college record, CPR certification, health exam, high school chemistry, high school foreign language, 3 years high school math, 3 years high school science, high school transcript, immunizations, minimum high school GPA of 2.5, minimum high school rank 40%, minimum GPA in nursing prerequisites of 2.25, prerequisite course work. Transfer students are accepted. *Application deadline:* 6/1 (fall), 11/1 (spring).
Advanced Placement Credit by examination available. Credit given for nursing courses completed elsewhere dependent upon specific evaluations.
Expenses (2012–13) *Tuition, state resident:* full-time $7898. *Tuition, nonresident:* full-time $17,444. *International tuition:* $17,444 full-time. *Room and board:* $9282 per academic year.
Contact Ms. Lynn C. Foster, Director of Student Affairs, Department of Nursing, Indiana State University, College of Nursing, Health, and Human Services, 749 Chestnut Street, Terre Haute, IN 47809. *Telephone:* 800-293-4842. *Fax:* 812-237-8022. *E-mail:* lynn.foster@indstate.edu.

GRADUATE PROGRAMS

Expenses (2012–13) *Tuition, state resident:* part-time $366 per credit hour. *Tuition, nonresident:* part-time $458 per credit hour. *Required fees:* part-time $550 per term.
Financial Aid 5 research assistantships (averaging $7,500 per year) were awarded; teaching assistantships, career-related internships or fieldwork and Federal Work-Study also available.
Contact Dr. Susan Eley, Chairperson, Advanced Practice Nursing, Department of Nursing, Indiana State University, Landsbaum Center for Health Education, 1433 No. 6 1/2 Street, Terre Haute, IN 47807. *Telephone:* 812-237-7916. *Fax:* 812-237-8939. *E-mail:* susan.eley@indstate.edu.

MASTER'S DEGREE PROGRAM
Degree MS
Available Programs Master's.
Concentrations Available Nursing administration; nursing education. *Nurse practitioner programs in:* family health.
Study Options Full-time and part-time.
Online Degree Options Yes (online only).
Program Entrance Requirements Minimum overall college GPA of 3.0, transcript of college record, CPR certification, written essay, immunizations, 3 letters of recommendation, prerequisite course work. *Application deadline:* 2/1 (fall), 9/1 (spring). *Application fee:* $35.
Advanced Placement Credit given for nursing courses completed elsewhere dependent upon specific evaluations.
Degree Requirements 48 total credit hours, thesis or project.

POST-MASTER'S PROGRAM
Areas of Study Nursing education. *Nurse practitioner programs in:* family health.

DOCTORAL DEGREE PROGRAM
Degree DNP
Available Programs Doctorate.
Areas of Study Advanced practice nursing.

Online Degree Options Yes (online only).
Program Entrance Requirements Clinical experience, minimum overall college GPA of 3.0, 3 letters of recommendation, MSN or equivalent, statistics course, writing sample. *Application deadline:* Applications may be processed on a rolling basis for some programs. *Application fee:* $35.
Degree Requirements 39 total credit hours, residency.

CONTINUING EDUCATION PROGRAM
Contact Ms. Esther Acree, Department of Nursing, Indiana State University, 749 Chestnut Street, Terre Haute, IN 47809. *Telephone:* 812-237-2320. *E-mail:* esther.acree@indstate.edu.

Indiana University Bloomington
Department of Nursing–Bloomington Division
Bloomington, Indiana

Founded in 1820
DEGREE • BSN
Nursing Program Faculty 25 (3.5% with doctorates).
Baccalaureate Enrollment 187 **Women** 97% **Men** 3% **Minority** 1%
Distance Learning Courses Available.
Nursing Student Activities Nursing Honor Society, Sigma Theta Tau, Student Nurses' Association.
Nursing Student Resources Academic advising; academic or career counseling; assistance for students with disabilities; campus computer network; computer lab; computer-assisted instruction; e-mail services; employment services for current students; interactive nursing skills videos; Internet; learning resource lab; library services; nursing audiovisuals; remedial services; resume preparation assistance; skills, simulation, or other laboratory; tutoring.
Library Facilities 8.9 million volumes (8,500 in nursing); 1,000 periodical subscriptions health-care related.

BACCALAUREATE PROGRAMS

Degree BSN
Available Programs Baccalaureate for Second Degree; Generic Baccalaureate; RN Baccalaureate.
Site Options Columbus , IN; Bedford, IN; Bloomington , IN.
Study Options Full-time.
Program Entrance Requirements Minimum overall college GPA of 2.5, transcript of college record, CPR certification, written essay, health exam, health insurance, high school chemistry, 3 years high school math, high school transcript, immunizations, interview, minimum GPA in nursing prerequisites of 2.7, prerequisite course work. Transfer students are accepted. *Application deadline:* 3/15 (fall).
Advanced Placement Credit by examination available. Credit given for nursing courses completed elsewhere dependent upon specific evaluations.
Contact *Telephone:* 812-855-2592. *Fax:* 812-855-6986.

Indiana University East
School of Nursing
Richmond, Indiana

http://www.iue.edu/nursing/
Founded in 1971
DEGREE • BSN
Nursing Program Faculty 15 (7% with doctorates).
Baccalaureate Enrollment 201 **Women** 92.5% **Men** 7.5% **Minority** 5% **International** 1%
Nursing Student Activities Sigma Theta Tau, Student Nurses' Association.
Nursing Student Resources Academic advising; academic or career counseling; assistance for students with disabilities; bookstore; campus computer network; career placement assistance; computer lab; computer-assisted instruction; daycare for children of students; e-mail services; externships; interactive nursing skills videos; Internet; learning resource lab; library services; nursing audiovisuals; placement services for program completers; remedial services; resume preparation assistance; skills, simulation, or other laboratory; tutoring; unpaid internships.
Library Facilities 67,036 volumes (5,039 in health, 3,418 in nursing); 435 periodical subscriptions (70 health-care related).

BACCALAUREATE PROGRAMS

Degree BSN
Available Programs ADN to Baccalaureate; Generic Baccalaureate; RN Baccalaureate.
Study Options Full-time.
Program Entrance Requirements Minimum overall college GPA of 2.7, transcript of college record, CPR certification, high school biology, high school chemistry, 3 years high school math, 3 years high school science, high school transcript, immunizations, minimum high school GPA of 2.0, minimum high school rank 50%, minimum GPA in nursing prerequisites of 2.0, prerequisite course work. Transfer students are accepted. *Application deadline:* 3/1 (fall).
Advanced Placement Credit by examination available. Credit given for nursing courses completed elsewhere dependent upon specific evaluations.
Contact *Telephone:* 765-973-8353. *Fax:* 765-973-8220.

Indiana University Kokomo
Indiana University School of Nursing
Kokomo, Indiana

Founded in 1945
DEGREE • BSN
Nursing Program Faculty 14 (43% with doctorates).
Baccalaureate Enrollment 235 **Women** 95% **Men** 5% **Minority** 1% **International** 1% **Part-time** 32%
Nursing Student Activities Sigma Theta Tau, Student Nurses' Association.
Nursing Student Resources Academic advising; academic or career counseling; assistance for students with disabilities; bookstore; campus computer network; career placement assistance; computer lab; computer-assisted instruction; daycare for children of students; e-mail services; employment services for current students; externships; interactive nursing skills videos; Internet; learning resource lab; library services; nursing audiovisuals; paid internships; remedial services; resume preparation assistance; skills, simulation, or other laboratory; tutoring.
Library Facilities 132,424 volumes (2,881 in health, 1,513 in nursing); 1,513 periodical subscriptions (75 health-care related).

BACCALAUREATE PROGRAMS

Degree BSN
Available Programs Accelerated RN Baccalaureate; Generic Baccalaureate.
Site Options Peru, IN; Marion, IN; Logansport, IN.
Study Options Full-time.
Program Entrance Requirements Minimum overall college GPA of 2.5, transcript of college record, CPR certification, high school biology, high school chemistry, 4 years high school math, high school transcript, immunizations, minimum high school GPA of 2.0, minimum high school rank 50%, minimum GPA in nursing prerequisites of 2.7, prerequisite course work. Transfer students are accepted.
Contact *Telephone:* 765-455-9384. *Fax:* 765-455-9421.

CONTINUING EDUCATION PROGRAM

Contact *Telephone:* 765-455-9384. *Fax:* 765-455-9421.

Indiana University Northwest
School of Nursing and Health Professions
Gary, Indiana

http://www.iun.edu/~nurse
Founded in 1959
DEGREE • BSN
Nursing Program Faculty 25 (15% with doctorates).
Baccalaureate Enrollment 178 **Women** 90% **Men** 10% **Minority** 30% **International** .6% **Part-time** 6%
Nursing Student Activities Sigma Theta Tau, Student Nurses' Association.
Nursing Student Resources Academic advising; academic or career counseling; assistance for students with disabilities; bookstore; campus computer network; career placement assistance; computer lab; computer-assisted instruction; daycare for children of students; e-mail services;

externships; interactive nursing skills videos; Internet; learning resource lab; library services; nursing audiovisuals; placement services for program completers; skills, simulation, or other laboratory; tutoring.
Library Facilities 251,508 volumes (42,000 in health, 15,000 in nursing); 1,541 periodical subscriptions (200 health-care related).

BACCALAUREATE PROGRAMS

Degree BSN
Available Programs Baccalaureate for Second Degree; Generic Baccalaureate; RN Baccalaureate.
Study Options Full-time.
Program Entrance Requirements Minimum overall college GPA of 2.5, transcript of college record, CPR certification, health exam, health insurance, high school biology, high school chemistry, high school foreign language, 4 years high school science, high school transcript, immunizations, minimum high school rank 25%, minimum GPA in nursing prerequisites, prerequisite course work. Transfer students are accepted.
Advanced Placement Credit given for nursing courses completed elsewhere dependent upon specific evaluations.
Contact *Telephone:* 219-980-6611. *Fax:* 219-980-6578.

Indiana University–Purdue University Fort Wayne
Department of Nursing
Fort Wayne, Indiana

http://www.ipfw.edu/nursing
Founded in 1917
DEGREES • BS • MS
Nursing Program Faculty 53 (19% with doctorates).
Baccalaureate Enrollment 339 **Women** 90% **Men** 10% **Minority** 14% **International** 2% **Part-time** 23%
Graduate Enrollment 56 **Women** 97% **Men** 3% **Minority** 10% **Part-time** 90%
Distance Learning Courses Available.
Nursing Student Activities Sigma Theta Tau, nursing club.
Nursing Student Resources Academic advising; academic or career counseling; assistance for students with disabilities; bookstore; campus computer network; career placement assistance; computer lab; computer-assisted instruction; daycare for children of students; e-mail services; employment services for current students; housing assistance; interactive nursing skills videos; Internet; learning resource lab; library services; nursing audiovisuals; placement services for program completers; remedial services; resume preparation assistance; skills, simulation, or other laboratory; tutoring.
Library Facilities 417,208 volumes (1,100 in health, 500 in nursing); 27,566 periodical subscriptions (120 health-care related).

BACCALAUREATE PROGRAMS

Degree BS
Available Programs Generic Baccalaureate; RN Baccalaureate.
Study Options Full-time and part-time.
Program Entrance Requirements Minimum overall college GPA of 2.5, transcript of college record, CPR certification, health exam, high school transcript, immunizations, minimum GPA in nursing prerequisites, professional liability insurance/malpractice insurance, prerequisite course work. Transfer students are accepted. *Application deadline:* 5/1 (fall), 12/1 (spring).
Advanced Placement Credit by examination available. Credit given for nursing courses completed elsewhere dependent upon specific evaluations.
Expenses (2012–13) *Tuition, state resident:* part-time $255 per credit. *Tuition, nonresident:* part-time $612 per credit.
Financial Aid 60% of baccalaureate students in nursing programs received some form of financial aid in 2011–12.
Contact Ms. Joanne Bauman, Nursing Advisor, Department of Nursing, Indiana University–Purdue University Fort Wayne, 2101 East Coliseum Boulevard, Fort Wayne, IN 46805. *Telephone:* 260-481-6282. *Fax:* 260-481-6482. *E-mail:* baumanj@ipfw.edu.

GRADUATE PROGRAMS

Expenses (2012–13) *Tuition, state resident:* part-time $314 per credit. *Tuition, nonresident:* part-time $711 per credit.

Financial Aid 46% of graduate students in nursing programs received some form of financial aid in 2011–12.

Contact Dr. Deb Poling, Director of Graduate Programs, Department of Nursing, Indiana University–Purdue University Fort Wayne, 2101 East Coliseum Boulevard, Fort Wayne, IN 46805. *Telephone:* 260-481-6276. *Fax:* 260-481-6276. *E-mail:* polingd@ipfw.edu.

MASTER'S DEGREE PROGRAM

Degree MS

Available Programs Master's.

Concentrations Available Nursing administration; nursing education. *Nurse practitioner programs in:* adult health, women's health.

Study Options Part-time.

Program Entrance Requirements Computer literacy, minimum overall college GPA of 3.0, transcript of college record, CPR certification, immunizations, 3 letters of recommendation, nursing research course, physical assessment course, professional liability insurance/malpractice insurance, prerequisite course work, resume, statistics course. *Application deadline:* 6/15 (fall), 4/15 (spring), 4/1 (summer). *Application fee:* $40.

Advanced Placement Credit by examination available. Credit given for nursing courses completed elsewhere dependent upon specific evaluations.

Degree Requirements 42 total credit hours, thesis or project.

POST-MASTER'S PROGRAM

Areas of Study Nursing administration.

Indiana University–Purdue University Indianapolis

School of Nursing
Indianapolis, Indiana

http://www.nursing.iupui.edu/
Founded in 1969

DEGREES • BSN • MSN • MSN/MPH • PHD

Nursing Program Faculty 182 (37% with doctorates).

Nursing Student Activities Sigma Theta Tau, Student Nurses' Association.

Nursing Student Resources Academic advising; academic or career counseling; assistance for students with disabilities; bookstore; campus computer network; career placement assistance; computer lab; computer-assisted instruction; e-mail services; employment services for current students; externships; housing assistance; interactive nursing skills videos; Internet; learning resource lab; library services; nursing audiovisuals; other; paid internships; remedial services; resume preparation assistance; skills, simulation, or other laboratory; tutoring; unpaid internships.

Library Facilities 1.5 million volumes (318,211 in health, 8,258 in nursing); 14,673 periodical subscriptions (1,951 health-care related).

BACCALAUREATE PROGRAMS

Degree BSN

Available Programs ADN to Baccalaureate; Accelerated Baccalaureate for Second Degree; Generic Baccalaureate; RN Baccalaureate.

Site Options Columbus, IN.

Study Options Full-time and part-time.

Program Entrance Requirements Minimum overall college GPA of 2.5, transcript of college record, CPR certification, health insurance, 2 years high school math, 1 year of high school science, high school transcript, immunizations, interview, minimum GPA in nursing prerequisites of 2.7, prerequisite course work. Transfer students are accepted.

Advanced Placement Credit by examination available. Credit given for nursing courses completed elsewhere dependent upon specific evaluations.

Contact *Telephone:* 317-274-2806. *Fax:* 317-274-2996.

GRADUATE PROGRAMS

Contact *Telephone:* 317-274-2806. *Fax:* 317-274-2996.

MASTER'S DEGREE PROGRAM

Degrees MSN; MSN/MPH

Available Programs Master's; RN to Master's.

Concentrations Available Nursing administration. *Clinical nurse specialist programs in:* acute care, adult health, community health, critical care, oncology, pediatric, psychiatric/mental health. *Nurse practitioner programs in:* acute care, adult health, family health, neonatal health, pediatric, women's health.

Study Options Full-time and part-time.

Program Entrance Requirements Clinical experience, computer literacy, minimum overall college GPA of 3.0, transcript of college record, written essay, immunizations, 3 letters of recommendation, physical assessment course, resume, statistics course.

Advanced Placement Credit given for nursing courses completed elsewhere dependent upon specific evaluations.

Degree Requirements 42 total credit hours, thesis or project.

POST-MASTER'S PROGRAM

Areas of Study Nursing administration. *Clinical nurse specialist programs in:* adult health, community health, pediatric, psychiatric/mental health. *Nurse practitioner programs in:* acute care, adult health, family health, neonatal health, pediatric, women's health.

DOCTORAL DEGREE PROGRAM

Degree PhD

Available Programs Doctorate; Post-Baccalaureate Doctorate.

Areas of Study Aging, bio-behavioral research, faculty preparation, family health, health policy, health promotion/disease prevention, health-care systems, human health and illness, information systems, nursing administration, nursing education, nursing policy, nursing research, nursing science, oncology.

Program Entrance Requirements Minimum overall college GPA of 3.0, interview by faculty committee, 3 letters of recommendation, scholarly papers, statistics course, vita, GRE General Test.

Degree Requirements 90 total credit hours, dissertation, oral exam, written exam, residency.

POSTDOCTORAL PROGRAM

Areas of Study Adolescent health, cancer care, chronic illness, family health, health promotion/disease prevention, individualized study, nursing informatics, nursing research, nursing science.

Postdoctoral Program Contact*Telephone:* 317-274-2806. *Fax:* 317-274-2996.

CONTINUING EDUCATION PROGRAM

Contact *Telephone:* 317-274-7779. *Fax:* 317-274-0012.

Indiana University South Bend

College of Health Sciences
South Bend, Indiana

http://www.iusb.edu/nursing/
Founded in 1922

DEGREES • BSN • MSN

Nursing Program Faculty 24 (30% with doctorates).

Baccalaureate Enrollment 175 **Women** 84% **Men** 16% **Minority** 11% **International** 2% **Part-time** 10%

Graduate Enrollment 36 **Women** 92% **Men** 8% **Minority** 20% **International** 8% **Part-time** 100%

Distance Learning Courses Available.

Nursing Student Activities Sigma Theta Tau, Student Nurses' Association.

Nursing Student Resources Academic advising; academic or career counseling; assistance for students with disabilities; bookstore; campus computer network; career placement assistance; computer lab; computer-assisted instruction; daycare for children of students; e-mail services; employment services for current students; externships; housing assistance; interactive nursing skills videos; Internet; learning resource lab; library services; nursing audiovisuals; placement services for program completers; resume preparation assistance; skills, simulation, or other laboratory; tutoring.

Library Facilities 300,202 volumes (4,300 in health, 2,300 in nursing); 1,937 periodical subscriptions (145 health-care related).

BACCALAUREATE PROGRAMS

Degree BSN

Available Programs Accelerated Baccalaureate for Second Degree; Generic Baccalaureate; RN Baccalaureate.

Study Options Full-time and part-time.

Program Entrance Requirements Minimum overall college GPA of 2.5, transcript of college record, CPR certification, written essay, health exam, high school biology, high school chemistry, high school transcript,

immunizations, minimum high school GPA of 2.0, minimum high school rank 50%, minimum GPA in nursing prerequisites of 2.7, prerequisite course work. Transfer students are accepted. *Application deadline:* 3/1 (fall), 10/1 (spring), 2/1 (summer).
Advanced Placement Credit given for nursing courses completed elsewhere dependent upon specific evaluations.
Expenses (2012–13) *Tuition, state resident:* full-time $6250; part-time $205 per hour. *Tuition, nonresident:* full-time $16,890; part-time $563 per hour. *International tuition:* $16,890 full-time. *Room and board:* room only: $2828 per academic year. *Required fees:* full-time $1735; part-time $60 per credit.
Financial Aid 65% of baccalaureate students in nursing programs received some form of financial aid in 2011–12.
Contact Office of Student Services, College of Health Sciences, Indiana University South Bend, 1700 Mishawaka Avenue, PO Box 7111, South Bend, IN 46634-7111. *Telephone:* 574-520-4571. *Fax:* 574-520-4461. *E-mail:* nursing@iusb.edu.

GRADUATE PROGRAMS

Expenses (2012–13) *Tuition, state resident:* full-time $5913; part-time $329 per credit hour. *Tuition, nonresident:* full-time $17,244; part-time $958 per credit hour. *International tuition:* $17,244 full-time. *Room and board:* room only: $3419 per academic year. *Required fees:* full-time $235; part-time $82 per credit.
Financial Aid 30% of graduate students in nursing programs received some form of financial aid in 2011–12.
Contact Dr. Roxanne Wolfram, NP, Director of Graduate Program in Nursing, College of Health Sciences, Indiana University South Bend, 1700 Mishawaka Avenue, PO Box 7111, South Bend, IN 46634-7111. *Telephone:* 574-520-4368. *Fax:* 574-520-4461. *E-mail:* rwolfram@ iusb.edu.

MASTER'S DEGREE PROGRAM

Degree MSN
Available Programs Master's.
Concentrations Available *Nurse practitioner programs in:* family health.
Study Options Part-time.
Program Entrance Requirements Clinical experience, computer literacy, minimum overall college GPA of 3.0, transcript of college record, CPR certification, written essay, immunizations, 3 letters of recommendation, nursing research course, physical assessment course, statistics course. *Application deadline:* 4/1 (fall). *Application fee:* $40.
Advanced Placement Credit given for nursing courses completed elsewhere dependent upon specific evaluations.
Degree Requirements 42 total credit hours, thesis or project.

Indiana University Southeast
Division of Nursing
New Albany, Indiana

http://www.ius.edu/nursing/
Founded in 1941
DEGREE • BSN
Nursing Program Faculty 23 (27% with doctorates).
Baccalaureate Enrollment 162 **Women** 92% **Men** 8% **Minority** 2% **International** 2%
Distance Learning Courses Available.
Nursing Student Activities Sigma Theta Tau, Student Nurses' Association.
Nursing Student Resources Academic advising; academic or career counseling; assistance for students with disabilities; bookstore; campus computer network; career placement assistance; computer lab; computer-assisted instruction; daycare for children of students; e-mail services; externships; housing assistance; interactive nursing skills videos; Internet; learning resource lab; library services; nursing audiovisuals; paid internships; remedial services; resume preparation assistance; skills, simulation, or other laboratory; tutoring.
Library Facilities 215,429 volumes (35 in health, 15 in nursing); 962 periodical subscriptions (35 health-care related).

BACCALAUREATE PROGRAMS

Degree BSN
Available Programs Generic Baccalaureate; RN Baccalaureate.

Study Options Full-time.
Program Entrance Requirements Transcript of college record, CPR certification, immunizations, minimum GPA in nursing prerequisites of 2.5, prerequisite course work. Transfer students are accepted.
Advanced Placement Credit given for nursing courses completed elsewhere dependent upon specific evaluations.
Contact *Telephone:* 812-941-2283. *Fax:* 812-941-2687.

Indiana Wesleyan University
School of Nursing
Marion, Indiana

http://www.indwes.edu/Academics/School-of-Nursing/
Founded in 1920
DEGREES • BSN • MSN
Nursing Program Faculty 210 (21% with doctorates).
Baccalaureate Enrollment 1,581 **Women** 93% **Men** 7% **Minority** 16% **Part-time** 9%
Graduate Enrollment 427 **Women** 95% **Men** 5% **Minority** 13% **Part-time** 10%
Distance Learning Courses Available.
Nursing Student Activities Nursing Honor Society, Sigma Theta Tau, Student Nurses' Association, nursing club.
Nursing Student Resources Academic advising; academic or career counseling; assistance for students with disabilities; bookstore; campus computer network; career placement assistance; computer lab; computer-assisted instruction; e-mail services; housing assistance; interactive nursing skills videos; Internet; learning resource lab; library services; nursing audiovisuals; remedial services; resume preparation assistance; skills, simulation, or other laboratory; tutoring.
Library Facilities 248,819 volumes (7,142 in health, 5,672 in nursing); 101,452 periodical subscriptions (160 health-care related).

BACCALAUREATE PROGRAMS

Degree BSN
Available Programs Accelerated Baccalaureate for Second Degree; Generic Baccalaureate; RN Baccalaureate.
Site Options Lexington, KY; Merrillville, IN; Louisville, KY.
Study Options Full-time and part-time.
Program Entrance Requirements Minimum overall college GPA of 2.75, transcript of college record, CPR certification, written essay, health exam, health insurance, high school biology, high school chemistry, high school foreign language, 3 years high school math, 3 years high school science, high school transcript, immunizations, minimum high school GPA of 2.8, minimum GPA in nursing prerequisites of 2.75, prerequisite course work. Transfer students are accepted. *Application deadline:* 5/30 (fall), 12/1 (spring).
Advanced Placement Credit given for nursing courses completed elsewhere dependent upon specific evaluations.
Contact *Telephone:* 765-677-2268. *Fax:* 765-677-2284.

GRADUATE PROGRAMS

Contact *Telephone:* 765-677-2045. *Fax:* 765-677-2380.

MASTER'S DEGREE PROGRAM

Degree MSN
Available Programs Master's.
Concentrations Available Nursing administration; nursing education. *Nurse practitioner programs in:* family health.
Site Options Lexington, KY; Merrillville, IN; Louisville, KY.
Study Options Full-time and part-time.
Online Degree Options Yes.
Program Entrance Requirements Clinical experience, minimum overall college GPA of 3.0, transcript of college record, written essay, immunizations, interview, 3 letters of recommendation, nursing research course, physical assessment course, resume, statistics course.
Advanced Placement Credit given for nursing courses completed elsewhere dependent upon specific evaluations.
Degree Requirements 41 total credit hours, thesis or project.

POST-MASTER'S PROGRAM

Areas of Study Nursing administration; nursing education. *Nurse practitioner programs in:* family health.

Marian University

School of Nursing
Indianapolis, Indiana

http://www.marian.edu/Nursing/Pages/default.aspx
Founded in 1851

DEGREE • BSN

Nursing Program Faculty 35
Baccalaureate Enrollment 480 **Women** 95% **Men** 5% **Minority** 15% **International** 2% **Part-time** 10%
Distance Learning Courses Available.
Nursing Student Activities Nursing Honor Society, Sigma Theta Tau, Student Nurses' Association.
Nursing Student Resources Academic advising; academic or career counseling; assistance for students with disabilities; bookstore; campus computer network; career placement assistance; computer lab; computer-assisted instruction; e-mail services; employment services for current students; interactive nursing skills videos; Internet; learning resource lab; library services; nursing audiovisuals; remedial services; resume preparation assistance; skills, simulation, or other laboratory; tutoring; unpaid internships.
Library Facilities 102,237 volumes (3,250 in health, 2,000 in nursing); 337 periodical subscriptions (116 health-care related).

BACCALAUREATE PROGRAMS

Degree BSN

Available Programs Accelerated Baccalaureate; Accelerated Baccalaureate for Second Degree; Accelerated RN Baccalaureate; Baccalaureate for Second Degree; Generic Baccalaureate; RN Baccalaureate.
Site Options Indianapolis, IN.
Study Options Full-time and part-time.
Online Degree Options Yes.
Program Entrance Requirements Minimum overall college GPA of 2.8, transcript of college record, CPR certification, health exam, health insurance, high school biology, high school chemistry, high school transcript, immunizations, minimum high school GPA of 2.3, minimum GPA in nursing prerequisites of 2.8, prerequisite course work. Transfer students are accepted. *Application deadline:* 7/15 (fall), 11/15 (winter), 12/15 (spring), 4/15 (summer). *Application fee:* $50.
Expenses (2012–13) *Tuition:* full-time $26,000; part-time $1200 per credit. *Required fees:* full-time $300; part-time $300 per term.
Financial Aid 97% of baccalaureate students in nursing programs received some form of financial aid in 2011–12.
Contact Ms. Marsha Schuler, Academic Advisor, School of Nursing, Marian University, 3200 Cold Spring Road, Indianapolis, IN 46222-1997. *Telephone:* 317-955-6157. *Fax:* 317-955-6135. *E-mail:* mschuler@marian.edu.

CONTINUING EDUCATION PROGRAM

Contact Jodie Freeland, Assistant Dean, Associate Professor, School of Nursing, Marian University, 3200 Cold Spring Road, Indianapolis, IN 46222. *Telephone:* 317-955-6145. *Fax:* 317-955-6135. *E-mail:* freeland@marian.edu.

Purdue University

School of Nursing
West Lafayette, Indiana

http://www.nursing.purdue.edu/
Founded in 1869

DEGREES • BS • DNP • MS

Nursing Program Faculty 60 (15% with doctorates).
Baccalaureate Enrollment 552 **Women** 94% **Men** 6% **Minority** 3% **International** .5% **Part-time** .06%
Graduate Enrollment 48 **Women** 96% **Men** 4% **Minority** 2% **Part-time** 50%
Nursing Student Activities Sigma Theta Tau, Student Nurses' Association.
Nursing Student Resources Academic advising; academic or career counseling; assistance for students with disabilities; bookstore; campus computer network; career placement assistance; computer lab; computer-assisted instruction; e-mail services; interactive nursing skills videos; Internet; learning resource lab; library services; nursing audiovisuals;

remedial services; resume preparation assistance; skills, simulation, or other laboratory; tutoring.
Library Facilities 5.2 million volumes (200,000 in health, 10,000 in nursing); 59,000 periodical subscriptions (1,000 health-care related).

BACCALAUREATE PROGRAMS

Degree BS
Available Programs ADN to Baccalaureate; Accelerated Baccalaureate for Second Degree; Baccalaureate for Second Degree; Generic Baccalaureate; RN Baccalaureate.
Site Options Indianapolis, IN.
Study Options Full-time and part-time.
Program Entrance Requirements Transcript of college record, CPR certification, health exam, health insurance, high school biology, high school chemistry, high school foreign language, 3 years high school math, 3 years high school science, high school transcript, immunizations, letters of recommendation, minimum high school GPA of 3.0. Transfer students are accepted.
Advanced Placement Credit by examination available. Credit given for nursing courses completed elsewhere dependent upon specific evaluations.
Contact *Telephone:* 765-494-1776. *Fax:* 765-494-0544.

GRADUATE PROGRAMS

Contact *Telephone:* 765-494-4015. *Fax:* 765-496-1800.

MASTER'S DEGREE PROGRAM
Degree MS
Available Programs Master's.
Concentrations Available *Nurse practitioner programs in:* adult health, pediatric.
Study Options Full-time and part-time.
Program Entrance Requirements Clinical experience, computer literacy, minimum overall college GPA of 3.0, transcript of college record, CPR certification, written essay, interview, 3 letters of recommendation, professional liability insurance/malpractice insurance, prerequisite course work, resume, statistics course.
Advanced Placement Credit given for nursing courses completed elsewhere dependent upon specific evaluations.
Degree Requirements 46 total credit hours, thesis or project.

POST-MASTER'S PROGRAM
Areas of Study *Nurse practitioner programs in:* adult health, pediatric.

DOCTORAL DEGREE PROGRAM
Degree DNP
Available Programs Doctorate.
Areas of Study Advanced practice nursing, aging, biology of health and illness, clinical practice, critical care, ethics, gerontology, health policy, health promotion/disease prevention, health-care systems, illness and transition, individualized study, information systems, nursing administration, nursing education, nursing policy, nursing research, nursing science, oncology, urban health, women's health.
Program Entrance Requirements Clinical experience, minimum overall college GPA of 3.0, interview by faculty committee, interview, letters of recommendation, MSN or equivalent, statistics course, vita, writing sample.
Degree Requirements 83 total credit hours, oral exam, residency.

CONTINUING EDUCATION PROGRAM

Contact *Telephone:* 765-494-4030. *Fax:* 765-494-6339.

Purdue University Calumet

School of Nursing
Hammond, Indiana

http://webs.purduecal.edu/nursing/
Founded in 1951

DEGREES • BS • MS

Nursing Program Faculty 39 (33% with doctorates).
Baccalaureate Enrollment 621 **Women** 84.5% **Men** 15.5% **Minority** 16.7% **Part-time** 61.5%
Graduate Enrollment 127 **Women** 93% **Men** 7% **Minority** 23% **International** 3% **Part-time** 94%
Distance Learning Courses Available.

Nursing Student Activities Sigma Theta Tau, Student Nurses' Association, nursing club.

Nursing Student Resources Academic advising; academic or career counseling; assistance for students with disabilities; bookstore; campus computer network; career placement assistance; computer lab; computer-assisted instruction; daycare for children of students; e-mail services; employment services for current students; externships; housing assistance; interactive nursing skills videos; Internet; learning resource lab; library services; nursing audiovisuals; other; paid internships; placement services for program completers; remedial services; resume preparation assistance; skills, simulation, or other laboratory; tutoring; unpaid internships.

Library Facilities 254,784 volumes (7,900 in health, 1,140 in nursing); 2,144 periodical subscriptions (610 health-care related).

BACCALAUREATE PROGRAMS

Degree BS
Available Programs Accelerated Baccalaureate for Second Degree; Accelerated RN Baccalaureate; Generic Baccalaureate; LPN to Baccalaureate.
Study Options Full-time and part-time.
Online Degree Options Yes.
Program Entrance Requirements Minimum overall college GPA of 2.5, transcript of college record, CPR certification, health exam, high school biology, high school chemistry, 3 years high school math, 4 years high school science, high school transcript, immunizations, minimum GPA in nursing prerequisites of 2.0, prerequisite course work. Transfer students are accepted. *Application deadline:* 2/1 (fall).
Advanced Placement Credit by examination available. Credit given for nursing courses completed elsewhere dependent upon specific evaluations.
Expenses (2011–12) *Tuition, state resident:* full-time $5712; part-time $204 per credit hour. *Tuition, nonresident:* full-time $13,689; part-time $489 per credit hour. *International tuition:* $13,689 full-time. *Room and board:* room only: $6048 per academic year. *Required fees:* full-time $1109; part-time $17 per credit.
Financial Aid 35% of baccalaureate students in nursing programs received some form of financial aid in 2010–11.
Contact Prof. Kathleen Ann Nix, Undergraduate Program Coordinator, School of Nursing, Purdue University Calumet, 2200 169th Street, Hammond, IN 46323-2094. *Telephone:* 219-989-2859. *Fax:* 219-989-2848. *E-mail:* nix@purduecal.edu.

GRADUATE PROGRAMS

Expenses (2011–12) *Tuition, state resident:* full-time $5437; part-time $259 per credit hour. *Tuition, nonresident:* full-time $11,975; part-time $570 per credit hour. *International tuition:* $11,975 full-time. *Room and board:* room only: $6048 per academic year. *Required fees:* full-time $352; part-time $17 per credit.
Financial Aid 50% of graduate students in nursing programs received some form of financial aid in 2010–11.
Contact Dr. Jane Walker, Graduate Program Coordinator, School of Nursing, Purdue University Calumet, 2200 169th Street, Hammond, IN 46323-2094. *Telephone:* 219-989-2815. *Fax:* 219-989-2848. *E-mail:* walkerj@calumet.purdue.edu.

MASTER'S DEGREE PROGRAM

Degree MS
Available Programs Master's.
Concentrations Available Nursing administration. *Clinical nurse specialist programs in:* adult health, critical care. *Nurse practitioner programs in:* family health.
Study Options Full-time and part-time.
Online Degree Options Yes.
Program Entrance Requirements Minimum overall college GPA of 3.0, transcript of college record, written essay, 3 letters of recommendation, physical assessment course, resume, statistics course. *Application deadline:* 2/15 (fall), 9/15 (spring), 2/15 (summer). *Application fee:* $55.
Advanced Placement Credit given for nursing courses completed elsewhere dependent upon specific evaluations.
Degree Requirements 45 total credit hours.

POST-MASTER'S PROGRAM

Areas of Study Nursing education. *Clinical nurse specialist programs in:* adult health, critical care. *Nurse practitioner programs in:* family health.

Purdue University North Central
Department of Nursing
Westville, Indiana

http://www.pnc.edu/depts/nu/index.html
Founded in 1967
DEGREE • BS
Nursing Program Faculty 34 (35% with doctorates).
Baccalaureate Enrollment 150 **Women** 97% **Men** 3% **Minority** 12% **Part-time** 87%
Distance Learning Courses Available.
Nursing Student Activities Nursing Honor Society, Student Nurses' Association.
Nursing Student Resources Academic advising; academic or career counseling; assistance for students with disabilities; bookstore; campus computer network; career placement assistance; computer lab; computer-assisted instruction; daycare for children of students; e-mail services; interactive nursing skills videos; Internet; learning resource lab; library services; nursing audiovisuals; placement services for program completers; resume preparation assistance; skills, simulation, or other laboratory; tutoring.
Library Facilities 87,848 volumes (1,100 in health, 560 in nursing); 42,367 periodical subscriptions (229 health-care related).

BACCALAUREATE PROGRAMS

Degree BS
Available Programs ADN to Baccalaureate; Accelerated Baccalaureate; Accelerated Baccalaureate for Second Degree; Baccalaureate for Second Degree; LPN to Baccalaureate; RN Baccalaureate.
Site Options Valparaiso, IN.
Study Options Full-time and part-time.
Program Entrance Requirements Minimum overall college GPA of 2.5, transcript of college record, CPR certification, health exam, health insurance, high school biology, high school chemistry, 3 years high school math, 3 years high school science, high school transcript, immunizations, minimum high school GPA of 2.5, minimum high school rank 50%, minimum GPA in nursing prerequisites of 2.5, professional liability insurance/malpractice insurance, prerequisite course work. Transfer students are accepted. *Application deadline:* 1/16 (fall), 8/16 (spring).
Advanced Placement Credit by examination available. Credit given for nursing courses completed elsewhere dependent upon specific evaluations.
Expenses (2012–13) *Tuition, state resident:* part-time $215 per credit hour. *Tuition, nonresident:* part-time $539 per credit hour.
Financial Aid 44% of baccalaureate students in nursing programs received some form of financial aid in 2011–12.
Contact Ms. Nicole Hartford, Professional Academic Advisor for Nursing, Department of Nursing, Purdue University North Central, 1401 South U.S. Highway 421, Westville, IN 46391. *Telephone:* 219-785-5439. *Fax:* 219-785-5495. *E-mail:* nursing@pnc.edu.

Saint Joseph's College
St. Elizabeth School of Nursing
Rensselaer, Indiana

http://www.steson.org
Founded in 1889
DEGREE • BSN
Nursing Program Faculty 30 (.07% with doctorates).
Baccalaureate Enrollment 250
Distance Learning Courses Available.
Nursing Student Activities Student Nurses' Association.
Nursing Student Resources Academic advising; assistance for students with disabilities; campus computer network; computer lab; computer-assisted instruction; e-mail services; interactive nursing skills videos; Internet; learning resource lab; library services; nursing audiovisuals; resume preparation assistance; skills, simulation, or other laboratory; tutoring.
Library Facilities 131,307 volumes; 13,262 periodical subscriptions.

BACCALAUREATE PROGRAMS

Degree BSN
Available Programs Accelerated Baccalaureate for Second Degree; RN Baccalaureate.

Site Options Lafayette, IN.

Study Options Full-time and part-time.

Program Entrance Requirements Minimum overall college GPA of 2.0, transcript of college record, CPR certification, written essay, health exam, health insurance, high school biology, high school chemistry, 3 years high school math, 2 years high school science, high school transcript, immunizations, 3 letters of recommendation, minimum high school GPA of 2.0, minimum high school rank 51%. Transfer students are accepted. *Application deadline:* Applications may be processed on a rolling basis for some programs. *Application fee:* $25.

Advanced Placement Credit given for nursing courses completed elsewhere dependent upon specific evaluations.

Expenses (2011–12) *Room and board:* $4030 per academic year.

Financial Aid 98% of baccalaureate students in nursing programs received some form of financial aid in 2010–11.

Contact Anita K. Reed, Coordinator of Admissions, St. Elizabeth School of Nursing, Saint Joseph's College, 1508 Tippecanoe Street, Lafayette, IN 47904. *Telephone:* 765-423-6400. *Fax:* 765-423-6383. *E-mail:* anita.reed@franciscanalliance.org.

Saint Mary's College
Department of Nursing
Notre Dame, Indiana

http://www3.saintmarys.edu/nursing
Founded in 1844

DEGREE • BS
Nursing Program Faculty 15 (9% with doctorates).

Baccalaureate Enrollment 240 **Women** 100% **Minority** 4%

Distance Learning Courses Available.

Nursing Student Activities Nursing Honor Society, Sigma Theta Tau, Student Nurses' Association.

Nursing Student Resources Academic advising; academic or career counseling; assistance for students with disabilities; bookstore; campus computer network; career placement assistance; computer lab; computer-assisted instruction; daycare for children of students; e-mail services; employment services for current students; externships; interactive nursing skills videos; Internet; learning resource lab; library services; nursing audiovisuals; paid internships; placement services for program completers; remedial services; resume preparation assistance; skills, simulation, or other laboratory; tutoring; unpaid internships.

Library Facilities 243,986 volumes (9,787 in health, 5,149 in nursing); 15,550 periodical subscriptions (70 health-care related).

BACCALAUREATE PROGRAMS
Degree BS
Available Programs Accelerated Baccalaureate; Generic Baccalaureate.
Site Options Goshen, IN; South Bend, IN.
Study Options Full-time.
Program Entrance Requirements Minimum overall college GPA of 3.0, transcript of college record, CPR certification, written essay, health exam, high school foreign language, 3 years high school math, 2 years high school science, high school transcript, immunizations, 2 letters of recommendation, minimum GPA in nursing prerequisites of 2.75. Transfer students are accepted. *Application deadline:* Applications may be processed on a rolling basis for some programs. *Application fee:* $30.

Advanced Placement Credit given for nursing courses completed elsewhere dependent upon specific evaluations.

Expenses (2012–13) *Tuition:* full-time $32,560; part-time $1290 per credit. *Room and board:* $5000 per academic year. *Required fees:* full-time $380.

Financial Aid 75% of baccalaureate students in nursing programs received some form of financial aid in 2011–12.

Contact Mrs. Mona Bowe, Vice President for Enrollment Management, Department of Nursing, Saint Mary's College, 124 LeMans, Notre Dame, IN 46556. *Telephone:* 574-284-4587. *Fax:* 574-284-4716. *E-mail:* mbowe@saintmarys.edu.

University of Evansville
Department of Nursing
Evansville, Indiana

http://www.evansville.edu/majors/nursing/
Founded in 1854

DEGREE • BSN
Nursing Program Faculty 11 (28% with doctorates).

Baccalaureate Enrollment 188 **Women** 86% **Men** 14% **Minority** 4% **International** 1% **Part-time** 20%

Distance Learning Courses Available.

Nursing Student Activities Sigma Theta Tau, Student Nurses' Association.

Nursing Student Resources Academic advising; academic or career counseling; assistance for students with disabilities; bookstore; campus computer network; career placement assistance; computer lab; computer-assisted instruction; e-mail services; employment services for current students; externships; housing assistance; interactive nursing skills videos; Internet; learning resource lab; library services; nursing audiovisuals; paid internships; placement services for program completers; remedial services; resume preparation assistance; skills, simulation, or other laboratory; tutoring; unpaid internships.

Library Facilities 282,681 volumes (11,000 in nursing); 550 periodical subscriptions (155 health-care related).

BACCALAUREATE PROGRAMS
Degree BSN
Available Programs Generic Baccalaureate; RN Baccalaureate.
Site Options Henderson, KY.
Study Options Full-time and part-time.
Program Entrance Requirements CPR certification, health exam, health insurance, high school chemistry, 3 years high school math, 2 years high school science, high school transcript, immunizations, minimum high school rank 67%, professional liability insurance/malpractice insurance. Transfer students are accepted. *Application deadline:* Applications may be processed on a rolling basis for some programs. *Application fee:* $35.

Advanced Placement Credit given for nursing courses completed elsewhere dependent upon specific evaluations.

Expenses (2012–13) *Tuition:* full-time $30,556; part-time $830 per credit hour. *International tuition:* $30,556 full-time. *Room and board:* $10,000 per academic year. *Required fees:* full-time $840; part-time $50 per term.

Financial Aid 100% of baccalaureate students in nursing programs received some form of financial aid in 2011–12.

Contact Dr. Amy M. Hall, Chair/Professor of Nursing, Department of Nursing, University of Evansville, 1800 Lincoln Avenue, Evansville, IN 47722. *Telephone:* 812-488-2414. *Fax:* 812-488-2717. *E-mail:* ah169@evansville.edu.

University of Indianapolis
School of Nursing
Indianapolis, Indiana

http://www.uindy.edu/
Founded in 1902

DEGREES • BSN • DNP • MSN • MSN/MALAS • MSN/MS • MSN/MSBA
Nursing Program Faculty 39 (50% with doctorates).

Baccalaureate Enrollment 353 **Women** 93.2% **Men** 6.8% **Minority** 6.5% **Part-time** 46%

Graduate Enrollment 248 **Women** 93.2% **Men** 6.8% **Minority** 12% **Part-time** 98%

Distance Learning Courses Available.

Nursing Student Activities Nursing Honor Society, Sigma Theta Tau, Student Nurses' Association.

Nursing Student Resources Academic advising; academic or career counseling; assistance for students with disabilities; bookstore; campus computer network; career placement assistance; computer lab; computer-assisted instruction; e-mail services; employment services for current students; externships; housing assistance; interactive nursing skills videos; Internet; learning resource lab; library services; nursing audiovisuals; other; paid internships; placement services for program completers;

remedial services; resume preparation assistance; skills, simulation, or other laboratory; tutoring; unpaid internships.
Library Facilities 173,363 volumes (15,600 in health, 1,000 in nursing); 1,015 periodical subscriptions (600 health-care related).

BACCALAUREATE PROGRAMS

Degree BSN
Available Programs ADN to Baccalaureate; Accelerated Baccalaureate for Second Degree; Generic Baccalaureate; RN Baccalaureate.
Site Options Indianapolis, IN.
Study Options Full-time and part-time.
Program Entrance Requirements Minimum overall college GPA of 2.82, transcript of college record, CPR certification, health exam, health insurance, high school biology, high school chemistry, 2 years high school math, 2 years high school science, high school transcript, immunizations, minimum GPA in nursing prerequisites of 2.0, prerequisite course work. Transfer students are accepted. *Application deadline:* 4/15 (fall), 10/15 (winter). *Application fee:* $25.
Advanced Placement Credit by examination available. Credit given for nursing courses completed elsewhere dependent upon specific evaluations.
Expenses (2012–13) *Tuition:* full-time $23,590; part-time $976 per credit hour. *International tuition:* $23,590 full-time. *Required fees:* full-time $400; part-time $150 per term.
Financial Aid 98% of baccalaureate students in nursing programs received some form of financial aid in 2011–12.
Contact Dr. Cheryl M. Martin, Director, BSN Program, School of Nursing, University of Indianapolis, 1400 East Hanna Avenue, Indianapolis, IN 46227-3697. *Telephone:* 317-788-3324. *Fax:* 317-788-3542. *E-mail:* martincm@uindy.edu.

GRADUATE PROGRAMS

Expenses (2012–13) *Tuition:* full-time $11,340; part-time $630 per credit hour. *International tuition:* $11,340 full-time.
Financial Aid 90% of graduate students in nursing programs received some form of financial aid in 2011–12.
Contact Dr. Anne Thomas, Director, Graduate Program, School of Nursing, University of Indianapolis, 1400 East Hanna Avenue, Indianapolis, IN 46227-3697. *Telephone:* 317-788-3206. *Fax:* 317-788-6208. *E-mail:* athomas@uindy.edu.

MASTER'S DEGREE PROGRAM

Degrees MSN; MSN/MALAS; MSN/MS; MSN/MSBA
Available Programs Accelerated Master's for Non-Nursing College Graduates; Master's.
Concentrations Available Nurse-midwifery; nursing administration; nursing education. *Nurse practitioner programs in:* adult health, family health, gerontology, neonatal health, primary care, women's health.
Site Options Indianapolis, IN.
Study Options Full-time and part-time.
Online Degree Options Yes.
Program Entrance Requirements Clinical experience, minimum overall college GPA of 3.0, transcript of college record, CPR certification, written essay, immunizations, interview, 3 letters of recommendation, nursing research course, professional liability insurance/malpractice insurance, prerequisite course work, resume, statistics course. *Application deadline:* 4/15 (fall). Applications may be processed on a rolling basis for some programs. *Application fee:* $60.
Advanced Placement Credit given for nursing courses completed elsewhere dependent upon specific evaluations.
Degree Requirements 39 total credit hours, thesis or project, comprehensive exam.

POST-MASTER'S PROGRAM

Areas of Study Nurse-midwifery; nursing administration; nursing education. *Nurse practitioner programs in:* adult health, family health, gerontology, neonatal health, primary care, women's health.

DOCTORAL DEGREE PROGRAM

Degree DNP
Available Programs Doctorate.
Areas of Study Advanced practice nursing, family health, gerontology, health-care systems, nursing administration, women's health.
Online Degree Options Yes (online only).
Program Entrance Requirements Clinical experience, minimum overall college GPA of 3.25, interview by faculty committee, 3 letters of recommendation, MSN or equivalent, statistics course, vita, writing sample. *Application deadline:* 4/15 (fall), 10/15 (winter). Applications

may be processed on a rolling basis for some programs. *Application fee:* $60.
Degree Requirements 35 total credit hours, residency.

University of Saint Francis
Department of Nursing
Fort Wayne, Indiana

http://www.sf.edu/nursing
Founded in 1890
DEGREES • BSN • MSN
Nursing Program Faculty 35 (5% with doctorates).
Baccalaureate Enrollment 263 **Women** 90.2% **Men** 9.8% **Minority** 7.2% **Part-time** 1.5%
Graduate Enrollment 119 **Women** 95% **Men** 5% **Minority** 5.8% **Part-time** 7.4%
Distance Learning Courses Available.
Nursing Student Activities Nursing Honor Society, Sigma Theta Tau, Student Nurses' Association.
Nursing Student Resources Academic advising; academic or career counseling; assistance for students with disabilities; bookstore; campus computer network; career placement assistance; computer lab; computer-assisted instruction; e-mail services; employment services for current students; externships; housing assistance; interactive nursing skills videos; Internet; learning resource lab; library services; nursing audiovisuals; paid internships; remedial services; resume preparation assistance; skills, simulation, or other laboratory; tutoring; unpaid internships.
Library Facilities 6,233 volumes in health, 3,376 volumes in nursing; 2,468 periodical subscriptions health-care related.

BACCALAUREATE PROGRAMS

Degree BSN
Available Programs ADN to Baccalaureate; Generic Baccalaureate; RN Baccalaureate.
Study Options Full-time and part-time.
Online Degree Options Yes.
Program Entrance Requirements Minimum overall college GPA of 2.7, transcript of college record, CPR certification, health exam, high school biology, high school chemistry, 1 year of high school math, high school transcript, immunizations, minimum high school GPA of 2.7, minimum GPA in nursing prerequisites of 2.7, prerequisite course work. Transfer students are accepted. *Application deadline:* 7/31 (fall), 11/18 (spring).
Advanced Placement Credit given for nursing courses completed elsewhere dependent upon specific evaluations.
Expenses (2012–13) *Tuition:* full-time $23,560; part-time $745 per credit hour. *International tuition:* $23,560 full-time. *Required fees:* full-time $880; part-time $21 per credit; part-time $125 per term.
Financial Aid 96% of baccalaureate students in nursing programs received some form of financial aid in 2011–12.
Contact Megan Winegarden, BSN Program Director, Department of Nursing, University of Saint Francis, 2701 Spring Street, Fort Wayne, IN 46808. *Telephone:* 260-399-7700 Ext. 8513. *Fax:* 260-399-8167. *E-mail:* mwinegarden@sf.edu.

GRADUATE PROGRAMS

Expenses (2012–13) *Tuition:* part-time $785 per credit hour.
Financial Aid 97% of graduate students in nursing programs received some form of financial aid in 2011–12. Federal Work-Study, scholarships, tuition waivers (full and partial), and unspecified assistantships available.
Contact Mindy Yoder, MSN Program Director, Department of Nursing, University of Saint Francis, 2701 Spring Street, Fort Wayne, IN 46808. *Telephone:* 260-399-7700 Ext. 8510. *Fax:* 260-399-8167. *E-mail:* myoder@sf.edu.

MASTER'S DEGREE PROGRAM

Degree MSN
Available Programs Master's; Master's for Nurses with Non-Nursing Degrees.
Concentrations Available *Nurse practitioner programs in:* family health.
Study Options Full-time and part-time.
Program Entrance Requirements Computer literacy, minimum overall college GPA of 3.2, transcript of college record, CPR certification, written essay, immunizations, interview, 3 letters of recommendation,

nursing research course, physical assessment course, resume, statistics course, GRE. *Application deadline:* 7/28 (fall), 4/14 (summer).
Advanced Placement Credit given for nursing courses completed elsewhere dependent upon specific evaluations.
Degree Requirements 48 total credit hours.

POST-MASTER'S PROGRAM

Areas of Study *Nurse practitioner programs in:* family health.

University of Southern Indiana
College of Nursing and Health Professions
Evansville, Indiana

http://health.usi.edu/
Founded in 1965
DEGREES • BSN • DNP • MSN
Nursing Program Faculty 42 (80% with doctorates).
Baccalaureate Enrollment 413 **Women** 90% **Men** 10% **Minority** 5% **International** 1% **Part-time** 26%
Graduate Enrollment 457 **Women** 93% **Men** 7% **Minority** 8% **Part-time** 72%
Distance Learning Courses Available.
Nursing Student Activities Sigma Theta Tau, Student Nurses' Association.
Nursing Student Resources Academic advising; academic or career counseling; assistance for students with disabilities; bookstore; campus computer network; career placement assistance; computer lab; computer-assisted instruction; daycare for children of students; e-mail services; employment services for current students; housing assistance; interactive nursing skills videos; Internet; learning resource lab; library services; nursing audiovisuals; placement services for program completers; remedial services; resume preparation assistance; skills, simulation, or other laboratory; tutoring; unpaid internships.
Library Facilities 361,999 volumes (9,200 in health, 1,500 in nursing); 36,103 periodical subscriptions (2,000 health-care related).

BACCALAUREATE PROGRAMS

Degree BSN
Available Programs Generic Baccalaureate; RN Baccalaureate.
Study Options Full-time.
Online Degree Options Yes.
Program Entrance Requirements Minimum overall college GPA of 3.0, transcript of college record, CPR certification, written essay, health exam, health insurance, high school transcript, immunizations, minimum GPA in nursing prerequisites of 2.0, professional liability insurance/malpractice insurance, prerequisite course work. Transfer students are accepted. *Application deadline:* 8/1 (fall).
Advanced Placement Credit given for nursing courses completed elsewhere dependent upon specific evaluations.
Expenses (2011–12) *Tuition, state resident:* full-time $6371; part-time $193 per credit hour. *Tuition, nonresident:* full-time $9570; part-time $290 per credit hour. *Room and board:* $7200; room only: $3840 per academic year. *Required fees:* full-time $500; part-time $15 per credit; part-time $250 per term.
Financial Aid 70% of baccalaureate students in nursing programs received some form of financial aid in 2010–11. *Gift aid (need-based):* Federal Pell, FSEOG, state, private, college/university gift aid from institutional funds, Federal Nursing. *Loans:* Federal Direct (Subsidized and Unsubsidized Stafford PLUS).*Work-study:* Federal Work-Study.*Financial aid application deadline:* 3/1.
Contact Dr. Ann H. White, Associate Dean, College of Nursing and Health Professions, University of Southern Indiana, 8600 University Boulevard, Evansville, IN 47712. *Telephone:* 812-465-1173. *Fax:* 812-465-7092. *E-mail:* awhite@usi.edu.

GRADUATE PROGRAMS

Expenses (2011–12) *Tuition, state resident:* full-time $6720; part-time $280 per credit hour. *Tuition, nonresident:* full-time $6720; part-time $280 per credit hour. *International tuition:* $6720 full-time. *Room and board:* $7200; room only: $3840 per academic year. *Required fees:* full-time $500; part-time $15 per credit; part-time $250 per term.
Financial Aid 45% of graduate students in nursing programs received some form of financial aid in 2010–11. Federal Work-Study, scholarships, tuition waivers (full and partial), and unspecified assistantships available. *Financial aid application deadline:* 3/1.

Contact Dr. Ann H. White, Associate Dean, College of Nursing and Health Professions, University of Southern Indiana, 8600 University Boulevard, Evansville, IN 47712. *Telephone:* 812-465-1173. *Fax:* 812-465-7092. *E-mail:* awhite@usi.edu.

MASTER'S DEGREE PROGRAM

Degree MSN
Available Programs Master's; RN to Master's.
Concentrations Available Nursing administration; nursing education. *Clinical nurse specialist programs in:* adult health. *Nurse practitioner programs in:* acute care, family health, psychiatric/mental health.
Study Options Full-time and part-time.
Online Degree Options Yes (online only).
Program Entrance Requirements Computer literacy, minimum overall college GPA of 3.0, transcript of college record, CPR certification, written essay, immunizations, 2 letters of recommendation, professional liability insurance/malpractice insurance, resume, statistics course. *Application deadline:* 2/15 (fall), 10/1 (winter). *Application fee:* $25.
Advanced Placement Credit given for nursing courses completed elsewhere dependent upon specific evaluations.
Degree Requirements 42 total credit hours.

POST-MASTER'S PROGRAM

Areas of Study Nursing administration; nursing education. *Clinical nurse specialist programs in:* adult health. *Nurse practitioner programs in:* acute care, family health, psychiatric/mental health.

DOCTORAL DEGREE PROGRAM

Degree DNP
Available Programs Doctorate.
Areas of Study Clinical practice, nursing administration.
Program Entrance Requirements Clinical experience, minimum overall college GPA of 3.25, 3 letters of recommendation, MSN or equivalent, vita, writing sample. *Application deadline:* 1/15 (fall). *Application fee:* $25.
Degree Requirements 78 total credit hours.

CONTINUING EDUCATION PROGRAM

Contact Peggy Graul, Coordinator of Continuing Education for Nursing and Health Professions, College of Nursing and Health Professions, University of Southern Indiana, 8600 University Boulevard, Evansville, IN 47712. *Telephone:* 812-465-1161. *Fax:* 812-465-7092. *E-mail:* pgraul@usi.edu.

Valparaiso University
College of Nursing
Valparaiso, Indiana

http://www.valpo.edu/nursing
Founded in 1859
DEGREES • BSN • MSN • MSN/MBA
Nursing Program Faculty 13 (38% with doctorates).
Baccalaureate Enrollment 310 **Women** 92% **Men** 8% **Minority** 12% **International** 2% **Part-time** 6%
Graduate Enrollment 34 **Women** 91% **Men** 9% **Minority** 12% **Part-time** 59%
Nursing Student Activities Sigma Theta Tau, Student Nurses' Association.
Nursing Student Resources Academic advising; academic or career counseling; assistance for students with disabilities; bookstore; campus computer network; career placement assistance; computer lab; computer-assisted instruction; e-mail services; employment services for current students; externships; housing assistance; interactive nursing skills videos; Internet; learning resource lab; library services; nursing audiovisuals; placement services for program completers; remedial services; resume preparation assistance; skills, simulation, or other laboratory; tutoring; unpaid internships.
Library Facilities 540,090 volumes (9,500 in health, 995 in nursing); 71,995 periodical subscriptions (1,000 health-care related).

BACCALAUREATE PROGRAMS

Degree BSN
Available Programs Accelerated Baccalaureate; Generic Baccalaureate; RN Baccalaureate.
Study Options Full-time and part-time.

Program Entrance Requirements Minimum overall college GPA of 3.0, transcript of college record, written essay, high school biology, high school chemistry, 2 years high school math, 4 years high school science, high school transcript, immunizations, minimum high school GPA of 2.0, minimum GPA in nursing prerequisites of 2.5. Transfer students are accepted.

Advanced Placement Credit by examination available. Credit given for nursing courses completed elsewhere dependent upon specific evaluations.

Contact *Telephone:* 219-464-5011. *Fax:* 219-464-6888.

GRADUATE PROGRAMS

Contact *Telephone:* 219-464-5289. *Fax:* 219-464-5425.

MASTER'S DEGREE PROGRAM
Degrees MSN; MSN/MBA
Available Programs Master's; RN to Master's.
Concentrations Available *Clinical nurse specialist programs in:* adult health, gerontology, women's health.
Study Options Full-time and part-time.
Program Entrance Requirements Minimum overall college GPA of 3.0, transcript of college record, CPR certification, written essay, immunizations, 2 letters of recommendation, nursing research course, physical assessment course, statistics course.
Advanced Placement Credit given for nursing courses completed elsewhere dependent upon specific evaluations.
Degree Requirements 36 total credit hours, thesis or project.

POST-MASTER'S PROGRAM
Areas of Study *Nurse practitioner programs in:* family health.

CONTINUING EDUCATION PROGRAM
Contact *Telephone:* 219-464-5291. *Fax:* 219-464-5425.

Vincennes University
Department of Nursing
Vincennes, Indiana

Founded in 1801
DEGREE • BSN

BACCALAUREATE PROGRAMS
Degree BSN
Available Programs RN Baccalaureate.
Contact *Telephone:* 812-888-8888.

IOWA

Allen College
Program in Nursing
Waterloo, Iowa

http://www.allencollege.edu/
Founded in 1989
DEGREES • BSN • DNP • MSN
Nursing Program Faculty 36 (28% with doctorates).
Baccalaureate Enrollment 327 **Women** 95% **Men** 5% **Minority** 3% **Part-time** 40%
Graduate Enrollment 158 **Women** 95% **Men** 5% **Minority** 3% **Part-time** 80%
Distance Learning Courses Available.
Nursing Student Activities Sigma Theta Tau, Student Nurses' Association, nursing club.
Nursing Student Resources Academic advising; academic or career counseling; campus computer network; career placement assistance; computer lab; computer-assisted instruction; e-mail services; externships; housing assistance; interactive nursing skills videos; Internet; library services; nursing audiovisuals; other; paid internships; placement services

for program completers; resume preparation assistance; skills, simulation, or other laboratory; tutoring.
Library Facilities 3,300 volumes (3,587 in health, 3,587 in nursing); 214 periodical subscriptions (240 health-care related).

BACCALAUREATE PROGRAMS
Degree BSN
Available Programs ADN to Baccalaureate; Accelerated Baccalaureate; Accelerated Baccalaureate for Second Degree; Accelerated RN Baccalaureate; Baccalaureate for Second Degree; Generic Baccalaureate; LPN to Baccalaureate; RN Baccalaureate.
Study Options Full-time and part-time.
Online Degree Options Yes.
Program Entrance Requirements Transcript of college record, CPR certification, health exam, immunizations, 1 letter of recommendation, minimum GPA in nursing prerequisites of 2.7, prerequisite course work. Transfer students are accepted. *Application deadline:* Applications may be processed on a rolling basis for some programs. *Application fee:* $50.
Advanced Placement Credit given for nursing courses completed elsewhere dependent upon specific evaluations.
Expenses (2012–13) *Tuition:* full-time $16,236; part-time $525 per credit hour. *International tuition:* $16,236 full-time. *Required fees:* full-time $1867; part-time $71 per credit; part-time $418 per term.
Financial Aid 81% of baccalaureate students in nursing programs received some form of financial aid in 2011–12.
Contact Ashlee Gilstrap, Student Services Education Secretary, Program in Nursing, Allen College, 1825 Logan Avenue, Waterloo, IA 50703. *Telephone:* 319-226-2014. *Fax:* 319-226-2010. *E-mail:* allencollegeadmissions@ihs.org.

GRADUATE PROGRAMS
Expenses (2012–13) *Tuition:* full-time $14,730; part-time $712 per credit hour. *International tuition:* $14,730 full-time. *Required fees:* full-time $836; part-time $71 per credit; part-time $275 per term.
Financial Aid 76% of graduate students in nursing programs received some form of financial aid in 2011–12. Institutionally sponsored loans, scholarships, and traineeships available. Aid available to part-time students. *Financial aid application deadline:* 8/15.
Contact Ashlee Gilstrap, Student Services Education Secretary, Program in Nursing, Allen College, 1825 Logan Avenue, Waterloo, IA 50703. *Telephone:* 319-226-2000. *Fax:* 319-226-2010. *E-mail:* allencollegeadmissions@ihs.org.

MASTER'S DEGREE PROGRAM
Degree MSN
Available Programs Master's; Master's for Nurses with Non-Nursing Degrees; RN to Master's.
Concentrations Available Nursing administration; nursing education. *Nurse practitioner programs in:* acute care, adult health, family health, gerontology, psychiatric/mental health.
Study Options Full-time and part-time.
Online Degree Options Yes.
Program Entrance Requirements Clinical experience, computer literacy, minimum overall college GPA of 3.0, transcript of college record, CPR certification, written essay, immunizations, interview, 3 letters of recommendation, nursing research course, professional liability insurance/malpractice insurance, prerequisite course work, resume, statistics course. *Application deadline:* Applications may be processed on a rolling basis for some programs. *Application fee:* $50.
Advanced Placement Credit given for nursing courses completed elsewhere dependent upon specific evaluations.
Degree Requirements 44 total credit hours, thesis or project.

POST-MASTER'S PROGRAM
Areas of Study Nursing administration; nursing education. *Nurse practitioner programs in:* acute care, adult health, family health, gerontology, psychiatric/mental health.

DOCTORAL DEGREE PROGRAM
Degree DNP
Available Programs Doctorate.
Online Degree Options Yes (online only).
Program Entrance Requirements Clinical experience, minimum overall college GPA of 3.25, interview by faculty committee, 3 letters of recommendation, MSN or equivalent, statistics course, vita, writing sample. *Application deadline:* Applications may be processed on a rolling basis for some programs. *Application fee:* $50.
Degree Requirements 33 total credit hours.

POSTDOCTORAL PROGRAM

Postdoctoral Program Contact Dr. Diane Young, Department Chair, MSN Program, Program in Nursing, Allen College, 1825 Logan Avenue, Waterloo, IA 50703. *Telephone:* 319-226-2047. *Fax:* 319-226-2070. *E-mail:* youngdm@ihs.org.

CONTINUING EDUCATION PROGRAM

Contact Dina Dowden, Continuing Education Coordinator, Program in Nursing, Allen College, 1825 Logan Avenue, Waterloo, IA 50703. *Telephone:* 319-226-2017. *Fax:* 319-226-2051. *E-mail:* dowdendk@ ihs.org.

Briar Cliff University
Department of Nursing
Sioux City, Iowa

http://www.briarcliff.edu/
Founded in 1930

DEGREES • BSN • MSN
Nursing Program Faculty 9 (33% with doctorates).
Baccalaureate Enrollment 125 **Women** 90% **Men** 10% **Minority** 5% **Part-time** 25%
Graduate Enrollment 50 **Women** 95% **Men** 5% **Minority** 5% **Part-time** 75%
Distance Learning Courses Available.
Nursing Student Activities Sigma Theta Tau, Student Nurses' Association, nursing club.
Nursing Student Resources Academic advising; academic or career counseling; assistance for students with disabilities; bookstore; campus computer network; career placement assistance; computer lab; computer-assisted instruction; e-mail services; employment services for current students; externships; interactive nursing skills videos; Internet; learning resource lab; library services; nursing audiovisuals; placement services for program completers; remedial services; resume preparation assistance; skills, simulation, or other laboratory; tutoring.
Library Facilities 82,007 volumes (7,954 in health, 266 in nursing); 151 periodical subscriptions (4,102 health-care related).

BACCALAUREATE PROGRAMS

Degree BSN
Available Programs ADN to Baccalaureate; Generic Baccalaureate; LPN to Baccalaureate; RN Baccalaureate.
Study Options Full-time and part-time.
Program Entrance Requirements Minimum overall college GPA of 2.75, transcript of college record, CPR certification, written essay, health exam, high school foreign language, high school transcript, immunizations, minimum GPA in nursing prerequisites of 2.75, prerequisite course work. Transfer students are accepted. *Application deadline:* 6/15 (fall), 7/1 (winter), 10/31 (spring), 4/1 (summer). Applications may be processed on a rolling basis for some programs. *Application fee:* $25.
Advanced Placement Credit given for nursing courses completed elsewhere dependent upon specific evaluations.
Expenses (2011–12) *Tuition:* full-time $23,600; part-time $780 per credit. *International tuition:* $23,600 full-time. *Room and board:* $7300; room only: $3622 per academic year. *Required fees:* full-time $1094; part-time $26 per credit.
Financial Aid 99% of baccalaureate students in nursing programs received some form of financial aid in 2010–11. *Gift aid (need-based):* Federal Pell, FSEOG, state, private, college/university gift aid from institutional funds. *Loans:* Federal Direct (Subsidized and Unsubsidized Stafford PLUS), Perkins, alternative loans, partnership loans, Minnesota SELF Loans.*Work-study:* Federal Work-Study, part-time campus jobs.*Financial aid application deadline:* 3/15.
Contact Dr. Richard A. Petersen, Department Chair and Associate Professor, Department of Nursing, Briar Cliff University, 3303 Rebecca Street, Sioux City, IA 51104. *Telephone:* 712-279-1662. *Fax:* 712-279-5299. *E-mail:* rick.petersen@briarcliff.edu.

GRADUATE PROGRAMS

Expenses (2011–12) *Tuition:* part-time $508 per credit. *Room and board:* $7300; room only: $3622 per academic year. *Required fees:* part-time $26 per credit.
Financial Aid 90% of graduate students in nursing programs received some form of financial aid in 2010–11.

Contact Dr. Richard A. Petersen, Department Chair and Associate Professor, Department of Nursing, Briar Cliff University, 3303 Rebecca Street, Sioux City, IA 51104. *Telephone:* 712-279-1662. *Fax:* 712-279-5299. *E-mail:* rick.petersen@briarcliff.edu.

MASTER'S DEGREE PROGRAM
Degree MSN
Available Programs Master's.
Concentrations Available Nursing education. *Nurse practitioner programs in:* family health.
Study Options Part-time.
Program Entrance Requirements Clinical experience, computer literacy, minimum overall college GPA of 3.0, transcript of college record, CPR certification, written essay, immunizations, 2 letters of recommendation, nursing research course, physical assessment course, resume, statistics course. *Application deadline:* 4/15 (fall). Applications may be processed on a rolling basis for some programs. *Application fee:* $25.
Advanced Placement Credit given for nursing courses completed elsewhere dependent upon specific evaluations.
Degree Requirements 40 total credit hours, thesis or project, comprehensive exam.

CONTINUING EDUCATION PROGRAM

Contact Dr. Richard A. Petersen, Chair and Associate Professor, Department of Nursing, Briar Cliff University, 3303 Rebecca Street, Sioux City, IA 51104. *Telephone:* 712-279-1662. *Fax:* 712-279-5299. *E-mail:* rick.petersen@briarcliff.edu.

Clarke University
Department of Nursing and Health
Dubuque, Iowa

http://www.clarke.edu/
Founded in 1843

DEGREES • BS • MSN
Nursing Program Faculty 18 (3% with doctorates).
Baccalaureate Enrollment 104 **Women** 92% **Men** 8% **Minority** 1% **International** 1% **Part-time** 9%
Graduate Enrollment 52 **Women** 99% **Men** 1% **Part-time** 35%
Nursing Student Activities Nursing Honor Society, Sigma Theta Tau, Student Nurses' Association.
Nursing Student Resources Academic advising; academic or career counseling; assistance for students with disabilities; bookstore; campus computer network; career placement assistance; computer lab; computer-assisted instruction; e-mail services; employment services for current students; externships; housing assistance; interactive nursing skills videos; Internet; learning resource lab; library services; nursing audiovisuals; paid internships; placement services for program completers; remedial services; resume preparation assistance; skills, simulation, or other laboratory; tutoring; unpaid internships.
Library Facilities 98,700 volumes (7,000 in health, 2,856 in nursing); 42,000 periodical subscriptions (124 health-care related).

BACCALAUREATE PROGRAMS

Degree BS
Available Programs Baccalaureate for Second Degree; Generic Baccalaureate; RN Baccalaureate.
Site Options Dubuque, IA.
Study Options Full-time and part-time.
Program Entrance Requirements Minimum overall college GPA of 2.75, transcript of college record, CPR certification, written essay, health exam, health insurance, high school chemistry, high school foreign language, high school math, high school transcript, immunizations, interview, 2 letters of recommendation, minimum high school GPA of 2.0, minimum GPA in nursing prerequisites of 1.67, professional liability insurance/malpractice insurance, prerequisite course work. Transfer students are accepted. *Application deadline:* Applications may be processed on a rolling basis for some programs.
Advanced Placement Credit given for nursing courses completed elsewhere dependent upon specific evaluations.
Contact *Telephone:* 563-588-8109. *Fax:* 563-588-8684.

GRADUATE PROGRAMS

Contact *Telephone:* 563-588-8109. *Fax:* 563-588-8684.

MASTER'S DEGREE PROGRAM

Degree MSN

Available Programs Master's.

Concentrations Available Nursing education. *Nurse practitioner programs in:* family health.

Study Options Full-time and part-time.

Program Entrance Requirements Computer literacy, minimum overall college GPA of 3.0, transcript of college record, CPR certification, written essay, immunizations, interview, 3 letters of recommendation, nursing research course, physical assessment course, prerequisite course work, resume, statistics course, GRE General Test or MAT. *Application deadline:* Applications may be processed on a rolling basis for some programs. *Application fee:* $35.

Advanced Placement Credit given for nursing courses completed elsewhere dependent upon specific evaluations.

Degree Requirements 37 total credit hours, thesis or project.

POST-MASTER'S PROGRAM

Areas of Study *Nurse practitioner programs in:* family health.

CONTINUING EDUCATION PROGRAM

Contact *Telephone:* 563-588-6378. *Fax:* 563-588-8684.

Coe College
Department of Nursing
Cedar Rapids, Iowa

Founded in 1851

DEGREE • BSN

Nursing Program Faculty 7 (86% with doctorates).

Baccalaureate Enrollment 50 **Women** 85% **Men** 15% **Minority** 2% **International** 1%

Nursing Student Activities Student Nurses' Association.

Nursing Student Resources Academic advising; academic or career counseling; assistance for students with disabilities; bookstore; campus computer network; career placement assistance; computer lab; e-mail services; employment services for current students; housing assistance; Internet; learning resource lab; library services; nursing audiovisuals; remedial services; resume preparation assistance; skills, simulation, or other laboratory; tutoring; unpaid internships.

Library Facilities 223,742 volumes (2,929 in health, 492 in nursing); 34,792 periodical subscriptions (34 health-care related).

BACCALAUREATE PROGRAMS

Degree BSN

Available Programs Generic Baccalaureate.

Study Options Full-time and part-time.

Program Entrance Requirements Minimum overall college GPA of 2.7, transcript of college record, CPR certification, written essay, health exam, health insurance, high school chemistry, high school transcript, immunizations, minimum high school GPA of 2.0, minimum GPA in nursing prerequisites of 2.7, prerequisite course work. Transfer students are accepted. *Application deadline:* 12/1 (fall). Applications may be processed on a rolling basis for some programs. *Application fee:* $50.

Advanced Placement Credit given for nursing courses completed elsewhere dependent upon specific evaluations.

Financial Aid 100% of baccalaureate students in nursing programs received some form of financial aid in 2011–12. *Gift aid (need-based):* Federal Pell, FSEOG, state, private, college/university gift aid from institutional funds, Federal Nursing, ROTC Scholarships. *Loans:* Federal Direct (Subsidized and Unsubsidized Stafford PLUS), Perkins, college/university.*Work-study:* Federal Work-Study, part-time campus jobs.*Financial aid application deadline (priority):* 3/1.

Contact Ms. Julie Staker, Dean of Admission, Department of Nursing, Coe College, 1220 First Avenue NE, Cedar Rapids, IA 52402. *Telephone:* 319-399-8046. *Fax:* 319-399-8816. *E-mail:* jstaker@coe.edu.

Dordt College
Nursing Program
Sioux Center, Iowa

Founded in 1955

DEGREE • BSN

Nursing Program Faculty 3

Library Facilities 175,000 volumes; 6,597 periodical subscriptions.

BACCALAUREATE PROGRAMS

Degree BSN

Available Programs Generic Baccalaureate.

Contact *Telephone:* 712-722-6000.

Grand View University
Division of Nursing
Des Moines, Iowa

http://www.grandview.edu

Founded in 1896

DEGREES • BSN • MS

Nursing Program Faculty 18 (33% with doctorates).

Baccalaureate Enrollment 200 **Women** 90% **Men** 10% **Minority** 15% **Part-time** 5%

Graduate Enrollment 6 **Women** 83% **Men** 17% **Part-time** 100%

Distance Learning Courses Available.

Nursing Student Activities Sigma Theta Tau, Student Nurses' Association.

Nursing Student Resources Academic advising; academic or career counseling; assistance for students with disabilities; bookstore; campus computer network; career placement assistance; computer lab; computer-assisted instruction; e-mail services; employment services for current students; externships; housing assistance; interactive nursing skills videos; Internet; learning resource lab; library services; nursing audiovisuals; placement services for program completers; remedial services; resume preparation assistance; skills, simulation, or other laboratory; tutoring; unpaid internships.

Library Facilities 135,448 volumes (5,672 in health, 4,061 in nursing); 27,077 periodical subscriptions (370 health-care related).

BACCALAUREATE PROGRAMS

Degree BSN

Available Programs Generic Baccalaureate; RN Baccalaureate.

Study Options Full-time and part-time.

Program Entrance Requirements Minimum overall college GPA of 2.75, transcript of college record, CPR certification, health exam, health insurance, high school chemistry, high school transcript, immunizations, 3 letters of recommendation, minimum GPA in nursing prerequisites of 2.75, prerequisite course work. Transfer students are accepted. *Application deadline:* 2/1 (fall), 10/1 (spring). Applications may be processed on a rolling basis for some programs.

Advanced Placement Credit by examination available. Credit given for nursing courses completed elsewhere dependent upon specific evaluations.

Contact *Telephone:* 515-263-2859. *Fax:* 515-263-6077.

GRADUATE PROGRAMS

Contact *Telephone:* 515-263-2859. *Fax:* 515-263-6077.

MASTER'S DEGREE PROGRAM

Degree MS

Available Programs Master's.

Concentrations Available Clinical nurse leader.

Study Options Part-time.

Program Entrance Requirements Clinical experience, computer literacy, minimum overall college GPA of 3.0, transcript of college record, CPR certification, written essay, immunizations, interview, 3 letters of recommendation, nursing research course, physical assessment course, professional liability insurance/malpractice insurance, prerequisite course work, resume, statistics course. *Application deadline:* 7/1 (fall). Applications may be processed on a rolling basis for some programs.

Degree Requirements 40 total credit hours, thesis or project.

CONTINUING EDUCATION PROGRAM

Contact *Telephone:* 515-263-2869. *Fax:* 515-263-6700.

Iowa Wesleyan College
Division of Nursing
Mount Pleasant, Iowa

http://www.iwc.edu/
Founded in 1842

DEGREE • BSN

Nursing Program Faculty 7 (29% with doctorates).
Baccalaureate Enrollment 80 **Women** 92% **Men** 8% **Minority** 7% **International** 1% **Part-time** 2%
Distance Learning Courses Available.
Nursing Student Activities Student Nurses' Association.
Nursing Student Resources Academic advising; academic or career counseling; assistance for students with disabilities; bookstore; campus computer network; career placement assistance; computer lab; computer-assisted instruction; e-mail services; employment services for current students; interactive nursing skills videos; Internet; learning resource lab; library services; nursing audiovisuals; remedial services; resume preparation assistance; skills, simulation, or other laboratory; tutoring; unpaid internships.
Library Facilities 83,956 volumes (500 in health, 300 in nursing); 113 periodical subscriptions (40 health-care related).

BACCALAUREATE PROGRAMS

Degree BSN
Available Programs ADN to Baccalaureate; Baccalaureate for Second Degree; Generic Baccalaureate; LPN to Baccalaureate; LPN to RN Baccalaureate; RN Baccalaureate.
Study Options Full-time and part-time.
Program Entrance Requirements Minimum overall college GPA of 2.25, transcript of college record, CPR certification, health exam, health insurance, high school transcript, immunizations, interview, minimum high school GPA of 2.25, minimum high school rank 50%, minimum GPA in nursing prerequisites of 2.25, professional liability insurance/malpractice insurance, prerequisite course work. Transfer students are accepted. *Application deadline:* 8/1 (fall). Applications may be processed on a rolling basis for some programs.
Expenses (2012–13) *Tuition:* full-time $24,300; part-time $610 per credit hour. *Room and board:* $3790; room only: $1570 per academic year. *Required fees:* full-time $150; part-time $150 per term.
Financial Aid 98% of baccalaureate students in nursing programs received some form of financial aid in 2011–12.
Contact Mr. Mark Petty, Dean for Admissions, Division of Nursing, Iowa Wesleyan College, 601 North Main Street, Mount Pleasant, IA 52641. *Telephone:* 800-582-2383 Ext. 6231. *Fax:* 319-385-6296. *E-mail:* mpetty@iwc.edu.

Luther College
Department of Nursing
Decorah, Iowa

http://nursing.luther.edu/
Founded in 1861

DEGREE • BA

Nursing Program Faculty 16 (25% with doctorates).
Baccalaureate Enrollment 130 **Women** 96% **Men** 4% **Minority** 3%
Nursing Student Activities Student Nurses' Association.
Nursing Student Resources Academic advising; academic or career counseling; assistance for students with disabilities; bookstore; campus computer network; career placement assistance; computer lab; computer-assisted instruction; e-mail services; Internet; learning resource lab; library services; nursing audiovisuals; placement services for program completers; remedial services; resume preparation assistance; skills, simulation, or other laboratory; tutoring; unpaid internships.
Library Facilities 332,977 volumes (4,324 in health, 3,337 in nursing); 688 periodical subscriptions (35 health-care related).

BACCALAUREATE PROGRAMS

Degree BA
Available Programs Generic Baccalaureate.
Site Options Rochester, MN.
Study Options Full-time and part-time.
Program Entrance Requirements Minimum overall college GPA of 2.75, transcript of college record, CPR certification, health exam, health insurance, 3 years high school math, 2 years high school science, high school transcript, immunizations, minimum high school rank 50%, minimum GPA in nursing prerequisites of 2.75, professional liability insurance/malpractice insurance, prerequisite course work. Transfer students are accepted.
Advanced Placement Credit given for nursing courses completed elsewhere dependent upon specific evaluations.
Expenses (2012–13) *Room and board:* $6610; room only: $3000 per academic year.
Financial Aid 98% of baccalaureate students in nursing programs received some form of financial aid in 2011–12. *Gift aid (need-based):* Federal Pell, FSEOG, state, private, college/university gift aid from institutional funds. *Loans:* Federal Direct (Subsidized and Unsubsidized Stafford PLUS), Perkins, college/university.*Work-study:* Federal Work-Study, part-time campus jobs.*Financial aid application deadline (priority):* 3/1.
Contact Ms. Ruth Green, Administrative Assistant, Department of Nursing, Luther College, 700 College Drive, Decorah, IA 52101. *Telephone:* 563-387-1057. *Fax:* 563-387-2149. *E-mail:* greenru@luther.edu.

CONTINUING EDUCATION PROGRAM

Contact Ms. Ruth Green, Administrative Assistant, Department of Nursing, Luther College, 700 College Drive, Decorah, IA 52101. *Telephone:* 563-387-1057. *Fax:* 563-387-2149. *E-mail:* greenru@luther.edu.

See display on next page and full description on page 490.

Mercy College of Health Sciences
Division of Nursing
Des Moines, Iowa

http://www.mchs.edu/
Founded in 1995

DEGREE • BSN

Nursing Program Faculty 22 (2% with doctorates).
Baccalaureate Enrollment 76 **Women** 98% **Men** 2% **Minority** 1% **Part-time** 98%
Nursing Student Activities Sigma Theta Tau, Student Nurses' Association.
Nursing Student Resources Academic advising; academic or career counseling; assistance for students with disabilities; campus computer network; career placement assistance; computer lab; computer-assisted instruction; daycare for children of students; e-mail services; employment services for current students; interactive nursing skills videos; Internet; learning resource lab; library services; nursing audiovisuals; placement services for program completers; skills, simulation, or other laboratory.
Library Facilities 32,785 volumes; 5,583 periodical subscriptions.

BACCALAUREATE PROGRAMS

Degree BSN
Available Programs ADN to Baccalaureate.
Study Options Full-time and part-time.
Program Entrance Requirements Minimum overall college GPA of 2.7, transcript of college record, CPR certification, health exam, high school biology, high school chemistry, high school transcript, immunizations, minimum GPA in nursing prerequisites of 2.7, prerequisite course work, RN licensure. Transfer students are accepted. *Application deadline:* Applications may be processed on a rolling basis for some programs. *Application fee:* $25.
Advanced Placement Credit given for nursing courses completed elsewhere dependent upon specific evaluations.
Contact *Telephone:* 515-643-3180. *Fax:* 515-643-6698.

Morningside College
Department of Nursing Education
Sioux City, Iowa

http://webs.morningside.edu/nursing/index.html
Founded in 1894

DEGREE • BSN
Nursing Program Faculty 12 (17% with doctorates).
Baccalaureate Enrollment 89 **Women** 91% **Men** 9% **Minority** 4% **Part-time** 9%
Nursing Student Activities Sigma Theta Tau, Student Nurses' Association.
Nursing Student Resources Academic advising; academic or career counseling; assistance for students with disabilities; bookstore; campus computer network; computer lab; computer-assisted instruction; e-mail services; employment services for current students; externships; housing assistance; interactive nursing skills videos; Internet; learning resource lab; library services; nursing audiovisuals; remedial services; resume preparation assistance; skills, simulation, or other laboratory; tutoring; unpaid internships.
Library Facilities 74,445 volumes (930 in health, 420 in nursing); 207 periodical subscriptions (275 health-care related).

BACCALAUREATE PROGRAMS

Degree BSN
Available Programs Baccalaureate for Second Degree; Generic Baccalaureate; International Nurse to Baccalaureate; LPN to Baccalaureate; RN Baccalaureate.
Study Options Full-time and part-time.
Program Entrance Requirements Minimum overall college GPA of 2.75, transcript of college record, CPR certification, high school transcript, immunizations, interview, minimum GPA in nursing prerequisites of 2.75, prerequisite course work. Transfer students are accepted. *Application deadline:* 8/15 (fall).
Advanced Placement Credit given for nursing courses completed elsewhere dependent upon specific evaluations.
Expenses (2012–13) *Tuition:* full-time $23,780; part-time $440 per credit. *International tuition:* $23,780 full-time. *Room and board:* $7620;

room only: $3900 per academic year. *Required fees:* full-time $1220; part-time $220 per term.
Financial Aid 99% of baccalaureate students in nursing programs received some form of financial aid in 2011–12. *Gift aid (need-based):* Federal Pell, FSEOG, state, private, college/university gift aid from institutional funds. *Loans:* Federal Direct (Subsidized and Unsubsidized Stafford PLUS), Perkins, college/university, private loans. *Work-study:* Federal Work-Study, part-time campus jobs. *Financial aid application deadline (priority):* 3/1.
Contact Dr. Mary B. Kovarna, Professor and Chair, Department of Nursing Education, Morningside College, 1501 Morningside Avenue, Sioux City, IA 51106-1751. *Telephone:* 712-274-5156. *Fax:* 712-274-5101. *E-mail:* kovarna@morningside.edu.

Mount Mercy University
Department of Nursing
Cedar Rapids, Iowa

http://www.mtmercy.edu/
Founded in 1928

DEGREES • BSN • MSN
Nursing Program Faculty 43 (14% with doctorates).
Baccalaureate Enrollment 243 **Women** 97% **Men** 3% **Minority** 3% **International** 2% **Part-time** 35%
Graduate Enrollment 41 **Women** 99% **Men** 1% **Minority** 1% **International** 1% **Part-time** 2%
Nursing Student Activities Sigma Theta Tau, Student Nurses' Association.
Nursing Student Resources Academic advising; academic or career counseling; assistance for students with disabilities; bookstore; campus computer network; career placement assistance; computer lab; computer-assisted instruction; e-mail services; employment services for current students; externships; housing assistance; interactive nursing skills videos; Internet; learning resource lab; library services; nursing audiovisuals; paid internships; placement services for program completers; remedial services; resume preparation assistance; skills, simulation, or other laboratory; tutoring; unpaid internships.

Library Facilities 132,216 volumes (5,400 in health, 1,475 in nursing); 2,613 periodical subscriptions (130 health-care related).

BACCALAUREATE PROGRAMS

Degree BSN

Available Programs ADN to Baccalaureate; Accelerated RN Baccalaureate; Generic Baccalaureate.

Study Options Full-time and part-time.

Program Entrance Requirements Minimum overall college GPA of 2.7, transcript of college record, CPR certification, health exam, health insurance, high school chemistry, 2 years high school math, 2 years high school science, high school transcript, immunizations, minimum high school rank 75%, minimum GPA in nursing prerequisites of 2.7, prerequisite course work. Transfer students are accepted. *Application deadline:* 5/31 (fall), 10/1 (winter), 10/1 (spring), 4/1 (summer).

Advanced Placement Credit by examination available. Credit given for nursing courses completed elsewhere dependent upon specific evaluations.

Expenses (2012–13) *Tuition:* full-time $25,400; part-time $698 per credit hour. *International tuition:* $25,400 full-time. *Room and board:* $5500; room only: $4000 per academic year. *Required fees:* full-time $500.

Financial Aid 90% of baccalaureate students in nursing programs received some form of financial aid in 2011–12. *Gift aid (need-based):* Federal Pell, FSEOG, state, private, college/university gift aid from institutional funds. *Loans:* Federal Direct (Subsidized and Unsubsidized Stafford PLUS), Perkins, state, college/university. *Work-study:* Federal Work-Study, part-time campus jobs. *Financial aid application deadline (priority):* 3/1.

Contact Dr. Mary P. Tarbox, Professor and Chair, Department of Nursing, Mount Mercy University, 1330 Elmhurst Drive NE, Cedar Rapids, IA 52402. *Telephone:* 800-248-4504 Ext. 6460. *Fax:* 319-368-6479. *E-mail:* mtarbox@mtmercy.edu.

GRADUATE PROGRAMS

Expenses (2012–13) *Tuition:* full-time $12,720; part-time $530 per credit hour. *International tuition:* $12,720 full-time. *Required fees:* full-time $200.

Financial Aid 50% of graduate students in nursing programs received some form of financial aid in 2011–12.

Contact Dr. Mary P. Tarbox, Chair, Department of Nursing, Mount Mercy University, 1330 Elmhurst Drive NE, Cedar Rapids, IA 52402. *Telephone:* 319-368-6471. *Fax:* 319-368-6479. *E-mail:* mtarbox@mtmercy.edu.

MASTER'S DEGREE PROGRAM

Degree MSN

Available Programs Master's.

Concentrations Available Health-care administration; nursing education. *Clinical nurse specialist programs in:* community health, public health.

Study Options Full-time and part-time.

Program Entrance Requirements Clinical experience, minimum overall college GPA of 3.0, transcript of college record, CPR certification, written essay, immunizations, 2 letters of recommendation, statistics course. *Application deadline:* Applications may be processed on a rolling basis for some programs.

Advanced Placement Credit given for nursing courses completed elsewhere dependent upon specific evaluations.

Degree Requirements 36 total credit hours, thesis or project.

CONTINUING EDUCATION PROGRAM

Contact Dr. Mary P. Tarbox, Department Chair, Department of Nursing, Mount Mercy University, 1330 Elmhurst Drive NE, Cedar Rapids, IA 52402. *Telephone:* 319-368-6471. *Fax:* 319-368-6479. *E-mail:* mtarbox@mtmercy.edu.

Northwestern College

Nursing Program
Orange City, Iowa

http://www.nwciowa.edu/nursing
Founded in 1882

DEGREE • BSN

Nursing Program Faculty 8 (12% with doctorates).

Baccalaureate Enrollment 58 **Women** 93% **Men** 7% **Part-time** 3%

Nursing Student Activities Nursing Honor Society, Sigma Theta Tau, Student Nurses' Association, nursing club.

Nursing Student Resources Academic advising; assistance for students with disabilities; bookstore; campus computer network; career placement assistance; computer lab; e-mail services; housing assistance; interactive nursing skills videos; Internet; learning resource lab; library services; nursing audiovisuals; placement services for program completers; remedial services; resume preparation assistance; skills, simulation, or other laboratory; tutoring.

Library Facilities 125,000 volumes; 615 periodical subscriptions.

BACCALAUREATE PROGRAMS

Degree BSN

Available Programs Generic Baccalaureate.

Study Options Full-time.

Program Entrance Requirements Transcript of college record, CPR certification, written essay, health exam, immunizations, minimum GPA in nursing prerequisites of 2.7, prerequisite course work. Transfer students are accepted. *Application deadline:* 4/10 (spring). *Application fee:* $550.

Advanced Placement Credit given for nursing courses completed elsewhere dependent upon specific evaluations.

Contact *Telephone:* 712-707-7086.

St. Ambrose University

Program in Nursing (BSN)
Davenport, Iowa

http://www.sau.edu/
Founded in 1882

DEGREES • BSN • MSN

Nursing Program Faculty 17 (35% with doctorates).

Baccalaureate Enrollment 266 **Women** 96% **Men** 4% **Minority** 7% **International** 2% **Part-time** 38%

Graduate Enrollment 14 **Women** 100% **Part-time** 100%

Nursing Student Activities Student Nurses' Association.

Nursing Student Resources Academic advising; academic or career counseling; assistance for students with disabilities; bookstore; campus computer network; career placement assistance; computer lab; e-mail services; employment services for current students; housing assistance; interactive nursing skills videos; Internet; learning resource lab; library services; nursing audiovisuals; resume preparation assistance; skills, simulation, or other laboratory; tutoring; unpaid internships.

Library Facilities 156,303 volumes (1,793 in health, 674 in nursing); 679 periodical subscriptions (157 health-care related).

BACCALAUREATE PROGRAMS

Degree BSN

Available Programs Generic Baccalaureate; RN Baccalaureate.

Study Options Full-time and part-time.

Program Entrance Requirements Minimum overall college GPA of 3.0, transcript of college record, CPR certification, health exam, health insurance, high school biology, high school chemistry, high school foreign language, 3 years high school math, high school transcript, immunizations, minimum GPA in nursing prerequisites of 3.0, prerequisite course work. Transfer students are accepted. *Application deadline:* 4/1 (fall), 10/25 (winter), 11/30 (spring), 4/15 (summer). Applications may be processed on a rolling basis for some programs. *Application fee:* $25.

Advanced Placement Credit by examination available. Credit given for nursing courses completed elsewhere dependent upon specific evaluations.

Expenses (2011–12) *Tuition:* full-time $25,730; part-time $798 per credit hour. *International tuition:* $25,730 full-time. *Room and board:* $3000 per academic year. *Required fees:* full-time $285; part-time $50 per term.

Financial Aid 90% of baccalaureate students in nursing programs received some form of financial aid in 2010–11.

Contact Prof. Dolores A. Hilden, PhD, Nursing Department, Program in Nursing (BSN), St. Ambrose University, 518 West Locust Street, Davenport, IA 52803. *Telephone:* 563-333-6076. *E-mail:* nursing@sau.edu.

GRADUATE PROGRAMS

Expenses (2011–12) *Tuition:* full-time $25,730; part-time $798 per credit hour. *Required fees:* part-time $50 per term.
Financial Aid 100% of graduate students in nursing programs received some form of financial aid in 2010–11.
Contact Ms. Kathryn M. McKnight, Director of MSN Program, Program in Nursing (BSN), St. Ambrose University, 1320 West Lombard Street, Davenport, IA 52804-2029. *Telephone:* 563-333-6069. *Fax:* 563-333-6063. *E-mail:* mcknightkathrynm@sau.edu.

MASTER'S DEGREE PROGRAM

Degree MSN
Available Programs Master's.
Concentrations Available Health-care administration; nursing administration.
Study Options Part-time.
Program Entrance Requirements Clinical experience, minimum overall college GPA of 3.0, transcript of college record, CPR certification, immunizations, 3 letters of recommendation, physical assessment course, resume, statistics course. *Application deadline:* 4/15 (fall). Applications may be processed on a rolling basis for some programs. *Application fee:* $25.
Advanced Placement Credit given for nursing courses completed elsewhere dependent upon specific evaluations.
Degree Requirements 37 total credit hours, thesis or project.

CONTINUING EDUCATION PROGRAM

Contact Dr. Dolores A. Hilden, Chairperson, Program in Nursing (BSN), St. Ambrose University, 1320 West Lombard Street, Davenport, IA 52804-2029. *Telephone:* 563-333-6076. *Fax:* 563-333-6063. *E-mail:* hildendoloresa@sau.edu.

University of Dubuque
School of Professional Programs
Dubuque, Iowa

http://www.dbq.edu/nursing/index.cfm
Founded in 1852
DEGREE • BSN
Nursing Program Faculty 8 (1% with doctorates).
Baccalaureate Enrollment 58 **Women** 86% **Men** 14% **Minority** 2%
Nursing Student Activities Student Nurses' Association.
Nursing Student Resources Academic advising; academic or career counseling; assistance for students with disabilities; bookstore; campus computer network; career placement assistance; computer lab; daycare for children of students; e-mail services; employment services for current students; interactive nursing skills videos; Internet; learning resource lab; library services; nursing audiovisuals; resume preparation assistance; skills, simulation, or other laboratory; tutoring; unpaid internships.
Library Facilities 183,336 volumes; 51,859 periodical subscriptions.

BACCALAUREATE PROGRAMS

Degree BSN
Available Programs RN Baccalaureate.
Study Options Full-time.
Program Entrance Requirements Transcript of college record, CPR certification, health exam, health insurance, immunizations, 2 letters of recommendation, minimum GPA in nursing prerequisites of 2.75, professional liability insurance/malpractice insurance, prerequisite course work. Transfer students are accepted.
Contact *Telephone:* 563-589-3000.

The University of Iowa
College of Nursing
Iowa City, Iowa

http://www.nursing.uiowa.edu/
Founded in 1847
DEGREES • BSN • MSN • MSN/MBA • MSN/MPH • PHD
Nursing Program Faculty 67 (63% with doctorates).
Baccalaureate Enrollment 618 **Women** 93% **Men** 7% **Minority** 6% **Part-time** 25%

Graduate Enrollment 258 **Women** 89% **Men** 11% **Minority** 4% **International** 7% **Part-time** 50%
Nursing Student Activities Sigma Theta Tau, Student Nurses' Association.
Nursing Student Resources Academic advising; academic or career counseling; assistance for students with disabilities; campus computer network; career placement assistance; computer lab; computer-assisted instruction; e-mail services; employment services for current students; Internet; learning resource lab; nursing audiovisuals; placement services for program completers; resume preparation assistance; skills, simulation, or other laboratory; tutoring.
Library Facilities 6.1 million volumes (273,469 in health); 106,486 periodical subscriptions (2,500 health-care related).

BACCALAUREATE PROGRAMS

Degree BSN
Available Programs Generic Baccalaureate; RN Baccalaureate.
Study Options Full-time and part-time.
Program Entrance Requirements Minimum overall college GPA of 2.7, transcript of college record, CPR certification, written essay, health exam, health insurance, high school biology, high school chemistry, high school foreign language, 3 years high school math, 3 years high school science, high school transcript, immunizations, minimum GPA in nursing prerequisites of 2.7, professional liability insurance/malpractice insurance, prerequisite course work. Transfer students are accepted.
Advanced Placement Credit given for nursing courses completed elsewhere dependent upon specific evaluations.
Contact *Telephone:* 319-335-7016. *Fax:* 319-384-4423.

GRADUATE PROGRAMS

Contact *Telephone:* 319-335-7021. *Fax:* 319-335-9990.

MASTER'S DEGREE PROGRAM

Degrees MSN; MSN/MBA; MSN/MPH
Available Programs Accelerated RN to Master's; Master's; Master's for Nurses with Non-Nursing Degrees.
Concentrations Available Nurse anesthesia; nursing administration; nursing education; nursing informatics. *Clinical nurse specialist programs in:* adult health, community health, gerontology, occupational health, psychiatric/mental health. *Nurse practitioner programs in:* adult health, family health, gerontology, neonatal health, pediatric, psychiatric/mental health.
Study Options Full-time and part-time.
Program Entrance Requirements Computer literacy, minimum overall college GPA of 3.0, transcript of college record, written essay, immunizations, 3 letters of recommendation, nursing research course, physical assessment course, professional liability insurance/malpractice insurance, prerequisite course work, resume, statistics course.
Advanced Placement Credit given for nursing courses completed elsewhere dependent upon specific evaluations.
Degree Requirements 33 total credit hours, thesis or project.

POST-MASTER'S PROGRAM

Areas of Study Nursing informatics. *Clinical nurse specialist programs in:* adult health, psychiatric/mental health. *Nurse practitioner programs in:* adult health, family health, gerontology, pediatric, psychiatric/mental health.

DOCTORAL DEGREE PROGRAM

Degree PhD
Available Programs Doctorate; Post-Baccalaureate Doctorate.
Areas of Study Aging, family health, gerontology, individualized study, information systems, nursing administration.
Program Entrance Requirements Minimum overall college GPA of 3.0, interview, 3 letters of recommendation, statistics course, vita, GRE General Test.
Degree Requirements 60 total credit hours, dissertation, oral exam, written exam, residency.

POSTDOCTORAL PROGRAM

Areas of Study Family health, nursing informatics, nursing interventions, outcomes.
Postdoctoral Program Contact *Telephone:* 319-335-7021. *Fax:* 319-335-9990.

CONTINUING EDUCATION PROGRAM

Contact *Telephone:* 319-335-7075. *Fax:* 319-335-9990.

Upper Iowa University
RN-BSN Nursing Program
Fayette, Iowa

http://www.uiu.edu/nursing/
Founded in 1857
DEGREE • BSN
Nursing Program Faculty 10
Library Facilities 74,813 volumes; 284 periodical subscriptions.

BACCALAUREATE PROGRAMS

Degree BSN
Available Programs RN Baccalaureate.
Site Options Cedar Rapids, IA; West Des Moines, IA.
Program Entrance Requirements Minimum overall college GPA of 2.5, transcript of college record, CPR certification, health exam, high school transcript, RN licensure. Transfer students are accepted.
Contact *Telephone:* 563-425-5357.

KANSAS

Baker University
School of Nursing
Topeka, Kansas

http://www.bakeru.edu/
Founded in 1858
DEGREE • BSN
Nursing Program Faculty 16 (25% with doctorates).
Baccalaureate Enrollment 167 **Women** 90% **Men** 10% **Minority** 11%
International 1% **Part-time** .1%
Nursing Student Activities Sigma Theta Tau, Student Nurses' Association.
Nursing Student Resources Academic advising; assistance for students with disabilities; campus computer network; computer lab; computer-assisted instruction; e-mail services; Internet; learning resource lab; library services; nursing audiovisuals; resume preparation assistance; skills, simulation, or other laboratory; tutoring.
Library Facilities 106,549 volumes (5,000 in health, 2,716 in nursing); 160 periodical subscriptions (414 health-care related).

BACCALAUREATE PROGRAMS

Degree BSN
Available Programs Generic Baccalaureate; RN Baccalaureate.
Study Options Full-time and part-time.
Program Entrance Requirements Transcript of college record, CPR certification, written essay, health exam, health insurance, high school transcript, immunizations, interview, minimum GPA in nursing prerequisites of 2.7, prerequisite course work. Transfer students are accepted. *Application deadline:* 12/1 (fall), 8/1 (spring).
Advanced Placement Credit given for nursing courses completed elsewhere dependent upon specific evaluations.
Expenses (2012–13) *Tuition:* full-time $15,550; part-time $518 per credit hour. *International tuition:* $15,550 full-time.
Financial Aid 87% of baccalaureate students in nursing programs received some form of financial aid in 2011–12.
Contact Ms. Cara Bonfiglio, Student Affairs Specialist, School of Nursing, Baker University, 1500 SW 10th Street, Topeka, KS 66604-1353. *Telephone:* 785-354-5850. *Fax:* 785-354-5832. *E-mail:* cbonfig@stormontvail.org.

Benedictine College
Department of Nursing
Atchison, Kansas

Founded in 1859
DEGREE • BSN
Library Facilities 207,316 volumes; 32,834 periodical subscriptions.

BACCALAUREATE PROGRAMS

Degree BSN
Available Programs Generic Baccalaureate.
Program Entrance Requirements Written essay, 2 letters of recommendation, minimum high school GPA of 2.75, prerequisite course work. *Application deadline:* 1/15 (fall).
Contact Lynne Connelly, Director of Nursing, Department of Nursing, Benedictine College, 1020 North 2nd Street, Atchison, KS 66002. *Telephone:* 913-360-7560. *E-mail:* lconnelly@benedictine.edu.

Bethel College
Department of Nursing
North Newton, Kansas

http://www.bethelks.edu/
Founded in 1887
DEGREE • BSN
Nursing Program Faculty 8
Baccalaureate Enrollment 42 **Women** 75% **Men** 25% **Minority** 30%
International 25% **Part-time** 1%
Distance Learning Courses Available.
Nursing Student Activities Nursing Honor Society, Sigma Theta Tau, Student Nurses' Association.
Nursing Student Resources Academic advising; academic or career counseling; assistance for students with disabilities; bookstore; campus computer network; computer lab; e-mail services; employment services for current students; housing assistance; Internet; learning resource lab; library services; nursing audiovisuals; resume preparation assistance; skills, simulation, or other laboratory; tutoring.
Library Facilities 5,690 volumes in health, 3,150 volumes in nursing; 445 periodical subscriptions health-care related.

BACCALAUREATE PROGRAMS

Degree BSN
Available Programs Generic Baccalaureate; LPN to Baccalaureate; RN Baccalaureate.
Study Options Full-time and part-time.
Online Degree Options Yes.
Program Entrance Requirements Minimum overall college GPA of 3.0, transcript of college record, CPR certification, written essay, health exam, health insurance, high school transcript, immunizations, interview, 2 letters of recommendation, minimum high school GPA of 2.75, minimum GPA in nursing prerequisites of 2.0, prerequisite course work. Transfer students are accepted. *Application deadline:* 2/1 (fall).
Advanced Placement Credit given for nursing courses completed elsewhere dependent upon specific evaluations.
Financial Aid 99% of baccalaureate students in nursing programs received some form of financial aid in 2010–11. *Gift aid (need-based):* Federal Pell, FSEOG, state, college/university gift aid from institutional funds. *Loans:* Federal Direct (Subsidized and Unsubsidized Stafford PLUS), Perkins. *Work-study:* Federal Work-Study, part-time campus jobs. *Financial aid application deadline (priority):* 4/1.
Contact Phyllis J. Miller, Director, Department of Nursing, Department of Nursing, Bethel College, 300 East 27th Street, North Newton, KS 67117. *Telephone:* 316-283-5295 Ext. 377. *Fax:* 316-284-5286. *E-mail:* pmiller@bethelks.edu.

Emporia State University
Newman Division of Nursing
Emporia, Kansas

http://www.emporia.edu/nursing
Founded in 1863
DEGREE • BSN
Nursing Program Faculty 12 (17% with doctorates).
Baccalaureate Enrollment 125 **Women** 94% **Men** 6% **Minority** 20%
International 2%
Nursing Student Activities Sigma Theta Tau, Student Nurses' Association.
Nursing Student Resources Academic advising; academic or career counseling; assistance for students with disabilities; bookstore; campus computer network; career placement assistance; computer lab; computer-assisted instruction; daycare for children of students; e-mail services;

employment services for current students; housing assistance; interactive nursing skills videos; Internet; learning resource lab; library services; nursing audiovisuals; placement services for program completers; remedial services; resume preparation assistance; skills, simulation, or other laboratory; tutoring.
Library Facilities 2.5 million volumes (53,197 in health, 2,200 in nursing); 41,417 periodical subscriptions (186 health-care related).

BACCALAUREATE PROGRAMS

Degree BSN
Available Programs ADN to Baccalaureate; Generic Baccalaureate; LPN to Baccalaureate; RN Baccalaureate.
Study Options Full-time.
Program Entrance Requirements Transcript of college record, written essay, minimum GPA in nursing prerequisites of 2.5, prerequisite course work. Transfer students are accepted. *Application deadline:* 5/1 (fall). *Application fee:* $25.
Advanced Placement Credit given for nursing courses completed elsewhere dependent upon specific evaluations.
Expenses (2012–13) *Tuition, area resident:* full-time $4102; part-time $137 per credit hour. *Tuition, state resident:* full-time $6154; part-time $205 per credit hour. *Tuition, nonresident:* full-time $15,156; part-time $505 per credit hour. *International tuition:* $15,156 full-time. *Room and board:* $7133 per academic year. *Required fees:* full-time $1170; part-time $140 per credit.
Financial Aid 90% of baccalaureate students in nursing programs received some form of financial aid in 2011–12. *Gift aid (need-based):* Federal Pell, FSEOG, state, private, college/university gift aid from institutional funds, Jones Foundation Grants. *Loans:* Perkins, Alaska Loans, alternative loans. *Work-study:* Federal Work-Study, part-time campus jobs. *Financial aid application deadline (priority):* 3/15.
Contact Dr. Jean M. DeDonder, Interim Chair and Associate Professor, Newman Division of Nursing, Emporia State University, Newman Division of Nursing, 1127 Chestnut Street, Emporia, KS 66801. *Telephone:* 620-343-6800 Ext. 5640. *Fax:* 620-341-7871. *E-mail:* jdedonde@emporia.edu.

Fort Hays State University
Department of Nursing
Hays, Kansas

http://www.fhsu.edu/nursing/
Founded in 1902
DEGREES • BSN • MSN • MSN/ED D
Nursing Program Faculty 20 (15% with doctorates).
Baccalaureate Enrollment 195 **Women** 91% **Men** 9% **Minority** 10% **Part-time** 52%
Graduate Enrollment 104 **Women** 95% **Men** 5% **Minority** 20% **Part-time** 87%
Distance Learning Courses Available.
Nursing Student Activities Sigma Theta Tau, Student Nurses' Association, nursing club.
Nursing Student Resources Academic advising; academic or career counseling; assistance for students with disabilities; bookstore; campus computer network; career placement assistance; computer lab; computer-assisted instruction; daycare for children of students; e-mail services; employment services for current students; housing assistance; interactive nursing skills videos; Internet; learning resource lab; library services; nursing audiovisuals; paid internships; placement services for program completers; remedial services; resume preparation assistance; skills, simulation, or other laboratory; tutoring.
Library Facilities 11,526 volumes in health, 2,378 volumes in nursing; 243 periodical subscriptions health-care related.

BACCALAUREATE PROGRAMS

Degree BSN
Available Programs Generic Baccalaureate; RN Baccalaureate.
Study Options Full-time and part-time.
Online Degree Options Yes.
Program Entrance Requirements Minimum overall college GPA of 2.5, transcript of college record, CPR certification, written essay, health exam, health insurance, high school transcript, immunizations, 2 letters of recommendation, minimum GPA in nursing prerequisites of 2.75, professional liability insurance/malpractice insurance, prerequisite course work, RN licensure. Transfer students are accepted. *Application deadline:* 3/1 (fall), 10/1 (spring).

Advanced Placement Credit by examination available. Credit given for nursing courses completed elsewhere dependent upon specific evaluations.
Expenses (2012–13) *Tuition, area resident:* part-time $141 per credit hour. *Tuition, state resident:* part-time $195 per credit hour. *Tuition, nonresident:* part-time $414 per credit hour. *Room and board:* $7003; room only: $3475 per academic year.
Financial Aid 75% of baccalaureate students in nursing programs received some form of financial aid in 2011–12.
Contact Mrs. Carolyn Insley, Coordinator of BSN Program, Department of Nursing, Fort Hays State University, 600 Park Street, Stroup Hall, Room 147, Hays, KS 67601-4099. *Telephone:* 785-628-4514. *Fax:* 785-628-4080. *E-mail:* cinsley@fhsu.edu.

GRADUATE PROGRAMS

Expenses (2012–13) *Tuition, area resident:* part-time $195 per credit hour. *Tuition, state resident:* part-time $276 per credit hour. *Tuition, nonresident:* part-time $494 per credit hour. *Room and board:* $7003; room only: $3475 per academic year.
Financial Aid 52% of graduate students in nursing programs received some form of financial aid in 2011–12. 1 teaching assistantship (averaging $5,000 per year) was awarded; research assistantships.
Contact Mrs. Janelle Harding, Assistant Professor, Department of Nursing, Fort Hays State University, 600 Park Street, Stroup Hall, Room 159, Hays, KS 67601-4099. *Telephone:* 785-628-4517. *Fax:* 785-628-4080. *E-mail:* jrharding@fhsu.edu.

MASTER'S DEGREE PROGRAM

Degrees MSN; MSN/Ed D
Available Programs Master's.
Concentrations Available Nursing administration; nursing education. *Nurse practitioner programs in:* family health.
Study Options Full-time and part-time.
Program Entrance Requirements Clinical experience, computer literacy, minimum overall college GPA of 3.0, transcript of college record, CPR certification, written essay, immunizations, 2 letters of recommendation, physical assessment course, professional liability insurance/malpractice insurance, prerequisite course work, statistics course, GRE General Test or MAT. *Application deadline:* 2/1 (fall), 9/1 (spring), 2/1 (summer).
Advanced Placement Credit given for nursing courses completed elsewhere dependent upon specific evaluations.
Degree Requirements 51 total credit hours, thesis or project, comprehensive exam.

POST-MASTER'S PROGRAM

Areas of Study Nursing administration; nursing education. *Nurse practitioner programs in:* family health.

Kansas Wesleyan University
Department of Nursing Education
Salina, Kansas

http://kwu.edu/academics/academic-departments/nursing
Founded in 1886
DEGREE • BSN
Nursing Program Faculty 8 (13% with doctorates).
Baccalaureate Enrollment 68 **Women** 91% **Men** 9% **Minority** 12% **International** 3% **Part-time** 2%
Nursing Student Activities Nursing club.
Nursing Student Resources Academic advising; academic or career counseling; assistance for students with disabilities; bookstore; campus computer network; career placement assistance; computer lab; computer-assisted instruction; e-mail services; employment services for current students; housing assistance; Internet; learning resource lab; library services; nursing audiovisuals; resume preparation assistance; skills, simulation, or other laboratory; tutoring.
Library Facilities 97,060 volumes (15,921 in health, 8,700 in nursing); 188 periodical subscriptions (1,123 health-care related).

BACCALAUREATE PROGRAMS

Degree BSN
Available Programs ADN to Baccalaureate; Generic Baccalaureate; RN Baccalaureate.
Study Options Full-time and part-time.

Program Entrance Requirements Minimum overall college GPA of 2.6, transcript of college record, health exam, high school transcript, immunizations, minimum GPA in nursing prerequisites of 2.6, prerequisite course work. Transfer students are accepted. *Application deadline:* Applications may be processed on a rolling basis for some programs.

Advanced Placement Credit by examination available. Credit given for nursing courses completed elsewhere dependent upon specific evaluations.

Contact *Telephone:* 785-827-5541 Ext. 2311. *Fax:* 785-827-0927.

MidAmerica Nazarene University
Division of Nursing
Olathe, Kansas

http://www.mnu.edu/
Founded in 1966
DEGREES • BSN • MSN
Nursing Program Faculty 55 (52% with doctorates).
Baccalaureate Enrollment 270
Graduate Enrollment 112
Distance Learning Courses Available.
Nursing Student Activities Nursing Honor Society, Student Nurses' Association, nursing club.
Nursing Student Resources Academic advising; academic or career counseling; assistance for students with disabilities; bookstore; campus computer network; career placement assistance; computer lab; computer-assisted instruction; e-mail services; employment services for current students; housing assistance; interactive nursing skills videos; Internet; learning resource lab; library services; nursing audiovisuals; remedial services; resume preparation assistance; skills, simulation, or other laboratory; tutoring; unpaid internships.
Library Facilities 106,268 volumes (1,903 in health, 547 in nursing); 275 periodical subscriptions (115 health-care related).

BACCALAUREATE PROGRAMS

Degree BSN
Available Programs ADN to Baccalaureate; Accelerated Baccalaureate; Accelerated Baccalaureate for Second Degree; Accelerated LPN to Baccalaureate; Accelerated RN Baccalaureate; Baccalaureate for Second Degree; Generic Baccalaureate; RN Baccalaureate.
Site Options Liberty, MO; Ottawa, KS.
Study Options Full-time and part-time.
Online Degree Options Yes.
Program Entrance Requirements Minimum overall college GPA of 2.6, transcript of college record, written essay, health insurance, high school transcript, immunizations, 2 letters of recommendation, minimum GPA in nursing prerequisites of 2.6, prerequisite course work. Transfer students are accepted. *Application deadline:* 10/1 (fall), 2/1 (spring).
Advanced Placement Credit by examination available. Credit given for nursing courses completed elsewhere dependent upon specific evaluations.
Financial Aid 80% of baccalaureate students in nursing programs received some form of financial aid in 2011–12.
Contact Dr. Susan G. Larson, Dean, School of Nursing and Health Science, Division of Nursing, MidAmerica Nazarene University, 2030 East College Way, Olathe, KS 66062-1899. *Telephone:* 913-971-3698. *Fax:* 913-971-3408. *E-mail:* slarson@mnu.edu.

GRADUATE PROGRAMS

Financial Aid 50% of graduate students in nursing programs received some form of financial aid in 2011–12.
Contact Dr. Karen D. Wiegman, Department Chair, Graduate Studies in Nursing, Division of Nursing, MidAmerica Nazarene University, 2030 East College Way, Olathe, KS 66062-1899. *Telephone:* 913-971-3081. *E-mail:* kdwiegman@mnu.edu.

MASTER'S DEGREE PROGRAM
Degree MSN
Available Programs Accelerated Master's; Master's.
Concentrations Available Health-care administration; nursing education.
Site Options Liberty, MO.

Study Options Full-time and part-time.
Program Entrance Requirements Transcript of college record, 2 letters of recommendation, prerequisite course work, statistics course. *Application deadline:* Applications may be processed on a rolling basis for some programs.
Advanced Placement Credit by examination available. Credit given for nursing courses completed elsewhere dependent upon specific evaluations.
Degree Requirements 36 total credit hours, thesis or project.

Newman University
Division of Nursing
Wichita, Kansas

http://www.newmanu.edu/
Founded in 1933
DEGREE • BSN
Nursing Program Faculty 23 (17% with doctorates).
Baccalaureate Enrollment 114 **Women** 93% **Men** 7% **Minority** 14.9% **International** 2.6% **Part-time** .01%
Graduate Enrollment 47 **Women** 46.8% **Men** 53.2% **Minority** .04%
Nursing Student Activities Sigma Theta Tau, nursing club.
Nursing Student Resources Academic advising; academic or career counseling; assistance for students with disabilities; bookstore; campus computer network; computer lab; computer-assisted instruction; e-mail services; Internet; learning resource lab; library services; nursing audiovisuals; remedial services; resume preparation assistance; skills, simulation, or other laboratory; tutoring.
Library Facilities 100,214 volumes (2,940 in health, 763 in nursing); 7,015 periodical subscriptions (769 health-care related).

BACCALAUREATE PROGRAMS

Degree BSN
Available Programs Generic Baccalaureate; LPN to Baccalaureate; RN Baccalaureate.
Study Options Full-time and part-time.
Online Degree Options Yes.
Program Entrance Requirements Minimum overall college GPA of 2.85, transcript of college record, CPR certification, written essay, health exam, health insurance, immunizations, interview, 2 letters of recommendation, minimum GPA in nursing prerequisites of 2.85, professional liability insurance/malpractice insurance, prerequisite course work. Transfer students are accepted. *Application deadline:* Applications may be processed on a rolling basis for some programs.
Advanced Placement Credit given for nursing courses completed elsewhere dependent upon specific evaluations.
Expenses (2012–13) *Tuition:* full-time $21,388; part-time $713 per credit hour. *International tuition:* $21,388 full-time. *Room and board:* $3200 per academic year. *Required fees:* full-time $502; part-time $15 per credit.
Financial Aid 43% of baccalaureate students in nursing programs received some form of financial aid in 2011–12.
Contact Dr. Bernadette M. Fetterolf, RN, Associate Dean, School of Nursing and Allied Health, Division of Nursing, Newman University, 3100 McCormick Avenue, Wichita, KS 67213-2097. *Telephone:* 316-942-4291 Ext. 2244. *Fax:* 316-942-4483. *E-mail:* fetterolfb@newmanu.edu.

GRADUATE PROGRAMS

Expenses (2012–13) *Tuition:* full-time $22,500; part-time $750 per credit hour. *Room and board:* $5600 per academic year. *Required fees:* full-time $500.
Financial Aid 100% of graduate students in nursing programs received some form of financial aid in 2011–12. *Application deadline:* 8/15.
Contact Ms. Sharon Niemann, Director, Master of Science in Nurse Anesthesia Program, Division of Nursing, Newman University, 3100 McCormick Avenue, Wichita, KS 67213-2097. *Telephone:* 316-942-4291 Ext. 2272. *Fax:* 316-942-4483. *E-mail:* niemanns@newmanu.edu.

MASTER'S DEGREE PROGRAM
Program Entrance Requirements MAT.

Pittsburg State University
Department of Nursing
Pittsburg, Kansas

http://www.pittstate.edu/nurs
Founded in 1903
DEGREES • BSN • MSN
Nursing Program Faculty 23 (25% with doctorates).
Baccalaureate Enrollment 142 **Women** 93% **Men** 7% **Minority** 100% **International** 1%
Graduate Enrollment 67 **Women** 90% **Men** 10% **Minority** 100% **International** 1%
Distance Learning Courses Available.
Nursing Student Activities Nursing Honor Society, Sigma Theta Tau, Student Nurses' Association.
Nursing Student Resources Academic advising; academic or career counseling; assistance for students with disabilities; bookstore; campus computer network; career placement assistance; computer lab; computer-assisted instruction; e-mail services; employment services for current students; externships; housing assistance; interactive nursing skills videos; Internet; learning resource lab; library services; nursing audiovisuals; placement services for program completers; resume preparation assistance; skills, simulation, or other laboratory; tutoring; unpaid internships.
Library Facilities 712,681 volumes (45,044 in nursing); 35,360 periodical subscriptions.

BACCALAUREATE PROGRAMS

Degree BSN
Available Programs Generic Baccalaureate; RN Baccalaureate.
Study Options Full-time and part-time.
Online Degree Options Yes.
Program Entrance Requirements Minimum overall college GPA of 2.5, transcript of college record, CPR certification, health exam, immunizations, 3 letters of recommendation, minimum GPA in nursing prerequisites of 2.5, professional liability insurance/malpractice insurance, prerequisite course work. Transfer students are accepted. *Application deadline:* 12/15 (fall). *Application fee:* $25.
Advanced Placement Credit by examination available. Credit given for nursing courses completed elsewhere dependent upon specific evaluations.
Contact *Telephone:* 620-235-4437. *Fax:* 620-235-4449.

GRADUATE PROGRAMS

Contact *Telephone:* 620-235-4431. *Fax:* 620-235-4449.

MASTER'S DEGREE PROGRAM
Degree MSN
Available Programs Master's.
Concentrations Available Clinical nurse leader; nursing administration; nursing education. *Clinical nurse specialist programs in:* family health. *Nurse practitioner programs in:* family health.
Study Options Full-time and part-time.
Program Entrance Requirements Clinical experience, minimum overall college GPA of 3.0, transcript of college record, CPR certification, written essay, immunizations, 3 letters of recommendation, nursing research course, physical assessment course, professional liability insurance/malpractice insurance, prerequisite course work, statistics course, GRE General Test. *Application deadline:* 3/15 (fall). *Application fee:* $50.
Advanced Placement Credit given for nursing courses completed elsewhere dependent upon specific evaluations.
Degree Requirements 47 total credit hours, thesis or project, comprehensive exam.

POST-MASTER'S PROGRAM
Areas of Study Clinical nurse leader; nursing administration; nursing education. *Clinical nurse specialist programs in:* family health. *Nurse practitioner programs in:* family health.

CONTINUING EDUCATION PROGRAM

Contact *Telephone:* 620-235-4434. *Fax:* 620-235-4449.

Southwestern College
Nursing Program
Winfield, Kansas

Founded in 1885
DEGREE • BSN
Nursing Program Faculty 6 (33% with doctorates).
Baccalaureate Enrollment 79
Nursing Student Activities Nursing Honor Society, Sigma Theta Tau, Student Nurses' Association, nursing club.
Nursing Student Resources Academic advising; academic or career counseling; assistance for students with disabilities; bookstore; campus computer network; career placement assistance; computer lab; computer-assisted instruction; e-mail services; externships; housing assistance; interactive nursing skills videos; Internet; learning resource lab; library services; nursing audiovisuals; paid internships; placement services for program completers; remedial services; resume preparation assistance; skills, simulation, or other laboratory; tutoring; unpaid internships.
Library Facilities 59,712 volumes; 140 periodical subscriptions.

BACCALAUREATE PROGRAMS

Degree BSN
Available Programs Accelerated RN Baccalaureate; Generic Baccalaureate; LPN to Baccalaureate; RN Baccalaureate.
Site Options Wichita, KS.
Study Options Full-time and part-time.
Online Degree Options Yes.
Program Entrance Requirements Transcript of college record, CPR certification, written essay, health exam, health insurance, high school transcript, immunizations, interview, minimum high school GPA of 2.75, minimum GPA in nursing prerequisites of 2.75, professional liability insurance/malpractice insurance, prerequisite course work. Transfer students are accepted.
Advanced Placement Credit given for nursing courses completed elsewhere dependent upon specific evaluations.
Contact *Telephone:* 620-229-6207. *Fax:* 620-229-6152 Ext. 6152.

Tabor College
Department of Nursing
Hillsboro, Kansas

http://www.tabor.edu/
Founded in 1908
DEGREE • BSN
Nursing Program Faculty 12
Baccalaureate Enrollment 71 **Women** 90% **Men** 10% **Minority** 10% **Part-time** 100%
Distance Learning Courses Available.
Nursing Student Activities Sigma Theta Tau.
Nursing Student Resources Academic advising; academic or career counseling; bookstore; campus computer network; computer lab; e-mail services; Internet; learning resource lab; library services; nursing audiovisuals; remedial services; resume preparation assistance; skills, simulation, or other laboratory; tutoring.
Library Facilities 77,175 volumes (240 in health, 140 in nursing); 142 periodical subscriptions (600 health-care related).

BACCALAUREATE PROGRAMS

Degree BSN
Available Programs ADN to Baccalaureate; Accelerated RN Baccalaureate.
Site Options Wichita, KS; Colby, KS; Larned, KS.
Study Options Full-time and part-time.
Online Degree Options Yes (online only).
Program Entrance Requirements Minimum overall college GPA of 2.5, transcript of college record, RN licensure. Transfer students are accepted. *Application deadline:* 8/31 (fall), 12/31 (spring), 4/30 (summer). Applications may be processed on a rolling basis for some programs. *Application fee:* $30.
Advanced Placement Credit by examination available. Credit given for nursing courses completed elsewhere dependent upon specific evaluations.
Contact *Telephone:* 316-729-6333 Ext. 206. *Fax:* 316-773-5436.

The University of Kansas
School of Nursing
Kansas City, Kansas

http://www.nursing.kumc.edu
Founded in 1866
DEGREES • BSN • MS • MS/MHSA • MS/MPH • PHD
Nursing Program Faculty 74 (58% with doctorates).
Baccalaureate Enrollment 260 **Women** 88% **Men** 12% **Minority** 11%
International 1% **Part-time** 10%
Graduate Enrollment 411 **Women** 93% **Men** 7% **Minority** 16% **International** 1% **Part-time** 93%
Distance Learning Courses Available.
Nursing Student Activities Nursing Honor Society, Sigma Theta Tau, Student Nurses' Association, nursing club.
Nursing Student Resources Academic advising; academic or career counseling; assistance for students with disabilities; bookstore; campus computer network; computer lab; computer-assisted instruction; e-mail services; employment services for current students; interactive nursing skills videos; Internet; learning resource lab; library services; nursing audiovisuals; remedial services; resume preparation assistance; skills, simulation, or other laboratory.
Library Facilities 5.1 million volumes (180,000 in health, 5,050 in nursing); 95,214 periodical subscriptions (6,500 health-care related).

BACCALAUREATE PROGRAMS

Degree BSN
Available Programs ADN to Baccalaureate; Generic Baccalaureate; RN Baccalaureate.
Study Options Full-time and part-time.
Program Entrance Requirements Minimum overall college GPA of 2.5, transcript of college record, CPR certification, written essay, health exam, health insurance, immunizations, 3 letters of recommendation, minimum GPA in nursing prerequisites of 2.5, prerequisite course work. Transfer students are accepted. *Application deadline:* 10/15 (fall). *Application fee:* $60.
Advanced Placement Credit given for nursing courses completed elsewhere dependent upon specific evaluations.
Expenses (2011–12) *Tuition, state resident:* part-time $246 per credit hour. *Tuition, nonresident:* part-time $646 per credit hour. *International tuition:* $646 full-time. *Required fees:* full-time $485.
Financial Aid 65% of baccalaureate students in nursing programs received some form of financial aid in 2010–11. *Gift aid (need-based):* Federal Pell, FSEOG, state, private, college/university gift aid from institutional funds, Federal Nursing. *Loans:* Federal Nursing Student Loans, Federal Direct (Subsidized and Unsubsidized Stafford PLUS), Perkins, college/university. *Work-study:* Federal Work-Study, part-time campus jobs. *Financial aid application deadline (priority):* 3/1.
Contact Debra J. Ford, PhD, Associate Dean of Student Affairs, School of Nursing, The University of Kansas, 3901 Rainbow Boulevard, Mail Stop 2029, Kansas City, KS 66160. *Telephone:* 913-588-1619. *Fax:* 913-588-1615. *E-mail:* dford@kumc.edu.

GRADUATE PROGRAMS

Expenses (2011–12) *Tuition, state resident:* part-time $304 per credit hour. *Tuition, nonresident:* part-time $726 per credit hour. *International tuition:* $726 full-time. *Required fees:* full-time $485.
Financial Aid 52% of graduate students in nursing programs received some form of financial aid in 2010–11. Research assistantships with full and partial tuition reimbursements available, teaching assistantships with full and partial tuition reimbursements available, traineeships available. *Financial aid application deadline:* 2/14.
Contact Debra J. Ford, PhD, Associate Dean, Student Affairs, School of Nursing, The University of Kansas, 3901 Rainbow Boulevard, Mail Stop 2029, Kansas City, KS 66160. *Telephone:* 913-588-1619. *Fax:* 913-588-1615. *E-mail:* dford@kumc.edu.

MASTER'S DEGREE PROGRAM

Degrees MS; MS/MHSA; MS/MPH
Available Programs Master's; RN to Master's.
Concentrations Available Health-care administration; nurse-midwifery; nursing administration; nursing informatics. *Clinical nurse specialist programs in:* adult health, gerontology. *Nurse practitioner programs in:* adult health, family health, gerontology, psychiatric/mental health.
Site Options Garden City, KS.

Study Options Full-time and part-time.
Online Degree Options Yes.
Program Entrance Requirements Clinical experience, minimum overall college GPA of 3.0, transcript of college record, CPR certification, immunizations, interview, 3 letters of recommendation, physical assessment course, resume, statistics course. *Application deadline:* 4/1 (fall), 9/1 (spring). *Application fee:* $60.
Degree Requirements 37 total credit hours, thesis or project, comprehensive exam.

POST-MASTER'S PROGRAM

Areas of Study Health-care administration; nurse-midwifery; nursing administration; nursing informatics. *Clinical nurse specialist programs in:* adult health, gerontology. *Nurse practitioner programs in:* adult health, family health, gerontology, psychiatric/mental health.

DOCTORAL DEGREE PROGRAM

Degree PhD
Available Programs Doctorate; Post-Baccalaureate Doctorate.
Areas of Study Nursing research.
Online Degree Options Yes.
Program Entrance Requirements Clinical experience, minimum overall college GPA of 3.5, interview by faculty committee, interview, 3 letters of recommendation, statistics course, vita, writing sample, GRE General Test. *Application deadline:* 12/1 (summer). *Application fee:* $60.
Degree Requirements 65 total credit hours, dissertation, oral exam, written exam, residency.

POSTDOCTORAL PROGRAM

Areas of Study Gerontology, nursing research, outcomes, self-care.
Postdoctoral Program Contact Dr. Marjorie J. Bott, Associate Dean, Research, School of Nursing, The University of Kansas, 3901 Rainbow Boulevard, Mail Stop 4043, Kansas City, KS 66160. *Telephone:* 913-588-1692. *E-mail:* mbott@kumc.edu.

CONTINUING EDUCATION PROGRAM

Contact Dr. Mary Gambino, Assistant Dean, Community Affairs, School of Nursing, The University of Kansas, 3901 Rainbow Boulevard, Mail Stop 4001, Kansas City, KS 66160. *Telephone:* 913-588-4488. *Fax:* 913-588-4486. *E-mail:* ceinfo@kumc.edu.

University of Saint Mary
Bachelor of Science in Nursing Program
Leavenworth, Kansas

http://www.stmary.edu/acad_nursing/default.asp
Founded in 1923
DEGREE • BSN
Nursing Program Faculty 22 (9% with doctorates).
Baccalaureate Enrollment 168 **Women** 93% **Men** 7% **Minority** 12.5%
International 3.5% **Part-time** 39%
Distance Learning Courses Available.
Nursing Student Activities Student Nurses' Association.
Nursing Student Resources Academic advising; academic or career counseling; bookstore; campus computer network; e-mail services; employment services for current students; Internet; learning resource lab; library services; nursing audiovisuals; placement services for program completers; resume preparation assistance; skills, simulation, or other laboratory; tutoring.
Library Facilities 120,366 volumes; 153 periodical subscriptions.

BACCALAUREATE PROGRAMS

Degree BSN
Available Programs Generic Baccalaureate; RN Baccalaureate.
Site Options Overland Park, KS.
Study Options Full-time.
Online Degree Options Yes (online only).
Program Entrance Requirements Minimum overall college GPA of 2.5, transcript of college record, CPR certification, written essay, health exam, health insurance, immunizations, 2 letters of recommendation, minimum GPA in nursing prerequisites of 2.5, prerequisite course work. Transfer students are accepted. *Application deadline:* 3/1 (fall). Applications may be processed on a rolling basis for some programs.
Contact *Telephone:* 913-758-4381. *Fax:* 913-758-4356.

Washburn University

School of Nursing
Topeka, Kansas

http://www.washburn.edu/academics/college-schools/nursing/index.html
Founded in 1865
DEGREES • BSN • MSN
Nursing Program Faculty 29 (24% with doctorates).

Baccalaureate Enrollment 315 **Women** 89% **Men** 11% **Minority** 10% **International** 1% **Part-time** 1%

Graduate Enrollment 51 **Women** 90% **Men** 10% **Minority** 1% **Part-time** 70%

Nursing Student Activities Sigma Theta Tau, Student Nurses' Association, nursing club.

Nursing Student Resources Academic advising; academic or career counseling; assistance for students with disabilities; bookstore; campus computer network; career placement assistance; computer lab; computer-assisted instruction; e-mail services; employment services for current students; interactive nursing skills videos; Internet; learning resource lab; library services; nursing audiovisuals; remedial services; resume preparation assistance; skills, simulation, or other laboratory; tutoring; unpaid internships.

Library Facilities 456,610 volumes (12,880 in health, 1,612 in nursing); 36,802 periodical subscriptions (84 health-care related).

BACCALAUREATE PROGRAMS

Degree BSN

Available Programs ADN to Baccalaureate; Baccalaureate for Second Degree; Generic Baccalaureate; LPN to Baccalaureate; RN Baccalaureate.

Study Options Full-time.

Program Entrance Requirements Minimum overall college GPA of 2.7, transcript of college record, CPR certification, written essay, health exam, health insurance, immunizations, interview, 2 letters of recommendation, minimum GPA in nursing prerequisites of 2.0, professional liability insurance/malpractice insurance, prerequisite course work. Transfer students are accepted.

Advanced Placement Credit by examination available. Credit given for nursing courses completed elsewhere dependent upon specific evaluations.

Contact *Telephone:* 785-231-1032 Ext. 1525. *Fax:* 785-231-1032.

GRADUATE PROGRAMS

Contact *Telephone:* 785-231-1010 Ext. 1533. *Fax:* 785-213-1032.

MASTER'S DEGREE PROGRAM

Degree MSN

Available Programs Master's.

Concentrations Available Nursing administration. *Nurse practitioner programs in:* adult health, family health.

Study Options Full-time and part-time.

Program Entrance Requirements Computer literacy, transcript of college record, CPR certification, written essay, immunizations, 2 letters of recommendation, nursing research course, physical assessment course, professional liability insurance/malpractice insurance, prerequisite course work, resume, statistics course. *Application deadline:* 3/15 (fall). *Application fee:* $35.

Degree Requirements 42 total credit hours, thesis or project.

POST-MASTER'S PROGRAM

Areas of Study Nursing education.

CONTINUING EDUCATION PROGRAM

Contact *Telephone:* 785-231-1010 Ext. 1526. *Fax:* 785-231-1032.

Wichita State University

School of Nursing
Wichita, Kansas

http://www.wichita.edu/nurs
Founded in 1895
DEGREES • BSN • DNP
Nursing Program Faculty 51 (25% with doctorates).
Baccalaureate Enrollment 251 **Women** 90% **Men** 10% **Minority** 21% **International** 4% **Part-time** 1%
Graduate Enrollment 150 **Women** 94% **Men** 6% **Minority** 6% **International** 1% **Part-time** 66%
Distance Learning Courses Available.
Nursing Student Activities Sigma Theta Tau, Student Nurses' Association.
Nursing Student Resources Academic advising; academic or career counseling; assistance for students with disabilities; bookstore; campus computer network; career placement assistance; computer lab; computer-assisted instruction; daycare for children of students; e-mail services; employment services for current students; housing assistance; interactive nursing skills videos; Internet; learning resource lab; library services; nursing audiovisuals; resume preparation assistance; skills, simulation, or other laboratory.
Library Facilities 1.9 million volumes (31,320 in health, 2,746 in nursing); 61,010 periodical subscriptions (406 health-care related).

BACCALAUREATE PROGRAMS

Degree BSN
Available Programs ADN to Baccalaureate; Accelerated Baccalaureate; Accelerated Baccalaureate for Second Degree; Generic Baccalaureate; LPN to RN Baccalaureate; RN Baccalaureate.
Site Options Derby, KS.
Study Options Full-time.
Online Degree Options Yes.
Program Entrance Requirements Minimum overall college GPA of 2.75, transcript of college record, CPR certification, written essay, health exam, health insurance, immunizations, interview, minimum GPA in nursing prerequisites of 2.0, professional liability insurance/malpractice insurance, prerequisite course work. Transfer students are accepted. *Application deadline:* 2/1 (fall), 9/1 (spring).
Advanced Placement Credit given for nursing courses completed elsewhere dependent upon specific evaluations.
Financial Aid 80% of baccalaureate students in nursing programs received some form of financial aid in 2010–11.
Contact Ms. Courtney Fleetwood, Senior Academic Advisor, School of Nursing, Wichita State University, 1845 Fairmount Street, Wichita, KS 67260-0041. *Telephone:* 316-978-5732. *Fax:* 316-978-3094. *E-mail:* courtney.fleetwood@wichita.edu.

GRADUATE PROGRAMS

Financial Aid 60% of graduate students in nursing programs received some form of financial aid in 2010–11.
Contact Dr. Alicia Huckstadt, Director, Graduate Program, School of Nursing, Wichita State University, 1845 Fairmount Street, Wichita, KS 67260-0041. *Telephone:* 316-978-3610. *Fax:* 316-978-3094. *E-mail:* alicia.huckstadt@wichita.edu.

MASTER'S DEGREE PROGRAM

Program Entrance Requirements *Application deadline:* Applications may be processed on a rolling basis for some programs. *Application fee:* $35.

DOCTORAL DEGREE PROGRAM

Degree DNP
Available Programs Doctorate; Post-Baccalaureate Doctorate.
Areas of Study Advanced practice nursing, clinical practice, critical care, faculty preparation, family health, health policy, health promotion/disease prevention, health-care systems, human health and illness, nursing administration, nursing education, nursing policy, nursing research, nursing science.
Program Entrance Requirements Clinical experience, minimum overall college GPA of 3.0, interview by faculty committee, interview, 2 letters of recommendation, statistics course, vita. *Application deadline:* 2/15 (fall), 10/15 (spring). *Application fee:* $35.
Degree Requirements 74 total credit hours, written exam, residency.

KENTUCKY

Bellarmine University

Donna and Allan Lansing School of Nursing and Health Sciences
Louisville, Kentucky

http://www.bellarmine.edu/
Founded in 1950

DEGREES • BSN • DNP • MSN • MSN/MBA

Nursing Program Faculty 85 (15% with doctorates).

Baccalaureate Enrollment 210 **Women** 88.8% **Men** 11.2% **Minority** 9.26% **International** .24% **Part-time** 18%

Graduate Enrollment 79 **Women** 92.8% **Men** 7.2% **Minority** 3.2% **Part-time** 89.6%

Nursing Student Activities Sigma Theta Tau, Student Nurses' Association.

Nursing Student Resources Academic advising; academic or career counseling; assistance for students with disabilities; bookstore; campus computer network; career placement assistance; computer lab; computer-assisted instruction; e-mail services; employment services for current students; externships; housing assistance; interactive nursing skills videos; Internet; learning resource lab; library services; nursing audiovisuals; paid internships; placement services for program completers; remedial services; resume preparation assistance; skills, simulation, or other laboratory; tutoring; unpaid internships.

Library Facilities 136,183 volumes (4,670 in health, 1,644 in nursing); 418 periodical subscriptions (93 health-care related).

BACCALAUREATE PROGRAMS

Degree BSN

Available Programs Accelerated Baccalaureate for Second Degree; Generic Baccalaureate; RN Baccalaureate.

Study Options Full-time and part-time.

Program Entrance Requirements Minimum overall college GPA of 2.5, transcript of college record, CPR certification, written essay, health exam, health insurance, high school biology, high school chemistry, 2 years high school math, 2 years high school science, high school transcript, immunizations, interview, minimum high school GPA of 2.75, minimum GPA in nursing prerequisites of 2.75, prerequisite course work. Transfer students are accepted. *Application deadline:* 8/15 (fall), 1/3 (winter), 1/3 (spring), 5/3 (summer). Applications may be processed on a rolling basis for some programs. *Application fee:* $25.

Advanced Placement Credit by examination available. Credit given for nursing courses completed elsewhere dependent upon specific evaluations.

Financial Aid 77% of baccalaureate students in nursing programs received some form of financial aid in 2011–12. *Gift aid (need-based):* Federal Pell, FSEOG, state, private, college/university gift aid from institutional funds. *Loans:* Federal Direct (Subsidized and Unsubsidized Stafford PLUS), Perkins, college/university. *Work-study:* Federal Work-Study, part-time campus jobs. *Financial aid application deadline (priority):* 3/1.

Contact Dr. Beverley Holland, BSN Department Chairperson, Donna and Allan Lansing School of Nursing and Health Sciences, Bellarmine University, 2001 Newburg Road, Miles Hall, #202, Louisville, KY 40205-0671. *Telephone:* 502-452-8279. *Fax:* 502-452-8058. *E-mail:* bholland@bellarmine.edu.

GRADUATE PROGRAMS

Financial Aid 77% of graduate students in nursing programs received some form of financial aid in 2011–12. Career-related internships or fieldwork and scholarships available.

Contact Ms. Julie Armstrong-Binnix, Marketing/Recruiter, Donna and Allan Lansing School of Nursing and Health Sciences, Bellarmine University, 2001 Newburg Road, Miles Hall, #201, Louisville, KY 40205-0671. *Telephone:* 502-452-8364. *Fax:* 502-452-8058. *E-mail:* julieab@bellarmine.edu.

MASTER'S DEGREE PROGRAM

Degrees MSN; MSN/MBA

Available Programs Master's; Master's for Nurses with Non-Nursing Degrees; RN to Master's.

Concentrations Available Nursing administration; nursing education.

Study Options Part-time.

Program Entrance Requirements Minimum overall college GPA of 2.75, transcript of college record, professional liability insurance/malpractice insurance, GRE General Test. *Application deadline:* 8/20 (fall), 1/5 (winter), 1/5 (spring), 5/1 (summer). Applications may be processed on a rolling basis for some programs. *Application fee:* $25.

Advanced Placement Credit given for nursing courses completed elsewhere dependent upon specific evaluations.

Degree Requirements 38 total credit hours, thesis or project.

POST-MASTER'S PROGRAM

Areas of Study *Nurse practitioner programs in:* family health.

DOCTORAL DEGREE PROGRAM

Degree DNP

Available Programs Doctorate for Nurses with Non-Nursing Degrees.

Areas of Study Advanced practice nursing, family health.

Program Entrance Requirements Minimum overall college GPA of 3.5, interview by faculty committee, 3 letters of recommendation, MSN or equivalent, vita, GRE General Test. *Application deadline:* 8/15 (fall), 1/5 (spring), 5/3 (summer). *Application fee:* $25.

Degree Requirements Residency.

CONTINUING EDUCATION PROGRAM

Contact Ms. Linda Bailey, Director, Continuing Education, Donna and Allan Lansing School of Nursing and Health Sciences, Bellarmine University, 2001 Newburg Road, Continuing Education Office, Louisville, KY 40205-0671. *Telephone:* 502-452-8161. *Fax:* 502-452-8203. *E-mail:* lbailey@bellarmine.edu.

Berea College

Department of Nursing
Berea, Kentucky

http://www.berea.edu/nur/
Founded in 1855

DEGREE • BSN

Nursing Program Faculty 9 (2% with doctorates).

Baccalaureate Enrollment 48 **Women** 90% **Men** 10% **Minority** 10% **International** 12.5%

Nursing Student Activities Student Nurses' Association.

Nursing Student Resources Academic advising; academic or career counseling; assistance for students with disabilities; bookstore; campus computer network; career placement assistance; computer lab; computer-assisted instruction; daycare for children of students; e-mail services; employment services for current students; externships; housing assistance; interactive nursing skills videos; Internet; learning resource lab; library services; nursing audiovisuals; paid internships; placement services for program completers; remedial services; resume preparation assistance; skills, simulation, or other laboratory; tutoring; unpaid internships.

Library Facilities 392,752 volumes; 1,438 periodical subscriptions.

BACCALAUREATE PROGRAMS

Degree BSN

Available Programs Generic Baccalaureate.

Study Options Full-time.

Program Entrance Requirements Minimum overall college GPA of 2.5, transcript of college record, CPR certification, written essay, high school transcript, immunizations, interview, 3 letters of recommendation, minimum high school GPA, minimum high school rank 15%, minimum GPA in nursing prerequisites of 2.5, prerequisite course work. Transfer students are accepted. *Application deadline:* Applications may be processed on a rolling basis for some programs.

Advanced Placement Credit given for nursing courses completed elsewhere dependent upon specific evaluations.

Contact *Telephone:* 859-985-3503.

Eastern Kentucky University
Department of Baccalaureate and Graduate Nursing
Richmond, Kentucky

http://www.bsn-gn.eku.edu/
Founded in 1906
DEGREES • BSN • MSN
Nursing Program Faculty 42 (40% with doctorates).
Baccalaureate Enrollment 500
Graduate Enrollment 200
Distance Learning Courses Available.
Nursing Student Activities Sigma Theta Tau, Student Nurses' Association.
Nursing Student Resources Academic advising; academic or career counseling; assistance for students with disabilities; bookstore; campus computer network; computer lab; computer-assisted instruction; e-mail services; housing assistance; interactive nursing skills videos; Internet; learning resource lab; library services; nursing audiovisuals; skills, simulation, or other laboratory.
Library Facilities 799,496 volumes; 2,901 periodical subscriptions.

BACCALAUREATE PROGRAMS

Degree BSN
Available Programs Accelerated RN Baccalaureate; Baccalaureate for Second Degree; Generic Baccalaureate; RN Baccalaureate.
Site Options Hazard, KY; Corbin, KY; Danville, KY.
Study Options Full-time and part-time.
Program Entrance Requirements Minimum overall college GPA of 2.5, CPR certification, immunizations, professional liability insurance/malpractice insurance, prerequisite course work. Transfer students are accepted.
Advanced Placement Credit given for nursing courses completed elsewhere dependent upon specific evaluations.
Contact *Telephone:* 859-622-1827. *Fax:* 859-622-1972.

GRADUATE PROGRAMS

Contact *Telephone:* 859-622-1838. *Fax:* 859-622-1972.

MASTER'S DEGREE PROGRAM
Degree MSN
Available Programs Master's.
Concentrations Available Nursing education. *Clinical nurse specialist programs in:* public health. *Nurse practitioner programs in:* family health, psychiatric/mental health.
Site Options Hazard, KY; Corbin, KY; Danville, KY.
Study Options Full-time and part-time.
Program Entrance Requirements Minimum overall college GPA of 2.75, transcript of college record, written essay, 3 letters of recommendation, statistics course.
Advanced Placement Credit given for nursing courses completed elsewhere dependent upon specific evaluations.
Degree Requirements 48 total credit hours, thesis or project, comprehensive exam.

Frontier Nursing University
Nursing Degree Programs
Hyden, Kentucky

Founded in 1939
DEGREES • DNP • MSN

GRADUATE PROGRAMS

Contact *Telephone:* 606-672-2312.

MASTER'S DEGREE PROGRAM
Degree MSN
Available Programs Accelerated AD/RN to Master's.

DOCTORAL DEGREE PROGRAM
Degree DNP
Available Programs Doctorate.

Kentucky Christian University
School of Nursing
Grayson, Kentucky

http://www.kcu.edu/template.php?area=academics&page=nursing/
Founded in 1919
DEGREE • BSN
Nursing Program Faculty 6 (20% with doctorates).
Baccalaureate Enrollment 63 **Women** 90% **Men** 10% **Minority** 1% **International** 1%
Nursing Student Activities Student Nurses' Association.
Nursing Student Resources Academic advising; assistance for students with disabilities; bookstore; campus computer network; computer lab; e-mail services; housing assistance; interactive nursing skills videos; Internet; learning resource lab; library services; nursing audiovisuals; other; remedial services; skills, simulation, or other laboratory.
Library Facilities 184,169 volumes (400 in health, 300 in nursing); 37,275 periodical subscriptions (200 health-care related).

BACCALAUREATE PROGRAMS

Degree BSN
Available Programs Generic Baccalaureate.
Study Options Full-time.
Program Entrance Requirements Transcript of college record, written essay, health exam, health insurance, high school transcript, immunizations, minimum GPA in nursing prerequisites of 2.5, prerequisite course work. Transfer students are accepted.
Contact *Telephone:* 606-474-3255. *Fax:* 606-474-3342.

CONTINUING EDUCATION PROGRAM

Contact *Telephone:* 606-474-3271. *Fax:* 606-474-3342.

Kentucky State University
School of Nursing
Frankfort, Kentucky

http://www.kysu.edu/
Founded in 1886
DEGREE • BSN
Nursing Program Faculty 18 (11% with doctorates).
Baccalaureate Enrollment 25
Nursing Student Activities Student Nurses' Association.
Nursing Student Resources Academic advising; academic or career counseling; assistance for students with disabilities; bookstore; campus computer network; career placement assistance; computer lab; computer-assisted instruction; e-mail services; externships; housing assistance; interactive nursing skills videos; Internet; learning resource lab; library services; nursing audiovisuals; other; placement services for program completers; remedial services; resume preparation assistance; skills, simulation, or other laboratory; tutoring.
Library Facilities 326,821 volumes; 864 periodical subscriptions.

BACCALAUREATE PROGRAMS

Degree BSN
Available Programs ADN to Baccalaureate.
Program Entrance Requirements Transfer students are accepted.
Contact *Telephone:* 502-597-6963. *Fax:* 502-597-5818.

Midway College
Program in Nursing (Baccalaureate)
Midway, Kentucky

http://www.midway.edu/academic-programs/nursing-science
Founded in 1847
DEGREE • BSN
Nursing Program Faculty 3 (33% with doctorates).
Baccalaureate Enrollment 70 **Women** 99% **Men** 1% **Minority** 20% **Part-time** 50%
Distance Learning Courses Available.

Nursing Student Activities Student Nurses' Association.
Nursing Student Resources Academic advising; academic or career counseling; assistance for students with disabilities; bookstore; campus computer network; career placement assistance; computer lab; computer-assisted instruction; e-mail services; externships; interactive nursing skills videos; Internet; learning resource lab; library services; nursing audiovisuals; placement services for program completers; remedial services; resume preparation assistance; skills, simulation, or other laboratory; tutoring; unpaid internships.
Library Facilities 96,236 volumes (1,200 in health, 800 in nursing); 250 periodical subscriptions (102 health-care related).

BACCALAUREATE PROGRAMS

Degree BSN
Available Programs ADN to Baccalaureate; Accelerated RN Baccalaureate; RN Baccalaureate.
Study Options Full-time and part-time.
Program Entrance Requirements Transfer students are accepted. *Application deadline:* 3/15 (fall), 3/15 (winter), 10/15 (spring), 3/15 (summer). Applications may be processed on a rolling basis for some programs. *Application fee:* $10.
Advanced Placement Credit given for nursing courses completed elsewhere dependent upon specific evaluations.
Expenses (2012–13) *Tuition:* full-time $530.
Financial Aid 100% of baccalaureate students in nursing programs received some form of financial aid in 2011–12.
Contact Dr. Barbara R. Kitchen, Chair, Nursing and Science Programs, Program in Nursing (Baccalaureate), Midway College, 512 East Stephens Street, Midway, KY 40347. *Telephone:* 859-846-5335. *Fax:* 859-846-5876. *E-mail:* bkitchen@midway.edu.

CONTINUING EDUCATION PROGRAM

Contact Dr. Barbara R. Kitchen, Chair, Nursing and Science Programs, Program in Nursing (Baccalaureate), Midway College, 512 East Stephens Street, Midway, KY 40347. *Telephone:* 859-846-5335. *Fax:* 859-846-5876. *E-mail:* bkitchen@midway.edu.

Morehead State University
Department of Nursing
Morehead, Kentucky

http://www.moreheadstate.edu/nursing
Founded in 1922
DEGREE • BSN
Nursing Program Faculty 52 (15% with doctorates).
Baccalaureate Enrollment 141 **Women** 84% **Men** 16% **Minority** 3% **Part-time** 5%
Distance Learning Courses Available.
Nursing Student Activities Student Nurses' Association.
Nursing Student Resources Academic advising; academic or career counseling; assistance for students with disabilities; bookstore; campus computer network; career placement assistance; computer lab; computer-assisted instruction; e-mail services; interactive nursing skills videos; Internet; learning resource lab; library services; nursing audiovisuals; remedial services; resume preparation assistance; skills, simulation, or other laboratory; tutoring.
Library Facilities 591,287 volumes (500,000 in health, 860 in nursing); 56,528 periodical subscriptions (286 health-care related).

BACCALAUREATE PROGRAMS

Degree BSN
Available Programs ADN to Baccalaureate; Generic Baccalaureate; RN Baccalaureate.
Site Options Prestonsburg, KY; Ashland, KY; Mt. Sterling, KY.
Study Options Full-time.
Online Degree Options Yes.
Program Entrance Requirements Minimum overall college GPA of 2.0, transcript of college record, CPR certification, immunizations, minimum GPA in nursing prerequisites of 3.0, prerequisite course work. Transfer students are accepted. *Application deadline:* 3/15 (fall).
Advanced Placement Credit by examination available. Credit given for nursing courses completed elsewhere dependent upon specific evaluations.
Expenses (2012–13) *Tuition, state resident:* full-time $7284; part-time $276 per credit hour. *Tuition, nonresident:* full-time $18,216; part-time

$690 per credit hour. *International tuition:* $18,216 full-time. *Room and board:* $7210; room only: $3630 per academic year. *Required fees:* full-time $650.
Financial Aid 80% of baccalaureate students in nursing programs received some form of financial aid in 2011–12. *Gift aid (need-based):* Federal Pell, FSEOG, state, private, college/university gift aid from institutional funds. *Loans:* Federal Direct (Subsidized and Unsubsidized Stafford PLUS), Perkins, college/university.*Work-study:* Federal Work-Study, part-time campus jobs.*Financial aid application deadline (priority):* 3/15.
Contact Ms. Carla June Aagaard, Academic Counseling Coordinator, Department of Nursing, Morehead State University, CHER 201A, Morehead, KY 40351. *Telephone:* 606-783-2641. *Fax:* 606-783-9211. *E-mail:* c.aagaard@moreheadstate.edu.

Murray State University
Program in Nursing
Murray, Kentucky

http://www.murraystate.edu/
Founded in 1922
DEGREES • BSN • MSN
Nursing Program Faculty 16 (47% with doctorates).
Baccalaureate Enrollment 206 **Women** 94% **Men** 6% **Minority** 3%
Graduate Enrollment 48 **Women** 85% **Men** 15%
Distance Learning Courses Available.
Nursing Student Activities Sigma Theta Tau, Student Nurses' Association.
Nursing Student Resources Academic advising; academic or career counseling; assistance for students with disabilities; bookstore; campus computer network; career placement assistance; computer lab; computer-assisted instruction; daycare for children of students; e-mail services; employment services for current students; externships; housing assistance; interactive nursing skills videos; Internet; learning resource lab; library services; nursing audiovisuals; placement services for program completers; remedial services; resume preparation assistance; skills, simulation, or other laboratory; tutoring; unpaid internships.
Library Facilities 933,382 volumes (4,060 in health, 2,160 in nursing); 1,381 periodical subscriptions (124 health-care related).

BACCALAUREATE PROGRAMS

Degree BSN
Available Programs Generic Baccalaureate; RN Baccalaureate.
Site Options Hopkinsville, KY; Paducah, KY; Madisonville, KY.
Study Options Full-time.
Program Entrance Requirements Transcript of college record, CPR certification, immunizations, minimum GPA in nursing prerequisites of 2.5, professional liability insurance/malpractice insurance, prerequisite course work. Transfer students are accepted. *Application deadline:* 5/1 (fall), 11/22 (spring).
Advanced Placement Credit by examination available. Credit given for nursing courses completed elsewhere dependent upon specific evaluations.
Contact *Telephone:* 270-809-2193. *Fax:* 270-809-6662.

GRADUATE PROGRAMS

Contact *Telephone:* 270-809-6671. *Fax:* 270-809-6662.

MASTER'S DEGREE PROGRAM
Degree MSN
Available Programs Master's.
Concentrations Available Nurse anesthesia. *Clinical nurse specialist programs in:* adult health, critical care, medical-surgical. *Nurse practitioner programs in:* family health.
Site Options Hopkinsville, KY; Paducah, KY; Madisonville, KY.
Study Options Full-time and part-time.
Program Entrance Requirements Clinical experience, minimum overall college GPA of 3.0, transcript of college record, CPR certification, immunizations, interview, 3 letters of recommendation, nursing research course, physical assessment course, professional liability insurance/malpractice insurance, prerequisite course work, statistics course, GRE General Test. *Application deadline:* 11/1 (fall).
Advanced Placement Credit given for nursing courses completed elsewhere dependent upon specific evaluations.
Degree Requirements 46 total credit hours.

POST-MASTER'S PROGRAM

Areas of Study Nurse anesthesia. *Clinical nurse specialist programs in:* adult health, critical care, medical-surgical. *Nurse practitioner programs in:* family health.

CONTINUING EDUCATION PROGRAM

Contact *Telephone:* 270-809-6674. *Fax:* 270-809-6662.

Northern Kentucky University
Department of Nursing
Highland Heights, Kentucky

http://www.nku.edu/majors/nursing.html
Founded in 1968
DEGREES • BSN • DNP • MSN
Nursing Program Faculty 100 (20% with doctorates).
Baccalaureate Enrollment 600 **Women** 93% **Men** 7% **Minority** 2% **International** 1% **Part-time** 50%
Graduate Enrollment 275 **Women** 95% **Men** 5% **Minority** 1% **Part-time** 90%
Distance Learning Courses Available.
Nursing Student Activities Sigma Theta Tau, Student Nurses' Association.
Nursing Student Resources Academic advising; academic or career counseling; assistance for students with disabilities; bookstore; campus computer network; career placement assistance; computer lab; computer-assisted instruction; daycare for children of students; e-mail services; employment services for current students; housing assistance; interactive nursing skills videos; Internet; learning resource lab; library services; nursing audiovisuals; resume preparation assistance; skills, simulation, or other laboratory; tutoring.
Library Facilities 892,212 volumes (6,380 in health, 3,500 in nursing); 813 periodical subscriptions (100 health-care related).

BACCALAUREATE PROGRAMS

Degree BSN
Available Programs Accelerated Baccalaureate for Second Degree; Generic Baccalaureate; RN Baccalaureate.
Study Options Full-time.
Program Entrance Requirements Minimum overall college GPA of 2.5, transcript of college record, CPR certification, health exam, health insurance, high school biology, high school chemistry, 3 years high school math, high school transcript, immunizations, minimum GPA in nursing prerequisites of 3.0, prerequisite course work. Transfer students are accepted. *Application deadline:* 1/15 (fall), 8/15 (spring).
Advanced Placement Credit by examination available. Credit given for nursing courses completed elsewhere dependent upon specific evaluations.
Expenses (2012–13) *Tuition, state resident:* full-time $3936; part-time $328 per credit hour. *Tuition, nonresident:* full-time $7872; part-time $656 per credit hour. *Room and board:* $7600; room only: $4200 per academic year. *Required fees:* full-time $250; part-time $125 per term.
Contact Dr. Carrie McCoy, Chair, Department of Nursing, Northern Kentucky University, Nunn Drive, AHC 303, Highland Heights, KY 41099. *Telephone:* 859-572-5248. *Fax:* 859-572-6098. *E-mail:* mccoy@nku.edu.

GRADUATE PROGRAMS

Expenses (2012–13) *Tuition, state resident:* part-time $510 per credit hour. *Tuition, nonresident:* part-time $765 per credit hour. *Room and board:* $7600; room only: $4200 per academic year. *Required fees:* part-time $45 per term.
Financial Aid 10% of graduate students in nursing programs received some form of financial aid in 2011–12.
Contact Dr. Jayne Lancaster, Interim Chair of Advanced Nursing Studies, Department of Nursing, Northern Kentucky University, HC 206, Highland Heights, KY 41099. *Telephone:* 859-572-7966. *Fax:* 859-572-1934. *E-mail:* lancasterj1@nku.edu.

MASTER'S DEGREE PROGRAM

Degree MSN
Available Programs Master's.
Concentrations Available Nursing administration; nursing education; nursing informatics. *Nurse practitioner programs in:* acute care, adult health, family health, pediatric.

Study Options Full-time and part-time.
Online Degree Options Yes.
Program Entrance Requirements Clinical experience, minimum overall college GPA of 3.0, transcript of college record, CPR certification, immunizations, 1 letter of recommendation, nursing research course, physical assessment course, professional liability insurance/malpractice insurance, prerequisite course work, resume, statistics course. *Application deadline:* 2/15 (fall), 10/15 (spring).
Advanced Placement Credit by examination available. Credit given for nursing courses completed elsewhere dependent upon specific evaluations.
Degree Requirements 42 total credit hours, thesis or project.

POST-MASTER'S PROGRAM

Areas of Study Nursing administration; nursing education. *Nurse practitioner programs in:* acute care, adult health, family health, pediatric, psychiatric/mental health.

DOCTORAL DEGREE PROGRAM

Degree DNP
Available Programs Doctorate.
Online Degree Options Yes.
Program Entrance Requirements Minimum overall college GPA of 3.0, 3 letters of recommendation, MSN or equivalent, statistics course, vita, writing sample. *Application deadline:* 2/15 (fall), 10/15 (spring).
Degree Requirements 36 total credit hours, dissertation.

CONTINUING EDUCATION PROGRAM

Contact Mary Gers, Director of Simulation and Technology, Department of Nursing, Northern Kentucky University, NKU, HC 303, Highland Heights, KY 41099. *Telephone:* 859-572-6322. *Fax:* 859-572-1934. *E-mail:* gersm@nku.edu.

Spalding University
School of Nursing
Louisville, Kentucky

http://www.spalding.edu/nursing
Founded in 1814
DEGREES • BSN • MSN
Nursing Program Faculty 33 (18% with doctorates).
Baccalaureate Enrollment 170 **Women** 94% **Men** 6% **Minority** 10% **International** 6%
Graduate Enrollment 56 **Women** 99.5% **Men** .5% **Minority** 2% **International** 3.4% **Part-time** 50%
Nursing Student Activities Sigma Theta Tau, Student Nurses' Association.
Nursing Student Resources Academic advising; academic or career counseling; assistance for students with disabilities; bookstore; campus computer network; career placement assistance; computer lab; computer-assisted instruction; e-mail services; employment services for current students; externships; interactive nursing skills videos; Internet; learning resource lab; library services; nursing audiovisuals; remedial services; resume preparation assistance; skills, simulation, or other laboratory; tutoring; unpaid internships.
Library Facilities 101,988 volumes (2,875 in health, 1,125 in nursing); 102 periodical subscriptions (367 health-care related).

BACCALAUREATE PROGRAMS

Degree BSN
Available Programs Accelerated Baccalaureate for Second Degree; Accelerated RN Baccalaureate; Generic Baccalaureate.
Study Options Full-time and part-time.
Program Entrance Requirements Minimum overall college GPA of 2.5, transcript of college record, CPR certification, health exam, health insurance, high school transcript, immunizations, minimum GPA in nursing prerequisites of 2.5, professional liability insurance/malpractice insurance, prerequisite course work. Transfer students are accepted.
Advanced Placement Credit given for nursing courses completed elsewhere dependent upon specific evaluations.
Contact *Telephone:* 502-585-7125. *Fax:* 502-588-7175.

GRADUATE PROGRAMS

Contact *Telephone:* 502-585-9911 Ext. 2332. *Fax:* 502-588-7175.

MASTER'S DEGREE PROGRAM

Degree MSN

Available Programs Accelerated RN to Master's; Master's.

Concentrations Available Nursing administration; nursing education. *Nurse practitioner programs in:* adult health, family health, pediatric.

Study Options Full-time and part-time.

Program Entrance Requirements Computer literacy, minimum overall college GPA of 3.0, transcript of college record, CPR certification, written essay, immunizations, interview, 2 letters of recommendation, physical assessment course, professional liability insurance/malpractice insurance, prerequisite course work, resume, statistics course, GRE General Test.

Advanced Placement Credit by examination available. Credit given for nursing courses completed elsewhere dependent upon specific evaluations.

Degree Requirements 53 total credit hours, thesis or project.

POST-MASTER'S PROGRAM

Areas of Study Nursing administration; nursing education. *Nurse practitioner programs in:* adult health, family health, pediatric.

CONTINUING EDUCATION PROGRAM

Contact *Telephone:* 502-585-9911 Ext. 2332. *Fax:* 502-588-7175.

Thomas More College

Program in Nursing
Crestview Hills, Kentucky

http://www.thomasmore.edu/
Founded in 1921

DEGREE • BSN

Nursing Program Faculty 7 (29% with doctorates).

Baccalaureate Enrollment 100 **Women** 92% **Men** 8% **Minority** .03% **International** .01%

Nursing Student Activities Student Nurses' Association.

Nursing Student Resources Academic advising; academic or career counseling; assistance for students with disabilities; bookstore; campus computer network; career placement assistance; computer lab; computer-assisted instruction; e-mail services; employment services for current students; externships; interactive nursing skills videos; Internet; learning resource lab; library services; nursing audiovisuals; other; placement services for program completers; remedial services; resume preparation assistance; skills, simulation, or other laboratory; tutoring.

Library Facilities 112,665 volumes (350 in health, 200 in nursing); 552 periodical subscriptions (50 health-care related).

BACCALAUREATE PROGRAMS

Degree BSN

Available Programs Generic Baccalaureate.

Study Options Full-time.

Program Entrance Requirements Transcript of college record, CPR certification, health exam, health insurance, high school transcript, immunizations, minimum GPA in nursing prerequisites of 2.75, professional liability insurance/malpractice insurance, prerequisite course work. Transfer students are accepted. *Application deadline:* 5/1 (fall). *Application fee:* $25.

Advanced Placement Credit given for nursing courses completed elsewhere dependent upon specific evaluations.

Financial Aid 90% of baccalaureate students in nursing programs received some form of financial aid in 2011–12. *Gift aid (need-based):* Federal Pell, FSEOG, state, private, college/university gift aid from institutional funds, Federal Nursing. *Loans:* Federal Nursing Student Loans, Federal Direct (Subsidized and Unsubsidized Stafford PLUS), Perkins, college/university.*Work-study:* Federal Work-Study, part-time campus jobs.*Financial aid application deadline (priority):* 3/15.

Contact Dr. Lisa Spangler Torok, Chair, Program in Nursing, Thomas More College, 333 Thomas More Parkway, Crestview Hills, KY 41017. *Telephone:* 859-344-3413. *Fax:* 859-344-3537. *E-mail:* lisa.spangler-torok@thomasmore.edu.

University of Kentucky

Graduate School Programs in the College of Nursing
Lexington, Kentucky

http://academics.uky.edu/ukcon/pub/Pages/Default.aspx
Founded in 1865

DEGREES • BSN • MSN • PHD

Nursing Program Faculty 65 (54% with doctorates).

Baccalaureate Enrollment 260 **Women** 97% **Men** 3% **Minority** 6% **Part-time** 14%

Graduate Enrollment 221 **Women** 92% **Men** 8% **Minority** 9% **International** 5% **Part-time** 35%

Nursing Student Activities Sigma Theta Tau, Student Nurses' Association.

Nursing Student Resources Academic advising; academic or career counseling; assistance for students with disabilities; bookstore; campus computer network; career placement assistance; computer lab; computer-assisted instruction; e-mail services; interactive nursing skills videos; Internet; learning resource lab; library services; nursing audiovisuals; skills, simulation, or other laboratory.

Library Facilities 105,793 volumes in health; 3,347 periodical subscriptions health-care related.

BACCALAUREATE PROGRAMS

Degree BSN

Available Programs Baccalaureate for Second Degree; Generic Baccalaureate; RN Baccalaureate.

Study Options Full-time and part-time.

Program Entrance Requirements Minimum overall college GPA of 2.5, transcript of college record, CPR certification, written essay, high school transcript, immunizations, minimum GPA in nursing prerequisites of 2.5, prerequisite course work. Transfer students are accepted.

Advanced Placement Credit by examination available. Credit given for nursing courses completed elsewhere dependent upon specific evaluations.

Contact *Telephone:* 859-323-5108. *Fax:* 859-323-1057.

GRADUATE PROGRAMS

Contact *Telephone:* 859-323-5108. *Fax:* 859-323-1057.

MASTER'S DEGREE PROGRAM

Degree MSN

Available Programs Master's; RN to Master's.

Concentrations Available Nurse case management; nursing administration. *Clinical nurse specialist programs in:* acute care, adult health, community health, critical care, gerontology, medical-surgical, oncology, parent-child, pediatric, perinatal, psychiatric/mental health, public health, women's health. *Nurse practitioner programs in:* acute care, adult health, family health, gerontology, pediatric, psychiatric/mental health.

Site Options Morehead, KY.

Study Options Full-time and part-time.

Program Entrance Requirements Clinical experience, minimum overall college GPA of 2.75, transcript of college record, written essay, interview, 3 letters of recommendation, physical assessment course, statistics course, GRE General Test.

Advanced Placement Credit given for nursing courses completed elsewhere dependent upon specific evaluations.

Degree Requirements 40 total credit hours, comprehensive exam.

POST-MASTER'S PROGRAM

Areas of Study Nurse case management. *Nurse practitioner programs in:* acute care, adult health, family health, gerontology, pediatric, psychiatric/mental health.

DOCTORAL DEGREE PROGRAM

Degree PhD

Available Programs Doctorate.

Areas of Study Nursing research.

Program Entrance Requirements Minimum overall college GPA of 3.3, interview, 3 letters of recommendation, MSN or equivalent, statistics course, writing sample, GRE General Test.

Degree Requirements 63 total credit hours, dissertation, oral exam, written exam, residency.

CONTINUING EDUCATION PROGRAM

Contact *Telephone:* 859-323-3851. *Fax:* 859-323-1057.

University of Louisville
School of Nursing
Louisville, Kentucky

http://www.louisville.edu/nursing
Founded in 1798
DEGREES • BSN • MSN • PHD
Nursing Program Faculty 72 (40% with doctorates).
Baccalaureate Enrollment 479 **Women** 89% **Men** 11% **Minority** 17%
International 1% **Part-time** 18%
Graduate Enrollment 137 **Women** 89% **Men** 11% **Minority** 18%
International 1% **Part-time** 48%
Distance Learning Courses Available.
Nursing Student Activities Sigma Theta Tau, Student Nurses' Association.
Nursing Student Resources Academic advising; academic or career counseling; assistance for students with disabilities; bookstore; campus computer network; career placement assistance; computer lab; computer-assisted instruction; e-mail services; employment services for current students; housing assistance; interactive nursing skills videos; Internet; learning resource lab; library services; nursing audiovisuals; skills, simulation, or other laboratory; tutoring.
Library Facilities 2.3 million volumes (253,595 in health, 2,806 in nursing); 81,310 periodical subscriptions (4,329 health-care related).

BACCALAUREATE PROGRAMS

Degree BSN
Available Programs Accelerated Baccalaureate for Second Degree; Generic Baccalaureate; RN Baccalaureate.
Site Options Owensboro, KY.
Study Options Full-time.
Online Degree Options Yes.
Program Entrance Requirements Minimum overall college GPA of 2.8, transcript of college record, CPR certification, written essay, health insurance, high school foreign language, 3 years high school math, 3 years high school science, high school transcript, immunizations, minimum high school GPA of 2.8, minimum GPA in nursing prerequisites of 2.8, professional liability insurance/malpractice insurance, prerequisite course work. Transfer students are accepted. *Application deadline:* 5/1 (fall), 9/15 (spring). *Application fee:* $40.
Advanced Placement Credit by examination available. Credit given for nursing courses completed elsewhere dependent upon specific evaluations.
Expenses (2012–13) *Tuition, state resident:* full-time $9466; part-time $395 per credit hour. *Tuition, nonresident:* full-time $22,950; part-time $957 per credit hour. *Room and board:* $5980; room only: $4520 per academic year. *Required fees:* full-time $1600.
Financial Aid 87% of baccalaureate students in nursing programs received some form of financial aid in 2011–12.
Contact Trish Hart, Director of Student Services, School of Nursing, University of Louisville, 555 South Floyd Street, Louisville, KY 40202. *Telephone:* 502-852-8298. *Fax:* 502-852-8783. *E-mail:* trish.hart@ louisville.edu.

GRADUATE PROGRAMS

Expenses (2012–13) *Tuition, state resident:* full-time $10,274; part-time $571 per credit hour. *Tuition, nonresident:* full-time $21,378; part-time $1188 per credit hour. *International tuition:* $21,378 full-time. *Room and board:* $5922 per academic year. *Required fees:* full-time $1600.
Financial Aid 87% of graduate students in nursing programs received some form of financial aid in 2011–12. 6 research assistantships with full tuition reimbursements available (averaging $20,000 per year), 6 teaching assistantships with full tuition reimbursements available (averaging $19,167 per year) were awarded; fellowships with full tuition reimbursements available, institutionally sponsored loans, scholarships, traineeships, and unspecified assistantships also available. Aid available to part-time students. *Financial aid application deadline:* 4/15.
Contact Dr. Rosalie Mainous, Associate Dean for Graduate Academic Affairs, School of Nursing, University of Louisville, 555 South Floyd Street, Louisville, KY 40292. *Telephone:* 502-852-8387. *Fax:* 502-852-8783. *E-mail:* rosalie.mainous@louisville.edu.

MASTER'S DEGREE PROGRAM

Degree MSN
Available Programs Master's.
Concentrations Available Nursing education. *Nurse practitioner programs in:* acute care, adult health, family health, neonatal health, psychiatric/mental health, women's health.
Study Options Full-time and part-time.
Program Entrance Requirements Clinical experience, minimum overall college GPA of 3.0, transcript of college record, CPR certification, written essay, immunizations, 2 letters of recommendation, professional liability insurance/malpractice insurance, GRE General Test. *Application deadline:* 4/1 (fall), 10/1 (spring). *Application fee:* $50.
Advanced Placement Credit given for nursing courses completed elsewhere dependent upon specific evaluations.
Degree Requirements 45 total credit hours.

POST-MASTER'S PROGRAM

Areas of Study *Nurse practitioner programs in:* acute care, adult health, family health, neonatal health, psychiatric/mental health, women's health.

DOCTORAL DEGREE PROGRAM

Degree PhD
Available Programs Doctorate; Post-Baccalaureate Doctorate.
Areas of Study Faculty preparation, health policy, individualized study, nursing research, nursing science.
Program Entrance Requirements Minimum overall college GPA of 3.0, interview by faculty committee, 3 letters of recommendation, vita, writing sample, GRE General Test. *Application deadline:* 2/1 (fall). *Application fee:* $50.
Degree Requirements Dissertation, written exam.

POSTDOCTORAL PROGRAM

Postdoctoral Program Contact Dr. Rosalie Mainous, Associate Dean for Graduate Academic Affairs, School of Nursing, University of Louisville, 555 South Floyd Street, Louisville, KY 40292. *Telephone:* 502-852-8387. *Fax:* 502-852-8783. *E-mail:* rosalie.mainous@ louisville.edu.

CONTINUING EDUCATION PROGRAM

Contact Dr. Deborah Thomas, Director, School of Nursing, University of Louisville, 555 South Floyd Street, K-3019, Louisville, KY 40292. *Telephone:* 502-852-8392. *Fax:* 502-852-8783. *E-mail:* dvthom01@ louisville.edu.

Western Kentucky University
School of Nursing
Bowling Green, Kentucky

http://www.wku.edu/nursing/
Founded in 1906
DEGREES • BSN • DNP • MSN
Nursing Program Faculty 50 (40% with doctorates).
Baccalaureate Enrollment 350 **Women** 89% **Men** 11% **Minority** 3%
Part-time 40%
Graduate Enrollment 150 **Women** 89% **Men** 11% **Minority** 2%
Distance Learning Courses Available.
Nursing Student Activities Nursing Honor Society, Sigma Theta Tau, Student Nurses' Association.
Nursing Student Resources Academic advising; academic or career counseling; assistance for students with disabilities; bookstore; campus computer network; career placement assistance; computer lab; computer-assisted instruction; e-mail services; employment services for current students; externships; housing assistance; interactive nursing skills videos; Internet; learning resource lab; library services; nursing audiovisuals; paid internships; placement services for program completers; remedial services; resume preparation assistance; skills, simulation, or other laboratory; tutoring; unpaid internships.
Library Facilities 1.9 million volumes (17,880 in health, 1,697 in nursing); 3,600 periodical subscriptions (217 health-care related).

BACCALAUREATE PROGRAMS

Degree BSN
Available Programs ADN to Baccalaureate; Baccalaureate for Second Degree; Generic Baccalaureate; RN Baccalaureate.
Study Options Full-time.

Program Entrance Requirements Minimum overall college GPA of 2.75, transcript of college record, CPR certification, health exam, health insurance, high school transcript, immunizations, minimum GPA in nursing prerequisites of 3.0, professional liability insurance/malpractice insurance, prerequisite course work. Transfer students are accepted. *Application deadline:* 1/15 (fall), 7/15 (spring).

Advanced Placement Credit by examination available. Credit given for nursing courses completed elsewhere dependent upon specific evaluations.

Expenses (2012–13) *Tuition, state resident:* full-time $9000; part-time $353 per credit hour. *Tuition, nonresident:* full-time $21,000; part-time $875 per credit hour. *Required fees:* full-time $800; part-time $400 per term.

Financial Aid 36% of baccalaureate students in nursing programs received some form of financial aid in 2011–12.

Contact Dr. Dawn Wright, Program Coordinator, School of Nursing, Western Kentucky University, 1906 College Heights Boulevard, Bowling Green, KY 42101-3576. *Telephone:* 270-745-3391. *Fax:* 270-745-3392. *E-mail:* dawn.wright@wku.edu.

GRADUATE PROGRAMS

Expenses (2012–13) *Tuition, area resident:* part-time $467 per credit hour. *Tuition, state resident:* part-time $583 per credit hour. *Tuition, nonresident:* part-time $583 per credit hour. *International tuition:* $962 full-time. *Required fees:* full-time $500.

Financial Aid 25% of graduate students in nursing programs received some form of financial aid in 2011–12. Research assistantships with partial tuition reimbursements available, teaching assistantships with partial tuition reimbursements available, Federal Work-Study, institutionally sponsored loans, traineeships, tuition waivers (partial), and unspecified assistantships available. Aid available to part-time students. *Financial aid application deadline:* 4/1.

Contact Dr. Beverly C. Siegrist, Professor, School of Nursing, Western Kentucky University, 1 Big Red Way, Academic Complex 108G, Bowling Green, KY 42101-3576. *Telephone:* 270-745-3490. *Fax:* 270-745-3392. *E-mail:* beverly.siegrist@wku.edu.

MASTER'S DEGREE PROGRAM

Degree MSN

Available Programs Accelerated Master's for Nurses with Non-Nursing Degrees; Master's.

Concentrations Available Nursing administration; nursing education.

Study Options Full-time and part-time.

Program Entrance Requirements Clinical experience, computer literacy, minimum overall college GPA of 2.75, transcript of college record, CPR certification, written essay, immunizations, interview, 3 letters of recommendation, nursing research course, physical assessment course, professional liability insurance/malpractice insurance, statistics course, GRE General Test. *Application deadline:* Applications may be processed on a rolling basis for some programs.

Advanced Placement Credit given for nursing courses completed elsewhere dependent upon specific evaluations.

Degree Requirements 45 total credit hours, thesis or project, comprehensive exam.

DOCTORAL DEGREE PROGRAM

Degree DNP

Available Programs Doctorate; Post-Baccalaureate Doctorate.

Areas of Study Advanced practice nursing, nursing administration.

Program Entrance Requirements Clinical experience, minimum overall college GPA of 2.75, interview by faculty committee, MSN or equivalent, statistics course, writing sample. *Application deadline:* Applications may be processed on a rolling basis for some programs. *Application fee:* $100.

Degree Requirements 42 total credit hours, written exam, residency.

CONTINUING EDUCATION PROGRAM

Contact Ms. Angela Drexler, School of Nursing, Western Kentucky University, 1 Big Red Way, Academic Complex 119, Bowling Green, KY 42101-3576. *Telephone:* 270-745-3762. *Fax:* 270-745-3392. *E-mail:* angelyn.drexler@wku.edu.

LOUISIANA

Dillard University
Division of Nursing
New Orleans, Louisiana

http://www.dillard.edu/index.php?option=com_content&view=article&id=106&Itemid=91

Founded in 1869

DEGREE • BSN
Nursing Program Faculty 13 (31% with doctorates).
Baccalaureate Enrollment 100 **Women** 98% **Men** 2% **Minority** 99% **International** 1%
Nursing Student Activities Nursing Honor Society, Sigma Theta Tau, Student Nurses' Association.
Nursing Student Resources Academic advising; academic or career counseling; assistance for students with disabilities; bookstore; campus computer network; career placement assistance; computer lab; computer-assisted instruction; e-mail services; externships; interactive nursing skills videos; Internet; learning resource lab; library services; nursing audiovisuals; paid internships; placement services for program completers; remedial services; resume preparation assistance; skills, simulation, or other laboratory; tutoring.
Library Facilities 105,128 volumes; 21 periodical subscriptions healthcare related.

BACCALAUREATE PROGRAMS

Degree BSN
Available Programs Generic Baccalaureate; LPN to Baccalaureate; LPN to RN Baccalaureate; RN Baccalaureate.
Study Options Full-time.
Program Entrance Requirements Minimum overall college GPA of 2.5, transcript of college record, CPR certification, health exam, health insurance, high school transcript, immunizations, minimum high school GPA of 2.5, minimum GPA in nursing prerequisites of 2.5, professional liability insurance/malpractice insurance, prerequisite course work. Transfer students are accepted. *Application deadline:* 3/1 (fall).
Expenses (2011–12) *Tuition:* full-time $13,650; part-time $569 per credit hour.
Financial Aid 99% of baccalaureate students in nursing programs received some form of financial aid in 2010–11. *Gift aid (need-based):* Federal Pell, FSEOG, state, private, college/university gift aid from institutional funds, United Negro College Fund, Federal Nursing. *Loans:* Federal Nursing Student Loans, Federal Direct (Subsidized and Unsubsidized Stafford PLUS), Perkins, alternative loans. *Work-study:* Federal Work-Study, part-time campus jobs. *Financial aid application deadline (priority):* 3/1.
Contact Dr. Lenetra L. Jefferson, School of Nursing, Division of Nursing, Dillard University, 2601 Gentilly Boulevard, New Orleans, LA 70122. *Telephone:* 504-816-4717. *Fax:* 504-816-4861. *E-mail:* ljefferson@dillard.edu.

CONTINUING EDUCATION PROGRAM

Contact Dr. Charlotte Hurst, PhD, Coordinator, Continuing Education, Division of Nursing, Dillard University, 2601 Gentilly Boulevard, PSB 102, New Orleans, LA 70122. *Telephone:* 504-816-4717. *Fax:* 504-816-4861. *E-mail:* churst@dillard.edu.

Grambling State University
School of Nursing
Grambling, Louisiana

Founded in 1901

DEGREES • BSN • MSN
Nursing Program Faculty 23 (20% with doctorates).
Baccalaureate Enrollment 600 **Women** 85% **Men** 15% **Minority** 68% **International** 9% **Part-time** 5%
Graduate Enrollment 41 **Women** 86% **Men** 14% **Minority** 66% **International** 12%
Distance Learning Courses Available.
Nursing Student Activities Student Nurses' Association.

Nursing Student Resources Academic advising; academic or career counseling; assistance for students with disabilities; bookstore; campus computer network; career placement assistance; computer lab; computer-assisted instruction; e-mail services; employment services for current students; interactive nursing skills videos; Internet; learning resource lab; library services; nursing audiovisuals; skills, simulation, or other laboratory; tutoring.
Library Facilities 322,995 volumes (10,000 in health, 5,000 in nursing); 1.2 million periodical subscriptions (65 health-care related).

BACCALAUREATE PROGRAMS

Degree BSN
Available Programs Generic Baccalaureate; LPN to RN Baccalaureate; RN Baccalaureate.
Study Options Full-time.
Program Entrance Requirements Transcript of college record, CPR certification, health exam, high school foreign language, 3 years high school math, 3 years high school science, high school transcript, immunizations, minimum high school GPA of 2.0, minimum GPA in nursing prerequisites of 2.75, professional liability insurance/malpractice insurance, prerequisite course work. Transfer students are accepted. *Application deadline:* 6/1 (fall), 12/1 (spring). *Application fee:* $20.
Advanced Placement Credit given for nursing courses completed elsewhere dependent upon specific evaluations.
Contact *Telephone:* 318-274-2528. *Fax:* 318-274-3491.

GRADUATE PROGRAMS

Contact *Telephone:* 318-274-2897. *Fax:* 318-274-3491.

MASTER'S DEGREE PROGRAM
Degree MSN
Available Programs Master's.
Concentrations Available Nursing education. *Clinical nurse specialist programs in:* adult health, maternity-newborn, pediatric. *Nurse practitioner programs in:* family health, pediatric.
Study Options Full-time and part-time.
Program Entrance Requirements Clinical experience, minimum overall college GPA of 3.0, transcript of college record, CPR certification, immunizations, interview, 3 letters of recommendation, physical assessment course, professional liability insurance/malpractice insurance, prerequisite course work, statistics course, GRE. *Application deadline:* 6/1 (fall). *Application fee:* $20.
Advanced Placement Credit given for nursing courses completed elsewhere dependent upon specific evaluations.
Degree Requirements 49 total credit hours, thesis or project, comprehensive exam.

POST-MASTER'S PROGRAM
Areas of Study *Nurse practitioner programs in:* family health.

Louisiana College
Department of Nursing
Pineville, Louisiana

http://www.lacollege.edu/
Founded in 1906
DEGREE • BSN
Nursing Program Faculty 6 (17% with doctorates).
Baccalaureate Enrollment 100
Nursing Student Activities Sigma Theta Tau, Student Nurses' Association.
Nursing Student Resources Academic advising; academic or career counseling; assistance for students with disabilities; bookstore; campus computer network; career placement assistance; computer lab; computer-assisted instruction; e-mail services; employment services for current students; externships; Internet; learning resource lab; library services; nursing audiovisuals; skills, simulation, or other laboratory; tutoring; unpaid internships.
Library Facilities 353,582 volumes (3,426 in health, 500 in nursing); 402 periodical subscriptions (142 health-care related).

BACCALAUREATE PROGRAMS

Degree BSN
Available Programs Generic Baccalaureate.
Study Options Full-time.

Program Entrance Requirements Minimum overall college GPA of 2.6, transcript of college record, CPR certification, health exam, health insurance, immunizations, interview, minimum high school GPA of 2.0, minimum high school rank 50%, minimum GPA in nursing prerequisites of 2.6, professional liability insurance/malpractice insurance, prerequisite course work. Transfer students are accepted.
Advanced Placement Credit given for nursing courses completed elsewhere dependent upon specific evaluations.
Contact *Telephone:* 318-487-7127. *Fax:* 318-487-7488.

Louisiana State University at Alexandria
Nursing Program
Alexandria, Louisiana

Founded in 1960
DEGREE • BSN
Library Facilities 166,340 volumes; 1,541 periodical subscriptions.

BACCALAUREATE PROGRAMS

Degree BSN
Available Programs RN Baccalaureate.
Program Entrance Requirements Minimum overall college GPA of 2.5, RN licensure.
Contact Admissions, Nursing Program, Louisiana State University at Alexandria, 8100 Highway 71 South, Alexandria, LA 71302. *Telephone:* 318-473-6417. *E-mail:* admissions@lsua.edu.

Louisiana State University Health Sciences Center
School of Nursing
New Orleans, Louisiana

http://nursing.lsuhsc.edu/
Founded in 1931
DEGREES • BSN • DNS • MN
Nursing Program Faculty 70 (33% with doctorates).
Baccalaureate Enrollment 766 Women 82.5% Men 17.5% Minority 19.45% International .65% Part-time 22.1%
Graduate Enrollment 305 Women 78.7% Men 21.3% Minority 22.6% International .32% Part-time 46%
Nursing Student Activities Nursing Honor Society, Sigma Theta Tau, Student Nurses' Association.
Nursing Student Resources Academic advising; academic or career counseling; assistance for students with disabilities; bookstore; campus computer network; computer lab; computer-assisted instruction; e-mail services; housing assistance; interactive nursing skills videos; Internet; learning resource lab; library services; nursing audiovisuals; skills, simulation, or other laboratory.
Library Facilities 215,938 volumes in health, 4,487 volumes in nursing; 4,913 periodical subscriptions (8,233 health-care related).

BACCALAUREATE PROGRAMS

Degree BSN
Available Programs Accelerated Baccalaureate for Second Degree; Generic Baccalaureate; RN Baccalaureate.
Study Options Full-time and part-time.
Program Entrance Requirements Minimum overall college GPA of 2.8, transcript of college record, interview, prerequisite course work. Transfer students are accepted. *Application deadline:* 1/15 (fall), 8/15 (spring). *Application fee:* $50.
Contact *Telephone:* 504-568-4180. *Fax:* 504-568-5853.

GRADUATE PROGRAMS

Contact *Telephone:* 504-568-4180. *Fax:* 504-568-5853.

MASTER'S DEGREE PROGRAM
Degree MN
Available Programs Master's.
Concentrations Available Health-care administration; nurse anesthesia; nursing administration; nursing education. *Clinical nurse specialist pro-*

grams in: adult health, community health, parent-child, psychiatric/mental health. *Nurse practitioner programs in:* neonatal health, primary care.
Study Options Full-time and part-time.
Program Entrance Requirements Clinical experience, minimum overall college GPA of 3.0, transcript of college record, CPR certification, interview, 3 letters of recommendation, statistics course, GRE General Test, MAT. *Application deadline:* 1/15 (fall), 8/15 (spring). *Application fee:* $100.
Degree Requirements 38 total credit hours.

DOCTORAL DEGREE PROGRAM

Degree DNS
Available Programs Doctorate.
Areas of Study Clinical practice, nursing education.
Program Entrance Requirements Clinical experience, minimum overall college GPA of 3.5, 3 letters of recommendation, MSN or equivalent, scholarly papers, writing sample, GRE General Test. *Application deadline:* 2/1 (fall), 9/1 (spring). *Application fee:* $50.
Degree Requirements 54 total credit hours, dissertation, oral exam.

POSTDOCTORAL PROGRAM

Postdoctoral Program Contact*Telephone:* 504-568-4107. *Fax:* 504-568-5853.

CONTINUING EDUCATION PROGRAM

Contact *Telephone:* 504-568-4106. *Fax:* 504-568-5853.

Loyola University New Orleans
School of Nursing
New Orleans, Louisiana

http://css.loyno.edu/nursing
Founded in 1912
DEGREES • BSN • DNP • MSN
Nursing Program Faculty 40 (100% with doctorates).
Baccalaureate Enrollment 25 **Women** 98% **Men** 2% **Minority** 22.7% **Part-time** 97.25%
Graduate Enrollment 490 **Women** 95% **Men** 5% **Minority** 36.5% **Part-time** 79.12%
Distance Learning Courses Available.
Nursing Student Activities Sigma Theta Tau.
Nursing Student Resources Academic advising; academic or career counseling; assistance for students with disabilities; bookstore; campus computer network; career placement assistance; computer lab; computer-assisted instruction; e-mail services; interactive nursing skills videos; Internet; learning resource lab; library services; nursing audiovisuals; skills, simulation, or other laboratory; tutoring.
Library Facilities 693,180 volumes (6,881 in health, 913 in nursing); 82,310 periodical subscriptions (6,716 health-care related).

BACCALAUREATE PROGRAMS

Degree BSN
Available Programs RN Baccalaureate.
Study Options Full-time and part-time.
Online Degree Options Yes (online only).
Program Entrance Requirements Minimum overall college GPA of 2.5, transcript of college record, written essay, immunizations, minimum GPA in nursing prerequisites of 2.0, professional liability insurance/malpractice insurance, RN licensure. Transfer students are accepted. *Application deadline:* Applications may be processed on a rolling basis for some programs. *Application fee:* $40.
Advanced Placement Credit by examination available. Credit given for nursing courses completed elsewhere dependent upon specific evaluations.
Expenses (2012–13) *Tuition:* full-time $11,568; part-time $482 per credit hour. *Required fees:* full-time $1096; part-time $548 per term.
Financial Aid 96% of baccalaureate students in nursing programs received some form of financial aid in 2011–12. *Gift aid (need-based):* Federal Pell, FSEOG, private, college/university gift aid from institutional funds. *Loans:* Perkins.*Work-study:* Federal Work-Study.*Financial aid application deadline:* 6/1(priority: 2/15).
Contact Dr. Ann Cary, Director, RN-BSN Coordinator and Professor, School of Nursing, Loyola University New Orleans, 6363 St. Charles Avenue, Campus Box 45, New Orleans, LA 70118. *Telephone:* 504-865-2579. *Fax:* 504-865-3254. *E-mail:* ahcary@loyno.edu.

GRADUATE PROGRAMS

Financial Aid 68% of graduate students in nursing programs received some form of financial aid in 2011–12. Traineeships and Incumbent Workers Training Program grants available. *Financial aid application deadline:* 5/1.
Contact Dr. Ann H. Cary, Director, School of Nursing, School of Nursing, Loyola University New Orleans, 6363 St. Charles Avenue, Campus Box 45, New Orleans, LA 70118. *Telephone:* 504-865-3142. *Fax:* 504-865-3254. *E-mail:* nursing@loyno.edu.

MASTER'S DEGREE PROGRAM

Degree MSN
Available Programs Master's; Master's for Nurses with Non-Nursing Degrees; RN to Master's.
Concentrations Available Health-care administration; nurse case management. *Nurse practitioner programs in:* adult health, family health.
Study Options Full-time and part-time.
Online Degree Options Yes.
Program Entrance Requirements Clinical experience, minimum overall college GPA of 3.0, transcript of college record, CPR certification, written essay, immunizations, interview, 3 letters of recommendation, nursing research course, professional liability insurance/malpractice insurance, prerequisite course work, statistics course. *Application deadline:* Applications may be processed on a rolling basis for some programs.
Advanced Placement Credit given for nursing courses completed elsewhere dependent upon specific evaluations.
Degree Requirements 36 total credit hours, comprehensive exam.

POST-MASTER'S PROGRAM

Areas of Study *Nurse practitioner programs in:* adult health, family health.

DOCTORAL DEGREE PROGRAM

Degree DNP
Available Programs Doctorate; Post-Baccalaureate Doctorate.
Areas of Study Advanced practice nursing, clinical practice, faculty preparation, family health, nursing administration, nursing research.
Online Degree Options Yes (online only).
Program Entrance Requirements Clinical experience, minimum overall college GPA of 3.2, interview by faculty committee, interview, 3 letters of recommendation, MSN or equivalent, statistics course, writing sample. *Application deadline:* 11/1 (fall), 2/1 (spring). *Application fee:* $75.
Degree Requirements 39 total credit hours, dissertation, written exam, residency.

McNeese State University
College of Nursing
Lake Charles, Louisiana

http://www.mcneese.edu/
Founded in 1939
DEGREES • BSN • MSN
Nursing Program Faculty 57 (18% with doctorates).
Baccalaureate Enrollment 1,075 **Women** 80% **Men** 20% **Minority** 24% **International** 2% **Part-time** 13%
Graduate Enrollment 84 **Women** 76% **Men** 24% **Minority** 20% **Part-time** 90%
Distance Learning Courses Available.
Nursing Student Activities Sigma Theta Tau, Student Nurses' Association.
Nursing Student Resources Academic advising; academic or career counseling; assistance for students with disabilities; bookstore; campus computer network; career placement assistance; computer lab; computer-assisted instruction; daycare for children of students; e-mail services; employment services for current students; housing assistance; interactive nursing skills videos; Internet; learning resource lab; library services; nursing audiovisuals; placement services for program completers; resume preparation assistance; skills, simulation, or other laboratory; tutoring.
Library Facilities 41,000 volumes in health, 27,500 volumes in nursing; 120 periodical subscriptions health-care related.

BACCALAUREATE PROGRAMS

Degree BSN

Available Programs ADN to Baccalaureate; Generic Baccalaureate; LPN to Baccalaureate; LPN to RN Baccalaureate.

Study Options Full-time and part-time.

Program Entrance Requirements Minimum overall college GPA of 2.7, transcript of college record, CPR certification, health exam, health insurance, high school transcript, immunizations, minimum high school GPA of 2.5, minimum GPA in nursing prerequisites of 2.7, prerequisite course work. Transfer students are accepted. *Application deadline:* 10/15 (fall), 3/10 (spring). *Application fee:* $30.

Advanced Placement Credit by examination available. Credit given for nursing courses completed elsewhere dependent upon specific evaluations.

Expenses (2011–12) *Tuition, state resident:* full-time $2466; part-time $1616 per semester. *Tuition, nonresident:* full-time $6672; part-time $3244 per semester. *International tuition:* $10,264 full-time. *Room and board:* $6900; room only: $4600 per academic year. *Required fees:* full-time $1092; part-time $64 per credit; part-time $546 per term.

Financial Aid 85% of baccalaureate students in nursing programs received some form of financial aid in 2010–11.

Contact Dr. Peggy L. Wolfe, Dean and Professor, College of Nursing, McNeese State University, PO Box 90415, Lake Charles, LA 70609-0415. *Telephone:* 337-475-5820. *Fax:* 337-475-5924. *E-mail:* pwolfe@mail.mcneese.edu.

GRADUATE PROGRAMS

Expenses (2011–12) *Tuition, state resident:* full-time $3730; part-time $1374 per semester. *Tuition, nonresident:* full-time $13,673; part-time $4364 per semester. *International tuition:* $10,263 full-time. *Room and board:* $6900; room only: $4600 per academic year. *Required fees:* full-time $1120; part-time $10 per credit; part-time $90 per term.

Financial Aid 38% of graduate students in nursing programs received some form of financial aid in 2010–11. *Application deadline:* 5/1.

Contact Dr. Valarie Waldmeier, MSN Coordinator, College of Nursing, McNeese State University, PO Box 90415, Lake Charles, LA 70609-0415. *Telephone:* 337-475-5753. *Fax:* 337-475-5702. *E-mail:* vwaldmei@mcneese.edu.

MASTER'S DEGREE PROGRAM

Degree MSN

Available Programs Master's.

Concentrations Available Nursing administration; nursing education. *Nurse practitioner programs in:* adult health, family health, psychiatric/mental health.

Site Options Baton Rouge, LA; Lafayette, LA; Lake Charles, LA.

Study Options Full-time and part-time.

Online Degree Options Yes (online only).

Program Entrance Requirements Minimum overall college GPA of 2.7, transcript of college record, written essay, immunizations, letters of recommendation, statistics course, GRE. *Application deadline:* 6/23 (fall), 11/18 (spring). *Application fee:* $20.

Advanced Placement Credit given for nursing courses completed elsewhere dependent upon specific evaluations.

Degree Requirements 42 total credit hours, thesis or project.

POST-MASTER'S PROGRAM

Areas of Study Nursing administration; nursing education. *Nurse practitioner programs in:* adult health, psychiatric/mental health.

CONTINUING EDUCATION PROGRAM

Contact Mrs. Patsy Trahan, Continuing Education Coordinator, College of Nursing, McNeese State University, PO Box 90415, Lake Charles, LA 70609-0415. *Telephone:* 337-475-5832. *Fax:* 337-475-5924. *E-mail:* ptrahan@mcneese.edu.

Nicholls State University
Department of Nursing
Thibodaux, Louisiana

http://www.nicholls.edu/nursing/
Founded in 1948

DEGREE • BSN

Nursing Program Faculty 19 (21% with doctorates).

Library Facilities 600,954 volumes; 11,149 periodical subscriptions.

BACCALAUREATE PROGRAMS

Degree BSN

Available Programs Generic Baccalaureate; LPN to Baccalaureate; RN Baccalaureate.

Program Entrance Requirements Minimum overall college GPA of 2.75, transcript of college record, minimum GPA in nursing prerequisites of 2.0, prerequisite course work. Transfer students are accepted.

Contact *Telephone:* 985-448-4696. *Fax:* 985-448-4932.

CONTINUING EDUCATION PROGRAM

Contact *Telephone:* 985-448-4696. *Fax:* 985-448-4932.

Northwestern State University of Louisiana
College of Nursing and Allied Health
Shreveport, Louisiana

http://www.nsula.edu/nursing
Founded in 1884

DEGREES • BSN • MSN

Nursing Program Faculty 54 (23% with doctorates).

Baccalaureate Enrollment 1,347 **Women** 85% **Men** 15% **Minority** 37% **Part-time** 35%

Graduate Enrollment 185 **Women** 92% **Men** 8% **Minority** 17% **International** 1% **Part-time** 92%

Distance Learning Courses Available.

Nursing Student Activities Sigma Theta Tau, Student Nurses' Association.

Nursing Student Resources Academic advising; academic or career counseling; assistance for students with disabilities; bookstore; campus computer network; computer lab; computer-assisted instruction; e-mail services; employment services for current students; interactive nursing skills videos; Internet; learning resource lab; library services; nursing audiovisuals; placement services for program completers; remedial services; skills, simulation, or other laboratory; tutoring.

Library Facilities 779,263 volumes (4,443 in health, 3,047 in nursing); 957 periodical subscriptions (1,360 health-care related).

BACCALAUREATE PROGRAMS

Degree BSN

Available Programs ADN to Baccalaureate; Generic Baccalaureate; LPN to Baccalaureate; RN Baccalaureate.

Site Options Alexandria, LA; Ferriday, LA.

Study Options Full-time and part-time.

Online Degree Options Yes.

Program Entrance Requirements Minimum overall college GPA of 2.0, transcript of college record, CPR certification, health exam, health insurance, high school transcript, immunizations, minimum GPA in nursing prerequisites of 2.7, prerequisite course work. Transfer students are accepted. *Application deadline:* 5/15 (fall), 8/15 (spring). *Application fee:* $20.

Advanced Placement Credit by examination available. Credit given for nursing courses completed elsewhere dependent upon specific evaluations.

Expenses (2012–13) *Tuition, state resident:* full-time $3939; part-time $110 per credit hour. *Tuition, nonresident:* full-time $7183; part-time $600 per credit hour. *International tuition:* $7183 full-time. *Required fees:* full-time $1275; part-time $425 per term.

Financial Aid 80% of baccalaureate students in nursing programs received some form of financial aid in 2011–12.

Contact Ms. Linda Copple, Coordinator, Baccalaureate Program, College of Nursing and Allied Health, Northwestern State University of Louisiana, 1800 Line Avenue, Shreveport, LA 71101. *Telephone:* 318-677-3100. *Fax:* 318-677-3127. *E-mail:* copplel@nsula.edu.

GRADUATE PROGRAMS

Expenses (2012–13) *Tuition, state resident:* full-time $8508; part-time $260 per credit hour. *Tuition, nonresident:* full-time $22,557; part-time $650 per credit hour. *International tuition:* $22,557 full-time. *Required fees:* full-time $1275; part-time $425 per term.

Financial Aid 25% of graduate students in nursing programs received some form of financial aid in 2011–12. Career-related internships or fieldwork and Federal Work-Study available. Aid available to part-time students. *Financial aid application deadline:* 5/1.

Contact Dr. Dana Roe, Coordinator, Graduate Studies and Research in Nursing, College of Nursing and Allied Health, Northwestern State University of Louisiana, 1800 Line Avenue, Shreveport, LA 71101. *Telephone:* 318-677-3100. *Fax:* 318-677-3127. *E-mail:* roed@nsula.edu.

MASTER'S DEGREE PROGRAM

Degree MSN

Available Programs Master's.

Concentrations Available Nursing administration; nursing education. *Clinical nurse specialist programs in:* adult health, critical care. *Nurse practitioner programs in:* acute care, family health, pediatric, women's health.

Site Options Alexandria, LA; Ferriday, LA.

Study Options Full-time and part-time.

Program Entrance Requirements Clinical experience, minimum overall college GPA of 3.0, transcript of college record, written essay, immunizations, 2 letters of recommendation, nursing research course, physical assessment course, professional liability insurance/malpractice insurance, prerequisite course work, statistics course, GRE General Test. *Application deadline:* 6/1 (fall). *Application fee:* $20.

Advanced Placement Credit given for nursing courses completed elsewhere dependent upon specific evaluations.

Degree Requirements 39 total credit hours, thesis or project, comprehensive exam.

POST-MASTER'S PROGRAM

Areas of Study *Nurse practitioner programs in:* acute care, family health, pediatric, women's health.

CONTINUING EDUCATION PROGRAM

Contact Ms. Heather Hayter, Lead Nurse Planner, College of Nursing and Allied Health, Northwestern State University of Louisiana, 1800 Line Avenue, Shreveport, LA 71101. *Telephone:* 318-677-3105. *Fax:* 318-677-3127. *E-mail:* hayterh@nsula.edu.

Our Lady of Holy Cross College
Division of Nursing
New Orleans, Louisiana

http://www.olhcc.edu/
Founded in 1916
DEGREE • BSN
Nursing Program Faculty 16 (32% with doctorates).
Baccalaureate Enrollment 168 **Women** 90% **Men** 10% **Minority** 15% **Part-time** 11%
Nursing Student Activities Sigma Theta Tau, Student Nurses' Association, nursing club.
Nursing Student Resources Academic advising; academic or career counseling; assistance for students with disabilities; bookstore; campus computer network; career placement assistance; computer lab; computer-assisted instruction; e-mail services; interactive nursing skills videos; Internet; learning resource lab; library services; nursing audiovisuals; remedial services; resume preparation assistance; skills, simulation, or other laboratory; tutoring.
Library Facilities 83,631 volumes (5,000 in health, 3,100 in nursing); 1,002 periodical subscriptions (103 health-care related).

BACCALAUREATE PROGRAMS

Degree BSN
Available Programs Generic Baccalaureate.
Study Options Full-time.
Program Entrance Requirements Minimum overall college GPA of 2.5, transcript of college record, CPR certification, written essay, health exam, health insurance, high school transcript, immunizations, 3 letters of recommendation, minimum high school GPA of 2.0, minimum GPA in nursing prerequisites of 2.5, professional liability insurance/malpractice insurance, prerequisite course work. Transfer students are accepted.
Advanced Placement Credit by examination available. Credit given for nursing courses completed elsewhere dependent upon specific evaluations.
Contact *Telephone:* 504-398-2215. *Fax:* 504-391-2421.

Our Lady of the Lake College
Division of Nursing
Baton Rouge, Louisiana

http://www.ololcollege.edu/
Founded in 1990
DEGREES • BSN • MSN
Nursing Program Faculty 38 (21% with doctorates).
Baccalaureate Enrollment 265 **Women** 85% **Men** 15% **Minority** 31% **Part-time** 19%
Graduate Enrollment 87 **Women** 45% **Men** 55% **Minority** 13%
Distance Learning Courses Available.
Nursing Student Activities Nursing Honor Society, Student Nurses' Association.
Nursing Student Resources Academic advising; academic or career counseling; assistance for students with disabilities; bookstore; campus computer network; career placement assistance; computer lab; computer-assisted instruction; e-mail services; employment services for current students; interactive nursing skills videos; Internet; learning resource lab; library services; nursing audiovisuals; paid internships; remedial services; resume preparation assistance; skills, simulation, or other laboratory; tutoring.
Library Facilities 10,000 volumes in health, 1,000 volumes in nursing; 215 periodical subscriptions (200 health-care related).

BACCALAUREATE PROGRAMS

Degree BSN
Available Programs ADN to Baccalaureate; Accelerated Baccalaureate for Second Degree; Generic Baccalaureate; LPN to Baccalaureate; RN Baccalaureate.
Study Options Full-time.
Online Degree Options Yes.
Program Entrance Requirements Minimum overall college GPA of 2.0, transcript of college record, CPR certification, written essay, health exam, health insurance, immunizations, minimum GPA in nursing prerequisites of 2.75, professional liability insurance/malpractice insurance, prerequisite course work. Transfer students are accepted. *Application deadline:* 1/15 (fall), 7/15 (spring). *Application fee:* $35.
Advanced Placement Credit given for nursing courses completed elsewhere dependent upon specific evaluations.
Expenses (2012–13) *Tuition:* full-time $12,614; part-time $394 per credit hour. *International tuition:* $12,614 full-time. *Required fees:* full-time $854; part-time $12 per credit; part-time $240 per term.
Financial Aid 94% of baccalaureate students in nursing programs received some form of financial aid in 2011–12.
Contact Dr. Phyllis LeBlanc, RN-BSN Program Director, Division of Nursing, Our Lady of the Lake College, 7500 Hennessy Boulevard, Baton Rouge, LA 70808. *Telephone:* 225-768-1793. *Fax:* 225-768-1760. *E-mail:* pleblanc@ololcollege.edu.

GRADUATE PROGRAMS

Expenses (2012–13) *Tuition:* full-time $30,638; part-time $851 per credit hour. *International tuition:* $30,638 full-time. *Required fees:* full-time $1358; part-time $12 per credit; part-time $513 per term.
Financial Aid 97% of graduate students in nursing programs received some form of financial aid in 2011–12.
Contact Dr. Jennifer Beck, Dean, School of Nursing, Division of Nursing, Our Lady of the Lake College, 7500 Hennessy Boulevard, Baton Rouge, LA 70808. *Telephone:* 225-768-1779. *Fax:* 225-768-1760. *E-mail:* jbeck@ololcollege.edu.

MASTER'S DEGREE PROGRAM

Degree MSN
Available Programs Master's.
Concentrations Available Nurse anesthesia; nursing administration; nursing education.
Study Options Full-time.
Program Entrance Requirements Clinical experience, minimum overall college GPA of 3.3, transcript of college record, interview, 3 letters of recommendation, nursing research course, physical assessment course, statistics course. *Application deadline:* 12/1 (fall), 7/15 (spring). *Application fee:* $35.
Advanced Placement Credit given for nursing courses completed elsewhere dependent upon specific evaluations.
Degree Requirements 80 total credit hours, thesis or project.

CONTINUING EDUCATION PROGRAM

Contact Ms. Shantelle Steib-Dennis, Director of Continuing Education, Division of Nursing, Our Lady of the Lake College, 7434 Perkins Road, Baton Rouge, LA 70808. *Telephone:* 225-768-1708. *Fax:* 225-214-1940. *E-mail:* Shantelle.Steib-dennis@ololcollege.edu.

Southeastern Louisiana University
School of Nursing
Hammond, Louisiana

http://www.selu.edu/acad_research/depts/nurs
Founded in 1925
DEGREES • BS • DNP • MSN
Nursing Program Faculty 62 (29% with doctorates).
Baccalaureate Enrollment 1,686 **Women** 84.4% **Men** 15.6% **Minority** 30.2% **International** 1.2% **Part-time** 17.6%
Graduate Enrollment 134 **Women** 87.3% **Men** 12.7% **Minority** 11.2% **Part-time** 85.1%
Distance Learning Courses Available.
Nursing Student Activities Nursing Honor Society, Sigma Theta Tau, Student Nurses' Association.
Nursing Student Resources Academic advising; academic or career counseling; assistance for students with disabilities; bookstore; campus computer network; career placement assistance; computer lab; computer-assisted instruction; e-mail services; employment services for current students; interactive nursing skills videos; Internet; learning resource lab; library services; nursing audiovisuals; other; resume preparation assistance; skills, simulation, or other laboratory; tutoring.
Library Facilities 732,536 volumes (19,210 in health, 5,545 in nursing); 3,779 periodical subscriptions (6,893 health-care related).

BACCALAUREATE PROGRAMS

Degree BS
Available Programs Accelerated Baccalaureate for Second Degree; Generic Baccalaureate; LPN to RN Baccalaureate; RN Baccalaureate.
Site Options Baton Rouge, LA.
Study Options Full-time and part-time.
Online Degree Options Yes.
Program Entrance Requirements CPR certification, health exam, high school biology, high school chemistry, 4 years high school math, 4 years high school science, high school transcript, immunizations, minimum high school GPA of 2.0. Transfer students are accepted. *Application deadline:* 7/15 (fall), 12/1 (spring), 5/1 (summer). Applications may be processed on a rolling basis for some programs. *Application fee:* $20.
Advanced Placement Credit given for nursing courses completed elsewhere dependent upon specific evaluations.
Expenses (2012–13) *Tuition, state resident:* full-time $3853; part-time $218 per credit hour. *Tuition, nonresident:* full-time $14,712; part-time $671 per credit hour. *International tuition:* $14,712 full-time. *Room and board:* $7020; room only: $4260 per academic year. *Required fees:* full-time $1389.
Financial Aid 82% of baccalaureate students in nursing programs received some form of financial aid in 2011–12. *Gift aid (need-based):* Federal Pell, FSEOG, state, private, college/university gift aid from institutional funds. *Loans:* Federal Direct (Subsidized and Unsubsidized Stafford PLUS), Perkins, college/university.*Work-study:* Federal Work-Study, part-time campus jobs.*Financial aid application deadline (priority):* 5/1.
Contact Dr. Eileen Creel, Department Head, School of Nursing, Southeastern Louisiana University, SLU 10835, Hammond, LA 70402. *Telephone:* 985-549-2156. *Fax:* 985-549-2869. *E-mail:* nursing@selu.edu.

GRADUATE PROGRAMS

Expenses (2012–13) *Tuition, state resident:* full-time $4486; part-time $318 per credit hour. *Tuition, nonresident:* full-time $15,344; part-time $921 per credit hour. *International tuition:* $15,344 full-time. *Room and board:* $7020; room only: $4260 per academic year. *Required fees:* full-time $1240.
Financial Aid 38% of graduate students in nursing programs received some form of financial aid in 2011–12. Federal Work-Study, institutionally sponsored loans, scholarships, traineeships, and unspecified assistantships available. Aid available to part-time students. *Financial aid application deadline:* 5/1.
Contact Dr. Lorinda Sealey, Graduate Nursing Program Coordinator, School of Nursing, Southeastern Louisiana University, SLU 10448, Hammond, LA 70402. *Telephone:* 985-549-5045. *Fax:* 985-549-5087. *E-mail:* vjohnson@selu.edu.

MASTER'S DEGREE PROGRAM
Degree MSN
Available Programs Master's.
Concentrations Available Nursing administration. *Nurse practitioner programs in:* family health, psychiatric/mental health.
Site Options Lafayette, LA; Lake Charles, LA.
Study Options Full-time and part-time.
Program Entrance Requirements Clinical experience, minimum overall college GPA of 2.7, transcript of college record, written essay, immunizations, letters of recommendation, physical assessment course, prerequisite course work, resume, statistics course, GRE (verbal and quantitative). *Application deadline:* 7/15 (fall), 12/1 (spring), 5/1 (summer). Applications may be processed on a rolling basis for some programs. *Application fee:* $20.
Advanced Placement Credit given for nursing courses completed elsewhere dependent upon specific evaluations.
Degree Requirements 39 total credit hours, thesis or project.

POST-MASTER'S PROGRAM
Areas of Study *Nurse practitioner programs in:* family health, psychiatric/mental health.

DOCTORAL DEGREE PROGRAM
Degree DNP
Available Programs Doctorate.
Site Options Lafayette, LA.
Program Entrance Requirements Minimum overall college GPA of 3.30, interview, 3 letters of recommendation, MSN or equivalent, vita. *Application deadline:* 7/15 (fall), 12/1 (spring), 5/1 (summer). Applications may be processed on a rolling basis for some programs. *Application fee:* $20.
Degree Requirements 39 total credit hours.

Southern University and Agricultural and Mechanical College
School of Nursing
Baton Rouge, Louisiana

http://www.subr.edu/
Founded in 1880
DEGREES • BSN • MSN • PHD
Nursing Program Faculty 36 (3% with doctorates).
Baccalaureate Enrollment 1,020 **Women** 91% **Men** 9% **Minority** 96% **International** 1% **Part-time** 12%
Nursing Student Activities Nursing Honor Society, Student Nurses' Association, nursing club.
Nursing Student Resources Academic advising; academic or career counseling; assistance for students with disabilities; bookstore; campus computer network; computer lab; computer-assisted instruction; e-mail services; interactive nursing skills videos; Internet; learning resource lab; library services; nursing audiovisuals; resume preparation assistance; skills, simulation, or other laboratory; tutoring.
Library Facilities 880,098 volumes (4,220 in health, 716 in nursing); 8,882 periodical subscriptions (114 health-care related).

BACCALAUREATE PROGRAMS

Degree BSN
Available Programs Generic Baccalaureate.
Study Options Full-time and part-time.
Program Entrance Requirements Minimum overall college GPA of 2.6, CPR certification, health exam, immunizations, minimum GPA in nursing prerequisites, prerequisite course work. Transfer students are accepted.
Contact *Telephone:* 225-771-3416. *Fax:* 225-771-2651.

GRADUATE PROGRAMS

Contact *Telephone:* 225-771-2663. *Fax:* 225-771-3547.

MASTER'S DEGREE PROGRAM
Degree MSN
Available Programs Master's.
Concentrations Available Health-care administration; nursing education. *Clinical nurse specialist programs in:* family health. *Nurse practitioner programs in:* family health.
Study Options Full-time and part-time.
Program Entrance Requirements Minimum overall college GPA of 3.0, transcript of college record, 3 letters of recommendation, physical assessment course, statistics course, GRE General Test.
Degree Requirements 46 total credit hours, thesis or project, comprehensive exam.

POST-MASTER'S PROGRAM
Areas of Study *Nurse practitioner programs in:* family health.

DOCTORAL DEGREE PROGRAM
Degree PhD
Areas of Study Advanced practice nursing, nursing education, nursing research, women's health.
Program Entrance Requirements Clinical experience, minimum overall college GPA of 3.2, interview by faculty committee, 3 letters of recommendation, MSN or equivalent, scholarly papers, statistics course, vita, writing sample, GRE General Test.
Degree Requirements 60 total credit hours, dissertation, written exam.

University of Louisiana at Lafayette
College of Nursing
Lafayette, Louisiana

http://www.nursing.louisiana.edu/
Founded in 1898
DEGREES • BSN • MSN
Nursing Program Faculty 47 (13% with doctorates).
Baccalaureate Enrollment 1,354 **Women** 83% **Men** 17% **Minority** 25% **Part-time** 10%
Distance Learning Courses Available.
Nursing Student Activities Nursing Honor Society, Sigma Theta Tau, Student Nurses' Association.
Nursing Student Resources Academic advising; academic or career counseling; assistance for students with disabilities; bookstore; campus computer network; career placement assistance; computer lab; computer-assisted instruction; daycare for children of students; e-mail services; employment services for current students; externships; housing assistance; interactive nursing skills videos; Internet; learning resource lab; library services; nursing audiovisuals; other; paid internships; placement services for program completers; remedial services; resume preparation assistance; skills, simulation, or other laboratory; tutoring; unpaid internships.
Library Facilities 1.1 million volumes (6,883 in health, 4,593 in nursing); 1,744 periodical subscriptions (184 health-care related).

BACCALAUREATE PROGRAMS

Degree BSN
Available Programs ADN to Baccalaureate; Accelerated Baccalaureate for Second Degree; Generic Baccalaureate; LPN to Baccalaureate.
Study Options Full-time and part-time.
Online Degree Options Yes.
Program Entrance Requirements Minimum overall college GPA of 2.8, transcript of college record, CPR certification, health exam, health insurance, high school biology, high school chemistry, high school foreign language, 2 years high school math, 3 years high school science, high school transcript, immunizations, minimum high school GPA of 2.0, minimum high school rank 25%, minimum GPA in nursing prerequisites of 2.0, prerequisite course work. Transfer students are accepted. *Application deadline:* 4/1 (fall), 11/2 (spring).
Advanced Placement Credit by examination available. Credit given for nursing courses completed elsewhere dependent upon specific evaluations.
Contact *Telephone:* 337-482-5604. *Fax:* 337-482-5700.

GRADUATE PROGRAMS

Contact *Telephone:* 337-482-5639. *Fax:* 337-482-5650.

MASTER'S DEGREE PROGRAM
Degree MSN
Available Programs Master's; RN to Master's.
Concentrations Available Health-care administration; nursing administration; nursing education. *Clinical nurse specialist programs in:* adult health, psychiatric/mental health. *Nurse practitioner programs in:* adult health, psychiatric/mental health.
Site Options Hammond, LA; Baton Rouge, LA; Lake Charles, LA.
Study Options Full-time and part-time.
Online Degree Options Yes (online only).
Program Entrance Requirements Minimum overall college GPA of 2.75, transcript of college record, immunizations, 3 letters of recommendation, physical assessment course, statistics course, GRE General Test. *Application deadline:* Applications may be processed on a rolling basis for some programs. *Application fee:* $25.
Advanced Placement Credit given for nursing courses completed elsewhere dependent upon specific evaluations.
Degree Requirements 38 total credit hours, thesis or project.

POST-MASTER'S PROGRAM
Areas of Study *Clinical nurse specialist programs in:* adult health, psychiatric/mental health. *Nurse practitioner programs in:* adult health, psychiatric/mental health.

CONTINUING EDUCATION PROGRAM
Contact *Telephone:* 337-482-5648. *Fax:* 337-482-5053.

University of Louisiana at Monroe
Nursing
Monroe, Louisiana

http://www.ulm.edu/nursing
Founded in 1931
DEGREE • BS
Nursing Program Faculty 29 (2% with doctorates).
Baccalaureate Enrollment 237 **Women** 85% **Men** 15% **Minority** 26% **International** 1% **Part-time** 20%
Distance Learning Courses Available.
Nursing Student Activities Sigma Theta Tau, Student Nurses' Association.
Nursing Student Resources Academic advising; academic or career counseling; assistance for students with disabilities; bookstore; campus computer network; computer lab; computer-assisted instruction; daycare for children of students; e-mail services; employment services for current students; interactive nursing skills videos; Internet; learning resource lab; library services; nursing audiovisuals; placement services for program completers; remedial services; resume preparation assistance; skills, simulation, or other laboratory; tutoring.
Library Facilities 629,606 volumes (20,924 in health, 3,000 in nursing); 95 periodical subscriptions (425 health-care related).

BACCALAUREATE PROGRAMS

Degree BS
Available Programs ADN to Baccalaureate; Generic Baccalaureate; LPN to Baccalaureate; RN Baccalaureate.
Study Options Full-time and part-time.
Online Degree Options Yes (online only).
Program Entrance Requirements Transcript of college record, CPR certification, health exam, health insurance, high school transcript, immunizations, minimum high school GPA of 2.0, minimum high school rank 50%, minimum GPA in nursing prerequisites of 2.8, professional liability insurance/malpractice insurance, prerequisite course work. Transfer students are accepted. *Application deadline:* 3/1 (fall), 9/1 (spring). *Application fee:* $50.
Advanced Placement Credit given for nursing courses completed elsewhere dependent upon specific evaluations.
Expenses (2011–12) *Tuition, state resident:* full-time $5102. *Tuition, nonresident:* full-time $13,047. *International tuition:* $12,902 full-time. *Required fees:* full-time $870.
Financial Aid 82% of baccalaureate students in nursing programs received some form of financial aid in 2010–11.

Contact Dr. Emily S. Doughty, Director, Nursing, University of Louisiana at Monroe, 700 University Avenue, Monroe, LA 71209-0460. *Telephone:* 318-342-1640. *Fax:* 318-342-1567. *E-mail:* doughty@ulm.edu.

CONTINUING EDUCATION PROGRAM

Contact Mrs. Shari Moreau, Coordinator of Continuing Education, Nursing, University of Louisiana at Monroe, 700 University Avenue, Monroe, LA 71209-0460. *Telephone:* 318-342-1640. *Fax:* 318-342-1567. *E-mail:* moreau@ulm.edu.

University of Phoenix–Louisiana Campus
College of Nursing
Metairie, Louisiana

Founded in 1976

DEGREE • BSN
Nursing Program Faculty 2 (50% with doctorates).
Baccalaureate Enrollment 9
Nursing Student Activities Sigma Theta Tau.
Nursing Student Resources Academic advising; academic or career counseling; assistance for students with disabilities; bookstore; campus computer network; computer lab; computer-assisted instruction; e-mail services; interactive nursing skills videos; Internet; learning resource lab; library services; nursing audiovisuals; remedial services; tutoring.
Library Facilities 16,781 periodical subscriptions (1,300 health-care related).

BACCALAUREATE PROGRAMS

Degree BSN
Available Programs Accelerated Baccalaureate; LPN to Baccalaureate.
Study Options Full-time.
Program Entrance Requirements Transcript of college record, CPR certification, immunizations, 1 letter of recommendation, RN licensure. Transfer students are accepted. *Application deadline:* Applications may be processed on a rolling basis for some programs.
Advanced Placement Credit by examination available. Credit given for nursing courses completed elsewhere dependent upon specific evaluations.
Contact *Telephone:* 504-461-8852.

MAINE

Husson University
School of Nursing
Bangor, Maine

http://www.husson.edu/
Founded in 1898

DEGREES • BSN • MSN
Nursing Program Faculty 13 (15% with doctorates).
Baccalaureate Enrollment 291 **Women** 93% **Men** 7% **Minority** 4%
Graduate Enrollment 49 **Women** 92% **Men** 8% **Part-time** 26%
Distance Learning Courses Available.
Nursing Student Activities Sigma Theta Tau, Student Nurses' Association, nursing club.
Nursing Student Resources Academic advising; academic or career counseling; assistance for students with disabilities; bookstore; campus computer network; career placement assistance; computer lab; computer-assisted instruction; e-mail services; employment services for current students; externships; interactive nursing skills videos; Internet; learning resource lab; library services; nursing audiovisuals; remedial services; resume preparation assistance; skills, simulation, or other laboratory; tutoring; unpaid internships.
Library Facilities 51,922 volumes (3,450 in health, 1,100 in nursing); 375 periodical subscriptions (183 health-care related).

BACCALAUREATE PROGRAMS

Degree BSN
Available Programs Generic Baccalaureate.
Study Options Full-time and part-time.
Program Entrance Requirements Minimum overall college GPA of 3.0, transcript of college record, written essay, health exam, health insurance, high school biology, high school chemistry, 2 years high school math, 2 years high school science, high school transcript, immunizations, 2 letters of recommendation, minimum high school GPA of 3.0, minimum GPA in nursing prerequisites of 3.0, prerequisite course work. Transfer students are accepted. *Application deadline:* Applications may be processed on a rolling basis for some programs. *Application fee:* $25.
Advanced Placement Credit by examination available. Credit given for nursing courses completed elsewhere dependent upon specific evaluations.
Expenses (2011–12) *Tuition:* full-time $14,105; part-time $455 per credit hour. *Required fees:* part-time $50 per credit.
Financial Aid 75% of baccalaureate students in nursing programs received some form of financial aid in 2010–11.
Contact Gloria Brawn, Administrative Assistant, Undergraduate Nursing Program, School of Nursing, Husson University, 1 College Circle, Bangor, ME 04401-2999. *Telephone:* 207-941-7058. *Fax:* 207-941-7198. *E-mail:* brawng@husson.edu.

GRADUATE PROGRAMS

Expenses (2011–12) *Tuition:* part-time $478 per credit hour. *Required fees:* part-time $50 per credit.
Financial Aid 67% of graduate students in nursing programs received some form of financial aid in 2010–11.
Contact Ms. Jeanne Harvey, Administrative Assistant, School of Nursing, Husson University, 1 College Circle, Bangor, ME 04401. *Telephone:* 207-941-7166. *Fax:* 207-941-7198. *E-mail:* harveyj@husson.edu.

MASTER'S DEGREE PROGRAM
Degree MSN
Available Programs Master's; Master's for Nurses with Non-Nursing Degrees.
Concentrations Available Nursing education. *Clinical nurse specialist programs in:* psychiatric/mental health. *Nurse practitioner programs in:* family health.
Site Options South Portland, ME; Presque Isle, ME.
Study Options Full-time and part-time.
Program Entrance Requirements Clinical experience, minimum overall college GPA of 3.0, transcript of college record, CPR certification, written essay, immunizations, interview, 3 letters of recommendation, physical assessment course, prerequisite course work, statistics course. *Application deadline:* Applications may be processed on a rolling basis for some programs. *Application fee:* $25.
Advanced Placement Credit by examination available. Credit given for nursing courses completed elsewhere dependent upon specific evaluations.
Degree Requirements 44 total credit hours, thesis or project.

POST-MASTER'S PROGRAM
Areas of Study Nursing education. *Clinical nurse specialist programs in:* psychiatric/mental health. *Nurse practitioner programs in:* family health, psychiatric/mental health.

Saint Joseph's College of Maine
Master of Science in Nursing Program
Standish, Maine

Founded in 1912

DEGREES • BSN • MSN • MSN/MHA
Nursing Program Faculty 65 (8% with doctorates).
Baccalaureate Enrollment 558 **Women** 95% **Men** 5% **Minority** 1% **Part-time** 48%
Graduate Enrollment 343 **Women** 93% **Men** 7% **Minority** 3% **Part-time** 100%
Distance Learning Courses Available.
Nursing Student Activities Sigma Theta Tau, Student Nurses' Association.
Nursing Student Resources Academic advising; academic or career counseling; assistance for students with disabilities; bookstore; campus computer network; computer lab; computer-assisted instruction; e-mail

services; interactive nursing skills videos; Internet; learning resource lab; library services; nursing audiovisuals; remedial services; resume preparation assistance; skills, simulation, or other laboratory; tutoring.
Library Facilities 85,000 volumes (4,114 in health, 409 in nursing); 45,141 periodical subscriptions (108 health-care related).

BACCALAUREATE PROGRAMS

Degree BSN
Available Programs Generic Baccalaureate; RN Baccalaureate.
Study Options Full-time and part-time.
Program Entrance Requirements Minimum overall college GPA of 2.0, transcript of college record, written essay, health exam, health insurance, high school biology, high school chemistry, 3 years high school math, 2 years high school science, high school transcript, immunizations, 1 letter of recommendation, minimum high school GPA of 2.0. *Application deadline:* 5/1 (spring). *Application fee:* $250.
Advanced Placement Credit given for nursing courses completed elsewhere dependent upon specific evaluations.
Contact *Telephone:* 207-893-7830. *Fax:* 207-892-7423.

GRADUATE PROGRAMS

Contact *Telephone:* 207-893-7956. *Fax:* 207-893-7520.

MASTER'S DEGREE PROGRAM

Degrees MSN; MSN/MHA
Available Programs Master's; Master's for Nurses with Non-Nursing Degrees; RN to Master's.
Concentrations Available Nursing administration; nursing education.
Study Options Full-time and part-time.
Online Degree Options Yes (online only).
Program Entrance Requirements Clinical experience, computer literacy, minimum overall college GPA of 3.0, transcript of college record, prerequisite course work, resume, MAT. *Application deadline:* Applications may be processed on a rolling basis for some programs.
Advanced Placement Credit given for nursing courses completed elsewhere dependent upon specific evaluations.
Degree Requirements 42 total credit hours, thesis or project.

CONTINUING EDUCATION PROGRAM

Contact *Telephone:* 207-893-7956. *Fax:* 207-893-7520.

University of Maine
School of Nursing
Orono, Maine

Founded in 1865
DEGREES • BSN • MSN
Nursing Program Faculty 20 (40% with doctorates).
Baccalaureate Enrollment 407 **Women** 90% **Men** 10% **Minority** .4% **International** .1% **Part-time** .5%
Graduate Enrollment 27 **Women** 99% **Men** 1% **Part-time** 50%
Distance Learning Courses Available.
Nursing Student Activities Sigma Theta Tau, Student Nurses' Association.
Nursing Student Resources Academic advising; academic or career counseling; assistance for students with disabilities; bookstore; campus computer network; computer lab; daycare for children of students; e-mail services; employment services for current students; housing assistance; interactive nursing skills videos; Internet; learning resource lab; library services; nursing audiovisuals; skills, simulation, or other laboratory; tutoring.
Library Facilities 1.1 million volumes (20,600 in health, 2,100 in nursing); 16,988 periodical subscriptions (3,750 health-care related).

BACCALAUREATE PROGRAMS

Degree BSN
Available Programs Generic Baccalaureate; RN Baccalaureate.
Site Options Presque Isle, ME; Augusta, ME; Portland, ME.
Study Options Full-time and part-time.
Program Entrance Requirements Minimum overall college GPA of 2.75, transcript of college record, CPR certification, written essay, health exam, high school biology, high school chemistry, high school foreign language, 3 years high school math, 3 years high school science, high school transcript, immunizations, interview, minimum high school rank 30%. Transfer students are accepted.

Advanced Placement Credit by examination available. Credit given for nursing courses completed elsewhere dependent upon specific evaluations.
Contact *Telephone:* 207-581-2588. *Fax:* 207-581-2585.

GRADUATE PROGRAMS

Contact *Telephone:* 207-581-2605. *Fax:* 207-581-2585.

MASTER'S DEGREE PROGRAM

Degree MSN
Available Programs Master's; RN to Master's.
Concentrations Available Health-care administration; nursing education. *Nurse practitioner programs in:* family health.
Study Options Full-time and part-time.
Program Entrance Requirements Clinical experience, minimum overall college GPA of 3.0, transcript of college record, CPR certification, written essay, immunizations, interview, 3 letters of recommendation, nursing research course, physical assessment course, statistics course, GRE General Test.
Advanced Placement Credit given for nursing courses completed elsewhere dependent upon specific evaluations.
Degree Requirements 47 total credit hours, thesis or project.

University of Maine at Fort Kent
Department of Nursing
Fort Kent, Maine

http://www.umfk.edu/
Founded in 1878
DEGREE • BSN
Nursing Program Faculty 6 (16% with doctorates).
Baccalaureate Enrollment 246 **Women** 90% **Men** 10% **Minority** 2% **International** 2% **Part-time** 63%
Distance Learning Courses Available.
Nursing Student Activities Nursing Honor Society, Student Nurses' Association, nursing club.
Nursing Student Resources Academic advising; academic or career counseling; assistance for students with disabilities; bookstore; campus computer network; career placement assistance; computer lab; computer-assisted instruction; e-mail services; employment services for current students; externships; housing assistance; interactive nursing skills videos; Internet; learning resource lab; library services; nursing audiovisuals; paid internships; placement services for program completers; remedial services; resume preparation assistance; skills, simulation, or other laboratory; tutoring; unpaid internships.
Library Facilities 160,000 volumes (3,386 in health, 2,425 in nursing); 41,000 periodical subscriptions (73 health-care related).

BACCALAUREATE PROGRAMS

Degree BSN
Available Programs Accelerated Baccalaureate; Generic Baccalaureate; RN Baccalaureate.
Study Options Full-time and part-time.
Online Degree Options Yes.
Program Entrance Requirements Minimum overall college GPA of 2.5, CPR certification, written essay, health exam, health insurance, high school chemistry, high school foreign language, high school math, high school transcript, immunizations, minimum GPA in nursing prerequisites of 2.5, prerequisite course work. Transfer students are accepted. *Application deadline:* 8/15 (fall), 1/10 (spring). *Application fee:* $40.
Advanced Placement Credit given for nursing courses completed elsewhere dependent upon specific evaluations.
Contact *Telephone:* 207-834-8607. *Fax:* 207-834-7577.

University of New England
Department of Nursing
Biddeford, Maine

http://www.une.edu/chp/nursing/
Founded in 1831
DEGREE • BSN
Nursing Program Faculty 16 (26% with doctorates).
Baccalaureate Enrollment 133 **Women** 73% **Men** 27% **Minority** 3%

Nursing Student Activities Nursing Honor Society, Sigma Theta Tau, Student Nurses' Association, nursing club.

Nursing Student Resources Academic advising; academic or career counseling; assistance for students with disabilities; bookstore; campus computer network; career placement assistance; computer lab; computer-assisted instruction; e-mail services; employment services for current students; housing assistance; interactive nursing skills videos; Internet; learning resource lab; library services; nursing audiovisuals; placement services for program completers; remedial services; resume preparation assistance; skills, simulation, or other laboratory; tutoring; unpaid internships.

Library Facilities 156,752 volumes (10,000 in health, 5,500 in nursing); 39,705 periodical subscriptions (1,300 health-care related).

BACCALAUREATE PROGRAMS

Degree BSN

Available Programs Accelerated RN Baccalaureate; Generic Baccalaureate; RN Baccalaureate.

Study Options Full-time and part-time.

Program Entrance Requirements Minimum overall college GPA of 3.0, transcript of college record, CPR certification, health exam, health insurance, high school biology, high school chemistry, 2 years high school math, 2 years high school science, high school transcript, immunizations, minimum high school GPA of 3.0, professional liability insurance/malpractice insurance. Transfer students are accepted. *Application deadline:* 2/15 (fall). *Application fee:* $100.

Advanced Placement Credit by examination available. Credit given for nursing courses completed elsewhere dependent upon specific evaluations.

Expenses (2011–12) *Tuition:* full-time $29,430; part-time $1040 per credit hour. *Room and board:* $12,020 per academic year. *Required fees:* full-time $1500.

Financial Aid 88% of baccalaureate students in nursing programs received some form of financial aid in 2010–11.

Contact Admissions Office, Department of Nursing, University of New England, 3 Hills Beach Road, Biddeford, ME 04005. *Telephone:* 207-602-2297. *E-mail:* admissions@une.edu.

CONTINUING EDUCATION PROGRAM

Contact Ms. Audrey Gup-Mathews, Director of Continuing Education, Department of Nursing, University of New England, 11 Hills Beach Road, Biddeford, ME 04005. *Telephone:* 207-602-2050. *Fax:* 207-602-5973.

University of Southern Maine
School of Nursing
Portland, Maine

http://www.usm.maine.edu/nursing
Founded in 1878
DEGREES • BS • DNP • MS • MS/MBA
Nursing Program Faculty 71 (21% with doctorates).
Baccalaureate Enrollment 420 **Women** 89% **Men** 11% **Minority** 11% **Part-time** 20%
Graduate Enrollment 103 **Women** 85% **Men** 15% **Minority** 6% **Part-time** 34%
Nursing Student Activities Sigma Theta Tau, Student Nurses' Association.
Nursing Student Resources Academic advising; academic or career counseling; assistance for students with disabilities; bookstore; campus computer network; computer lab; computer-assisted instruction; e-mail services; interactive nursing skills videos; Internet; learning resource lab; library services; nursing audiovisuals; remedial services; resume preparation assistance; skills, simulation, or other laboratory; tutoring.
Library Facilities 469,292 volumes (18,042 in health, 622 in nursing); 1,177 periodical subscriptions (230 health-care related).

BACCALAUREATE PROGRAMS

Degree BS

Available Programs ADN to Baccalaureate; Accelerated Baccalaureate for Second Degree; Generic Baccalaureate; RN Baccalaureate.

Site Options Lewiston, ME.

Study Options Full-time and part-time.

Program Entrance Requirements Minimum overall college GPA of 3.0, transcript of college record, written essay, high school biology, high school chemistry, 3 years high school math, 2 years high school science, high school transcript, immunizations, 2 letters of recommendation, minimum high school GPA of 3.0. Transfer students are accepted. *Application deadline:* 1/15 (fall). *Application fee:* $40.

Advanced Placement Credit by examination available. Credit given for nursing courses completed elsewhere dependent upon specific evaluations.

Expenses (2012–13) *Tuition, state resident:* full-time $7590; part-time $253 per credit hour. *Tuition, nonresident:* full-time $19,950; part-time $665 per credit hour. *International tuition:* $19,950 full-time. *Room and board:* $9130 per academic year. *Required fees:* full-time $2000; part-time $28 per credit; part-time $650 per term.

Financial Aid 96% of baccalaureate students in nursing programs received some form of financial aid in 2011–12.

Contact Ms. Brenda D. Webster, Coordinator of Nursing Student Services, School of Nursing, University of Southern Maine, PO Box 9300, Portland, ME 04104-9300. *Telephone:* 207-780-4802. *Fax:* 207-228-8177. *E-mail:* bwebster@usm.maine.edu.

GRADUATE PROGRAMS

Expenses (2012–13) *Tuition, state resident:* full-time $9120; part-time $380 per credit hour. *Tuition, nonresident:* full-time $24,624; part-time $1026 per credit hour. *International tuition:* $24,624 full-time. *Room and board:* $9130 per academic year. *Required fees:* full-time $1052; part-time $28 per credit; part-time $526 per term.

Financial Aid 90% of graduate students in nursing programs received some form of financial aid in 2011–12. 5 research assistantships with tuition reimbursements available (averaging $3,375 per year), 3 teaching assistantships with tuition reimbursements available (averaging $3,375 per year) were awarded; career-related internships or fieldwork, Federal Work-Study, scholarships, traineeships, tuition waivers (full and partial), and unspecified assistantships also available. Aid available to part-time students. *Financial aid application deadline:* 2/15.

Contact Ms. Brenda D. Webster, Coordinator of Nursing Student Services, School of Nursing, University of Southern Maine, PO Box 9300, Portland, ME 04104-9300. *Telephone:* 207-780-4802. *Fax:* 207-228-8177. *E-mail:* bwebster@usm.maine.edu.

MASTER'S DEGREE PROGRAM

Degrees MS; MS/MBA

Available Programs Master's; Master's for Non-Nursing College Graduates; Master's for Nurses with Non-Nursing Degrees; RN to Master's.

Concentrations Available Clinical nurse leader; nursing administration; nursing education. *Nurse practitioner programs in:* adult health, family health, psychiatric/mental health.

Study Options Full-time and part-time.

Program Entrance Requirements Minimum overall college GPA of 3.0, transcript of college record, written essay, 2 letters of recommendation, physical assessment course, prerequisite course work, statistics course, GRE General Test or MAT. *Application deadline:* 4/1 (fall), 10/1 (spring), 11/1 (summer). *Application fee:* $50.

Advanced Placement Credit given for nursing courses completed elsewhere dependent upon specific evaluations.

Degree Requirements 54 total credit hours.

POST-MASTER'S PROGRAM

Areas of Study *Nurse practitioner programs in:* adult health, family health, psychiatric/mental health.

DOCTORAL DEGREE PROGRAM

Degree DNP

Available Programs Doctorate.

Areas of Study Clinical practice, ethics, health policy, health-care systems, nursing policy.

Program Entrance Requirements Clinical experience, minimum overall college GPA of 3.25, interview by faculty committee, 3 letters of recommendation, MSN or equivalent, statistics course, vita, writing sample, GRE. *Application deadline:* 3/15 (fall). *Application fee:* $65.

Degree Requirements 43 total credit hours, residency.

CONTINUING EDUCATION PROGRAM

Contact Professional and Continuing Education, School of Nursing, University of Southern Maine, USM Professional and Continuing Education, PO Box 9300, Portland, ME 04104-9300. *Telephone:* 207-780-5900. *E-mail:* pce@usm.maine.edu.

MARYLAND

Bowie State University
Department of Nursing
Bowie, Maryland

http://www.bowiestate.edu/academics/departments/nursing
Founded in 1865
DEGREES • BSN • MSN
Nursing Program Faculty 20 (35% with doctorates).
Baccalaureate Enrollment 225 **Women** 88% **Men** 12% **Minority** 93% **International** 5% **Part-time** 25%
Graduate Enrollment 43 **Women** 87% **Men** 13% **Minority** 93% **International** 47% **Part-time** 5%
Distance Learning Courses Available.
Nursing Student Activities Nursing Honor Society, Student Nurses' Association.
Nursing Student Resources Academic advising; academic or career counseling; assistance for students with disabilities; bookstore; campus computer network; computer lab; computer-assisted instruction; housing assistance; interactive nursing skills videos; Internet; library services; nursing audiovisuals; skills, simulation, or other laboratory; tutoring.
Library Facilities 285,815 volumes; 770 periodical subscriptions.

BACCALAUREATE PROGRAMS

Degree BSN
Available Programs Accelerated Baccalaureate; Generic Baccalaureate; RN Baccalaureate.
Study Options Full-time.
Program Entrance Requirements Minimum overall college GPA of 2.75, transcript of college record, health exam, health insurance, high school biology, high school chemistry, 4 years high school math, 4 years high school science, high school transcript, immunizations, minimum high school GPA of 3.0, minimum GPA in nursing prerequisites of 2.75, prerequisite course work. Transfer students are accepted. *Application deadline:* 3/31 (fall).
Advanced Placement Credit given for nursing courses completed elsewhere dependent upon specific evaluations.
Contact *Telephone:* 301-860-3202. *Fax:* 301-860-3222.

GRADUATE PROGRAMS

Contact *Telephone:* 301-860-3202. *Fax:* 301-860-3222.

MASTER'S DEGREE PROGRAM
Degree MSN
Available Programs Master's.
Concentrations Available Nursing education. *Nurse practitioner programs in:* family health.
Study Options Full-time and part-time.
Program Entrance Requirements Clinical experience, minimum overall college GPA of 2.5, CPR certification, written essay, immunizations, 3 letters of recommendation, physical assessment course, professional liability insurance/malpractice insurance, resume, statistics course. *Application deadline:* 11/30 (fall), 4/30 (spring). Applications may be processed on a rolling basis for some programs.
Advanced Placement Credit by examination available. Credit given for nursing courses completed elsewhere dependent upon specific evaluations.
Degree Requirements 45 total credit hours, comprehensive exam.

Coppin State University
Helene Fuld School of Nursing
Baltimore, Maryland

http://www.coppin.edu/nursing
Founded in 1900
DEGREES • BSN • MSN
Nursing Program Faculty 45 (18% with doctorates).
Baccalaureate Enrollment 529 **Women** 91% **Men** 9% **Minority** 99% **International** 2% **Part-time** 33%

Graduate Enrollment 32 **Women** 94% **Men** 6% **Minority** 94% **Part-time** 22%
Distance Learning Courses Available.
Nursing Student Activities Nursing Honor Society, Sigma Theta Tau, Student Nurses' Association.
Nursing Student Resources Academic advising; academic or career counseling; assistance for students with disabilities; bookstore; campus computer network; career placement assistance; computer lab; computer-assisted instruction; e-mail services; externships; interactive nursing skills videos; Internet; learning resource lab; library services; nursing audiovisuals; other; placement services for program completers; remedial services; resume preparation assistance; skills, simulation, or other laboratory; tutoring; unpaid internships.
Library Facilities 134,983 volumes (1,339 in health, 1,298 in nursing); 665 periodical subscriptions (132 health-care related).

BACCALAUREATE PROGRAMS

Degree BSN
Available Programs Accelerated RN Baccalaureate; Baccalaureate for Second Degree; Generic Baccalaureate; RN Baccalaureate.
Site Options Baltimore, MD.
Study Options Full-time and part-time.
Program Entrance Requirements Written essay, health exam, high school biology, high school chemistry, high school foreign language, 3 years high school math, 2 years high school science, high school transcript, immunizations, 3 letters of recommendation, minimum high school GPA of 2.5, minimum GPA in nursing prerequisites of 2.5. Transfer students are accepted.
Contact *Telephone:* 410-951-3988. *Fax:* 410-400-5978.

GRADUATE PROGRAMS

Contact *Telephone:* 410-951-3988. *Fax:* 410-400-5978.

MASTER'S DEGREE PROGRAM
Degree MSN
Available Programs Master's.
Concentrations Available *Nurse practitioner programs in:* family health.
Site Options Baltimore, MD.
Study Options Full-time and part-time.
Program Entrance Requirements Clinical experience, computer literacy, minimum overall college GPA of 3.0, transcript of college record, CPR certification, written essay, immunizations, interview, 3 letters of recommendation, nursing research course, physical assessment course, statistics course.
Advanced Placement Credit given for nursing courses completed elsewhere dependent upon specific evaluations.
Degree Requirements 48 total credit hours, thesis or project, comprehensive exam.

POST-MASTER'S PROGRAM
Areas of Study *Nurse practitioner programs in:* family health.

Frostburg State University
Nursing Department
Frostburg, Maryland

Founded in 1898
DEGREE • BSN
Library Facilities 345,691 volumes; 3,899 periodical subscriptions.

BACCALAUREATE PROGRAMS

Degree BSN
Available Programs RN Baccalaureate.
Study Options Part-time.
Online Degree Options Yes (online only).
Program Entrance Requirements Prerequisite course work, RN licensure. *Application deadline:* 4/1 (summer).
Contact Roxanne Weighley, Nursing Department, Nursing Department, Frostburg State University, 101 Braddock Road, Frostburg, MD 21532-2303. *Telephone:* 301-687-4141. *E-mail:* rmweighley@frostburg.edu.

The Johns Hopkins University
School of Nursing
Baltimore, Maryland

http://nursing.jhu.edu
Founded in 1876
DEGREES • BS • DNP • MSN • MSN/MBA • MSN/MPH • MSN/PHD • PHD
Nursing Program Faculty 222 (32% with doctorates).
Baccalaureate Enrollment 477 **Women** 91.6% **Men** 8.4% **Minority** 25.2% **International** 1.3% **Part-time** 14.3%
Graduate Enrollment 380 **Women** 91.3% **Men** 8.7% **Minority** 25.3% **International** 5.3% **Part-time** 69.2%
Distance Learning Courses Available.
Nursing Student Activities Nursing Honor Society, Sigma Theta Tau, Student Nurses' Association, nursing club.
Nursing Student Resources Academic advising; academic or career counseling; assistance for students with disabilities; bookstore; campus computer network; career placement assistance; computer lab; computer-assisted instruction; e-mail services; employment services for current students; housing assistance; Internet; learning resource lab; library services; nursing audiovisuals; other; resume preparation assistance; skills, simulation, or other laboratory; tutoring.

BACCALAUREATE PROGRAMS

Degree BS
Available Programs Accelerated Baccalaureate; Accelerated Baccalaureate for Second Degree.
Study Options Full-time and part-time.
Program Entrance Requirements Minimum overall college GPA of 3.0, transcript of college record, CPR certification, written essay, health exam, health insurance, immunizations, interview, 3 letters of recommendation, minimum GPA in nursing prerequisites of 3.0, prerequisite course work. Transfer students are accepted. *Application deadline:* 1/15 (fall), 11/15 (summer). *Application fee:* $75.
Advanced Placement Credit by examination available. Credit given for nursing courses completed elsewhere dependent upon specific evaluations.
Financial Aid 90% of baccalaureate students in nursing programs received some form of financial aid in 2011–12. *Gift aid (need-based):* Federal Pell, FSEOG, state, private, college/university gift aid from institutional funds. *Loans:* Federal Direct (Subsidized and Unsubsidized Stafford PLUS), Perkins, college/university. *Work-study:* Federal Work-Study. *Financial aid application deadline:* 3/1.
Contact Office of Admissions and Student Services, School of Nursing, The Johns Hopkins University, 525 North Wolfe Street, Baltimore, MD 21205-2110. *Telephone:* 410-955-7548. *Fax:* 410-614-7086. *E-mail:* jhuson@jhu.edu.

GRADUATE PROGRAMS

Financial Aid 68% of graduate students in nursing programs received some form of financial aid in 2011–12. 6 fellowships with partial tuition reimbursements available (averaging $23,272 per year) were awarded; research assistantships with full tuition reimbursements available, teaching assistantships with full tuition reimbursements available, career-related internships or fieldwork, Federal Work-Study, scholarships, traineeships, and tuition waivers (partial) also available. Aid available to part-time students. *Financial aid application deadline:* 3/1.
Contact Office of Admissions and Student Services, School of Nursing, The Johns Hopkins University, 525 North Wolfe Street, Baltimore, MD 21205-2110. *Telephone:* 410-955-7548. *Fax:* 410-614-7086. *E-mail:* jhuson@jhu.edu.

MASTER'S DEGREE PROGRAM

Degrees MSN; MSN/MBA; MSN/MPH; MSN/PhD
Available Programs Master's.
Concentrations Available Health-care administration; nurse case management; nurse-midwifery; nursing administration. *Clinical nurse specialist programs in:* acute care, adult health, gerontology, pediatric. *Nurse practitioner programs in:* acute care, adult health, family health, gerontology, pediatric, primary care.
Study Options Full-time and part-time.
Online Degree Options Yes.
Program Entrance Requirements Clinical experience, computer literacy, minimum overall college GPA of 3.0, transcript of college record, CPR certification, written essay, immunizations, interview, 3 letters of recommendation, nursing research course, physical assessment course, prerequisite course work, resume, statistics course. *Application deadline:* 12/1 (fall), 9/1 (spring), 1/15 (summer). Applications may be processed on a rolling basis for some programs. *Application fee:* $75.
Advanced Placement Credit by examination available. Credit given for nursing courses completed elsewhere dependent upon specific evaluations.
Degree Requirements 36 total credit hours, thesis or project.

POST-MASTER'S PROGRAM

Areas of Study Nursing education. *Nurse practitioner programs in:* acute care, adult health, family health, gerontology, pediatric, primary care.

DOCTORAL DEGREE PROGRAM

Degree DNP
Available Programs Doctorate.
Areas of Study Advanced practice nursing, clinical practice, community health, critical care, family health, forensic nursing, gerontology, health policy, health promotion/disease prevention, health-care systems, human health and illness, illness and transition, individualized study, information systems, maternity-newborn, neuro-behavior, nurse case management, nursing administration, nursing education, nursing policy, nursing research, nursing science, oncology, urban health, women's health.
Program Entrance Requirements Minimum overall college GPA of 3.0, clinical experience, interview, 3 letters of recommendation, MSN or equivalent, statistics course, vita, writing sample. *Application deadline:* 1/1 (summer). *Application fee:* $100.
Degree Requirements 42 total credit hours, Capstone project.

DOCTORAL DEGREE PROGRAM

Degree PhD
Available Programs Doctorate.
Areas of Study Addiction/substance abuse, advanced practice nursing, aging, bio-behavioral research, biology of health and illness, clinical practice, community health, critical care, family health, forensic nursing, gerontology, health policy, health promotion/disease prevention, health-care systems, human health and illness, illness and transition, individualized study, information systems, nurse case management, nursing research, nursing science, oncology, urban health, women's health.
Program Entrance Requirements Clinical experience, minimum overall college GPA of 3.0, interview, 3 letters of recommendation, MSN or equivalent, scholarly papers, statistics course, vita, writing sample, GRE (for PhD). *Application deadline:* 3/1 (fall), 9/1 (spring). *Application fee:* $100.
Degree Requirements Dissertation, oral exam, written exam.

POSTDOCTORAL PROGRAM

Areas of Study Health promotion/disease prevention, individualized study, vulnerable population.
Postdoctoral Program Contact Office of Admissions and Student Services, School of Nursing, The Johns Hopkins University, 525 North Wolfe Street, Baltimore, MD 21205-2110. *Telephone:* 410-955-7548. *Fax:* 410-614-7086. *E-mail:* jhuson@jhu.edu.

CONTINUING EDUCATION PROGRAM

Contact David Newton, Executive Director, Professional Programs, School of Nursing, The Johns Hopkins University, 525 North Wolfe Street, Baltimore, MD 21205-2110. *Telephone:* 410-502-3335. *Fax:* 443-769-1232. *E-mail:* son-professionalprgm@jhu.edu.

See display on next page and full description on page 486.

Notre Dame of Maryland University
Department of Nursing
Baltimore, Maryland

http://www.ndm.edu/academics/departments-and-programs/nursing/
Founded in 1873
DEGREE • BS
Nursing Program Faculty 5 (60% with doctorates).
Nursing Student Resources Library services.
Library Facilities 999,295 volumes; 42,427 periodical subscriptions.

BACCALAUREATE PROGRAMS

Degree BS
Available Programs Accelerated RN Baccalaureate; RN Baccalaureate.
Site Options Frederick, MD; Aberdeen, MD.
Study Options Full-time and part-time.
Program Entrance Requirements Minimum overall college GPA of 2.5, transcript of college record, interview, minimum GPA in nursing prerequisites of 2.0, prerequisite course work, RN licensure. Transfer students are accepted.
Advanced Placement Credit by examination available. Credit given for nursing courses completed elsewhere dependent upon specific evaluations.
Contact *Telephone:* 410-532-5500.

Salisbury University
Program in Nursing
Salisbury, Maryland

http://www.salisbury.edu/nursing
Founded in 1925
DEGREES • BS • DNP • MS
Nursing Program Faculty 53 (85% with doctorates).
Baccalaureate Enrollment 570 **Women** 92% **Men** 8% **Minority** 23% **International** .5% **Part-time** 4%
Graduate Enrollment 50 **Women** 94% **Men** 6% **Minority** 16% **Part-time** 62%
Distance Learning Courses Available.
Nursing Student Activities Nursing Honor Society, Sigma Theta Tau, Student Nurses' Association.
Nursing Student Resources Academic advising; academic or career counseling; assistance for students with disabilities; bookstore; campus computer network; career placement assistance; computer lab; computer-assisted instruction; e-mail services; employment services for current students; externships; housing assistance; interactive nursing skills videos; Internet; learning resource lab; library services; nursing audiovisuals; paid internships; placement services for program completers; remedial services; resume preparation assistance; skills, simulation, or other laboratory; tutoring; unpaid internships.

Library Facilities 287,084 volumes (8,945 in health, 1,380 in nursing); 1,093 periodical subscriptions (75 health-care related).

BACCALAUREATE PROGRAMS

Degree BS
Available Programs ADN to Baccalaureate; Accelerated Baccalaureate for Second Degree; Generic Baccalaureate; RN Baccalaureate.
Study Options Full-time and part-time.
Program Entrance Requirements Minimum overall college GPA of 3.0, transcript of college record, CPR certification, health exam, high school biology, high school chemistry, 2 years high school math, high school transcript, immunizations, minimum GPA in nursing prerequisites of 3.0, prerequisite course work. Transfer students are accepted. *Application deadline:* 2/1 (winter). *Application fee:* $45.
Expenses (2012–13) *Tuition, state resident:* full-time $5576. *Tuition, nonresident:* full-time $13,922. *Room and board:* $10,500; room only: $6350 per academic year. *Required fees:* full-time $2124.
Financial Aid 75% of baccalaureate students in nursing programs received some form of financial aid in 2011–12.
Contact Dr. Lisa A. Seldomridge, Chair and Professor, Department of Nursing, Program in Nursing, Salisbury University, 1101 Camden Avenue, Salisbury, MD 21801. *Telephone:* 410-543-6413. *Fax:* 410-548-3313. *E-mail:* laseldomridge@salisbury.edu.

GRADUATE PROGRAMS

Expenses (2012–13) *Tuition, state resident:* part-time $584 per credit. *Tuition, nonresident:* part-time $742 per credit. *Required fees:* part-time $77 per credit.
Financial Aid Career-related internships or fieldwork, institutionally sponsored loans, scholarships, and unspecified assistantships available.
Contact Dr. Mary T. Parsons, Director, Graduate and Second Degree Programs, Program in Nursing, Salisbury University, 1101 Camden Avenue, Salisbury, MD 21801. *Telephone:* 410-543-6416. *Fax:* 410-548-3313. *E-mail:* mtparsons@salisbury.edu.

MASTER'S DEGREE PROGRAM
Degree MS
Available Programs Master's; RN to Master's.
Concentrations Available Health-care administration; nursing education. *Nurse practitioner programs in:* family health.
Study Options Full-time and part-time.

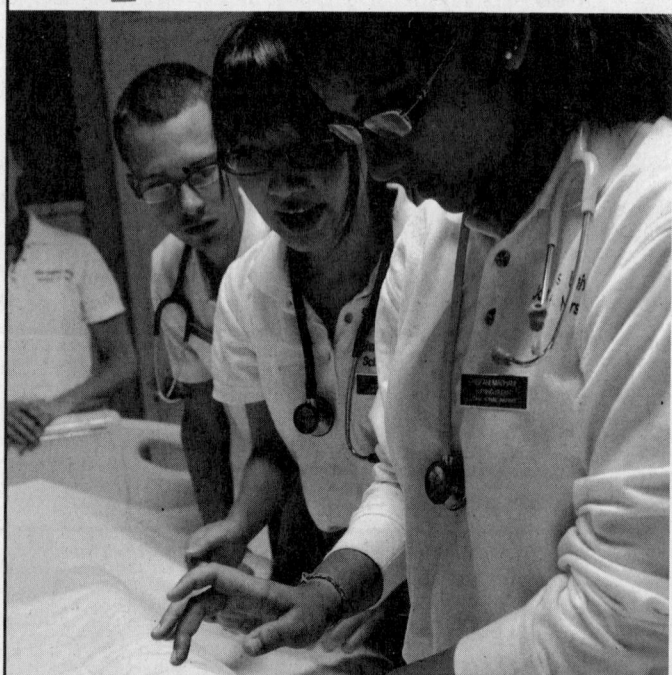

Program Entrance Requirements Minimum overall college GPA of 3.0, transcript of college record, CPR certification, written essay, immunizations, interview, 2 letters of recommendation, nursing research course, physical assessment course, professional liability insurance/malpractice insurance, prerequisite course work, resume, statistics course. *Application deadline:* Applications may be processed on a rolling basis for some programs. *Application fee:* $45.

Advanced Placement Credit given for nursing courses completed elsewhere dependent upon specific evaluations.

Degree Requirements 45 total credit hours, thesis or project.

POST-MASTER'S PROGRAM
Areas of Study Health-care administration; nursing education. *Nurse practitioner programs in:* family health.

DOCTORAL DEGREE PROGRAM
Degree DNP

Available Programs Doctorate.

Areas of Study Advanced practice nursing, biology of health and illness, clinical practice, community health, family health, gerontology, health policy, health promotion/disease prevention, health-care systems, individualized study, information systems, nursing policy, women's health.

Program Entrance Requirements Clinical experience, minimum overall college GPA of 3.5, interview, 3 letters of recommendation, MSN or equivalent, statistics course, vita, writing sample. *Application deadline:* 5/1 (fall). Applications may be processed on a rolling basis for some programs. *Application fee:* $45.

Degree Requirements 38 total credit hours, dissertation.

Stevenson University
Nursing Division
Stevenson, Maryland

http://www.stevenson.edu/academics/nursing/index.asp
Founded in 1952

DEGREES • BS • MS
Nursing Program Faculty 50 (30% with doctorates).

Baccalaureate Enrollment 700 **Women** 94% **Men** 6% **Minority** 25% **Part-time** 52%

Graduate Enrollment 150 **Women** 95% **Men** 5% **Minority** 30% **Part-time** 100%

Distance Learning Courses Available.

Nursing Student Activities Sigma Theta Tau, Student Nurses' Association, nursing club.

Nursing Student Resources Academic advising; academic or career counseling; assistance for students with disabilities; bookstore; campus computer network; career placement assistance; computer lab; computer-assisted instruction; e-mail services; employment services for current students; externships; interactive nursing skills videos; Internet; learning resource lab; library services; nursing audiovisuals; placement services for program completers; remedial services; resume preparation assistance; skills, simulation, or other laboratory; tutoring.

Library Facilities 81,802 volumes (3,301 in health, 776 in nursing); 1,058 periodical subscriptions (635 health-care related).

BACCALAUREATE PROGRAMS
Degree BS

Available Programs ADN to Baccalaureate; Accelerated RN Baccalaureate; Baccalaureate for Second Degree; Generic Baccalaureate; RN Baccalaureate.

Site Options Eastern shore, MD; southern state, MD; Baltimore, MD.

Study Options Full-time and part-time.

Online Degree Options Yes (online only).

Program Entrance Requirements Minimum overall college GPA of 3.0, transcript of college record, written essay, health exam, health insurance, high school biology, high school chemistry, 2 years high school math, high school transcript, immunizations, interview, minimum high school GPA of 3.0, minimum GPA in nursing prerequisites of 3.0. Transfer students are accepted. *Application deadline:* 2/1 (spring).

Advanced Placement Credit by examination available. Credit given for nursing courses completed elsewhere dependent upon specific evaluations.

Expenses (2012–13) *Tuition:* full-time $23,562; part-time $596 per credit. *Room and board:* $11,888; room only: $7888 per academic year. *Required fees:* full-time $1748.

Financial Aid 85% of baccalaureate students in nursing programs received some form of financial aid in 2011–12.

Contact Dr. Denise Seigart, Associate Dean for Nursing Education, Nursing Division, Stevenson University, 1525 Greenspring Valley Road, Stevenson, MD 21153-0641. *Telephone:* 443-334-2821. *Fax:* 443-334-2148. *E-mail:* dseigart@stevenson.edu.

GRADUATE PROGRAMS
Expenses (2012–13) *Tuition:* part-time $560 per credit.

Financial Aid 20% of graduate students in nursing programs received some form of financial aid in 2011–12.

Contact Dr. Judith Feustle, Associate Dean, GPS Nursing, Nursing Division, Stevenson University, Garrison Hall, 100 Campus Circle, Owings MIlls, MD 21117. *Telephone:* 443-352-4292. *Fax:* 443-394-0538. *E-mail:* jfeustle@stevenson.edu.

MASTER'S DEGREE PROGRAM
Degree MS

Available Programs Accelerated Master's; Accelerated RN to Master's; RN to Master's.

Concentrations Available Health-care administration; nursing administration; nursing education.

Site Options Eastern shore, MD; southern state, MD; Baltimore, MD.

Study Options Part-time.

Online Degree Options Yes (online only).

Program Entrance Requirements Computer literacy, minimum overall college GPA of 3.0, transcript of college record, immunizations, letters of recommendation, nursing research course.

Advanced Placement Credit given for nursing courses completed elsewhere dependent upon specific evaluations.

Degree Requirements 36 total credit hours, thesis or project.

Towson University
Department of Nursing
Towson, Maryland

http://www.towson.edu/nursing
Founded in 1866

DEGREES • BS • MS
Nursing Program Faculty 81 (15% with doctorates).

Baccalaureate Enrollment 366 **Women** 88% **Men** 12% **Minority** 25% **Part-time** 10%

Graduate Enrollment 118 **Women** 92% **Men** 8% **Minority** 22% **Part-time** 60%

Distance Learning Courses Available.

Nursing Student Activities Sigma Theta Tau, Student Nurses' Association.

Nursing Student Resources Academic advising; academic or career counseling; assistance for students with disabilities; bookstore; campus computer network; career placement assistance; computer lab; computer-assisted instruction; daycare for children of students; e-mail services; housing assistance; interactive nursing skills videos; Internet; learning resource lab; library services; nursing audiovisuals; remedial services; resume preparation assistance; skills, simulation, or other laboratory; tutoring.

Library Facilities 734,559 volumes (16,393 in health, 1,450 in nursing); 9,245 periodical subscriptions (715 health-care related).

BACCALAUREATE PROGRAMS
Degree BS

Available Programs Generic Baccalaureate; RN Baccalaureate.

Site Options Hagerstown, MD.

Study Options Full-time and part-time.

Program Entrance Requirements Minimum overall college GPA of 3.0, transcript of college record, CPR certification, health exam, health insurance, immunizations, prerequisite course work. Transfer students are accepted. *Application deadline:* 1/15 (fall), 8/15 (spring). *Application fee:* $50.

Advanced Placement Credit given for nursing courses completed elsewhere dependent upon specific evaluations.

Expenses (2012–13) *Tuition, state resident:* full-time $5660; part-time $246 per unit. *Tuition, nonresident:* full-time $17,282; part-time $723 per unit. *International tuition:* $17,282 full-time. *Required fees:* full-time $2472; part-time $103 per credit.

Financial Aid *Gift aid (need-based):* Federal Pell, FSEOG, state, private, college/university gift aid from institutional funds. *Loans:* Federal Direct

(Subsidized and Unsubsidized Stafford PLUS), Perkins. *Work-study:* Federal Work-Study, part-time campus jobs. *Financial aid application deadline (priority):* 2/15.

Contact Ms. Brook R. Necker, Admissions and Retention Coordinator, Department of Nursing, Towson University, 8000 York Road, Towson, MD 21252-0001. *Telephone:* 410-704-4170. *E-mail:* bnecker@towson.edu.

GRADUATE PROGRAMS

Expenses (2012–13) *Tuition, state resident:* part-time $351 per unit. *Tuition, nonresident:* part-time $737 per unit. *Required fees:* part-time $102 per credit.

Financial Aid 15% of graduate students in nursing programs received some form of financial aid in 2011–12.

Contact Dr. Kathleen Ogle, Graduate Program Director, Department of Nursing, Towson University, 8000 York Road, Towson, MD 21252-0001. *Telephone:* 410-704-4389. *Fax:* 410-704-4325. *E-mail:* kogle@towson.edu.

MASTER'S DEGREE PROGRAM

Degree MS

Available Programs Master's.

Concentrations Available Health-care administration; nursing education.

Site Options Hagerstown, MD.

Study Options Full-time and part-time.

Program Entrance Requirements Minimum overall college GPA of 3.0, transcript of college record, nursing research course, physical assessment course, resume, statistics course. *Application deadline:* 8/1 (fall), 12/1 (spring), 5/1 (summer). Applications may be processed on a rolling basis for some programs. *Application fee:* $50.

Advanced Placement Credit given for nursing courses completed elsewhere dependent upon specific evaluations.

Degree Requirements 36 total credit hours.

POST-MASTER'S PROGRAM

Areas of Study Health-care administration; nursing education.

University of Maryland, Baltimore
Master's Program in Nursing
Baltimore, Maryland

http://nursing.umaryland.edu/
Founded in 1807

DEGREES • BSN • DNP • MS • MSN/MBA • MSN/MPH • PHD

Nursing Program Faculty 216 (57% with doctorates).

Baccalaureate Enrollment 594 **Women** 84% **Men** 16% **Minority** 38% **International** 3% **Part-time** 23%

Graduate Enrollment 1,119 **Women** 88% **Men** 12% **Minority** 35% **International** 2% **Part-time** 66%

Distance Learning Courses Available.

Nursing Student Activities Nursing Honor Society, Sigma Theta Tau, Student Nurses' Association.

Nursing Student Resources Academic advising; academic or career counseling; assistance for students with disabilities; bookstore; campus computer network; career placement assistance; computer lab; computer-assisted instruction; e-mail services; interactive nursing skills videos; Internet; learning resource lab; library services; nursing audiovisuals; remedial services; skills, simulation, or other laboratory; tutoring.

Library Facilities 360,000 volumes in health, 60 volumes in nursing; 2,400 periodical subscriptions health-care related.

BACCALAUREATE PROGRAMS

Degree BSN

Available Programs ADN to Baccalaureate; Generic Baccalaureate; RN Baccalaureate.

Site Options Baltimore-Shady Grove, MD.

Study Options Full-time and part-time.

Online Degree Options Yes.

Program Entrance Requirements Minimum overall college GPA of 3.0, transcript of college record, CPR certification, written essay, health exam, health insurance, immunizations, 2 letters of recommendation,

minimum GPA in nursing prerequisites of 3.0, prerequisite course work. *Application deadline:* 2/1 (fall), 9/1 (spring). *Application fee:* $50.

Advanced Placement Credit by examination available.

Expenses (2012–13) *Tuition, state resident:* full-time $7498; part-time $496 per credit. *Tuition, nonresident:* full-time $27,012; part-time $697 per credit. *International tuition:* $27,012 full-time. *Required fees:* full-time $1675.

Financial Aid 61% of baccalaureate students in nursing programs received some form of financial aid in 2011–12.

Contact Mr. Kevin Nies, Associate Director of Admissions, Master's Program in Nursing, University of Maryland, Baltimore, 655 West Lombard Street, Room 102G, Baltimore, MD 21201. *Telephone:* 410-706-1281. *Fax:* 410-706-7238. *E-mail:* nies@son.umaryland.edu.

GRADUATE PROGRAMS

Expenses (2012–13) *Tuition, state resident:* full-time $27,000; part-time $600 per credit. *Tuition, nonresident:* full-time $48,330; part-time $1074 per credit. *International tuition:* $48,330 full-time. *Required fees:* full-time $1265.

Financial Aid 53% of graduate students in nursing programs received some form of financial aid in 2011–12. Fellowships, research assistantships, teaching assistantships, career-related internships or fieldwork and traineeships available. Aid available to part-time students. *Financial aid application deadline:* 2/15.

Contact Mr. Kevin Nies, Assistant Director of Admissions, Master's Program in Nursing, University of Maryland, Baltimore, 655 West Lombard Street, Room 505, Baltimore, MD 21201-1579. *Telephone:* 410-706-1281. *Fax:* 410-706-7832. *E-mail:* knies@son.umaryland.edu.

MASTER'S DEGREE PROGRAM

Degrees MS; MSN/MBA; MSN/MPH

Available Programs Accelerated Master's for Non-Nursing College Graduates; Master's; RN to Master's.

Concentrations Available Clinical nurse leader; nurse anesthesia; nursing administration; nursing informatics. *Clinical nurse specialist programs in:* acute care, community health, critical care. *Nurse practitioner programs in:* acute care, adult health, family health, gerontology, pediatric, primary care, psychiatric/mental health.

Site Options Baltimore-Shady Grove, MD.

Study Options Full-time and part-time.

Online Degree Options Yes.

Program Entrance Requirements Computer literacy, minimum overall college GPA of 3.0, transcript of college record, CPR certification, written essay, immunizations, interview, 2 letters of recommendation, nursing research course, physical assessment course, professional liability insurance/malpractice insurance, prerequisite course work, resume, statistics course. *Application deadline:* 2/1 (fall), 9/1 (spring). *Application fee:* $50.

Advanced Placement Credit given for nursing courses completed elsewhere dependent upon specific evaluations.

Degree Requirements 36–45 total credits, thesis or project, scholarly paper.

POST-MASTER'S PROGRAM

Areas of Study Nursing administration; nursing education; nursing informatics. *Clinical nurse specialist programs in:* community health, pediatric, public health. *Nurse practitioner programs in:* acute care, adult health, family health, gerontology, pediatric, primary care, psychiatric/mental health.

DOCTORAL DEGREE PROGRAM

Degree DNP

Available Programs Doctorate; Doctorate for Nurses with Non-Nursing Degrees; Post-Baccalaureate Doctorate.

Areas of Study Advanced practice nursing, aging, community health, critical care, family health, gerontology, health policy, information systems, nursing administration, nursing policy.

Program Entrance Requirements Clinical experience, minimum overall college GPA of 3.0, interview by faculty committee, 3 letters of recommendation, MSN or equivalent, statistics course, vita. *Application deadline:* 2/15 (fall). *Application fee:* $50.

Degree Requirements 38 total credit hours, oral exam.

DOCTORAL DEGREE PROGRAM

Degree PhD

Available Programs Doctorate, Post-Baccalaureate Doctorate.

Areas of Study Addiction/substance abuse, aging, bio-behavioral research, biology of health and illness, critical care, faculty preparation, gerontology, health promotion/disease prevention, illness and transition, individualized study, information systems, neuro-behavior, nursing administration, nursing education, nursing research, nursing science, oncology.

Program Entrance Requirements Minimum overall college GPA of 3.5, interview, interview by faculty committee, 3 letters of recommendation, MSN or equivalent, statistics course, vita. *Application deadline:* 2/15 (fall). *Application fee:* $50.

Degree Requirements 60 total credit hours, dissertation, oral exam, residency, written exam.

CONTINUING EDUCATION PROGRAM

Contact Sonia Smith, Program Coordinator, Master's Program in Nursing, University of Maryland, Baltimore, 655 West Lombard Street, Room 311G, Baltimore, MD 21201-1579. *Telephone:* 410-706-3768. *E-mail:* Ssmith@son.umaryland.edu.

Washington Adventist University
Nursing Department
Takoma Park, Maryland

http://www.wau.edu/
Founded in 1904

DEGREE • BS
Nursing Program Faculty 8 (14% with doctorates).
Baccalaureate Enrollment 240 **Women** 90% **Men** 10% **Minority** 75% **International** 1% **Part-time** 10%
Nursing Student Activities Student Nurses' Association, nursing club.
Nursing Student Resources Academic advising; academic or career counseling; bookstore; campus computer network; computer lab; e-mail services; externships; interactive nursing skills videos; Internet; learning resource lab; library services; nursing audiovisuals; remedial services; skills, simulation, or other laboratory; tutoring; unpaid internships.

BACCALAUREATE PROGRAMS

Degree BS
Available Programs Accelerated RN Baccalaureate; Generic Baccalaureate.
Study Options Full-time.
Program Entrance Requirements Minimum overall college GPA of 2.75, transcript of college record, CPR certification, written essay, health exam, immunizations, interview, 2 letters of recommendation, minimum GPA in nursing prerequisites of 2.75, prerequisite course work. Transfer students are accepted.
Advanced Placement Credit given for nursing courses completed elsewhere dependent upon specific evaluations.
Contact *Telephone:* 301-891-4144. *Fax:* 301-891-4191.

MASSACHUSETTS

American International College
Division of Nursing
Springfield, Massachusetts

http://www.aic.edu/academics/hs/nursing
Founded in 1885

DEGREES • BSN • MSN
Nursing Program Faculty 11 (27% with doctorates).
Baccalaureate Enrollment 410 **Women** 87% **Men** 13% **Minority** 34% **Part-time** 5%
Graduate Enrollment 21 **Women** 95% **Men** 5% **Minority** 38% **Part-time** 100%
Distance Learning Courses Available.
Nursing Student Activities Nursing Honor Society, Sigma Theta Tau, Student Nurses' Association.
Nursing Student Resources Academic advising; academic or career counseling; assistance for students with disabilities; bookstore; campus computer network; career placement assistance; computer lab; e-mail services; employment services for current students; externships; housing assistance; interactive nursing skills videos; Internet; learning resource lab; library services; nursing audiovisuals; other; placement services for program completers; remedial services; resume preparation assistance; skills, simulation, or other laboratory; tutoring; unpaid internships.
Library Facilities 70,741 volumes (750 in health, 275 in nursing); 7,211 periodical subscriptions (50 health-care related).

BACCALAUREATE PROGRAMS

Degree BSN
Available Programs ADN to Baccalaureate; Generic Baccalaureate; RN Baccalaureate.
Study Options Full-time and part-time.
Program Entrance Requirements Minimum overall college GPA of 2.50, transcript of college record, health exam, health insurance, high school biology, high school chemistry, 3 years high school math, 2 years high school science, high school transcript, immunizations, minimum high school GPA of 2.5, minimum GPA in nursing prerequisites of 2.5, professional liability insurance/malpractice insurance, prerequisite course work. Transfer students are accepted. *Application deadline:* 2/15 (fall). *Application fee:* $25.
Advanced Placement Credit by examination available. Credit given for nursing courses completed elsewhere dependent upon specific evaluations.
Expenses (2012–13) *Tuition:* full-time $29,158; part-time $601 per credit hour. *International tuition:* $29,158 full-time. *Room and board:* $11,710; room only: $6086 per academic year. *Required fees:* full-time $1452.
Financial Aid 99% of baccalaureate students in nursing programs received some form of financial aid in 2011–12. *Gift aid (need-based):* Federal Pell, FSEOG, state, private, college/university gift aid from institutional funds. *Loans:* Federal Direct (Subsidized and Unsubsidized Stafford PLUS), Perkins. *Work-study:* Federal Work-Study, part-time campus jobs. *Financial aid application deadline (priority):* 5/1.
Contact Ms. Janelle Holmboe, Admission Services, Division of Nursing, American International College, 1000 State Street, Springfield, MA 01109. *Telephone:* 413-205-3201. *Fax:* 413-205-3275. *E-mail:* janelle.holmboe@aic.edu.

GRADUATE PROGRAMS

Expenses (2012–13) *Tuition:* part-time $549 per credit hour. *Room and board:* $11,710; room only: $6086 per academic year. *Required fees:* part-time $25 per term.
Financial Aid 62% of graduate students in nursing programs received some form of financial aid in 2011–12.
Contact Ms. Diane Mendez, Director of Graduate Admissions, Division of Nursing, American International College, 1000 State Street, Springfield, MA 01109. *Telephone:* 413-205-3703. *Fax:* 413-205-3201. *E-mail:* diane.mendez@aic.edu.

MASTER'S DEGREE PROGRAM
Degree MSN
Available Programs Master's.
Concentrations Available Nursing administration; nursing education.
Study Options Full-time and part-time.
Online Degree Options Yes (online only).
Program Entrance Requirements Clinical experience, minimum overall college GPA of 3.0, transcript of college record, CPR certification, immunizations, interview, 2 letters of recommendation, professional liability insurance/malpractice insurance, prerequisite course work, resume. *Application deadline:* Applications may be processed on a rolling basis for some programs. *Application fee:* $50.
Advanced Placement Credit given for nursing courses completed elsewhere dependent upon specific evaluations.
Degree Requirements 36 total credit hours, thesis or project.

Anna Maria College
Department of Nursing
Paxton, Massachusetts

http://www.annamaria.edu/
Founded in 1946

DEGREE • BSN
Nursing Program Faculty 6 (16% with doctorates).
Baccalaureate Enrollment 32 **Women** 94% **Men** 6% **Minority** 6% **Part-time** 100%
Nursing Student Activities Sigma Theta Tau.

Nursing Student Resources Academic advising; academic or career counseling; assistance for students with disabilities; bookstore; campus computer network; career placement assistance; computer lab; e-mail services; employment services for current students; Internet; learning resource lab; library services; nursing audiovisuals; placement services for program completers; remedial services; resume preparation assistance; skills, simulation, or other laboratory; tutoring; unpaid internships.

Library Facilities 3,000 volumes in health, 400 volumes in nursing; 22 periodical subscriptions health-care related.

BACCALAUREATE PROGRAMS

Degree BSN

Available Programs ADN to Baccalaureate; RN Baccalaureate.

Study Options Part-time.

Program Entrance Requirements Minimum overall college GPA of 2.5, transcript of college record, interview, 1 letter of recommendation, minimum high school GPA of 2.5, minimum GPA in nursing prerequisites of 2.5, RN licensure. Transfer students are accepted. *Application deadline:* Applications may be processed on a rolling basis for some programs. *Application fee:* $40.

Advanced Placement Credit by examination available. Credit given for nursing courses completed elsewhere dependent upon specific evaluations.

Contact *Telephone:* 508-829-3316 Ext. 316. *Fax:* 508-849-3343 Ext. 371.

CONTINUING EDUCATION PROGRAM

Contact *Telephone:* 508-849-3316 Ext. 316. *Fax:* 508-849-3343 Ext. 371.

Boston College

William F. Connell School of Nursing
Chestnut Hill, Massachusetts

http://www.bc.edu/nursing
Founded in 1863

DEGREES • BS • MS • MSN/MA • MSN/MBA • MSN/PHD • PHD

Nursing Program Faculty 127 (35% with doctorates).

Baccalaureate Enrollment 391 **Women** 96% **Men** 4% **Minority** 24% **International** .3%

Graduate Enrollment 296 **Women** 91% **Men** 9% **Minority** 16% **International** 2% **Part-time** 42%

Nursing Student Activities Nursing Honor Society, Sigma Theta Tau, Student Nurses' Association.

Nursing Student Resources Academic advising; academic or career counseling; assistance for students with disabilities; bookstore; campus computer network; career placement assistance; computer lab; computer-assisted instruction; e-mail services; employment services for current students; externships; housing assistance; interactive nursing skills videos; Internet; learning resource lab; library services; nursing audiovisuals; other; placement services for program completers; remedial services; resume preparation assistance; skills, simulation, or other laboratory; tutoring; unpaid internships.

Library Facilities 2.7 million volumes (65,000 in health, 20,000 in nursing); 256,702 periodical subscriptions (5,395 health-care related).

BACCALAUREATE PROGRAMS

Degree BS

Available Programs Generic Baccalaureate.

Study Options Full-time.

Program Entrance Requirements Transcript of college record, written essay, health exam, health insurance, high school biology, high school chemistry, high school foreign language, 4 years high school math, 3 years high school science, high school transcript, immunizations, 2 letters of recommendation. Transfer students are accepted. *Application deadline:* 1/1 (fall), 11/1 (winter). *Application fee:* $70.

Advanced Placement Credit given for nursing courses completed elsewhere dependent upon specific evaluations.

Expenses (2012–13) *Tuition:* full-time $43,140. *Room and board:* $12,608; room only: $7790 per academic year. *Required fees:* full-time $1496.

Financial Aid 77% of baccalaureate students in nursing programs received some form of financial aid in 2011–12.

Contact Ms. Christine Murphy, Undergraduate Program Assistant, William F. Connell School of Nursing, Boston College, 140 Commonwealth Avenue, Cushing Hall 202D, Chestnut Hill, MA 02467-3812. *Telephone:* 617-552-4925. *Fax:* 617-552-0745. *E-mail:* christine.murphy.1@bc.edu.

GRADUATE PROGRAMS

Expenses (2012–13) *Tuition:* part-time $1120 per credit hour. *Room and board:* $12,608; room only: $7790 per academic year.

Financial Aid 77% of graduate students in nursing programs received some form of financial aid in 2011–12. 9 fellowships with full tuition reimbursements available (averaging $15,300 per year), 7 teaching assistantships (averaging $13,612 per year) were awarded; research assistantships, Federal Work-Study, institutionally sponsored loans, scholarships, traineeships, tuition waivers (partial), and unspecified assistantships also available. Aid available to part-time students. *Financial aid application deadline:* 3/1.

Contact Ms. Marybeth Crowley, Graduate Programs Office, William F. Connell School of Nursing, Boston College, 140 Commonwealth Avenue, Cushing Hall, Chestnut Hill, MA 02467-3812. *Telephone:* 617-552-4928. *Fax:* 617-552-2121. *E-mail:* csongrad@bc.edu.

MASTER'S DEGREE PROGRAM

Degrees MS; MSN/MA; MSN/MBA; MSN/PhD

Available Programs Accelerated Master's; Accelerated Master's for Non-Nursing College Graduates; Accelerated Master's for Nurses with Non-Nursing Degrees; Master's; RN to Master's.

Concentrations Available Nurse anesthesia. *Clinical nurse specialist programs in:* adult health, community health, forensic nursing, gerontology, palliative care, pediatric, psychiatric/mental health. *Nurse practitioner programs in:* adult health, family health, gerontology, pediatric, psychiatric/mental health, women's health.

Study Options Full-time and part-time.

Program Entrance Requirements Minimum overall college GPA of 3.0, transcript of college record, written essay, 3 letters of recommendation, statistics course. *Application deadline:* 4/30 (fall), 9/15 (spring). Applications may be processed on a rolling basis for some programs. *Application fee:* $40.

Advanced Placement Credit given for nursing courses completed elsewhere dependent upon specific evaluations.

Degree Requirements 45 total credit hours, comprehensive exam.

POST-MASTER'S PROGRAM

Areas of Study Nurse anesthesia; nursing education. *Clinical nurse specialist programs in:* adult health, community health, forensic nursing, gerontology, palliative care, pediatric, psychiatric/mental health. *Nurse practitioner programs in:* adult health, family health, gerontology, pediatric, psychiatric/mental health, women's health.

DOCTORAL DEGREE PROGRAM

Degree PhD

Available Programs Doctorate; Post-Baccalaureate Doctorate.

Areas of Study Addiction/substance abuse, advanced practice nursing, aging, bio-behavioral research, biology of health and illness, clinical practice, community health, ethics, family health, forensic nursing, gerontology, health promotion/disease prevention, human health and illness, illness and transition, individualized study, maternity-newborn, neurobehavior, nurse case management, nursing research, nursing science, oncology, urban health, women's health.

Program Entrance Requirements Minimum overall college GPA of 3.0, interview by faculty committee, interview, 3 letters of recommendation, MSN or equivalent, statistics course, vita, writing sample, GRE General Test. *Application deadline:* 12/31 (fall). *Application fee:* $40.

Degree Requirements 46 total credit hours, dissertation, oral exam, written exam.

CONTINUING EDUCATION PROGRAM

Contact Dr. Jean Weyman, Assistant Dean, Continuing Education, William F. Connell School of Nursing, Boston College, 140 Commonwealth Avenue, Service Building, 211F, Chestnut Hill, MA 02467-3812. *Telephone:* 617-552-4256. *Fax:* 617-552-0745. *E-mail:* jean.weyman@bc.edu.

Curry College
Division of Nursing
Milton, Massachusetts

http://www.curry.edu/
Founded in 1879
DEGREES • BS • MSN
Nursing Program Faculty 48 (33% with doctorates).
Baccalaureate Enrollment 611 **Women** 92% **Men** 8% **Minority** 15% **Part-time** 48%
Graduate Enrollment 31 **Women** 97% **Men** 3% **Minority** 20% **Part-time** 100%
Nursing Student Activities Sigma Theta Tau, Student Nurses' Association.
Nursing Student Resources Academic advising; academic or career counseling; assistance for students with disabilities; bookstore; campus computer network; career placement assistance; computer lab; computer-assisted instruction; daycare for children of students; e-mail services; employment services for current students; housing assistance; interactive nursing skills videos; Internet; learning resource lab; library services; nursing audiovisuals; placement services for program completers; remedial services; resume preparation assistance; skills, simulation, or other laboratory; tutoring.
Library Facilities 154,100 volumes (5,867 in health, 4,589 in nursing); 47,600 periodical subscriptions (162 health-care related).

BACCALAUREATE PROGRAMS

Degree BS
Available Programs Accelerated Baccalaureate for Second Degree; Generic Baccalaureate; RN Baccalaureate; RPN to Baccalaureate.
Site Options Boston, MA; Plymouth, MA.
Study Options Full-time.
Program Entrance Requirements Written essay, health exam, health insurance, high school biology, high school chemistry, high school foreign language, 4 years high school math, 4 years high school science, high school transcript, immunizations, 1 letter of recommendation, minimum high school GPA of 2.75, minimum GPA in nursing prerequisites of 3.0. Transfer students are accepted. *Application deadline:* 4/1 (fall). Applications may be processed on a rolling basis for some programs. *Application fee:* $50.
Advanced Placement Credit by examination available. Credit given for nursing courses completed elsewhere dependent upon specific evaluations.
Contact *Telephone:* 800-669-0686. *Fax:* 617-333-2114.

GRADUATE PROGRAMS

Contact *Telephone:* 617-333-2243. *Fax:* 617-333-6680.

MASTER'S DEGREE PROGRAM
Degree MSN
Available Programs Master's; RN to Master's.
Concentrations Available Clinical nurse leader.
Site Options Boston, MA.
Program Entrance Requirements Minimum overall college GPA of 3.0, transcript of college record, written essay, immunizations, 2 letters of recommendation, nursing research course, physical assessment course, resume, statistics course. *Application deadline:* Applications may be processed on a rolling basis for some programs. *Application fee:* $50.
Degree Requirements 37 total credit hours, thesis or project.

Elms College
Division of Nursing
Chicopee, Massachusetts

http://www.elms.edu/
Founded in 1928
DEGREES • BS • MSN
Nursing Program Faculty 13 (46% with doctorates).
Baccalaureate Enrollment 200 **Women** 87% **Men** 13% **Minority** 11% **Part-time** 35%
Graduate Enrollment 42 **Women** 97% **Men** 3% **Minority** 5% **Part-time** 50%
Nursing Student Activities Nursing Honor Society, Sigma Theta Tau, Student Nurses' Association.

Nursing Student Resources Academic advising; academic or career counseling; assistance for students with disabilities; bookstore; campus computer network; career placement assistance; computer lab; computer-assisted instruction; e-mail services; employment services for current students; externships; interactive nursing skills videos; Internet; learning resource lab; library services; nursing audiovisuals; resume preparation assistance; skills, simulation, or other laboratory; tutoring.
Library Facilities 3,832 volumes in health, 3,000 volumes in nursing; 130 periodical subscriptions·health-care related.

BACCALAUREATE PROGRAMS

Degree BS
Available Programs Generic Baccalaureate; RN Baccalaureate.
Study Options Full-time and part-time.
Program Entrance Requirements Minimum overall college GPA of 2.5, transcript of college record, CPR certification, written essay, health exam, health insurance, high school biology, high school chemistry, high school transcript, immunizations, interview, 2 letters of recommendation, minimum high school GPA of 3.3, minimum high school rank 25%, minimum GPA in nursing prerequisites of 2.5, professional liability insurance/malpractice insurance. Transfer students are accepted. *Application deadline:* Applications may be processed on a rolling basis for some programs. *Application fee:* $30.
Advanced Placement Credit given for nursing courses completed elsewhere dependent upon specific evaluations.
Contact *Telephone:* 413-265-2237. *Fax:* 413-265-2335.

GRADUATE PROGRAMS

Contact *Telephone:* 413-265-2455.

MASTER'S DEGREE PROGRAM
Degree MSN
Available Programs Master's; RN to Master's.
Concentrations Available Nursing administration; nursing education.
Study Options Full-time and part-time.
Program Entrance Requirements Minimum overall college GPA of 3.0, transcript of college record, CPR certification, written essay, immunizations, interview, 2 letters of recommendation, professional liability insurance/malpractice insurance, resume. *Application deadline:* Applications may be processed on a rolling basis for some programs. *Application fee:* $30.
Degree Requirements 36 total credit hours, thesis or project.

Emmanuel College
Department of Nursing
Boston, Massachusetts

http://www.emmanuel.edu/x11602.xml
Founded in 1919
DEGREES • BS • MS
Nursing Program Faculty 22 (37% with doctorates).
Baccalaureate Enrollment 166 **Women** 92% **Men** 8% **Minority** 16% **Part-time** 99%
Graduate Enrollment 35 **Women** 89% **Men** 11% **Minority** 20% **Part-time** 94%
Distance Learning Courses Available.
Nursing Student Activities Sigma Theta Tau.
Nursing Student Resources Academic advising; academic or career counseling; assistance for students with disabilities; bookstore; campus computer network; computer lab; computer-assisted instruction; e-mail services; interactive nursing skills videos; Internet; library services; nursing audiovisuals; resume preparation assistance; skills, simulation, or other laboratory; tutoring.
Library Facilities 150,000 volumes (2,438 in health, 647 in nursing); 2,100 periodical subscriptions (10,532 health-care related).

BACCALAUREATE PROGRAMS

Degree BS
Available Programs RN Baccalaureate.
Site Options Woburn, MA; Boston, MA.
Study Options Full-time and part-time.
Program Entrance Requirements Transcript of college record, written essay, interview, 2 letters of recommendation, RN licensure. Transfer students are accepted. *Application deadline:* Applications may be processed on a rolling basis for some programs.

Advanced Placement Credit by examination available. Credit given for nursing courses completed elsewhere dependent upon specific evaluations.

Expenses (2012–13) *Tuition:* part-time $1772 per course. *International tuition:* $10,632 full-time.

Financial Aid 45% of baccalaureate students in nursing programs received some form of financial aid in 2011–12. *Gift aid (need-based):* Federal Pell, FSEOG, state, private, college/university gift aid from institutional funds. *Loans:* Federal Direct (Subsidized and Unsubsidized Stafford PLUS), Perkins, state.*Work-study:* Federal Work-Study, part-time campus jobs.*Financial aid application deadline (priority):* 2/15.

Contact Dr. Mary Diane Arathuzik, Chair and Associate Professor, Department of Nursing, Emmanuel College, 400 The Fenway, Boston, MA 02115. *Telephone:* 617-735-9945. *Fax:* 617-507-0434. *E-mail:* arathuzi@emmanuel.edu.

GRADUATE PROGRAMS

Expenses (2012–13) *Tuition:* part-time $2518 per course. *International tuition:* $15,108 full-time.

Financial Aid 32% of graduate students in nursing programs received some form of financial aid in 2011–12.

Contact Dr. Mary Diane Arathuzik, Chair and Associate Professor of Nursing, Department of Nursing, Emmanuel College, 400 The Fenway, Boston, MA 02115. *Telephone:* 617-735-9845. *Fax:* 617-507-0434. *E-mail:* arathuzi@emmanuel.edu.

MASTER'S DEGREE PROGRAM

Degree MS

Available Programs Master's.

Concentrations Available Nursing administration; nursing education.

Site Options Boston, MA.

Study Options Full-time and part-time.

Program Entrance Requirements Clinical experience, minimum overall college GPA of 3.0, transcript of college record, written essay, 2 letters of recommendation, resume. *Application deadline:* 4/30 (fall).

Advanced Placement Credit given for nursing courses completed elsewhere dependent upon specific evaluations.

Degree Requirements 36 total credit hours, comprehensive exam.

See display below and full description on page 482.

Endicott College
Major in Nursing
Beverly, Massachusetts

http://www.endicott.edu/

Founded in 1939

DEGREES • BS • MSN

Nursing Program Faculty 27 (25% with doctorates).

Baccalaureate Enrollment 170 **Women** 95% **Men** 5% **Minority** 2% **Part-time** 20%

Graduate Enrollment 25 **Women** 97% **Men** 3% **Minority** 1%

Distance Learning Courses Available.

Nursing Student Activities Nursing Honor Society, Sigma Theta Tau, Student Nurses' Association.

Nursing Student Resources Academic advising; academic or career counseling; assistance for students with disabilities; bookstore; campus computer network; career placement assistance; computer lab; computer-assisted instruction; e-mail services; externships; interactive nursing skills videos; Internet; learning resource lab; library services; nursing audiovisuals; resume preparation assistance; skills, simulation, or other laboratory; tutoring; unpaid internships.

Library Facilities 116,875 volumes (2,828 in health, 624 in nursing); 77,487 periodical subscriptions (55 health-care related).

BACCALAUREATE PROGRAMS

Degree BS

Available Programs Generic Baccalaureate; RN Baccalaureate.

Site Options Beverly, MA.

Study Options Full-time.

Program Entrance Requirements Minimum overall college GPA of 2.5, transcript of college record, written essay, health exam, health insurance, high school biology, high school chemistry, 3 years high school math, 2 years high school science, high school transcript, immunizations, 1 letter of recommendation, minimum high school GPA of 2.5, minimum high school rank 50%, minimum GPA in nursing prerequisites of 2.5. Transfer students are accepted.

Advanced Placement Credit given for nursing courses completed elsewhere dependent upon specific evaluations.

Financial Aid 88% of baccalaureate students in nursing programs received some form of financial aid in 2011–12.
Contact Mr. Thomas J. Redman, Vice President for Admissions and Financial Aid, Major in Nursing, Endicott College, 376 Hale Street, Beverly, MA 01915. *Telephone:* 978-232-2005. *Fax:* 978-232-2500. *E-mail:* admissio@endicott.edu.

GRADUATE PROGRAMS

Contact Dr. Kelly L. Fisher, Dean, School of Nursing, Major in Nursing, Endicott College, 375 Hale Street, Beverly, MA 01915. *E-mail:* kfisher@endicott.edu.

MASTER'S DEGREE PROGRAM

Degree MSN
Available Programs Master's.
Concentrations Available Nursing administration; nursing education.
Site Options Beverly, MA.
Study Options Full-time and part-time.
Program Entrance Requirements Clinical experience, transcript of college record, written essay, letters of recommendation, statistics course.
Advanced Placement Credit given for nursing courses completed elsewhere dependent upon specific evaluations.
Degree Requirements 33 total credit hours, thesis or project.

CONTINUING EDUCATION PROGRAM

Contact Dr. Kelly Fisher, Dean, School of Nursing, Major in Nursing, Endicott College, 376 Hale Street, Beverly, MA 01915. *Telephone:* 978-232-2328. *Fax:* 978-232-3100. *E-mail:* kfisher@endicott.edu.

Fitchburg State University
Department of Nursing
Fitchburg, Massachusetts

http://www.fitchburgstate.edu/academics/academic-departments/department-homepage-nursing/
Founded in 1894
DEGREES • BS • MS
Nursing Program Faculty 16 (31% with doctorates).
Baccalaureate Enrollment 197 **Women** 93% **Men** 7% **Minority** 8% **Part-time** 11%
Graduate Enrollment 16 **Women** 100% **Part-time** 100%
Distance Learning Courses Available.
Nursing Student Activities Sigma Theta Tau, Student Nurses' Association.
Nursing Student Resources Academic advising; academic or career counseling; assistance for students with disabilities; bookstore; campus computer network; career placement assistance; computer lab; computer-assisted instruction; e-mail services; employment services for current students; housing assistance; interactive nursing skills videos; Internet; learning resource lab; library services; nursing audiovisuals; remedial services; resume preparation assistance; skills, simulation, or other laboratory; tutoring; unpaid internships.
Library Facilities 208,450 volumes; 3,050 periodical subscriptions.

BACCALAUREATE PROGRAMS

Degree BS
Available Programs Accelerated LPN to Baccalaureate; Generic Baccalaureate; RN Baccalaureate.
Study Options Full-time.
Online Degree Options Yes.
Program Entrance Requirements Transcript of college record, written essay, health insurance, high school biology, high school chemistry, high school foreign language, 3 years high school math, 3 years high school science, high school transcript, immunizations, minimum high school GPA of 3.0, minimum GPA in nursing prerequisites of 2.5. Transfer students are accepted. *Application deadline:* 1/1 (fall). Applications may be processed on a rolling basis for some programs. *Application fee:* $25.
Expenses (2012–13) *Tuition, state resident:* full-time $970; part-time $40 per credit. *Tuition, nonresident:* full-time $7050; part-time $294 per credit. *Room and board:* $8602; room only: $5652 per academic year.
Financial Aid 76% of baccalaureate students in nursing programs received some form of financial aid in 2011–12.
Contact Ms. Kay Reynolds, Director of Admissions, Department of Nursing, Fitchburg State University, 160 Pearl Street, Fitchburg, MA

01420-2697. *Telephone:* 978-665-3144. *Fax:* 978-665-4540. *E-mail:* admissions@fitchburgstate.edu.

GRADUATE PROGRAMS

Expenses (2012–13) *Tuition, state resident:* part-time $218 per credit. *Tuition, nonresident:* part-time $218 per credit.
Financial Aid 11% of graduate students in nursing programs received some form of financial aid in 2011–12.
Contact Dr. Robert Dumas, Chairperson, Forensic Nursing Program, Department of Nursing, Fitchburg State University, 160 Pearl Street, Fitchburg, MA 01420-2697. *Telephone:* 978-665-3026. *Fax:* 978-665-4501. *E-mail:* rdumas@fitchburgstate.edu.

MASTER'S DEGREE PROGRAM

Degree MS
Available Programs Master's; Master's for Nurses with Non-Nursing Degrees.
Concentrations Available *Clinical nurse specialist programs in:* forensic nursing.
Study Options Part-time.
Online Degree Options Yes (online only).
Program Entrance Requirements Clinical experience, computer literacy, minimum overall college GPA of 2.8, transcript of college record, written essay, immunizations, 3 letters of recommendation, nursing research course, physical assessment course, prerequisite course work, resume, statistics course. *Application deadline:* Applications may be processed on a rolling basis for some programs. *Application fee:* $25.
Degree Requirements 36 total credit hours, thesis or project.

POST-MASTER'S PROGRAM

Areas of Study *Clinical nurse specialist programs in:* forensic nursing.

Framingham State University
Department of Nursing
Framingham, Massachusetts

http://www.framingham.edu/nursing
Founded in 1839
DEGREES • BS • MSN
Nursing Program Faculty 8 (75% with doctorates).
Baccalaureate Enrollment 74 **Women** 85% **Men** 15% **Minority** 33% **International** 2% **Part-time** 90%
Graduate Enrollment 58 **Women** 98% **Men** 2% **Minority** 3% **International** 1% **Part-time** 100%
Nursing Student Activities Sigma Theta Tau.
Nursing Student Resources Academic advising; academic or career counseling; assistance for students with disabilities; bookstore; campus computer network; career placement assistance; computer lab; computer-assisted instruction; daycare for children of students; e-mail services; employment services for current students; housing assistance; interactive nursing skills videos; Internet; learning resource lab; library services; nursing audiovisuals; placement services for program completers; remedial services; resume preparation assistance; skills, simulation, or other laboratory; tutoring.
Library Facilities 212,555 volumes (5,338 in health, 5,338 in nursing); 212 periodical subscriptions (1,200 health-care related).

BACCALAUREATE PROGRAMS

Degree BS
Available Programs ADN to Baccalaureate.
Study Options Full-time and part-time.
Program Entrance Requirements Minimum overall college GPA of 3.0, transcript of college record, written essay, RN licensure. Transfer students are accepted. *Application deadline:* Applications may be processed on a rolling basis for some programs. *Application fee:* $50.
Advanced Placement Credit by examination available. Credit given for nursing courses completed elsewhere dependent upon specific evaluations.
Contact *Telephone:* 508-626-4713. *Fax:* 508-626-4746.

GRADUATE PROGRAMS

Contact *Telephone:* 508-626-4713. *Fax:* 508-626-4746.

MASTER'S DEGREE PROGRAM

Degree MSN

Available Programs Master's.

Concentrations Available Nursing administration; nursing education.

Study Options Part-time.

Program Entrance Requirements Minimum overall college GPA of 3.0, transcript of college record, written essay, interview, 3 letters of recommendation, nursing research course, resume, statistics course. *Application deadline:* 6/1 (fall). Applications may be processed on a rolling basis for some programs. *Application fee:* $50.

Degree Requirements 36 total credit hours, thesis or project.

CONTINUING EDUCATION PROGRAM

Contact *Telephone:* 508-626-4713. *Fax:* 508-626-4746.

Massachusetts College of Pharmacy and Health Sciences
School of Nursing
Boston, Massachusetts

http://www.mcphs.edu/

Founded in 1823

DEGREE • BSN

Nursing Program Faculty 16 (44% with doctorates).

Baccalaureate Enrollment 358 **Women** 66.3% **Men** 33.7% **Minority** 35% **International** 3%

Distance Learning Courses Available.

Nursing Student Activities Nursing Honor Society, Sigma Theta Tau, Student Nurses' Association, nursing club.

Nursing Student Resources Academic advising; academic or career counseling; assistance for students with disabilities; bookstore; campus computer network; career placement assistance; computer lab; computer-assisted instruction; e-mail services; employment services for current students; housing assistance; interactive nursing skills videos; Internet; learning resource lab; library services; nursing audiovisuals; remedial services; resume preparation assistance; skills, simulation, or other laboratory; tutoring.

Library Facilities 17,400 volumes in health, 1,200 volumes in nursing; 10,000 periodical subscriptions health-care related.

BACCALAUREATE PROGRAMS

Degree BSN

Available Programs Accelerated Baccalaureate; Accelerated Baccalaureate for Second Degree.

Site Options Manchester , NH; Worcester , MA.

Study Options Full-time.

Program Entrance Requirements Minimum overall college GPA of 2.5, written essay, high school biology, high school chemistry, 3 years high school math, 2 years high school science, high school transcript, 2 letters of recommendation, prerequisite course work. Transfer students are accepted. *Application deadline:* 2/1 (fall), 10/1 (spring). *Application fee:* $70.

Contact *Telephone:* 800-225-5506.

CONTINUING EDUCATION PROGRAM

Contact *Telephone:* 617-735-1080.

MGH Institute of Health Professions
School of Nursing
Boston, Massachusetts

http://www.mghihp.edu/academics/nursing/

Founded in 1977

DEGREES • BSN • DNP • MS

Nursing Program Faculty 51 (55% with doctorates).

Baccalaureate Enrollment 171 **Women** 85% **Men** 15% **Minority** 22% **International** 1%

Graduate Enrollment 408 **Women** 87% **Men** 13% **Minority** 21% **International** .05% **Part-time** 18%

Distance Learning Courses Available.

Nursing Student Activities Nursing Honor Society, Student Nurses' Association.

Nursing Student Resources Academic advising; academic or career counseling; assistance for students with disabilities; bookstore; campus computer network; career placement assistance; computer lab; computer-assisted instruction; daycare for children of students; e-mail services; interactive nursing skills videos; Internet; learning resource lab; library services; nursing audiovisuals; remedial services; resume preparation assistance; skills, simulation, or other laboratory; tutoring.

Library Facilities 35,000 volumes in health, 15,000 volumes in nursing; 1,600 periodical subscriptions health-care related.

BACCALAUREATE PROGRAMS

Degree BSN

Available Programs Accelerated Baccalaureate.

Site Options Boston, MA.

Study Options Full-time.

Program Entrance Requirements Transcript of college record, written essay, health insurance, immunizations, 3 letters of recommendation, minimum GPA in nursing prerequisites of 3.0, prerequisite course work. Transfer students are accepted. *Application deadline:* 7/1 (spring), 11/1 (summer). *Application fee:* $100.

Advanced Placement Credit by examination available. Credit given for nursing courses completed elsewhere dependent upon specific evaluations.

Expenses (2012–13) *Tuition:* full-time $46,500. *International tuition:* $46,500 full-time. *Required fees:* full-time $1800.

Financial Aid 89% of baccalaureate students in nursing programs received some form of financial aid in 2011–12.

Contact Admissions, School of Nursing, MGH Institute of Health Professions, 36 1st Avenue, Boston, MA 02129. *Telephone:* 617-726-3140. *Fax:* 617-726-8010. *E-mail:* admissions@mghihp.edu.

GRADUATE PROGRAMS

Expenses (2012–13) *Tuition:* full-time $52,416; part-time $1092 per credit. *International tuition:* $52,416 full-time. *Required fees:* full-time $1800.

Financial Aid 72% of graduate students in nursing programs received some form of financial aid in 2011–12. 4 research assistantships (averaging $1,200 per year), 17 teaching assistantships (averaging $1,200 per year) were awarded; career-related internships or fieldwork, scholarships, traineeships, and unspecified assistantships also available. Aid available to part-time students. *Financial aid application deadline:* 4/1.

Contact Office of Admissions, School of Nursing, MGH Institute of Health Professions, PO Box 6357, Boston, MA 02114. *Telephone:* 617-726-3140. *Fax:* 617-726-8010. *E-mail:* admissions@mghihp.edu.

MASTER'S DEGREE PROGRAM

Degree MS

Available Programs Master's; Master's for Non-Nursing College Graduates; Master's for Nurses with Non-Nursing Degrees; RN to Master's.

Concentrations Available Nursing education. *Clinical nurse specialist programs in:* acute care, adult health, family health, gerontology, pediatric, psychiatric/mental health. *Nurse practitioner programs in:* acute care, adult health, family health, gerontology, pediatric, primary care, psychiatric/mental health, women's health.

Site Options Boston, MA.

Study Options Full-time and part-time.

Program Entrance Requirements Minimum overall college GPA of 3.0, transcript of college record, CPR certification, written essay, immunizations, 3 letters of recommendation, professional liability insurance/malpractice insurance, prerequisite course work, resume, statistics course, GRE General Test. *Application deadline:* 1/10 (fall). *Application fee:* $100.

Advanced Placement Credit by examination available. Credit given for nursing courses completed elsewhere dependent upon specific evaluations.

Degree Requirements 91 total credit hours, thesis or project.

POST-MASTER'S PROGRAM

Areas of Study *Clinical nurse specialist programs in:* psychiatric/mental health. *Nurse practitioner programs in:* acute care, adult health, gerontology, pediatric, primary care, psychiatric/mental health, women's health.

DOCTORAL DEGREE PROGRAM

Degree DNP

Available Programs Doctorate; Doctorate for Nurses with Non-Nursing Degrees.

Site Options Boston, MA.

Program Entrance Requirements Minimum overall college GPA of 3.0, interview by faculty committee, 3 letters of recommendation, MSN or equivalent, vita. *Application deadline:* 6/1 (fall). Applications may be processed on a rolling basis for some programs. *Application fee:* $100.
Degree Requirements 43 total credit hours, residency.

Northeastern University
School of Nursing
Boston, Massachusetts

http://www.northeastern.edu/bouve/nursing/index.html
Founded in 1898
DEGREES • BSN • DNP • MS
Distance Learning Courses Available.
Library Facilities 1.4 million volumes; 130,151 periodical subscriptions.

BACCALAUREATE PROGRAMS

Degree BSN
Available Programs Generic Baccalaureate.
Contact Undergraduate Admissions, School of Nursing, Northeastern University, 360 Huntington Avenue, 150 Richards Hall, Boston, MA 02115. *Telephone:* 617-373-2200. *Fax:* 617-373-8780. *E-mail:* admissions@neu.edu.

GRADUATE PROGRAMS

Financial Aid Fellowships, research assistantships, teaching assistantships, career-related internships or fieldwork, institutionally sponsored loans, scholarships, traineeships, tuition waivers (full and partial), and unspecified assistantships available.
Contact Ms. Molly Schnabel, Director of Graduate Admissions and Student Services, School of Nursing, Northeastern University, 360 Huntington Avenue, 123 Behrakis Health Sciences Building, Boston, MA 02115. *Telephone:* 617-373-3501. *Fax:* 617-373-4701. *E-mail:* bouvegrad@neu.edu.

MASTER'S DEGREE PROGRAM
Degree MS
Available Programs Master's.
Program Entrance Requirements GRE General Test.

DOCTORAL DEGREE PROGRAM
Degree DNP
Available Programs Post-Baccalaureate Doctorate.

CONTINUING EDUCATION PROGRAM

Contact Bouve College of Health Sciences, School of Nursing, Northeastern University, 360 Huntington Avenue, 123 Behrakis Health Sciences Building, Boston, MA 02115. *Telephone:* 617-373-2708. *E-mail:* bouvegrad@neu.edu.

Regis College
School of Nursing, Science and Health Professions
Weston, Massachusetts

http://www.regiscollege.edu/grad
Founded in 1927
DEGREES • BSN • DNP • MSN
Nursing Program Faculty 36 (75% with doctorates).
Baccalaureate Enrollment 78
Graduate Enrollment 600 **Women** 90% **Men** 10%
Nursing Student Activities Sigma Theta Tau, Student Nurses' Association, nursing club.
Nursing Student Resources Academic advising; academic or career counseling; assistance for students with disabilities; bookstore; campus computer network; computer lab; e-mail services; Internet; learning resource lab; library services; nursing audiovisuals; resume preparation assistance; skills, simulation, or other laboratory; tutoring.
Library Facilities 134,109 volumes (6,300 in health, 4,700 in nursing); 424 periodical subscriptions (228 health-care related).

BACCALAUREATE PROGRAMS

Degree BSN
Available Programs ADN to Baccalaureate; Accelerated Baccalaureate; Accelerated Baccalaureate for Second Degree; Accelerated RN Baccalaureate; Baccalaureate for Second Degree; Generic Baccalaureate; RN Baccalaureate.
Site Options Medford, MA; Brighton, MA; Boston, MA.
Study Options Full-time.
Program Entrance Requirements Written essay, health exam, health insurance, high school foreign language, 3 years high school math, 2 years high school science, high school transcript, immunizations, 2 letters of recommendation, minimum high school GPA of 3.0, minimum high school rank 40%, minimum GPA in nursing prerequisites. Transfer students are accepted. *Application deadline:* Applications may be processed on a rolling basis for some programs. *Application fee:* $50.
Advanced Placement Credit by examination available. Credit given for nursing courses completed elsewhere dependent upon specific evaluations.
Expenses (2012–13) *Tuition:* full-time $33,000; part-time $660 per credit. *Room and board:* $11,000 per academic year.
Financial Aid 85% of baccalaureate students in nursing programs received some form of financial aid in 2011–12.
Contact Dr. Antionette Hays, Dean, School of Nursing and Health Professions, School of Nursing, Science and Health Professions, Regis College, 235 Wellesley Street, Weston, MA 02493. *Telephone:* 781-768-7090. *Fax:* 781-768-7071. *E-mail:* antoinette.hays@regiscollege.edu.

GRADUATE PROGRAMS

Expenses (2012–13) *Tuition:* full-time $33,000; part-time $915 per credit. *International tuition:* $33,000 full-time. *Room and board:* $11,000 per academic year.
Financial Aid 52% of graduate students in nursing programs received some form of financial aid in 2011–12. 13 research assistantships were awarded; Federal Work-Study, scholarships, traineeships, and unspecified assistantships also available. Aid available to part-time students.
Contact Ms. Claudia C. Pouravelis, Director of Graduate Admission, School of Nursing, Science and Health Professions, Regis College, 235 Wellesley Street, Weston, MA 02493. *Telephone:* 781-768-7058. *Fax:* 781-768-7071. *E-mail:* claudia.pouravelis@regiscollege.edu.

MASTER'S DEGREE PROGRAM
Degree MSN
Available Programs Accelerated AD/RN to Master's; Accelerated Master's; Accelerated Master's for Non-Nursing College Graduates; Accelerated Master's for Nurses with Non-Nursing Degrees; Accelerated RN to Master's; Master's; Master's for Non-Nursing College Graduates; Master's for Nurses with Non-Nursing Degrees; RN to Master's.
Concentrations Available Clinical nurse leader; health-care administration; nurse case management; nursing administration; nursing education; nursing informatics. *Clinical nurse specialist programs in:* acute care. *Nurse practitioner programs in:* adult health, family health, pediatric, primary care, psychiatric/mental health, women's health.
Site Options Medford, MA; Brighton, MA; Boston, MA.
Study Options Full-time and part-time.
Program Entrance Requirements Computer literacy, minimum overall college GPA of 3.0, transcript of college record, CPR certification, written essay, immunizations, interview, 3 letters of recommendation, physical assessment course, professional liability insurance/malpractice insurance, prerequisite course work, resume, statistics course, GRE General Test or MAT. *Application deadline:* Applications may be processed on a rolling basis for some programs. *Application fee:* $50.
Advanced Placement Credit by examination available. Credit given for nursing courses completed elsewhere dependent upon specific evaluations.
Degree Requirements 44 total credit hours, thesis or project.

POST-MASTER'S PROGRAM
Areas of Study Clinical nurse leader; health-care administration; nurse case management; nursing administration; nursing education. *Nurse practitioner programs in:* adult health, family health, pediatric, primary care, psychiatric/mental health, women's health.

DOCTORAL DEGREE PROGRAM
Degree DNP
Available Programs Doctorate; Post-Baccalaureate Doctorate.
Areas of Study Gerontology, health policy, nursing administration, nursing education, nursing policy.
Program Entrance Requirements Clinical experience, minimum overall college GPA of 3.5, interview by faculty committee, interview, 2

letters of recommendation, MSN or equivalent, statistics course, vita, writing sample, MAT or GRE if GPA from master's lower than 3.5. *Application deadline:* Applications may be processed on a rolling basis for some programs. *Application fee:* $75.
Degree Requirements 50 total credit hours.

CONTINUING EDUCATION PROGRAM

Contact Dr. Claudia Pouravelis, Associate Dean of Graduate Affairs, School of Nursing, Science and Health Professions, Regis College, 235 Wellesley Street, Weston, MA 02493. *Telephone:* 781-768-7058. *Fax:* 781-768-7089. *E-mail:* claudia.pouravelis@regiscollege.edu.

Salem State University
Program in Nursing
Salem, Massachusetts

http://www.salemstate.edu/
Founded in 1854
DEGREES • BSN • MSN • MSN/MBA
Nursing Program Faculty 100 (25% with doctorates).
Distance Learning Courses Available.
Nursing Student Activities Nursing Honor Society, Sigma Theta Tau, Student Nurses' Association.
Nursing Student Resources Academic advising; academic or career counseling; assistance for students with disabilities; bookstore; campus computer network; career placement assistance; computer lab; computer-assisted instruction; daycare for children of students; e-mail services; employment services for current students; externships; housing assistance; interactive nursing skills videos; Internet; learning resource lab; library services; nursing audiovisuals; paid internships; remedial services; resume preparation assistance; skills, simulation, or other laboratory; tutoring.
Library Facilities 297,889 volumes (2,000 in health; 1,600 in nursing); 58,079 periodical subscriptions (50 health-care related).

BACCALAUREATE PROGRAMS

Degree BSN
Available Programs ADN to Baccalaureate; Accelerated Baccalaureate for Second Degree; Generic Baccalaureate; International Nurse to Baccalaureate; LPN to Baccalaureate; LPN to RN Baccalaureate.
Site Options Haverhill, MA.
Study Options Full-time.
Program Entrance Requirements Minimum overall college GPA of 3.5, transcript of college record, CPR certification, health exam, health insurance, high school biology, high school chemistry, 3 years high school math, 2 years high school science, high school transcript, immunizations, interview, minimum high school GPA of 3.5, professional liability insurance/malpractice insurance. Transfer students are accepted. *Application deadline:* 2/1 (fall), 10/1 (spring), 4/1 (summer). Applications may be processed on a rolling basis for some programs. *Application fee:* $40.
Advanced Placement Credit by examination available. Credit given for nursing courses completed elsewhere dependent upon specific evaluations.
Expenses (2011–12) *Tuition, state resident:* full-time $910; part-time $38 per credit hour. *Tuition, nonresident:* full-time $7050; part-time $294 per credit hour. *International tuition:* $7050 full-time. *Room and board:* $13,000; room only: $9540 per academic year. *Required fees:* part-time $282 per credit; part-time $845 per term.
Financial Aid 60% of baccalaureate students in nursing programs received some form of financial aid in 2010–11.
Contact Dr. Mary Dunn, Assistant Dean of Admissions, Program in Nursing, Salem State University, 352 Lafayette Street, Salem, MA 01970. *Telephone:* 978-542-6200. *E-mail:* admissions@salemstate.edu.

GRADUATE PROGRAMS

Expenses (2011–12) *Tuition, state resident:* full-time $2520; part-time $140 per credit hour. *Tuition, nonresident:* full-time $4140; part-time $230 per credit hour. *International tuition:* $4140 full-time. *Room and board:* $12,740; room only: $9540 per academic year. *Required fees:* full-time $2100; part-time $175 per credit; part-time $525 per term.
Financial Aid 25% of graduate students in nursing programs received some form of financial aid in 2010–11. Career-related internships or fieldwork, Federal Work-Study, scholarships, and unspecified assistant-

ships available. Aid available to part-time students. *Financial aid application deadline:* 5/1.
Contact Dr. Kathleen Skrabut, Coordinator, Graduate Program, Program in Nursing, Salem State University, 352 Lafayette Street, Salem, MA 01970. *Telephone:* 978-542-7018. *Fax:* 978-542-2016. *E-mail:* kskrabut@salemstate.edu.

MASTER'S DEGREE PROGRAM

Degrees MSN; MSN/MBA
Available Programs Accelerated Master's for Non-Nursing College Graduates; Master's; Master's for Nurses with Non-Nursing Degrees.
Concentrations Available Clinical nurse leader; nursing administration; nursing education. *Clinical nurse specialist programs in:* community health, public health, rehabilitation. *Nurse practitioner programs in:* women's health.
Study Options Full-time and part-time.
Program Entrance Requirements Clinical experience, computer literacy, minimum overall college GPA of 3.0, transcript of college record, CPR certification, written essay, immunizations, interview, 3 letters of recommendation, professional liability insurance/malpractice insurance, resume, statistics course, GRE or MAT. *Application deadline:* 3/1 (fall), 10/1 (winter), 10/1 (spring), 3/1 (summer). Applications may be processed on a rolling basis for some programs. *Application fee:* $50.
Advanced Placement Credit given for nursing courses completed elsewhere dependent upon specific evaluations.
Degree Requirements 39 total credit hours, thesis or project.

CONTINUING EDUCATION PROGRAM

Contact Dr. Mary A. Farrell, Coordinator, Program in Nursing, Salem State University, 352 Lafayette Street, Salem, MA 01970. *Telephone:* 978-542-6805. *Fax:* 978-542-2016. *E-mail:* mfarrell@salemstate.edu.

Simmons College
School of Nursing and Health Sciences
Boston, Massachusetts

http://www.simmons.edu/snhs/
Founded in 1899
DEGREES • BS • DNP • MS
Nursing Program Faculty 138 (19% with doctorates).
Baccalaureate Enrollment 538 **Women** 100% **Minority** 18% **International** 3% **Part-time** 13%
Graduate Enrollment 269 **Women** 95% **Men** 5% **Minority** 13% **International** 2% **Part-time** 66%
Distance Learning Courses Available.
Nursing Student Activities Nursing Honor Society, Sigma Theta Tau, Student Nurses' Association, nursing club.
Nursing Student Resources Academic advising; academic or career counseling; assistance for students with disabilities; bookstore; campus computer network; career placement assistance; computer lab; computer-assisted instruction; e-mail services; employment services for current students; housing assistance; interactive nursing skills videos; Internet; learning resource lab; library services; nursing audiovisuals; placement services for program completers; remedial services; resume preparation assistance; skills, simulation, or other laboratory; tutoring; unpaid internships.
Library Facilities 261,832 volumes (3,159 in health; 1,643 in nursing); 73,188 periodical subscriptions (801 health-care related).

BACCALAUREATE PROGRAMS

Degree BS
Available Programs ADN to Baccalaureate; Accelerated Baccalaureate; Accelerated Baccalaureate for Second Degree; Baccalaureate for Second Degree; Generic Baccalaureate; LPN to Baccalaureate; RN Baccalaureate.
Site Options South Shore, MA.
Study Options Full-time and part-time.
Program Entrance Requirements Transcript of college record, written essay, health exam, health insurance, high school biology, high school chemistry, high school foreign language, 4 years high school math, 3 years high school science, high school transcript, immunizations, 2 letters of recommendation, minimum GPA in nursing prerequisites of 3.0, prerequisite course work. Transfer students are accepted. *Application deadline:* 2/1 (fall), 11/1 (spring). *Application fee:* $55.
Advanced Placement Credit given for nursing courses completed elsewhere dependent upon specific evaluations.

Expenses (2012–13) *Tuition:* full-time $36,596; part-time $1144 per credit hour. *International tuition:* $36,596 full-time. *Room and board:* $13,140 per academic year. *Required fees:* full-time $1000; part-time $500 per term.
Financial Aid 85% of baccalaureate students in nursing programs received some form of financial aid in 2011–12.
Contact Ms. Catherine C. Capolupo, Assistant Vice President, Marketing and Admission, School of Nursing and Health Sciences, Simmons College, 300 The Fenway, Boston, MA 02115. *Telephone:* 617-521-2051. *Fax:* 617-521-3190. *E-mail:* ugadm@simmons.edu.

GRADUATE PROGRAMS

Expenses (2012–13) *Tuition:* part-time $1164 per credit hour. *Room and board:* $14,720 per academic year.
Financial Aid 70% of graduate students in nursing programs received some form of financial aid in 2011–12.
Contact Ms. Carmen Fortin, Assistant Dean, Director of Admission, School of Nursing and Health Sciences, Simmons College, 300 The Fenway, Boston, MA 02115. *Telephone:* 617-521-2605. *Fax:* 617-521-3137. *E-mail:* carmen.fortin@simmons.edu.

MASTER'S DEGREE PROGRAM
Degree MS
Available Programs Accelerated Master's; Accelerated Master's for Non-Nursing College Graduates; Accelerated Master's for Nurses with Non-Nursing Degrees; Master's; RN to Master's.
Concentrations Available Nursing administration. *Nurse practitioner programs in:* family health, primary care.
Site Options South Shore, MA; Boston (Longwood Medical Area), MA.
Study Options Part-time.
Program Entrance Requirements Clinical experience, computer literacy, minimum overall college GPA of 3.0, transcript of college record, written essay, 3 letters of recommendation, physical assessment course, prerequisite course work, resume, statistics course. *Application deadline:* 6/1 (fall), 11/1 (spring), 1/10 (summer). *Application fee:* $50.
Degree Requirements 98 total credit hours, thesis or project.

POST-MASTER'S PROGRAM
Areas of Study *Nurse practitioner programs in:* family health, oncology.

DOCTORAL DEGREE PROGRAM
Degree DNP
Available Programs Doctorate.
Areas of Study Clinical practice.
Program Entrance Requirements Clinical experience, minimum overall college GPA of 3.0, 3 letters of recommendation, MSN or equivalent, statistics course, vita, writing sample. *Application deadline:* 6/1 (fall), 11/1 (spring). *Application fee:* $50.
Degree Requirements 36 total credit hours.

University of Massachusetts Amherst
School of Nursing
Amherst, Massachusetts

http://www.umass.edu/nursing
Founded in 1863
DEGREES • BS • MS • PHD
Nursing Program Faculty 65 (40% with doctorates).
Baccalaureate Enrollment 441 **Women** 90% **Men** 10% **Minority** 19% **International** 3% **Part-time** 1%
Graduate Enrollment 234 **Women** 91% **Men** 9% **Minority** 13% **International** 1% **Part-time** 79%
Distance Learning Courses Available.
Nursing Student Activities Sigma Theta Tau, Student Nurses' Association.
Nursing Student Resources Academic advising; academic or career counseling; bookstore; campus computer network; career placement assistance; computer lab; computer-assisted instruction; e-mail services; employment services for current students; housing assistance; interactive nursing skills videos; Internet; learning resource lab; library services; nursing audiovisuals; resume preparation assistance; skills, simulation, or other laboratory; tutoring; unpaid internships.

Library Facilities 3.9 million volumes (363,696 in health, 41,844 in nursing); 81,772 periodical subscriptions (4,088 health-care related).

BACCALAUREATE PROGRAMS
Degree BS
Available Programs Accelerated Baccalaureate for Second Degree; Accelerated RN Baccalaureate; Generic Baccalaureate.
Study Options Full-time.
Online Degree Options Yes.
Program Entrance Requirements Minimum overall college GPA of 3.0, transcript of college record, CPR certification, written essay, health exam, health insurance, high school foreign language, 3 years high school math, 3 years high school science, high school transcript, immunizations, 1 letter of recommendation, minimum high school GPA of 3.5, minimum GPA in nursing prerequisites of 2.5, professional liability insurance/malpractice insurance, prerequisite course work. *Application deadline:* 1/15 (fall). *Application fee:* $70.
Advanced Placement Credit given for nursing courses completed elsewhere dependent upon specific evaluations.
Financial Aid 86% of baccalaureate students in nursing programs received some form of financial aid in 2011–12. *Gift aid (need-based):* Federal Pell, FSEOG, state, private, college/university gift aid from institutional funds. *Loans:* Federal Direct (Subsidized and Unsubsidized Stafford PLUS), Perkins. *Work-study:* Federal Work-Study. *Financial aid application deadline (priority):* 3/1.
Contact Ms. Elizabeth Theroux, Academic Secretary, Undergraduate Nursing Education, School of Nursing, University of Massachusetts Amherst, 024 Skinner Hall, 651 North Pleasant Street, Amherst, MA 01003-9304. *Telephone:* 413-545-5096. *Fax:* 413-577-2550. *E-mail:* etheroux@acad.umass.edu.

GRADUATE PROGRAMS
Financial Aid 38% of graduate students in nursing programs received some form of financial aid in 2011–12. Fellowships with full and partial tuition reimbursements available, research assistantships with full and partial tuition reimbursements available, teaching assistantships with full and partial tuition reimbursements available, career-related internships or fieldwork, Federal Work-Study, scholarships, traineeships, tuition waivers (full and partial), and unspecified assistantships available. Aid available to part-time students. *Financial aid application deadline:* 2/1.
Contact Ms. Karen Ayotte, Academic Services Graduate Program Assistant, School of Nursing, University of Massachusetts Amherst, 125 Skinner Hall, 651 North Pleasant Street, Amherst, MA 01003-9299. *Telephone:* 413-545-1302. *Fax:* 413-577-2550. *E-mail:* kayotte@nursing.umass.edu.

MASTER'S DEGREE PROGRAM
Degree MS
Available Programs Master's.
Concentrations Available Clinical nurse leader.
Study Options Full-time and part-time.
Online Degree Options Yes (online only).
Program Entrance Requirements Minimum overall college GPA of 3.0, transcript of college record, CPR certification, written essay, immunizations, 2 letters of recommendation, physical assessment course, professional liability insurance/malpractice insurance, prerequisite course work, statistics course, GRE General Test. *Application deadline:* 12/15 (fall). Applications may be processed on a rolling basis for some programs. *Application fee:* $65.
Advanced Placement Credit given for nursing courses completed elsewhere dependent upon specific evaluations.
Degree Requirements 37 total credit hours.

DOCTORAL DEGREE PROGRAM
Degree PhD
Available Programs Doctorate; Post-Baccalaureate Doctorate.
Areas of Study Faculty preparation, health promotion/disease prevention, health-care systems, individualized study, nursing education, nursing research, nursing science.
Program Entrance Requirements Minimum overall college GPA of 3.2, interview, 2 letters of recommendation, MSN or equivalent, scholarly papers, statistics course, vita, writing sample, GRE General Test. *Application deadline:* 12/15 (fall). Applications may be processed on a rolling basis for some programs. *Application fee:* $65.
Degree Requirements 57 total credit hours, dissertation, oral exam, written exam, residency.

CONTINUING EDUCATION PROGRAM

Contact Ms. Karen Ayotte, Academic Services Graduate Program Assistant, School of Nursing, University of Massachusetts Amherst, 104 Skinner Hall, 651 North Pleasant Street, Amherst, MA 01003-9299. *Telephone:* 413-545-1302. *Fax:* 413-577-2550. *E-mail:* kayotte@nursing.umass.edu.

University of Massachusetts Boston

College of Nursing and Health Sciences
Boston, Massachusetts

http://www.umb.edu/
Founded in 1964

DEGREES · BS · DNP · MS · PHD

Nursing Program Faculty 127 (30% with doctorates).

Baccalaureate Enrollment 1,325 **Women** 86% **Men** 14% **Minority** 40% **International** .4% **Part-time** 50%

Graduate Enrollment 209 **Women** 92.4% **Men** 7.6% **Minority** 20% **International** 2% **Part-time** 70%

Distance Learning Courses Available.

Nursing Student Activities Sigma Theta Tau, Student Nurses' Association.

Nursing Student Resources Academic advising; academic or career counseling; assistance for students with disabilities; bookstore; campus computer network; career placement assistance; computer lab; computer-assisted instruction; daycare for children of students; e-mail services; employment services for current students; housing assistance; interactive nursing skills videos; Internet; learning resource lab; library services; nursing audiovisuals; other; paid internships; remedial services; resume preparation assistance; skills, simulation, or other laboratory; tutoring.

Library Facilities 600,000 volumes (3,700 in health, 1,911 in nursing); 75,000 periodical subscriptions (4,815 health-care related).

BACCALAUREATE PROGRAMS

Degree BS

Available Programs Accelerated Baccalaureate for Second Degree; Generic Baccalaureate; RN Baccalaureate.

Study Options Full-time and part-time.

Online Degree Options Yes.

Program Entrance Requirements Minimum overall college GPA of 3.0, transcript of college record, written essay, health insurance, 3 years high school math, high school transcript, immunizations, 2 letters of recommendation, minimum high school GPA of 3.0, minimum GPA in nursing prerequisites of 2.7. Transfer students are accepted. *Application deadline:* 2/1 (fall), 11/1 (spring). *Application fee:* $60.

Advanced Placement Credit given for nursing courses completed elsewhere dependent upon specific evaluations.

Expenses (2012–13) *Tuition, state resident:* full-time $1714; part-time $72 per credit. *Tuition, nonresident:* full-time $9758; part-time $407 per credit. *International tuition:* $9758 full-time. *Required fees:* part-time $300 per term.

Financial Aid 70% of baccalaureate students in nursing programs received some form of financial aid in 2011–12. *Gift aid (need-based):* Federal Pell, FSEOG, state, private, college/university gift aid from institutional funds, TEACH Grants. *Loans:* Federal Direct (Subsidized and Unsubsidized Stafford PLUS), Perkins. *Work-study:* Federal Work-Study. *Financial aid application deadline (priority):* 3/1.

Contact Mr. Jon Hutton, Director of Enrollment Information Services, College of Nursing and Health Sciences, University of Massachusetts Boston, 100 Morrissey Boulevard, Boston, MA 02125. *Telephone:* 617-287-6000. *Fax:* 617-287-5999. *E-mail:* enrollment.information@umb.edu.

GRADUATE PROGRAMS

Expenses (2012–13) *Tuition, state resident:* full-time $2590; part-time $108 per credit. *Tuition, nonresident:* full-time $9758; part-time $407 per credit. *International tuition:* $9758 full-time. *Required fees:* part-time $400 per term.

Financial Aid 35% of graduate students in nursing programs received some form of financial aid in 2011–12. 3 research assistantships with full tuition reimbursements available (averaging $13,000 per year), 13 teaching assistantships with full tuition reimbursements available (averaging $13,000 per year) were awarded; career-related internships or fieldwork, Federal Work-Study, and unspecified assistantships also available. Aid available to part-time students. *Financial aid application deadline:* 3/1.

Contact Mr. Jon Hutton, Director of Enrollment Information Services, College of Nursing and Health Sciences, University of Massachusetts Boston, 100 Morrissey Boulevard, Boston, MA 02125. *Telephone:* 617-287-6000. *Fax:* 617-287-6040. *E-mail:* enrollment.information@umb.edu.

MASTER'S DEGREE PROGRAM

Degree MS

Available Programs Master's.

Concentrations Available *Clinical nurse specialist programs in:* acute care, adult health, critical care, gerontology. *Nurse practitioner programs in:* adult health, family health, gerontology.

Study Options Full-time and part-time.

Program Entrance Requirements Clinical experience, minimum overall college GPA of 3.0, transcript of college record, written essay, immunizations, 3 letters of recommendation, physical assessment course, statistics course. *Application deadline:* 3/15 (fall), 10/15 (spring). *Application fee:* $60.

Advanced Placement Credit given for nursing courses completed elsewhere dependent upon specific evaluations.

Degree Requirements 48 total credit hours, thesis or project.

POST-MASTER'S PROGRAM

Areas of Study Clinical nurse leader; nursing education. *Clinical nurse specialist programs in:* acute care, adult health, critical care, gerontology. *Nurse practitioner programs in:* acute care, adult health, family health, gerontology.

DOCTORAL DEGREE PROGRAM

Degree DNP

Available Programs Doctorate.

Areas of Study Advanced practice nursing.

Online Degree Options Yes (online only).

Program Entrance Requirements Minimum overall college GPA of 3.2, clinical experience, 3 letters of recommendation, MSN or equivalent, statistics course, vita, writing sample. *Application deadline:* 5/1 (fall), 12/1 (winter). *Application fee:* $60.

Degree Requirements 39 total credit hours, Capstone project, residency.

DOCTORAL DEGREE PROGRAM

Degree PhD

Available Programs Doctorate; Post-Baccalaureate Doctorate.

Areas of Study Health policy, health promotion/disease prevention.

Online Degree Options Yes.

Program Entrance Requirements Clinical experience, minimum overall college GPA of 3.3, interview by faculty committee, interview, 3 letters of recommendation, MSN or equivalent, statistics course, vita, writing sample, GRE General Test. *Application deadline:* 2/15 (fall). Applications may be processed on a rolling basis for some programs. *Application fee:* $60.

Degree Requirements 60 total credit hours, dissertation, oral exam, written exam, residency.

POSTDOCTORAL PROGRAM

Areas of Study Cancer care, nursing research.

Postdoctoral Program Contact Dr. Laura L. Hayman, Associate Dean for Research, College of Nursing and Health Sciences, University of Massachusetts Boston, Boston, MA 02125. *Telephone:* 617-287-7504. *E-mail:* laura.hayman@umb.edu.

CONTINUING EDUCATION PROGRAM

Contact Ms. Wanda Willard, Director of Credit Programs, College of Nursing and Health Sciences, University of Massachusetts Boston, 100 Morrissey Boulevard, Wheatley Building, 2nd Floor, Boston, MA 02125-3393. *Telephone:* 617-287-7874. *Fax:* 617-287-7922. *E-mail:* wanda.willard@umb.edu.

University of Massachusetts Dartmouth

College of Nursing
North Dartmouth, Massachusetts

http://www.umassd.edu/nursing
Founded in 1895

DEGREES • BSN • MS • PHD

Nursing Program Faculty 52 (33% with doctorates).

Nursing Student Activities Sigma Theta Tau, Student Nurses' Association, nursing club.

Nursing Student Resources Academic advising; academic or career counseling; assistance for students with disabilities; bookstore; campus computer network; career placement assistance; computer lab; computer-assisted instruction; daycare for children of students; e-mail services; employment services for current students; externships; housing assistance; interactive nursing skills videos; Internet; learning resource lab; library services; nursing audiovisuals; placement services for program completers; resume preparation assistance; skills, simulation, or other laboratory; tutoring; unpaid internships.

Library Facilities 457,879 volumes; 2,017 periodical subscriptions.

BACCALAUREATE PROGRAMS

Degree BSN

Available Programs Generic Baccalaureate; RN Baccalaureate.

Site Options Fall River, MA.

Study Options Full-time and part-time.

Program Entrance Requirements Transcript of college record, CPR certification, written essay, health exam, health insurance, high school biology, high school chemistry, high school foreign language, 3 years high school math, 3 years high school science, high school transcript, immunizations, letters of recommendation, minimum high school GPA of 3.0, minimum high school rank 66%, professional liability insurance/malpractice insurance. Transfer students are accepted.

Advanced Placement Credit by examination available. Credit given for nursing courses completed elsewhere dependent upon specific evaluations.

Contact *Telephone:* 508-999-8605. *Fax:* 508-999-8755.

GRADUATE PROGRAMS

Contact *Telephone:* 508-999-8251.

MASTER'S DEGREE PROGRAM

Degree MS

Available Programs Master's.

Concentrations Available *Clinical nurse specialist programs in:* adult health, community health. *Nurse practitioner programs in:* adult health.

Study Options Full-time and part-time.

Program Entrance Requirements Clinical experience, computer literacy, minimum overall college GPA of 3.0, transcript of college record, CPR certification, written essay, immunizations, interview, 3 letters of recommendation, nursing research course, physical assessment course, professional liability insurance/malpractice insurance, statistics course, GRE General Test.

Advanced Placement Credit given for nursing courses completed elsewhere dependent upon specific evaluations.

Degree Requirements 39 total credit hours, thesis or project.

POST-MASTER'S PROGRAM

Areas of Study *Nurse practitioner programs in:* adult health.

DOCTORAL DEGREE PROGRAM

Degree PhD

Available Programs Doctorate.

Areas of Study Nursing education.

Program Entrance Requirements Clinical experience, minimum overall college GPA of 3.3, 3 letters of recommendation, MSN or equivalent, statistics course, vita, writing sample, GRE General Test.

Degree Requirements 52 total credit hours.

CONTINUING EDUCATION PROGRAM

Contact *Telephone:* 508-999-8591.

University of Massachusetts Lowell

Department of Nursing
Lowell, Massachusetts

http://www.uml.edu/SHE/Nursing/default.aspx
Founded in 1894

DEGREES • BS • DNP • MS • PHD

Nursing Program Faculty 50 (42% with doctorates).

Baccalaureate Enrollment 500 **Women** 90% **Men** 10% **Minority** 27% **Part-time** 14%

Graduate Enrollment 133 **Women** 95% **Men** 5% **Minority** 5% **International** .1% **Part-time** 72%

Distance Learning Courses Available.

Nursing Student Activities Nursing Honor Society, Sigma Theta Tau, Student Nurses' Association, nursing club.

Nursing Student Resources Academic advising; academic or career counseling; assistance for students with disabilities; bookstore; campus computer network; career placement assistance; computer lab; computer-assisted instruction; e-mail services; employment services for current students; housing assistance; interactive nursing skills videos; Internet; learning resource lab; library services; nursing audiovisuals; other; placement services for program completers; resume preparation assistance; skills, simulation, or other laboratory; tutoring.

Library Facilities 298,756 volumes (29,100 in health, 4,465 in nursing); 45,105 periodical subscriptions (350 health-care related).

BACCALAUREATE PROGRAMS

Degree BS

Available Programs Generic Baccalaureate; RN Baccalaureate.

Study Options Full-time.

Program Entrance Requirements Minimum overall college GPA of 2.7, transcript of college record, CPR certification, health exam, health insurance, high school chemistry, high school foreign language, 3 years high school math, 3 years high school science, high school transcript, immunizations, minimum high school GPA of 3.25, minimum GPA in nursing prerequisites of 2.7, professional liability insurance/malpractice insurance. Transfer students are accepted. *Application deadline:* 11/1 (fall), 1/1 (winter). Applications may be processed on a rolling basis for some programs. *Application fee:* $50.

Advanced Placement Credit by examination available.

Expenses (2012–13) *Tuition, state resident:* full-time $11,847. *Tuition, nonresident:* full-time $24,896. *Room and board:* $10,282 per academic year.

Financial Aid 68% of baccalaureate students in nursing programs received some form of financial aid in 2011–12.

Contact Office of Undergraduate Admissions, Department of Nursing, University of Massachusetts Lowell, 883 Broadway Street, Suite 110, Lowell, MA 01854-3931. *Telephone:* 978-934-3931. *E-mail:* admissions@uml.edu.

GRADUATE PROGRAMS

Expenses (2012–13) *Tuition, state resident:* full-time $11,228; part-time $535 per credit hour. *Tuition, nonresident:* full-time $20,773.

Financial Aid 50% of graduate students in nursing programs received some form of financial aid in 2011–12. 37 fellowships with tuition reimbursements available, 10 teaching assistantships with full tuition reimbursements available were awarded; research assistantships with full tuition reimbursements available, career-related internships or fieldwork, Federal Work-Study, institutionally sponsored loans, scholarships, and traineeships also available. Aid available to part-time students. *Financial aid application deadline:* 4/1.

Contact Dr. Mary Aruda, Coordinator of MS/DNP Program, Department of Nursing, University of Massachusetts Lowell, 3 Solomont Way, Suite 2, Lowell, MA 01854-5126. *Telephone:* 978-934-4097. *Fax:* 978-934-2015. *E-mail:* mary_aruda@uml.edu.

MASTER'S DEGREE PROGRAM

Degree MS

Available Programs Accelerated Master's; Accelerated RN to Master's; Master's.

Concentrations Available *Clinical nurse specialist programs in:* family health, psychiatric/mental health. *Nurse practitioner programs in:* family health, gerontology, psychiatric/mental health.

Study Options Full-time and part-time.

Program Entrance Requirements Computer literacy, minimum overall college GPA of 3.0, transcript of college record, CPR certification, written essay, immunizations, interview, 3 letters of recommendation, statistics course, GRE General Test. *Application deadline:* Applications may be processed on a rolling basis for some programs. *Application fee:* $50.
Advanced Placement Credit given for nursing courses completed elsewhere dependent upon specific evaluations.
Degree Requirements 42 total credit hours, thesis or project.

POST-MASTER'S PROGRAM
Areas of Study *Clinical nurse specialist programs in:* psychiatric/mental health.

DOCTORAL DEGREE PROGRAM
Degree DNP
Available Programs Doctorate.
Areas of Study Advanced practice nursing.
Program Entrance Requirements Minimum overall college GPA of 3.0, interview, interview by faculty committee, letters of recommendation, MSN or equivalent, statistics course, vita. *Application deadline:* 11/1 (fall), 4/1 (spring). Applications may be processed on a rolling basis for some programs. *Application fee:* $50.
Degree Requirements 33 total credit hours, scholarly project.

DOCTORAL DEGREE PROGRAM
Degree PhD
Available Programs Doctorate.
Areas of Study Health promotion/disease prevention.
Program Entrance Requirements Minimum overall college GPA of 3.4, interview by faculty committee, interview, 3 letters of recommendation, MSN or equivalent, scholarly papers, statistics course, writing sample, GRE General Test. *Application deadline:* Applications may be processed on a rolling basis for some programs.
Degree Requirements 48 total credit hours, dissertation, oral exam, written exam. 2 qualifying papers, one in theory and one in methods.

University of Massachusetts Worcester
Graduate School of Nursing
Worcester, Massachusetts

http://www.umassmed.edu/gsn/
Founded in 1962
DEGREES • MS • PHD
Nursing Program Faculty 51 (40% with doctorates).
Graduate Enrollment 174 **Women** 87% **Men** 13% **Minority** 23% **International** 1% **Part-time** 4%
Distance Learning Courses Available.
Nursing Student Activities Sigma Theta Tau, Student Nurses' Association.
Nursing Student Resources Academic advising; academic or career counseling; assistance for students with disabilities; bookstore; campus computer network; computer lab; computer-assisted instruction; e-mail services; interactive nursing skills videos; Internet; learning resource lab; library services; nursing audiovisuals; skills, simulation, or other laboratory; unpaid internships.
Library Facilities 207,500 volumes in health, 1,173 volumes in nursing; 5,400 periodical subscriptions health-care related.

GRADUATE PROGRAMS
Contact *Telephone:* 508-856-5756. *Fax:* 508-856-5756.

MASTER'S DEGREE PROGRAM
Degree MS
Available Programs Accelerated Master's for Non-Nursing College Graduates; Master's.
Concentrations Available Nursing education. *Nurse practitioner programs in:* acute care, family health, gerontology, primary care.
Site Options Shrewsbury, MA; Worcester, MA.
Study Options Full-time and part-time.
Program Entrance Requirements Clinical experience, computer literacy, minimum overall college GPA of 3.0, transcript of college record, CPR certification, written essay, immunizations, interview, 3 letters of recommendation, physical assessment course, prerequisite course work,

resume, statistics course, GRE General Test. *Application deadline:* 3/15 (fall). Applications may be processed on a rolling basis for some programs.
Advanced Placement Credit given for nursing courses completed elsewhere dependent upon specific evaluations.
Degree Requirements 42 total credit hours.

POST-MASTER'S PROGRAM
Areas of Study Nursing education. *Nurse practitioner programs in:* acute care, gerontology, primary care.

DOCTORAL DEGREE PROGRAM
Degree PhD
Available Programs Doctorate.
Areas of Study Advanced practice nursing, bio-behavioral research, clinical practice, critical care, family health, health promotion/disease prevention, human health and illness, illness and transition, nursing research, nursing science, oncology.
Site Options Worcester, MA.
Program Entrance Requirements Minimum overall college GPA of 3.0, interview by faculty committee, interview, 3 letters of recommendation, MSN or equivalent, scholarly papers, statistics course, vita, writing sample, GRE General Test. *Application deadline:* 3/15 (fall). Applications may be processed on a rolling basis for some programs.
Degree Requirements 57 total credit hours, dissertation, oral exam, written exam.

CONTINUING EDUCATION PROGRAM
Contact *Telephone:* 508-856-3488. *Fax:* 508-856-6552.

Worcester State University
Department of Nursing
Worcester, Massachusetts

http://www.worcester.edu/
Founded in 1874
DEGREES • BS • MS
Nursing Program Faculty 45 (50% with doctorates).
Baccalaureate Enrollment 287 **Women** 90% **Men** 10% **Minority** 10%
Graduate Enrollment 80 **Women** 70% **Men** 30% **Minority** 30% **Part-time** 100%
Nursing Student Activities Nursing Honor Society, Sigma Theta Tau, Student Nurses' Association, nursing club.
Nursing Student Resources Academic advising; academic or career counseling; assistance for students with disabilities; bookstore; campus computer network; career placement assistance; computer lab; computer-assisted instruction; e-mail services; employment services for current students; externships; housing assistance; interactive nursing skills videos; Internet; learning resource lab; library services; nursing audiovisuals; paid internships; remedial services; resume preparation assistance; skills, simulation, or other laboratory; tutoring; unpaid internships.
Library Facilities 203,856 volumes (5,400 in health, 500 in nursing); 300 periodical subscriptions (385 health-care related).

BACCALAUREATE PROGRAMS
Degree BS
Available Programs Generic Baccalaureate; RN Baccalaureate.
Study Options Full-time.
Program Entrance Requirements Transcript of college record, high school foreign language, 3 years high school math, 3 years high school science, high school transcript, minimum high school GPA of 3.2. *Application deadline:* 1/15 (fall). Applications may be processed on a rolling basis for some programs. *Application fee:* $40.
Advanced Placement Credit by examination available.
Expenses (2012–13) *Tuition, state resident:* full-time $970; part-time $130 per credit hour. *Tuition, nonresident:* full-time $1455. *International tuition:* $1455 full-time. *Room and board:* $10,500; room only: $7380 per academic year. *Required fees:* part-time $299 per credit; part-time $3594 per term.
Financial Aid 80% of baccalaureate students in nursing programs received some form of financial aid in 2011–12.
Contact Mr. Joseph Dicarlo, Director, Admissions, Department of Nursing, Worcester State University, 486 Chandler Street, Worcester, MA 01602. *Telephone:* 508-929-8040. *Fax:* 508-929-8183. *E-mail:* Joseph.Dicarlo@worcester.edu.

GRADUATE PROGRAMS

Expenses (2012–13) *Tuition, state resident:* part-time ·$150 per credit. *Tuition, nonresident:* part-time $150 per credit. *Required fees:* part-time $114 per credit.
Financial Aid 50% of graduate students in nursing programs received some form of financial aid in 2011–12.
Contact Dr. Stephanie Chalupka, Associate Dean for Nursing, Department of Nursing, Worcester State University, 486 Chandler Street, Worcester, MA 01602. *Telephone:* 508-929-8129. *Fax:* 508-929-8168. *E-mail:* schalupka@worcester.edu.

MASTER'S DEGREE PROGRAM

Degree MS
Available Programs Master's; Master's for Nurses with Non-Nursing Degrees; RN to Master's.
Concentrations Available Nursing education. *Clinical nurse specialist programs in:* community health, public health.
Study Options Full-time and part-time.
Program Entrance Requirements Clinical experience, computer literacy, minimum overall college GPA of 3.0, transcript of college record, CPR certification, written essay, immunizations, 2 letters of recommendation, nursing research course, professional liability insurance/malpractice insurance, prerequisite course work, resume, statistics course. *Application deadline:* 4/1 (fall), 11/1 (winter). Applications may be processed on a rolling basis for some programs. *Application fee:* $40.
Degree Requirements 42 total credit hours, thesis or project.

POST-MASTER'S PROGRAM

Areas of Study Nursing education.

CONTINUING EDUCATION PROGRAM

Contact Ms. Gina Fleury, RN, Continuing Education Coordinator, Department of Nursing, Worcester State University, 486 Chandler Street, Worcester, MA 01602. *Telephone:* 508-929-8683. *E-mail:* gfleury@worcester.edu.

MICHIGAN

Andrews University
Department of Nursing
Berrien Springs, Michigan

Founded in 1874
DEGREES • BS • MS
Nursing Program Faculty 11 (50% with doctorates).
Baccalaureate Enrollment 106
Graduate Enrollment 10
Nursing Student Activities Nursing Honor Society, Sigma Theta Tau, Student Nurses' Association.
Nursing Student Resources Academic advising; academic or career counseling; assistance for students with disabilities; bookstore; campus computer network; career placement assistance; computer lab; computer-assisted instruction; daycare for children of students; e-mail services; employment services for current students; externships; housing assistance; interactive nursing skills videos; Internet; learning resource lab; library services; nursing audiovisuals; paid internships; placement services for program completers; remedial services; resume preparation assistance; skills, simulation, or other laboratory; tutoring; unpaid internships.
Library Facilities 645,172 volumes (77,000 in health, 500 in nursing); 44,500 periodical subscriptions (700 health-care related).

BACCALAUREATE PROGRAMS

Degree BS
Available Programs ADN to Baccalaureate; Generic Baccalaureate.
Study Options Full-time.
Program Entrance Requirements Minimum overall college GPA of 2.5, transcript of college record, health exam, high school transcript, immunizations, minimum GPA in nursing prerequisites of 2.5. Transfer students are accepted.
Contact *Telephone:* 269-471-3192. *Fax:* 269-471-3454.

GRADUATE PROGRAMS

Contact *Telephone:* 269-471-3337. *Fax:* 269-471-3454.

MASTER'S DEGREE PROGRAM

Degree MS
Available Programs Master's.
Concentrations Available Nursing education.
Study Options Part-time.
Program Entrance Requirements Minimum overall college GPA of 3.0, transcript of college record, CPR certification, immunizations, 3 letters of recommendation, GRE.
Degree Requirements 38 total credit hours, thesis or project.

POST-MASTER'S PROGRAM

Areas of Study Nursing education.

Calvin College
Department of Nursing
Grand Rapids, Michigan

http://www.calvin.edu/academic/nursing
Founded in 1876
DEGREE • BSN
Nursing Program Faculty 20 (20% with doctorates).
Baccalaureate Enrollment 120 **Women** 95% **Men** 5% **Minority** 10% **International** 10%
Nursing Student Activities Sigma Theta Tau, Student Nurses' Association, nursing club.
Nursing Student Resources Academic advising; academic or career counseling; assistance for students with disabilities; bookstore; campus computer network; career placement assistance; computer lab; computer-assisted instruction; e-mail services; employment services for current students; externships; housing assistance; interactive nursing skills videos; Internet; learning resource lab; library services; nursing audiovisuals; paid internships; placement services for program completers; remedial services; resume preparation assistance; skills, simulation, or other laboratory; tutoring.
Library Facilities 1.3 million volumes; 32,052 periodical subscriptions.

BACCALAUREATE PROGRAMS

Degree BSN
Available Programs Generic Baccalaureate.
Site Options Grand Rapids, MI.
Study Options Full-time.
Program Entrance Requirements Minimum overall college GPA of 2.5, transcript of college record, CPR certification, health exam, health insurance, immunizations, 2 letters of recommendation, minimum GPA in nursing prerequisites of 2.5, professional liability insurance/malpractice insurance, prerequisite course work. Transfer students are accepted.
Contact *Telephone:* 616-526-6268. *Fax:* 616-526-8567.

Davenport University
Division of Nursing
Grand Rapids, Michigan

Founded in 1866
DEGREE • BSN
Nursing Program Faculty 40
Baccalaureate Enrollment 215 **Women** 94% **Men** 6% **Minority** 30% **Part-time** 17%
Distance Learning Courses Available.
Nursing Student Activities Student Nurses' Association.
Nursing Student Resources Academic advising; academic or career counseling; assistance for students with disabilities; bookstore; campus computer network; career placement assistance; computer lab; computer-assisted instruction; e-mail services; employment services for current students; externships; housing assistance; interactive nursing skills videos; Internet; learning resource lab; library services; nursing audiovisuals; placement services for program completers; remedial services; resume preparation assistance; skills, simulation, or other laboratory; tutoring.
Library Facilities 74,714 volumes (100 in health, 50 in nursing); 219 periodical subscriptions (20 health-care related).

BACCALAUREATE PROGRAMS

Degree BSN
Available Programs ADN to Baccalaureate; Generic Baccalaureate; RN Baccalaureate.
Site Options Midland, MI; Warren, MI.
Study Options Full-time and part-time.
Online Degree Options Yes.
Program Entrance Requirements Minimum overall college GPA of 3.5, transcript of college record, CPR certification, written essay, health exam, health insurance, high school biology, high school chemistry, 2 years high school math, 3 years high school science, high school transcript, immunizations, 2 letters of recommendation, minimum high school GPA of 3.5, minimum GPA in nursing prerequisites. Transfer students are accepted. *Application deadline:* 1/31 (fall).
Advanced Placement Credit by examination available. Credit given for nursing courses completed elsewhere dependent upon specific evaluations.
Contact *Telephone:* 616-451-3511. *Fax:* 616-732-1145.

Davenport University
Bachelor of Science in Nursing Program
Kalamazoo, Michigan

Founded in 1977
DEGREE • BSN

BACCALAUREATE PROGRAMS

Degree BSN
Available Programs Generic Baccalaureate; RN Baccalaureate.
Contact *Telephone:* 616-871-3977. *Fax:* 616-554-5225.

Eastern Michigan University
School of Nursing
Ypsilanti, Michigan

http://www.emich.edu/nursing
Founded in 1849
DEGREES • BSN • MSN
Nursing Program Faculty 53 (28% with doctorates).
Baccalaureate Enrollment 338 **Women** 87% **Men** 13% **Minority** 30% **International** 2% **Part-time** 58%
Graduate Enrollment 40 **Women** 98% **Men** 2% **Minority** 32% **International** 2% **Part-time** 95%
Nursing Student Activities Sigma Theta Tau, Student Nurses' Association.
Nursing Student Resources Academic advising; academic or career counseling; assistance for students with disabilities; bookstore; campus computer network; career placement assistance; computer lab; computer-assisted instruction; daycare for children of students; e-mail services; employment services for current students; housing assistance; interactive nursing skills videos; Internet; learning resource lab; library services; nursing audiovisuals; placement services for program completers; remedial services; resume preparation assistance; skills, simulation, or other laboratory; tutoring.
Library Facilities 1.1 million volumes (24,200 in health, 5,300 in nursing); 24,607 periodical subscriptions (1,600 health-care related).

BACCALAUREATE PROGRAMS

Degree BSN
Available Programs Baccalaureate for Second Degree; Generic Baccalaureate; RN Baccalaureate.
Site Options Livonia, MI; Monroe, MI; Jackson, MI; Brighton, MI; Detroit, MI.
Study Options Full-time and part-time.
Program Entrance Requirements Transcript of college record, CPR certification, health exam, health insurance, immunizations, minimum GPA in nursing prerequisites of 3.0, prerequisite course work, RN licensure. Transfer students are accepted.
Advanced Placement Credit given for nursing courses completed elsewhere dependent upon specific evaluations.
Contact *Telephone:* 734-487-2340. *Fax:* 734-487-6946.

GRADUATE PROGRAMS

Contact *Telephone:* 734-487-3275. *Fax:* 734-487-6946.

MASTER'S DEGREE PROGRAM
Degree MSN
Available Programs Master's.
Concentrations Available *Clinical nurse specialist programs in:* adult health.
Site Options Livonia, MI; Monroe, MI.
Program Entrance Requirements Clinical experience, minimum overall college GPA of 2.5, transcript of college record, CPR certification, written essay, immunizations, interview, 3 letters of recommendation, physical assessment course, statistics course.
Degree Requirements 40 total credit hours, thesis or project.

Ferris State University
School of Nursing
Big Rapids, Michigan

http://www.ferris.edu/homepage.htm
Founded in 1884
DEGREES • BSN • MSN • MSN/MBA
Nursing Program Faculty 24 (20% with doctorates).
Baccalaureate Enrollment 510 **Women** 87% **Men** 13% **Minority** 7% **Part-time** 72%
Graduate Enrollment 81 **Women** 95% **Men** 5% **Minority** 4% **Part-time** 98%
Distance Learning Courses Available.
Nursing Student Activities Sigma Theta Tau, Student Nurses' Association, nursing club.
Nursing Student Resources Academic advising; academic or career counseling; assistance for students with disabilities; bookstore; campus computer network; career placement assistance; computer lab; computer-assisted instruction; daycare for children of students; e-mail services; employment services for current students; housing assistance; interactive nursing skills videos; Internet; library services; nursing audiovisuals; resume preparation assistance; skills, simulation, or other laboratory; tutoring.
Library Facilities 424,107 volumes (12,177 in health, 785 in nursing); 69,328 periodical subscriptions (515 health-care related).

BACCALAUREATE PROGRAMS

Degree BSN
Available Programs Accelerated Baccalaureate for Second Degree; Accelerated RN Baccalaureate; Baccalaureate for Second Degree; RN Baccalaureate.
Site Options Greenville, MI; Traverse City, MI; Grand Rapids, MI.
Study Options Full-time.
Online Degree Options Yes.
Program Entrance Requirements Minimum overall college GPA of 2.7, transcript of college record, CPR certification, health insurance, immunizations, minimum GPA in nursing prerequisites of 2.7, prerequisite course work. Transfer students are accepted. *Application deadline:* 4/15 (spring).
Advanced Placement Credit by examination available. Credit given for nursing courses completed elsewhere dependent upon specific evaluations.
Expenses (2012–13) *Tuition, area resident:* full-time $10,710. *Tuition, state resident:* full-time $16,080. *Tuition, nonresident:* full-time $16,080. *International tuition:* $17,190 full-time. *Room and board:* $9344 per academic year. *Required fees:* full-time $2025.
Financial Aid 87% of baccalaureate students in nursing programs received some form of financial aid in 2011–12. *Gift aid (need-based):* Federal Pell, FSEOG, state, private, college/university gift aid from institutional funds. *Loans:* Federal Nursing Student Loans, Federal Direct (Subsidized and Unsubsidized Stafford PLUS), Perkins, college/university, alternative loans. *Work-study:* Federal Work-Study, part-time campus jobs. *Financial aid application deadline (priority):* 2/15.
Contact Dr. Julie A. Coon, EdD, Director, School of Nursing, School of Nursing, Ferris State University, 200 Ferris Drive, VFS 400-A, Big Rapids, MI 49307. *Telephone:* 231-591-2267. *Fax:* 231-591-2325. *E-mail:* coonj@ferris.edu.

GRADUATE PROGRAMS

Expenses (2012–13) *Tuition, area resident:* part-time $485 per credit hour. *Tuition, state resident:* part-time $728 per credit hour. *Tuition, nonresident:* part-time $728 per credit hour. *Room and board:* $9344 per academic year.

Financial Aid 20% of graduate students in nursing programs received some form of financial aid in 2011–12.

Contact Dr. Susan Owens, MSN Program Coordinator, School of Nursing, Ferris State University, 200 Ferris Drive, VFS 300-A, Big Rapids, MI 49307. *Telephone:* 231-591-2290. *Fax:* 231-591-2325. *E-mail:* owenss3@ferris.edu.

MASTER'S DEGREE PROGRAM

Degrees MSN; MSN/MBA

Available Programs Accelerated AD/RN to Master's; Accelerated RN to Master's; Master's; RN to Master's.

Concentrations Available Nursing administration; nursing education; nursing informatics.

Study Options Full-time and part-time.

Online Degree Options Yes (online only).

Program Entrance Requirements Clinical experience, minimum overall college GPA of 3.0, transcript of college record, written essay, immunizations, 3 letters of recommendation, resume. *Application deadline:* 8/1 (fall), 12/1 (winter), 12/2 (spring).

Advanced Placement Credit given for nursing courses completed elsewhere dependent upon specific evaluations.

Degree Requirements 36 total credit hours, thesis or project, comprehensive exam.

Finlandia University
College of Professional Studies
Hancock, Michigan

http://www.finlandia.edu/
Founded in 1896
DEGREE • BSN

Nursing Program Faculty 14 (7% with doctorates).

Baccalaureate Enrollment 86 **Women** 85% **Men** 15% **Minority** 2% **Part-time** 7%

Distance Learning Courses Available.

Nursing Student Activities Student Nurses' Association, nursing club.

Nursing Student Resources Academic advising; academic or career counseling; assistance for students with disabilities; bookstore; campus computer network; career placement assistance; computer lab; computer-assisted instruction; e-mail services; interactive nursing skills videos; Internet; learning resource lab; library services; nursing audiovisuals; placement services for program completers; remedial services; resume preparation assistance; skills, simulation, or other laboratory; tutoring.

Library Facilities 68,803 volumes (4,601 in health, 2,316 in nursing); 997 periodical subscriptions (97 health-care related).

BACCALAUREATE PROGRAMS

Degree BSN

Available Programs Generic Baccalaureate; RN Baccalaureate.

Study Options Full-time.

Online Degree Options Yes.

Program Entrance Requirements Minimum overall college GPA of 2.5, transcript of college record, CPR certification, health exam, high school biology, high school chemistry, 1 year of high school math, 2 years high school science, high school transcript, immunizations, minimum high school GPA of 2.5, minimum GPA in nursing prerequisites of 2.5, prerequisite course work. Transfer students are accepted. *Application deadline:* Applications may be processed on a rolling basis for some programs.

Advanced Placement Credit given for nursing courses completed elsewhere dependent upon specific evaluations.

Contact *Telephone:* 906-487-7274.

Grand Valley State University
Kirkhof College of Nursing
Allendale, Michigan

http://www.gvsu.edu/kcon
Founded in 1960
DEGREES • BSN • DNP • MSN

Nursing Program Faculty 85 (38% with doctorates).

Baccalaureate Enrollment 376 **Women** 88% **Men** 12% **Minority** 4% **Part-time** 38%

Graduate Enrollment 84 **Women** 87% **Men** 13% **Minority** 9% **International** 1% **Part-time** 59%

Distance Learning Courses Available.

Nursing Student Activities Sigma Theta Tau, Student Nurses' Association.

Nursing Student Resources Academic advising; academic or career counseling; assistance for students with disabilities; bookstore; campus computer network; career placement assistance; computer lab; computer-assisted instruction; daycare for children of students; e-mail services; employment services for current students; housing assistance; interactive nursing skills videos; Internet; learning resource lab; library services; nursing audiovisuals; remedial services; resume preparation assistance; skills, simulation, or other laboratory; tutoring.

Library Facilities 1.1 million volumes (19,156 in health, 1,448 in nursing); 1,531 periodical subscriptions (4,617 health-care related).

BACCALAUREATE PROGRAMS

Degree BSN

Available Programs ADN to Baccalaureate; Baccalaureate for Second Degree; Generic Baccalaureate; RN Baccalaureate.

Site Options Grand Rapids, MI.

Study Options Full-time and part-time.

Program Entrance Requirements Minimum overall college GPA of 3.0, transcript of college record, CPR certification, health exam, health insurance, immunizations, interview, minimum GPA in nursing prerequisites of 3.0, prerequisite course work. Transfer students are accepted. *Application deadline:* 3/1 (fall), 8/31 (winter).

Advanced Placement Credit given for nursing courses completed elsewhere dependent upon specific evaluations.

Expenses (2012–13) *Tuition, state resident:* full-time $10,078; part-time $420 per credit hour. *Tuition, nonresident:* full-time $14,568; part-time $607 per credit hour. *International tuition:* $14,568 full-time. *Room and board:* $7920; room only: $5400 per academic year. *Required fees:* full-time $204; part-time $17 per credit.

Financial Aid 80% of baccalaureate students in nursing programs received some form of financial aid in 2011–12. *Gift aid (need-based):* Federal Pell, FSEOG, state, private, college/university gift aid from institutional funds. *Loans:* Federal Nursing Student Loans, Federal Direct (Subsidized and Unsubsidized Stafford PLUS), Perkins. *Work-study:* Federal Work-Study, part-time campus jobs. *Financial aid application deadline (priority):* 3/1.

Contact Ms. Kristin Norton, Director of Student Services, Kirkhof College of Nursing, Grand Valley State University, Cook-DeVos Center for Health Sciences, 301 Michigan Street NE, Room 322, Grand Rapids, MI 49503-3314. *Telephone:* 616-331-5637. *Fax:* 616-331-2510. *E-mail:* nortonkr@gvsu.edu.

GRADUATE PROGRAMS

Expenses (2012–13) *Tuition, state resident:* part-time $557 per credit hour. *Tuition, nonresident:* part-time $740 per credit hour. *International tuition:* $740 full-time. *Room and board:* $7920; room only: $5400 per academic year.

Financial Aid 78% of graduate students in nursing programs received some form of financial aid in 2011–12. 14 fellowships (averaging $3,207 per year), 9 research assistantships with full and partial tuition reimbursements available (averaging $8,053 per year) were awarded; career-related internships or fieldwork, Federal Work-Study, institutionally sponsored loans, and traineeships also available. *Financial aid application deadline:* 2/15.

Contact Ms. Linda Buck, Student Services Coordinator, Kirkhof College of Nursing, Grand Valley State University, Cook-DeVos Center for Health Sciences, 301 Michigan Street NE, Room 318, Grand Rapids, MI 49503-3314. *Telephone:* 616-331-5785. *Fax:* 616-331-2510. *E-mail:* buckli@gvsu.edu.

MASTER'S DEGREE PROGRAM
Degree MSN

Available Programs Master's.
Concentrations Available Clinical nurse leader.
Site Options Grand Rapids, MI.
Study Options Full-time and part-time.
Program Entrance Requirements Minimum overall college GPA of 3.0, transcript of college record, CPR certification, written essay, immunizations, interview, resume, GRE. *Application deadline:* 2/1 (fall). *Application fee:* $30.
Advanced Placement Credit given for nursing courses completed elsewhere dependent upon specific evaluations.
Degree Requirements 41 total credit hours, thesis or project.

DOCTORAL DEGREE PROGRAM

Degree DNP
Available Programs Post-Baccalaureate Doctorate.
Areas of Study Advanced practice nursing, nursing administration.
Site Options Grand Rapids, MI.
Program Entrance Requirements Minimum overall college GPA of 3.0, interview by faculty committee, vita, writing sample. *Application deadline:* 2/1 (fall). *Application fee:* $30.
Degree Requirements 94 total credit hours, dissertation.

CONTINUING EDUCATION PROGRAM

Contact Ms. Grace Hoyer, Academic Community Liaison, Kirkhof College of Nursing, Grand Valley State University, Cook-DeVos Center for Health Sciences, 301 Michigan Street NE, Room 350, Grand Rapids, MI 49503-3314. *Telephone:* 616-331-3558. *Fax:* 616-331-2510. *E-mail:* hoyerg@gvsu.edu.

Hope College
Department of Nursing
Holland, Michigan

Founded in 1866
DEGREE • BSN
Nursing Program Faculty 13 (30% with doctorates).
Baccalaureate Enrollment 135 **Women** 90% **Men** 10% **Minority** 10%
Nursing Student Activities Sigma Theta Tau, Student Nurses' Association.
Nursing Student Resources Academic advising; academic or career counseling; assistance for students with disabilities; bookstore; campus computer network; career placement assistance; computer lab; computer-assisted instruction; e-mail services; employment services for current students; externships; housing assistance; interactive nursing skills videos; Internet; learning resource lab; library services; nursing audiovisuals; remedial services; resume preparation assistance; skills, simulation, or other laboratory; tutoring; unpaid internships.
Library Facilities 374,504 volumes; 8,651 periodical subscriptions.

BACCALAUREATE PROGRAMS

Degree BSN
Available Programs Generic Baccalaureate.
Study Options Full-time and part-time.
Program Entrance Requirements Minimum overall college GPA of 3.0, transcript of college record, written essay, 2 letters of recommendation. Transfer students are accepted. *Application deadline:* 10/1 (fall), 2/1 (winter).
Contact Nursing Contact, Department of Nursing, Hope College, 35 East 12th Street, Holland, MI 49422-9000. *Telephone:* 616-395-7420. *Fax:* 616-395-7163. *E-mail:* nursing@hope.edu.

Lake Superior State University
Department of Nursing
Sault Sainte Marie, Michigan

http://www.lssu.edu/nursing/
Founded in 1946
DEGREE • BSN
Nursing Program Faculty 20 (15% with doctorates).
Baccalaureate Enrollment 115 **Women** 90% **Men** 10% **Minority** 10%
International 3%
Distance Learning Courses Available.

Nursing Student Activities Nursing Honor Society, Student Nurses' Association, nursing club.
Nursing Student Resources Academic advising; academic or career counseling; assistance for students with disabilities; bookstore; campus computer network; career placement assistance; computer lab; computer-assisted instruction; daycare for children of students; e-mail services; employment services for current students; interactive nursing skills videos; Internet; learning resource lab; library services; nursing audiovisuals; placement services for program completers; remedial services; resume preparation assistance; skills, simulation, or other laboratory; tutoring.
Library Facilities 200,449 volumes (5,246 in health, 942 in nursing); 850 periodical subscriptions (1,196 health-care related).

BACCALAUREATE PROGRAMS

Degree BSN
Available Programs ADN to Baccalaureate; Generic Baccalaureate; LPN to Baccalaureate; LPN to RN Baccalaureate; RN Baccalaureate; RPN to Baccalaureate.
Site Options Escanaba, MI; Petoskey, MI.
Study Options Full-time and part-time.
Program Entrance Requirements Minimum overall college GPA of 2.5, transcript of college record, CPR certification, health exam, health insurance, high school biology, high school chemistry, high school transcript, immunizations, 1 letter of recommendation, minimum high school GPA of 2.0, minimum GPA in nursing prerequisites of 2.5, professional liability insurance/malpractice insurance, prerequisite course work. Transfer students are accepted. *Application deadline:* 2/1 (fall), 10/1 (spring).
Advanced Placement Credit given for nursing courses completed elsewhere dependent upon specific evaluations.
Contact *Telephone:* 906-635-2446. *Fax:* 906-635-2266.

Madonna University
College of Nursing and Health
Livonia, Michigan

http://www.madonna.edu/
Founded in 1947
DEGREES • BSN • DNP • MSN • MSN/MBA
Nursing Program Faculty 71 (26% with doctorates).
Baccalaureate Enrollment 395 **Women** 87% **Men** 13% **Minority** 15% **International** 1% **Part-time** 32%
Graduate Enrollment 283 **Women** 90% **Men** 10% **Minority** 25% **International** 5% **Part-time** 96%
Distance Learning Courses Available.
Nursing Student Activities Sigma Theta Tau, Student Nurses' Association.
Nursing Student Resources Academic advising; academic or career counseling; assistance for students with disabilities; bookstore; campus computer network; career placement assistance; computer lab; computer-assisted instruction; e-mail services; interactive nursing skills videos; Internet; learning resource lab; library services; nursing audiovisuals; remedial services; resume preparation assistance; skills, simulation, or other laboratory; tutoring.
Library Facilities 108,000 volumes (3,632 in health); 515 periodical subscriptions (2,778 health-care related).

BACCALAUREATE PROGRAMS

Degree BSN
Available Programs ADN to Baccalaureate; Generic Baccalaureate; LPN to Baccalaureate; RN Baccalaureate.
Study Options Full-time and part-time.
Program Entrance Requirements Minimum overall college GPA of 2.75, transcript of college record, written essay, high school biology, high school chemistry, 1 year of high school math. Transfer students are accepted. *Application deadline:* 1/31 (fall), 7/31 (winter). *Application fee:* $25.
Advanced Placement Credit by examination available. Credit given for nursing courses completed elsewhere dependent upon specific evaluations.
Expenses (2012–13) *Tuition:* full-time $16,700; part-time $562 per credit hour. *International tuition:* $19,000 full-time. *Room and board:* $9134; room only: $3516 per academic year. *Required fees:* full-time $350.

Financial Aid 75% of baccalaureate students in nursing programs received some form of financial aid in 2011–12.

Contact Ms. Lauren Stemberger, Pre-Nursing Admissions Officer, College of Nursing and Health, Madonna University, 36600 Schoolcraft Road, Livonia, MI 48150-1173. *Telephone:* 734-432-5346. *E-mail:* lstemberger@madonna.edu.

GRADUATE PROGRAMS

Expenses (2012–13) *Tuition:* full-time $10,296; part-time $572 per credit hour. *International tuition:* $12,375 full-time. *Room and board:* $8000; room only: $5100 per academic year. *Required fees:* full-time $250; part-time $60 per term.

Financial Aid 20% of graduate students in nursing programs received some form of financial aid in 2011–12.

Contact Mr. Sandro Faber-Bermudez, Admissions Officer, Graduate Nursing program, College of Nursing and Health, Madonna University, 36600 Schoolcraft Road, Livonia, MI 48150-1173. *Telephone:* 734-432-5407. *Fax:* 734-432-5463. *E-mail:* sfaber-bermudez@madonna.edu.

MASTER'S DEGREE PROGRAM

Degrees MSN; MSN/MBA

Available Programs Master's.

Concentrations Available Nursing administration. *Nurse practitioner programs in:* acute care, adult health, primary care.

Study Options Full-time and part-time.

Program Entrance Requirements Clinical experience, computer literacy, minimum overall college GPA of 3.0, transcript of college record, written essay, interview, 2 letters of recommendation, nursing research course, physical assessment course, prerequisite course work, resume, statistics course. *Application deadline:* 2/1 (fall), 9/30 (winter), 2/1 (spring), 2/1 (summer). *Application fee:* $25.

Degree Requirements 48 total credit hours.

POST-MASTER'S PROGRAM

Areas of Study Nursing administration; nursing education. *Nurse practitioner programs in:* acute care, adult health, primary care.

DOCTORAL DEGREE PROGRAM

Degree DNP

Available Programs Doctorate.

Areas of Study Advanced practice nursing, individualized study, nursing administration.

Program Entrance Requirements Clinical experience, minimum overall college GPA of 3.0, interview by faculty committee, interview, 3 letters of recommendation, MSN or equivalent, scholarly papers, vita, writing sample. *Application deadline:* 3/1 (fall). *Application fee:* $25.

Degree Requirements 36 total credit hours, oral exam, written exam, residency.

CONTINUING EDUCATION PROGRAM

Contact Dr. Susan Hasenau, Coordinator of Nursing Continuing Education, College of Nursing and Health, Madonna University, 36600 Schoolcraft Road, Livonia, MI 48150-1173. *Telephone:* 734-432-5863. *Fax:* 734-432-5463. *E-mail:* shasenau@madonna.edu.

Michigan State University

College of Nursing
East Lansing, Michigan

http://www.nursing.msu.edu/
Founded in 1855
DEGREES • BSN • MSN • PHD
Nursing Program Faculty 93 (42% with doctorates).
Baccalaureate Enrollment 340 **Women** 84.7% **Men** 15.3% **Minority** 8.7% **International** .3% **Part-time** 11.8%
Graduate Enrollment 181 **Women** 91.2% **Men** 8.8% **Minority** 7.8% **International** 1.1% **Part-time** 57.5%
Distance Learning Courses Available.
Nursing Student Activities Sigma Theta Tau, Student Nurses' Association.
Nursing Student Resources Academic advising; academic or career counseling; assistance for students with disabilities; bookstore; campus computer network; career placement assistance; computer lab; computer-assisted instruction; daycare for children of students; e-mail services;

employment services for current students; externships; housing assistance; interactive nursing skills videos; Internet; learning resource lab; library services; nursing audiovisuals; placement services for program completers; remedial services; resume preparation assistance; skills, simulation, or other laboratory; tutoring.

Library Facilities 6.7 million volumes (272,697 in health, 5,579 in nursing); 172,144 periodical subscriptions (7,151 health-care related).

BACCALAUREATE PROGRAMS

Degree BSN

Available Programs Accelerated Baccalaureate for Second Degree; Generic Baccalaureate; RN Baccalaureate.

Study Options Full-time.

Online Degree Options Yes.

Program Entrance Requirements Minimum overall college GPA of 2.75, transcript of college record, written essay, 2 letters of recommendation, minimum GPA in nursing prerequisites of 2.75, prerequisite course work. Transfer students are accepted. *Application deadline:* 3/1 (fall), 10/1 (spring), 12/15 (summer).

Advanced Placement Credit given for nursing courses completed elsewhere dependent upon specific evaluations.

Financial Aid 78% of baccalaureate students in nursing programs received some form of financial aid in 2011–12.

Contact Office of Student Support Services, College of Nursing, Michigan State University, C120, 1355 Bogue Street, East Lansing, MI 48824-1317. *Telephone:* 517-353-4827. *Fax:* 517-432-8251. *E-mail:* nurse@hc.msu.edu.

GRADUATE PROGRAMS

Financial Aid 79% of graduate students in nursing programs received some form of financial aid in 2011–12. 1 research assistantship with tuition reimbursement available (averaging $6,110 per year), 2 teaching assistantships with tuition reimbursements available (averaging $7,076 per year) were awarded.

Contact Ms. Nikki O'Brien, Program Advisor, College of Nursing, Michigan State University, C120, 1355 Bogue Street, East Lansing, MI 48824-1317. *Telephone:* 517-353-4827. *Fax:* 517-432-8251. *E-mail:* obrienni@msu.edu.

MASTER'S DEGREE PROGRAM

Degree MSN

Available Programs Master's.

Concentrations Available Nurse anesthesia. *Clinical nurse specialist programs in:* adult health. *Nurse practitioner programs in:* adult health, family health, gerontology.

Study Options Full-time and part-time.

Online Degree Options Yes.

Program Entrance Requirements Clinical experience, minimum overall college GPA of 3.0, transcript of college record, CPR certification, written essay, immunizations, interview, 3 letters of recommendation, prerequisite course work, resume, statistics course. *Application deadline:* 2/1 (fall), 3/15 (spring). Applications may be processed on a rolling basis for some programs.

Degree Requirements Thesis or project.

POST-MASTER'S PROGRAM

Areas of Study *Clinical nurse specialist programs in:* adult health. *Nurse practitioner programs in:* adult health, family health, gerontology.

DOCTORAL DEGREE PROGRAM

Degree PhD

Available Programs Doctorate; Post-Baccalaureate Doctorate.

Areas of Study Family health, health promotion/disease prevention, human health and illness, individualized study, nursing research.

Program Entrance Requirements Minimum overall college GPA of 3.0, interview by faculty committee, interview, 3 letters of recommendation, statistics course, vita, writing sample. *Application deadline:* 12/1 (fall). Applications may be processed on a rolling basis for some programs.

Degree Requirements 72 total credit hours, dissertation, written exam.

CONTINUING EDUCATION PROGRAM

Contact Katie Kessler, Director of Professional Education, College of Nursing, Michigan State University, A103, 1355 Bogue Street, East Lansing, MI 48824-1317. *Telephone:* 517-355-8539. *Fax:* 517-432-8131. *E-mail:* kathleen.kessler@hc.msu.edu.

Northern Michigan University
College of Nursing and Allied Health Science
Marquette, Michigan

http://webb.nmu.edu/Nursing/
Founded in 1899
DEGREES • BSN • MSN
Nursing Program Faculty 16 (69% with doctorates).
Baccalaureate Enrollment 221 **Women** 81% **Men** 19% **Minority** 4% **Part-time** 7%
Graduate Enrollment 16 **Women** 81% **Men** 19% **Part-time** 100%
Distance Learning Courses Available.
Nursing Student Activities Sigma Theta Tau, Student Nurses' Association.
Nursing Student Resources Academic advising; academic or career counseling; assistance for students with disabilities; bookstore; campus computer network; career placement assistance; computer lab; computer-assisted instruction; e-mail services; employment services for current students; housing assistance; interactive nursing skills videos; Internet; learning resource lab; library services; nursing audiovisuals; other; paid internships; remedial services; resume preparation assistance; skills, simulation, or other laboratory; tutoring.
Library Facilities 32,879 volumes in health, 2,733 volumes in nursing; 5,000 periodical subscriptions health-care related.

BACCALAUREATE PROGRAMS
Degree BSN
Available Programs Accelerated Baccalaureate; Generic Baccalaureate; LPN to Baccalaureate; RN Baccalaureate.
Study Options Full-time.
Program Entrance Requirements Minimum overall college GPA of 2.75, transcript of college record, CPR certification, health exam, high school transcript, immunizations, minimum GPA in nursing prerequisites of 2.0, prerequisite course work. Transfer students are accepted. *Application deadline:* 2/1 (fall), 10/1 (winter).
Advanced Placement Credit by examination available. Credit given for nursing courses completed elsewhere dependent upon specific evaluations.
Contact *Telephone:* 906-227-2834. *Fax:* 906-227-1658.

GRADUATE PROGRAMS
Contact *Telephone:* 906-227-2488. *Fax:* 906-227-1658.

MASTER'S DEGREE PROGRAM
Degree MSN
Available Programs Master's.
Concentrations Available *Nurse practitioner programs in:* family health.
Study Options Part-time.
Program Entrance Requirements Clinical experience, computer literacy, minimum overall college GPA of 3.0, transcript of college record, CPR certification, written essay, immunizations, 2 letters of recommendation, physical assessment course, professional liability insurance/malpractice insurance, GRE General Test. *Application deadline:* 2/1 (fall).
Advanced Placement Credit given for nursing courses completed elsewhere dependent upon specific evaluations.
Degree Requirements 45 total credit hours, thesis or project, comprehensive exam.

POST-MASTER'S PROGRAM
Areas of Study *Nurse practitioner programs in:* family health.

CONTINUING EDUCATION PROGRAM
Contact *Telephone:* 906-227-2044. *Fax:* 906-227-2928.

Oakland University
School of Nursing
Rochester, Michigan

http://www2.oakland.edu/nursing
Founded in 1957
DEGREES • BSN • MSN
Nursing Program Faculty 44 (50% with doctorates).

Baccalaureate Enrollment 462 **Women** 89% **Men** 11% **Minority** 12% **Part-time** 29%
Graduate Enrollment 123 **Women** 79% **Men** 21% **Minority** 11% **International** 1% **Part-time** 35%
Nursing Student Activities Nursing Honor Society, Sigma Theta Tau, Student Nurses' Association.
Nursing Student Resources Academic advising; academic or career counseling; assistance for students with disabilities; bookstore; campus computer network; career placement assistance; computer lab; computer-assisted instruction; e-mail services; employment services for current students; externships; housing assistance; interactive nursing skills videos; Internet; learning resource lab; library services; nursing audiovisuals; paid internships; placement services for program completers; remedial services; resume preparation assistance; skills, simulation, or other laboratory; tutoring; unpaid internships.
Library Facilities 856,760 volumes (12,652 in health, 2,780 in nursing); 20,490 periodical subscriptions (375 health-care related).

BACCALAUREATE PROGRAMS
Degree BSN
Available Programs Generic Baccalaureate; RN Baccalaureate.
Site Options Royal Oak, MI.
Study Options Full-time and part-time.
Program Entrance Requirements Minimum overall college GPA of 3.0, transcript of college record, CPR certification, health exam, high school biology, high school chemistry, 2 years high school math, 1 year of high school science, high school transcript, immunizations, minimum high school GPA of 3.0, minimum GPA in nursing prerequisites of 3.0, professional liability insurance/malpractice insurance, prerequisite course work. Transfer students are accepted.
Advanced Placement Credit given for nursing courses completed elsewhere dependent upon specific evaluations.
Contact *Telephone:* 248-370-4065. *Fax:* 248-370-4279.

GRADUATE PROGRAMS
Contact *Telephone:* 248-370-4082. *Fax:* 248-370-2996.

MASTER'S DEGREE PROGRAM
Degree MSN
Available Programs Master's.
Concentrations Available Nurse anesthesia; nursing education. *Nurse practitioner programs in:* adult health, family health, gerontology.
Site Options Royal Oak, MI.
Study Options Full-time and part-time.
Program Entrance Requirements Clinical experience, minimum overall college GPA of 3.0, transcript of college record, CPR certification, written essay, immunizations, interview, 2 letters of recommendation, professional liability insurance/malpractice insurance, prerequisite course work, GRE General Test.
Advanced Placement Credit given for nursing courses completed elsewhere dependent upon specific evaluations.
Degree Requirements 45 total credit hours, thesis or project.

POST-MASTER'S PROGRAM
Areas of Study Nurse anesthesia; nursing education. *Nurse practitioner programs in:* adult health, family health, gerontology.

CONTINUING EDUCATION PROGRAM
Contact *Telephone:* 248-370-4013. *Fax:* 248-370-4279.

The Robert B. Miller College
School of Nursing
Battle Creek, Michigan

DEGREE • BSN

BACCALAUREATE PROGRAMS
Degree BSN
Available Programs RN Baccalaureate.
Study Options Full-time and part-time.
Program Entrance Requirements Minimum overall college GPA of 2.5, RN licensure.
Contact Nursing Program, School of Nursing, The Robert B. Miller College, 450 North Avenue, Battle Creek, MI 49017-3397. *Telephone:* 269-660-8021. *Fax:* 269-565-2180. *E-mail:* info@millercollege.edu.

Rochester College
School of Nursing
Rochester Hills, Michigan

http://www.rc.edu
Founded in 1959
DEGREE • BSN
Baccalaureate Enrollment 42
Distance Learning Courses Available.
Nursing Student Resources Academic advising; academic or career counseling; assistance for students with disabilities; bookstore; campus computer network; career placement assistance; computer lab; computer-assisted instruction; e-mail services; externships; housing assistance; interactive nursing skills videos; Internet; learning resource lab; library services; nursing audiovisuals; remedial services; resume preparation assistance; skills, simulation, or other laboratory; tutoring; unpaid internships.
Library Facilities 55,000 volumes; 200 periodical subscriptions.

BACCALAUREATE PROGRAMS

Degree BSN
Available Programs Generic Baccalaureate; RN Baccalaureate.
Study Options Full-time.
Program Entrance Requirements Minimum overall college GPA of 3.0, transcript of college record, written essay, interview, minimum GPA in nursing prerequisites of 3.0, prerequisite course work. Transfer students are accepted. *Application deadline:* 6/1 (fall).
Expenses (2012–13) *Tuition:* full-time $8000; part-time $500 per credit. *Room and board:* $8000 per academic year. *Required fees:* full-time $300.
Financial Aid 75% of baccalaureate students in nursing programs received some form of financial aid in 2011–12.
Contact Mrs. Jaime M. Sinutko, Director of Nursing, School of Nursing, Rochester College, 800 West Avon Road, Rochester Hills, MI 48085. *Telephone:* 248-218-2283. *E-mail:* jsinutko@rc.edu.

Saginaw Valley State University
Crystal M. Lange College of Health and Human Services
University Center, Michigan

http://www.svsu.edu/collegeofhealthhumanservices
Founded in 1963
DEGREES • BSN • DNP • MSN
Nursing Program Faculty 18 (50% with doctorates).
Baccalaureate Enrollment 384 **Women** 80% **Men** 20%
Graduate Enrollment 95 **Women** 92% **Men** 8% **Part-time** 100%
Nursing Student Activities Sigma Theta Tau, Student Nurses' Association.
Nursing Student Resources Academic advising; academic or career counseling; assistance for students with disabilities; bookstore; campus computer network; career placement assistance; computer lab; computer-assisted instruction; e-mail services; employment services for current students; externships; interactive nursing skills videos; Internet; learning resource lab; library services; nursing audiovisuals; remedial services; resume preparation assistance; skills, simulation, or other laboratory; tutoring.
Library Facilities 241,661 volumes; 23,741 periodical subscriptions.

BACCALAUREATE PROGRAMS

Degree BSN
Available Programs ADN to Baccalaureate; Accelerated Baccalaureate for Second Degree; Baccalaureate for Second Degree; Generic Baccalaureate; RN Baccalaureate.
Study Options Full-time and part-time.
Program Entrance Requirements Minimum overall college GPA of 2.5, transcript of college record, CPR certification, health exam, immunizations, interview, minimum GPA in nursing prerequisites of 2.5, professional liability insurance/malpractice insurance, prerequisite course work. Transfer students are accepted. *Application deadline:* 4/15 (fall), 10/15 (winter).
Advanced Placement Credit by examination available. Credit given for nursing courses completed elsewhere dependent upon specific evaluations.

Expenses (2012–13) *Tuition, state resident:* full-time $6145. *Tuition, nonresident:* full-time $14,900. *Required fees:* full-time $200.
Contact Dr. Sally Decker, Nursing Department Chair, Crystal M. Lange College of Health and Human Services, Saginaw Valley State University, 7400 Bay Road, H 226, University Center, MI 48710-0001. *Telephone:* 989-964-4098. *Fax:* 989-964-4925. *E-mail:* decker@svsu.edu.

GRADUATE PROGRAMS

Expenses (2012–13) *Tuition, state resident:* full-time $7420. *Tuition, nonresident:* full-time $14,165. *Required fees:* full-time $800.
Financial Aid Federal Work-Study and scholarships available.
Contact Dr. Karen Brown-Fackler, MSN Coordinator, Crystal M. Lange College of Health and Human Services, Saginaw Valley State University, 7400 Bay Road, H 219, University Center, MI 48710-0001. *Telephone:* 989-964-2185. *Fax:* 989-964-4925. *E-mail:* kmbrown4@svsu.edu.

MASTER'S DEGREE PROGRAM

Degree MSN
Available Programs Accelerated AD/RN to Master's; Master's; RN to Master's.
Concentrations Available Clinical nurse leader; nursing administration; nursing education. *Clinical nurse specialist programs in:* family health. *Nurse practitioner programs in:* family health.
Site Options Gaylord, MI.
Study Options Part-time.
Program Entrance Requirements Clinical experience, minimum overall college GPA of 3.0, transcript of college record, CPR certification, written essay, immunizations, interview, 3 letters of recommendation, professional liability insurance/malpractice insurance, resume, statistics course, GRE. *Application deadline:* Applications may be processed on a rolling basis for some programs.
Advanced Placement Credit given for nursing courses completed elsewhere dependent upon specific evaluations.
Degree Requirements 39 total credit hours, thesis or project.

POST-MASTER'S PROGRAM

Areas of Study Nursing administration; nursing education.

DOCTORAL DEGREE PROGRAM

Degree DNP
Available Programs Doctorate.
Program Entrance Requirements interview, letters of recommendation, vita. *Application deadline:* Applications may be processed on a rolling basis for some programs.

CONTINUING EDUCATION PROGRAM

Contact CE Coordinator, Crystal M. Lange College of Health and Human Services, Saginaw Valley State University, 7400 Bay Road, University Center, MI 48710-0001. *Telephone:* 989-964-4595. *Fax:* 989-964-4925.

Siena Heights University
Nursing Program
Adrian, Michigan

http://www.sienaheights.edu/
Founded in 1919
DEGREE • BSN
Nursing Program Faculty 7 (10% with doctorates).
Baccalaureate Enrollment 80 **Women** 90% **Men** 10% **Minority** 5% **International** 5% **Part-time** 20%
Distance Learning Courses Available.
Nursing Student Activities Student Nurses' Association.
Nursing Student Resources Academic advising; academic or career counseling; bookstore; campus computer network; computer lab; computer-assisted instruction; e-mail services; interactive nursing skills videos; Internet; learning resource lab; library services; skills, simulation, or other laboratory; tutoring.
Library Facilities 142,000 volumes (200 in health, 80 in nursing); 300 periodical subscriptions (150 health-care related).

BACCALAUREATE PROGRAMS

Degree BSN
Available Programs Generic Baccalaureate; RN Baccalaureate.
Study Options Full-time.

Program Entrance Requirements Minimum overall college GPA of 3.0, transcript of college record, CPR certification, written essay, health exam, health insurance, high school transcript, immunizations, interview, minimum GPA in nursing prerequisites of 3.0, professional liability insurance/malpractice insurance, prerequisite course work. Transfer students are accepted. *Application deadline:* 10/1 (fall).

Expenses (2011–12) *Tuition:* full-time $19,934; part-time $410 per credit hour. *International tuition:* $19,934 full-time. *Room and board:* $7890; room only: $4000 per academic year. *Required fees:* full-time $1220.

Financial Aid 90% of baccalaureate students in nursing programs received some form of financial aid in 2010–11.

Contact Miss Sara Johnson, Director of Admissions, Nursing Program, Siena Heights University, 1247 East Siena Heights Drive, Adrian, MI 49221. *Telephone:* 517-264-7180. *E-mail:* sjohnson@sienaheights.edu.

Spring Arbor University
Program in Nursing
Spring Arbor, Michigan

http://www.arbor.edu/bsn
Founded in 1873

DEGREES • BSN • MSN • MSN/MBA
Nursing Program Faculty 19 (12% with doctorates).
Baccalaureate Enrollment 272 **Women** 92% **Men** 8% **Minority** 9%
International 1% **Part-time** 70%
Graduate Enrollment 56 **Women** 92% **Men** 8% **Minority** 5%
Distance Learning Courses Available.
Nursing Student Resources Academic advising; assistance for students with disabilities; bookstore; campus computer network; career placement assistance; computer-assisted instruction; e-mail services; Internet; library services; nursing audiovisuals; other; tutoring.
Library Facilities 115,987 volumes (1,000 in health, 350 in nursing); 523 periodical subscriptions (25 health-care related).

BACCALAUREATE PROGRAMS

Degree BSN
Available Programs ADN to Baccalaureate.
Site Options Traverse City, MI; Dearborn, MI; Grand Rapids, MI; Lambertville, MI; Lansing, MI; Kalamazoo, MI; Battle Creek, MI; Gaylord, MI; Jackson, MI.
Program Entrance Requirements Minimum overall college GPA of 2.5, transcript of college record, written essay, high school biology, high school chemistry, 1 year of high school math, 2 years high school science, high school transcript, minimum GPA in nursing prerequisites of 2.5, RN licensure. Transfer students are accepted. *Application deadline:* Applications may be processed on a rolling basis for some programs. *Application fee:* $40.
Financial Aid 84% of baccalaureate students in nursing programs received some form of financial aid in 2010–11.
Contact Mr. Alvin V. Kauffman, Director of Nursing, Program in Nursing, Spring Arbor University, 106 East Main Street, Suite #3, Spring Arbor, MI 49283-9799. *Telephone:* 517-750-6579. *Fax:* 517-750-6602. *E-mail:* alvin.kauffman@arbor.edu.

GRADUATE PROGRAMS

Financial Aid 68% of graduate students in nursing programs received some form of financial aid in 2010–11.
Contact Mr. Jim Madden, Senior Admission Specialist, Program in Nursing, Spring Arbor University, 3497 South 9th Street, Suite A, Kalamazoo, MI 49009-9501. *Telephone:* 800-930-9754 Ext. 4058. *Fax:* 269-372-1840. *E-mail:* jmadden@arbor.edu.

MASTER'S DEGREE PROGRAM

Degrees MSN; MSN/MBA
Available Programs Master's.
Concentrations Available Nursing education. *Nurse practitioner programs in:* adult health, gerontology.
Study Options Full-time.
Online Degree Options Yes (online only).
Program Entrance Requirements Computer literacy, minimum overall college GPA of 3.0, transcript of college record, written essay, interview, 2 letters of recommendation, nursing research course, prerequisite course work, statistics course. *Application deadline:* 7/1 (fall). *Application fee:* $40.
Degree Requirements 62 total credit hours, thesis or project.

University of Detroit Mercy
McAuley School of Nursing
Detroit, Michigan

http://www.udmercy.edu/healthprof/nursing/
Founded in 1877

DEGREES • BSN • MSN
Nursing Program Faculty 80
Baccalaureate Enrollment 933 **Women** 88% **Men** 12% **Minority** 24%
International 6% **Part-time** 46%
Graduate Enrollment 132 **Women** 95% **Men** 5% **Minority** 27% **International** 2% **Part-time** 96%
Distance Learning Courses Available.
Nursing Student Activities Sigma Theta Tau, Student Nurses' Association.
Nursing Student Resources Academic advising; academic or career counseling; bookstore; campus computer network; career placement assistance; computer lab; computer-assisted instruction; e-mail services; Internet; learning resource lab; library services; nursing audiovisuals; other; paid internships; placement services for program completers; remedial services; resume preparation assistance; skills, simulation, or other laboratory; tutoring.
Library Facilities 32,330 volumes in health, 3,404 volumes in nursing; 2,670 periodical subscriptions health-care related.

BACCALAUREATE PROGRAMS

Degree BSN
Available Programs Accelerated Baccalaureate for Second Degree; Generic Baccalaureate; RN Baccalaureate.
Site Options Dearborn, MI; Grand Rapids, MI; Wayne, MI.
Study Options Full-time and part-time.
Program Entrance Requirements Minimum overall college GPA of 2.5, transcript of college record, CPR certification, health exam, health insurance, high school biology, high school chemistry, 2 years high school math, 2 years high school science, high school transcript, immunizations, minimum high school GPA of 2.5, minimum GPA in nursing prerequisites of 2.5, prerequisite course work. Transfer students are accepted.
Advanced Placement Credit given for nursing courses completed elsewhere dependent upon specific evaluations.
Contact *Telephone:* 313-993-1245. *Fax:* 313-993-3325.

GRADUATE PROGRAMS

Contact *Telephone:* 313-993-6423. *Fax:* 313-993-6175.

MASTER'S DEGREE PROGRAM

Degree MSN
Available Programs Accelerated AD/RN to Master's; Master's; Master's for Nurses with Non-Nursing Degrees.
Concentrations Available Nursing administration; nursing education. *Nurse practitioner programs in:* family health.
Study Options Full-time and part-time.
Program Entrance Requirements Clinical experience, minimum overall college GPA of 3.0, transcript of college record, CPR certification, immunizations, interview, 3 letters of recommendation, resume.
Degree Requirements 50 total credit hours.

POST-MASTER'S PROGRAM

Areas of Study Nursing administration; nursing education. *Nurse practitioner programs in:* family health.

University of Michigan
School of Nursing
Ann Arbor, Michigan

http://www.nursing.umich.edu/
Founded in 1817

DEGREES • BSN • MS • MSN/MBA • MSN/MPH • PHD
Nursing Program Faculty 130 (66% with doctorates).
Baccalaureate Enrollment 618 **Women** 90% **Men** 10% **Minority** 20%
International 3% **Part-time** 13%
Graduate Enrollment 240 **Women** 95% **Men** 5% **Minority** 30% **International** 11% **Part-time** 40%
Distance Learning Courses Available.

Nursing Student Activities Nursing Honor Society, Sigma Theta Tau, Student Nurses' Association, nursing club.

Nursing Student Resources Academic advising; academic or career counseling; assistance for students with disabilities; bookstore; campus computer network; career placement assistance; computer lab; computer-assisted instruction; daycare for children of students; e-mail services; employment services for current students; externships; housing assistance; interactive nursing skills videos; Internet; learning resource lab; library services; nursing audiovisuals; paid internships; placement services for program completers; remedial services; resume preparation assistance; skills, simulation, or other laboratory; tutoring; unpaid internships.

Library Facilities 12.4 million volumes (1.2 million in nursing); 151,854 periodical subscriptions.

BACCALAUREATE PROGRAMS

Degree BSN
Available Programs Accelerated Baccalaureate for Second Degree; Generic Baccalaureate; RN Baccalaureate.
Site Options Kalamazoo, MI; Traverse City, MI.
Study Options Full-time and part-time.
Program Entrance Requirements Minimum overall college GPA of 3.0, transcript of college record, written essay, high school chemistry, 2 years high school math, 2 years high school science, high school transcript, minimum high school GPA of 3.0, prerequisite course work. Transfer students are accepted. *Application deadline:* 2/1 (fall). Applications may be processed on a rolling basis for some programs. *Application fee:* $80.
Advanced Placement Credit given for nursing courses completed elsewhere dependent upon specific evaluations.
Contact *Telephone:* 734-647-1443. *Fax:* 734-936-0740.

GRADUATE PROGRAMS

Contact *Telephone:* 734-764-7188. *Fax:* 734-647-1419.

MASTER'S DEGREE PROGRAM

Degrees MS; MSN/MBA; MSN/MPH
Available Programs Accelerated RN to Master's; Master's; RN to Master's.
Concentrations Available Health-care administration; nurse-midwifery; nursing administration; nursing informatics. *Clinical nurse specialist programs in:* community health, gerontology, home health care, medical-surgical, occupational health, psychiatric/mental health. *Nurse practitioner programs in:* acute care, adult health, family health, gerontology, pediatric, primary care, psychiatric/mental health.
Study Options Full-time and part-time.
Program Entrance Requirements Computer literacy, minimum overall college GPA of 3.0, transcript of college record, written essay, interview, 3 letters of recommendation, resume, GRE General Test (if undergraduate GPA less than 3.25). *Application deadline:* 2/1 (fall). Applications may be processed on a rolling basis for some programs. *Application fee:* $80.
Advanced Placement Credit given for nursing courses completed elsewhere dependent upon specific evaluations.
Degree Requirements 37 total credit hours, thesis or project.

POST-MASTER'S PROGRAM

Areas of Study Health-care administration; nurse-midwifery; nursing administration; nursing informatics. *Clinical nurse specialist programs in:* community health, gerontology, home health care, medical-surgical, occupational health, psychiatric/mental health, women's health. *Nurse practitioner programs in:* acute care, adult health, family health, gerontology, pediatric, primary care, psychiatric/mental health, women's health.

DOCTORAL DEGREE PROGRAM

Degree PhD
Available Programs Doctorate; Post-Baccalaureate Doctorate.
Areas of Study Advanced practice nursing, aging, bio-behavioral research, biology of health and illness, community health, critical care, ethics, family health, gerontology, health policy, health promotion/disease prevention, health-care systems, individualized study, information systems, neuro-behavior, nursing administration, nursing policy, nursing research, nursing science, women's health.
Program Entrance Requirements Minimum overall college GPA of 3.0, interview, 3 letters of recommendation, scholarly papers, vita, writing sample, GRE General Test. *Application deadline:* 12/11 (fall). *Application fee:* $80.

Degree Requirements 50 total credit hours, dissertation, oral exam, written exam, residency.

POSTDOCTORAL PROGRAM

Areas of Study Addiction/substance abuse, aging, chronic illness, community health, family health, gerontology, health promotion/disease prevention, individualized study, information systems, neuro-behavior, nursing interventions, nursing research, nursing science, vulnerable population, women's health.
Postdoctoral Program Contact *Telephone:* 734-764-9454. *Fax:* 734-763-6668.

University of Michigan–Flint
Department of Nursing
Flint, Michigan

http://www.umflint.edu/nursing
Founded in 1956
DEGREES • BSN • DAP • DNP • MSN
Nursing Program Faculty 104 (19% with doctorates).
Baccalaureate Enrollment 494 **Women** 80.57% **Men** 19.43% **Minority** 14.37% **International** 1.21% **Part-time** 54.9%
Graduate Enrollment 157 **Women** 88.54% **Men** 11.46% **Minority** 14.65% **International** 1.27% **Part-time** 72%
Distance Learning Courses Available.
Nursing Student Activities Nursing Honor Society, Sigma Theta Tau, Student Nurses' Association, nursing club.
Nursing Student Resources Academic advising; academic or career counseling; assistance for students with disabilities; bookstore; campus computer network; career placement assistance; computer lab; computer-assisted instruction; daycare for children of students; e-mail services; employment services for current students; externships; housing assistance; interactive nursing skills videos; Internet; library services; nursing audiovisuals; remedial services; resume preparation assistance; skills, simulation, or other laboratory; tutoring.
Library Facilities 353,617 volumes (16,552 in health, 1,709 in nursing); 559 periodical subscriptions (204 health-care related).

BACCALAUREATE PROGRAMS

Degree BSN
Available Programs Accelerated Baccalaureate for Second Degree; Generic Baccalaureate; RN Baccalaureate.
Site Options Lansing, MI; Detroit, MI; Alpena Community College/Alpena, MI; Flint, MI.
Study Options Full-time.
Online Degree Options Yes.
Program Entrance Requirements Minimum overall college GPA of 3.0, transcript of college record, CPR certification, written essay, health exam, health insurance, immunizations, 2 letters of recommendation, minimum high school GPA of 3.0, minimum GPA in nursing prerequisites of 3.0, prerequisite course work. Transfer students are accepted. *Application deadline:* 1/10 (fall), 9/1 (winter). *Application fee:* $30.
Advanced Placement Credit given for nursing courses completed elsewhere upon specific evaluations.
Expenses (2012–13) *Tuition, state resident:* full-time $10,224. *Tuition, nonresident:* full-time $20,436. *International tuition:* $20,436 full-time. *Room and board:* $7506 per academic year. *Required fees:* full-time $542.
Financial Aid 77% of baccalaureate students in nursing programs received some form of financial aid in 2011–12.
Contact Ms. Karin Anderson, Senior Secretary, Department of Nursing, University of Michigan–Flint, 303 East Kearsley Street, 2180 William S. White, Flint, MI 48502-1950. *Telephone:* 810-762-3420. *Fax:* 810-766-6851. *E-mail:* karinan@umflint.edu.

GRADUATE PROGRAMS

Expenses (2012–13) *Tuition, state resident:* full-time $7748. *Tuition, nonresident:* full-time $11,616. *International tuition:* $11,616 full-time. *Room and board:* $7506 per academic year. *Required fees:* full-time $412.
Financial Aid 67% of graduate students in nursing programs received some form of financial aid in 2011–12.
Contact Ms. Karin Anderson, Senior Secretary, Department of Nursing, University of Michigan–Flint, 303 East Kearsley Street, 2180 William S. White, Flint, MI 48502-1950. *Telephone:* 810-762-3420. *Fax:* 810-766-6851. *E-mail:* karinan@umflint.edu.

MASTER'S DEGREE PROGRAM
Degree MSN
Available Programs Accelerated RN to Master's; RN to Master's.
Concentrations Available Nurse anesthesia. *Nurse practitioner programs in:* adult health.
Site Options Flint, MI.
Study Options Full-time.
Online Degree Options Yes.
Program Entrance Requirements Minimum overall college GPA of 3.2, transcript of college record, written essay, 3 letters of recommendation, resume. *Application deadline:* 8/1 (fall), 10/1 (winter). *Application fee:* $55.
Advanced Placement Credit given for nursing courses completed elsewhere dependent upon specific evaluations.
Degree Requirements 43 total credit hours.

DOCTORAL DEGREE PROGRAM
Degree DAP
Available Programs Doctorate.
Areas of Study Anesthesia.
Online Degree Options Yes (online only).
Program Entrance Requirements Minimum overall college GPA of 3.0, interview, 3 letters of recommendation, MSN or equivalent. *Application deadline:* 5/1 (fall). *Application fee:* $55.
Degree Requirements 32 total credit hours.

Degree DNP
Available Programs Doctorate.
Areas of Study Advanced practice nursing, family health, gerontology.
Site Options Flint, MI.
Online Degree Options Yes (online only).
Program Entrance Requirements Clinical experience, minimum overall college GPA of 3.2, interview, 3 letters of recommendation, MSN or equivalent, statistics course, vita. *Application deadline:* 3/1 (fall). *Application fee:* $55.
Degree Requirements 31 total credit hours.

University of Phoenix–Metro Detroit Campus
College of Nursing
Southfield, Michigan

DEGREES • BSN • MSN
Nursing Program Faculty 15 (33% with doctorates).
Baccalaureate Enrollment 18 **Women** 94.4% **Men** 5.6% **Minority** 38.9%
Graduate Enrollment 4 **Women** 100%
Nursing Student Activities Sigma Theta Tau.
Nursing Student Resources Academic advising; academic or career counseling; assistance for students with disabilities; bookstore; campus computer network; computer lab; computer-assisted instruction; e-mail services; interactive nursing skills videos; Internet; learning resource lab; library services; nursing audiovisuals; skills, simulation, or other laboratory; tutoring.
Library Facilities 1,759 volumes; 692 periodical subscriptions (1,300 health-care related).

BACCALAUREATE PROGRAMS
Degree BSN
Available Programs Accelerated Baccalaureate.
Site Options Livonia, MI; Ann Arbor, MI; Southfield, MI.
Study Options Full-time.
Program Entrance Requirements Transcript of college record, CPR certification, immunizations, 1 letter of recommendation, RN licensure. Transfer students are accepted. *Application deadline:* Applications may be processed on a rolling basis for some programs.
Advanced Placement Credit by examination available. Credit given for nursing courses completed elsewhere dependent upon specific evaluations.
Contact *Telephone:* 800-834-2438.

GRADUATE PROGRAMS
Contact *Telephone:* 800-834-2438.

MASTER'S DEGREE PROGRAM
Degree MSN

Available Programs Master's.
Concentrations Available Health-care administration; nursing administration; nursing education.
Site Options Livonia, MI; Ann Arbor, MI; Southfield, MI.
Study Options Full-time.
Program Entrance Requirements Clinical experience, computer literacy, minimum overall college GPA of 2.5, transcript of college record. *Application deadline:* Applications may be processed on a rolling basis for some programs. *Application fee:* $45.
Advanced Placement Credit given for nursing courses completed elsewhere dependent upon specific evaluations.
Degree Requirements 39 total credit hours, thesis or project.

University of Phoenix–West Michigan Campus
College of Health and Human Services
Walker, Michigan

Founded in 2000
Nursing Program Faculty 2
Nursing Student Activities Sigma Theta Tau.
Nursing Student Resources Academic advising; academic or career counseling; assistance for students with disabilities; bookstore; computer lab; computer-assisted instruction; e-mail services; interactive nursing skills videos; Internet; learning resource lab; library services; nursing audiovisuals; remedial services; resume preparation assistance; skills, simulation, or other laboratory.
Library Facilities 16,781 periodical subscriptions (1,300 health-care related).

Wayne State University
College of Nursing
Detroit, Michigan

http://www.nursing.wayne.edu/
Founded in 1868

DEGREES • BSN • DNP • MSN
Nursing Program Faculty 93 (45% with doctorates).
Baccalaureate Enrollment 208 **Women** 81% **Men** 19% **Minority** 21% **International** 1% **Part-time** 16%
Graduate Enrollment 420 **Women** 91% **Men** 9% **Minority** 28% **International** 5% **Part-time** 67%
Distance Learning Courses Available.
Nursing Student Activities Nursing Honor Society, Sigma Theta Tau, Student Nurses' Association, nursing club.
Nursing Student Resources Academic advising; academic or career counseling; assistance for students with disabilities; bookstore; campus computer network; career placement assistance; computer lab; computer-assisted instruction; e-mail services; employment services for current students; interactive nursing skills videos; Internet; learning resource lab; library services; nursing audiovisuals; placement services for program completers; resume preparation assistance; skills, simulation, or other laboratory; tutoring.
Library Facilities 4 million volumes (156,000 in health, 6,600 in nursing); 17,032 periodical subscriptions (5,000 health-care related).

BACCALAUREATE PROGRAMS
Degree BSN
Available Programs Accelerated Baccalaureate for Second Degree; Generic Baccalaureate.
Study Options Full-time and part-time.
Program Entrance Requirements Minimum overall college GPA of 2.0, transcript of college record, interview, minimum GPA in nursing prerequisites of 2.5, prerequisite course work. Transfer students are accepted. *Application deadline:* 3/31 (fall). *Application fee:* $50.
Expenses (2012–13) *Tuition, area resident:* full-time $15,734; part-time $543 per credit hour. *Tuition, state resident:* full-time $28,983; part-time $999 per credit hour. *Tuition, nonresident:* full-time $28,983; part-time $999 per credit hour. *International tuition:* $28,983 full-time. *Room and board:* $8813 per academic year. *Required fees:* full-time $1215.
Financial Aid 86% of baccalaureate students in nursing programs received some form of financial aid in 2011–12.

Contact Office of Student Affairs, College of Nursing, Wayne State University, 5557 Cass Avenue, Detroit, MI 48202. *Telephone:* 313-577-4082. *Fax:* 313-577-6949.

GRADUATE PROGRAMS

Expenses (2012–13) *Tuition, state resident:* full-time $12,520; part-time $969 per credit hour. *Tuition, nonresident:* full-time $20,248; part-time $1613 per credit hour. *International tuition:* $20,248 full-time. *Room and board:* $8813 per academic year. *Required fees:* full-time $890.

Financial Aid 68% of graduate students in nursing programs received some form of financial aid in 2011–12. 2 fellowships with tuition reimbursements available (averaging $13,708 per year), 1 research assistantship with tuition reimbursement available (averaging $17,391 per year), 4 teaching assistantships with tuition reimbursements available (averaging $27,103 per year) were awarded; Federal Work-Study, institutionally sponsored loans, scholarships, traineeships, and unspecified assistantships also available. Aid available to part-time students.

Contact Office of Student Affairs, College of Nursing, Wayne State University, 5557 Cass Avenue, Detroit, MI 48202. *Telephone:* 313-577-4082. *Fax:* 313-577-6949.

MASTER'S DEGREE PROGRAM

Degree MSN

Available Programs Master's.

Concentrations Available Nurse-midwifery. *Clinical nurse specialist programs in:* acute care, community health, critical care, psychiatric/mental health. *Nurse practitioner programs in:* acute care, gerontology, neonatal health, pediatric, primary care, psychiatric/mental health, women's health.

Study Options Full-time and part-time.

Program Entrance Requirements Minimum overall college GPA of 3.0, transcript of college record, written essay, 3 letters of recommendation, resume. *Application deadline:* 7/1 (fall), 11/1 (winter), 4/1 (spring), 4/1 (summer).

Advanced Placement Credit given for nursing courses completed elsewhere dependent upon specific evaluations.

Degree Requirements 47 total credit hours.

POST-MASTER'S PROGRAM

Areas of Study Nurse-midwifery; nursing education. *Clinical nurse specialist programs in:* psychiatric/mental health. *Nurse practitioner programs in:* acute care, gerontology, pediatric, primary care, psychiatric/mental health, women's health.

DOCTORAL DEGREE PROGRAM

Degree DNP

Available Programs Doctorate; Post-Baccalaureate Doctorate.

Areas of Study Advanced practice nursing, clinical practice.

Program Entrance Requirements Clinical experience, minimum overall college GPA of 3.0, interview by faculty committee, interview, 2 letters of recommendation, vita, writing sample, GRE General Test (for PhD applicants; DNP applicants may choose the GRE exception but must submit a writing sample). *Application deadline:* 1/15 (fall). Applications may be processed on a rolling basis for some programs. *Application fee:* $50.

Degree Requirements 90 total credit hours, written exam, residency.

POSTDOCTORAL PROGRAM

Areas of Study Adolescent health, community health, individualized study, self-care.

Postdoctoral Program Contact Mr. Dennis Ross, Academic Services Officer, College of Nursing, Wayne State University, 5557 Cass Avenue, Detroit, MI 48202. *Telephone:* 313-577-4082. *Fax:* 313-577-6949. *E-mail:* nursinginfo@wayne.edu.

CONTINUING EDUCATION PROGRAM

Contact Office of the Dean, College of Nursing, Wayne State University, 5557 Cass Avenue, Detroit, MI 48202. *Telephone:* 313-577-4070. *E-mail:* nursinginfo@wayne.edu.

Western Michigan University
College of Health and Human Services
Kalamazoo, Michigan

Founded in 1903

DEGREES • BSN • MSN

Nursing Program Faculty 38 (26% with doctorates).
Baccalaureate Enrollment 383 **Women** 85% **Men** 15% **Minority** 11% **International** 1% **Part-time** 21%
Graduate Enrollment 7 **Women** 85% **Men** 15% **Minority** 15% **Part-time** 100%
Nursing Student Activities Sigma Theta Tau, Student Nurses' Association.
Nursing Student Resources Academic advising; academic or career counseling; assistance for students with disabilities; bookstore; campus computer network; career placement assistance; computer lab; computer-assisted instruction; daycare for children of students; e-mail services; employment services for current students; externships; housing assistance; interactive nursing skills videos; Internet; learning resource lab; library services; nursing audiovisuals; placement services for program completers; remedial services; resume preparation assistance; skills, simulation, or other laboratory.
Library Facilities 2.2 million volumes (766 in nursing); 52,673 periodical subscriptions (362 health-care related).

BACCALAUREATE PROGRAMS

Degree BSN

Available Programs ADN to Baccalaureate; Generic Baccalaureate.

Site Options St. Joseph, MI.

Study Options Full-time and part-time.

Program Entrance Requirements Minimum overall college GPA of 3.0, transcript of college record, CPR certification, high school biology, high school chemistry, 3 years high school math, 3 years high school science, high school transcript, immunizations, minimum high school GPA of 3.0, minimum GPA in nursing prerequisites of 3.0, prerequisite course work. Transfer students are accepted. *Application deadline:* Applications may be processed on a rolling basis for some programs. *Application fee:* $35.

Advanced Placement Credit given for nursing courses completed elsewhere dependent upon specific evaluations.

Financial Aid 43% of baccalaureate students in nursing programs received some form of financial aid in 2010–11.

Contact Mrs. Marsha Ann Mahan, Student Advisor, College of Health and Human Services, Western Michigan University, 1903 West Michigan Avenue, Kalamazoo, MI 49008. *Telephone:* 269-387-8150. *Fax:* 269-387-8170. *E-mail:* marsha.mahan@wmich.edu.

GRADUATE PROGRAMS

Financial Aid 100% of graduate students in nursing programs received some form of financial aid in 2010–11. 2 fellowships (averaging $4,056 per year), 8 research assistantships (averaging $9,839 per year), 14 teaching assistantships (averaging $4,802 per year) were awarded; Federal Work-Study also available. *Financial aid application deadline:* 2/15.

Contact Dr. Linda H. Zoeller, Director and Professor, College of Health and Human Services, Western Michigan University, 1903 West Michigan Avenue, Kalamazoo, MI 49008-5345. *Telephone:* 269-387-8162. *E-mail:* linda.zoeller@wmich.edu.

MASTER'S DEGREE PROGRAM

Degree MSN

Available Programs Master's.

Concentrations Available Nursing administration; nursing education.

Site Options St. Joseph, MI.

Study Options Part-time.

Program Entrance Requirements Minimum overall college GPA of 3.4, transcript of college record, interview, 3 letters of recommendation, resume. *Application deadline:* Applications may be processed on a rolling basis for some programs. *Application fee:* $40.

Degree Requirements 36 total credit hours, thesis or project, comprehensive exam.

CONTINUING EDUCATION PROGRAM

Contact Ms. Marsha Ann Mahan, Student Advisor, College of Health and Human Services, Western Michigan University, 1903 West Michigan

Avenue, Kalamazoo, MI 49008-5345. *Telephone:* 269-387-8150. *E-mail:* marsha.mahan@wmich.edu.

MINNESOTA

Augsburg College
Program in Nursing
Minneapolis, Minnesota

http://www.augsburg.edu/nursing
Founded in 1869
DEGREES • BS • MA
Nursing Program Faculty 9 (50% with doctorates).
Baccalaureate Enrollment 169 **Women** 83% **Men** 17% **Part-time** 89%
Graduate Enrollment 42 **Women** 100% **Minority** 2% **Part-time** 90%
Nursing Student Resources Academic advising; academic or career counseling; assistance for students with disabilities; bookstore; campus computer network; computer lab; computer-assisted instruction; e-mail services; Internet; library services; tutoring.
Library Facilities 146,433 volumes (1,550 in health, 200 in nursing); 754 periodical subscriptions (70 health-care related).

BACCALAUREATE PROGRAMS

Degree BS
Available Programs ADN to Baccalaureate.
Site Options Rochester, MN; Saint Paul, MN.
Study Options Full-time and part-time.
Program Entrance Requirements Minimum overall college GPA of 2.5, transcript of college record, CPR certification, written essay, high school transcript, immunizations, letters of recommendation, prerequisite course work, RN licensure. Transfer students are accepted.
Contact *Telephone:* 612-330-1101. *Fax:* 612-330-1784.

GRADUATE PROGRAMS

Contact *Telephone:* 612-330-1101. *Fax:* 612-330-1784.

MASTER'S DEGREE PROGRAM
Degree MA
Available Programs Master's.
Concentrations Available *Clinical nurse specialist programs in:* community health.
Site Options Rochester, MN; Saint Paul, MN.
Study Options Full-time and part-time.
Program Entrance Requirements Computer literacy, minimum overall college GPA of 3.0, transcript of college record, written essay, immunizations, 3 letters of recommendation, prerequisite course work, statistics course.
Advanced Placement Credit given for nursing courses completed elsewhere dependent upon specific evaluations.
Degree Requirements 48 total credit hours, thesis or project.

Bemidji State University
Department of Nursing
Bemidji, Minnesota

http://www.bemidjistate.edu/academics/departments/nursing/
Founded in 1919
DEGREE • BS
Nursing Program Faculty 5 (60% with doctorates).
Baccalaureate Enrollment 62 **Women** 95% **Men** 5% **Minority** 3% **Part-time** 68%
Distance Learning Courses Available.
Nursing Student Resources Academic advising; academic or career counseling; assistance for students with disabilities; bookstore; campus computer network; career placement assistance; computer lab; computer-assisted instruction; daycare for children of students; e-mail services; employment services for current students; housing assistance; Internet; library services; nursing audiovisuals; remedial services; tutoring.

Library Facilities 9,000 volumes in health, 1,000 volumes in nursing; 300 periodical subscriptions health-care related.

BACCALAUREATE PROGRAMS

Degree BS
Available Programs Generic Baccalaureate; RN Baccalaureate.
Study Options Full-time and part-time.
Program Entrance Requirements Minimum overall college GPA, transcript of college record, immunizations, professional liability insurance/malpractice insurance, RN licensure. Transfer students are accepted.
Contact *Telephone:* 218-755-3892. *Fax:* 218-755-4402.

CONTINUING EDUCATION PROGRAM

Contact *Telephone:* 218-755-3892. *Fax:* 218-755-4402.

Bethel University
Department of Nursing
St. Paul, Minnesota

http://cas.bethel.edu/dept/nursing/index-2
Founded in 1871
DEGREES • BSN • MA
Nursing Program Faculty 36 (40% with doctorates).
Baccalaureate Enrollment 283 **Women** 93.6% **Men** 6.4% **Minority** 11%
Graduate Enrollment 66 **Women** 97% **Men** 3% **Minority** 9.1%
Distance Learning Courses Available.
Nursing Student Activities Sigma Theta Tau, nursing club.
Nursing Student Resources Academic advising; academic or career counseling; assistance for students with disabilities; bookstore; campus computer network; career placement assistance; computer lab; computer-assisted instruction; daycare for children of students; e-mail services; employment services for current students; interactive nursing skills videos; Internet; learning resource lab; library services; nursing audiovisuals; paid internships; placement services for program completers; remedial services; resume preparation assistance; skills, simulation, or other laboratory; tutoring.
Library Facilities 205,073 volumes (4,900 in nursing); 40,664 periodical subscriptions (1,006 health-care related).

BACCALAUREATE PROGRAMS

Degree BSN
Available Programs Generic Baccalaureate; RN Baccalaureate.
Site Options Brooklyn Park, MN.
Study Options Full-time and part-time.
Program Entrance Requirements Minimum overall college GPA of 2.5, transcript of college record, CPR certification, written essay, health exam, health insurance, high school transcript, immunizations, interview, 2 letters of recommendation, minimum GPA in nursing prerequisites of 2.5, professional liability insurance/malpractice insurance, prerequisite course work. Transfer students are accepted. *Application deadline:* 9/15 (fall).
Advanced Placement Credit given for nursing courses completed elsewhere dependent upon specific evaluations.
Contact *Telephone:* 651-638-6455. *Fax:* 651-635-1965.

GRADUATE PROGRAMS

Contact *Telephone:* 651-635-8080. *Fax:* 651-635-1965.

MASTER'S DEGREE PROGRAM
Degree MA
Available Programs Master's.
Concentrations Available Nursing administration; nursing education.
Study Options Full-time and part-time.
Program Entrance Requirements Clinical experience, computer literacy, minimum overall college GPA of 3.0, transcript of college record, written essay, immunizations, interview, 3 letters of recommendation, professional liability insurance/malpractice insurance, resume, statistics course, MAT. *Application deadline:* Applications may be processed on a rolling basis for some programs. *Application fee:* $25.
Advanced Placement Credit given for nursing courses completed elsewhere dependent upon specific evaluations.
Degree Requirements 43 total credit hours, thesis or project.

Capella University
Nursing Programs
Minneapolis, Minnesota

Founded in 1993
DEGREES • BSN • DNP • MSN

BACCALAUREATE PROGRAMS

Degree BSN
Available Programs RN Baccalaureate.
Program Entrance Requirements RN licensure. *Application fee:* $50.
Contact Nursing Program, Nursing Programs, Capella University, 225 South 6th Street, 9th Floor, Minneapolis, MN 55402. *Telephone:* 866-283-7921. *Fax:* 612-337-5396.

GRADUATE PROGRAMS

Contact Nursing Program, Nursing Programs, Capella University, 225 South 6th Street, 9th Floor, Minneapolis, MN 55402. *Telephone:* 866-283-7921. *Fax:* 612-337-5396.

MASTER'S DEGREE PROGRAM

Degree MSN
Available Programs Accelerated RN to Master's; Master's.
Concentrations Available Nursing administration; nursing education. *Clinical nurse specialist programs in:* gerontology.
Program Entrance Requirements Minimum overall college GPA of 3.0. *Application fee:* $50.

DOCTORAL DEGREE PROGRAM

Degree DNP
Available Programs Doctorate.
Areas of Study Nursing administration.
Program Entrance Requirements Minimum overall college GPA of 3.0. *Application fee:* $50.

College of Saint Benedict
Department of Nursing
Saint Joseph, Minnesota

http://www.csbsju.edu/nursing/
Founded in 1887
DEGREE • BS
Nursing Program Faculty 17 (50% with doctorates).
Baccalaureate Enrollment 161 **Women** 90% **Men** 10% **Minority** 8% **International** 1% **Part-time** 1%
Nursing Student Activities Nursing Honor Society, Sigma Theta Tau, Student Nurses' Association, nursing club.
Nursing Student Resources Academic advising; academic or career counseling; assistance for students with disabilities; bookstore; campus computer network; career placement assistance; computer lab; computer-assisted instruction; e-mail services; employment services for current students; interactive nursing skills videos; Internet; learning resource lab; library services; nursing audiovisuals; paid internships; placement services for program completers; remedial services; resume preparation assistance; skills, simulation, or other laboratory; tutoring; unpaid internships.
Library Facilities 640,538 volumes (7,300 in health, 700 in nursing); 33,108 periodical subscriptions (335 health-care related).

BACCALAUREATE PROGRAMS

Degree BS
Available Programs Generic Baccalaureate.
Study Options Full-time.
Program Entrance Requirements Transcript of college record, CPR certification, health exam, immunizations, minimum GPA in nursing prerequisites of 2.75, professional liability insurance/malpractice insurance, prerequisite course work. Transfer students are accepted. *Application deadline:* 5/1 (fall).
Advanced Placement Credit given for nursing courses completed elsewhere dependent upon specific evaluations.
Expenses (2012–13) *Tuition:* full-time $35,298; part-time $1471 per credit. *International tuition:* $35,298 full-time. *Room and board:* $9272; room only: $4464 per academic year. *Required fees:* full-time $1300.

Financial Aid 96% of baccalaureate students in nursing programs received some form of financial aid in 2011–12. *Gift aid (need-based):* Federal Pell, FSEOG, state, private, college/university gift aid from institutional funds. *Loans:* Federal Direct (Subsidized and Unsubsidized Stafford PLUS), Perkins, state, private loans. *Work-study:* Federal Work-Study, part-time campus jobs. *Financial aid application deadline (priority):* 3/15.
Contact Dr. Carie Ann Braun, Associate Professor and Chair, Department of Nursing, College of Saint Benedict, 37 College Avenue South, St. Joseph, MN 56374. *Telephone:* 320-363-5223. *Fax:* 320-363-6099. *E-mail:* cbraun@csbsju.edu.

The College of St. Scholastica
Department of Nursing
Duluth, Minnesota

http://www.css.edu/nursing.xml
Founded in 1912
DEGREES • BS • DNP • MA
Nursing Program Faculty 36 (50% with doctorates).
Baccalaureate Enrollment 635 **Women** 87% **Men** 13% **Minority** 12% **International** 1% **Part-time** 25%
Graduate Enrollment 183 **Women** 93% **Men** 7% **Minority** 13% **International** 1% **Part-time** 74%
Distance Learning Courses Available.
Nursing Student Activities Sigma Theta Tau, Student Nurses' Association.
Nursing Student Resources Academic advising; academic or career counseling; assistance for students with disabilities; bookstore; campus computer network; career placement assistance; computer lab; computer-assisted instruction; e-mail services; Internet; learning resource lab; library services; nursing audiovisuals; paid internships; placement services for program completers; resume preparation assistance; skills, simulation, or other laboratory; tutoring; unpaid internships.
Library Facilities 118,042 volumes (7,280 in health, 1,150 in nursing); 55,088 periodical subscriptions (291 health-care related).

BACCALAUREATE PROGRAMS

Degree BS
Available Programs ADN to Baccalaureate; Accelerated Baccalaureate for Second Degree; Generic Baccalaureate.
Site Options St. Cloud, MN; Duluth, MN.
Study Options Full-time.
Online Degree Options Yes.
Program Entrance Requirements Minimum overall college GPA of 3.0, transcript of college record, CPR certification, health exam, health insurance, high school transcript, immunizations, minimum GPA in nursing prerequisites of 2.0, prerequisite course work. Transfer students are accepted. *Application deadline:* 9/20 (fall).
Expenses (2012–13) *Tuition:* full-time $30,208; part-time $943 per credit. *Room and board:* $8040; room only: $4088 per academic year. *Required fees:* full-time $320; part-time $160 per term.
Financial Aid 98% of baccalaureate students in nursing programs received some form of financial aid in 2011–12. *Gift aid (need-based):* Federal Pell, FSEOG, state, private, college/university gift aid from institutional funds. *Loans:* Federal Nursing Student Loans, Federal Direct (Subsidized and Unsubsidized Stafford PLUS), Perkins, state, private loans. *Work-study:* Federal Work-Study, part-time campus jobs. *Financial aid application deadline (priority):* 3/1.
Contact Ms. Paula Byrne, Chair, Department of Traditional Undergraduate Nursing, Department of Nursing, The College of St. Scholastica, 1200 Kenwood Avenue, Duluth, MN 55811. *Telephone:* 218-723-6020. *Fax:* 218-733-2221. *E-mail:* pbyrne@css.edu.

GRADUATE PROGRAMS

Expenses (2012–13) *Tuition:* part-time $740 per credit. *Room and board:* $8040; room only: $4088 per academic year. *Required fees:* part-time $100 per term.
Financial Aid 90% of graduate students in nursing programs received some form of financial aid in 2011–12. Scholarships and traineeships available. Aid available to part-time students.
Contact Dr. Sally Fauchald, Chair, Graduate Nursing Department, Department of Nursing, The College of St. Scholastica, 1200 Kenwood Avenue, Duluth, MN 55811. *Telephone:* 218-723-6590. *Fax:* 218-733-2221. *E-mail:* sfauchal@css.edu.

MASTER'S DEGREE PROGRAM
Degree MA
Available Programs Master's.
Concentrations Available *Clinical nurse specialist programs in:* adult health, gerontology. *Nurse practitioner programs in:* adult health, family health, gerontology, psychiatric/mental health.
Site Options St. Cloud, MN; Duluth, MN.
Study Options Full-time and part-time.
Program Entrance Requirements Clinical experience, computer literacy, minimum overall college GPA of 3.0, transcript of college record, CPR certification, written essay, immunizations, interview, 3 letters of recommendation, nursing research course, physical assessment course, professional liability insurance/malpractice insurance, resume, statistics course, GRE General Test. *Application deadline:* 3/1 (spring). *Application fee:* $50.
Advanced Placement Credit given for nursing courses completed elsewhere dependent upon specific evaluations.
Degree Requirements 47 total credit hours, thesis or project.

POST-MASTER'S PROGRAM
Areas of Study Nursing informatics. *Clinical nurse specialist programs in:* adult health, gerontology. *Nurse practitioner programs in:* adult health, family health, gerontology, psychiatric/mental health.

DOCTORAL DEGREE PROGRAM
Degree DNP
Available Programs Doctorate; Post-Baccalaureate Doctorate.
Areas of Study Advanced practice nursing, gerontology, health policy, nursing education, nursing policy.
Site Options St. Cloud, MN; Duluth, MN.
Program Entrance Requirements Clinical experience, minimum overall college GPA of 3.0, interview by faculty committee, 3 letters of recommendation, MSN or equivalent, vita, writing sample. *Application deadline:* 3/1 (spring). *Application fee:* $50.
Degree Requirements 30 total credit hours, dissertation.

POSTDOCTORAL PROGRAM
Postdoctoral Program Contact Dr. Carleen A. Maynard, Chair, Graduate Nursing Department, Department of Nursing, The College of St. Scholastica, 1200 Kenwood Avenue, Duluth, MN 55811. *Telephone:* 218-723-6452. *Fax:* 218-733-2295. *E-mail:* cmaynard@css.edu.

Concordia College
Department of Nursing
Moorhead, Minnesota

http://www.cord.edu/Academics/Nursing/index.php
Founded in 1891
DEGREES • BA • MS
Nursing Program Faculty 6 (33% with doctorates).
Baccalaureate Enrollment 75
Graduate Enrollment 2 **Women** 100%
Nursing Student Activities Sigma Theta Tau, Student Nurses' Association.
Nursing Student Resources Academic advising; academic or career counseling; assistance for students with disabilities; bookstore; campus computer network; career placement assistance; computer lab; computer-assisted instruction; e-mail services; employment services for current students; externships; housing assistance; interactive nursing skills videos; Internet; learning resource lab; library services; nursing audiovisuals; paid internships; placement services for program completers; remedial services; resume preparation assistance; skills, simulation, or other laboratory; tutoring; unpaid internships.
Library Facilities 337,352 volumes (2,135 in health, 837 in nursing); 3,907 periodical subscriptions (81 health-care related).

BACCALAUREATE PROGRAMS
Degree BA
Available Programs Accelerated Baccalaureate for Second Degree; Generic Baccalaureate.
Study Options Full-time.
Program Entrance Requirements Minimum overall college GPA of 2.9, transcript of college record, CPR certification, health exam, health insurance, immunizations, interview, 2 letters of recommendation, minimum GPA in nursing prerequisites of 2.7, professional liability insurance/malpractice insurance, prerequisite course work. Transfer students are accepted.
Advanced Placement Credit by examination available. Credit given for nursing courses completed elsewhere dependent upon specific evaluations.
Contact *Telephone:* 218-299-3879. *Fax:* 218-299-4309.

GRADUATE PROGRAMS
Contact *Telephone:* 218-299-3879. *Fax:* 218-299-4309.

MASTER'S DEGREE PROGRAM
Degree MS
Available Programs Master's.
Concentrations Available Nursing education.
Study Options Full-time and part-time.
Program Entrance Requirements Computer literacy, minimum overall college GPA of 3.0, transcript of college record, written essay, interview, 3 letters of recommendation.
Advanced Placement Credit given for nursing courses completed elsewhere dependent upon specific evaluations.
Degree Requirements 36 total credit hours, thesis or project, comprehensive exam.

Crown College
Nursing Department
St. Bonifacius, Minnesota

http://www.crown.edu/
Founded in 1916
DEGREE • BSN
Nursing Program Faculty 6
Baccalaureate Enrollment 20 **Women** 100% **International** 10%
Distance Learning Courses Available.
Nursing Student Activities Student Nurses' Association.
Nursing Student Resources Academic advising; academic or career counseling; assistance for students with disabilities; bookstore; campus computer network; computer lab; computer-assisted instruction; e-mail services; employment services for current students; housing assistance; interactive nursing skills videos; Internet; learning resource lab; library services; nursing audiovisuals; remedial services; resume preparation assistance; skills, simulation, or other laboratory; tutoring; unpaid internships.
Library Facilities 148,561 volumes; 29,308 periodical subscriptions.

BACCALAUREATE PROGRAMS
Degree BSN
Available Programs Generic Baccalaureate.
Site Options Owatonna, MN.
Study Options Full-time.
Program Entrance Requirements CPR certification, written essay, health exam, immunizations, 2 letters of recommendation, minimum high school GPA, minimum GPA in nursing prerequisites of 2.5, prerequisite course work. Transfer students are accepted. *Application deadline:* 2/1 (spring).
Contact *Telephone:* 952-446-4482.

Globe University–Woodbury
Bachelor of Science in Nursing
Woodbury, Minnesota

http://www.globeuniversity.edu/
Founded in 1885
DEGREE • BS
Nursing Program Faculty 16
Baccalaureate Enrollment 135
Nursing Student Activities Student Nurses' Association.
Nursing Student Resources Academic advising; academic or career counseling; assistance for students with disabilities; bookstore; campus computer network; career placement assistance; computer lab; computer-assisted instruction; e-mail services; employment services for current students; interactive nursing skills videos; Internet; learning resource lab; library services; nursing audiovisuals; placement services for program

completers; remedial services; resume preparation assistance; skills, simulation, or other laboratory; tutoring; unpaid internships.
Library Facilities 8,069 volumes; 63,753 periodical subscriptions.

BACCALAUREATE PROGRAMS

Degree BS
Available Programs Generic Baccalaureate.
Study Options Full-time and part-time.
Program Entrance Requirements Minimum overall college GPA of 2.75, transcript of college record, CPR certification, written essay, health exam, high school biology, high school chemistry, 2 years high school science, high school transcript, immunizations, interview, 2 letters of recommendation, minimum high school GPA of 2.75, minimum high school rank 60%, minimum GPA in nursing prerequisites of 2.75, prerequisite course work. Transfer students are accepted. *Application deadline:* Applications may be processed on a rolling basis for some programs. *Application fee:* $50.
Advanced Placement Credit given for nursing courses completed elsewhere dependent upon specific evaluations.
Contact *Telephone:* 612-798-3762.

Gustavus Adolphus College
Department of Nursing
St. Peter, Minnesota

http://www.gustavus.edu/
Founded in 1862
DEGREE • BA
Nursing Program Faculty 9 (20% with doctorates).
Baccalaureate Enrollment 76 **Women** 92% **Men** 8% **Minority** 8% **International** 4%
Nursing Student Activities Sigma Theta Tau, Student Nurses' Association.
Nursing Student Resources Academic advising; academic or career counseling; assistance for students with disabilities; bookstore; campus computer network; career placement assistance; computer lab; computer-assisted instruction; e-mail services; employment services for current students; housing assistance; interactive nursing skills videos; Internet; learning resource lab; library services; nursing audiovisuals; paid internships; remedial services; resume preparation assistance; skills, simulation, or other laboratory; tutoring; unpaid internships.
Library Facilities 357,186 volumes; 23,619 periodical subscriptions.

BACCALAUREATE PROGRAMS

Degree BA
Available Programs Generic Baccalaureate.
Study Options Full-time.
Program Entrance Requirements Minimum overall college GPA of 2.7, transcript of college record, written essay, high school transcript, immunizations, interview, minimum GPA in nursing prerequisites, prerequisite course work. Transfer students are accepted.
Contact *Telephone:* 507-933-6126. *Fax:* 507-933-6153.

Herzing University
Nursing Program
Minneapolis, Minnesota

Founded in 1961
DEGREE • BSN

BACCALAUREATE PROGRAMS

Degree BSN
Available Programs Generic Baccalaureate.
Contact Nursing Information, Nursing Program, Herzing University, 5700 West Broadway, Crystal, MN 55428. *Telephone:* 763-535-3000. *Fax:* 763-535-9205. *E-mail:* mpl-info@herzing.edu.

Metropolitan State University
College of Health, Community and Professional Studies
St. Paul, Minnesota

http://www.metrostate.edu/
Founded in 1971
DEGREES • BSN • MSN
Nursing Program Faculty 22 (18% with doctorates).
Baccalaureate Enrollment 230 **Women** 91% **Men** 9% **Minority** 9% **Part-time** 96%
Graduate Enrollment 40 **Women** 95% **Men** 5% **Minority** 8% **Part-time** 23%
Nursing Student Activities Sigma Theta Tau, Student Nurses' Association.
Nursing Student Resources Academic advising; academic or career counseling; assistance for students with disabilities; bookstore; campus computer network; computer lab; e-mail services; externships; Internet; library services; skills, simulation, or other laboratory.

BACCALAUREATE PROGRAMS

Degree BSN
Site Options Minneapolis, MN.
Study Options Full-time and part-time.
Program Entrance Requirements Minimum overall college GPA of 2.5, transcript of college record, health insurance, immunizations, minimum GPA in nursing prerequisites of 3.0, professional liability insurance/malpractice insurance, prerequisite course work. Transfer students are accepted.
Advanced Placement Credit given for nursing courses completed elsewhere dependent upon specific evaluations.
Contact *Telephone:* 651-793-1379. *Fax:* 651-793-1382.

GRADUATE PROGRAMS

Contact *Telephone:* 651-793-1378. *Fax:* 651-793-1382.

MASTER'S DEGREE PROGRAM
Degree MSN
Available Programs Master's for Nurses with Non-Nursing Degrees; RN to Master's.
Concentrations Available Nursing administration. *Nurse practitioner programs in:* adult health, family health.
Study Options Full-time and part-time.
Program Entrance Requirements Clinical experience, computer literacy, minimum overall college GPA of 3.0, transcript of college record, written essay, immunizations, interview, 3 letters of recommendation, professional liability insurance/malpractice insurance, resume, statistics course, GRE General Test.
Advanced Placement Credit given for nursing courses completed elsewhere dependent upon specific evaluations.
Degree Requirements 42 total credit hours, thesis or project.

POST-MASTER'S PROGRAM
Areas of Study *Nurse practitioner programs in:* adult health, family health.

Minnesota Intercollegiate Nursing Consortium
Minnesota Intercollegiate Nursing Consortium
Northfield, Minnesota

http://www.stolaf.edu/depts/nursing/
DEGREE • BA
Nursing Program Faculty 11 (45% with doctorates).
Baccalaureate Enrollment 95 **Women** 86% **Men** 14% **Minority** 11% **International** 1%
Nursing Student Activities Sigma Theta Tau, Student Nurses' Association.
Nursing Student Resources Academic advising; academic or career counseling; assistance for students with disabilities; bookstore; campus computer network; career placement assistance; computer lab; computer-assisted instruction; e-mail services; employment services for current students; externships; interactive nursing skills videos; Internet; learning

resource lab; library services; nursing audiovisuals; paid internships; remedial services; resume preparation assistance; skills, simulation, or other laboratory; tutoring; unpaid internships.

BACCALAUREATE PROGRAMS

Degree BA
Available Programs Generic Baccalaureate.
Site Options St. Peter, MN; Northfield, MN.
Study Options Full-time.
Program Entrance Requirements Minimum overall college GPA of 2.85, transcript of college record, CPR certification, written essay, health exam, health insurance, immunizations, interview, minimum GPA in nursing prerequisites of 2.7, prerequisite course work. Transfer students are accepted. *Application deadline:* 11/15 (fall).
Advanced Placement Credit given for nursing courses completed elsewhere dependent upon specific evaluations.
Expenses (2011–12) *Tuition:* full-time $36,625. *International tuition:* $36,625 full-time. *Room and board:* $8750; room only: $4855 per academic year. *Required fees:* full-time $1350; part-time $675 per term.
Contact Dr. Rita S. Glazebrook, Director, Minnesota Intercollegiate Nursing Consortium, 1520 St. Olaf Avenue, Northfield, MN 55057-1098. *Telephone:* 507-786-3265. *Fax:* 507-786-3733. *E-mail:* glazebro@stolaf.edu.

Minnesota State University Mankato

School of Nursing
Mankato, Minnesota

http://www.mnsu.edu/nursing/
Founded in 1868
DEGREES • BS • DNP • MSN • MSN/MS
Nursing Program Faculty 48 (21% with doctorates).
Baccalaureate Enrollment 292 **Women** 90% **Men** 10% **Minority** 9% **International** 1% **Part-time** 1%
Graduate Enrollment 60 **Women** 96% **Men** 4% **Part-time** 48%
Distance Learning Courses Available.
Nursing Student Activities Nursing Honor Society, Sigma Theta Tau, Student Nurses' Association.
Nursing Student Resources Academic advising; academic or career counseling; assistance for students with disabilities; bookstore; campus computer network; career placement assistance; computer lab; computer-assisted instruction; daycare for children of students; e-mail services; employment services for current students; Internet; learning resource lab; library services; nursing audiovisuals; paid internships; placement services for program completers; resume preparation assistance; skills, simulation, or other laboratory; tutoring.
Library Facilities 1.2 million volumes (35,852 in health, 1,500 in nursing); 20,000 periodical subscriptions (156 health-care related).

BACCALAUREATE PROGRAMS

Degree BS
Available Programs Accelerated Baccalaureate for Second Degree; Generic Baccalaureate; RN Baccalaureate.
Study Options Full-time and part-time.
Program Entrance Requirements Minimum overall college GPA of 2.5, transcript of college record, health exam, health insurance, minimum GPA in nursing prerequisites of 2.0, prerequisite course work. Transfer students are accepted.
Advanced Placement Credit by examination available. Credit given for nursing courses completed elsewhere dependent upon specific evaluations.
Contact *Telephone:* 507-389-6828. *Fax:* 507-389-6516.

GRADUATE PROGRAMS

Contact *Telephone:* 507-389-1317. *Fax:* 507-389-6516.

MASTER'S DEGREE PROGRAM

Degrees MSN; MSN/MS
Available Programs Accelerated RN to Master's; Master's; Master's for Nurses with Non-Nursing Degrees; RN to Master's.
Concentrations Available Nursing education. *Clinical nurse specialist programs in:* adult health, family health, pediatric. *Nurse practitioner programs in:* family health.
Study Options Full-time and part-time.

Program Entrance Requirements Clinical experience, computer literacy, minimum overall college GPA of 3.0, transcript of college record, CPR certification, written essay, immunizations, 3 letters of recommendation, nursing research course, professional liability insurance/malpractice insurance, prerequisite course work, resume, statistics course.
Advanced Placement Credit given for nursing courses completed elsewhere dependent upon specific evaluations.
Degree Requirements 53 total credit hours, thesis or project.

POST-MASTER'S PROGRAM

Areas of Study Nursing education. *Clinical nurse specialist programs in:* family health. *Nurse practitioner programs in:* family health.

DOCTORAL DEGREE PROGRAM

Degree DNP
Available Programs Doctorate.
Degree Requirements 36 total credit hours.

CONTINUING EDUCATION PROGRAM

Contact *Telephone:* 507-389-5194. *Fax:* 507-389-6516.

Minnesota State University Moorhead

School of Nursing and Healthcare Leadership
Moorhead, Minnesota

http://www.mnstate.edu/snhl/
Founded in 1885
DEGREES • BSN • MS
Nursing Program Faculty 11 (36% with doctorates).
Baccalaureate Enrollment 212 **Women** 95% **Men** 5% **Minority** 3% **Part-time** 12%
Graduate Enrollment 43 **Women** 97% **Men** 3% **Minority** 6% **Part-time** 90%
Distance Learning Courses Available.
Nursing Student Activities Sigma Theta Tau, Student Nurses' Association.
Nursing Student Resources Academic advising; academic or career counseling; assistance for students with disabilities; bookstore; campus computer network; career placement assistance; computer lab; computer-assisted instruction; daycare for children of students; e-mail services; employment services for current students; Internet; library services; nursing audiovisuals; placement services for program completers; remedial services; resume preparation assistance; tutoring; unpaid internships.
Library Facilities 5,560 volumes in health, 824 volumes in nursing; 50 periodical subscriptions health-care related.

BACCALAUREATE PROGRAMS

Degree BSN
Available Programs ADN to Baccalaureate; RN Baccalaureate.
Online Degree Options Yes (online only).
Program Entrance Requirements CPR certification, written essay, high school transcript, immunizations, 2 letters of recommendation, RN licensure. Transfer students are accepted. *Application deadline:* 3/15 (fall), 10/1 (spring).
Expenses (2011–12) *Tuition, state resident:* part-time $300 per credit. *Tuition, nonresident:* part-time $300 per credit.
Financial Aid 60% of baccalaureate students in nursing programs received some form of financial aid in 2010–11. *Gift aid (need-based):* Federal Pell, FSEOG, state, private, college/university gift aid from institutional funds. *Loans:* Federal Direct (Subsidized and Unsubsidized Stafford PLUS), Perkins, state, alternative loans.*Work-study:* Federal Work-Study, part-time campus jobs.*Financial aid application deadline (priority):* 2/15.
Contact Dr. Barbara Matthees, Professor, School of Nursing and Healthcare Leadership, Minnesota State University Moorhead, 1104 7th Avenue South, Moorhead, MN 56563. *Telephone:* 218-477-2695. *Fax:* 218-477-5990. *E-mail:* matthees@mnstate.edu.

GRADUATE PROGRAMS

Expenses (2011–12) *Tuition, state resident:* part-time $400 per credit. *Tuition, nonresident:* part-time $400 per credit.
Financial Aid 66% of graduate students in nursing programs received some form of financial aid in 2010–11.

Contact Dr. Barbara Matthees, Professor, School of Nursing and Healthcare Leadership, Minnesota State University Moorhead, 1104 7th Avenue South, Moorhead, MN 56563. *Telephone:* 218-477-2695. *Fax:* 218-477-5990. *E-mail:* matthees@mnstate.edu.

MASTER'S DEGREE PROGRAM

Degree MS

Available Programs Master's.

Concentrations Available Nursing education. *Clinical nurse specialist programs in:* adult health, gerontology.

Study Options Full-time and part-time.

Online Degree Options Yes (online only).

Program Entrance Requirements Computer literacy, minimum overall college GPA of 3.0, transcript of college record, written essay, interview, 3 letters of recommendation, resume, statistics course. *Application deadline:* Applications may be processed on a rolling basis for some programs.

Advanced Placement Credit given for nursing courses completed elsewhere dependent upon specific evaluations.

Degree Requirements 45 total credit hours, thesis or project.

St. Catherine University
Department of Nursing
St. Paul, Minnesota

http://www.stkate.edu/schools/soh/
Founded in 1905
DEGREES • BS • DNP • MA
Nursing Program Faculty 61 (39% with doctorates).

Baccalaureate Enrollment 308 **Women** 97% **Men** 3% **Minority** 30.5% **International** .6% **Part-time** 35%

Graduate Enrollment 121 **Women** 98% **Men** 2% **Minority** 17% **International** .8% **Part-time** 20%

Distance Learning Courses Available.

Nursing Student Activities Nursing Honor Society, Sigma Theta Tau, Student Nurses' Association.

Nursing Student Resources Academic advising; academic or career counseling; assistance for students with disabilities; bookstore; campus computer network; career placement assistance; computer lab; computer-assisted instruction; daycare for children of students; e-mail services; employment services for current students; housing assistance; interactive nursing skills videos; Internet; learning resource lab; library services; nursing audiovisuals; paid internships; remedial services; resume preparation assistance; skills, simulation, or other laboratory; tutoring; unpaid internships.

Library Facilities 71,500 volumes in health, 18,200 volumes in nursing; 4,600 periodical subscriptions health-care related.

BACCALAUREATE PROGRAMS

Degree BS

Available Programs Baccalaureate for Second Degree; Generic Baccalaureate; RN Baccalaureate.

Study Options Full-time.

Program Entrance Requirements Minimum overall college GPA of 2.75, transcript of college record, CPR certification, written essay, health insurance, immunizations, 2 letters of recommendation, minimum GPA in nursing prerequisites of 2.75, prerequisite course work. Transfer students are accepted. *Application deadline:* 10/1 (fall).

Expenses (2012–13) *Tuition:* part-time $1028 per credit. *Room and board:* $4001; room only: $2245 per academic year.

Financial Aid 83% of baccalaureate students in nursing programs received some form of financial aid in 2011–12. *Gift aid (need-based):* Federal Pell, FSEOG, state, private, college/university gift aid from institutional funds. *Loans:* Federal Nursing Student Loans, Federal Direct (Subsidized and Unsubsidized Stafford PLUS), Perkins, state, alternative loans.*Work-study:* Federal Work-Study, part-time campus jobs.*Financial aid application deadline (priority):* 4/15.

Contact Dr. Vicki Schug, Baccalaureate Program Director, Department of Nursing, St. Catherine University, 2004 Randolph Avenue, St. Paul, MN 55105. *Telephone:* 651-690-6940. *Fax:* 651-690-6941. *E-mail:* vlschug@stkate.edu.

GRADUATE PROGRAMS

Expenses (2012–13) *Tuition:* part-time $834 per credit. *International tuition:* $834 full-time. *Room and board:* $4001; room only: $2245 per academic year. *Required fees:* part-time $30 per term.

Financial Aid 52% of graduate students in nursing programs received some form of financial aid in 2011–12.

Contact Kathleen Smith, Graduate Programs Director, Department of Nursing, St. Catherine University, 2004 Randolph Avenue, #4250, St. Paul, MN 55105. *Telephone:* 651-690-6580. *Fax:* 651-690-6941. *E-mail:* ksmith@stkate.edu.

MASTER'S DEGREE PROGRAM

Degree MA

Available Programs Master's.

Concentrations Available Nursing education. *Nurse practitioner programs in:* adult health, gerontology, neonatal health, pediatric.

Study Options Full-time and part-time.

Program Entrance Requirements Clinical experience, minimum overall college GPA of 3.0, transcript of college record, CPR certification, written essay, immunizations, interview, 3 letters of recommendation, professional liability insurance/malpractice insurance, resume, statistics course. *Application deadline:* 1/15 (winter).

Advanced Placement Credit given for nursing courses completed elsewhere dependent upon specific evaluations.

Degree Requirements 38 total credit hours, thesis or project.

POST-MASTER'S PROGRAM

Areas of Study Nursing education. *Nurse practitioner programs in:* adult health, gerontology, neonatal health, pediatric.

DOCTORAL DEGREE PROGRAM

Degree DNP

Available Programs Doctorate.

Areas of Study Advanced practice nursing, health policy, health-care systems.

Program Entrance Requirements Minimum overall college GPA of 3.0, interview by faculty committee, interview, 3 letters of recommendation, MSN or equivalent, statistics course, vita, writing sample. *Application deadline:* 1/15 (winter).

Degree Requirements 33 total credit hours, dissertation.

St. Cloud State University
Department of Nursing Science
St. Cloud, Minnesota

Founded in 1869
DEGREE • BS
Nursing Program Faculty 12 (25% with doctorates).

Baccalaureate Enrollment 111

Nursing Student Activities Nursing club.

Nursing Student Resources Academic advising; academic or career counseling; assistance for students with disabilities; bookstore; campus computer network; career placement assistance; computer lab; computer-assisted instruction; daycare for children of students; e-mail services; interactive nursing skills videos; Internet; learning resource lab; library services; nursing audiovisuals; remedial services; resume preparation assistance; skills, simulation, or other laboratory; tutoring; unpaid internships.

Library Facilities 947,787 volumes (18,000 in health, 750 in nursing); 955 periodical subscriptions (100 health-care related).

BACCALAUREATE PROGRAMS

Degree BS

Available Programs Generic Baccalaureate.

Study Options Full-time.

Program Entrance Requirements Minimum overall college GPA of 2.75, transcript of college record, CPR certification, health exam, immunizations, 2 letters of recommendation, minimum GPA in nursing prerequisites of 2.75, prerequisite course work.

Contact *Telephone:* 320-308-1749.

Saint Mary's University of Minnesota

B.S. in Nursing
Winona, Minnesota

Founded in 1912

DEGREE • BS

Library Facilities 241,470 volumes; 39,650 periodical subscriptions.

BACCALAUREATE PROGRAMS

Degree BS

Available Programs RN Baccalaureate.

Program Entrance Requirements Transcript of college record, written essay, interview, letters of recommendation, RN licensure. *Application fee:* $25.

Contact Admissions Office, B.S. in Nursing, Saint Mary's University of Minnesota, 2500 Park Avenue, Minneapolis, MN 55404. *Telephone:* 612-728-5100. *E-mail:* tc-admission@smumn.edu.

St. Olaf College

Department of Nursing
Northfield, Minnesota

http://www.stolaf.edu/depts/nursing/
Founded in 1874

DEGREE • BA

Nursing Program Faculty 5 (40% with doctorates).
Baccalaureate Enrollment 46 **Women** 80% **Men** 20% **Minority** 13% **International** 4%
Nursing Student Activities Sigma Theta Tau, Student Nurses' Association.
Nursing Student Resources Academic advising; academic or career counseling; assistance for students with disabilities; bookstore; campus computer network; career placement assistance; computer lab; computer-assisted instruction; e-mail services; employment services for current students; externships; interactive nursing skills videos; Internet; learning resource lab; library services; nursing audiovisuals; paid internships; placement services for program completers; remedial services; resume preparation assistance; skills, simulation, or other laboratory; tutoring; unpaid internships.
Library Facilities 759,931 volumes; 33,632 periodical subscriptions.

BACCALAUREATE PROGRAMS

Degree BA

Available Programs Generic Baccalaureate.
Site Options St. Peter, MN.
Study Options Full-time.
Program Entrance Requirements Minimum overall college GPA of 2.85, transcript of college record, CPR certification, written essay, health exam, health insurance, immunizations, interview, minimum GPA in nursing prerequisites of 2.7, prerequisite course work. Transfer students are accepted. *Application deadline:* 11/15 (fall).
Advanced Placement Credit given for nursing courses completed elsewhere dependent upon specific evaluations.
Expenses (2012–13) *Tuition:* full-time $48,650. *Room and board:* $9090; room only: $4260 per academic year. *Required fees:* full-time $1475.
Financial Aid 43% of baccalaureate students in nursing programs received some form of financial aid in 2011–12. *Gift aid (need-based):* Federal Pell, FSEOG, state, private, college/university gift aid from institutional funds. *Loans:* Federal Nursing Student Loans, Federal Direct (Subsidized and Unsubsidized Stafford PLUS), Perkins, state, college/university. *Work-study:* Federal Work-Study, part-time campus jobs. *Financial aid application deadline:* 3/1(priority: 2/1).
Contact Dr. Diana Odland Neal, Chair, Department of Nursing, St. Olaf College, 1520 St. Olaf Avenue, Northfield, MN 55057-1098. *Telephone:* 507-786-3349. *Fax:* 507-786-3733. *E-mail:* neal@stolaf.edu.

University of Minnesota, Twin Cities Campus

School of Nursing
Minneapolis, Minnesota

http://www.nursing.umn.edu/
Founded in 1851

DEGREES • BSN • DNP • PHD

Nursing Program Faculty 85 (90% with doctorates).
Baccalaureate Enrollment 392 **Women** 87% **Men** 13% **Minority** 20% **Part-time** 8%
Graduate Enrollment 512 **Women** 88% **Men** 12% **Minority** 13% **International** 5% **Part-time** 44%
Distance Learning Courses Available.
Nursing Student Activities Nursing Honor Society, Sigma Theta Tau, Student Nurses' Association, nursing club.
Nursing Student Resources Academic advising; academic or career counseling; assistance for students with disabilities; bookstore; campus computer network; computer lab; computer-assisted instruction; daycare for children of students; e-mail services; employment services for current students; housing assistance; Internet; learning resource lab; library services; skills, simulation, or other laboratory.
Library Facilities 5.7 million volumes (4,000 in health, 1,500 in nursing); 45,000 periodical subscriptions (4,800 health-care related).

BACCALAUREATE PROGRAMS

Degree BSN

Available Programs Generic Baccalaureate.
Site Options Rochester, MN.
Study Options Full-time.
Program Entrance Requirements Minimum overall college GPA of 2.8, transcript of college record, CPR certification, written essay, health exam, health insurance, immunizations, minimum GPA in nursing prerequisites of 2.8, prerequisite course work. Transfer students are accepted. *Application deadline:* 2/1 (fall). *Application fee:* $60.
Expenses (2012–13) *Tuition, state resident:* full-time $12,100; part-time $6030 per semester. *Tuition, nonresident:* full-time $17,300; part-time $8655 per semester. *International tuition:* $17,300 full-time. *Room and board:* $12,000; room only: $9000 per academic year. *Required fees:* full-time $1456.
Financial Aid 73% of baccalaureate students in nursing programs received some form of financial aid in 2011–12.
Contact Office of Student Services, School of Nursing, University of Minnesota, Twin Cities Campus, 5-160 Weaver-Densford Hall, 308 Harvard Street SE, Minneapolis, MN 55455-0213. *Telephone:* 612-625-7980. *Fax:* 612-625-7727. *E-mail:* sonstudentinfo@umn.edu.

GRADUATE PROGRAMS

Expenses (2012–13) *Tuition, state resident:* full-time $22,000; part-time $11,000 per semester. *Tuition, nonresident:* full-time $22,000; part-time $11,000 per semester. *International tuition:* $22,000 full-time. *Room and board:* $12,000; room only: $9000 per academic year. *Required fees:* full-time $6550; part-time $3070 per term.
Financial Aid Fellowships, research assistantships, teaching assistantships, career-related internships or fieldwork and traineeships available.
Contact Office of Student Services, School of Nursing, University of Minnesota, Twin Cities Campus, 5-160 Weaver-Densford Hall, 308 Harvard Street SE, Minneapolis, MN 55455-0213. *Telephone:* 612-625-7980. *Fax:* 612-625-7727. *E-mail:* sonstudentinfo@umn.edu.

DOCTORAL DEGREE PROGRAM

Degree DNP

Available Programs Doctorate, Doctorate for Nurses with Non-Nursing Degrees, Post-Baccalaureate Doctorate.
Areas of Study Advanced practice nursing, community health, gerontology, information systems, maternity-newborn, women's health.
Program Entrance Requirements Minimum overall college GPA of 3.0, interview, interview by faculty committee, 2 letters of recommendation, writing sample, vita. *Application deadline:* 3/1 (fall). Applications may be processed on a rolling basis for some programs. *Application fee:* $60.
Degree Requirements 30-60 total credit hours, project and thesis presentation.

DOCTORAL DEGREE PROGRAM

Degree PhD
Available Programs Doctorate; Doctorate for Nurses with Non-Nursing Degrees; Post-Baccalaureate Doctorate.
Program Entrance Requirements Minimum overall college GPA of 3.0, interview by faculty committee, interview, 2 letters of recommendation, vita, writing sample, GRE General Test. *Application deadline:* 3/1 (fall). Applications may be processed on a rolling basis for some programs. *Application fee:* $60.
Degree Requirements 60 total credit hours, dissertation, oral exam, written exam.

CONTINUING EDUCATION PROGRAM

Contact Office of Student Services, School of Nursing, University of Minnesota, Twin Cities Campus, 5-160 Weaver-Densford Hall, 308 Harvard Street SE, Minneapolis, MN 55455-0213. *Telephone:* 612-625-7980. *Fax:* 612-625-7727. *E-mail:* sonstudentinfo@umn.edu.

Walden University
Nursing Programs
Minneapolis, Minnesota

http://www.waldenu.edu/Colleges-and-Schools/College-of-Health-Sciences/School-of-Nursing.htm
Founded in 1970
DEGREES • BSN • DNP • MSN
Nursing Program Faculty 213 (100% with doctorates).
Baccalaureate Enrollment 1,048 **Women** 93% **Men** 7% **Minority** 27% **International** 2% **Part-time** 81%
Graduate Enrollment 6,501 **Women** 92% **Men** 8% **Minority** 35% **International** 2% **Part-time** 23%
Distance Learning Courses Available.
Nursing Student Activities Nursing Honor Society.
Nursing Student Resources Academic advising; academic or career counseling; assistance for students with disabilities; bookstore; campus computer network; career placement assistance; e-mail services; library services; nursing audiovisuals; placement services for program completers; remedial services; resume preparation assistance; tutoring.
Library Facilities 196,355 volumes; 29 periodical subscriptions (6,689 health-care related).

BACCALAUREATE PROGRAMS

Degree BSN
Available Programs RN Baccalaureate.
Study Options Full-time and part-time.
Online Degree Options Yes (online only).
Program Entrance Requirements Transcript of college record, high school transcript, prerequisite course work, RN licensure. Transfer students are accepted. *Application deadline:* Applications may be processed on a rolling basis for some programs. *Application fee:* $50.
Expenses (2012–13) *Tuition:* full-time $10,440; part-time $290 per credit. *International tuition:* $10,440 full-time. *Required fees:* full-time $285; part-time $95 per term.
Contact Dr. Karen Ouzts, Program Director, Nursing Programs, Walden University, 100 Washington Avenue South, Suite 900, Minneapolis, MN 55401. *Telephone:* 720-383-1356. *E-mail:* karen.ouzts@waldenu.edu.

GRADUATE PROGRAMS

Expenses (2012–13) *Tuition:* part-time $395 per credit.
Contact Dr. Vincent Hall, Program Director, Nursing Programs, Walden University, 100 Washington Avenue South, Suite 900, Minneapolis, MN 55401. *E-mail:* vincent.hall@waldenu.edu.

MASTER'S DEGREE PROGRAM

Degree MSN
Available Programs Master's; RN to Master's.
Concentrations Available Nursing administration; nursing education; nursing informatics. *Nurse practitioner programs in:* family health, gerontology.
Study Options Full-time and part-time.
Online Degree Options Yes (online only).
Program Entrance Requirements Minimum overall college GPA of 2.5, transcript of college record. *Application deadline:* Applications may be processed on a rolling basis for some programs. *Application fee:* $50.
Degree Requirements 56 total credit hours, thesis or project.

POST-MASTER'S PROGRAM

Areas of Study Nursing administration; nursing education; nursing informatics.

DOCTORAL DEGREE PROGRAM

Degree DNP
Available Programs Doctorate.
Online Degree Options Yes (online only).
Program Entrance Requirements Minimum overall college GPA of 3.0, MSN or equivalent. *Application deadline:* Applications may be processed on a rolling basis for some programs. *Application fee:* $50.
Degree Requirements 53 total credit hours.

Winona State University
College of Nursing and Health Sciences
Winona, Minnesota

http://www.winona.edu/nursing/
Founded in 1858
DEGREES • BS • DNP • MS
Nursing Program Faculty 39 (46% with doctorates).
Baccalaureate Enrollment 400 **Women** 94% **Men** 6% **Minority** 3% **International** 2% **Part-time** 13%
Graduate Enrollment 110 **Women** 89% **Men** 11% **Minority** 5% **International** 1% **Part-time** 65%
Distance Learning Courses Available.
Nursing Student Activities Sigma Theta Tau, Student Nurses' Association, nursing club.
Nursing Student Resources Academic advising; academic or career counseling; assistance for students with disabilities; bookstore; campus computer network; career placement assistance; computer lab; computer-assisted instruction; daycare for children of students; e-mail services; employment services for current students; externships; housing assistance; Internet; learning resource lab; library services; nursing audiovisuals; paid internships; placement services for program completers; remedial services; resume preparation assistance; skills, simulation, or other laboratory; tutoring.
Library Facilities 320,353 volumes (6,132 in health, 3,920 in nursing); 36,660 periodical subscriptions (413 health-care related).

BACCALAUREATE PROGRAMS

Degree BS
Available Programs Generic Baccalaureate; RN Baccalaureate.
Site Options Rochester, MN.
Study Options Full-time and part-time.
Program Entrance Requirements Minimum overall college GPA of 3.0, transcript of college record, CPR certification, health exam, health insurance, immunizations, minimum GPA in nursing prerequisites of 3.3, professional liability insurance/malpractice insurance, prerequisite course work. Transfer students are accepted. *Application deadline:* 11/1 (fall), 1/31 (spring).
Contact *Telephone:* 507-457-5120. *Fax:* 507-457-5550.

GRADUATE PROGRAMS

Contact *Telephone:* 507-285-7135. *Fax:* 507-292-5127.

MASTER'S DEGREE PROGRAM

Degree MS
Available Programs Master's; Master's for Nurses with Non-Nursing Degrees; RN to Master's.
Concentrations Available Nursing administration; nursing education. *Clinical nurse specialist programs in:* adult health. *Nurse practitioner programs in:* adult health, family health.
Site Options Rochester, MN.
Study Options Full-time and part-time.
Program Entrance Requirements Clinical experience, computer literacy, minimum overall college GPA of 3.0, transcript of college record, CPR certification, written essay, immunizations, interview, 3 letters of recommendation, nursing research course, physical assessment course, professional liability insurance/malpractice insurance, statistics course, GRE (if GPA less than 3.0). *Application deadline:* 12/1 (fall). *Application fee:* $20.
Advanced Placement Credit given for nursing courses completed elsewhere dependent upon specific evaluations.
Degree Requirements 43 total credit hours, thesis or project.

POST-MASTER'S PROGRAM

Areas of Study Nursing administration; nursing education. *Clinical nurse specialist programs in:* adult health. *Nurse practitioner programs in:* adult health, family health.

DOCTORAL DEGREE PROGRAM

Degree DNP
Available Programs Doctorate.
Areas of Study Advanced practice nursing, faculty preparation, nursing administration.
Site Options Rochester, MN.
Online Degree Options Yes (online only).
Program Entrance Requirements Clinical experience, minimum overall college GPA of 3.0, 2 letters of recommendation, MSN or equivalent, statistics course, vita, writing sample. *Application deadline:* 3/15 (spring). *Application fee:* $20.
Degree Requirements 36 total credit hours, oral exam.

MISSISSIPPI

Alcorn State University
School of Nursing
Natchez, Mississippi

http://www.alcorn.edu/nursing/
Founded in 1871
DEGREES • BSN • MSN
Nursing Program Faculty 21 (29% with doctorates).
Baccalaureate Enrollment 63 **Women** 88.8% **Men** 11.2% **Minority** 42.8% **Part-time** 7.9%
Graduate Enrollment 53 **Women** 89.3% **Men** 10.7% **Minority** 35.7% **Part-time** 78.6%
Distance Learning Courses Available.
Nursing Student Activities Nursing Honor Society, Sigma Theta Tau, Student Nurses' Association.
Nursing Student Resources Academic advising; campus computer network; computer lab; housing assistance; learning resource lab; library services; nursing audiovisuals; paid internships; skills, simulation, or other laboratory.
Library Facilities 366,116 volumes (2,082 in health, 1,385 in nursing); 63,478 periodical subscriptions (30 health-care related).

BACCALAUREATE PROGRAMS

Degree BSN
Available Programs Generic Baccalaureate; LPN to RN Baccalaureate; RN Baccalaureate.
Study Options Full-time.
Online Degree Options Yes.
Program Entrance Requirements Minimum overall college GPA of 2.5, transcript of college record, health exam, immunizations, minimum high school GPA of 2.5, professional liability insurance/malpractice insurance, prerequisite course work. Transfer students are accepted. *Application deadline:* 12/19 (fall).
Contact *Telephone:* 601-304-4305. *Fax:* 601-304-4398.

GRADUATE PROGRAMS

Contact *Telephone:* 601-304-4303. *Fax:* 601-304-4398.

MASTER'S DEGREE PROGRAM

Degree MSN
Available Programs Master's.
Concentrations Available Nursing education. *Nurse practitioner programs in:* family health.
Study Options Full-time and part-time.
Online Degree Options Yes.
Program Entrance Requirements Computer literacy, minimum overall college GPA of 3.0, transcript of college record, written essay, 2 letters of recommendation, statistics course. *Application deadline:* 7/15 (fall). *Application fee:* $10.
Advanced Placement Credit given for nursing courses completed elsewhere dependent upon specific evaluations.
Degree Requirements 43 total credit hours, thesis or project.

POST-MASTER'S PROGRAM

Areas of Study Nursing education. *Nurse practitioner programs in:* family health.

Delta State University
School of Nursing
Cleveland, Mississippi

http://nursing.deltastate.edu/
Founded in 1924
DEGREES • BSN • MSN
Nursing Program Faculty 18 (50% with doctorates).
Baccalaureate Enrollment 99 **Women** 89% **Men** 11% **Minority** 25% **Part-time** 14%
Graduate Enrollment 50 **Women** 86% **Men** 14% **Minority** 22% **Part-time** 44%
Distance Learning Courses Available.
Nursing Student Activities Sigma Theta Tau, Student Nurses' Association.
Nursing Student Resources Academic advising; academic or career counseling; assistance for students with disabilities; bookstore; campus computer network; career placement assistance; computer lab; computer-assisted instruction; daycare for children of students; e-mail services; externships; housing assistance; interactive nursing skills videos; Internet; learning resource lab; library services; nursing audiovisuals; other; remedial services; resume preparation assistance; skills, simulation, or other laboratory; tutoring.
Library Facilities 440,565 volumes (5,000 in health, 1,000 in nursing); 25,270 periodical subscriptions (120 health-care related).

BACCALAUREATE PROGRAMS

Degree BSN
Available Programs ADN to Baccalaureate; Generic Baccalaureate.
Site Options Greenville, MS; Clarksdale, MS.
Study Options Full-time and part-time.
Program Entrance Requirements Transcript of college record, CPR certification, health exam, health insurance, immunizations, 3 letters of recommendation, minimum GPA in nursing prerequisites of 2.5, professional liability insurance/malpractice insurance, prerequisite course work. Transfer students are accepted. *Application deadline:* 3/1 (fall), 2/1 (summer).
Advanced Placement Credit given for nursing courses completed elsewhere dependent upon specific evaluations.
Expenses (2012–13) *Tuition, state resident:* full-time $5724; part-time $239 per credit hour. *Tuition, nonresident:* full-time $14,820; part-time $618 per credit hour. *International tuition:* $14,820 full-time. *Room and board:* $6568; room only: $3976 per academic year. *Required fees:* full-time $1356; part-time $57 per credit; part-time $678 per term.
Financial Aid 95% of baccalaureate students in nursing programs received some form of financial aid in 2011–12.
Contact Dr. Vicki L. Bingham, Chair of Academic Programs, School of Nursing, Delta State University, PO Box 3343, Cleveland, MS 38733. *Telephone:* 662-846-4255. *Fax:* 662-846-4267. *E-mail:* vbingham@deltastate.edu.

GRADUATE PROGRAMS

Expenses (2012–13) *Tuition, state resident:* full-time $5724; part-time $318 per credit hour. *Tuition, nonresident:* full-time $14,820; part-time $823 per credit hour. *International tuition:* $14,820 full-time. *Room and board:* $6568; room only: $3976 per academic year. *Required fees:* full-time $543; part-time $25 per credit; part-time $271 per term.
Financial Aid 70% of graduate students in nursing programs received some form of financial aid in 2011–12. Research assistantships, career-related internships or fieldwork, Federal Work-Study, and institutionally sponsored loans available. *Financial aid application deadline:* 6/1.
Contact Dr. Vicki L. Bingham, Chair of Academic Programs, School of Nursing, Delta State University, PO Box 3343, Cleveland, MS 38733. *Telephone:* 662-846-4255. *Fax:* 662-846-4267. *E-mail:* vbingham@deltastate.edu.

MASTER'S DEGREE PROGRAM

Degree MSN
Available Programs Master's; Master's for Nurses with Non-Nursing Degrees.

Concentrations Available Nursing administration; nursing education. *Nurse practitioner programs in:* family health, gerontology, psychiatric/mental health.

Study Options Full-time and part-time.

Online Degree Options Yes (online only).

Program Entrance Requirements Clinical experience, computer literacy, minimum overall college GPA of 3.0, transcript of college record, CPR certification, written essay, immunizations, interview, 3 letters of recommendation, nursing research course, physical assessment course, professional liability insurance/malpractice insurance, prerequisite course work, resume, statistics course, GRE General Test. *Application deadline:* 4/1 (fall).

Advanced Placement Credit given for nursing courses completed elsewhere dependent upon specific evaluations.

Degree Requirements 44 total credit hours, thesis or project, comprehensive exam.

POST-MASTER'S PROGRAM

Areas of Study Nursing administration; nursing education. *Nurse practitioner programs in:* family health, gerontology, psychiatric/mental health.

Mississippi College
School of Nursing
Clinton, Mississippi

http://www.mc.edu/
Founded in 1826
DEGREE • BSN
Nursing Program Faculty 20 (30% with doctorates).
Baccalaureate Enrollment 143 **Women** 85% **Men** 15% **Minority** 38% **International** 3% **Part-time** 9%
Distance Learning Courses Available.
Nursing Student Activities Sigma Theta Tau, Student Nurses' Association, nursing club.
Nursing Student Resources Academic advising; academic or career counseling; assistance for students with disabilities; bookstore; campus computer network; career placement assistance; computer lab; computer-assisted instruction; e-mail services; employment services for current students; externships; housing assistance; interactive nursing skills videos; Internet; learning resource lab; library services; nursing audiovisuals; paid internships; placement services for program completers; remedial services; resume preparation assistance; skills, simulation, or other laboratory; tutoring; unpaid internships.
Library Facilities 430,447 volumes (42,000 in health, 8,000 in nursing); 38,267 periodical subscriptions (290 health-care related).

BACCALAUREATE PROGRAMS

Degree BSN
Available Programs Generic Baccalaureate; RN Baccalaureate.
Study Options Full-time and part-time.
Program Entrance Requirements Minimum overall college GPA of 2.5, transcript of college record, CPR certification, health exam, high school biology, high school chemistry, high school transcript, immunizations, 2 letters of recommendation, minimum GPA in nursing prerequisites of 2.5, professional liability insurance/malpractice insurance, prerequisite course work. Transfer students are accepted. *Application deadline:* 2/1 (fall), 9/1 (spring), 4/1 (summer).
Advanced Placement Credit given for nursing courses completed elsewhere dependent upon specific evaluations.
Expenses (2012–13) *Tuition:* full-time $13,720; part-time $430 per credit hour. *International tuition:* $13,720 full-time. *Room and board:* $7800 per academic year. *Required fees:* full-time $1000; part-time $400 per term.
Financial Aid 93% of baccalaureate students in nursing programs received some form of financial aid in 2011–12.
Contact Dr. Mary Jean Padgett, Dean, School of Nursing, Mississippi College, Box 4037, 200 South Capitol Street, Clinton, MS 39058. *Telephone:* 601-925-3278. *Fax:* 601-925-3379. *E-mail:* padgett@mc.edu.

Mississippi University for Women
College of Nursing and Speech Language Pathology
Columbus, Mississippi

http://www.muw.edu/nursing
Founded in 1884
DEGREES • BSN • MSN
Nursing Program Faculty 58 (30% with doctorates).
Baccalaureate Enrollment 492 **Women** 80% **Men** 20% **Minority** 30% **International** 1% **Part-time** 1%
Graduate Enrollment 45 **Women** 90% **Men** 10% **Minority** 15% **Part-time** 1%
Distance Learning Courses Available.
Nursing Student Activities Sigma Theta Tau, Student Nurses' Association.
Nursing Student Resources Academic advising; academic or career counseling; assistance for students with disabilities; bookstore; campus computer network; career placement assistance; computer lab; computer-assisted instruction; daycare for children of students; e-mail services; employment services for current students; externships; housing assistance; interactive nursing skills videos; Internet; learning resource lab; library services; nursing audiovisuals; paid internships; placement services for program completers; remedial services; resume preparation assistance; skills, simulation, or other laboratory; tutoring; unpaid internships.
Library Facilities 25,959 volumes (27,440 in health, 26,420 in nursing); 4,341 periodical subscriptions (236 health-care related).

BACCALAUREATE PROGRAMS

Degree BSN
Available Programs ADN to Baccalaureate; Generic Baccalaureate.
Site Options Tupelo, MS.
Study Options Full-time.
Online Degree Options Yes.
Program Entrance Requirements Minimum overall college GPA of 2.75, transcript of college record, CPR certification, health exam, health insurance, immunizations, minimum GPA in nursing prerequisites of 2.75, professional liability insurance/malpractice insurance, prerequisite course work. Transfer students are accepted. *Application deadline:* 1/15 (fall).
Advanced Placement Credit given for nursing courses completed elsewhere dependent upon specific evaluations.
Expenses (2012–13) *Tuition, state resident:* full-time $5316; part-time $222 per credit hour. *Tuition, nonresident:* full-time $14,484; part-time $604 per credit hour. *International tuition:* $14,484 full-time. *Room and board:* $6076; room only: $3539 per academic year. *Required fees:* full-time $250; part-time $125 per term.
Financial Aid 90% of baccalaureate students in nursing programs received some form of financial aid in 2011–12.
Contact Dr. Tammie McCoy, Baccalaureate Nursing Department Chair, College of Nursing and Speech Language Pathology, Mississippi University for Women, 1100 College Street, MUW-910, Columbus, MS 39701-5800. *Telephone:* 662-329-7301. *Fax:* 662-329-8559. *E-mail:* tmccoy@nsgslp.muw.edu.

GRADUATE PROGRAMS

Expenses (2012–13) *Tuition, state resident:* full-time $5316; part-time $296 per credit hour. *Tuition, nonresident:* full-time $14,484; part-time $604 per credit hour. *International tuition:* $14,484 full-time. *Room and board:* $6076; room only: $3539 per academic year. *Required fees:* full-time $1000.
Financial Aid 80% of graduate students in nursing programs received some form of financial aid in 2011–12. Fellowships, Federal Work-Study, institutionally sponsored loans, and traineeships available. *Financial aid application deadline:* 4/1.
Contact Dr. Johnnie Sue Wijewardane, Graduate Nursing Program Department Chair, College of Nursing and Speech Language Pathology, Mississippi University for Women, 1100 College Street, MUW-910, Columbus, MS 39701-5800. *Telephone:* 662-329-7323. *Fax:* 662-329-7372. *E-mail:* jscw@nsgslp.muw.edu.

MASTER'S DEGREE PROGRAM

Degree MSN
Available Programs Master's.
Concentrations Available *Nurse practitioner programs in:* family health, gerontology, pediatric, psychiatric/mental health.

Study Options Full-time.
Program Entrance Requirements Clinical experience, computer literacy, minimum overall college GPA of 3.0, transcript of college record, CPR certification, written essay, immunizations, interview, 3 letters of recommendation, nursing research course, physical assessment course, professional liability insurance/malpractice insurance, prerequisite course work, resume, statistics course, GRE General Test. *Application deadline:* 4/1 (fall). *Application fee:* $25.
Advanced Placement Credit given for nursing courses completed elsewhere dependent upon specific evaluations.
Degree Requirements 39 total credit hours, thesis or project, comprehensive exam.

POST-MASTER'S PROGRAM
Areas of Study *Nurse practitioner programs in:* family health, gerontology, pediatric, psychiatric/mental health.

University of Mississippi Medical Center
Program in Nursing
Jackson, Mississippi

http://son.umc.edu/
Founded in 1955
DEGREES • BSN • MSN • PHD
Nursing Program Faculty 66 (56% with doctorates).
Baccalaureate Enrollment 290 **Women** 85.7% **Men** 14.3% **Minority** 14% **Part-time** 9%
Graduate Enrollment 258 **Women** 91% **Men** 9% **Minority** 16% **Part-time** 45%
Distance Learning Courses Available.
Nursing Student Activities Nursing Honor Society, Sigma Theta Tau, Student Nurses' Association, nursing club.
Nursing Student Resources Academic advising; academic or career counseling; assistance for students with disabilities; bookstore; campus computer network; computer lab; computer-assisted instruction; e-mail services; employment services for current students; externships; interactive nursing skills videos; Internet; learning resource lab; library services; nursing audiovisuals; remedial services; skills, simulation, or other laboratory; tutoring; unpaid internships.
Library Facilities 310,016 volumes (72,557 in health, 8,170 in nursing); 2,732 periodical subscriptions (4,180 health-care related).

BACCALAUREATE PROGRAMS

Degree BSN
Available Programs ADN to Baccalaureate; Accelerated Baccalaureate for Second Degree; Generic Baccalaureate.
Site Options Oxford, MS.
Study Options Full-time and part-time.
Program Entrance Requirements Minimum overall college GPA of 2.5, transcript of college record, CPR certification, health exam, health insurance, immunizations, minimum GPA in nursing prerequisites of 2.5, professional liability insurance/malpractice insurance, prerequisite course work. Transfer students are accepted. *Application deadline:* 1/15 (spring). *Application fee:* $25.
Advanced Placement Credit given for nursing courses completed elsewhere dependent upon specific evaluations.
Expenses (2012–13) *Tuition, state resident:* full-time $9423; part-time $262 per credit hour. *Tuition, nonresident:* part-time $416 per credit hour. *Required fees:* full-time $600.
Financial Aid 78% of baccalaureate students in nursing programs received some form of financial aid in 2011–12.
Contact Dr. Patricia A. Waltman, Associate Dean for Academic Affairs, Program in Nursing, University of Mississippi Medical Center, 2500 North State Street, Jackson, MS 39216-4505. *Telephone:* 601-984-6211. *Fax:* 601-815-9309. *E-mail:* pwaltman@son.umsmed.edu.

GRADUATE PROGRAMS

Expenses (2012–13) *Tuition, state resident:* full-time $9423; part-time $349 per credit hour. *Tuition, nonresident:* full-time $24,398; part-time $555 per credit hour.
Financial Aid 80% of graduate students in nursing programs received some form of financial aid in 2011–12. Institutionally sponsored loans and traineeships available. Aid available to part-time students. *Financial aid application deadline:* 4/1.

Contact Dr. Marcia Rachel, Associate Dean for Graduate Studies, Program in Nursing, University of Mississippi Medical Center, 2500 North State Street, Jackson, MS 39216-4505. *Telephone:* 601-984-6228. *Fax:* 601-815-4067. *E-mail:* mrachel@umc.edu.

MASTER'S DEGREE PROGRAM
Degree MSN
Available Programs Accelerated AD/RN to Master's; Master's; RN to Master's.
Concentrations Available Nursing administration; nursing education. *Nurse practitioner programs in:* acute care, family health, gerontology, psychiatric/mental health.
Study Options Full-time and part-time.
Program Entrance Requirements Computer literacy, minimum overall college GPA of 3.0, transcript of college record, CPR certification, immunizations, 3 letters of recommendation, professional liability insurance/malpractice insurance, resume, statistics course, GRE. *Application deadline:* 10/15 (fall), 2/15 (winter), 3/31 (spring). Applications may be processed on a rolling basis for some programs. *Application fee:* $25.
Advanced Placement Credit given for nursing courses completed elsewhere dependent upon specific evaluations.
Degree Requirements 40 total credit hours, comprehensive exam.

POST-MASTER'S PROGRAM
Areas of Study Nursing administration; nursing education. *Nurse practitioner programs in:* acute care, family health, gerontology, psychiatric/mental health.

DOCTORAL DEGREE PROGRAM
Degree PhD
Available Programs Doctorate.
Areas of Study Bio-behavioral research, health policy, health promotion/disease prevention, health-care systems, human health and illness, nursing research, nursing science.
Program Entrance Requirements Minimum overall college GPA of 3.0, interview by faculty committee, interview, letters of recommendation, MSN or equivalent, statistics course, vita, GRE. *Application deadline:* 5/1 (fall). *Application fee:* $25.
Degree Requirements 60 total credit hours, dissertation, oral exam, written exam, residency.

CONTINUING EDUCATION PROGRAM

Contact Dr. Renee Williams, Director of Continuing Education, Program in Nursing, University of Mississippi Medical Center, 2500 North State Street, Jackson, MS 39216-4505. *Telephone:* 601-984-6227. *Fax:* 601-984-6214. *E-mail:* rwilliams@son.umsmed.edu.

University of Southern Mississippi
School of Nursing
Hattiesburg, Mississippi

http://www.usm.edu/nursing/
Founded in 1910
DEGREES • BSN • MSN • PHD
Nursing Program Faculty 57 (49% with doctorates).
Baccalaureate Enrollment 416 **Women** 81% **Men** 19% **Minority** 19% **Part-time** 2%
Graduate Enrollment 143 **Women** 84% **Men** 16% **Minority** 24% **Part-time** 25%
Distance Learning Courses Available.
Nursing Student Activities Nursing Honor Society, Sigma Theta Tau, Student Nurses' Association.
Nursing Student Resources Academic advising; academic or career counseling; assistance for students with disabilities; bookstore; campus computer network; career placement assistance; computer lab; computer-assisted instruction; e-mail services; externships; housing assistance; interactive nursing skills videos; Internet; learning resource lab; library services; nursing audiovisuals; remedial services; resume preparation assistance; skills, simulation, or other laboratory; tutoring.
Library Facilities 1.2 million volumes; 33,307 periodical subscriptions (170 health-care related).

BACCALAUREATE PROGRAMS

Degree BSN
Available Programs ADN to Baccalaureate; Generic Baccalaureate.

Site Options Meridian, MS; Long Beach, MS.
Study Options Full-time and part-time.
Online Degree Options Yes.
Program Entrance Requirements Minimum overall college GPA of 2.5, transcript of college record, CPR certification, written essay, health exam, health insurance, high school transcript, immunizations, minimum GPA in nursing prerequisites of 2.5, professional liability insurance/malpractice insurance, prerequisite course work. Transfer students are accepted. *Application deadline:* 2/1 (fall), 9/1 (spring).
Expenses (2012–13) *Tuition, state resident:* full-time $6336; part-time $244 per credit. *Tuition, nonresident:* full-time $8112; part-time $576 per credit. *International tuition:* $8112 full-time. *Room and board:* $8388; room only: $5618 per academic year. *Required fees:* full-time $800; part-time $75 per credit.
Financial Aid 85% of baccalaureate students in nursing programs received some form of financial aid in 2011–12.
Contact Cindy Sheffield, Assistant to the Dean for Academic/Advisement Records, School of Nursing, University of Southern Mississippi, 118 College Drive, Box 5095, Hattiesburg, MS 39406-5095. *Telephone:* 601-266-5454. *Fax:* 601-266-5711. *E-mail:* cynthia.sheffield@usm.edu.

GRADUATE PROGRAMS

Expenses (2012–13) *Tuition, state resident:* full-time $5834; part-time $325 per credit. *Tuition, nonresident:* full-time $13,790; part-time $767 per credit. *International tuition:* $13,790 full-time. *Required fees:* full-time $300; part-time $50 per credit.
Financial Aid 85% of graduate students in nursing programs received some form of financial aid in 2011–12. 14 research assistantships with full tuition reimbursements available (averaging $12,577 per year), teaching assistantships (averaging $12,000 per year) were awarded; Federal Work-Study, institutionally sponsored loans, scholarships, traineeships, and unspecified assistantships also available. *Financial aid application deadline:* 3/15.
Contact Ms. Cynthia Sheffield, Assistant to the Dean for Academic/Advisement Records, School of Nursing, University of Southern Mississippi, 118 College Drive, Box 5095, Hattiesburg, MS 39406-5095. *Telephone:* 601-266-5454. *Fax:* 601-266-5711. *E-mail:* Cynthia.Sheffield@usm.edu.

MASTER'S DEGREE PROGRAM

Degree MSN
Available Programs Master's; RN to Master's.
Concentrations Available Nursing administration. *Nurse practitioner programs in:* family health, gerontology, psychiatric/mental health.
Site Options Meridian, MS; Long Beach, MS.
Study Options Full-time and part-time.
Program Entrance Requirements Minimum overall college GPA of 3.0, transcript of college record, CPR certification, immunizations, 3 letters of recommendation, professional liability insurance/malpractice insurance, statistics course, GRE General Test. *Application deadline:* 2/1 (fall), 9/1 (spring).
Degree Requirements 45 total credit hours, thesis or project, comprehensive exam.

POST-MASTER'S PROGRAM

Areas of Study Nursing administration. *Nurse practitioner programs in:* family health, gerontology, psychiatric/mental health.

DOCTORAL DEGREE PROGRAM

Degree PhD
Available Programs Doctorate; Post-Baccalaureate Doctorate.
Program Entrance Requirements Clinical experience, minimum overall college GPA of 3.5, interview by faculty committee, 3 letters of recommendation, MSN or equivalent, statistics course, vita, writing sample, GRE General Test. *Application deadline:* 2/1 (fall).
Degree Requirements 72 total credit hours, dissertation, written exam.

William Carey University
School of Nursing
Hattiesburg, Mississippi

http://wmcarey.edu/
Founded in 1906
DEGREES • BSN • MSN • PHD
Nursing Program Faculty 25 (40% with doctorates).

Baccalaureate Enrollment 214 **Women** 85% **Men** 15% **Minority** 36% **International** .5% **Part-time** 26%
Graduate Enrollment 91 **Women** 89% **Men** 11% **Minority** 41% **Part-time** 45%
Distance Learning Courses Available.
Nursing Student Activities Sigma Theta Tau, Student Nurses' Association.
Nursing Student Resources Academic advising; academic or career counseling; assistance for students with disabilities; bookstore; campus computer network; computer lab; computer-assisted instruction; e-mail services; interactive nursing skills videos; Internet; learning resource lab; library services; nursing audiovisuals; resume preparation assistance; skills, simulation, or other laboratory; tutoring.
Library Facilities 450 volumes in health, 450 volumes in nursing; 50 periodical subscriptions health-care related.

BACCALAUREATE PROGRAMS

Degree BSN
Available Programs ADN to Baccalaureate; Generic Baccalaureate.
Site Options Biloxi, MS; New Orleans, LA.
Study Options Full-time and part-time.
Program Entrance Requirements Minimum overall college GPA of 2.75, transcript of college record, CPR certification, health exam, high school transcript, immunizations, minimum GPA in nursing prerequisites, professional liability insurance/malpractice insurance, prerequisite course work. Transfer students are accepted. *Application deadline:* 2/22 (fall), 8/10 (spring). *Application fee:* $40.
Advanced Placement Credit given for nursing courses completed elsewhere dependent upon specific evaluations.
Expenses (2012–13) *Tuition:* part-time $335 per contact hour. *Room and board:* room only: $1800 per academic year. *Required fees:* part-time $250 per term.
Financial Aid 90% of baccalaureate students in nursing programs received some form of financial aid in 2011–12.
Contact Dr. Janet K. Williams, Dean, School of Nursing, William Carey University, 498 Tuscan Avenue, Box 8, Hattiesburg, MS 39401. *Telephone:* 601-318-6478. *Fax:* 601-318-6446. *E-mail:* jwilliams@wmcarey.edu.

GRADUATE PROGRAMS

Expenses (2012–13) *Tuition:* part-time $310 per contact hour. *International tuition:* $310 full-time. *Required fees:* full-time $1000; part-time $50 per credit.
Financial Aid 50% of graduate students in nursing programs received some form of financial aid in 2011–12.
Contact Dr. Marilyn McLeod Cooksey, Associate Dean of Graduate Studies, School of Nursing, William Carey University, 498 Tuscan Avenue, Hattiesburg, MS 39401. *Telephone:* 601-318-6478. *E-mail:* mcooksey@wmcarey.edu.

MASTER'S DEGREE PROGRAM

Degree MSN
Available Programs Master's.
Concentrations Available Nursing education.
Site Options Biloxi, MS.
Study Options Full-time and part-time.
Program Entrance Requirements Computer literacy, minimum overall college GPA of 3.0, transcript of college record, CPR certification, written essay, immunizations, 2 letters of recommendation, nursing research course, professional liability insurance/malpractice insurance, prerequisite course work, resume. *Application deadline:* 8/15 (fall), 2/15 (spring). Applications may be processed on a rolling basis for some programs. *Application fee:* $30.
Advanced Placement Credit given for nursing courses completed elsewhere dependent upon specific evaluations.
Degree Requirements 35 total credit hours, thesis or project.

DOCTORAL DEGREE PROGRAM

Degree PhD
Available Programs Doctorate.
Areas of Study Nursing education.
Program Entrance Requirements Minimum overall college GPA of 3.5, 3 letters of recommendation, MSN or equivalent, statistics course, vita, writing sample. *Application deadline:* 6/22 (fall). Applications may be processed on a rolling basis for some programs. *Application fee:* $390.
Degree Requirements 56 total credit hours, dissertation, written exam.

MISSOURI

Avila University
School of Nursing
Kansas City, Missouri

http://www.avila.edu/nursing
Founded in 1916
DEGREE • BSN
Nursing Program Faculty 15 (13% with doctorates).
Baccalaureate Enrollment 106 **Women** 85% **Men** 15% **Minority** 16%
Part-time .02%
Nursing Student Activities Student Nurses' Association.
Nursing Student Resources Academic advising; academic or career counseling; assistance for students with disabilities; bookstore; campus computer network; career placement assistance; computer lab; computer-assisted instruction; e-mail services; externships; interactive nursing skills videos; Internet; learning resource lab; library services; nursing audiovisuals; remedial services; resume preparation assistance; skills, simulation, or other laboratory; tutoring.
Library Facilities 80,845 volumes (675 in health, 475 in nursing); 22,464 periodical subscriptions (60 health-care related).

BACCALAUREATE PROGRAMS
Degree BSN
Available Programs Generic Baccalaureate.
Study Options Full-time.
Program Entrance Requirements Minimum overall college GPA of 2.7, transcript of college record, CPR certification, written essay, health exam, health insurance, immunizations, interview, minimum GPA in nursing prerequisites of 2.0, prerequisite course work. Transfer students are accepted. *Application deadline:* 1/10 (fall). *Application fee:* $45.
Advanced Placement Credit given for nursing courses completed elsewhere dependent upon specific evaluations.
Expenses (2012–13) *Tuition:* full-time $23,100; part-time $600 per credit hour. *International tuition:* $23,100 full-time. *Room and board:* $7000; room only: $4000 per academic year. *Required fees:* full-time $850.
Financial Aid 98% of baccalaureate students in nursing programs received some form of financial aid in 2011–12.
Contact Office of Admissions, School of Nursing, Avila University, 11901 Wornall Road, Kansas City, MO 64145-1698. *Telephone:* 816-501-2400. *Fax:* 816-501-2453. *E-mail:* admissions@avila.edu.

Central Methodist University
College of Liberal Arts and Sciences
Fayette, Missouri

http://www.centralmethodist.edu/
Founded in 1854
DEGREES • BN • MSN
Nursing Program Faculty 7
Library Facilities 97,793 volumes; 316 periodical subscriptions.

BACCALAUREATE PROGRAMS
Degree BN
Available Programs Generic Baccalaureate.
Program Entrance Requirements Written essay, health exam, high school biology, high school chemistry, immunizations, minimum high school GPA of 2.75, prerequisite course work. Transfer students are accepted.
Contact *Telephone:* 660-248-6359.

GRADUATE PROGRAMS
Contact *Telephone:* 573-220-1378.

MASTER'S DEGREE PROGRAM
Degree MSN
Available Programs Master's.
Program Entrance Requirements CPR certification, written essay, immunizations, prerequisite course work, statistics course.

Chamberlain College of Nursing
Chamberlain College of Nursing
St. Louis, Missouri

http://www.chamberlain.edu/
Founded in 1889
DEGREE • BSN
Nursing Program Faculty 80 (21% with doctorates).
Distance Learning Courses Available.
Nursing Student Activities Student Nurses' Association.
Nursing Student Resources Academic advising; academic or career counseling; assistance for students with disabilities; bookstore; campus computer network; career placement assistance; computer lab; computer-assisted instruction; e-mail services; employment services for current students; housing assistance; Internet; learning resource lab; library services; nursing audiovisuals; placement services for program completers; skills, simulation, or other laboratory; tutoring.
Library Facilities 3,287 volumes in health, 957 volumes in nursing; 182 periodical subscriptions health-care related.

BACCALAUREATE PROGRAMS
Degree BSN
Available Programs ADN to Baccalaureate; Accelerated RN Baccalaureate; Generic Baccalaureate; LPN to RN Baccalaureate; RN Baccalaureate.
Site Options Columbus, OH; Phoenix, AZ; Addison, IL.
Study Options Full-time.
Online Degree Options Yes (online only).
Program Entrance Requirements Minimum overall college GPA of 2.75, transcript of college record, written essay, health exam, health insurance, high school biology, high school chemistry, 3 years high school math, 3 years high school science, high school transcript, immunizations, interview, minimum high school GPA of 2.75, minimum high school rank 33%. Transfer students are accepted.
Advanced Placement Credit by examination available. Credit given for nursing courses completed elsewhere dependent upon specific evaluations.
Contact *Telephone:* 800-942-4310 Ext. 1. *Fax:* 314-768-3044.

College of the Ozarks
Armstrong McDonald School of Nursing
Point Lookout, Missouri

http://www.cofo.edu/
Founded in 1906
DEGREE • BSN
Nursing Program Faculty 8 (38% with doctorates).
Baccalaureate Enrollment 61 **Women** 83.8% **Men** 16.2% **Minority** 3.2% **International** 1.61%
Nursing Student Activities Nursing club.
Nursing Student Resources Academic advising; academic or career counseling; assistance for students with disabilities; bookstore; campus computer network; career placement assistance; computer lab; computer-assisted instruction; daycare for children of students; e-mail services; employment services for current students; externships; housing assistance; interactive nursing skills videos; Internet; learning resource lab; library services; nursing audiovisuals; paid internships; placement services for program completers; remedial services; resume preparation assistance; skills, simulation, or other laboratory; tutoring; unpaid internships.
Library Facilities 108,128 volumes (1,225 in health, 861 in nursing); 370 periodical subscriptions (68 health-care related).

BACCALAUREATE PROGRAMS
Degree BSN
Available Programs Generic Baccalaureate.
Study Options Full-time and part-time.
Program Entrance Requirements Minimum overall college GPA of 2.5, transcript of college record, health exam, 2 years high school math, high school transcript, immunizations, interview, 2 letters of recommendation, minimum high school GPA of 3.0, minimum high school rank 51%, minimum GPA in nursing prerequisites of 2.5, professional liability insurance/malpractice insurance, prerequisite course work. Transfer students are accepted. *Application deadline:* 10/1 (fall), 3/1 (spring).

Expenses (2012–13) *Tuition:* part-time $310 per credit hour. *Room and board:* $5900; room only: $3000 per academic year.

Financial Aid 100% of baccalaureate students in nursing programs received some form of financial aid in 2011–12. *Gift aid (need-based):* Federal Pell, FSEOG, state, private, college/university gift aid from institutional funds. *Loans:* alternative loans. *Work-study:* Federal Work-Study, part-time campus jobs. *Financial aid application deadline (priority):* 2/15.

Contact Mrs. Deborah J. Lyon, Office Manager, Armstrong McDonald School of Nursing, College of the Ozarks, PO Box 17, Point Lookout, MO 65726. *Telephone:* 417-690-2421. *Fax:* 417-690-2422. *E-mail:* dlyon@cofo.edu.

Cox College
Department of Nursing
Springfield, Missouri

Founded in 1994

DEGREES • BSN • MSN

Nursing Program Faculty 61 (10% with doctorates).
Baccalaureate Enrollment 240 **Women** 87% **Men** 13% **Minority** 5% **Part-time** 80%
Graduate Enrollment 83 **Women** 92% **Men** 8%
Distance Learning Courses Available.
Nursing Student Activities Nursing Honor Society, Student Nurses' Association, nursing club.
Nursing Student Resources Academic advising; academic or career counseling; assistance for students with disabilities; bookstore; campus computer network; career placement assistance; computer lab; computer-assisted instruction; daycare for children of students; e-mail services; employment services for current students; externships; housing assistance; interactive nursing skills videos; Internet; learning resource lab; library services; nursing audiovisuals; placement services for program completers; remedial services; resume preparation assistance; skills, simulation, or other laboratory; tutoring.
Library Facilities 29,750 volumes (5,500 in health, 1,900 in nursing); 249 periodical subscriptions (250 health-care related).

BACCALAUREATE PROGRAMS

Degree BSN
Available Programs ADN to Baccalaureate; Accelerated Baccalaureate; Accelerated Baccalaureate for Second Degree; Baccalaureate for Second Degree; Generic Baccalaureate; LPN to Baccalaureate; LPN to RN Baccalaureate; RN Baccalaureate.
Site Options Springfield, MO.
Study Options Full-time.
Online Degree Options Yes (online only).
Program Entrance Requirements Minimum overall college GPA of 3.0, transcript of college record, CPR certification, high school transcript, immunizations, interview, minimum high school GPA of 3.0, minimum GPA in nursing prerequisites of 3.0, professional liability insurance/malpractice insurance, prerequisite course work, RN licensure. Transfer students are accepted. *Application deadline:* 1/15 (fall), 8/15 (spring). *Application fee:* $45.
Advanced Placement Credit given for nursing courses completed elsewhere dependent upon specific evaluations.
Expenses (2011–12) *Tuition:* part-time $348 per semester. *Required fees:* part-time $40 per credit; part-time $105 per term.
Financial Aid 80% of baccalaureate students in nursing programs received some form of financial aid in 2010–11. *Gift aid (need-based):* Federal Pell, FSEOG, state, private, college/university gift aid from institutional funds, United Negro College Fund, Federal Nursing. *Loans:* Federal Direct (Subsidized and Unsubsidized Stafford PLUS). *Work-study:* Federal Work-Study. *Financial aid application deadline (priority):* 4/1.
Contact Ms. Lindy Biglieni, Director of Admissions, Department of Nursing, Cox College, 1423 North Jefferson Avenue, Springfield, MO 65802. *Telephone:* 417-269-3401. *Fax:* 417-269-3586. *E-mail:* lbiglie@coxcollege.edu.

GRADUATE PROGRAMS

Expenses (2011–12) *Tuition:* part-time $464 per credit hour. *Required fees:* part-time $40 per credit; part-time $105 per term.
Contact Lindy Biglieni, Director of Admissions, Department of Nursing, Cox College, 1423 North Jefferson Avenue, Springfield, MO 65802. *Telephone:* 417-269-3401. *E-mail:* admissions@coxcollege.edu.

MASTER'S DEGREE PROGRAM

Degree MSN
Available Programs Master's; RN to Master's.
Concentrations Available Clinical nurse leader; nursing education. *Clinical nurse specialist programs in:* family health.
Site Options Springfield, MO.
Study Options Full-time and part-time.
Online Degree Options Yes (online only).
Program Entrance Requirements Clinical experience, computer literacy, minimum overall college GPA of 3.0, transcript of college record, CPR certification, written essay, immunizations, interview, letters of recommendation, resume. *Application deadline:* 3/1 (fall). *Application fee:* $45.
Degree Requirements 42 total credit hours, thesis or project.

CONTINUING EDUCATION PROGRAM

Contact Michelle Jacobs, Professional Advancement Director, Department of Nursing, Cox College, 1423 North Jefferson Avenue, Springfield, MO 65802. *Telephone:* 417-269-5062. *E-mail:* michelle.jacobs@coxcollege.edu.

Culver-Stockton College
Blessing–Rieman College of Nursing
Canton, Missouri

http://www.culver.edu/

See description of programs under Blessing–Rieman College of Nursing (Quincy, Illinois).

Goldfarb School of Nursing at Barnes-Jewish College
Goldfarb School of Nursing at Barnes-Jewish College
St. Louis, Missouri

Founded in 1902

DEGREES • BSN • MSN • PHD

Nursing Program Faculty 51 (45% with doctorates).
Baccalaureate Enrollment 635 **Women** 90% **Men** 10% **Minority** 19% **International** 1% **Part-time** 2%
Graduate Enrollment 185 **Women** 81% **Men** 19% **Minority** 28% **International** 1% **Part-time** 54%
Distance Learning Courses Available.
Nursing Student Activities Nursing Honor Society, Sigma Theta Tau, Student Nurses' Association, nursing club.
Nursing Student Resources Academic advising; academic or career counseling; assistance for students with disabilities; bookstore; campus computer network; career placement assistance; computer lab; computer-assisted instruction; e-mail services; employment services for current students; externships; housing assistance; interactive nursing skills videos; Internet; learning resource lab; library services; nursing audiovisuals; placement services for program completers; remedial services; resume preparation assistance; skills, simulation, or other laboratory; tutoring.
Library Facilities 1,125 volumes (13,000 in health, 8,200 in nursing); 47 periodical subscriptions (250 health-care related).

BACCALAUREATE PROGRAMS

Degree BSN
Available Programs ADN to Baccalaureate; Accelerated Baccalaureate; Accelerated Baccalaureate for Second Degree; Generic Baccalaureate; RN Baccalaureate.
Site Options Town and Country, MO.
Study Options Full-time.
Program Entrance Requirements Minimum overall college GPA of 3.0, transcript of college record, CPR certification, health exam, high school biology, high school transcript, immunizations, minimum high school GPA of 3.0, minimum GPA in nursing prerequisites of 3.0, prerequisite course work. Transfer students are accepted. *Application deadline:* 8/15 (fall), 12/15 (spring), 4/1 (summer). Applications may be processed on a rolling basis for some programs. *Application fee:* $50.

Advanced Placement Credit by examination available. Credit given for nursing courses completed elsewhere dependent upon specific evaluations.

Expenses (2012–13) *Tuition:* full-time $25,520; part-time $633 per credit hour. *International tuition:* $25,520 full-time. *Required fees:* full-time $900; part-time $20 per credit; part-time $150 per term.

Financial Aid 95% of baccalaureate students in nursing programs received some form of financial aid in 2011–12. *Gift aid (need-based):* Federal Pell, FSEOG, state, private, college/university gift aid from institutional funds. *Loans:* Federal Direct (Subsidized and Unsubsidized Stafford PLUS).*Work-study:* Federal Work-Study.*Financial aid application deadline (priority):* 4/1.

Contact Dr. Connie Koch, Associate Dean for Academic Programs, Goldfarb School of Nursing at Barnes-Jewish College, 4483 Duncan, MS #90-36-697, St. Louis, MO 63110-1091. *Telephone:* 314-362-6289. *Fax:* 314-362-0984. *E-mail:* ckoch@bjc.org.

GRADUATE PROGRAMS

Expenses (2012–13) *Tuition:* full-time $15,120; part-time $660 per credit hour. *International tuition:* $15,120 full-time. *Required fees:* full-time $300; part-time $15 per credit; part-time $50 per term.

Financial Aid 80% of graduate students in nursing programs received some form of financial aid in 2011–12.

Contact Dr. Connie Koch, Associate Dean for Academic Programs, Goldfarb School of Nursing at Barnes-Jewish College, 4483 Duncan, MS #90-36-697, St. Louis, MO 63110-1091. *Telephone:* 314-362-6289. *Fax:* 314-362-0984. *E-mail:* ckoch@bjc.org.

MASTER'S DEGREE PROGRAM

Degree MSN

Available Programs Master's.

Concentrations Available Health-care administration; nurse anesthesia; nursing administration; nursing education. *Nurse practitioner programs in:* acute care, adult health.

Study Options Full-time and part-time.

Program Entrance Requirements Clinical experience, computer literacy, minimum overall college GPA of 3.0, transcript of college record, CPR certification, immunizations, 2 letters of recommendation, nursing research course, physical assessment course, resume, statistics course. *Application deadline:* 8/20 (fall), 12/15 (spring), 4/15 (summer). Applications may be processed on a rolling basis for some programs. *Application fee:* $50.

Advanced Placement Credit given for nursing courses completed elsewhere dependent upon specific evaluations.

Degree Requirements 34 total credit hours, thesis or project.

POST-MASTER'S PROGRAM

Areas of Study Health-care administration; nursing administration; nursing education. *Nurse practitioner programs in:* acute care, adult health.

DOCTORAL DEGREE PROGRAM

Degree PhD

Available Programs Doctorate.

Areas of Study Clinical practice, nursing administration, nursing education.

Program Entrance Requirements Minimum overall college GPA of 3.0, interview by faculty committee, 3 letters of recommendation, MSN or equivalent, statistics course, vita, writing sample. *Application deadline:* 7/15 (fall). Applications may be processed on a rolling basis for some programs. *Application fee:* $50.

Degree Requirements 111 total credit hours, dissertation, oral exam, written exam, residency.

Graceland University

School of Nursing
Independence, Missouri

http://www.graceland.edu/nursing
Founded in 1895
DEGREES • BSN • DNP • MSN
Nursing Program Faculty 23 (56% with doctorates).
Baccalaureate Enrollment 136 **Women** 84.6% **Men** 15.4% **Minority** 4.4% **International** 1.5% **Part-time** 5.1%
Graduate Enrollment 477 **Women** 89.5% **Men** 10.5% **Minority** 9.9% **Part-time** 43.2%

Distance Learning Courses Available.

Nursing Student Activities Nursing Honor Society, Sigma Theta Tau, Student Nurses' Association, nursing club.

Nursing Student Resources Academic advising; academic or career counseling; assistance for students with disabilities; bookstore; campus computer network; computer lab; computer-assisted instruction; e-mail services; housing assistance; interactive nursing skills videos; Internet; learning resource lab; library services; nursing audiovisuals; resume preparation assistance; skills, simulation, or other laboratory; tutoring.

Library Facilities 143,989 volumes (1,902 in health, 790 in nursing); 903 periodical subscriptions (2,815 health-care related).

BACCALAUREATE PROGRAMS

Degree BSN

Available Programs ADN to Baccalaureate; Accelerated Baccalaureate; Generic Baccalaureate; RN Baccalaureate.

Site Options Independence, MO.

Study Options Full-time and part-time.

Program Entrance Requirements Minimum overall college GPA of 2.5, transcript of college record, written essay, health exam, high school chemistry, high school transcript, immunizations, interview, 2 letters of recommendation, minimum high school GPA of 2.5, minimum GPA in nursing prerequisites of 2.0, prerequisite course work. Transfer students are accepted. *Application deadline:* 11/30 (fall). *Application fee:* $50.

Advanced Placement Credit given for nursing courses completed elsewhere dependent upon specific evaluations.

Expenses (2012–13) *Tuition:* full-time $22,780; part-time $710 per credit hour. *International tuition:* $22,780 full-time. *Required fees:* full-time $1675; part-time $837 per term.

Financial Aid 36% of baccalaureate students in nursing programs received some form of financial aid in 2011–12. *Gift aid (need-based):* Federal Pell, FSEOG, state, private, college/university gift aid from institutional funds. *Loans:* Federal Direct (Subsidized and Unsubsidized Stafford PLUS), Perkins, state, college/university.*Work-study:* Federal Work-Study, part-time campus jobs.*Financial aid application deadline:* Continuous.

Contact Ms. Laurie Hale, Admissions Counselor, School of Nursing, Graceland University, 1401 West Truman Road, Independence, MO 64050-3434. *Telephone:* 800-423-4675. *Fax:* 816-833-2990. *E-mail:* lhale@graceland.edu.

GRADUATE PROGRAMS

Expenses (2012–13) *Tuition:* part-time $625 per credit hour.

Financial Aid 72% of graduate students in nursing programs received some form of financial aid in 2011–12.

Contact Ms. Jill Whitworth, Program Consultant, School of Nursing, Graceland University, 1401 West Truman Road, Independence, MO 64050-3434. *Telephone:* 816-423-4712. *Fax:* 816-833-2990. *E-mail:* jwhitwor@graceland.edu.

MASTER'S DEGREE PROGRAM

Degree MSN

Available Programs Master's; RN to Master's.

Concentrations Available Nursing education. *Nurse practitioner programs in:* family health.

Site Options Independence, MO.

Study Options Full-time and part-time.

Online Degree Options Yes (online only).

Program Entrance Requirements Clinical experience, minimum overall college GPA of 3.0, transcript of college record, written essay, 3 letters of recommendation, nursing research course, physical assessment course, prerequisite course work, statistics course. *Application deadline:* 6/1 (fall), 10/1 (winter), 2/1 (spring). *Application fee:* $50.

Advanced Placement Credit given for nursing courses completed elsewhere dependent upon specific evaluations.

Degree Requirements 47 total credit hours, thesis or project, comprehensive exam.

POST-MASTER'S PROGRAM

Areas of Study Nursing education. *Nurse practitioner programs in:* family health.

DOCTORAL DEGREE PROGRAM

Degree DNP

Available Programs Doctorate.

Areas of Study Advanced practice nursing, family health, health policy, health promotion/disease prevention, health-care systems, human health and illness, nursing policy, nursing science.

Site Options Independence, MO.

Online Degree Options Yes (online only).
Program Entrance Requirements Minimum overall college GPA of 3.2, 3 letters of recommendation, MSN or equivalent, writing sample. *Application deadline:* 5/15 (fall). *Application fee:* $50.
Degree Requirements 31 total credit hours, dissertation, residency.

Lincoln University
Department of Nursing
Jefferson City, Missouri

http://www.lincolnu.edu/web/dept.-of-nursing-science/nursing-science
Founded in 1866
DEGREE • BSN
Distance Learning Courses Available.
Nursing Student Resources Academic advising; academic or career counseling; assistance for students with disabilities; bookstore; campus computer network; computer lab; e-mail services; Internet; library services; remedial services; tutoring.
Library Facilities 222,797 volumes; 202 periodical subscriptions.

BACCALAUREATE PROGRAMS

Degree BSN
Available Programs RN Baccalaureate.
Contact Dr. Connie Hamacher, Department Head of Nursing Science, Department of Nursing, Lincoln University, 820 Chestnut, Elliff Hall, Room 100, Jefferson City, MO 65101. *Telephone:* 573-681-5421. *E-mail:* nursing@lincolnu.edu.

Maryville University of Saint Louis
Nursing Program, School of Health Professions
St. Louis, Missouri

http://www.maryville.edu/academics-hp-nursing.htm
Founded in 1872
DEGREES • BSN • DNP • MSN
Nursing Program Faculty 65 (4% with doctorates).
Baccalaureate Enrollment 463 **Women** 95% **Men** 5% **Minority** 10% **International** 1% **Part-time** 45%
Graduate Enrollment 116 **Women** 92% **Men** 8% **Minority** 14% **Part-time** 79%
Nursing Student Activities Sigma Theta Tau, Student Nurses' Association.
Nursing Student Resources Academic advising; academic or career counseling; assistance for students with disabilities; bookstore; campus computer network; career placement assistance; computer lab; computer-assisted instruction; e-mail services; externships; interactive nursing skills videos; Internet; learning resource lab; library services; nursing audiovisuals; paid internships; remedial services; resume preparation assistance; skills, simulation, or other laboratory; tutoring.
Library Facilities 251,035 volumes (8,680 in health, 1,464 in nursing); 62,337 periodical subscriptions (4,315 health-care related).

BACCALAUREATE PROGRAMS

Degree BSN
Available Programs Accelerated Baccalaureate; Accelerated RN Baccalaureate; Generic Baccalaureate; LPN to Baccalaureate; RN Baccalaureate.
Study Options Full-time and part-time.
Program Entrance Requirements Minimum overall college GPA of 2.75, transcript of college record, health exam, high school transcript, immunizations, minimum high school GPA of 2.75, minimum GPA in nursing prerequisites of 2.75. Transfer students are accepted. *Application deadline:* 12/15 (fall). Applications may be processed on a rolling basis for some programs.
Advanced Placement Credit given for nursing courses completed elsewhere dependent upon specific evaluations.
Contact *Telephone:* 314-529-9453. *Fax:* 314-529-9495.

Contact *Telephone:* 314-529-9453. *Fax:* 314-529-9495.

MASTER'S DEGREE PROGRAM
Degree MSN
Available Programs Accelerated RN to Master's; Master's; RN to Master's.
Concentrations Available Nursing education. *Nurse practitioner programs in:* adult health, family health.
Study Options Full-time and part-time.
Program Entrance Requirements Minimum overall college GPA of 3.0, transcript of college record, written essay, 3 letters of recommendation, resume, statistics course. *Application deadline:* Applications may be processed on a rolling basis for some programs.
Advanced Placement Credit by examination available. Credit given for nursing courses completed elsewhere dependent upon specific evaluations.
Degree Requirements 42 total credit hours, thesis or project.

DOCTORAL DEGREE PROGRAM
Degree DNP
Available Programs Doctorate.
Areas of Study Advanced practice nursing, ethics, health policy, nursing research.
Program Entrance Requirements Minimum overall college GPA of 3.5, 3 letters of recommendation, MSN or equivalent, vita, writing sample. *Application deadline:* Applications may be processed on a rolling basis for some programs.
Degree Requirements 30 total credit hours.

Missouri Southern State University
Department of Nursing
Joplin, Missouri

http://www.mssu.edu/academics/technology/nursing/
Founded in 1937
DEGREES • BSN • MSN
Nursing Program Faculty 10 (10% with doctorates).
Baccalaureate Enrollment 107 **Women** 79.44% **Men** 20.56% **Minority** 12.15%
Graduate Enrollment 49 **Women** 96% **Men** 4% **Minority** 8% **Part-time** 31%
Distance Learning Courses Available.
Nursing Student Activities Nursing Honor Society, Student Nurses' Association.
Nursing Student Resources Academic advising; academic or career counseling; assistance for students with disabilities; bookstore; campus computer network; career placement assistance; computer lab; computer-assisted instruction; daycare for children of students; e-mail services; employment services for current students; housing assistance; interactive nursing skills videos; Internet; learning resource lab; library services; nursing audiovisuals; remedial services; resume preparation assistance; skills, simulation, or other laboratory; tutoring.
Library Facilities 4,872 volumes in health, 4,470 volumes in nursing; 4,412 periodical subscriptions health-care related.

BACCALAUREATE PROGRAMS

Degree BSN
Available Programs ADN to Baccalaureate; Baccalaureate for Second Degree; Generic Baccalaureate; LPN to Baccalaureate; RN Baccalaureate.
Study Options Full-time.
Program Entrance Requirements Transcript of college record, CPR certification, health exam, health insurance, immunizations, minimum GPA in nursing prerequisites of 2.5, professional liability insurance/malpractice insurance, prerequisite course work, RN licensure. Transfer students are accepted. *Application deadline:* 1/31 (fall). *Application fee:* $50.
Advanced Placement Credit by examination available. Credit given for nursing courses completed elsewhere dependent upon specific evaluations.
Expenses (2011–12) *Tuition, state resident:* full-time $5053. *Tuition, nonresident:* full-time $10,106. *International tuition:* $10,106 full-time.

Room and board: $5320; room only: $5160 per academic year. Required fees: full-time $3829.

Financial Aid 77% of baccalaureate students in nursing programs received some form of financial aid in 2010–11. *Gift aid (need-based):* Federal Pell, FSEOG, state, private, college/university gift aid from institutional funds, Teach Grants. *Loans:* Federal Direct (Subsidized and Unsubsidized Stafford PLUS), Perkins.*Work-study:* Federal Work-Study, part-time campus jobs.*Financial aid application deadline (priority):* 4/1.

Contact Dr. J. Mari Beth Linder, Director, Department of Nursing, Missouri Southern State University, Health Sciences Building, Room 243, 3950 East Newman Road, Joplin, MO 64801-1595. *Telephone:* 417-625-9322. *Fax:* 417-625-3186. *E-mail:* linder-m@mssu.edu.

GRADUATE PROGRAMS

Expenses (2011–12) *Tuition, area resident:* full-time $6764; part-time $322 per credit hour. *Room and board:* $5320; room only: $5160 per academic year.

Contact Dr. Mari Beth Linder, Director, Department of Nursing, Missouri Southern State University, Health Sciences Building, Room 243, 3950 East Newman Road, Joplin, MO 64801. *Telephone:* 417-625-9322. *Fax:* 417-625-3186. *E-mail:* linder-m@mssu.edu.

MASTER'S DEGREE PROGRAM

Degree MSN

Available Programs Master's.

Concentrations Available Nursing education. *Clinical nurse specialist programs in:* family health.

Study Options Full-time and part-time.

Program Entrance Requirements Minimum overall college GPA of 3.0, transcript of college record, resume. *Application deadline:* 12/1 (fall). *Application fee:* $35.

Degree Requirements 42 total credit hours.

Missouri State University
Department of Nursing
Springfield, Missouri

http://www.missouristate.edu/nursing
Founded in 1905

DEGREES • BSN • DNP • MSN

Nursing Program Faculty 14 (36% with doctorates).

Baccalaureate Enrollment 210 **Women** 90% **Men** 10% **Minority** 4% **International** 1% **Part-time** 25%

Graduate Enrollment 51 **Women** 97% **Men** 3% **Minority** 2% **Part-time** 40%

Distance Learning Courses Available.

Nursing Student Activities Sigma Theta Tau, Student Nurses' Association.

Nursing Student Resources Academic advising; academic or career counseling; assistance for students with disabilities; bookstore; campus computer network; career placement assistance; computer lab; computer-assisted instruction; daycare for children of students; e-mail services; employment services for current students; externships; housing assistance; interactive nursing skills videos; Internet; learning resource lab; library services; nursing audiovisuals; paid internships; placement services for program completers; remedial services; resume preparation assistance; skills, simulation, or other laboratory; tutoring; unpaid internships.

Library Facilities 1.6 million volumes (10,500 in health, 3,516 in nursing); 4,330 periodical subscriptions (370 health-care related).

BACCALAUREATE PROGRAMS

Degree BSN

Available Programs ADN to Baccalaureate; Accelerated RN Baccalaureate; Generic Baccalaureate; LPN to Baccalaureate; RN Baccalaureate.

Study Options Full-time.

Online Degree Options Yes.

Program Entrance Requirements Minimum overall college GPA of 2.75, transcript of college record, CPR certification, written essay, health insurance, immunizations, prerequisite course work. Transfer students are accepted. *Application deadline:* 1/31 (summer). *Application fee:* $50.

Advanced Placement Credit given for nursing courses completed elsewhere dependent upon specific evaluations.

Expenses (2012–13) *Tuition, state resident:* full-time $6264; part-time $200 per credit hour. *Tuition, nonresident:* full-time $12,610; part-time $412 per credit hour. *International tuition:* $12,610 full-time. *Room and*

---

board: $7204; room only: $5768 per academic year. *Required fees:* full-time $1228.

Financial Aid 65% of baccalaureate students in nursing programs received some form of financial aid in 2011–12.

Contact Dr. Kathryn L. Hope, Head, Department of Nursing, Department of Nursing, Missouri State University, 901 South National Avenue, Springfield, MO 65897. *Telephone:* 417-836-5310. *Fax:* 417-836-5484. *E-mail:* kathrynhope@missouristate.edu.

GRADUATE PROGRAMS

Expenses (2012–13) *Tuition, state resident:* full-time $4356; part-time $242 per credit hour. *Tuition, nonresident:* full-time $8712; part-time $484 per credit hour. *International tuition:* $8712 full-time. *Room and board:* $7204; room only: $5768 per academic year. *Required fees:* full-time $778.

Financial Aid 25% of graduate students in nursing programs received some form of financial aid in 2011–12. Federal Work-Study, institutionally sponsored loans, scholarships, and unspecified assistantships available. *Financial aid application deadline:* 3/31.

Contact Dr. Kathryn L. Hope, Head, Department of Nursing, Department of Nursing, Missouri State University, 901 South National Avenue, Springfield, MO 65897. *Telephone:* 417-836-5310. *Fax:* 417-836-5484. *E-mail:* kathrynhope@missouristate.edu.

MASTER'S DEGREE PROGRAM

Degree MSN

Available Programs Accelerated AD/RN to Master's; Master's; RN to Master's.

Concentrations Available Nursing education. *Nurse practitioner programs in:* family health.

Study Options Full-time and part-time.

Online Degree Options Yes (online only).

Program Entrance Requirements Computer literacy, minimum overall college GPA of 3.0, transcript of college record, CPR certification, written essay, immunizations, interview, nursing research course, physical assessment course, professional liability insurance/malpractice insurance, prerequisite course work, statistics course, GRE General Test. *Application deadline:* 2/15 (fall). *Application fee:* $50.

Advanced Placement Credit given for nursing courses completed elsewhere dependent upon specific evaluations.

Degree Requirements 51 total credit hours, thesis or project, comprehensive exam.

POST-MASTER'S PROGRAM

Areas of Study Nursing education. *Nurse practitioner programs in:* family health.

DOCTORAL DEGREE PROGRAM

Degree DNP

Available Programs Doctorate; Post-Baccalaureate Doctorate.

Areas of Study Advanced practice nursing, health-care systems.

Online Degree Options Yes.

Program Entrance Requirements Clinical experience, minimum overall college GPA of 3.25, interview by faculty committee, interview, statistics course, vita, writing sample. *Application deadline:* 12/1 (summer). *Application fee:* $50.

Degree Requirements 29 total credit hours, oral exam.

CONTINUING EDUCATION PROGRAM

Contact Virginia Cordova, Program Coordinator, Department of Nursing, Missouri State University, 901 South National Avenue, Department of Continuing Education, Springfield, MO 65897. *Telephone:* 417-836-6660. *Fax:* 417-836-7674. *E-mail:* virginiacordova@missouristate.edu.

Missouri Western State University
Department of Nursing
St. Joseph, Missouri

http://www.missouriwestern.edu/nursing
Founded in 1915

DEGREES • BSN • MSN

Nursing Program Faculty 35 (23% with doctorates).

Baccalaureate Enrollment 200 **Women** 86% **Men** 14% **Minority** 4% **Part-time** 7%

Graduate Enrollment 17 **Women** 100% **Part-time** 100%

Distance Learning Courses Available.

Nursing Student Activities Sigma Theta Tau, Student Nurses' Association.

Nursing Student Resources Academic advising; academic or career counseling; assistance for students with disabilities; bookstore; campus computer network; career placement assistance; computer lab; computer-assisted instruction; e-mail services; employment services for current students; interactive nursing skills videos; Internet; learning resource lab; library services; nursing audiovisuals; placement services for program completers; remedial services; resume preparation assistance; skills, simulation, or other laboratory; tutoring; unpaid internships.

Library Facilities 224,131 volumes; 3,214 periodical subscriptions (29 health-care related).

BACCALAUREATE PROGRAMS

Degree BSN

Available Programs ADN to Baccalaureate; Generic Baccalaureate.

Site Options Kansas City, MO.

Study Options Full-time.

Program Entrance Requirements Minimum overall college GPA of 2.7, transcript of college record, CPR certification, written essay, health insurance, high school transcript, immunizations, minimum GPA in nursing prerequisites of 2.7, prerequisite course work. Transfer students are accepted. *Application deadline:* 1/15 (fall), 7/31 (spring). *Application fee:* $45.

Advanced Placement Credit by examination available. Credit given for nursing courses completed elsewhere dependent upon specific evaluations.

Expenses (2012–13) *Tuition, state resident:* part-time $189 per credit. *Tuition, nonresident:* part-time $372 per credit. *Room and board:* $9036 per academic year.

Financial Aid 88% of baccalaureate students in nursing programs received some form of financial aid in 2011–12. *Gift aid (need-based):* Federal Pell, FSEOG, state, private, college/university gift aid from institutional funds. *Loans:* Federal Direct (Subsidized and Unsubsidized Stafford PLUS), Perkins. *Work-study:* Federal Work-Study, part-time campus jobs. *Financial aid application deadline:* Continuous.

Contact Rebecca Boettcher, Admissions/Advisement Counselor, Department of Nursing, Missouri Western State University, 4525 Downs Drive, Murphy Hall 309, St. Joseph, MO 64507. *Telephone:* 816-271-4415. *Fax:* 816-271-5849. *E-mail:* rboettcher@missouriwestern.edu.

GRADUATE PROGRAMS

Expenses (2012–13) *Tuition, state resident:* part-time $281 per credit hour. *Tuition, nonresident:* part-time $540 per credit hour.

Financial Aid 78% of graduate students in nursing programs received some form of financial aid in 2011–12.

Contact Dr. Kathleen E. O'Connor, Associate Professor and Chairperson, Department of Nursing, Missouri Western State University, 4525 Downs Drive, St. Joseph, MO 64507. *Telephone:* 816-271-4415. *Fax:* 816-271-5849. *E-mail:* koconnor5@missouriwestern.edu.

MASTER'S DEGREE PROGRAM

Degree MSN

Available Programs Master's.

Concentrations Available Health-care administration.

Study Options Part-time.

Program Entrance Requirements Minimum overall college GPA of 2.75, transcript of college record, written essay, interview, nursing research course, prerequisite course work, statistics course. *Application deadline:* 7/15 (fall), 10/15 (spring). *Application fee:* $30.

Degree Requirements 36 total credit hours, thesis or project.

CONTINUING EDUCATION PROGRAM

Contact Rebecca Boettcher, Admissions/Advisement Counselor, Department of Nursing, Missouri Western State University, 4525 Downs Drive, Murphy Hall 309, St. Joseph, MO 64507. *Telephone:* 816-271-4415. *Fax:* 816-271-5849. *E-mail:* rboettcher@missouriwestern.edu.

Research College of Nursing
College of Nursing
Kansas City, Missouri

http://www.researchcollege.edu/
Founded in 1980
DEGREES • BSN • MSN
Nursing Program Faculty 37 (16% with doctorates).
Baccalaureate Enrollment 306 **Women** 92% **Men** 8% **Minority** 7%
Graduate Enrollment 118 **Women** 95% **Men** 5% **Minority** 13% **Part-time** 90%
Distance Learning Courses Available.
Nursing Student Activities Sigma Theta Tau, Student Nurses' Association.
Nursing Student Resources Academic advising; academic or career counseling; bookstore; campus computer network; career placement assistance; computer lab; computer-assisted instruction; daycare for children of students; e-mail services; housing assistance; Internet; learning resource lab; library services; resume preparation assistance; skills, simulation, or other laboratory; tutoring.
Library Facilities 150,000 volumes; 675 periodical subscriptions.

BACCALAUREATE PROGRAMS

Degree BSN

Available Programs Accelerated Baccalaureate; Accelerated Baccalaureate for Second Degree; Baccalaureate for Second Degree; Generic Baccalaureate.

Study Options Full-time.

Program Entrance Requirements Transcript of college record, high school chemistry, 3 years high school math, 2 years high school science, high school transcript, minimum high school rank 50%, minimum GPA in nursing prerequisites of 2.7. Transfer students are accepted. *Application deadline:* 2/15 (spring). *Application fee:* $20.

Advanced Placement Credit given for nursing courses completed elsewhere dependent upon specific evaluations.

Expenses (2012–13) *Tuition:* full-time $29,100. *Room and board:* $7500; room only: $3600 per academic year. *Required fees:* full-time $370.

Financial Aid 90% of baccalaureate students in nursing programs received some form of financial aid in 2011–12.

Contact Ms. Leslie Ann Mendenhall, Director of Transfer and Graduate Admissions, College of Nursing, Research College of Nursing, 2525 East Meyer Boulevard, Kansas City, MO 64132-1199. *Telephone:* 816-995-2820. *Fax:* 816-995-2813. *E-mail:* leslie.mendenhall@researchcollege.edu.

GRADUATE PROGRAMS

Expenses (2012–13) *Tuition:* part-time $445 per credit. *Required fees:* part-time $25 per credit.

Financial Aid 15% of graduate students in nursing programs received some form of financial aid in 2011–12.

Contact Ms. Leslie Ann Mendenhall, Director of Transfer and Graduate Admissions, College of Nursing, Research College of Nursing, 2525 East Meyer Boulevard, Kansas City, MO 64132-1199. *Telephone:* 816-995-2820. *Fax:* 816-995-2813. *E-mail:* leslie.mendenhall@researchcollege.edu.

MASTER'S DEGREE PROGRAM
Degree MSN
Available Programs Master's; RN to Master's.
Concentrations Available Clinical nurse leader; nursing administration; nursing education. *Nurse practitioner programs in:* adult health, family health.
Study Options Full-time and part-time.
Online Degree Options Yes.
Program Entrance Requirements Minimum overall college GPA of 3.0, transcript of college record, written essay, interview, 3 letters of recommendation, physical assessment course, resume, statistics course. *Application deadline:* 8/1 (spring). *Application fee:* $50.
Advanced Placement Credit given for nursing courses completed elsewhere dependent upon specific evaluations.
Degree Requirements 45 total credit hours, thesis or project.

POST-MASTER'S PROGRAM
Areas of Study Clinical nurse leader; nursing administration; nursing education. *Nurse practitioner programs in:* adult health, family health.

Saint Louis University
School of Nursing
St. Louis, Missouri

http://nursing.slu.edu/
Founded in 1818
DEGREES • BSN • DNP • MN/MPH • MSN • PHD
Nursing Program Faculty 53 (60% with doctorates).
Baccalaureate Enrollment 589 **Women** 91% **Men** 9% **Minority** 14%
International 1% **Part-time** 8%
Graduate Enrollment 575 **Women** 91% **Men** 9% **Minority** 15% **Part-time** 70%
Distance Learning Courses Available.
Nursing Student Activities Sigma Theta Tau, Student Nurses' Association.
Nursing Student Resources Academic advising; academic or career counseling; assistance for students with disabilities; bookstore; campus computer network; career placement assistance; computer lab; e-mail services; employment services for current students; housing assistance; interactive nursing skills videos; Internet; library services; nursing audiovisuals; remedial services; resume preparation assistance; skills, simulation, or other laboratory; tutoring; unpaid internships.
Library Facilities 1.9 million volumes (275,000 in health, 4,800 in nursing); 13,049 periodical subscriptions (7,661 health-care related).

BACCALAUREATE PROGRAMS

Degree BSN
Available Programs Accelerated Baccalaureate; Accelerated Baccalaureate for Second Degree; Generic Baccalaureate; RN Baccalaureate.
Site Options St. Louis, MO.
Study Options Full-time and part-time.
Online Degree Options Yes.
Program Entrance Requirements Minimum overall college GPA of 3.4, transcript of college record, health exam, high school biology, high school chemistry, high school transcript, immunizations, minimum high school GPA of 3.2. Transfer students are accepted. *Application deadline:* 12/1 (fall).
Advanced Placement Credit by examination available. Credit given for nursing courses completed elsewhere dependent upon specific evaluations.
Expenses (2012–13) *Tuition:* full-time $34,740. *Room and board:* $10,000 per academic year. *Required fees:* full-time $506.
Financial Aid 97% of baccalaureate students in nursing programs received some form of financial aid in 2011–12.
Contact Mr. Scott Ragsdale, Recruitment Specialist, School of Nursing, Saint Louis University, 3525 Caroline Street, St. Louis, MO 63104. *Telephone:* 314-977-8995. *Fax:* 314-977-8949. *E-mail:* sragsda2@slu.edu.

GRADUATE PROGRAMS

Expenses (2012–13) *Tuition:* part-time $1010 per credit hour.
Financial Aid 50% of graduate students in nursing programs received some form of financial aid in 2011–12. 2 research assistantships (averaging $10,250 per year), 5 teaching assistantships with full tuition reimbursements available (averaging $11,000 per year) were awarded; Federal Work-Study, scholarships, traineeships, tuition waivers, and unspecified assistantships also available. Aid available to part-time students. *Financial aid application deadline:* 6/1.
Contact Dr. Mary Lee Barron, Advanced Practice Program Director, School of Nursing, Saint Louis University, 3525 Caroline Street, St. Louis, MO 63104. *Telephone:* 314-977-8978. *Fax:* 314-977-8949. *E-mail:* barronml@slu.edu.

MASTER'S DEGREE PROGRAM
Degrees MN/MPH; MSN
Available Programs Accelerated Master's for Non-Nursing College Graduates; Master's; Master's for Nurses with Non-Nursing Degrees.
Concentrations Available Nursing education. *Nurse practitioner programs in:* acute care, adult health, family health, gerontology, pediatric, psychiatric/mental health.
Site Options St. Louis, MO.
Study Options Full-time and part-time.
Online Degree Options Yes (online only).
Program Entrance Requirements Minimum overall college GPA of 3.2, transcript of college record, CPR certification, immunizations, 3 letters of recommendation, resume. *Application deadline:* 4/1 (fall), 9/1 (spring). *Application fee:* $55.
Advanced Placement Credit given for nursing courses completed elsewhere dependent upon specific evaluations.
Degree Requirements 39 total credit hours, comprehensive exam.

POST-MASTER'S PROGRAM
Areas of Study Nursing education. *Nurse practitioner programs in:* acute care, adult health, family health, gerontology, pediatric, psychiatric/mental health.

DOCTORAL DEGREE PROGRAM
Degree DNP
Available Programs Doctorate.
Areas of Study Advanced practice nursing.
Online Degree Options Yes (online only).
Program Entrance Requirements Minimum overall college GPA of 3.25, 3 letters of recommendation, MSN or equivalent, statistics course, vita, writing sample. *Application deadline:* 3/15 (fall). Applications may be processed on a rolling basis for some programs. *Application fee:* $40.
Degree Requirements 28 total credit hours, dissertation.

DOCTORAL DEGREE PROGRAM
Degree PhD
Available Programs Doctorate.
Areas of Study Advanced practice nursing, nursing research.
Site Options St. Louis, MO.
Program Entrance Requirements Minimum overall college GPA of 3.25, 3 letters of recommendation, MSN or equivalent, statistics course, vita, writing sample, GRE General Test. *Application deadline:* 4/1 (fall), 11/1 (spring), 4/1 (summer). Applications may be processed on a rolling basis for some programs. *Application fee:* $55.
Degree Requirements 69 total credit hours, dissertation, oral exam, written exam, residency.

CONTINUING EDUCATION PROGRAM

Contact Mrs. Cathi Slinkard, Continuing Education Director, School of Nursing, Saint Louis University, 3525 Caroline Street, St. Louis, MO 63104. *Telephone:* 314-977-1909. *Fax:* 314-977-8949. *E-mail:* cslinkar@slu.edu.

Saint Luke's College of Health Sciences
Nursing College
Kansas City, Missouri

http://www.saintlukescollege.edu/
Founded in 1903
DEGREE • BSN
Nursing Program Faculty 17 (18% with doctorates).
Baccalaureate Enrollment 115 **Women** 95% **Men** 5% **Minority** 10%
International 1% **Part-time** 12%
Nursing Student Activities Student Nurses' Association.
Nursing Student Resources Academic advising; assistance for students with disabilities; bookstore; campus computer network; career placement assistance; computer lab; computer-assisted instruction; e-mail services; employment services for current students; interactive nursing skills videos; Internet; learning resource lab; library services; nursing audiovisuals; paid internships; skills, simulation, or other laboratory; tutoring.

BACCALAUREATE PROGRAMS

Degree BSN
Available Programs Generic Baccalaureate.
Site Options Kansas City, MO.
Study Options Full-time and part-time.
Program Entrance Requirements Transcript of college record, CPR certification, written essay, health exam, health insurance, high school transcript, immunizations, interview, 3 letters of recommendation, minimum GPA in nursing prerequisites of 2.7, prerequisite course work. Transfer students are accepted.
Advanced Placement Credit given for nursing courses completed elsewhere dependent upon specific evaluations.
Contact *Telephone:* 816-932-2367.

Southeast Missouri State University

Department of Nursing
Cape Girardeau, Missouri

http://www.semo.edu/nursing
Founded in 1873
DEGREES • BSN • MSN
Nursing Program Faculty 30 (45% with doctorates).
Baccalaureate Enrollment 495 **Women** 95% **Men** 5% **Minority** 7% **International** 3% **Part-time** 20%
Graduate Enrollment 50 **Women** 80% **Men** 20% **Minority** 2% **Part-time** 65%
Distance Learning Courses Available.
Nursing Student Activities Sigma Theta Tau, Student Nurses' Association.
Nursing Student Resources Academic advising; academic or career counseling; assistance for students with disabilities; bookstore; campus computer network; computer lab; computer-assisted instruction; e-mail services; employment services for current students; externships; housing assistance; interactive nursing skills videos; Internet; learning resource lab; library services; nursing audiovisuals; remedial services; resume preparation assistance; skills, simulation, or other laboratory; tutoring.
Library Facilities 434,408 volumes (450,750 in health, 16,145 in nursing); 61,161 periodical subscriptions (75 health-care related).

BACCALAUREATE PROGRAMS

Degree BSN
Available Programs Accelerated Baccalaureate for Second Degree; Generic Baccalaureate; RN Baccalaureate.
Site Options Poplar Bluff, MO; Sikeston, MO; Kennett, MO.
Study Options Full-time.
Online Degree Options Yes.
Program Entrance Requirements Minimum overall college GPA of 2.5, transcript of college record, CPR certification, health exam, health insurance, immunizations, minimum GPA in nursing prerequisites of 2.5, professional liability insurance/malpractice insurance, prerequisite course work. Transfer students are accepted. *Application deadline:* 3/1 (fall), 10/1 (spring).
Advanced Placement Credit given for nursing courses completed elsewhere dependent upon specific evaluations.
Contact *Telephone:* 573-651-2956. *Fax:* 573-651-2142.

GRADUATE PROGRAMS

Contact *Telephone:* 573-651-2871. *Fax:* 573-651-2142.

MASTER'S DEGREE PROGRAM
Degree MSN
Available Programs Master's.
Concentrations Available Nursing education. *Clinical nurse specialist programs in:* adult health. *Nurse practitioner programs in:* family health.
Site Options Poplar Bluff, MO; Sikeston, MO; Kennett, MO.
Study Options Full-time and part-time.
Program Entrance Requirements Clinical experience, minimum overall college GPA of 3.0, transcript of college record, CPR certification, written essay, immunizations, 2 letters of recommendation, physical assessment course, professional liability insurance/malpractice insurance, prerequisite course work, resume, statistics course.
Degree Requirements 45 total credit hours, thesis or project.

POST-MASTER'S PROGRAM
Areas of Study *Nurse practitioner programs in:* family health.

Southwest Baptist University

College of Nursing
Bolivar, Missouri

http://www.sbuniv.edu/collegeofnursing
Founded in 1878
DEGREES • BSN • MSN
Nursing Program Faculty 12 (25% with doctorates).

Baccalaureate Enrollment 143 **Women** 87.5% **Men** 12.5% **Minority** 2.1% **Part-time** 82.5%
Graduate Enrollment 31 **Women** 96.8% **Men** 3.2% **Part-time** 74.1%
Distance Learning Courses Available.
Nursing Student Activities Nursing Honor Society, Student Nurses' Association.
Nursing Student Resources Academic advising; bookstore; campus computer network; computer lab; computer-assisted instruction; e-mail services; interactive nursing skills videos; Internet; learning resource lab; library services; nursing audiovisuals; skills, simulation, or other laboratory.
Library Facilities 222,145 volumes (4,042 in health, 3,602 in nursing); 32,160 periodical subscriptions (41,500 health-care related).

BACCALAUREATE PROGRAMS

Degree BSN
Available Programs RN Baccalaureate.
Site Options Springfield, MO.
Study Options Full-time and part-time.
Program Entrance Requirements Minimum overall college GPA of 2.5, transcript of college record, CPR certification, high school transcript, immunizations, letters of recommendation, minimum GPA in nursing prerequisites of 2.5, professional liability insurance/malpractice insurance, prerequisite course work, RN licensure. Transfer students are accepted. *Application deadline:* 8/15 (fall), 1/1 (winter), 1/15 (spring), 6/1 (summer). Applications may be processed on a rolling basis for some programs.
Advanced Placement Credit given for nursing courses completed elsewhere dependent upon specific evaluations.
Expenses (2012–13) *Tuition:* full-time $7440; part-time $310 per credit hour. *International tuition:* $7440 full-time. *Room and board:* $6350; room only: $3150 per academic year. *Required fees:* full-time $910; part-time $600 per credit.
Financial Aid 70% of baccalaureate students in nursing programs received some form of financial aid in 2011–12. *Gift aid (need-based):* Federal Pell, FSEOG, state, private, college/university gift aid from institutional funds. *Loans:* Federal Nursing Student Loans, Federal Direct (Subsidized and Unsubsidized Stafford PLUS), Perkins, state, alternative loans. *Work-study:* Federal Work-Study. *Financial aid application deadline (priority):* 3/15.
Contact Ms. Dana Hunt, Director, BSN Program, College of Nursing, Southwest Baptist University, 4431 South Fremont Avenue, Springfield, MO 65804. *Telephone:* 417-820-5060. *Fax:* 417-887-4847. *E-mail:* dhunt@sbuniv.edu.

GRADUATE PROGRAMS

Expenses (2012–13) *Tuition:* full-time $9600; part-time $400 per credit hour. *International tuition:* $9600 full-time. *Required fees:* full-time $1820.
Financial Aid 60% of graduate students in nursing programs received some form of financial aid in 2011–12.
Contact Dr. Martha Cheryl Baker, Dean, College of Nursing, Southwest Baptist University, 4431 South Fremont Avenue, Springfield, MO 65804. *Telephone:* 417-820-5058. *Fax:* 417-887-4847. *E-mail:* mbaker@sbuniv.edu.

MASTER'S DEGREE PROGRAM
Degree MSN
Available Programs Master's.
Concentrations Available Nursing administration; nursing education.
Site Options Springfield, MO.
Study Options Full-time and part-time.
Online Degree Options Yes.
Program Entrance Requirements Computer literacy, minimum overall college GPA of 3.0, transcript of college record, CPR certification, written essay, immunizations, letters of recommendation, nursing research course, physical assessment course, professional liability insurance/malpractice insurance, statistics course. *Application deadline:* 7/15 (fall), 1/1 (spring). Applications may be processed on a rolling basis for some programs. *Application fee:* $30.
Advanced Placement Credit given for nursing courses completed elsewhere dependent upon specific evaluations.
Degree Requirements 36 total credit hours, thesis or project, comprehensive exam.

Truman State University
Program in Nursing
Kirksville, Missouri

http://nursing.truman.edu/
Founded in 1867
DEGREE • BSN
Nursing Program Faculty 11 (18% with doctorates).
Baccalaureate Enrollment 172 **Women** 94% **Men** 6% **Minority** 5% **International** 5% **Part-time** 1%
Nursing Student Activities Nursing Honor Society, Sigma Theta Tau, Student Nurses' Association, nursing club.
Nursing Student Resources Academic advising; academic or career counseling; assistance for students with disabilities; bookstore; campus computer network; career placement assistance; computer lab; computer-assisted instruction; e-mail services; employment services for current students; externships; interactive nursing skills videos; Internet; learning resource lab; library services; nursing audiovisuals; paid internships; remedial services; resume preparation assistance; skills, simulation, or other laboratory; tutoring; unpaid internships.
Library Facilities 508,801 volumes (6,923 in health, 1,654 in nursing); 3,439 periodical subscriptions (900 health-care related).

BACCALAUREATE PROGRAMS

Degree BSN
Available Programs Generic Baccalaureate.
Study Options Full-time.
Program Entrance Requirements Minimum overall college GPA of 2.75, transcript of college record, written essay, high school biology, high school chemistry, high school foreign language, 3 years high school math, 3 years high school science, high school transcript, immunizations, minimum high school GPA of 3.3, minimum GPA in nursing prerequisites of 3.0. Transfer students are accepted.
Contact *Telephone:* 660-785-4557. *Fax:* 660-785-7424.

University of Central Missouri
Department of Nursing
Warrensburg, Missouri

http://www.ucmo.edu/nursing
Founded in 1871
DEGREES • BS • MS
Nursing Program Faculty 17 (35% with doctorates).
Baccalaureate Enrollment 146 **Women** 96% **Men** 4% **Minority** 8% **International** 3%
Graduate Enrollment 153 **Women** 94% **Men** 6% **Minority** 7% **International** 2% **Part-time** 97%
Distance Learning Courses Available.
Nursing Student Activities Nursing club.
Nursing Student Resources Academic advising; academic or career counseling; assistance for students with disabilities; bookstore; campus computer network; career placement assistance; computer lab; computer-assisted instruction; daycare for children of students; e-mail services; employment services for current students; externships; housing assistance; interactive nursing skills videos; Internet; learning resource lab; library services; nursing audiovisuals; placement services for program completers; remedial services; resume preparation assistance; skills, simulation, or other laboratory; tutoring.
Library Facilities 1.3 million volumes (17,000 in health, 1,000 in nursing); 835 periodical subscriptions (300 health-care related).

BACCALAUREATE PROGRAMS

Degree BS
Available Programs ADN to Baccalaureate; Generic Baccalaureate; RN Baccalaureate.
Site Options Lee's Summit, MO; Warrensburg, MO.
Study Options Full-time.
Online Degree Options Yes.
Program Entrance Requirements Minimum overall college GPA of 2.75, minimum GPA in nursing prerequisites of 2.0, prerequisite course work. Transfer students are accepted. *Application deadline:* 1/1 (fall), 7/1 (spring). *Application fee:* $45.

Advanced Placement Credit by examination available. Credit given for nursing courses completed elsewhere dependent upon specific evaluations.
Expenses (2012–13) *Tuition, state resident:* full-time $7147; part-time $238 per credit hour. *Tuition, nonresident:* full-time $13,435; part-time $448 per credit hour. *International tuition:* $13,435 full-time. *Room and board:* $6173; room only: $4888 per academic year. *Required fees:* full-time $400.
Financial Aid 89% of baccalaureate students in nursing programs received some form of financial aid in 2011–12.
Contact Dr. Julie Ann Clawson, Chair, Department of Nursing, University of Central Missouri, 600 South College, UHC 106A, Warrensburg, MO 64093. *Telephone:* 660-543-4775. *Fax:* 660-543-8304. *E-mail:* clawson@ucmo.edu.

GRADUATE PROGRAMS

Expenses (2012–13) *Tuition, state resident:* full-time $3603; part-time $300 per credit hour. *Tuition, nonresident:* full-time $6863; part-time $572 per credit hour. *International tuition:* $6863 full-time. *Room and board:* $6173; room only: $4888 per academic year.
Financial Aid 70% of graduate students in nursing programs received some form of financial aid in 2011–12.
Contact Dr. Joseph Vaughn, Dean, Department of Nursing, University of Central Missouri, Graduate Studies, WDE 1800, Warrensburg, MO 64093. *Telephone:* 660-543-4621. *E-mail:* vaughn@ucmo.edu.

MASTER'S DEGREE PROGRAM
Degree MS
Available Programs Master's.
Concentrations Available Nursing education. *Nurse practitioner programs in:* family health.
Site Options Lee's Summit, MO; Warrensburg, MO.
Study Options Part-time.
Online Degree Options Yes (online only).
Program Entrance Requirements Clinical experience, minimum overall college GPA of 3.0, transcript of college record, CPR certification, immunizations, professional liability insurance/malpractice insurance. *Application deadline:* 2/15 (fall), 9/15 (spring), 2/15 (summer). Applications may be processed on a rolling basis for some programs.
Advanced Placement Credit given for nursing courses completed elsewhere dependent upon specific evaluations.
Degree Requirements 32 total credit hours, thesis or project.

University of Missouri
Sinclair School of Nursing
Columbia, Missouri

http://nursing.missouri.edu/
Founded in 1839
DEGREES • BSN • MSN • MSN/PHD • PHD
Baccalaureate Enrollment 380 **Women** 90% **Men** 10% **Minority** 6% **International** 3% **Part-time** 31%
Graduate Enrollment 200 **Women** 95% **Men** 5% **Minority** 8% **International** 2% **Part-time** 77%
Distance Learning Courses Available.
Nursing Student Activities Nursing Honor Society, Sigma Theta Tau, Student Nurses' Association, nursing club.
Nursing Student Resources Academic advising; academic or career counseling; assistance for students with disabilities; bookstore; campus computer network; career placement assistance; computer lab; computer-assisted instruction; daycare for children of students; e-mail services; employment services for current students; externships; housing assistance; interactive nursing skills videos; Internet; learning resource lab; library services; nursing audiovisuals; paid internships; remedial services; resume preparation assistance; skills, simulation, or other laboratory; tutoring; unpaid internships.
Library Facilities 3.6 million volumes (114,580 in health, 6,416 in nursing); 45,438 periodical subscriptions.

BACCALAUREATE PROGRAMS

Degree BSN
Available Programs ADN to Baccalaureate; Accelerated Baccalaureate; Accelerated Baccalaureate for Second Degree; Generic Baccalaureate; RN Baccalaureate.
Study Options Full-time and part-time.

Online Degree Options Yes.
Program Entrance Requirements Minimum overall college GPA of 2.5, transcript of college record, CPR certification, high school biology, high school chemistry, 4 years high school math, 3 years high school science, high school transcript, immunizations, interview, minimum GPA in nursing prerequisites of 2.5, prerequisite course work. Transfer students are accepted.
Advanced Placement Credit by examination available. Credit given for nursing courses completed elsewhere dependent upon specific evaluations.
Contact *Telephone:* 573-882-0277. *Fax:* 573-884-4544.

GRADUATE PROGRAMS

Contact *Telephone:* 573-882-0277.

MASTER'S DEGREE PROGRAM
Degrees MSN; MSN/PhD
Available Programs Master's.
Concentrations Available Nursing administration; nursing education. *Clinical nurse specialist programs in:* acute care, adult health, cardiovascular, community health, critical care, home health care, maternity-newborn, oncology, palliative care, pediatric, public health, rehabilitation, school health, women's health. *Nurse practitioner programs in:* family health, gerontology, pediatric, primary care, psychiatric/mental health.
Study Options Full-time and part-time.
Online Degree Options Yes (online only).
Program Entrance Requirements Computer literacy, minimum overall college GPA of 3.0, transcript of college record, CPR certification, immunizations, interview, 2 letters of recommendation, nursing research course, prerequisite course work, statistics course, GRE General Test.
Advanced Placement Credit given for nursing courses completed elsewhere dependent upon specific evaluations.
Degree Requirements 43 total credit hours, comprehensive exam.

POST-MASTER'S PROGRAM
Areas of Study Nursing administration; nursing education. *Clinical nurse specialist programs in:* acute care, adult health, cardiovascular, community health, critical care, home health care, maternity-newborn, oncology, palliative care, pediatric, public health, rehabilitation, school health, women's health. *Nurse practitioner programs in:* family health, gerontology, pediatric, primary care, psychiatric/mental health.

DOCTORAL DEGREE PROGRAM
Degree PhD
Available Programs Doctorate; Post-Baccalaureate Doctorate.
Areas of Study Aging, family health, gerontology, health promotion/disease prevention, health-care systems, human health and illness, nursing research, oncology, women's health.
Program Entrance Requirements Minimum overall college GPA of 3.5, interview by faculty committee, 3 letters of recommendation, vita, writing sample.
Degree Requirements 72 total credit hours, dissertation, oral exam, written exam, residency.

CONTINUING EDUCATION PROGRAM

Contact *Telephone:* 573-882-0215. *Fax:* 573-884-4544.

University of Missouri–Kansas City
School of Nursing
Kansas City, Missouri

http://www.umkc.edu/nursing
Founded in 1929
DEGREES • BSN • MSN • PHD
Nursing Program Faculty 48 (44% with doctorates).
Baccalaureate Enrollment 462 **Women** 90% **Men** 10% **Minority** 19% **International** .01% **Part-time** 27%
Graduate Enrollment 381 **Women** 93% **Men** 7% **Minority** 10% **Part-time** 87%
Distance Learning Courses Available.
Nursing Student Activities Sigma Theta Tau, Student Nurses' Association.

Nursing Student Resources Academic advising; academic or career counseling; assistance for students with disabilities; bookstore; campus computer network; career placement assistance; computer lab; computer-assisted instruction; e-mail services; employment services for current students; housing assistance; interactive nursing skills videos; Internet; learning resource lab; library services; nursing audiovisuals; other; placement services for program completers; remedial services; resume preparation assistance; skills, simulation, or other laboratory; tutoring.
Library Facilities 1.6 million volumes (111,108 in health, 15,000 in nursing); 49,032 periodical subscriptions (60,000 health-care related).

BACCALAUREATE PROGRAMS

Degree BSN
Available Programs Accelerated Baccalaureate; Generic Baccalaureate; RN Baccalaureate.
Study Options Full-time.
Program Entrance Requirements Minimum overall college GPA of 2.75, transcript of college record, CPR certification, written essay, health insurance, high school foreign language, 4 years high school math, 4 years high school science, high school transcript, immunizations, 1 letter of recommendation, minimum GPA in nursing prerequisites of 2.75, professional liability insurance/malpractice insurance, prerequisite course work. Transfer students are accepted. *Application deadline:* 1/31 (fall).
Contact *Telephone:* 816-235-1740. *Fax:* 816-235-6593.

GRADUATE PROGRAMS

Contact *Telephone:* 816-235-1740. *Fax:* 816-235-6593.

MASTER'S DEGREE PROGRAM
Degree MSN
Available Programs Master's.
Concentrations Available Nursing education. *Nurse practitioner programs in:* adult health, family health, neonatal health, pediatric, women's health.
Site Options Joplin, MO; St. Joseph, MO.
Study Options Full-time and part-time.
Program Entrance Requirements Clinical experience, computer literacy, minimum overall college GPA of 3.2, transcript of college record, CPR certification, written essay, immunizations, 3 letters of recommendation, physical assessment course, professional liability insurance/malpractice insurance, resume, statistics course. *Application deadline:* 12/1 (fall), 12/1 (summer). *Application fee:* $35.
Degree Requirements 43 total credit hours.

POST-MASTER'S PROGRAM
Areas of Study Nursing education. *Nurse practitioner programs in:* adult health, family health, neonatal health, pediatric, women's health.

DOCTORAL DEGREE PROGRAM
Degree PhD
Available Programs Doctorate; Post-Baccalaureate Doctorate.
Areas of Study Health promotion/disease prevention, health-care systems.
Program Entrance Requirements Minimum overall college GPA of 3.5, interview by faculty committee, interview, 3 letters of recommendation, MSN or equivalent, vita, writing sample, GRE. *Application deadline:* 2/1 (summer). *Application fee:* $35.
Degree Requirements 61 total credit hours, dissertation, oral exam, written exam, residency.

CONTINUING EDUCATION PROGRAM

Contact *Telephone:* 816-235-6463. *Fax:* 816-235-1701.

University of Missouri–St. Louis
College of Nursing
St. Louis, Missouri

http://www.umsl.edu/divisions/nursing/
Founded in 1963
DEGREES • BSN • DNP • MSN
Nursing Program Faculty 83 (25% with doctorates).
Baccalaureate Enrollment 843 **Women** 85% **Men** 15% **Minority** 25% **Part-time** 33%
Graduate Enrollment 227 **Women** 94% **Men** 6% **Minority** 17% **Part-time** 100%

Distance Learning Courses Available.

Nursing Student Activities Nursing Honor Society, Sigma Theta Tau, Student Nurses' Association.

Nursing Student Resources Academic advising; academic or career counseling; assistance for students with disabilities; bookstore; campus computer network; career placement assistance; computer lab; computer-assisted instruction; daycare for children of students; e-mail services; employment services for current students; externships; interactive nursing skills videos; Internet; learning resource lab; library services; nursing audiovisuals; resume preparation assistance; skills, simulation, or other laboratory; tutoring; unpaid internships.

Library Facilities 1.2 million volumes (90,905 in health, 18,413 in nursing); 2,940 periodical subscriptions (7,190 health-care related).

BACCALAUREATE PROGRAMS

Degree BSN

Available Programs Accelerated Baccalaureate; Baccalaureate for Second Degree; Generic Baccalaureate; RN Baccalaureate.

Site Options Bridgeton, MO; Creve Coeur, MO; St. Louis, MO; St. Charles, MO.

Study Options Full-time and part-time.

Online Degree Options Yes.

Program Entrance Requirements Minimum overall college GPA of 2.5, transcript of college record, CPR certification, health exam, 4 years high school math, 3 years high school science, high school transcript, immunizations, minimum high school GPA of 2.5, minimum GPA in nursing prerequisites, professional liability insurance/malpractice insurance. Transfer students are accepted. *Application deadline:* 2/1 (fall), 10/1 (spring). *Application fee:* $35.

Advanced Placement Credit given for nursing courses completed elsewhere dependent upon specific evaluations.

Expenses (2012–13) *Tuition, state resident:* full-time $7968; part-time $266 per credit hour. *Tuition, nonresident:* full-time $21,537; part-time $718 per credit hour. *International tuition:* $21,537 full-time. *Room and board:* $8690; room only: $3490 per academic year. *Required fees:* full-time $1346.

Financial Aid 77% of baccalaureate students in nursing programs received some form of financial aid in 2011–12.

Contact Dr. Sandra J. Lindquist, Associate Dean for the Undergraduate Program, College of Nursing, University of Missouri–St. Louis, One University Boulevard, 233 Nursing Administration Building, St. Louis, MO 63121-4499. *Telephone:* 314-516-6066. *Fax:* 314-516-7519. *E-mail:* sandy_lindquist@umsl.edu.

GRADUATE PROGRAMS

Expenses (2012–13) *Tuition, state resident:* full-time $8364; part-time $349 per credit hour. *Tuition, nonresident:* full-time $21,595; part-time $900 per credit hour. *International tuition:* $21,595 full-time. *Room and board:* $8690; room only: $3490 per academic year. *Required fees:* full-time $1268.

Financial Aid 55% of graduate students in nursing programs received some form of financial aid in 2011–12. 3 research assistantships with full and partial tuition reimbursements available (averaging $12,339 per year) were awarded. *Financial aid application deadline:* 4/1.

Contact Dr. Nancy Magnuson, Acting Associate Dean for Advanced Nursing Education, College of Nursing, University of Missouri–St. Louis, One University Boulevard, Nursing Administration Building, St. Louis, MO 63121-4499. *Telephone:* 314-516-6066. *Fax:* 314-516-7519. *E-mail:* magnusonn@umsl.edu.

MASTER'S DEGREE PROGRAM

Degree MSN

Available Programs Master's.

Concentrations Available Nursing education. *Nurse practitioner programs in:* adult health, family health, neonatal health, pediatric, women's health.

Site Options Park Hills, MO; Town & Country, MO; St. Charles, MO.

Study Options Full-time and part-time.

Online Degree Options Yes.

Program Entrance Requirements Clinical experience, minimum overall college GPA of 3.0, transcript of college record, CPR certification, immunizations, 2 letters of recommendation, physical assessment course, statistics course. *Application deadline:* 2/15 (fall), 10/1 (spring). *Application fee:* $35.

Advanced Placement Credit given for nursing courses completed elsewhere dependent upon specific evaluations.

Degree Requirements 43 total credit hours.

POST-MASTER'S PROGRAM

Areas of Study *Nurse practitioner programs in:* adult health, family health, pediatric, women's health.

DOCTORAL DEGREE PROGRAM

Degree DNP

Available Programs Doctorate.

Areas of Study Advanced practice nursing.

Program Entrance Requirements Minimum overall college GPA of 3.0, interview, 2 letters of recommendation, MSN or equivalent, statistics course, writing sample, GRE. *Application deadline:* 4/1 (fall). *Application fee:* $35.

Degree Requirements 30 total credit hours, dissertation.

CONTINUING EDUCATION PROGRAM

Contact Vanessa Loyd, Director of Continuing Education and Outreach, College of Nursing, University of Missouri–St. Louis, One University Boulevard, St. Louis, MO 63121-4400. *Telephone:* 314-516-6066. *Fax:* 314-516-6730. *E-mail:* loydv@umsl.edu.

Webster University
Department of Nursing
St. Louis, Missouri

http://www.webster.edu/depts/artsci/nursing/nursing.html

Founded in 1915

DEGREES • BSN • MSN

Nursing Program Faculty 12 (72% with doctorates).

Baccalaureate Enrollment 150 **Women** 93% **Men** 7% **Minority** 14% **International** 1% **Part-time** 90%

Graduate Enrollment 75 **Women** 90% **Men** 10% **Minority** 20% **International** 10% **Part-time** 100%

Nursing Student Activities Nursing Honor Society, Sigma Theta Tau.

Nursing Student Resources Academic advising; academic or career counseling; assistance for students with disabilities; bookstore; campus computer network; career placement assistance; computer lab; e-mail services; employment services for current students; Internet; learning resource lab; library services; nursing audiovisuals; placement services for program completers; remedial services; resume preparation assistance; skills, simulation, or other laboratory; tutoring.

Library Facilities 284,852 volumes (7,030 in health, 3,114 in nursing); 1,509 periodical subscriptions (108 health-care related).

BACCALAUREATE PROGRAMS

Degree BSN

Available Programs ADN to Baccalaureate; RN Baccalaureate.

Site Options Kansas City, MO.

Program Entrance Requirements Minimum overall college GPA of 2.5, transcript of college record, immunizations, interview, prerequisite course work, RN licensure. Transfer students are accepted.

Contact *Telephone:* 314-968-7483. *Fax:* 314-963-6101.

GRADUATE PROGRAMS

Contact *Telephone:* 314-968-7483. *Fax:* 314-963-6101.

MASTER'S DEGREE PROGRAM

Degree MSN

Available Programs Master's; RN to Master's.

Concentrations Available Nursing administration; nursing education. *Clinical nurse specialist programs in:* family health.

Site Options Kansas City, MO.

Study Options Part-time.

Program Entrance Requirements Clinical experience, computer literacy, minimum overall college GPA of 3.0, transcript of college record, written essay, immunizations, interview, 3 letters of recommendation, nursing research course, physical assessment course, resume, statistics course.

Advanced Placement Credit given for nursing courses completed elsewhere dependent upon specific evaluations.

Degree Requirements 36 total credit hours, thesis or project.

William Jewell College
Department of Nursing
Liberty, Missouri

http://www.jewell.edu/
Founded in 1849
DEGREE • BS
Nursing Program Faculty 36 (25% with doctorates).
Baccalaureate Enrollment 150 **Women** 89% **Men** 11% **Minority** 3% **International** 1%
Nursing Student Activities Nursing Honor Society, Sigma Theta Tau, Student Nurses' Association.
Nursing Student Resources Academic advising; academic or career counseling; assistance for students with disabilities; bookstore; campus computer network; career placement assistance; computer lab; computer-assisted instruction; e-mail services; employment services for current students; externships; housing assistance; interactive nursing skills videos; Internet; learning resource lab; library services; nursing audiovisuals; paid internships; placement services for program completers; resume preparation assistance; skills, simulation, or other laboratory; tutoring; unpaid internships.
Library Facilities 172,159 volumes (4,000 in health, 1,000 in nursing); 747 periodical subscriptions (250 health-care related).

BACCALAUREATE PROGRAMS

Degree BS
Available Programs Accelerated Baccalaureate; Generic Baccalaureate.
Study Options Full-time.
Program Entrance Requirements Minimum overall college GPA of 2.7, transcript of college record, CPR certification, written essay, health insurance, high school foreign language, high school transcript, immunizations, interview, 2 letters of recommendation, minimum high school GPA of 3.0, minimum GPA in nursing prerequisites of 2.7, professional liability insurance/malpractice insurance, prerequisite course work. Transfer students are accepted. *Application deadline:* 6/1 (spring), 8/1 (summer). *Application fee:* $25.
Advanced Placement Credit given for nursing courses completed elsewhere dependent upon specific evaluations.
Contact *Telephone:* 816-415-5072. *Fax:* 816-415-5024.

MONTANA

Carroll College
Department of Nursing
Helena, Montana

http://www.carroll.edu/
Founded in 1909
DEGREE • BS
Nursing Program Faculty 18 (5% with doctorates).
Baccalaureate Enrollment 119 **Women** 87% **Men** 13% **Minority** 1% **Part-time** 3%
Nursing Student Activities Nursing Honor Society, Sigma Theta Tau, Student Nurses' Association, nursing club.
Nursing Student Resources Academic advising; academic or career counseling; assistance for students with disabilities; bookstore; campus computer network; career placement assistance; computer lab; computer-assisted instruction; e-mail services; employment services for current students; externships; housing assistance; interactive nursing skills videos; Internet; learning resource lab; library services; nursing audiovisuals; paid internships; placement services for program completers; remedial services; resume preparation assistance; skills, simulation, or other laboratory; tutoring; unpaid internships.
Library Facilities 3,250 volumes in health, 3,200 volumes in nursing; 2 periodical subscriptions health-care related.

BACCALAUREATE PROGRAMS

Degree BS
Available Programs Generic Baccalaureate.
Study Options Full-time.

Program Entrance Requirements Minimum overall college GPA of 2.75, transcript of college record, written essay, health insurance, high school transcript, immunizations, minimum GPA in nursing prerequisites of 2.75, prerequisite course work. Transfer students are accepted. *Application deadline:* 3/1 (spring).
Expenses (2012–13) *Tuition:* full-time $26,004; part-time $1094 per credit. *International tuition:* $26,004 full-time. *Room and board:* $8062; room only: $4292 per academic year. *Required fees:* full-time $1265; part-time $640 per term.
Financial Aid 95% of baccalaureate students in nursing programs received some form of financial aid in 2011–12. *Gift aid (need-based):* Federal Pell, FSEOG, state, private, college/university gift aid from institutional funds. *Loans:* Federal Direct (Subsidized and Unsubsidized Stafford PLUS), Perkins, private loans. *Work-study:* Federal Work-Study, part-time campus jobs. *Financial aid application deadline (priority):* 3/1.
Contact Ms. Cynthia Thornquist, Director of Admissions and Enrollment, Department of Nursing, Carroll College, 1601 North Benton Avenue, Helena, MT 59625. *Telephone:* 406-447-4384. *Fax:* 406-447-4533. *E-mail:* cthornqu@carroll.edu.

Montana State University
College of Nursing
Bozeman, Montana

http://www.montana.edu/nursing
Founded in 1893
DEGREES • BSN • DNP • MN
Nursing Program Faculty 115 (22% with doctorates).
Baccalaureate Enrollment 884 **Women** 87.6% **Men** 12.4% **Minority** 16.2% **International** .01% **Part-time** 17.4%
Graduate Enrollment 81 **Women** 93.8% **Men** 6.2% **Minority** 6.1% **Part-time** 55.5%
Distance Learning Courses Available.
Nursing Student Activities Sigma Theta Tau, Student Nurses' Association.
Nursing Student Resources Academic advising; academic or career counseling; assistance for students with disabilities; bookstore; campus computer network; career placement assistance; computer lab; computer-assisted instruction; daycare for children of students; e-mail services; employment services for current students; housing assistance; Internet; library services; nursing audiovisuals; paid internships; placement services for program completers; remedial services; resume preparation assistance; skills, simulation, or other laboratory; tutoring; unpaid internships.
Library Facilities 817 volumes (80,389 in health, 11,535 in nursing); 14,958 periodical subscriptions (1,690 health-care related).

BACCALAUREATE PROGRAMS

Degree BSN
Available Programs Accelerated Baccalaureate for Second Degree; Baccalaureate for Second Degree; Generic Baccalaureate; LPN to Baccalaureate.
Site Options Billings, MT; Great Falls, MT; Missoula, MT.
Study Options Full-time and part-time.
Program Entrance Requirements Minimum overall college GPA of 2.75, transcript of college record, CPR certification, health insurance, high school transcript, immunizations, minimum high school GPA of 2.5, minimum high school rank 50%, minimum GPA in nursing prerequisites of 2.75, prerequisite course work. Transfer students are accepted. *Application deadline:* 7/1 (fall), 12/1 (spring), 5/1 (summer). Applications may be processed on a rolling basis for some programs. *Application fee:* $30.
Advanced Placement Credit by examination available. Credit given for nursing courses completed elsewhere dependent upon specific evaluations.
Expenses (2012–13) *Tuition, state resident:* full-time $5330; part-time $222 per credit. *Tuition, nonresident:* full-time $18,598; part-time $774 per credit. *International tuition:* $18,598 full-time. *Required fees:* full-time $1760; part-time $120 per credit; part-time $880 per term.
Financial Aid 70% of baccalaureate students in nursing programs received some form of financial aid in 2011–12.
Contact Ms. Melissa Gutzman, Undergraduate Student Services Coordinator, College of Nursing, Montana State University, 111 Sherrick Hall, PO Box 173560, Bozeman, MT 59717-3560. *Telephone:* 406-994-3783. *Fax:* 406-994-6020. *E-mail:* melissak@montana.edu.

GRADUATE PROGRAMS

Expenses (2012–13) *Tuition, state resident:* full-time $6396; part-time $266 per credit. *Tuition, nonresident:* full-time $19,664; part-time $819 per credit. *International tuition:* $19,664 full-time. *Required fees:* full-time $2697; part-time $159 per credit; part-time $1348 per term.
Financial Aid 70% of graduate students in nursing programs received some form of financial aid in 2011–12. 8 teaching assistantships with partial tuition reimbursements available (averaging $7,050 per year) were awarded; scholarships, traineeships, and tuition waivers (partial) also available. *Financial aid application deadline:* 3/1.
Contact Ms. Lynn Taylor, Graduate Program Assistant, College of Nursing, Montana State University, 122 Sherrick Hall, PO Box 173560, Bozeman, MT 59717-3560. *Telephone:* 406-994-3500. *Fax:* 406-994-6020. *E-mail:* lynnt@montana.edu.

MASTER'S DEGREE PROGRAM

Degree MN
Available Programs Master's.
Concentrations Available Clinical nurse leader. *Nurse practitioner programs in:* family health, psychiatric/mental health.
Site Options Billings, MT; Great Falls, MT; Missoula, MT.
Study Options Full-time and part-time.
Program Entrance Requirements Computer literacy, minimum overall college GPA of 3.0, transcript of college record, CPR certification, written essay, immunizations, interview, 3 letters of recommendation, nursing research course, physical assessment course, prerequisite course work, statistics course, GRE General Test. *Application deadline:* 2/15 (fall). *Application fee:* $60.
Advanced Placement Credit given for nursing courses completed elsewhere dependent upon specific evaluations.
Degree Requirements 35 total credit hours, thesis or project, comprehensive exam.

POST-MASTER'S PROGRAM

Areas of Study Nursing education. *Nurse practitioner programs in:* family health, psychiatric/mental health.

DOCTORAL DEGREE PROGRAM

Degree DNP
Available Programs Doctorate; Post-Baccalaureate Doctorate.
Areas of Study Advanced practice nursing.
Program Entrance Requirements Minimum overall college GPA of 3.0, interview by faculty committee, 3 letters of recommendation, statistics course, vita, writing sample. *Application deadline:* 2/15 (fall). *Application fee:* $60.
Degree Requirements 65 total credit hours.

Montana State University–Northern

College of Nursing
Havre, Montana

http://www.msun.edu/academics/nursing
Founded in 1929
DEGREE • BSN
Nursing Program Faculty 12 (8% with doctorates).
Baccalaureate Enrollment 53 **Women** 96% **Men** 4% **Part-time** 92%
Distance Learning Courses Available.
Nursing Student Activities Nursing club.
Nursing Student Resources Academic advising; academic or career counseling; assistance for students with disabilities; bookstore; campus computer network; career placement assistance; computer lab; computer-assisted instruction; e-mail services; employment services for current students; housing assistance; interactive nursing skills videos; Internet; learning resource lab; library services; nursing audiovisuals; remedial services; resume preparation assistance; skills, simulation, or other laboratory; tutoring.
Library Facilities 2,600 volumes in health, 1,300 volumes in nursing; 40 periodical subscriptions health-care related.

BACCALAUREATE PROGRAMS

Degree BSN
Available Programs ADN to Baccalaureate; RN Baccalaureate.
Site Options Great Falls, MT; Lewistown, MT.
Study Options Full-time and part-time.

Online Degree Options Yes (online only).
Program Entrance Requirements Minimum overall college GPA of 2.25, transcript of college record, CPR certification, health exam, health insurance, immunizations, professional liability insurance/malpractice insurance, prerequisite course work, RN licensure. Transfer students are accepted. *Application deadline:* 8/1 (fall), 1/10 (winter), 5/2 (summer). Applications may be processed on a rolling basis for some programs. *Application fee:* $30.
Advanced Placement Credit given for nursing courses completed elsewhere dependent upon specific evaluations.
Contact *Telephone:* 406-265-4196 Ext. 4196. *Fax:* 406-265-3772.

Salish Kootenai College

Nursing Department
Pablo, Montana

Founded in 1977
DEGREE • BS
Nursing Program Faculty 7
Nursing Student Activities Nursing club.
Nursing Student Resources Academic advising; academic or career counseling; bookstore; computer lab; daycare for children of students; employment services for current students; Internet; library services.
Library Facilities 24,000 volumes; 200 periodical subscriptions.

BACCALAUREATE PROGRAMS

Degree BS
Available Programs RN Baccalaureate.
Study Options Full-time and part-time.
Program Entrance Requirements Transcript of college record, CPR certification, health exam, health insurance, high school biology, high school chemistry, 2 years high school math, 2 years high school science, high school transcript, immunizations, minimum high school GPA of 2.5, professional liability insurance/malpractice insurance, prerequisite course work, RN licensure.
Contact *Telephone:* 406-275-4800.

University of Great Falls

B.S. in Nursing Degree Completion Program
Great Falls, Montana

Founded in 1932
DEGREE • BSN

BACCALAUREATE PROGRAMS

Degree BSN
Available Programs RN Baccalaureate.
Study Options Part-time.
Program Entrance Requirements Transcript of college record, prerequisite course work. *Application deadline:* 4/5 (fall).
Expenses (2012–13) *Tuition:* part-time $453 per credit hour.
Contact Nicole Brandt, RN to BSN Admission Liaison, B.S. in Nursing Degree Completion Program, University of Great Falls, 1301 20th Street South, Great Falls, MT 59405. *Telephone:* 406-791-5234. *E-mail:* rn2bsn@ugf.edu.

NEBRASKA

BryanLGH College of Health Sciences

School of Nursing
Lincoln, Nebraska

http://www.bryanhealth.com/collegeofhealthsciences
DEGREES • BSN • MS
Nursing Program Faculty 29 (10% with doctorates).

Baccalaureate Enrollment 417 **Women** 90.4% **Men** 9.6% **Minority** 7.9% **Part-time** 45.56%
Graduate Enrollment 47 **Women** 59.6% **Men** 40.4% **Minority** 10.64% **Part-time** 10.6%
Distance Learning Courses Available.
Nursing Student Activities Sigma Theta Tau, Student Nurses' Association.
Nursing Student Resources Academic advising; academic' or career counseling; assistance for students with disabilities; bookstore; campus computer network; career placement assistance; computer lab; computer-assisted instruction; e-mail services; employment services for current students; housing assistance; Internet; learning resource lab; library services; nursing audiovisuals; remedial services; resume preparation assistance; skills, simulation, or other laboratory; tutoring.
Library Facilities 4,000 volumes in health, 3,000 volumes in nursing; 20,000 periodical subscriptions health-care related.

BACCALAUREATE PROGRAMS

Degree BSN
Available Programs Generic Baccalaureate; RN Baccalaureate.
Study Options Full-time.
Program Entrance Requirements Minimum overall college GPA of 2.0, transcript of college record, CPR certification, written essay, health insurance, high school chemistry, high school foreign language, 3 years high school math, 3 years high school science, high school transcript, immunizations, interview, 3 letters of recommendation, minimum high school GPA of 2.75, minimum GPA in nursing prerequisites of 2.0, professional liability insurance/malpractice insurance. Transfer students are accepted. *Application deadline:* 2/1 (fall), 6/1 (spring). *Application fee:* $40.
Advanced Placement Credit given for nursing courses completed elsewhere dependent upon specific evaluations.
Financial Aid 64% of baccalaureate students in nursing programs received some form of financial aid in 2010–11.
Contact Kelli Backman, Director of Enrollment, School of Nursing, BryanLGH College of Health Sciences, 5035 Everett Street, Lincoln, NE 68505. *Telephone:* 402-481-8698. *Fax:* 402-481-8621. *E-mail:* kelli.backman@bryanlgh.org.

GRADUATE PROGRAMS

Financial Aid 93% of graduate students in nursing programs received some form of financial aid in 2010–11.
Contact Dr. Sharon Hadenfeldt, RN, Dean of Graduate Studies, School of Nursing, BryanLGH College of Health Sciences, 5035 Everett Street, Lincoln, NE 68506. *Telephone:* 402-481-8606. *Fax:* 402-481-8404. *E-mail:* sharon.hadenfeldt@bryanlgh.org.

MASTER'S DEGREE PROGRAM

Degree MS
Available Programs Master's.
Concentrations Available Nurse anesthesia; nursing education.
Study Options Full-time.
Program Entrance Requirements Clinical experience, computer literacy, minimum overall college GPA of 3.0, transcript of college record, CPR certification, written essay, immunizations, interview, 4 letters of recommendation, prerequisite course work, resume. *Application deadline:* 10/30 (fall). *Application fee:* $75.
Degree Requirements 71 total credit hours, thesis or project.

Clarkson College
Master of Science in Nursing Program
Omaha, Nebraska

http://www.clarksoncollege.edu/academics/nursing/
Founded in 1888
DEGREES • BSN • MSN
Nursing Program Faculty 42 (6% with doctorates).
Baccalaureate Enrollment 500 **Women** 90% **Men** 10% **Minority** 10% **Part-time** 15%
Graduate Enrollment 200 **Women** 90% **Men** 10% **Minority** 10% **Part-time** 50%
Distance Learning Courses Available.
Nursing Student Activities Sigma Theta Tau, Student Nurses' Association.
Nursing Student Resources Academic advising; academic or career counseling; assistance for students with disabilities; bookstore; campus computer network; career placement assistance; computer lab; computer-assisted instruction; daycare for children of students; e-mail services; employment services for current students; interactive nursing skills videos; Internet; learning resource lab; library services; nursing audiovisuals; placement services for program completers; resume preparation assistance; skills, simulation, or other laboratory; tutoring.
Library Facilities 8,807 volumes (7,500 in health, 2,200 in nursing); 262 periodical subscriptions (600 health-care related).

BACCALAUREATE PROGRAMS

Degree BSN
Available Programs ADN to Baccalaureate; Accelerated RN Baccalaureate; Baccalaureate for Second Degree; Generic Baccalaureate; LPN to Baccalaureate; LPN to RN Baccalaureate; RN Baccalaureate.
Study Options Full-time and part-time.
Online Degree Options Yes.
Program Entrance Requirements Minimum overall college GPA of 2.5, transcript of college record, CPR certification, written essay, health exam, health insurance, 2 years high school math, 2 years high school science, high school transcript, immunizations, minimum high school GPA of 2.5, minimum high school rank 50%. Transfer students are accepted. *Application fee:* $35.
Advanced Placement Credit given for nursing courses completed elsewhere dependent upon specific evaluations.
Contact *Telephone:* 402-552-3100. *Fax:* 402-552-6057.

GRADUATE PROGRAMS

Contact *Telephone:* 800-647-5500. *Fax:* 402-552-6057.

MASTER'S DEGREE PROGRAM

Degree MSN
Available Programs Master's; RN to Master's.
Concentrations Available Health-care administration; nurse anesthesia; nursing administration; nursing education. *Nurse practitioner programs in:* adult health, family health.
Study Options Full-time and part-time.
Online Degree Options Yes (online only).
Program Entrance Requirements Clinical experience, minimum overall college GPA of 3.0, transcript of college record, written essay, 2 letters of recommendation, resume. *Application deadline:* 7/1 (fall), 11/15 (spring), 4/1 (summer). *Application fee:* $35.
Advanced Placement Credit given for nursing courses completed elsewhere dependent upon specific evaluations.
Degree Requirements 46 total credit hours, thesis or project.

POST-MASTER'S PROGRAM

Areas of Study Health-care administration; nurse anesthesia; nursing administration; nursing education. *Nurse practitioner programs in:* adult health, family health.

CONTINUING EDUCATION PROGRAM

Contact *Telephone:* 402-552-3100. *Fax:* 402-552-6057.

College of Saint Mary
Division of Health Care Professions
Omaha, Nebraska

Founded in 1923
DEGREE • BSN
Nursing Program Faculty 18 (6% with doctorates).
Baccalaureate Enrollment 45 **Women** 100% **Minority** 10% **Part-time** 65%
Graduate Enrollment 8
Nursing Student Activities Nursing Honor Society, Sigma Theta Tau, Student Nurses' Association, nursing club.
Nursing Student Resources Academic advising; academic or career counseling; bookstore; campus computer network; career placement assistance; computer lab; computer-assisted instruction; e-mail services; interactive nursing skills videos; Internet; learning resource lab; library services; nursing audiovisuals; other; placement services for program completers; resume preparation assistance; skills, simulation, or other laboratory; tutoring.
Library Facilities 88,503 volumes; 178 periodical subscriptions (100 health-care related).

BACCALAUREATE PROGRAMS

Degree BSN
Available Programs ADN to Baccalaureate; Generic Baccalaureate.
Study Options Full-time and part-time.
Program Entrance Requirements Minimum overall college GPA of 2.5, transcript of college record, CPR certification, health exam, immunizations, 2 letters of recommendation, minimum high school GPA, minimum GPA in nursing prerequisites of 2.5, prerequisite course work. Transfer students are accepted.
Advanced Placement Credit given for nursing courses completed elsewhere dependent upon specific evaluations.
Contact *Telephone:* 402-399-2658. *Fax:* 402-399-2654.

GRADUATE PROGRAMS

Contact *Telephone:* 402-399-2482. *Fax:* 402-399-2414.

Creighton University
School of Nursing
Omaha, Nebraska

http://www.creighton.edu/nursing/
Founded in 1878
DEGREES • BSN • DNP • MSN
Nursing Program Faculty 54 (46% with doctorates).
Baccalaureate Enrollment 548 **Women** 90.7% **Men** 9.3% **Minority** 20.4% **International** .3% **Part-time** 3.2%
Graduate Enrollment 165 **Women** 95.8% **Men** 4.2% **Minority** 7.9% **Part-time** 54.5%
Distance Learning Courses Available.
Nursing Student Activities Nursing Honor Society, Sigma Theta Tau, Student Nurses' Association.
Nursing Student Resources Academic advising; academic or career counseling; assistance for students with disabilities; bookstore; campus computer network; career placement assistance; computer lab; computer-assisted instruction; daycare for children of students; e-mail services; employment services for current students; Internet; learning resource lab; library services; nursing audiovisuals; remedial services; resume preparation assistance; skills, simulation, or other laboratory; tutoring; unpaid internships.
Library Facilities 882,402 volumes (184,619 in health, 3,861 in nursing); 52,522 periodical subscriptions (10,376 health-care related).

BACCALAUREATE PROGRAMS

Degree BSN
Available Programs Accelerated Baccalaureate for Second Degree; Generic Baccalaureate; RN Baccalaureate.
Site Options Hastings, NE.
Study Options Full-time and part-time.
Online Degree Options Yes.
Program Entrance Requirements Minimum overall college GPA of 2.0, transcript of college record, written essay, health exam, health insurance, high school chemistry, 3 years high school math, 2 years high school science, high school transcript, immunizations, 1 letter of recommendation, minimum high school GPA of 3.0, minimum high school rank 50%. Transfer students are accepted. *Application deadline:* Applications may be processed on a rolling basis for some programs. *Application fee:* $50.
Advanced Placement Credit given for nursing courses completed elsewhere dependent upon specific evaluations.
Contact *Telephone:* 402-280-2067. *Fax:* 402-280-2045.

GRADUATE PROGRAMS

Contact *Telephone:* 402-280-2067. *Fax:* 402-280-2045.

MASTER'S DEGREE PROGRAM
Degree MSN
Available Programs Master's.
Concentrations Available Clinical nurse leader; nursing administration; nursing education. *Clinical nurse specialist programs in:* adult health, cardiovascular, family health, gerontology, maternity-newborn, oncology, pediatric. *Nurse practitioner programs in:* acute care, adult health, family health, gerontology, neonatal health, oncology, pediatric, psychiatric/mental health.
Site Options Hastings, NE.

Study Options Full-time and part-time.
Program Entrance Requirements Clinical experience, minimum overall college GPA of 3.0, transcript of college record, CPR certification, written essay, immunizations, 3 letters of recommendation, physical assessment course, prerequisite course work, resume, statistics course. *Application deadline:* Applications may be processed on a rolling basis for some programs. *Application fee:* $50.
Advanced Placement Credit given for nursing courses completed elsewhere dependent upon specific evaluations.
Degree Requirements 36 total credit hours, thesis or project.

POST-MASTER'S PROGRAM
Areas of Study Clinical nurse leader; nursing administration; nursing education. *Clinical nurse specialist programs in:* adult health, cardiovascular, family health, gerontology, maternity-newborn, oncology, pediatric. *Nurse practitioner programs in:* acute care, adult health, family health, gerontology, neonatal health, oncology, pediatric, psychiatric/mental health.

DOCTORAL DEGREE PROGRAM
Degree DNP
Available Programs Doctorate; Post-Baccalaureate Doctorate.
Areas of Study Advanced practice nursing, clinical practice, critical care, family health, gerontology, health promotion/disease prevention, maternity-newborn, neuro-behavior, nursing administration, nursing education, oncology.
Site Options Hastings, NE.
Program Entrance Requirements Clinical experience, minimum overall college GPA of 3.0, 3 letters of recommendation, statistics course, vita. *Application deadline:* Applications may be processed on a rolling basis for some programs. *Application fee:* $50.
Degree Requirements 32 total credit hours, residency.

Midland University
Department of Nursing
Fremont, Nebraska

http://www.midlandu.edu/
Founded in 1883
DEGREE • BSN
Nursing Program Faculty 12 (25% with doctorates).
Baccalaureate Enrollment 130 **Women** 93% **Men** 7% **Minority** 4% **International** 3% **Part-time** 9%
Distance Learning Courses Available.
Nursing Student Activities Sigma Theta Tau, Student Nurses' Association.
Nursing Student Resources Academic advising; academic or career counseling; assistance for students with disabilities; bookstore; campus computer network; career placement assistance; computer lab; computer-assisted instruction; e-mail services; employment services for current students; housing assistance; interactive nursing skills videos; Internet; learning resource lab; library services; nursing audiovisuals; paid internships; placement services for program completers; remedial services; resume preparation assistance; skills, simulation, or other laboratory; tutoring; unpaid internships.
Library Facilities 110,000 volumes (4,700 in health, 2,000 in nursing); 900 periodical subscriptions (550 health-care related).

BACCALAUREATE PROGRAMS

Degree BSN
Available Programs ADN to Baccalaureate; Generic Baccalaureate; LPN to RN Baccalaureate; RN Baccalaureate.
Site Options Columbus, NE.
Study Options Full-time and part-time.
Program Entrance Requirements Minimum overall college GPA of 2.5, transcript of college record, CPR certification, written essay, health exam, high school transcript, immunizations, interview, 2 letters of recommendation, minimum GPA in nursing prerequisites of 2.5, prerequisite course work. Transfer students are accepted. *Application deadline:* 3/1 (spring). Applications may be processed on a rolling basis for some programs.
Advanced Placement Credit given for nursing courses completed elsewhere dependent upon specific evaluations.
Contact *Telephone:* 402-941-6505. *Fax:* 402-941-6513.

Nebraska Methodist College
Department of Nursing
Omaha, Nebraska

http://www.methodistcollege.edu/
Founded in 1891
DEGREES • BSN • MSN
Nursing Program Faculty 35 (26% with doctorates).
Baccalaureate Enrollment 537 **Women** 92% **Men** 8% **Minority** 9% **International** 1% **Part-time** 39%
Graduate Enrollment 93 **Women** 98% **Men** 2% **Minority** 3% **Part-time** 33%
Distance Learning Courses Available.
Nursing Student Activities Nursing Honor Society, Sigma Theta Tau, Student Nurses' Association.
Nursing Student Resources Academic advising; academic or career counseling; assistance for students with disabilities; bookstore; campus computer network; career placement assistance; computer lab; computer-assisted instruction; e-mail services; employment services for current students; interactive nursing skills videos; Internet; learning resource lab; library services; nursing audiovisuals; remedial services; resume preparation assistance; skills, simulation, or other laboratory; tutoring.
Library Facilities 10,300 volumes (4,500 in health, 1,700 in nursing); 164 periodical subscriptions (13,600 health-care related).

BACCALAUREATE PROGRAMS
Degree BSN
Available Programs Accelerated Baccalaureate for Second Degree; Accelerated RN Baccalaureate; Generic Baccalaureate; LPN to Baccalaureate; LPN to RN Baccalaureate; RN Baccalaureate.
Study Options Full-time and part-time.
Program Entrance Requirements Minimum overall college GPA of 2.5, transcript of college record, written essay, high school biology, high school chemistry, 2 years high school math, 2 years high school science, high school transcript, interview, minimum high school GPA of 2.5, minimum GPA in nursing prerequisites of 2.5. Transfer students are accepted. *Application deadline:* Applications may be processed on a rolling basis for some programs. *Application fee:* $25.
Advanced Placement Credit given for nursing courses completed elsewhere dependent upon specific evaluations.
Expenses (2012–13) *Tuition:* full-time $15,450; part-time $515 per credit hour. *International tuition:* $15,450 full-time. *Room and board:* room only: $5274 per academic year. *Required fees:* full-time $630; part-time $315 per term.
Financial Aid 96% of baccalaureate students in nursing programs received some form of financial aid in 2011–12.
Contact Dr. Linda Hughes, Dean of Nursing, Department of Nursing, Nebraska Methodist College, 720 North 87th Street, Omaha, NE 68114-2852. *Telephone:* 402-354-7049. *Fax:* 402-354-7130. *E-mail:* Linda.Hughes@methodistcollege.edu.

GRADUATE PROGRAMS
Expenses (2012–13) *Tuition:* full-time $11,952; part-time $664 per credit hour. *International tuition:* $11,952 full-time. *Room and board:* $9556; room only: $6020 per academic year. *Required fees:* full-time $450; part-time $225 per term.
Financial Aid 82% of graduate students in nursing programs received some form of financial aid in 2011–12.
Contact Dr. Linda Foley, Director, Graduate Nursing, Department of Nursing, Nebraska Methodist College, 720 North 87th Street, Omaha, NE 68114-2852. *Telephone:* 402-354-7050. *Fax:* 402-354-7130. *E-mail:* linda.foley@methodistcollege.edu.

MASTER'S DEGREE PROGRAM
Degree MSN
Available Programs Master's; Master's for Nurses with Non-Nursing Degrees; RN to Master's.
Concentrations Available Nursing administration; nursing education.
Study Options Full-time and part-time.
Online Degree Options Yes (online only).
Program Entrance Requirements Computer literacy, minimum overall college GPA of 3.0, transcript of college record, CPR certification, written essay, immunizations, interview, 2 letters of recommendation, nursing research course, physical assessment course, prerequisite course work, resume, statistics course. *Application deadline:* Applications may be processed on a rolling basis for some programs. *Application fee:* $25.
Advanced Placement Credit given for nursing courses completed elsewhere dependent upon specific evaluations.
Degree Requirements 36 total credit hours, thesis or project.

POST-MASTER'S PROGRAM
Areas of Study Nursing administration; nursing education.

CONTINUING EDUCATION PROGRAM
Contact Jillian Plymesser, Online Program Coordinator, Department of Nursing, Nebraska Methodist College, 720 North 87th Street, Omaha, NE 68114-2852. *Telephone:* 402-354-7129. *E-mail:* jillian.plymesser@methodistcollege.edu.

Nebraska Wesleyan University
Department of Nursing
Lincoln, Nebraska

http://www.nebrwesleyan.edu/
Founded in 1887
DEGREES • BSN • MSN
Nursing Program Faculty 15 (50% with doctorates).
Baccalaureate Enrollment 87 **Women** 92% **Men** 8% **Minority** 7% **International** 11% **Part-time** 40%
Graduate Enrollment 54 **Women** 96% **Men** 4% **Minority** 12% **International** 2% **Part-time** 50%
Distance Learning Courses Available.
Nursing Student Activities Sigma Theta Tau.
Nursing Student Resources Academic advising; academic or career counseling; assistance for students with disabilities; bookstore; campus computer network; career placement assistance; computer lab; e-mail services; Internet; library services; nursing audiovisuals; resume preparation assistance; unpaid internships.
Library Facilities 225,771 volumes (5,000 in health, 3,700 in nursing); 1,551 periodical subscriptions (470 health-care related).

BACCALAUREATE PROGRAMS
Degree BSN
Available Programs ADN to Baccalaureate; Accelerated RN Baccalaureate; International Nurse to Baccalaureate; RN Baccalaureate.
Site Options Omaha, NE.
Study Options Full-time and part-time.
Program Entrance Requirements Transfer students are accepted. *Application deadline:* Applications may be processed on a rolling basis for some programs. *Application fee:* $100.
Advanced Placement Credit by examination available. Credit given for nursing courses completed elsewhere dependent upon specific evaluations.
Contact *Telephone:* 800-541-3818 Ext. 2330. *Fax:* 402-465-2479.

GRADUATE PROGRAMS
Contact *Telephone:* 402-465-2336. *Fax:* 402-465-2179.

MASTER'S DEGREE PROGRAM
Degree MSN
Available Programs Accelerated AD/RN to Master's; Accelerated Master's; Accelerated RN to Master's; Master's; RN to Master's.
Concentrations Available Nursing administration; nursing education.
Site Options Omaha, NE.
Study Options Full-time and part-time.
Program Entrance Requirements Clinical experience, computer literacy, minimum overall college GPA of 3.0, transcript of college record, written essay, immunizations, 2 letters of recommendation, nursing research course, resume, statistics course. *Application deadline:* 8/1 (fall), 12/10 (spring). Applications may be processed on a rolling basis for some programs. *Application fee:* $100.
Advanced Placement Credit by examination available. Credit given for nursing courses completed elsewhere dependent upon specific evaluations.
Degree Requirements 40 total credit hours, thesis or project, comprehensive exam.

POST-MASTER'S PROGRAM
Areas of Study Nursing administration; nursing education.

Union College
Division of Health Sciences
Lincoln, Nebraska

http://www.ucollege.edu/
Founded in 1891
DEGREE • BSN
Nursing Program Faculty 12
Baccalaureate Enrollment 173 **Women** 82% **Men** 18% **Minority** 10%
International 5.2% **Part-time** 12.7%
Nursing Student Activities Sigma Theta Tau, nursing club.
Nursing Student Resources Academic advising; academic or career counseling; assistance for students with disabilities; bookstore; campus computer network; career placement assistance; computer lab; computer-assisted instruction; e-mail services; employment services for current students; externships; interactive nursing skills videos; Internet; learning resource lab; library services; nursing audiovisuals; placement services for program completers; remedial services; resume preparation assistance; skills, simulation, or other laboratory; tutoring; unpaid internships.
Library Facilities 176,653 volumes (450 in health, 350 in nursing); 32,990 periodical subscriptions (50 health-care related).

BACCALAUREATE PROGRAMS
Degree BSN
Available Programs ADN to Baccalaureate; Generic Baccalaureate; LPN to Baccalaureate.
Study Options Full-time and part-time.
Program Entrance Requirements Minimum overall college GPA of 2.75, transcript of college record, CPR certification, written essay, health exam, health insurance, high school transcript, immunizations, 3 letters of recommendation, minimum GPA in nursing prerequisites of 2.75, professional liability insurance/malpractice insurance, prerequisite course work. Transfer students are accepted. *Application deadline:* 3/1 (fall), 10/1 (spring). *Application fee:* $25.
Advanced Placement Credit by examination available. Credit given for nursing courses completed elsewhere dependent upon specific evaluations.
Financial Aid 83% of baccalaureate students in nursing programs received some form of financial aid in 2010–11.
Contact Ms. Sherri Gregory, Admission and Progression Coordinator, Division of Health Sciences, Union College, 3800 South 48th Street, Lincoln, NE 68506. *Telephone:* 402-486-2600 Ext. 2343. *Fax:* 402-486-2582. *E-mail:* shgregor@ucollege.edu.

University of Nebraska Medical Center
College of Nursing
Omaha, Nebraska

http://www.unmc.edu/nursing/
Founded in 1869
DEGREES • BSN • MSN • PHD
Nursing Program Faculty 112 (60% with doctorates).
Baccalaureate Enrollment 600
Graduate Enrollment 300
Nursing Student Activities Nursing Honor Society, Sigma Theta Tau, Student Nurses' Association, nursing club.
Nursing Student Resources Academic advising; academic or career counseling; assistance for students with disabilities; bookstore; campus computer network; career placement assistance; computer lab; computer-assisted instruction; daycare for children of students; e-mail services; employment services for current students; externships; housing assistance; interactive nursing skills videos; Internet; learning resource lab; library services; nursing audiovisuals; other; paid internships; placement services for program completers; remedial services; resume preparation assistance; skills, simulation, or other laboratory; tutoring.
Library Facilities 251,347 volumes (240,000 in health, 3,500 in nursing); 7,603 periodical subscriptions (2,200 health-care related).

BACCALAUREATE PROGRAMS
Degree BSN

Available Programs ADN to Baccalaureate; Accelerated Baccalaureate; Accelerated Baccalaureate for Second Degree; Accelerated RN Baccalaureate; Baccalaureate for Second Degree; Generic Baccalaureate; International Nurse to Baccalaureate; LPN to Baccalaureate; LPN to RN Baccalaureate; RN Baccalaureate; RPN to Baccalaureate.
Study Options Full-time.
Program Entrance Requirements Minimum overall college GPA of 2.5, transcript of college record, CPR certification, health insurance, high school transcript, immunizations, 2 letters of recommendation, prerequisite course work. Transfer students are accepted.
Advanced Placement Credit by examination available. Credit given for nursing courses completed elsewhere dependent upon specific evaluations.
Contact *Telephone:* 402-559-5184.

GRADUATE PROGRAMS
Contact *Telephone:* 402-559-5184.

MASTER'S DEGREE PROGRAM
Degree MSN
Available Programs Master's; Master's for Non-Nursing College Graduates; RN to Master's.
Concentrations Available Health-care administration; nurse case management; nursing administration; nursing education; nursing informatics. *Clinical nurse specialist programs in:* acute care, adult health, cardiovascular, community health, critical care, family health, gerontology, maternity-newborn, medical-surgical, oncology, parent-child, pediatric, perinatal, psychiatric/mental health, public health, women's health. *Nurse practitioner programs in:* acute care, adult health, community health, family health, gerontology, neonatal health, oncology, pediatric, primary care, psychiatric/mental health, women's health.
Study Options Full-time and part-time.
Program Entrance Requirements Computer literacy, minimum overall college GPA of 3.0, transcript of college record, CPR certification, immunizations, interview, 3 letters of recommendation, nursing research course, statistics course.
Advanced Placement Credit given for nursing courses completed elsewhere dependent upon specific evaluations.
Degree Requirements 45 total credit hours.

POST-MASTER'S PROGRAM
Areas of Study Health-care administration; nurse case management; nursing administration; nursing education; nursing informatics. *Clinical nurse specialist programs in:* acute care, adult health, cardiovascular, community health, critical care, family health, gerontology, maternity-newborn, medical-surgical, oncology, parent-child, pediatric, perinatal, psychiatric/mental health, public health, women's health. *Nurse practitioner programs in:* acute care, adult health, community health, family health, gerontology, neonatal health, oncology, pediatric, primary care, psychiatric/mental health, women's health.

DOCTORAL DEGREE PROGRAM
Degree PhD
Available Programs Doctorate; Doctorate for Nurses with Non-Nursing Degrees; Post-Baccalaureate Doctorate.
Areas of Study Advanced practice nursing, aging, bio-behavioral research, biology of health and illness, clinical practice, community health, critical care, faculty preparation, family health, gerontology, health policy, health promotion/disease prevention, health-care systems, human health and illness, illness and transition, individualized study, information systems, maternity-newborn, neuro-behavior, nurse case management, nursing administration, nursing policy, nursing research, nursing science, oncology, women's health.
Program Entrance Requirements Minimum overall college GPA of 3.2, interview by faculty committee, interview, 3 letters of recommendation, scholarly papers, statistics course, vita, writing sample.
Degree Requirements Dissertation, oral exam, written exam.

POSTDOCTORAL PROGRAM
Postdoctoral Program Contact *Telephone:* 402-559-7457. *Fax:* 410-706-0945.

CONTINUING EDUCATION PROGRAM
Contact *Telephone:* 402-559-7487.

NEVADA

Great Basin College
BSN Program
Elko, Nevada

http://www.gbcnv.edu/programs/BS-NUR.html
Founded in 1967

DEGREE • BSN
Nursing Program Faculty 6 (33% with doctorates).
Baccalaureate Enrollment 38 **Women** 95% **Men** 5% **Minority** 35%
Distance Learning Courses Available.
Nursing Student Activities Nursing club.
Nursing Student Resources Academic advising; academic or career counseling; assistance for students with disabilities; bookstore; campus computer network; computer lab; computer-assisted instruction; daycare for children of students; e-mail services; employment services for current students; Internet; learning resource lab; library services; nursing audio-visuals; resume preparation assistance; skills, simulation, or other laboratory.
Library Facilities 113,341 volumes; 142 periodical subscriptions.

BACCALAUREATE PROGRAMS

Degree BSN
Available Programs ADN to Baccalaureate; RN Baccalaureate.
Online Degree Options Yes.
Program Entrance Requirements CPR certification, written essay, health exam, health insurance, immunizations, 3 letters of recommendation, minimum GPA in nursing prerequisites of 3.0, prerequisite course work, RN licensure.
Expenses (2011–12) *Tuition, area resident:* part-time $113 per credit. *Tuition, state resident:* full-time $3700. *Required fees:* part-time $15 per credit.
Financial Aid 35% of baccalaureate students in nursing programs received some form of financial aid in 2010–11. *Gift aid (need-based):* Federal Pell, FSEOG, state, private, college/university gift aid from institutional funds. *Loans:* college/university.*Work-study:* Federal Work-Study, part-time campus jobs.*Financial aid application deadline (priority):* 5/13.
Contact Program Information, BSN Program, Great Basin College, 1500 College Parkway, Elko, NV 89801. *Telephone:* 775-738-8493.

Nevada State College at Henderson
Nursing Program
Henderson, Nevada

http://www.nsc.nevada.edu/83.asp
Founded in 2002

DEGREE • BSN
Nursing Program Faculty 31 (16% with doctorates).
Baccalaureate Enrollment 312 **Women** 86% **Men** 14% **Minority** 34% **Part-time** 66%
Distance Learning Courses Available.
Nursing Student Activities Sigma Theta Tau, Student Nurses' Association.
Nursing Student Resources Academic advising; academic or career counseling; assistance for students with disabilities; bookstore; campus computer network; computer lab; computer-assisted instruction; e-mail services; interactive nursing skills videos; Internet; learning resource lab; library services; nursing audiovisuals; skills, simulation, or other laboratory; tutoring.
Library Facilities 16,016 volumes (1,075 in health, 647 in nursing); 47 periodical subscriptions (4,981 health-care related).

BACCALAUREATE PROGRAMS

Degree BSN
Available Programs Accelerated Baccalaureate for Second Degree; Generic Baccalaureate; RN Baccalaureate.
Study Options Full-time and part-time.
Online Degree Options Yes.

Program Entrance Requirements Minimum overall college GPA of 2.5, transcript of college record, CPR certification, health exam, health insurance, high school transcript, immunizations, minimum GPA in nursing prerequisites of 3.25, prerequisite course work. Transfer students are accepted. *Application deadline:* 3/15 (fall), 9/15 (spring).
Advanced Placement Credit given for nursing courses completed elsewhere dependent upon specific evaluations.
Expenses (2011–12) *Tuition, area resident:* full-time $4300; part-time $149 per credit. *Tuition, nonresident:* full-time $14,500; part-time $273 per credit. *Required fees:* full-time $2000.
Financial Aid 54% of baccalaureate students in nursing programs received some form of financial aid in 2010–11.
Contact Adeste Sipin, Academic Advisor, Nursing Program, Nevada State College at Henderson, 1125 Nevada State Drive, Henderson, NV 89002. *Telephone:* 702-992-2638. *Fax:* 702-992-2058. *E-mail:* adeste.sipin@nsc.nevada.edu.

Roseman University of Health Sciences
College of Nursing
Henderson, Nevada

http://www.roseman.edu/

DEGREE • BSN
Nursing Program Faculty 52 (25% with doctorates).
Baccalaureate Enrollment 205 **Women** 78% **Men** 22% **Minority** 57%
Distance Learning Courses Available.
Nursing Student Activities Nursing Honor Society, Student Nurses' Association.
Nursing Student Resources Academic advising; academic or career counseling; assistance for students with disabilities; campus computer network; career placement assistance; computer lab; computer-assisted instruction; e-mail services; interactive nursing skills videos; Internet; learning resource lab; library services; nursing audiovisuals; remedial services; resume preparation assistance; skills, simulation, or other laboratory; unpaid internships.

BACCALAUREATE PROGRAMS

Degree BSN
Available Programs Accelerated Baccalaureate; Accelerated Baccalaureate for Second Degree; Generic Baccalaureate.
Site Options South Jordan, UT; Las Vegas, NV.
Study Options Full-time.
Program Entrance Requirements Transcript of college record, written essay, health exam, health insurance, immunizations, interview, minimum GPA in nursing prerequisites of 2.75, prerequisite course work. Transfer students are accepted. *Application deadline:* 5/1 (fall), 10/1 (spring). Applications may be processed on a rolling basis for some programs. *Application fee:* $100.
Advanced Placement Credit given for nursing courses completed elsewhere dependent upon specific evaluations.
Expenses (2012–13) *Tuition:* full-time $22,875. *International tuition:* $22,875 full-time. *Required fees:* full-time $1480.
Financial Aid 90% of baccalaureate students in nursing programs received some form of financial aid in 2011–12.
Contact Ms. Imelda R. Revuelto, Recruitment, Admissions, and Enrollment Coordinator, College of Nursing, Roseman University of Health Sciences, 11 Sunset Way, Henderson, NV 89014. *Telephone:* 702-968-2075. *Fax:* 702-968-2097. *E-mail:* irevuelto@roseman.edu.

Touro University
School of Nursing
Henderson, Nevada

DEGREES • BSN • DNP • MSN
Nursing Program Faculty 10 (60% with doctorates).
Baccalaureate Enrollment 31 **Women** 77.5% **Men** 22.5% **Minority** 41.9%
Graduate Enrollment 6 **Women** 83% **Men** 17% **Minority** 70% **Part-time** 100%
Distance Learning Courses Available.
Nursing Student Activities Sigma Theta Tau, Student Nurses' Association.

Nursing Student Resources Academic advising; assistance for students with disabilities; bookstore; campus computer network; computer lab; computer-assisted instruction; e-mail services; interactive nursing skills videos; Internet; learning resource lab; library services; nursing audiovisuals; remedial services; skills, simulation, or other laboratory; tutoring.
Library Facilities 86 volumes in health; 6,002 periodical subscriptions health-care related.

BACCALAUREATE PROGRAMS

Degree BSN
Available Programs ADN to Baccalaureate; Generic Baccalaureate; RN Baccalaureate.
Study Options Full-time.
Online Degree Options Yes.
Program Entrance Requirements Minimum overall college GPA of 3.0, transcript of college record, CPR certification, health exam, health insurance, immunizations, minimum GPA in nursing prerequisites of 3.0, prerequisite course work, RN licensure. Transfer students are accepted. *Application deadline:* 7/30 (fall), 12/31 (spring). Applications may be processed on a rolling basis for some programs. *Application fee:* $50.
Advanced Placement Credit given for nursing courses completed elsewhere dependent upon specific evaluations.
Expenses (2012–13) *Tuition, area resident:* full-time $18,240. *Required fees:* full-time $1600.
Financial Aid 90% of baccalaureate students in nursing programs received some form of financial aid in 2011–12.
Contact Oscar Espinoza-Parra, Director of Admissions, School of Nursing, Touro University, 874 American Pacific Drive, Henderson, NV 89014. *Telephone:* 702-777-1751. *Fax:* 702-777-1752. *E-mail:* oscar.parra@tun.touro.edu.

GRADUATE PROGRAMS

Expenses (2012–13) *Tuition, state resident:* part-time $600 per credit.
Financial Aid 90% of graduate students in nursing programs received some form of financial aid in 2011–12.
Contact Dr. Douglas Turner, Graduate Coordinator, School of Nursing, Touro University, 874 American Pacific Drive, Henderson, NV 89014. *Telephone:* 702-777-3997. *Fax:* 702-777-1752. *E-mail:* douglas.turner@tun.touro.edu.

MASTER'S DEGREE PROGRAM

Degree MSN
Available Programs Master's.
Concentrations Available Nursing education.
Study Options Full-time and part-time.
Online Degree Options Yes (online only).
Program Entrance Requirements Clinical experience, computer literacy, minimum overall college GPA of 3.0, transcript of college record, CPR certification, 2 letters of recommendation, statistics course. *Application deadline:* Applications may be processed on a rolling basis for some programs. *Application fee:* $50.
Advanced Placement Credit given for nursing courses completed elsewhere dependent upon specific evaluations.
Degree Requirements 36 total credit hours, thesis or project, comprehensive exam.

DOCTORAL DEGREE PROGRAM

Degree DNP
Available Programs Doctorate.
Areas of Study Individualized study.
Online Degree Options Yes (online only).
Program Entrance Requirements Clinical experience, minimum overall college GPA of 3.0, 3 letters of recommendation, MSN or equivalent, statistics course, vita, writing sample. *Application deadline:* Applications may be processed on a rolling basis for some programs. *Application fee:* $50.
Degree Requirements 39 total credit hours, oral exam, residency.

University of Nevada, Las Vegas
School of Nursing
Las Vegas, Nevada

http://nursing.unlv.edu/
Founded in 1957
DEGREES • BSN • DNP • MSN • PHD
Nursing Program Faculty 31 (55% with doctorates).

Baccalaureate Enrollment 169 **Women** 80% **Men** 20% **Minority** 52% **International** .01%
Graduate Enrollment 134 **Women** 92% **Men** 8% **Minority** 12% **International** .01% **Part-time** 58%
Distance Learning Courses Available.
Nursing Student Activities Nursing Honor Society, Sigma Theta Tau, Student Nurses' Association.
Nursing Student Resources Academic advising; academic or career counseling; assistance for students with disabilities; bookstore; campus computer network; career placement assistance; computer lab; computer-assisted instruction; daycare for children of students; e-mail services; employment services for current students; interactive nursing skills videos; Internet; learning resource lab; library services; nursing audiovisuals; remedial services; resume preparation assistance; skills, simulation, or other laboratory; tutoring.
Library Facilities 35,800 volumes in health, 12,000 volumes in nursing; 305 periodical subscriptions health-care related.

BACCALAUREATE PROGRAMS

Degree BSN
Available Programs Accelerated Baccalaureate; Generic Baccalaureate.
Study Options Full-time.
Program Entrance Requirements Minimum overall college GPA of 3.0, transcript of college record, CPR certification, health exam, health insurance, high school transcript, immunizations, minimum GPA in nursing prerequisites of 3.0, prerequisite course work. Transfer students are accepted. *Application deadline:* Applications may be processed on a rolling basis for some programs.
Advanced Placement Credit by examination available. Credit given for nursing courses completed elsewhere dependent upon specific evaluations.
Expenses (2012–13) *Tuition, state resident:* full-time $4481; part-time $187 per credit. *Tuition, nonresident:* full-time $18,076. *International tuition:* $18,151 full-time. *Room and board:* $3720; room only: $2322 per academic year. *Required fees:* full-time $1200.
Financial Aid 67% of baccalaureate students in nursing programs received some form of financial aid in 2011–12. *Gift aid (need-based):* Federal Pell, FSEOG, state, private, college/university gift aid from institutional funds. *Loans:* Federal Nursing Student Loans, Federal Direct (Subsidized and Unsubsidized Stafford PLUS), Perkins, state, college/university.*Work-study:* Federal Work-Study, part-time campus jobs.*Financial aid application deadline (priority):* 2/1.
Contact Ms. Cheryl Perna, Undergraduate Coordinator, School of Nursing, University of Nevada, Las Vegas, 4505 Maryland Parkway, Las Vegas, NV 89154-3018. *Telephone:* 702-895-0167. *Fax:* 702-895-4807. *E-mail:* cheryl.perna@unlv.edu.

GRADUATE PROGRAMS

Expenses (2012–13) *Tuition, state resident:* full-time $9414; part-time $523 per credit hour. *Tuition, nonresident:* full-time $23,009. *International tuition:* $24,687 full-time. *Room and board:* $3720; room only: $2320 per academic year. *Required fees:* full-time $658; part-time $14 per credit; part-time $91 per term.
Financial Aid 40% of graduate students in nursing programs received some form of financial aid in 2011–12. 3 teaching assistantships with partial tuition reimbursements available (averaging $9,334 per year) were awarded; institutionally sponsored loans, scholarships, and unspecified assistantships also available. *Financial aid application deadline:* 3/1.
Contact Dr. Michelle Giddings, Coordinator, MSN Program, School of Nursing, University of Nevada, Las Vegas, 4505 Maryland Parkway, Box 453018, Las Vegas, NV 89154-3018. *Telephone:* 702-895-3404. *Fax:* 702-895-4807. *E-mail:* michelle.giddings@unlv.edu.

MASTER'S DEGREE PROGRAM

Degree MSN
Available Programs Master's.
Concentrations Available Nursing education. *Nurse practitioner programs in:* family health.
Study Options Full-time and part-time.
Online Degree Options Yes (online only).
Program Entrance Requirements Clinical experience, computer literacy, minimum overall college GPA of 3.0, transcript of college record, CPR certification, written essay, immunizations, interview, 2 letters of recommendation, nursing research course, professional liability insurance/malpractice insurance, prerequisite course work, resume, statistics course. *Application deadline:* 2/1 (spring). *Application fee:* $60.
Advanced Placement Credit given for nursing courses completed elsewhere dependent upon specific evaluations.
Degree Requirements 46 total credit hours, thesis or project.

POST-MASTER'S PROGRAM

Areas of Study Nursing education. *Nurse practitioner programs in:* family health.

DOCTORAL DEGREE PROGRAM

Degree DNP
Available Programs Doctorate.
Areas of Study Advanced practice nursing, nursing administration.
Online Degree Options Yes (online only).
Program Entrance Requirements Minimum overall college GPA of 3.5, clinical experience, interview by faculty committee, 3 letters of recommendation, MSN or equivalent, vita. *Application deadline:* Applications are processed on a rolling basis. *Application fee:* $60.
Degree Requirements 39 total credit hours, DNP scholarly project, residency.

DOCTORAL DEGREE PROGRAM

Degree PhD
Available Programs Doctorate.
Areas of Study Community health, nursing education.
Online Degree Options Yes (online only).
Program Entrance Requirements Clinical experience, minimum overall college GPA of 3.5, interview by faculty committee, 2 letters of recommendation, MSN or equivalent, statistics course, vita, writing sample, GRE General Test. *Application deadline:* 3/15 (spring). Applications may be processed on a rolling basis for some programs. *Application fee:* $60.
Degree Requirements 62 total credit hours, dissertation, oral exam, written exam.

CONTINUING EDUCATION PROGRAM

Contact Dr. Lori Candela, Continuing Education Coordinator, School of Nursing, University of Nevada, Las Vegas, 4505 Maryland Parkway, Las Vegas, NV 89154-3018. *Telephone:* 702-895-2443. *Fax:* 702-895-4807. *E-mail:* Lori.Candela@unlv.edu.

University of Nevada, Reno
Orvis School of Nursing
Reno, Nevada

http://www.unr.edu/nursing
Founded in 1874
DEGREES • BSN • DNP • MSN • MSN/MPH
Nursing Program Faculty 30 (65% with doctorates).
Baccalaureate Enrollment 144 **Women** 60% **Men** 40% **Minority** 16% **International** 5%
Graduate Enrollment 67 **Women** 90% **Men** 10% **Minority** 1% **Part-time** 90%
Distance Learning Courses Available.
Nursing Student Activities Nursing Honor Society, Sigma Theta Tau, Student Nurses' Association.
Nursing Student Resources Academic advising; academic or career counseling; assistance for students with disabilities; bookstore; campus computer network; career placement assistance; computer lab; computer-assisted instruction; e-mail services; housing assistance; Internet; learning resource lab; library services; nursing audiovisuals; resume preparation assistance; skills, simulation, or other laboratory.
Library Facilities 1.2 million volumes (5,000 in health, 3,000 in nursing); 25,360 periodical subscriptions (172 health-care related).

BACCALAUREATE PROGRAMS

Degree BSN
Available Programs ADN to Baccalaureate; Accelerated Baccalaureate; Generic Baccalaureate; RN Baccalaureate.
Site Options Reno , NV.
Study Options Full-time.
Program Entrance Requirements Transcript of college record, CPR certification, written essay, health exam, health insurance, immunizations, interview, minimum GPA in nursing prerequisites of 3.0, professional liability insurance/malpractice insurance, prerequisite course work. Transfer students are accepted. *Application deadline:* 2/11 (fall), 9/17 (spring).
Advanced Placement Credit given for nursing courses completed elsewhere dependent upon specific evaluations.
Expenses (2012–13) *Tuition, area resident:* full-time $3491; part-time $204 per credit. *Tuition, state resident:* full-time $4661; part-time $282

per credit. *Tuition, nonresident:* full-time $10,467. *International tuition:* $11,407 full-time. *Room and board:* $9769; room only: $5290 per academic year. *Required fees:* full-time $1000.
Financial Aid 50% of baccalaureate students in nursing programs received some form of financial aid in 2011–12.
Contact Mary Ann Lambert, Coordinator, Undergraduate Program, Orvis School of Nursing, University of Nevada, Reno, Mail Stop 134, Reno, NV 89557. *Telephone:* 775-682-7150. *Fax:* 775-784-4262. *E-mail:* lambert@unr.edu.

GRADUATE PROGRAMS

Expenses (2012–13) *Tuition, state resident:* part-time $239 per credit. *Tuition, nonresident:* part-time $171 per credit. *Room and board:* $6200; room only: $4750 per academic year. *Required fees:* part-time $25 per credit; part-time $232 per term.
Financial Aid 30% of graduate students in nursing programs received some form of financial aid in 2011–12. Research assistantships with partial tuition reimbursements available, teaching assistantships with partial tuition reimbursements available, Federal Work-Study, institutionally sponsored loans, scholarships, and unspecified assistantships available. *Financial aid application deadline:* 3/1.
Contact Dr. Stephanie DeBoor, Coordinator, Graduate Program, Orvis School of Nursing, University of Nevada, Reno, Pennington Health Sciences Building, Reno, NV 89557-0134. *Telephone:* 775-682-7156. *Fax:* 775-784-4262. *E-mail:* deboors2@unr.edu.

MASTER'S DEGREE PROGRAM

Degrees MSN; MSN/MPH
Available Programs Master's.
Concentrations Available Clinical nurse leader; nursing education. *Nurse practitioner programs in:* family health.
Site Options Reno, NV.
Study Options Full-time and part-time.
Program Entrance Requirements Clinical experience, computer literacy, minimum overall college GPA of 3.0, transcript of college record, CPR certification, written essay, immunizations, 3 letters of recommendation, physical assessment course, professional liability insurance/malpractice insurance, prerequisite course work, resume, statistics course. *Application deadline:* 3/1 (fall). *Application fee:* $60.
Advanced Placement Credit given for nursing courses completed elsewhere dependent upon specific evaluations.
Degree Requirements 37 total credit hours, thesis or project, comprehensive exam.

POST-MASTER'S PROGRAM

Areas of Study Clinical nurse leader; nursing education. *Nurse practitioner programs in:* family health.

DOCTORAL DEGREE PROGRAM

Degree DNP
Available Programs Doctorate.
Areas of Study Advanced practice nursing, nursing administration.
Online Degree Options Yes (online only).
Program Entrance Requirements Clinical experience, minimum overall college GPA of 3.5, 2 letters of recommendation, MSN or equivalent, vita, writing sample. *Application deadline:* 3/15 (fall).
Degree Requirements 39 total credit hours, written exam, residency.

NEW HAMPSHIRE

Colby-Sawyer College
Department of Nursing
New London, New Hampshire

http://www.colby-sawyer.edu/nursing/index.html
Founded in 1837
DEGREE • BSN
Nursing Program Faculty 14 (.14% with doctorates).
Baccalaureate Enrollment 169 **Women** 93% **Men** 7% **Minority** 4% **International** 1% **Part-time** 1%
Nursing Student Activities Nursing Honor Society, Student Nurses' Association.

Nursing Student Resources Academic advising; academic or career counseling; assistance for students with disabilities; bookstore; campus computer network; career placement assistance; computer lab; computer-assisted instruction; e-mail services; employment services for current students; housing assistance; interactive nursing skills videos; Internet; learning resource lab; library services; nursing audiovisuals; remedial services; resume preparation assistance; skills, simulation, or other laboratory; tutoring; unpaid internships.
Library Facilities 93,696 volumes (12,050 in health, 760 in nursing); 27,072 periodical subscriptions (135 health-care related).

BACCALAUREATE PROGRAMS

Degree BSN
Available Programs Generic Baccalaureate.
Study Options Full-time and part-time.
Program Entrance Requirements Minimum overall college GPA of 2.7, transcript of college record, CPR certification, written essay, health exam, health insurance, high school biology, high school chemistry, high school foreign language, 3 years high school math, 3 years high school science, high school transcript, immunizations, 2 letters of recommendation, minimum high school GPA of 2.75, minimum GPA in nursing prerequisites of 2.7, prerequisite course work. Transfer students are accepted. *Application deadline:* Applications may be processed on a rolling basis for some programs.
Advanced Placement Credit by examination available. Credit given for nursing courses completed elsewhere dependent upon specific evaluations.
Contact *Telephone:* 603-526-3795. *Fax:* 603-526-3159.

Franklin Pierce University
Master of Science in Nursing
Rindge, New Hampshire

http://www.franklinpierce.edu/
Founded in 1962
DEGREES • BS • MSN
Nursing Program Faculty 4 (50% with doctorates).
Baccalaureate Enrollment 110 **Women** 97% **Men** 3% **Minority** 3% **Part-time** 100%
Graduate Enrollment 24 **Women** 96% **Men** 4% **Minority** 8% **Part-time** 100%
Distance Learning Courses Available.
Nursing Student Resources Academic advising; assistance for students with disabilities; bookstore; campus computer network; computer lab; library services.
Library Facilities 144,770 volumes; 30,093 periodical subscriptions (200 health-care related).

BACCALAUREATE PROGRAMS

Degree BS
Available Programs ADN to Baccalaureate; RN Baccalaureate.
Site Options Concord, NH; Lebanon, NH; Portsmouth, NH.
Study Options Part-time.
Program Entrance Requirements RN licensure. Transfer students are accepted. *Application deadline:* Applications may be processed on a rolling basis for some programs.
Advanced Placement Credit by examination available.
Contact *Telephone:* 603-433-2000 Ext. 2000. *Fax:* 603-899-1067 Ext. 1067.

GRADUATE PROGRAMS

Contact *Telephone:* 603-322-2000. *Fax:* 603-899-1067.

MASTER'S DEGREE PROGRAM
Degree MSN
Available Programs Master's; Master's for Nurses with Non-Nursing Degrees; RN to Master's.
Concentrations Available Nursing administration; nursing education.
Site Options Concord, NH; Lebanon, NH; Portsmouth, NH.
Study Options Part-time.
Program Entrance Requirements Computer literacy, minimum overall college GPA of 2.8, transcript of college record, written essay, interview, 3 letters of recommendation, resume, statistics course. *Application deadline:* Applications may be processed on a rolling basis for some programs.

Degree Requirements 34 total credit hours, thesis or project.

Rivier University
Division of Nursing
Nashua, New Hampshire

http://www.rivier.edu/
Founded in 1933
DEGREES • BS • MS
Nursing Program Faculty 33 (18% with doctorates).
Baccalaureate Enrollment 623 **Women** 94% **Men** 6% **Minority** 9% **Part-time** 37%
Graduate Enrollment 97 **Women** 95% **Men** 5% **Minority** 7% **Part-time** 92%
Distance Learning Courses Available.
Nursing Student Activities Nursing Honor Society, Sigma Theta Tau, Student Nurses' Association.
Nursing Student Resources Academic advising; academic or career counseling; assistance for students with disabilities; bookstore; campus computer network; career placement assistance; computer lab; computer-assisted instruction; e-mail services; employment services for current students; externships; housing assistance; interactive nursing skills videos; Internet; learning resource lab; library services; nursing audiovisuals; other; placement services for program completers; remedial services; resume preparation assistance; skills, simulation, or other laboratory; tutoring.
Library Facilities 178,669 volumes (3,777 in health, 1,170 in nursing); 230 periodical subscriptions (4,000 health-care related).

BACCALAUREATE PROGRAMS

Degree BS
Available Programs ADN to Baccalaureate; Generic Baccalaureate; LPN to Baccalaureate; LPN to RN Baccalaureate; RN Baccalaureate.
Study Options Full-time and part-time.
Online Degree Options Yes.
Program Entrance Requirements Minimum overall college GPA, transcript of college record, written essay, health exam, health insurance, high school chemistry, high school foreign language, high school math, high school science, high school transcript, immunizations, 2 letters of recommendation, minimum high school GPA, minimum high school rank, prerequisite course work. Transfer students are accepted. *Application deadline:* Applications may be processed on a rolling basis for some programs. *Application fee:* $25.
Advanced Placement Credit by examination available. Credit given for nursing courses completed elsewhere dependent upon specific evaluations.
Expenses (2012–13) *Tuition:* full-time $26,430; part-time $881 per credit. *Room and board:* $10,118 per academic year. *Required fees:* full-time $350.
Contact Anne Parks, Senior Associate Director of Admissions, Division of Nursing, Rivier University, 420 South Main Street, Nashua, NH 03060-5086. *Telephone:* 603-897-8515. *Fax:* 603-897-8808. *E-mail:* aparks@rivier.edu.

GRADUATE PROGRAMS

Expenses (2012–13) *Tuition:* full-time $15,858; part-time $881 per credit. *Required fees:* full-time $150.
Contact Pamela A. Slawinowski, Assistant to Program Director, Division of Nursing, Rivier University, 420 South Main Street, Nashua, NH 03060-5086. *Telephone:* 603-897-8528. *Fax:* 603-897-8884. *E-mail:* pslawinowski@rivier.edu.

MASTER'S DEGREE PROGRAM
Degree MS
Available Programs Master's; Master's for Nurses with Non-Nursing Degrees; RN to Master's.
Concentrations Available Nursing education. *Clinical nurse specialist programs in:* family health, psychiatric/mental health. *Nurse practitioner programs in:* family health, psychiatric/mental health.
Study Options Full-time and part-time.
Program Entrance Requirements Clinical experience, minimum overall college GPA of 3.0, transcript of college record, written essay, immunizations, interview, 2 letters of recommendation, resume, statistics course, GRE, MAT. *Application deadline:* Applications may be processed on a rolling basis for some programs. *Application fee:* $25.

Advanced Placement Credit by examination available. Credit given for nursing courses completed elsewhere dependent upon specific evaluations.

Degree Requirements 43 total credit hours, thesis or project.

POST-MASTER'S PROGRAM

Areas of Study Nursing education. *Clinical nurse specialist programs in:* psychiatric/mental health. *Nurse practitioner programs in:* family health, psychiatric/mental health.

Saint Anselm College
Department of Nursing
Manchester, New Hampshire

http://www.anselm.edu/Academics/Majors-and-Departments/Nursing.htm

Founded in 1889

DEGREE • BSN

Nursing Program Faculty 21 (33% with doctorates).

Baccalaureate Enrollment 331 Women 97% Men 3%

Nursing Student Activities Sigma Theta Tau, Student Nurses' Association, nursing club.

Nursing Student Resources Academic advising; academic or career counseling; assistance for students with disabilities; bookstore; campus computer network; career placement assistance; computer lab; computer-assisted instruction; e-mail services; employment services for current students; externships; housing assistance; interactive nursing skills videos; Internet; learning resource lab; library services; nursing audiovisuals; resume preparation assistance; skills, simulation, or other laboratory; tutoring.

Library Facilities 222,000 volumes (6,346 in health); 1,900 periodical subscriptions (4,575 health-care related).

BACCALAUREATE PROGRAMS

Degree BSN

Available Programs RN Baccalaureate.

Study Options Full-time and part-time.

Program Entrance Requirements Transcript of college record, written essay, health exam, health insurance, high school biology, high school chemistry, high school foreign language, 3 years high school math, 3 years high school science, high school transcript, immunizations, 2 letters of recommendation, professional liability insurance/malpractice insurance. *Application deadline:* 11/15 (fall). *Application fee:* $55.

Advanced Placement Credit by examination available. Credit given for nursing courses completed elsewhere dependent upon specific evaluations.

Expenses (2012–13) *Tuition:* full-time $32,710. *Room and board:* $12,380 per academic year. *Required fees:* full-time $3165.

Financial Aid 95% of baccalaureate students in nursing programs received some form of financial aid in 2011–12. *Gift aid (need-based):* Federal Pell, FSEOG, state, private, college/university gift aid from institutional funds. *Loans:* Federal Direct (Subsidized and Unsubsidized Stafford PLUS), Perkins.*Work-study:* Federal Work-Study, part-time campus jobs.*Financial aid application deadline:* 3/15(priority: 3/15).

Contact Mr. Eric Nichols, Director of Admission, Department of Nursing, Saint Anselm College, 100 Saint Anselm Drive, Manchester, NH 03102-1310. *Telephone:* 603-641-7500. *Fax:* 603-641-7550. *E-mail:* enichols@anselm.edu.

CONTINUING EDUCATION PROGRAM

Contact Sharon George, Dean of Nursing, Department of Nursing, Saint Anselm College, 100 Saint Anselm Drive, #1745, Manchester, NH 03102-1310. *Telephone:* 603-641-7084. *Fax:* 603-641-7089. *E-mail:* sgeorge@anselm.edu.

University of New Hampshire
Department of Nursing
Durham, New Hampshire

http://www.unh.edu/nursing

Founded in 1866

DEGREES • BS • MS

Nursing Program Faculty 13 (75% with doctorates).

Baccalaureate Enrollment 268 Women 91% Men 9% Minority 1%

Graduate Enrollment 54 Women 95% Men 5% Minority 1%

Nursing Student Activities Nursing Honor Society, Sigma Theta Tau, Student Nurses' Association.

Nursing Student Resources Academic advising; academic or career counseling; assistance for students with disabilities; bookstore; campus computer network; computer lab; computer-assisted instruction; daycare for children of students; e-mail services; housing assistance; interactive nursing skills videos; Internet; learning resource lab; nursing audiovisuals; paid internships; resume preparation assistance; skills, simulation, or other laboratory; tutoring.

Library Facilities 1.6 million volumes; 64,222 periodical subscriptions.

BACCALAUREATE PROGRAMS

Degree BS

Available Programs Generic Baccalaureate; RN Baccalaureate.

Study Options Full-time and part-time.

Program Entrance Requirements High school transcript, prerequisite course work. Transfer students are accepted.

Contact *Telephone:* 603-862-4715. *Fax:* 603-862-4771.

GRADUATE PROGRAMS

Contact *Telephone:* 603-862-2285. *Fax:* 603-862-4771.

MASTER'S DEGREE PROGRAM

Degree MS

Available Programs Master's; Master's for Nurses with Non-Nursing Degrees.

Concentrations Available *Clinical nurse specialist programs in:* adult health. *Nurse practitioner programs in:* adult health, family health.

Program Entrance Requirements GRE General Test or MAT.

Degree Requirements 45 total credit hours, thesis or project, comprehensive exam.

POST-MASTER'S PROGRAM

Areas of Study *Clinical nurse specialist programs in:* adult health. *Nurse practitioner programs in:* adult health, family health.

NEW JERSEY

Bloomfield College
Division of Nursing
Bloomfield, New Jersey

http://www.bloomfield.edu/

Founded in 1868

DEGREE • BS

Nursing Program Faculty 18 (33% with doctorates).

Baccalaureate Enrollment 172 Women 91% Men 9% Minority 65% International 3% Part-time 24%

Nursing Student Activities Student Nurses' Association.

Nursing Student Resources Academic advising; academic or career counseling; assistance for students with disabilities; bookstore; campus computer network; career placement assistance; computer lab; computer-assisted instruction; e-mail services; employment services for current students; interactive nursing skills videos; Internet; learning resource lab; library services; nursing audiovisuals; other; placement services for program completers; remedial services; resume preparation assistance; skills, simulation, or other laboratory; tutoring.

Library Facilities 57,793 volumes (2,000 in health, 1,600 in nursing); 460 periodical subscriptions (44 health-care related).

BACCALAUREATE PROGRAMS

Degree BS

Available Programs Generic Baccalaureate; RN Baccalaureate.

Study Options Full-time and part-time.

Program Entrance Requirements Transcript of college record, CPR certification, health exam, immunizations, minimum GPA in nursing prerequisites of 2.5, prerequisite course work. Transfer students are accepted. *Application deadline:* 5/1 (fall). *Application fee:* $40.

Advanced Placement Credit by examination available. Credit given for nursing courses completed elsewhere dependent upon specific evaluations.

Expenses (2012–13) *Tuition:* full-time $23,850; part-time $2980 per course. *International tuition:* $23,850 full-time. *Room and board:* $10,700 per academic year. *Required fees:* full-time $1200; part-time $150 per credit.

Financial Aid 93% of baccalaureate students in nursing programs received some form of financial aid in 2011–12. *Gift aid (need-based):* Federal Pell, FSEOG, state, private, college/university gift aid from institutional funds. *Loans:* Federal Direct (Subsidized and Unsubsidized Stafford PLUS).*Work-study:* Federal Work-Study, part-time campus jobs.*Financial aid application deadline:* 6/1(priority: 3/15).

Contact Dr. Neddie Serra, Chair, Division of Nursing, Bloomfield College, Bloomfield, NJ 07003. *Telephone:* 973-748-9000 Ext. 120. *Fax:* 973-743-3998. *E-mail:* neddie_serra@bloomfield.edu.

Caldwell College

Nursing Programs
Caldwell, New Jersey

http://www.caldwell.edu/

Founded in 1939

DEGREE • BSN

Nursing Program Faculty 13 (24% with doctorates).

Baccalaureate Enrollment 150

Nursing Student Activities Student Nurses' Association, nursing club.

Nursing Student Resources Academic advising; academic or career counseling; assistance for students with disabilities; bookstore; campus computer network; computer lab; computer-assisted instruction; e-mail services; employment services for current students; housing assistance; Internet; learning resource lab; library services; nursing audiovisuals; paid internships; remedial services; skills, simulation, or other laboratory; tutoring.

Library Facilities 178,400 volumes (4,794 in health, 97 in nursing); 422 periodical subscriptions (5,215 health-care related).

BACCALAUREATE PROGRAMS

Degree BSN

Available Programs Baccalaureate for Second Degree; Generic Baccalaureate; RN Baccalaureate.

Study Options Full-time and part-time.

Program Entrance Requirements Minimum overall college GPA of 2.75, transcript of college record, CPR certification, written essay, health exam, health insurance, high school biology, high school chemistry, high school foreign language, 4 years high school math, 3 years high school science, high school transcript, immunizations, 2 letters of recommendation, minimum high school GPA of 2.75, minimum GPA in nursing prerequisites of 2.75, professional liability insurance/malpractice insurance, prerequisite course work. Transfer students are accepted. *Application deadline:* Applications may be processed on a rolling basis for some programs. *Application fee:* $40.

Advanced Placement Credit by examination available.

Expenses (2012–13) *Tuition:* full-time $26,900; part-time $738 per credit. *Room and board:* $12,066 per academic year. *Required fees:* full-time $900; part-time $150 per term.

Contact Ms. Michelle Perez, Academic Advisor, Nursing Programs, Caldwell College, 120 Bloomfield Avenue, Caldwell, NJ 07006. *Telephone:* 973-618-3339. *E-mail:* miperez@caldwell.edu.

The College of New Jersey

School of Nursing, Health and Exercise Science
Ewing, New Jersey

http://nursing.pages.tcnj.edu/

Founded in 1855

DEGREES • BSN • MSN

Nursing Program Faculty 16 (38% with doctorates).

Baccalaureate Enrollment 286 **Women** 90% **Men** 10% **Minority** 38% **Part-time** 3%

Graduate Enrollment 25 **Women** 88% **Men** 12% **Minority** 24% **Part-time** 88%

Nursing Student Activities Sigma Theta Tau, Student Nurses' Association.

Nursing Student Resources Academic advising; academic or career counseling; assistance for students with disabilities; bookstore; campus computer network; career placement assistance; computer lab; computer-assisted instruction; daycare for children of students; e-mail services; employment services for current students; externships; interactive nursing skills videos; Internet; learning resource lab; library services; nursing audiovisuals; paid internships; resume preparation assistance; skills, simulation, or other laboratory; tutoring; unpaid internships.

Library Facilities 694,144 volumes (30,000 in health, 18,800 in nursing); 73,733 periodical subscriptions (228 health-care related).

BACCALAUREATE PROGRAMS

Degree BSN

Available Programs Generic Baccalaureate; RN Baccalaureate.

Study Options Full-time and part-time.

Program Entrance Requirements Written essay, health exam, high school transcript, immunizations. Transfer students are accepted. *Application deadline:* 1/15 (fall), 11/15 (spring). *Application fee:* $75.

Advanced Placement Credit by examination available. Credit given for nursing courses completed elsewhere dependent upon specific evaluations.

Expenses (2012–13) *Tuition, state resident:* full-time $10,102; part-time $358 per credit hour. *Tuition, nonresident:* full-time $20,254; part-time $717 per credit hour. *International tuition:* $20,254 full-time. *Room and board:* $10,998; room only: $8006 per academic year. *Required fees:* full-time $4600; part-time $170 per credit.

Financial Aid 80% of baccalaureate students in nursing programs received some form of financial aid in 2011–12. *Gift aid (need-based):* Federal Pell, FSEOG, state, private, college/university gift aid from institutional funds. *Loans:* Federal Nursing Student Loans, Federal Direct (Subsidized and Unsubsidized Stafford PLUS), Perkins.*Work-study:* Federal Work-Study.*Financial aid application deadline (priority):* 3/1.

Contact Antonino Scarpati, Assistant Dean for Student Services, School of Nursing, Health and Exercise Science, The College of New Jersey, PO Box 7718, 2000 Pennington Road, Ewing, NJ 08628-0718. *Telephone:* 609-771-2669. *Fax:* 609-637-5159. *E-mail:* roger@tcnj.edu.

GRADUATE PROGRAMS

Expenses (2012–13) *Tuition, state resident:* full-time $11,616; part-time $645 per credit hour. *Tuition, nonresident:* full-time $18,321; part-time $1018 per credit hour. *International tuition:* $18,321 full-time. *Required fees:* full-time $3206; part-time $159 per credit.

Financial Aid 48% of graduate students in nursing programs received some form of financial aid in 2011–12. Tuition waivers (partial) and unspecified assistantships available. *Financial aid application deadline:* 5/1.

Contact Dr. Claire Lindberg, Chair, Division of Advanced Nursing Education and Practice, School of Nursing, Health and Exercise Science, The College of New Jersey, PO Box 7718, 2000 Pennington Road, Ewing, NJ 08628-0718. *Telephone:* 609-771-2591. *Fax:* 609-637-5159. *E-mail:* lindberg@tcnj.edu.

MASTER'S DEGREE PROGRAM

Degree MSN

Available Programs Master's; Master's for Nurses with Non-Nursing Degrees; RN to Master's.

Concentrations Available Clinical nurse leader. *Clinical nurse specialist programs in:* adult health. *Nurse practitioner programs in:* adult health, family health, neonatal health, school health.

Study Options Full-time and part-time.

Program Entrance Requirements Computer literacy, minimum overall college GPA of 3.0, transcript of college record, written essay, immunizations, interview, 3 letters of recommendation, physical assessment course, statistics course, GRE General Test. *Application deadline:* 2/1 (fall), 2/1 (summer). *Application fee:* $75.

Advanced Placement Credit given for nursing courses completed elsewhere dependent upon specific evaluations.

Degree Requirements 47 total credit hours, comprehensive exam.

POST-MASTER'S PROGRAM

Areas of Study Nursing administration. *Clinical nurse specialist programs in:* adult health. *Nurse practitioner programs in:* adult health, family health, neonatal health.

College of Saint Elizabeth
Department of Nursing
Morristown, New Jersey

http://www.cse.edu/academics/academic-areas/health-wellness/nursing/
Founded in 1899

DEGREE • BSN

Nursing Program Faculty 13 (25% with doctorates).
Baccalaureate Enrollment 231 **Women** 95% **Men** 5% **Minority** 48% **Part-time** 99%
Nursing Student Activities Nursing Honor Society, Sigma Theta Tau, nursing club.
Nursing Student Resources Academic advising; academic or career counseling; assistance for students with disabilities; bookstore; campus computer network; career placement assistance; computer lab; computer-assisted instruction; e-mail services; employment services for current students; interactive nursing skills videos; Internet; learning resource lab; library services; nursing audiovisuals; other; remedial services; resume preparation assistance; skills, simulation, or other laboratory; tutoring.
Library Facilities 119,438 volumes (4,246 in health, 702 in nursing); 977 periodical subscriptions (194 health-care related).

BACCALAUREATE PROGRAMS

Degree BSN
Available Programs ADN to Baccalaureate; Accelerated RN Baccalaureate; International Nurse to Baccalaureate; RN Baccalaureate.
Site Options Randolph, NJ; Elizabeth , NJ; Hoboken, NJ.
Study Options Part-time.
Program Entrance Requirements Minimum overall college GPA of 2.0, transcript of college record, CPR certification, health exam, immunizations, prerequisite course work, RN licensure. Transfer students are accepted.
Advanced Placement Credit by examination available. Credit given for nursing courses completed elsewhere dependent upon specific evaluations.
Contact *Telephone:* 973-290-4056. *Fax:* 973-290-4177.

CONTINUING EDUCATION PROGRAM

Contact *Telephone:* 973-290-4073. *Fax:* 973-290-4177.

Fairleigh Dickinson University, Metropolitan Campus
Henry P. Becton School of Nursing and Allied Health
Teaneck, New Jersey

http://fduinfo.com/depts/ucnah.php
Founded in 1942

DEGREES • BSN • DNP • MSN

Nursing Program Faculty 22 (70% with doctorates).
Baccalaureate Enrollment 379 **Women** 88% **Men** 12% **Minority** 55% **International** 1% **Part-time** 26%
Graduate Enrollment 468 **Women** 86% **Men** 14% **Minority** 60% **International** 2% **Part-time** 95%
Distance Learning Courses Available.
Nursing Student Activities Nursing Honor Society, Sigma Theta Tau, Student Nurses' Association.
Nursing Student Resources Academic advising; academic or career counseling; assistance for students with disabilities; bookstore; campus computer network; career placement assistance; computer lab; computer-assisted instruction; e-mail services; employment services for current students; externships; housing assistance; interactive nursing skills videos; Internet; learning resource lab; library services; nursing audiovisuals; other; placement services for program completers; remedial services; resume preparation assistance; skills, simulation, or other laboratory; tutoring; unpaid internships.
Library Facilities 2,336 volumes in health, 2,336 volumes in nursing; 1,526 periodical subscriptions health-care related.

BACCALAUREATE PROGRAMS

Degree BSN
Available Programs Accelerated Baccalaureate for Second Degree; Generic Baccalaureate; RN Baccalaureate.
Site Options Teaneck, NJ; Morristown, NJ; Summit, NJ.
Study Options Full-time.
Program Entrance Requirements Minimum overall college GPA of 3.0, transcript of college record, CPR certification, health exam, health insurance, high school biology, high school chemistry, 2 years high school math, 2 years high school science, high school transcript, immunizations, 2 letters of recommendation, professional liability insurance/malpractice insurance. Transfer students are accepted. *Application deadline:* Applications may be processed on a rolling basis for some programs. *Application fee:* $40.
Advanced Placement Credit given for nursing courses completed elsewhere dependent upon specific evaluations.
Expenses (2012–13) *Tuition:* full-time $32,852; part-time $907 per credit. *International tuition:* $32,852 full-time. *Room and board:* $12,406; room only: $8336 per academic year. *Required fees:* full-time $904; part-time $16 per credit; part-time $188 per term.
Financial Aid 94% of baccalaureate students in nursing programs received some form of financial aid in 2011–12.
Contact Ms. Sylvia Cabassa, Associate Director, Undergraduate Nursing, Henry P. Becton School of Nursing and Allied Health, Fairleigh Dickinson University, Metropolitan Campus, 1000 River Road, H-DH4-02, Teaneck, NJ 07666-1914. *Telephone:* 201-692-2880. *Fax:* 201-692-2388. *E-mail:* scabassa@fdu.edu.

GRADUATE PROGRAMS

Expenses (2012–13) *Tuition:* full-time $20,340; part-time $1130 per credit. *International tuition:* $20,340 full-time. *Room and board:* $12,406; room only: $8336 per academic year. *Required fees:* full-time $940; part-time $16 per credit; part-time $188 per term.
Financial Aid 91% of graduate students in nursing programs received some form of financial aid in 2011–12.
Contact Dr. Elizabeth S. Parietti, Associate Director of Graduate Programs, Henry P. Becton School of Nursing and Allied Health, Fairleigh Dickinson University, Metropolitan Campus, 1000 River Road, H-DH4-02, Teaneck, NJ 07666-1914. *Telephone:* 201-692-2881. *Fax:* 201-692-2388. *E-mail:* parietti@fdu.edu.

MASTER'S DEGREE PROGRAM

Degree MSN
Available Programs Accelerated RN to Master's; Master's; RN to Master's.
Concentrations Available Nursing administration; nursing education; nursing informatics. *Nurse practitioner programs in:* adult health, family health, gerontology, psychiatric/mental health.
Site Options Teaneck, NJ; Morristown, NJ; Summit, NJ.
Study Options Full-time and part-time.
Online Degree Options Yes.
Program Entrance Requirements Clinical experience, minimum overall college GPA of 3.0, transcript of college record, CPR certification, immunizations, 2 letters of recommendation, nursing research course, physical assessment course, professional liability insurance/malpractice insurance, resume, statistics course. *Application deadline:* Applications may be processed on a rolling basis for some programs. *Application fee:* $40.
Advanced Placement Credit given for nursing courses completed elsewhere dependent upon specific evaluations.
Degree Requirements 30 total credit hours, thesis or project.

POST-MASTER'S PROGRAM

Areas of Study Nursing administration; nursing education; nursing informatics. *Nurse practitioner programs in:* adult health, family health, gerontology, psychiatric/mental health.

DOCTORAL DEGREE PROGRAM

Degree DNP

Available Programs Doctorate.

Areas of Study Advanced practice nursing, clinical practice, health policy, health-care systems, human health and illness, information systems, nursing administration, nursing policy, nursing research, nursing science.

Program Entrance Requirements Clinical experience, minimum overall college GPA of 3.5, interview by faculty committee, interview, 3 letters of recommendation, MSN or equivalent, vita, writing sample. *Application deadline:* Applications may be processed on a rolling basis for some programs. *Application fee:* $40.

Degree Requirements 36 total credit hours, dissertation, oral exam, residency.

CONTINUING EDUCATION PROGRAM

Contact Mrs. Marian L. Rutherford, RN, Administrator for Clinical Affairs, Henry P. Becton School of Nursing and Allied Health, Fairleigh Dickinson University, Metropolitan Campus, 1000 River Road, H-DH4-02, Teaneck, NJ 07666-1914. *Telephone:* 201-692-2520. *Fax:* 201-692-2388. *E-mail:* marian@fdu.edu.

Felician College
Division of Nursing and Health Management
Lodi, New Jersey

http://www.felician.edu/
Founded in 1942
DEGREES • BSN • MA/MSM • MSN
Nursing Program Faculty 25 (32% with doctorates).
Baccalaureate Enrollment 512 **Women** 92% **Men** 8% **Minority** 32% **International** 2% **Part-time** 20%
Graduate Enrollment 93 **Women** 89% **Men** 11% **Minority** 33% **Part-time** 88%
Distance Learning Courses Available.
Nursing Student Activities Nursing Honor Society, Sigma Theta Tau, Student Nurses' Association.
Nursing Student Resources Academic advising; academic or career counseling; assistance for students with disabilities; bookstore; campus computer network; career placement assistance; computer lab; computer-assisted instruction; daycare for children of students; e-mail services; interactive nursing skills videos; Internet; learning resource lab; library services; nursing audiovisuals; placement services for program completers; remedial services; resume preparation assistance; skills, simulation, or other laboratory; tutoring.
Library Facilities 158,728 volumes (12,519 in health, 12,519 in nursing); 22,575 periodical subscriptions (21 health-care related).

BACCALAUREATE PROGRAMS

Degree BSN
Available Programs Accelerated Baccalaureate for Second Degree; Generic Baccalaureate.
Site Options East Orange, NJ; Long Branch, NJ; Edison, NJ.
Study Options Full-time and part-time.
Program Entrance Requirements Minimum overall college GPA of 3.0, transcript of college record, written essay, health exam, health insurance, high school biology, high school chemistry, 2 years high school math, 2 years high school science, high school transcript, immunizations, minimum high school GPA of 3.0, minimum GPA in nursing prerequisites of 2.8, professional liability insurance/malpractice insurance. Transfer students are accepted. *Application deadline:* 8/15 (fall), 1/10 (spring). Applications may be processed on a rolling basis for some programs. *Application fee:* $30.
Advanced Placement Credit by examination available. Credit given for nursing courses completed elsewhere dependent upon specific evaluations.
Contact *Telephone:* 201-559-6131. *Fax:* 201-559-6138.

GRADUATE PROGRAMS

Contact *Telephone:* 201-559-6077. *Fax:* 201-559-6138.

MASTER'S DEGREE PROGRAM
Degrees MA/MSM; MSN
Available Programs Accelerated RN to Master's; Master's.
Concentrations Available Nursing administration; nursing education. *Nurse practitioner programs in:* adult health, family health.
Study Options Full-time and part-time.

Online Degree Options Yes.

Program Entrance Requirements Clinical experience, computer literacy, minimum overall college GPA of 3.0, transcript of college record, CPR certification, written essay, immunizations, 2 letters of recommendation, nursing research course, physical assessment course, professional liability insurance/malpractice insurance, prerequisite course work, statistics course. *Application deadline:* Applications may be processed on a rolling basis for some programs. *Application fee:* $40.

Advanced Placement Credit given for nursing courses completed elsewhere dependent upon specific evaluations.

Degree Requirements 46 total credit hours, thesis or project.

POST-MASTER'S PROGRAM
Areas of Study Nursing administration; nursing education. *Nurse practitioner programs in:* adult health, family health.

Kean University
Department of Nursing
Union, New Jersey

http://www.kean.edu/KU/School-of-Nursing
Founded in 1855
DEGREES • BSN • MSN • MSN/MPA
Nursing Program Faculty 31 (32% with doctorates).
Baccalaureate Enrollment 313 **Women** 93% **Men** 7% **Minority** 45% **International** 35% **Part-time** 90%
Graduate Enrollment 102 **Women** 93% **Men** 7% **Minority** 40% **International** 20% **Part-time** 95%
Nursing Student Activities Nursing Honor Society, Sigma Theta Tau, nursing club.
Nursing Student Resources Academic advising; academic or career counseling; assistance for students with disabilities; bookstore; campus computer network; career placement assistance; computer lab; computer-assisted instruction; daycare for children of students; e-mail services; employment services for current students; housing assistance; interactive nursing skills videos; Internet; learning resource lab; library services; nursing audiovisuals; placement services for program completers; remedial services; resume preparation assistance; tutoring.
Library Facilities 335,655 volumes; 37,256 periodical subscriptions.

BACCALAUREATE PROGRAMS

Degree BSN
Available Programs ADN to Baccalaureate; RN Baccalaureate.
Site Options Branchburg, NJ; Toms River, NJ.
Study Options Full-time and part-time.
Program Entrance Requirements Minimum overall college GPA of 2.0, written essay, 2 letters of recommendation, prerequisite course work, RN licensure. Transfer students are accepted. *Application deadline:* Applications may be processed on a rolling basis for some programs.
Advanced Placement Credit by examination available. Credit given for nursing courses completed elsewhere dependent upon specific evaluations.
Contact *Telephone:* 908-737-3390. *Fax:* 908-737-3393.

GRADUATE PROGRAMS

Contact *Telephone:* 908-737-3390. *Fax:* 908-737-3393.

MASTER'S DEGREE PROGRAM
Degrees MSN; MSN/MPA
Available Programs Accelerated Master's for Nurses with Non-Nursing Degrees; Master's; Master's for Nurses with Non-Nursing Degrees.
Concentrations Available Health-care administration; nursing administration. *Clinical nurse specialist programs in:* community health, school health.
Site Options Toms River, NJ.
Study Options Full-time and part-time.
Program Entrance Requirements Clinical experience, computer literacy, minimum overall college GPA of 3.0, transcript of college record, written essay, immunizations, interview, 2 letters of recommendation, nursing research course, physical assessment course, professional liability insurance/malpractice insurance, statistics course.
Advanced Placement Credit given for nursing courses completed elsewhere dependent upon specific evaluations.
Degree Requirements 36 total credit hours, thesis or project.

Monmouth University
Marjorie K. Unterberg School of Nursing
West Long Branch, New Jersey

http://www.monmouth.edu/
Founded in 1933
DEGREES • BSN • MSN
Nursing Program Faculty 17 (67% with doctorates).
Baccalaureate Enrollment 71 **Women** 93% **Men** 7% **Minority** 23%
Part-time 98%
Graduate Enrollment 245 **Women** 97% **Men** 3% **Minority** 25% **International** .08% **Part-time** 92%
Distance Learning Courses Available.
Nursing Student Activities Sigma Theta Tau, Student Nurses' Association.
Nursing Student Resources Academic advising; academic or career counseling; assistance for students with disabilities; bookstore; campus computer network; career placement assistance; computer lab; computer-assisted instruction; e-mail services; employment services for current students; interactive nursing skills videos; Internet; learning resource lab; library services; nursing audiovisuals; paid internships; remedial services; resume preparation assistance; skills, simulation, or other laboratory; tutoring.
Library Facilities 286,000 volumes (250,000 in health, 25,000 in nursing); 43,200 periodical subscriptions (98 health-care related).

BACCALAUREATE PROGRAMS

Degree BSN
Available Programs ADN to Baccalaureate; RN Baccalaureate.
Site Options Red Bank, NJ; Freehold, NJ.
Study Options Full-time and part-time.
Program Entrance Requirements Transcript of college record, health exam, immunizations, 2 letters of recommendation, minimum GPA in nursing prerequisites of 2.0, professional liability insurance/malpractice insurance, prerequisite course work, RN licensure. Transfer students are accepted. *Application deadline:* 7/15 (fall), 11/15 (spring), 5/1 (summer). Applications may be processed on a rolling basis for some programs. *Application fee:* $50.
Advanced Placement Credit by examination available. Credit given for nursing courses completed elsewhere dependent upon specific evaluations.
Contact *Telephone:* 732-571-3443. *Fax:* 732-263-5131.

GRADUATE PROGRAMS

Contact *Telephone:* 732-571-3443. *Fax:* 732-263-5131.

MASTER'S DEGREE PROGRAM
Degree MSN
Available Programs Master's; Master's for Nurses with Non-Nursing Degrees; RN to Master's.
Concentrations Available Nursing administration; nursing education. *Clinical nurse specialist programs in:* forensic nursing, school health. *Nurse practitioner programs in:* adult health, family health, psychiatric/mental health.
Site Options Edison, NJ.
Study Options Full-time and part-time.
Program Entrance Requirements Minimum overall college GPA of 2.75, transcript of college record, immunizations, 2 letters of recommendation, professional liability insurance/malpractice insurance. *Application deadline:* 7/15 (fall), 11/15 (spring), 5/1 (summer). Applications may be processed on a rolling basis for some programs. *Application fee:* $50.
Advanced Placement Credit by examination available. Credit given for nursing courses completed elsewhere dependent upon specific evaluations.
Degree Requirements 42 total credit hours.

POST-MASTER'S PROGRAM
Areas of Study Nursing administration; nursing education. *Clinical nurse specialist programs in:* forensic nursing, school health. *Nurse practitioner programs in:* adult health, family health, psychiatric/mental health.

CONTINUING EDUCATION PROGRAM

Contact *Telephone:* 732-571-3694. *Fax:* 732-263-5131.

New Jersey City University
Department of Nursing
Jersey City, New Jersey

https://www.njcu.edu/nursing/
Founded in 1927
DEGREE • BSN
Nursing Program Faculty 10 (70% with doctorates).
Baccalaureate Enrollment 125 **Women** 85% **Men** 15% **Minority** 75%
International 15% **Part-time** 40%
Nursing Student Activities Nursing Honor Society, Sigma Theta Tau, Student Nurses' Association.
Nursing Student Resources Academic advising; academic or career counseling; assistance for students with disabilities; bookstore; campus computer network; computer lab; computer-assisted instruction; daycare for children of students; e-mail services; interactive nursing skills videos; Internet; learning resource lab; library services; nursing audiovisuals; remedial services; skills, simulation, or other laboratory.
Library Facilities 319,360 volumes; 25,214 periodical subscriptions.

BACCALAUREATE PROGRAMS

Degree BSN
Available Programs Accelerated Baccalaureate for Second Degree; RN Baccalaureate.
Site Options Wall Township, NJ; East Orange, NJ.
Study Options Full-time.
Program Entrance Requirements Minimum overall college GPA of 3.0, transcript of college record, CPR certification, written essay, health exam, immunizations, 2 letters of recommendation, professional liability insurance/malpractice insurance, prerequisite course work, RN licensure. Transfer students are accepted. *Application deadline:* 5/15 (fall), 3/15 (summer). *Application fee:* $35.
Advanced Placement Credit by examination available. Credit given for nursing courses completed elsewhere dependent upon specific evaluations.
Financial Aid 40% of baccalaureate students in nursing programs received some form of financial aid in 2010–11. *Gift aid (need-based):* Federal Pell, FSEOG, state, college/university gift aid from institutional funds. *Loans:* Federal Direct (Subsidized and Unsubsidized Stafford PLUS). *Work-study:* Federal Work-Study. *Financial aid application deadline (priority):* 4/15.
Contact Dr. Debra Scardaville, PhD, Associate Professor, Department of Nursing, New Jersey City University, 2039 Kennedy Boulevard, R404, Jersey City, NJ 07305. *Telephone:* 201-200-2511. *Fax:* 201-200-3222. *E-mail:* dscardavil@njcu.edu.

Ramapo College of New Jersey
Master of Science in Nursing Program
Mahwah, New Jersey

http://ww2.ramapo.edu/nursing/
Founded in 1969
DEGREES • BSN • MSN
Nursing Program Faculty 29 (20% with doctorates).
Baccalaureate Enrollment 435 **Women** 90% **Men** 10% **Minority** 35%
International 7% **Part-time** 15%
Graduate Enrollment 41 **Women** 95% **Men** 5% **Minority** 17% **Part-time** 90%
Distance Learning Courses Available.
Nursing Student Activities Nursing Honor Society, Student Nurses' Association.
Nursing Student Resources Academic advising; academic or career counseling; assistance for students with disabilities; bookstore; campus computer network; career placement assistance; computer lab; computer-assisted instruction; e-mail services; employment services for current students; externships; housing assistance; interactive nursing skills videos; Internet; learning resource lab; library services; nursing audiovisuals; placement services for program completers; remedial services; resume preparation assistance; skills, simulation, or other laboratory; tutoring; unpaid internships.
Library Facilities 298,364 volumes (3,500 in nursing); 488 periodical subscriptions (200 health-care related).

BACCALAUREATE PROGRAMS

Degree BSN
Available Programs Generic Baccalaureate; RN Baccalaureate.
Site Options Englewood, NJ.
Study Options Full-time.
Online Degree Options Yes.
Program Entrance Requirements CPR certification, health exam, 3 years high school science, immunizations, minimum high school GPA of 2.5, minimum high school rank 20%, professional liability insurance/malpractice insurance. Transfer students are accepted. *Application deadline:* 3/1 (fall), 3/1 (spring). Applications may be processed on a rolling basis for some programs. *Application fee:* $60.
Advanced Placement Credit given for nursing courses completed elsewhere dependent upon specific evaluations.
Contact *Telephone:* 201-684-7737. *Fax:* 201-684-7934.

GRADUATE PROGRAMS

Contact *Telephone:* 201-684-7737. *Fax:* 201-684-7934.

MASTER'S DEGREE PROGRAM

Degree MSN
Available Programs Master's.
Concentrations Available Nursing education.
Study Options Full-time and part-time.
Online Degree Options Yes (online only).
Program Entrance Requirements Clinical experience, computer literacy, minimum overall college GPA of 3.0, transcript of college record, CPR certification, 2 letters of recommendation, nursing research course, professional liability insurance/malpractice insurance, statistics course. *Application deadline:* Applications may be processed on a rolling basis for some programs. *Application fee:* $60.
Advanced Placement Credit given for nursing courses completed elsewhere dependent upon specific evaluations.
Degree Requirements 32 total credit hours.

POST-MASTER'S PROGRAM

Areas of Study Nursing education.

CONTINUING EDUCATION PROGRAM

Contact *Telephone:* 201-684-7206. *Fax:* 201-684-7954.

The Richard Stockton College of New Jersey

Program in Nursing
Pomona, New Jersey

http://www.stockton.edu
Founded in 1969

DEGREES • BSN • MSN

Nursing Program Faculty 6 (66% with doctorates).
Baccalaureate Enrollment 69 **Women** 98% **Men** 2% **Minority** 10% **Part-time** 80%
Graduate Enrollment 20 **Women** 90% **Men** 10% **Minority** 15% **Part-time** 95%
Nursing Student Activities Sigma Theta Tau.
Nursing Student Resources Academic advising; academic or career counseling; assistance for students with disabilities; bookstore; campus computer network; computer lab; computer-assisted instruction; daycare for children of students; e-mail services; housing assistance; Internet; learning resource lab; library services; nursing audiovisuals; resume preparation assistance; skills, simulation, or other laboratory; tutoring.
Library Facilities 308,800 volumes (9,761 in health, 1,258 in nursing); 47,250 periodical subscriptions (83 health-care related).

BACCALAUREATE PROGRAMS

Degree BSN
Available Programs RN Baccalaureate.
Study Options Full-time and part-time.
Program Entrance Requirements Transfer students are accepted.
Advanced Placement Credit given for nursing courses completed elsewhere dependent upon specific evaluations.
Contact *Telephone:* 609-652-4837.

GRADUATE PROGRAMS

Contact *Telephone:* 609-652-4501.

MASTER'S DEGREE PROGRAM

Degree MSN
Concentrations Available *Nurse practitioner programs in:* adult health.
Study Options Full-time and part-time.
Program Entrance Requirements Clinical experience, computer literacy, minimum overall college GPA of 3.0, transcript of college record, CPR certification, written essay, immunizations, 2 letters of recommendation, nursing research course, physical assessment course, professional liability insurance/malpractice insurance, statistics course.
Advanced Placement Credit given for nursing courses completed elsewhere dependent upon specific evaluations.
Degree Requirements 42 total credit hours, thesis or project.

Rowan University

RN to BSN Program
Glassboro, New Jersey

Founded in 1923

DEGREE • BSN

Library Facilities 438,135 volumes; 50,883 periodical subscriptions.

BACCALAUREATE PROGRAMS

Degree BSN
Available Programs RN Baccalaureate.
Study Options Part-time.
Program Entrance Requirements Minimum overall college GPA of 2.75, transcript of college record, prerequisite course work, RN licensure. *Application fee:* $65.
Contact Admissions, RN to BSN Program, Rowan University, 201 Mullica Hill Road, Glassboro, NJ 08028. *Telephone:* 856-256-5435. *E-mail:* cgceenrollement@rowan.edu.

Rutgers School of Nursing–Camden

Rutgers School of Nursing–Camden
Camden, New Jersey

http://nursing.camden.rutgers.edu/

DEGREE • BS

Nursing Program Faculty 35 (20% with doctorates).
Baccalaureate Enrollment 252 **Women** 84% **Men** 16% **Minority** 41% **Part-time** 22%
Distance Learning Courses Available.
Nursing Student Activities Sigma Theta Tau, Student Nurses' Association.
Nursing Student Resources Academic advising; academic or career counseling; assistance for students with disabilities; bookstore; campus computer network; computer lab; computer-assisted instruction; e-mail services; employment services for current students; externships; housing assistance; interactive nursing skills videos; Internet; learning resource lab; library services; nursing audiovisuals; remedial services; resume preparation assistance; skills, simulation, or other laboratory; tutoring.

BACCALAUREATE PROGRAMS

Degree BS
Available Programs Accelerated RN Baccalaureate; Generic Baccalaureate; RN Baccalaureate.
Site Options Atlantic City, NJ; Blackwood, NJ.
Study Options Full-time.
Program Entrance Requirements Written essay, health insurance, 2 years high school math, high school transcript, minimum high school GPA of 3.0. Transfer students are accepted. *Application deadline:* 3/12 (fall).
Contact Mahirym Holguin, Administrative Assistant, Rutgers School of Nursing–Camden, 311 North Fifth Street, Armitage Hall, Room 407, Camden, NJ 08102. *Telephone:* 856-225-6226. *Fax:* 856-225-6250. *E-mail:* nursecam@camden.rutgers.edu.

Rutgers, The State University of New Jersey, College of Nursing

Rutgers, The State University of New Jersey, College of Nursing
Newark, New Jersey

http://www.rutgers.edu/
Founded in 1956
DEGREES • BS • MS • MS/MPH • PHD
Nursing Program Faculty 31 (80% with doctorates).
Baccalaureate Enrollment 567 **Women** 90% **Men** 10% **Minority** 52% **International** 1% **Part-time** 20%
Graduate Enrollment 176 **Women** 98% **Men** 2% **Minority** 30% **Part-time** 90%
Distance Learning Courses Available.
Nursing Student Activities Sigma Theta Tau, Student Nurses' Association, nursing club.
Nursing Student Resources Academic advising; academic or career counseling; assistance for students with disabilities; bookstore; campus computer network; career placement assistance; computer lab; computer-assisted instruction; e-mail services; employment services for current students; externships; housing assistance; interactive nursing skills videos; Internet; learning resource lab; library services; nursing audiovisuals; paid internships; remedial services; resume preparation assistance; skills, simulation, or other laboratory; tutoring; unpaid internships.
Library Facilities 6.4 million volumes; 28,934 periodical subscriptions.

BACCALAUREATE PROGRAMS

Degree BS
Available Programs Accelerated Baccalaureate for Second Degree; Baccalaureate for Second Degree; Generic Baccalaureate; RN Baccalaureate.
Site Options Freehold, NJ; New Brunswick, NJ.
Study Options Full-time and part-time.
Program Entrance Requirements Minimum overall college GPA of 3.2, transcript of college record, health exam, high school biology, high school chemistry, 3 years high school math, 2 years high school science, high school transcript, immunizations, minimum high school GPA of 3.2, minimum high school rank, professional liability insurance/malpractice insurance. Transfer students are accepted. *Application deadline:* 12/1 (fall). *Application fee:* $65.
Advanced Placement Credit by examination available. Credit given for nursing courses completed elsewhere dependent upon specific evaluations.
Contact *Telephone:* 973-353-5205.

GRADUATE PROGRAMS

Contact *Telephone:* 973-353-5060. *Fax:* 973-353-1277.

MASTER'S DEGREE PROGRAM
Degrees MS; MS/MPH
Available Programs Master's.
Concentrations Available *Clinical nurse specialist programs in:* adult health, community health, oncology, parent-child, psychiatric/mental health. *Nurse practitioner programs in:* acute care, adult health, family health, pediatric, psychiatric/mental health, women's health.
Site Options Freehold, NJ; Camden, NJ.
Study Options Full-time and part-time.
Program Entrance Requirements Minimum overall college GPA of 3.0, transcript of college record, written essay, immunizations, 3 letters of recommendation, physical assessment course, professional liability insurance/malpractice insurance, resume, statistics course. *Application deadline:* 6/1 (fall), 10/1 (spring). *Application fee:* $65.
Advanced Placement Credit given for nursing courses completed elsewhere dependent upon specific evaluations.
Degree Requirements 42 total credit hours.

POST-MASTER'S PROGRAM
Areas of Study Nursing education. *Clinical nurse specialist programs in:* adult health, community health, oncology, parent-child, psychiatric/mental health. *Nurse practitioner programs in:* acute care, adult health, family health, pediatric, psychiatric/mental health, women's health.

DOCTORAL DEGREE PROGRAM
Degree PhD
Available Programs Doctorate.
Areas of Study Nursing research.
Program Entrance Requirements Minimum overall college GPA of 3.2, interview by faculty committee, 3 letters of recommendation, MSN or equivalent, scholarly papers, statistics course, vita, writing sample. *Application deadline:* 3/15 (fall). *Application fee:* $65.
Degree Requirements 59 total credit hours, dissertation, written exam, residency.

CONTINUING EDUCATION PROGRAM

Contact *Telephone:* 973-353-1061. *Fax:* 973-353-1700.

Saint Peter's University

Nursing Program
Jersey City, New Jersey

http://www.saintpeters.edu/
Founded in 1872
DEGREES • BSN • MSN
Nursing Program Faculty 15 (73% with doctorates).
Baccalaureate Enrollment 161 **Women** 85% **Men** 15% **Minority** 40%
Graduate Enrollment 55 **Women** 99% **Men** 1% **Minority** 45%
Distance Learning Courses Available.
Nursing Student Activities Nursing Honor Society, Sigma Theta Tau, Student Nurses' Association.
Nursing Student Resources Academic advising; academic or career counseling; assistance for students with disabilities; bookstore; campus computer network; career placement assistance; computer lab; computer-assisted instruction; e-mail services; externships; interactive nursing skills videos; Internet; learning resource lab; library services; nursing audiovisuals; remedial services; resume preparation assistance; skills, simulation, or other laboratory; tutoring.
Library Facilities 7,200 volumes in health; 1,586 periodical subscriptions health-care related.

BACCALAUREATE PROGRAMS

Degree BSN
Available Programs ADN to Baccalaureate; Generic Baccalaureate; RN Baccalaureate.
Site Options Englewood Cliffs, NJ.
Study Options Full-time.
Program Entrance Requirements Minimum overall college GPA of 2.7, transcript of college record, written essay, high school biology, high school chemistry, high school foreign language, 3 years high school math, 3 years high school science, high school transcript, immunizations, 2 letters of recommendation, minimum high school GPA of 3.0. Transfer students are accepted. *Application deadline:* Applications may be processed on a rolling basis for some programs.
Contact *Telephone:* 201-761-7113. *Fax:* 201-761-7105.

GRADUATE PROGRAMS

Contact *Telephone:* 201-761-6272. *Fax:* 201-761-6271.

MASTER'S DEGREE PROGRAM
Degree MSN
Available Programs Master's; Master's for Nurses with Non-Nursing Degrees.
Concentrations Available Nurse case management; nursing administration. *Nurse practitioner programs in:* adult health.
Site Options Englewood Cliffs, NJ.
Study Options Part-time.
Program Entrance Requirements Clinical experience, minimum overall college GPA of 3.0, transcript of college record, written essay, immunizations, 3 letters of recommendation, nursing research course, physical assessment course, professional liability insurance/malpractice insurance, statistics course. *Application deadline:* 8/25 (fall), 10/24 (winter), 12/15 (spring), 5/5 (summer). *Application fee:* $40.
Degree Requirements 39 total credit hours, thesis or project.

POST-MASTER'S PROGRAM
Areas of Study *Nurse practitioner programs in:* adult health.

Seton Hall University

College of Nursing
South Orange, New Jersey

http://nursing.shu.edu/
Founded in 1856

DEGREES • BSN • DNP • MSN • MSN/MA • MSN/MBA

Nursing Program Faculty 43 (50% with doctorates).
Baccalaureate Enrollment 730 **Women** 89% **Men** 11% **Minority** 43% **International** 1% **Part-time** 10%
Graduate Enrollment 190 **Women** 87% **Men** 13% **Minority** 17% **Part-time** 46%
Distance Learning Courses Available.
Nursing Student Activities Sigma Theta Tau, Student Nurses' Association.
Nursing Student Resources Academic advising; academic or career counseling; assistance for students with disabilities; bookstore; campus computer network; career placement assistance; computer lab; computer-assisted instruction; e-mail services; externships; housing assistance; interactive nursing skills videos; Internet; learning resource lab; library services; nursing audiovisuals; paid internships; remedial services; resume preparation assistance; skills, simulation, or other laboratory; tutoring.
Library Facilities 506,042 volumes; 1,475 periodical subscriptions.

BACCALAUREATE PROGRAMS

Degree BSN
Available Programs Accelerated Baccalaureate for Second Degree; Baccalaureate for Second Degree; Generic Baccalaureate; RN Baccalaureate.
Site Options Camden, NJ; Brick/Toms River, NJ; Lakewood, NJ.
Study Options Full-time and part-time.
Program Entrance Requirements Minimum overall college GPA of 3.0, transcript of college record, CPR certification, written essay, high school biology, high school chemistry, high school foreign language, 3 years high school math, 2 years high school science, high school transcript, minimum high school GPA of 3.0, professional liability insurance/malpractice insurance. Transfer students are accepted.
Contact *Telephone:* 973-761-9291. *Fax:* 973-761-9607.

GRADUATE PROGRAMS

Contact *Telephone:* 973-761-9291. *Fax:* 973-761-9607.

MASTER'S DEGREE PROGRAM

Degrees MSN; MSN/MA; MSN/MBA
Available Programs Accelerated Master's for Nurses with Non-Nursing Degrees; Master's; Master's for Nurses with Non-Nursing Degrees; RN to Master's.
Concentrations Available Clinical nurse leader; health-care administration; nurse case management; nursing administration; nursing education. *Clinical nurse specialist programs in:* school health. *Nurse practitioner programs in:* adult health, gerontology, pediatric, school health.
Study Options Full-time and part-time.
Online Degree Options Yes (online only).
Program Entrance Requirements Clinical experience, computer literacy, minimum overall college GPA of 3.0, transcript of college record, CPR certification, written essay, immunizations, interview, 2 letters of recommendation, nursing research course, physical assessment course, professional liability insurance/malpractice insurance, prerequisite course work, resume, statistics course. *Application deadline:* Applications may be processed on a rolling basis for some programs.
Advanced Placement Credit by examination available. Credit given for nursing courses completed elsewhere dependent upon specific evaluations.
Degree Requirements 43 total credit hours, thesis or project.

POST-MASTER'S PROGRAM

Areas of Study Health-care administration; nurse case management; nursing administration; nursing education. *Nurse practitioner programs in:* adult health, gerontology, pediatric, school health.

DOCTORAL DEGREE PROGRAM

Degree DNP
Available Programs Doctorate; Post-Baccalaureate Doctorate.
Areas of Study Advanced practice nursing, nursing administration, nursing research.

Program Entrance Requirements Clinical experience, minimum overall college GPA of 3.0, interview, 2 letters of recommendation, MSN or equivalent, scholarly papers, statistics course, vita, writing sample, GRE (waived for students with GPA of 3.5 or higher).
Degree Requirements 46 total credit hours, dissertation.

Thomas Edison State College

W. Cary Edwards School of Nursing
Trenton, New Jersey

http://www.tesc.edu/nursing
Nursing program founded in 1983

DEGREES • ACCELERATED 2ND DEGREE BSN • RN-BSN • RN-BSN/MSN • BSN-MSN

Nursing Student Resources Students in the W. Cary Edwards School of Nursing have the opportunity to earn degrees through traditional and non-traditional methods, which take into consideration the individual needs and interests of each student. All post-licensure nursing courses are designed and delivered online. Students in these courses communicate with fellow students and mentors, who guide students in the course and grade assignments and exams in an asynchronous environment, which allows for a flexible learning schedule. Students may earn credit toward a degree by demonstrating college-level knowledge through testing and assessment of prior learning; by transfer credit for courses taken through other regionally accredited institutions; through the College's e-Pack® courses; and for licenses, certificates, and courses taken at work or through military training, if approved and recommended for academic credit.
W. Cary Edwards School of Nursing Mentors The School utilizes mentors, who are off-site nurse educators from a variety of nursing education and service settings to develop, implement, and evaluate the program. All mentors have a minimum of a master's degree in nursing, with approximately 77% prepared at the doctoral level and many tenured at their home institution. With its courses offered by distance learning, the School has the opportunity to draw nurse educators from across the country, resulting in a diverse and experienced group of online nurse mentors. The W. Cary Edwards School of Nursing programs are accredited by the National League for Nursing Accrediting Commission (NLNAC) and the Commission on Collegiate Nursing Education (CCNE) and approved by the New Jersey Board of Nursing.

BACHELOR'S AND MASTER'S DEGREE PROGRAMS

Degrees Accelerated 2nd Degree BSN • RN-BSN • RN-BSN/MSN • BSN-MSN
Master's degree has three specialties: Nurse Educator, Nursing Informatics and **Nursing Administration**
ACCELERATED 2ND DEGREE BSN PROGRAM A one-year, 120-credit degree program designed for adults who already possess a bachelor's degree (non-nursing) completed prior to admission and who are interested in becoming registered nurses. The program includes 60 credits of professional nursing completed both online and on ground at Thomas Edison State College in Trenton, NJ. The Accelerated 2nd Degree BSN Program prepares graduates for the National Council Licensure Examination for Registered Nurses (NCLEX-RN). Due to the rigorous nature of this full-time program, outside employment is not recommended.
RN-BSN/MSN DEGREE PROGRAMS The online RN-BSN/MSN degree programs are designed for experienced registered nurses (RNs) who want an alternative to campus-based instruction. Three options are offered: BSN (Bachelor of Science in Nursing), BSNM (Bachelor of Science in Nursing and Master of Science in Nursing), and MSN (Master of Science in Nursing). Three nursing specialties are offered in the MSN degree: Nurse Educator, Nursing Informatics, and Nursing Administration.
Study Options Self-paced RN-BSN and RN-BSN/MSN programs; online nursing courses offered quarterly; multiple options for credit earning; no time limit for RN-BSN and RN-BSN/MSN degree completion; no residency requirement with maximum flexibility in transfer credit.
CERTIFICATE PROGRAMS Three 12–18 credit graduate nursing certificate programs—Nurse Educator; Nursing Informatics; and Nursing Administration—are available to RNs with a master's degree in another area of nursing specialty.
Program Entrance Requirements For the **Accelerated 2nd Degree BSN Program**, admission requirements include a bachelor's degree from a regionally accredited college or university completed prior to admission

with an earned cumulative GPA of 3.0 or higher, all science prerequisites completed within five years prior to admission, a grade of B or better in all prerequisite science and math courses, completed general education and nursing prerequisites prior to admission, a criminal background check, drug screen, health and immunization verification, malpractice and health insurance, and CPR certification.

For the **RN-BSN** and **RN-BSN/MSN,** admission is open and rolling. RNs can enroll any day of the year. In addition to the documentation of their current RN license valid in the United States, all applicants must submit a completed online application with $75 fee, and have official transcripts of all completed course work sent to the Office of the Registrar (undergraduate students) or Office of Admissions for graduate students. Up to 80 credits may be accepted from a community college, and up to 60 credits, will be awarded to diploma graduates based on current licensure. There is no age restriction on credits transferred in to meet general education requirements or lower-division nursing requirements. Any upper-division nursing credits accepted for transfer must be from an accredited baccalaureate or higher degree nursing program, and newer than 10 years if completed prior to application to the W. Cary Edwards School of Nursing.

All credits used in the nursing requirement must have a grade equivalent of C or better. All previously completed graduate credits transferred in to meet MSN degree and graduate certificate requirements must be newer than seven years at the time of enrollment in the W. Cary Edwards School of Nursing, have a grade equivalent of B or better, and be from a **regionally accredited college or university or recognized foreign institution**. Applicants to the BSN/MSN (BSNM) program will be enrolled in the MSN degree on certification for graduation from the BSN degree. Up to 9 graduate credits required in the BSN degree may be applied to the MSN degree requirements.

Expenses (2012–13) *Accelerated 2nd Degree BSN Program Tuition,* $29,900. *RN-BSN Tuition, state resident:* $379 per credit. RN-BSN *Tuition, nonresident:* $464 per credit; $576 for the *MSN degree and Graduate Nursing Certificate Programs.*

Financial Aid 9.6% of the RNs in the undergraduate nursing program and 7% in the graduate nursing program received some form of financial aid in 2011–2012.

Contact Thomas Edison State College, 101 W. State St., Trenton, NJ 08608-1176. *Telephone*: 888-442-8372. *E-mail*: nursinginfo@tesc.edu.

University of Medicine and Dentistry of New Jersey

School of Nursing
Newark, New Jersey

http://sn.umdnj.edu/
Founded in 1970

DEGREES • BSN • DNP • MSN • MSN/MPH

Nursing Program Faculty 171 (30% with doctorates).
Baccalaureate Enrollment 493 **Women** 85% **Men** 15% **Minority** 48%
Graduate Enrollment 720 **Women** 80% **Men** 20% **Minority** 30% **Part-time** 80%
Distance Learning Courses Available.
Nursing Student Activities Nursing Honor Society, Sigma Theta Tau, Student Nurses' Association.
Nursing Student Resources Academic advising; academic or career counseling; assistance for students with disabilities; bookstore; campus computer network; computer lab; computer-assisted instruction; daycare for children of students; e-mail services; housing assistance; interactive nursing skills videos; Internet; learning resource lab; library services; nursing audiovisuals; remedial services; resume preparation assistance; skills, simulation, or other laboratory; tutoring.
Library Facilities 263,451 volumes (92,000 in health, 3,300 in nursing); 6,325 periodical subscriptions (4,500 health-care related).

BACCALAUREATE PROGRAMS

Degree BSN
Available Programs Accelerated Baccalaureate for Second Degree; RN Baccalaureate.
Site Options Stratford, NJ.

Study Options Full-time and part-time.
Program Entrance Requirements Minimum overall college GPA of 3.25, transcript of college record, CPR certification, written essay, health exam, health insurance, immunizations, 3 letters of recommendation, minimum GPA in nursing prerequisites of 2.75, prerequisite course work. *Application deadline:* 5/20 (fall), 11/1 (spring), 3/15 (summer). Applications may be processed on a rolling basis for some programs. *Application fee:* $45.
Advanced Placement Credit given for nursing courses completed elsewhere dependent upon specific evaluations.
Financial Aid 82% of baccalaureate students in nursing programs received some form of financial aid in 2011–12.
Contact Ms. Angie Pichardo, Admissions Coordinator, School of Nursing, University of Medicine and Dentistry of New Jersey, 65 Bergen Street, Newark, NJ 07101. *Telephone:* 973-972-5336. *E-mail:* picharan@umdnj.edu.

GRADUATE PROGRAMS

Financial Aid 32% of graduate students in nursing programs received some form of financial aid in 2011–12. Teaching assistantships, institutionally sponsored loans and scholarships available. Aid available to part-time students. *Financial aid application deadline:* 5/1.
Contact Ms. Angie Pichardo, Admissions Coordinator, School of Nursing, University of Medicine and Dentistry of New Jersey, 65 Bergen Street, SSB 1130, Newark, NJ 07101. *Telephone:* 973-972-5336. *Fax:* 973-972-7904. *E-mail:* picharan@umdnj.edu.

MASTER'S DEGREE PROGRAM

Degrees MSN; MSN/MPH
Available Programs Master's; Master's for Nurses with Non-Nursing Degrees; RN to Master's.
Concentrations Available Clinical nurse leader; nurse anesthesia; nurse-midwifery; nursing education; nursing informatics. *Nurse practitioner programs in:* acute care, adult health, family health, gerontology, psychiatric/mental health, women's health.
Site Options Voorhees, NJ; Somers Point, NJ; Stratford, NJ.
Study Options Full-time and part-time.
Online Degree Options Yes.
Program Entrance Requirements Clinical experience, minimum overall college GPA of 3.0, transcript of college record, CPR certification, 2 letters of recommendation, physical assessment course, prerequisite course work, resume, statistics course, GRE. *Application deadline:* 7/1 (fall), 11/1 (spring), 3/15 (summer). Applications may be processed on a rolling basis for some programs. *Application fee:* $50.
Advanced Placement Credit given for nursing courses completed elsewhere dependent upon specific evaluations.
Degree Requirements 40 total credit hours.

POST-MASTER'S PROGRAM

Areas of Study Clinical nurse leader; nurse-midwifery; nursing informatics. *Nurse practitioner programs in:* acute care, adult health, family health, gerontology, psychiatric/mental health, women's health.

DOCTORAL DEGREE PROGRAM

Degree DNP
Available Programs Doctorate; Doctorate for Nurses with Non-Nursing Degrees; Post-Baccalaureate Doctorate.
Areas of Study Clinical practice, nursing administration.
Site Options Stratford, NJ.
Program Entrance Requirements Clinical experience, minimum overall college GPA of 3.0, interview by faculty committee, interview, 2 letters of recommendation, MSN or equivalent, statistics course, vita, writing sample. *Application deadline:* 7/1 (fall), 11/1 (spring). Applications may be processed on a rolling basis for some programs. *Application fee:* $50.
Degree Requirements 32 total credit hours, dissertation.

CONTINUING EDUCATION PROGRAM

Contact Dr. Donna Cill, Assistant Dean and Director of the Center for Lifelong Learning, School of Nursing, University of Medicine and Dentistry of New Jersey, 65 Bergen Street, Room 1132-A, Newark, NJ 07101-1709. *Telephone:* 973-972-9793. *Fax:* 973-972-7904. *E-mail:* cilldm@umdnj.edu.

William Paterson University of New Jersey
Department of Nursing
Wayne, New Jersey

http://www.wpunj.edu/
Founded in 1855
DEGREES • BSN • DNP • MSN
Nursing Program Faculty 29 (64% with doctorates).
Baccalaureate Enrollment 400 **Women** 82% **Men** 18% **Minority** 55% **International** 5% **Part-time** 25%
Graduate Enrollment 52 **Women** 95% **Men** 5% **Minority** 20% **International** 5% **Part-time** 90%
Distance Learning Courses Available.
Nursing Student Activities Sigma Theta Tau, Student Nurses' Association.
Nursing Student Resources Academic advising; academic or career counseling; assistance for students with disabilities; bookstore; campus computer network; career placement assistance; computer lab; computer-assisted instruction; daycare for children of students; e-mail services; employment services for current students; housing assistance; interactive nursing skills videos; Internet; learning resource lab; library services; nursing audiovisuals; placement services for program completers; remedial services; resume preparation assistance; skills, simulation, or other laboratory; tutoring.
Library Facilities 338,573 volumes (15,000 in health, 12,700 in nursing); 6,569 periodical subscriptions (150 health-care related).

BACCALAUREATE PROGRAMS
Degree BSN
Available Programs ADN to Baccalaureate; Accelerated Baccalaureate for Second Degree; Generic Baccalaureate; LPN to Baccalaureate; RN Baccalaureate.
Study Options Full-time.
Program Entrance Requirements Minimum overall college GPA of 2.5, transcript of college record, CPR certification, health exam, health insurance, high school biology, high school chemistry, 1 year of high school math, 2 years high school science, high school transcript, immunizations, minimum high school GPA of 3.25, professional liability insurance/malpractice insurance, prerequisite course work. Transfer students are accepted. *Application deadline:* 5/1 (fall). Applications may be processed on a rolling basis for some programs. *Application fee:* $50.
Contact *Telephone:* 973-720-2673. *Fax:* 973-720-2668.

GRADUATE PROGRAMS
Contact *Telephone:* 973-720-3511. *Fax:* 973-720-3517.

MASTER'S DEGREE PROGRAM
Degree MSN
Available Programs Master's; Master's for Nurses with Non-Nursing Degrees.
Concentrations Available Nursing administration; nursing education. *Clinical nurse specialist programs in:* community health. *Nurse practitioner programs in:* adult health, family health.
Site Options Englewood, NJ; Paramus, NJ.
Study Options Full-time and part-time.
Program Entrance Requirements Computer literacy, minimum overall college GPA of 3.0, transcript of college record, CPR certification, written essay, 2 letters of recommendation, nursing research course, physical assessment course, professional liability insurance/malpractice insurance, resume, statistics course, GRE General Test. *Application deadline:* Applications may be processed on a rolling basis for some programs. *Application fee:* $50.
Advanced Placement Credit given for nursing courses completed elsewhere dependent upon specific evaluations.
Degree Requirements 42 total credit hours, thesis or project.

POST-MASTER'S PROGRAM
Areas of Study *Clinical nurse specialist programs in:* school health. *Nurse practitioner programs in:* adult health, family health.

DOCTORAL DEGREE PROGRAM
Degree DNP
Available Programs Doctorate.
Areas of Study Advanced practice nursing, clinical practice, health-care systems, individualized study.

Program Entrance Requirements Clinical experience, minimum overall college GPA of 3.3, interview by faculty committee, letters of recommendation, MSN or equivalent, statistics course, vita, writing sample. *Application deadline:* 4/15 (fall). *Application fee:* $75.
Degree Requirements 42 total credit hours.

NEW MEXICO

Eastern New Mexico University
Department of Allied Health–Nursing
Portales, New Mexico

http://liberal-arts.enmu.edu/health/nursing/index.shtml
Founded in 1934
DEGREE • BSN
Nursing Program Faculty 7 (1% with doctorates).
Baccalaureate Enrollment 243 **Women** 90% **Men** 10% **Minority** 45% **International** 5% **Part-time** 95%
Distance Learning Courses Available.
Nursing Student Activities Nursing Honor Society.
Nursing Student Resources Academic advising; academic or career counseling; assistance for students with disabilities; bookstore; campus computer network; career placement assistance; computer lab; computer-assisted instruction; e-mail services; housing assistance; Internet; library services; other; resume preparation assistance; tutoring.
Library Facilities 799,277 volumes (100 in health, 50 in nursing); 65,559 periodical subscriptions (15 health-care related).

BACCALAUREATE PROGRAMS
Degree BSN
Available Programs RPN to Baccalaureate.
Study Options Full-time and part-time.
Online Degree Options Yes (online only).
Program Entrance Requirements Minimum overall college GPA of 2.0, transcript of college record, CPR certification, high school chemistry, immunizations, interview, 3 letters of recommendation, minimum high school GPA of 2.5, minimum GPA in nursing prerequisites of 2.0, professional liability insurance/malpractice insurance, prerequisite course work, RN licensure. Transfer students are accepted. *Application deadline:* 9/4 (fall), 9/4 (winter), 1/19 (spring), 6/1 (summer).
Advanced Placement Credit given for nursing courses completed elsewhere dependent upon specific evaluations.
Expenses (2011–12) *Tuition, state resident:* full-time $2073; part-time $173 per credit hour. *Tuition, nonresident:* full-time $4829; part-time $402 per credit hour. *International tuition:* $4829 full-time. *Room and board:* $745; room only: $425 per academic year.
Financial Aid 10% of baccalaureate students in nursing programs received some form of financial aid in 2010–11.
Contact Dr. Leslie Paternoster, Nursing Program Director, Department of Allied Health–Nursing, Eastern New Mexico University, 1500 South Avenue K, Station 12, Portales, NM 88130. *Telephone:* 575-562-2773. *Fax:* 575-562-2293. *E-mail:* leslie.paternoster@enmu.edu.

New Mexico Highlands University
Department of Nursing
Las Vegas, New Mexico

http://www.nmhu.edu/nursing
Founded in 1893
DEGREE • BSN
Nursing Program Faculty 3 (75% with doctorates).
Baccalaureate Enrollment 51 **Women** 90% **Men** 10% **Minority** 67% **Part-time** 80%
Distance Learning Courses Available.
Nursing Student Resources Academic advising; academic or career counseling; assistance for students with disabilities; bookstore; campus computer network; career placement assistance; e-mail services; housing assistance; Internet; library services; nursing audiovisuals; placement services for program completers; resume preparation assistance; tutoring.

Library Facilities 437,323 volumes (500 in nursing); 43,235 periodical subscriptions.

BACCALAUREATE PROGRAMS

Degree BSN
Available Programs RN Baccalaureate.
Online Degree Options Yes (online only).
Program Entrance Requirements Minimum overall college GPA of 2.5, minimum GPA in nursing prerequisites of 2.0, RN licensure. *Application deadline:* 6/15 (fall).
Advanced Placement Credit given for nursing courses completed elsewhere dependent upon specific evaluations.
Expenses (2012–13) *Tuition, state resident:* full-time $3504; part-time $146 per credit hour. *Tuition, nonresident:* full-time $5671; part-time $236 per credit hour. *International tuition:* $7231 full-time. *Room and board:* $7160; room only: $3990 per academic year. *Required fees:* full-time $20.
Financial Aid 3% of baccalaureate students in nursing programs received some form of financial aid in 2011–12. *Gift aid (need-based):* Federal Pell, FSEOG, state, private, college/university gift aid from institutional funds. *Loans:* Federal Direct (Subsidized and Unsubsidized Stafford PLUS), Perkins.*Work-study:* Federal Work-Study, part-time campus jobs.*Financial aid application deadline:* Continuous.
Contact Ms. Susan M. Martin, Recruiter/Advisor Coordinator, RN-BSN Program, Department of Nursing, New Mexico Highlands University, Box 9000, Las Vegas, NM 87701. *Telephone:* 505-426-2116. *Fax:* 505-426-2109. *E-mail:* smmartin@nmhu.edu.

New Mexico State University
School of Nursing
Las Cruces, New Mexico

http://www.nmsu.edu/~nursing
Founded in 1888
DEGREES • BSN • MSN • PHD
Nursing Program Faculty 35 (37% with doctorates).
Baccalaureate Enrollment 171 Women 84% Men 16% Minority 49% International 1% Part-time 15%
Graduate Enrollment 116 Women 88% Men 12% Minority 24% International 1% Part-time 25%
Distance Learning Courses Available.
Nursing Student Activities Sigma Theta Tau, Student Nurses' Association.
Nursing Student Resources Academic advising; academic or career counseling; assistance for students with disabilities; bookstore; campus computer network; computer lab; computer-assisted instruction; daycare for children of students; e-mail services; housing assistance; interactive nursing skills videos; Internet; learning resource lab; library services; nursing audiovisuals; paid internships; remedial services; skills, simulation, or other laboratory; tutoring.
Library Facilities 1.8 million volumes (33,000 in health, 17,500 in nursing); 61,374 periodical subscriptions (620 health-care related).

BACCALAUREATE PROGRAMS

Degree BSN
Available Programs Generic Baccalaureate; RN Baccalaureate.
Site Options Carlsbad, NM; Alamagordo, NM; Grants, NM.
Study Options Full-time.
Online Degree Options Yes.
Program Entrance Requirements Minimum overall college GPA of 3.0, transcript of college record, CPR certification, health insurance, immunizations, minimum GPA in nursing prerequisites of 3.0, prerequisite course work. Transfer students are accepted.
Advanced Placement Credit given for nursing courses completed elsewhere dependent upon specific evaluations.
Financial Aid 82% of baccalaureate students in nursing programs received some form of financial aid in 2010–11. *Gift aid (need-based):* Federal Pell, FSEOG, state, private, college/university gift aid from institutional funds. *Loans:* Federal Direct (Subsidized and Unsubsidized Stafford PLUS), Perkins, state.*Work-study:* Federal Work-Study, part-time campus jobs.*Financial aid application deadline (priority):* 3/1.
Contact Andrea Kasuiba, Advising Coordinator, School of Nursing, New Mexico State University, PO Box 30001, MSC 3185, Las Cruces, NM 88003-8001. *Telephone:* 575-646-2164. *Fax:* 505-646-6166. *E-mail:* andreaK@ad.nmsu.edu.

GRADUATE PROGRAMS

Financial Aid 73% of graduate students in nursing programs received some form of financial aid in 2010–11. 1 teaching assistantship (averaging $28,242 per year) was awarded; fellowships, research assistantships, career-related internships or fieldwork, Federal Work-Study, scholarships, and traineeships also available. *Financial aid application deadline:* 3/1.
Contact Dr. Kathleen M. Huttlinger, Interim Associate Director for Graduate Studies, School of Nursing, New Mexico State University, PO Box 30001, MSC 3185, Las Cruces, NM 88003-8001. *Telephone:* 505-646-8170. *Fax:* 505-646-2167. *E-mail:* huttlin@nmsu.edu.

MASTER'S DEGREE PROGRAM

Degree MSN
Available Programs Master's; Master's for Nurses with Non-Nursing Degrees.
Concentrations Available Nursing administration.
Study Options Full-time and part-time.
Online Degree Options Yes (online only).
Program Entrance Requirements Minimum overall college GPA of 3.0, transcript of college record, CPR certification, written essay, immunizations, 3 letters of recommendation, resume, statistics course, NCLEX exam.
Advanced Placement Credit given for nursing courses completed elsewhere dependent upon specific evaluations.
Degree Requirements 38 total credit hours, comprehensive exam.

DOCTORAL DEGREE PROGRAM

Degree PhD
Available Programs Doctorate.
Areas of Study Nursing research.
Online Degree Options Yes (online only).
Program Entrance Requirements Minimum overall college GPA of 3.0, interview by faculty committee, 3 letters of recommendation, MSN or equivalent, statistics course, vita, writing sample, NCLEX exam.
Degree Requirements 60 total credit hours, dissertation, oral exam, written exam.

CONTINUING EDUCATION PROGRAM

Contact Dr. Mary H. Sizemore, Local Monitoring Program Chair, School of Nursing, New Mexico State University, PO Box 30001, MSC 3185, Las Cruces, NM 88003-8001. *Telephone:* 505-646-3812. *Fax:* 505-646-2167. *E-mail:* masizemo@nmsu.edu.

Northern New Mexico College
College of Nursing and Health Sciences
Española, New Mexico

Founded in 1909
DEGREE • BSN
Library Facilities 18,065 volumes; 222 periodical subscriptions.

BACCALAUREATE PROGRAMS

Degree BSN
Available Programs RN Baccalaureate.
Program Entrance Requirements RN licensure.
Contact Director, RN to BSN Program, College of Nursing and Health Sciences, Northern New Mexico College, 921 North Paseo de Oate, Espanola, NM 87532. *Telephone:* 505-747-2278. *E-mail:* nklebanoff@nnmc.edu.

University of New Mexico
College of Nursing
Albuquerque, New Mexico

http://www.unm.edu/
Founded in 1889
DEGREES • BSN • MSN • MSN/MPH • PHD
Nursing Program Faculty 59 (56% with doctorates).
Baccalaureate Enrollment 229 Women 87% Men 13% Minority 55% Part-time 37%

Graduate Enrollment 171 **Women** 92% **Men** 8% **Minority** 37% **Part-time** 61%

Distance Learning Courses Available.

Nursing Student Activities Sigma Theta Tau, Student Nurses' Association.

Nursing Student Resources Academic advising; assistance for students with disabilities; bookstore; campus computer network; career placement assistance; computer lab; computer-assisted instruction; daycare for children of students; e-mail services; housing assistance; interactive nursing skills videos; Internet; learning resource lab; library services; nursing audiovisuals; remedial services; skills, simulation, or other laboratory.

Library Facilities 4.2 million volumes (139,930 in health, 12,000 in nursing); 70,043 periodical subscriptions (1,800 health-care related).

BACCALAUREATE PROGRAMS

Degree BSN

Available Programs Accelerated Baccalaureate for Second Degree; Generic Baccalaureate; RN Baccalaureate.

Study Options Full-time.

Program Entrance Requirements Minimum overall college GPA of 3.0, transcript of college record, written essay, 2 letters of recommendation, minimum GPA in nursing prerequisites of 3.0, prerequisite course work. Transfer students are accepted. *Application deadline:* 2/15 (fall), 9/15 (spring). *Application fee:* $50.

Advanced Placement Credit given for nursing courses completed elsewhere dependent upon specific evaluations.

Expenses (2012–13) *Tuition, state resident:* part-time $425 per credit hour. *Tuition, nonresident:* part-time $1035 per credit hour. *Room and board:* room only: $7250 per academic year. *Required fees:* part-time $360 per term.

Financial Aid 60% of baccalaureate students in nursing programs received some form of financial aid in 2011–12. *Gift aid (need-based):* Federal Pell, FSEOG, state, private, college/university gift aid from institutional funds, United Negro College Fund, Federal Nursing. *Loans:* Federal Nursing Student Loans, Federal Direct (Subsidized and Unsubsidized Stafford PLUS), Perkins, state, college/university. *Work-study:* Federal Work-Study, part-time campus jobs. *Financial aid application deadline (priority):* 3/1.

Contact Ms. Ann Marie Oechsler, Director of Student Services, College of Nursing, University of New Mexico, 1 University of New Mexico, MSC09 5350, Albuquerque, NM 87131-0001. *Telephone:* 505-272-4223. *Fax:* 505-272-3970. *E-mail:* aoechsler@salud.unm.edu.

GRADUATE PROGRAMS

Expenses (2012–13) *Tuition, state resident:* part-time $503 per credit hour. *Tuition, nonresident:* part-time $1112 per credit hour. *Room and board:* room only: $7250 per academic year. *Required fees:* part-time $500 per term.

Financial Aid 40% of graduate students in nursing programs received some form of financial aid in 2011–12. 10 fellowships (averaging $10,863 per year), 2 research assistantships with partial tuition reimbursements available (averaging $6,183 per year), 14 teaching assistantships with partial tuition reimbursements available (averaging $7,276 per year) were awarded; institutionally sponsored loans, scholarships, traineeships, and unspecified assistantships also available. Aid available to part-time students. *Financial aid application deadline:* 3/1.

Contact Ms. Karen Wells, Senior Academic Advisor, College of Nursing, University of New Mexico, 1 University of New Mexico, MSC09 5350, NRPH Building, Room 152, Albuquerque, NM 87131-0001. *Telephone:* 505-272-4223. *Fax:* 505-272-3970. *E-mail:* kwells@salud.unm.edu.

MASTER'S DEGREE PROGRAM

Degrees MSN; MSN/MPH

Available Programs Master's.

Concentrations Available Nurse-midwifery; nursing administration; nursing education. *Nurse practitioner programs in:* acute care, family health, pediatric.

Study Options Full-time and part-time.

Online Degree Options Yes (online only).

Program Entrance Requirements Clinical experience, minimum overall college GPA of 3.0, transcript of college record, interview, 3 letters of recommendation, resume. *Application deadline:* 2/15 (fall), 10/15 (spring). *Application fee:* $50.

Advanced Placement Credit given for nursing courses completed elsewhere dependent upon specific evaluations.

Degree Requirements 32 total credit hours, thesis or project, comprehensive exam.

POST-MASTER'S PROGRAM

Areas of Study Nurse-midwifery; nursing administration; nursing education. *Nurse practitioner programs in:* acute care, family health, pediatric.

DOCTORAL DEGREE PROGRAM

Degree PhD

Available Programs Doctorate.

Areas of Study Health policy, nursing research.

Online Degree Options Yes.

Program Entrance Requirements Clinical experience, minimum overall college GPA of 3.0, interview by faculty committee, 3 letters of recommendation, MSN or equivalent, vita, writing sample. *Application deadline:* 2/15 (summer). *Application fee:* $50.

Degree Requirements 69 total credit hours, dissertation.

University of Phoenix–New Mexico Campus
College of Nursing
Albuquerque, New Mexico

DEGREES • BSN • MSN • MSN/ED D

Nursing Program Faculty 18 (13% with doctorates).

Baccalaureate Enrollment 24 **Women** 100% **Minority** 33.3%

Graduate Enrollment 14 **Women** 100% **Minority** 21.43%

Nursing Student Activities Sigma Theta Tau.

Nursing Student Resources Academic advising; academic or career counseling; assistance for students with disabilities; bookstore; campus computer network; computer lab; computer-assisted instruction; e-mail services; interactive nursing skills videos; Internet; learning resource lab; library services; nursing audiovisuals; remedial services; skills, simulation, or other laboratory; tutoring.

Library Facilities 16,781 periodical subscriptions (1,300 health-care related).

BACCALAUREATE PROGRAMS

Degree BSN

Available Programs Accelerated Baccalaureate.

Site Options Santa Fe, NM; Santa Teresa, NM.

Study Options Full-time.

Program Entrance Requirements Transcript of college record, CPR certification, immunizations, 1 letter of recommendation, RN licensure. Transfer students are accepted.

Advanced Placement Credit by examination available. Credit given for nursing courses completed elsewhere dependent upon specific evaluations.

Contact *Telephone:* 505-821-4800.

GRADUATE PROGRAMS

Contact *Telephone:* 505-821-4800.

MASTER'S DEGREE PROGRAM

Degrees MSN; MSN/Ed D

Available Programs Master's.

Concentrations Available Nursing administration; nursing education.

Site Options Santa Fe, NM; Santa Teresa, NM.

Study Options Full-time.

Online Degree Options Yes.

Program Entrance Requirements Clinical experience, computer literacy, minimum overall college GPA of 2.5, transcript of college record. *Application deadline:* Applications may be processed on a rolling basis for some programs. *Application fee:* $45.

Advanced Placement Credit given for nursing courses completed elsewhere dependent upon specific evaluations.

Degree Requirements 39 total credit hours, thesis or project.

Western New Mexico University
Nursing Department
Silver City, New Mexico

Founded in 1893
DEGREE • BSN
Nursing Program Faculty 14 (7% with doctorates).
Baccalaureate Enrollment 85 **Women** 91% **Men** 9% **Minority** 39%
Part-time 88%
Distance Learning Courses Available.
Nursing Student Activities Student Nurses' Association.
Nursing Student Resources Academic advising; assistance for students with disabilities; bookstore; campus computer network; computer lab; computer-assisted instruction; e-mail services; Internet; learning resource lab; library services; nursing audiovisuals; skills, simulation, or other laboratory; tutoring.
Library Facilities 245,146 volumes (4,980 in health, 4,900 in nursing); 236 periodical subscriptions (14 health-care related).

BACCALAUREATE PROGRAMS
Degree BSN
Available Programs RN Baccalaureate.
Study Options Full-time.
Online Degree Options Yes (online only).
Program Entrance Requirements Minimum overall college GPA of 2.5, transcript of college record, CPR certification, immunizations, prerequisite course work, RN licensure. Transfer students are accepted. *Application deadline:* 7/15 (fall), 7/15 (winter), 11/15 (spring), 4/15 (summer). Applications may be processed on a rolling basis for some programs.
Expenses (2012–13) *Tuition, state resident:* full-time $4315; part-time $180 per credit hour. *Tuition, nonresident:* full-time $12,514. *Room and board:* $8630; room only: $4550 per academic year. *Required fees:* full-time $720; part-time $30 per credit.
Financial Aid 40% of baccalaureate students in nursing programs received some form of financial aid in 2011–12.
Contact Ms. Cindy Andrews, BSN Advisor, Nursing Department, Western New Mexico University, PO Box 680, Silver City, NM 88062. *Telephone:* 575-538-6976. *Fax:* 575-538-6961. *E-mail:* andrewsc2@wnmu.edu.

NEW YORK

Adelphi University
School of Nursing
Garden City, New York

http://www.adelphi.edu/
Founded in 1896
DEGREES • BS • MS • MS/MBA • PHD
Nursing Program Faculty 163 (24% with doctorates).
Baccalaureate Enrollment 1,128 **Women** 87% **Men** 13% **Minority** 44% **Part-time** 20%
Graduate Enrollment 138 **Women** 94% **Men** 6% **Minority** 53% **Part-time** 96%
Distance Learning Courses Available.
Nursing Student Activities Nursing Honor Society, Sigma Theta Tau, Student Nurses' Association, nursing club.
Nursing Student Resources Academic advising; academic or career counseling; assistance for students with disabilities; bookstore; campus computer network; career placement assistance; computer lab; computer-assisted instruction; daycare for children of students; e-mail services; employment services for current students; externships; housing assistance; interactive nursing skills videos; Internet; learning resource lab; library services; nursing audiovisuals; paid internships; placement services for program completers; remedial services; resume preparation assistance; skills, simulation, or other laboratory; tutoring; unpaid internships.
Library Facilities 602,901 volumes (29,918 in health, 2,666 in nursing); 70,641 periodical subscriptions (364 health-care related).

BACCALAUREATE PROGRAMS
Degree BS
Available Programs Accelerated Baccalaureate for Second Degree; Generic Baccalaureate; RN Baccalaureate.
Site Options Sayville, NY; Poughkeepsie, NY; Manhattan, NY.
Study Options Full-time.
Program Entrance Requirements Minimum overall college GPA of 3.0, transcript of college record, written essay, health exam, high school foreign language, 3 years high school math, 3 years high school science, high school transcript, immunizations, interview, 2 letters of recommendation, minimum high school GPA of 3.0, minimum GPA in nursing prerequisites of 2.7. Transfer students are accepted. *Application deadline:* Applications may be processed on a rolling basis for some programs. *Application fee:* $40.
Advanced Placement Credit given for nursing courses completed elsewhere dependent upon specific evaluations.
Expenses (2012–13) *Tuition:* full-time $29,550; part-time $875 per credit hour. *International tuition:* $29,550 full-time. *Room and board:* $13,460; room only: $10,760 per academic year. *Required fees:* full-time $2000; part-time $1000 per term.
Financial Aid 90% of baccalaureate students in nursing programs received some form of financial aid in 2011–12.
Contact Mrs. Christine Murphy, Director of Admissions, School of Nursing, Adelphi University, One South Avenue, Levermore Hall, Garden City, NY 11530. *Telephone:* 516-877-3050. *E-mail:* murphy2@adelphi.edu.

GRADUATE PROGRAMS
Expenses (2012–13) *Tuition:* part-time $960 per credit hour. *Room and board:* $13,460; room only: $10,760 per academic year. *Required fees:* part-time $400 per term.
Financial Aid 50% of graduate students in nursing programs received some form of financial aid in 2011–12. 13 research assistantships (averaging $4,011 per year) were awarded; career-related internships or fieldwork, unspecified assistantships, and graduate achievement awards also available. Aid available to part-time students. *Financial aid application deadline:* 2/15.
Contact Mrs. Christine Murphy, Director of Admissions, School of Nursing, Adelphi University, One South Avenue, Levermore Hall, Garden City, NY 11530. *Telephone:* 516-877-3050. *Fax:* 516-877-3039. *E-mail:* murphy2@adelphi.edu.

MASTER'S DEGREE PROGRAM
Degrees MS; MS/MBA
Available Programs Master's.
Concentrations Available Health-care administration; nursing administration; nursing education. *Nurse practitioner programs in:* adult health.
Study Options Full-time and part-time.
Program Entrance Requirements Clinical experience, computer literacy, minimum overall college GPA of 3.0, transcript of college record, CPR certification, written essay, immunizations, interview, 2 letters of recommendation, nursing research course, professional liability insurance/malpractice insurance, resume, statistics course. *Application deadline:* 3/1 (fall). Applications may be processed on a rolling basis for some programs. *Application fee:* $50.
Advanced Placement Credit given for nursing courses completed elsewhere dependent upon specific evaluations.
Degree Requirements 42 total credit hours, thesis or project, comprehensive exam.

POST-MASTER'S PROGRAM
Areas of Study Health-care administration; nursing administration; nursing education. *Nurse practitioner programs in:* adult health.

DOCTORAL DEGREE PROGRAM
Degree PhD
Available Programs Doctorate.
Areas of Study Faculty preparation, health-care systems, nursing administration, nursing education, nursing research.
Program Entrance Requirements Minimum overall college GPA of 3.5, interview by faculty committee, interview, 3 letters of recommendation, MSN or equivalent, statistics course, vita, writing sample, GRE. *Application deadline:* 2/15 (fall). *Application fee:* $50.
Degree Requirements 54 total credit hours, dissertation, oral exam, written exam.

CONTINUING EDUCATION PROGRAM

Contact Mrs. Karen Pappas, Director of Continuing Education, School of Nursing, Adelphi University, One South Avenue, Garden City, NY 11530. *Telephone:* 516-877-4554. *E-mail:* pappas@adelphi.edu.

See display below and full description on page 474.

See display below and full description on page 474.

Binghamton University, State University of New York

Decker School of Nursing
Binghamton, New York

http://dson.binghamton.edu/
Founded in 1946

DEGREES • BS • DNP • MS • PHD
Nursing Program Faculty 58 (40% with doctorates).
Baccalaureate Enrollment 354
Graduate Enrollment 191
Distance Learning Courses Available.
Nursing Student Activities Sigma Theta Tau, Student Nurses' Association.
Nursing Student Resources Academic advising; assistance for students with disabilities; campus computer network; computer lab; e-mail services; Internet; learning resource lab; library services; skills, simulation, or other laboratory.
Library Facilities 2.4 million volumes (7,000 in health); 93,414 periodical subscriptions (9,300 health-care related).

BACCALAUREATE PROGRAMS

Degree BS
Available Programs Accelerated RN Baccalaureate; Generic Baccalaureate.
Study Options Full-time and part-time.
Program Entrance Requirements Minimum overall college GPA of 2.7, transcript of college record, CPR certification, written essay, health exam, high school biology, high school chemistry, high school foreign language, 3 years high school math, 2 years high school science, high school transcript, 2 letters of recommendation, minimum high school GPA of 3.0, prerequisite course work. Transfer students are accepted. *Application deadline:* Applications may be processed on a rolling basis for some programs. *Application fee:* $50.
Advanced Placement Credit by examination available. Credit given for nursing courses completed elsewhere dependent upon specific evaluations.
Expenses (2011–12) *Tuition, area resident:* full-time $5270; part-time $325 per credit. *Tuition, nonresident:* full-time $13,380. *Required fees:* part-time $3904 per term.
Financial Aid *Gift aid (need-based):* Federal Pell, FSEOG, state, private, college/university gift aid from institutional funds. *Loans:* Federal Nursing Student Loans, Federal Direct (Subsidized and Unsubsidized Stafford PLUS), Perkins, college/university. *Work-study:* Federal Work-Study. *Financial aid application deadline (priority):* 2/1.
Contact Ms. Fran Srnka-Debnar, Clinical Instructor and Coordinator, Student Services, Decker School of Nursing, Binghamton University, State University of New York, PO Box 6000, Binghamton, NY 13902. *Telephone:* 607-777-4954. *Fax:* 607-777-4440. *E-mail:* fsrnka@binghamton.edu.

GRADUATE PROGRAMS

Expenses (2011–12) *Tuition, area resident:* full-time $10,282; part-time $370 per credit hour. *Tuition, nonresident:* full-time $16,572; part-time $632 per credit hour. *International tuition:* $16,572 full-time. *Required fees:* full-time $1412; part-time $90 per credit; part-time $706 per term.
Financial Aid 45% of graduate students in nursing programs received some form of financial aid in 2010–11. 4 fellowships with partial tuition reimbursements available (averaging $8,250 per year), 1 research assistantship with full tuition reimbursement available (averaging $10,000 per year), 8 teaching assistantships with full tuition reimbursements available (averaging $10,000 per year) were awarded; career-related internships or fieldwork, Federal Work-Study, institutionally sponsored loans, traineeships, tuition waivers (full and partial), and unspecified assistantships also available. *Financial aid application deadline:* 2/15.
Contact Ms. Jennie Orton, Assistant to the Director of Graduate Programs, Decker School of Nursing, Binghamton University, State University of New York, PO Box 6000, Binghamton, NY 13902-6000. *Telephone:* 607-777-4614. *Fax:* 607-777-4440. *E-mail:* jorton@binghamton.edu.

MASTER'S DEGREE PROGRAM

Degree MS

Available Programs Master's.

Concentrations Available Nursing administration; nursing education. *Clinical nurse specialist programs in:* community health, family health, gerontology, psychiatric/mental health. *Nurse practitioner programs in:* community health, family health, gerontology, psychiatric/mental health.

Study Options Full-time and part-time.

Program Entrance Requirements Computer literacy, minimum overall college GPA of 3.0, transcript of college record, written essay, 2 letters of recommendation, resume, statistics course, GRE General Test. *Application deadline:* 6/15 (fall), 11/15 (spring). Applications may be processed on a rolling basis for some programs. *Application fee:* $60.

Advanced Placement Credit given for nursing courses completed elsewhere dependent upon specific evaluations.

Degree Requirements 48 total credit hours, thesis or project, comprehensive exam.

POST-MASTER'S PROGRAM

Areas of Study *Nurse practitioner programs in:* community health, family health, gerontology, psychiatric/mental health.

DOCTORAL DEGREE PROGRAM

Degree DNP

Available Programs Doctorate, Post-Baccalaureate Doctorate.

Areas of Study Community health, family health, gerontology, psychiatric/mental health.

Online Degree Options Yes (Post-MS to DNP is online).

Program Entrance Requirements Minimum overall college GPA of 3.0. Application requirements differ between programs; please contact school for complete requirements. *Application deadline:* 6/1 (fall). Applications may be processed on a rolling basis for some programs. *Application fee:* $60.

Degree Requirements 77 credits for Post-BS to DNP, 38 credits for Post-MS to DNP, dissertation, oral exam, residency, written exam.

DOCTORAL DEGREE PROGRAM

Degree PhD

Available Programs Doctorate; Post-Baccalaureate Doctorate.

Areas of Study Nursing research.

Online Degree Options Yes.

Program Entrance Requirements Clinical experience, minimum overall college GPA of 3.0, interview by faculty committee, interview, 3 letters of recommendation, MSN or equivalent, scholarly papers, statistics course, vita, writing sample. *Application deadline:* 6/15 (fall), 11/15 (spring). Applications may be processed on a rolling basis for some programs. *Application fee:* $60.

Degree Requirements 55 total credit hours, dissertation, written exam.

CONTINUING EDUCATION PROGRAM

Contact Dean's Office, Decker School of Nursing, Binghamton University, State University of New York, PO Box 6000, Binghamton, NY 13902-6000. *Telephone:* 607-777-4954. *Fax:* 607-777-4440.

The College at Brockport, State University of New York

Department of Nursing
Brockport, New York

http://www.brockport.edu/
Founded in 1867

DEGREE • BSN

Nursing Program Faculty 24 (50% with doctorates).

Baccalaureate Enrollment 200 **Women** 93% **Men** 7% **Minority** 15% **International** 2% **Part-time** 9%

Distance Learning Courses Available.

Nursing Student Activities Nursing Honor Society, Sigma Theta Tau, Student Nurses' Association.

Nursing Student Resources Academic advising; academic or career counseling; assistance for students with disabilities; bookstore; campus computer network; career placement assistance; computer lab; computer-assisted instruction; daycare for children of students; e-mail services; interactive nursing skills videos; Internet; learning resource lab; library services; nursing audiovisuals; remedial services; resume preparation assistance; skills, simulation, or other laboratory; tutoring.

Library Facilities 18,952 volumes in health, 1,065 volumes in nursing; 257 periodical subscriptions health-care related.

BACCALAUREATE PROGRAMS

Degree BSN

Available Programs ADN to Baccalaureate; Generic Baccalaureate.

Site Options Rochester, NY.

Study Options Full-time and part-time.

Program Entrance Requirements Minimum overall college GPA of 2.75, transcript of college record, CPR certification, health exam, health insurance, high school transcript, immunizations, minimum GPA in nursing prerequisites of 2.0, prerequisite course work. Transfer students are accepted. *Application deadline:* 1/20 (fall).

Advanced Placement Credit given for nursing courses completed elsewhere dependent upon specific evaluations.

Expenses (2011–12) *Tuition, state resident:* full-time $5270; part-time $220 per contact hour. *Tuition, nonresident:* full-time $14,320; part-time $597 per contact hour. *International tuition:* $14,320 full-time. *Room and board:* $9200; room only: $6040 per academic year. *Required fees:* full-time $1235; part-time $51 per credit.

Financial Aid 66% of baccalaureate students in nursing programs received some form of financial aid in 2010–11. *Gift aid (need-based):* Federal Pell, FSEOG, state, private, college/university gift aid from institutional funds. *Loans:* Federal Nursing Student Loans, Federal Direct (Subsidized and Unsubsidized Stafford PLUS), Perkins, alternative loans. *Work-study:* Federal Work-Study, part-time campus jobs. *Financial aid application deadline (priority):* 3/15.

Contact Dr. Kathleen Peterson, Chairperson, Department of Nursing, The College at Brockport, State University of New York, 350 New Campus Drive, Brockport, NY 14420-2988. *Telephone:* 585-395-2355. *Fax:* 585-395-5312. *E-mail:* kpeterso@brockport.edu.

College of Mount Saint Vincent

Department of Nursing
Riverdale, New York

http://www.mountsaintvincent.edu/408.htm
Founded in 1911

DEGREES • BS • MSN

Nursing Program Faculty 30 (90% with doctorates).

Baccalaureate Enrollment 520 **Women** 80% **Men** 20% **Minority** 80% **International** 10% **Part-time** 10%

Graduate Enrollment 100 **Women** 90% **Men** 10% **Minority** 80% **International** 10% **Part-time** 100%

Nursing Student Activities Sigma Theta Tau, Student Nurses' Association.

Nursing Student Resources Academic advising; academic or career counseling; bookstore; campus computer network; computer lab; computer-assisted instruction; e-mail services; employment services for current students; housing assistance; interactive nursing skills videos; Internet; learning resource lab; library services; nursing audiovisuals; paid internships; remedial services; resume preparation assistance; skills, simulation, or other laboratory; tutoring.

Library Facilities 110,924 volumes (5,304 in nursing); 19,823 periodical subscriptions.

BACCALAUREATE PROGRAMS

Degree BS

Available Programs Baccalaureate for Second Degree; Generic Baccalaureate; International Nurse to Baccalaureate; LPN to Baccalaureate; LPN to RN Baccalaureate.

Site Options Manhattan, NY.

Study Options Full-time and part-time.

Program Entrance Requirements Minimum overall college GPA of 2.7, transcript of college record, CPR certification, written essay, health exam, health insurance, high school biology, high school chemistry, high school foreign language, 3 years high school math, 3 years high school science, high school transcript, immunizations, 1 letter of recommendation, minimum high school GPA of 2.7, minimum GPA in nursing prerequisites of 3.0, prerequisite course work. Transfer students are accepted. *Application deadline:* 8/1 (fall), 1/5 (spring). Applications may be processed on a rolling basis for some programs. *Application fee:* $35.

Financial Aid 90% of baccalaureate students in nursing programs received some form of financial aid in 2010–11.

Contact Ms. Harriet Rothman, Recruitment and Advisement Coordinator, Department of Nursing, College of Mount Saint Vincent,

6301 Riverdale Avenue, Riverdale, NY 10471-1093. *Telephone:* 718-405-3365. *Fax:* 718-405-3286. *E-mail:* nursing@mountsaintvincent.edu.

GRADUATE PROGRAMS

Financial Aid 90% of graduate students in nursing programs received some form of financial aid in 2010–11. Career-related internships or fieldwork available. *Financial aid application deadline:* 6/1.
Contact Dr. Carol Vicino, Director, Graduate Program of Nursing, Department of Nursing, College of Mount Saint Vincent, 6301 Riverdale Avenue, Riverdale, NY 10471-1093. *Telephone:* 718-405-3351. *Fax:* 718-405-3286. *E-mail:* carol.vicino@mountsaintvincent.edu.

MASTER'S DEGREE PROGRAM
Degree MSN
Available Programs Master's.

The College of New Rochelle
School of Nursing
New Rochelle, New York

Founded in 1904
DEGREES • BSN • MS
Nursing Program Faculty 15 (75% with doctorates).
Baccalaureate Enrollment 521 **Women** 90% **Men** 10% **Minority** 67% **International** 1% **Part-time** 50%
Graduate Enrollment 121 **Women** 90% **Men** 10% **Minority** 18% **International** 1% **Part-time** 100%
Nursing Student Activities Nursing Honor Society, Sigma Theta Tau, Student Nurses' Association, nursing club.
Nursing Student Resources Academic advising; academic or career counseling; assistance for students with disabilities; bookstore; campus computer network; career placement assistance; computer lab; computer-assisted instruction; e-mail services; housing assistance; interactive nursing skills videos; Internet; learning resource lab; library services; nursing audiovisuals; other; remedial services; resume preparation assistance; skills, simulation, or other laboratory; tutoring.
Library Facilities 220,000 volumes (8,700 in health, 8,700 in nursing); 1,450 periodical subscriptions (165 health-care related).

BACCALAUREATE PROGRAMS

Degree BSN
Available Programs Accelerated Baccalaureate for Second Degree; Accelerated RN Baccalaureate; Baccalaureate for Second Degree; Generic Baccalaureate; RN Baccalaureate.
Site Options Bronx, NY.
Study Options Full-time and part-time.
Program Entrance Requirements Transcript of college record, CPR certification, written essay, health exam, health insurance, high school biology, high school chemistry, high school transcript, immunizations. Transfer students are accepted. *Application deadline:* 3/1 (fall), 10/1 (spring). *Application fee:* $35.
Advanced Placement Credit by examination available. Credit given for nursing courses completed elsewhere dependent upon specific evaluations.
Contact *Telephone:* 914-654-5803. *Fax:* 914-654-5994.

GRADUATE PROGRAMS

Contact *Telephone:* 914-654-5803. *Fax:* 914-654-5994.

MASTER'S DEGREE PROGRAM
Degree MS
Available Programs Master's; RN to Master's.
Concentrations Available Health-care administration; nursing administration; nursing education. *Nurse practitioner programs in:* family health.
Site Options New Rochelle, NY.
Study Options Full-time and part-time.
Program Entrance Requirements Clinical experience, minimum overall college GPA of 3.0, transcript of college record, written essay, immunizations, interview, 2 letters of recommendation, physical assessment course, professional liability insurance/malpractice insurance, resume, statistics course. *Application fee:* $35.
Advanced Placement Credit given for nursing courses completed elsewhere dependent upon specific evaluations.

Degree Requirements 40 total credit hours, thesis or project.

POST-MASTER'S PROGRAM
Areas of Study Health-care administration; nursing administration; nursing education. *Clinical nurse specialist programs in:* palliative care. *Nurse practitioner programs in:* family health.

College of Staten Island of the City University of New York
Department of Nursing
Staten Island, New York

http://www.csi.cuny.edu/nursing
Founded in 1955
DEGREES • BS • MS
Nursing Program Faculty 61 (23% with doctorates).
Baccalaureate Enrollment 182 **Women** 87% **Men** 13% **Minority** 40% **Part-time** 74%
Graduate Enrollment 52 **Women** 99% **Men** 1% **Minority** 43% **International** 7% **Part-time** 93%
Nursing Student Activities Nursing Honor Society, Sigma Theta Tau.
Nursing Student Resources Academic advising; academic or career counseling; assistance for students with disabilities; bookstore; campus computer network; career placement assistance; computer lab; computer-assisted instruction; daycare for children of students; e-mail services; externships; Internet; learning resource lab; library services; nursing audiovisuals; remedial services; resume preparation assistance; skills, simulation, or other laboratory; tutoring.
Library Facilities 3,700 volumes in health, 1,500 volumes in nursing; 4,900 periodical subscriptions health-care related.

BACCALAUREATE PROGRAMS

Degree BS
Available Programs RN Baccalaureate.
Site Options Brooklyn, NY.
Study Options Full-time and part-time.
Program Entrance Requirements Minimum overall college GPA of 2.5, transcript of college record, CPR certification, health exam, health insurance, high school transcript, immunizations, minimum GPA in nursing prerequisites, professional liability insurance/malpractice insurance, prerequisite course work, RN licensure. Transfer students are accepted. *Application fee:* $65.
Advanced Placement Credit given for nursing courses completed elsewhere dependent upon specific evaluations.
Contact *Telephone:* 718-982-3810. *Fax:* 718-982-3813.

GRADUATE PROGRAMS

Contact *Telephone:* 718-982-3845. *Fax:* 718-982-3813.

MASTER'S DEGREE PROGRAM
Degree MS
Available Programs Master's.
Concentrations Available *Clinical nurse specialist programs in:* adult health, gerontology. *Nurse practitioner programs in:* adult health, gerontology.
Site Options Brooklyn, NY.
Study Options Full-time and part-time.
Program Entrance Requirements Clinical experience, minimum overall college GPA of 3.0, transcript of college record, written essay, immunizations, interview, 2 letters of recommendation, nursing research course, physical assessment course, professional liability insurance/malpractice insurance, prerequisite course work, statistics course. *Application deadline:* Applications may be processed on a rolling basis for some programs. *Application fee:* $65.
Advanced Placement Credit given for nursing courses completed elsewhere dependent upon specific evaluations.
Degree Requirements 48 total credit hours, thesis or project.

POST-MASTER'S PROGRAM
Areas of Study *Nurse practitioner programs in:* adult health, gerontology.

Columbia University
School of Nursing
New York, New York

http://www.nursing.columbia.edu/
Founded in 1754
DEGREES • BS • MS • MSN/MBA • MSN/MPH • PHD
Nursing Program Faculty 68 (73% with doctorates).
Baccalaureate Enrollment 171 **Women** 92% **Men** 8% **Minority** 30% **International** 1%
Graduate Enrollment 438 **Women** 92% **Men** 8% **Minority** 33% **International** 2% **Part-time** 62%
Nursing Student Activities Sigma Theta Tau, nursing club.
Nursing Student Resources Academic advising; academic or career counseling; assistance for students with disabilities; bookstore; campus computer network; computer lab; computer-assisted instruction; daycare for children of students; e-mail services; employment services for current students; housing assistance; interactive nursing skills videos; Internet; learning resource lab; library services; resume preparation assistance; skills, simulation, or other laboratory.
Library Facilities 9.5 million volumes (469,000 in health, 8,220 in nursing); 117,264 periodical subscriptions.

BACCALAUREATE PROGRAMS
Degree BS
Available Programs Accelerated Baccalaureate; Accelerated Baccalaureate for Second Degree.
Study Options Full-time.
Program Entrance Requirements Transcript of college record, written essay, 3 letters of recommendation, prerequisite course work. *Application deadline:* 11/15 (summer). *Application fee:* $65.
Expenses (2011–12) *Tuition:* full-time $70,560. *International tuition:* $70,560 full-time. *Required fees:* full-time $1911.
Financial Aid 98% of baccalaureate students in nursing programs received some form of financial aid in 2010–11. *Gift aid (need-based):* Federal Pell, FSEOG, state, private, college/university gift aid from institutional funds. *Loans:* Perkins, alternative loans. *Work-study:* Federal Work-Study, part-time campus jobs. *Financial aid application deadline:* 3/1.
Contact Office of Admissions, School of Nursing, Columbia University, 617 West 168th Street, Suite 134, New York, NY 10032. *Telephone:* 212-305-5756. *Fax:* 212-305-3680. *E-mail:* nursing@columbia.edu.

GRADUATE PROGRAMS
Expenses (2011–12) *Tuition:* part-time $1248 per credit. *Required fees:* full-time $1911; part-time $225 per term.
Financial Aid 98% of graduate students in nursing programs received some form of financial aid in 2010–11. Research assistantships, teaching assistantships, Federal Work-Study and institutionally sponsored loans available. Aid available to part-time students.
Contact Office of Admissions, School of Nursing, Columbia University, 630 West 168th Street, Box 6, New York, NY 10032. *Telephone:* 212-305-5756. *Fax:* 212-305-3680. *E-mail:* nursing@columbia.edu.

MASTER'S DEGREE PROGRAM
Degrees MS; MSN/MBA; MSN/MPH
Available Programs Accelerated Master's for Non-Nursing College Graduates; Master's; Master's for Non-Nursing College Graduates.
Concentrations Available Nurse anesthesia; nurse-midwifery. *Nurse practitioner programs in:* acute care, adult health, family health, gerontology, oncology, pediatric, psychiatric/mental health, women's health.
Study Options Full-time and part-time.
Program Entrance Requirements Clinical experience, minimum overall college GPA of 3.0, transcript of college record, written essay, interview, 3 letters of recommendation, physical assessment course, prerequisite course work, resume, statistics course, GRE General Test. *Application deadline:* 4/16 (fall), 1/15 (summer). *Application fee:* $65.
Advanced Placement Credit by examination available. Credit given for nursing courses completed elsewhere dependent upon specific evaluations.
Degree Requirements 45 total credit hours, thesis or project, comprehensive exam.

POST-MASTER'S PROGRAM
Areas of Study Nurse anesthesia. *Nurse practitioner programs in:* acute care, adult health, family health, gerontology, oncology, pediatric, psychiatric/mental health, women's health.

DOCTORAL DEGREE PROGRAM
Degree PhD
Available Programs Doctorate; Doctorate for Nurses with Non-Nursing Degrees; Post-Baccalaureate Doctorate.
Areas of Study Addiction/substance abuse, advanced practice nursing, clinical practice, information systems, maternity-newborn, nursing education, nursing research, nursing science.
Program Entrance Requirements Minimum overall college GPA of 3.0, interview by faculty committee, interview, 3 letters of recommendation, statistics course, vita, writing sample, GRE General Test. *Application deadline:* 1/2 (fall). *Application fee:* $75.
Degree Requirements 60 total credit hours, dissertation, written exam.

POSTDOCTORAL PROGRAM
Areas of Study Nursing informatics, nursing research.
Postdoctoral Program Contact Sarah Cook, Vice Dean, School of Nursing, Columbia University, 630 West 168th Street, Box 6, New York, NY 10032. *Telephone:* 212-305-3582. *Fax:* 212-305-1116. *E-mail:* ssc3@columbia.edu.

CONTINUING EDUCATION PROGRAM
Contact Sarah Cook, Vice Dean, School of Nursing, Columbia University, 630 West 168th Street, Box 6, New York, NY 10032. *Telephone:* 212-305-3582. *Fax:* 212-305-1116. *E-mail:* ssc3@columbia.edu.

Concordia College–New York
Nursing Program
Bronxville, New York

http://www.concordia-ny.edu/
Founded in 1881
DEGREE • BS
Nursing Program Faculty 6 (50% with doctorates).
Baccalaureate Enrollment 40 **Women** 80% **Men** 20% **Minority** 48% **International** 2%
Nursing Student Activities Student Nurses' Association.
Nursing Student Resources Academic advising; academic or career counseling; assistance for students with disabilities; bookstore; campus computer network; career placement assistance; computer lab; computer-assisted instruction; e-mail services; housing assistance; interactive nursing skills videos; Internet; learning resource lab; library services; nursing audiovisuals; resume preparation assistance; skills, simulation, or other laboratory; tutoring.
Library Facilities 71,500 volumes; 467 periodical subscriptions.

BACCALAUREATE PROGRAMS
Degree BS
Available Programs Accelerated Baccalaureate for Second Degree; Generic Baccalaureate.
Study Options Full-time.
Program Entrance Requirements Minimum overall college GPA of 3.2, transcript of college record, written essay, health exam, health insurance, high school biology, high school chemistry, 3 years high school science, high school transcript, immunizations, interview, 2 letters of recommendation, minimum high school GPA, minimum GPA in nursing prerequisites of 3.0, professional liability insurance/malpractice insurance, prerequisite course work. Transfer students are accepted. *Application deadline:* 4/1 (winter). *Application fee:* $50.
Advanced Placement Credit given for nursing courses completed elsewhere dependent upon specific evaluations.
Contact *Telephone:* 914-337-9300.

Daemen College
Department of Nursing
Amherst, New York

http://www.daemen.edu/
Founded in 1947
DEGREES • BS • DNP • MS
Nursing Program Faculty 24 (75% with doctorates).
Baccalaureate Enrollment 250 **Women** 96% **Men** 4% **Minority** 3% **International** 2% **Part-time** 15%

Graduate Enrollment 170 **Women** 96% **Men** 4% **Minority** 8% **International** 6% **Part-time** 90%
Distance Learning Courses Available.
Nursing Student Activities Sigma Theta Tau, nursing club.
Nursing Student Resources Academic advising; academic or career counseling; assistance for students with disabilities; bookstore; campus computer network; career placement assistance; computer lab; computer-assisted instruction; e-mail services; Internet; learning resource lab; library services; nursing audiovisuals; placement services for program completers; remedial services; resume preparation assistance; skills, simulation, or other laboratory; tutoring.
Library Facilities 181,410 volumes (10,000 in health, 4,000 in nursing); 53,175 periodical subscriptions (250 health-care related).

BACCALAUREATE PROGRAMS

Degree BS
Available Programs ADN to Baccalaureate; Accelerated RN Baccalaureate; International Nurse to Baccalaureate; RN Baccalaureate.
Site Options Jamestown, NY; Olean, NY.
Study Options Full-time and part-time.
Program Entrance Requirements Minimum overall college GPA of 2.0, transcript of college record, 2 years high school math, 2 years high school science, high school transcript, immunizations, minimum high school GPA of 3.0, minimum GPA in nursing prerequisites of 2.0. Transfer students are accepted. *Application deadline:* Applications may be processed on a rolling basis for some programs. *Application fee:* $25.
Advanced Placement Credit given for nursing courses completed elsewhere dependent upon specific evaluations.
Expenses (2012–13) *Tuition:* full-time $11,310; part-time $375 per credit hour. *International tuition:* $11,310 full-time. *Room and board:* $10,400 per academic year. *Required fees:* full-time $255; part-time $43 per credit.
Financial Aid 100% of baccalaureate students in nursing programs received some form of financial aid in 2011–12.
Contact Dr. Mary Lou Rusin, Professor and Chair, Department of Nursing, Daemen College, 4380 Main Street, Amherst, NY 14226. *Telephone:* 716-839-8387. *Fax:* 716-839-8403. *E-mail:* mrusin@daemen.edu.

GRADUATE PROGRAMS

Expenses (2012–13) *Tuition:* full-time $15,480; part-time $860 per credit hour. *International tuition:* $15,480 full-time. *Room and board:* $10,400 per academic year.
Financial Aid 75% of graduate students in nursing programs received some form of financial aid in 2011–12. Institutionally sponsored loans and scholarships available. *Financial aid application deadline:* 2/15.
Contact Dr. Mary Lou Rusin, Professor and Chair, Department of Nursing, Daemen College, 4380 Main Street, Amherst, NY 14226. *Telephone:* 716-839-8387. *Fax:* 716-839-8403. *E-mail:* mrusin@daemen.edu.

MASTER'S DEGREE PROGRAM

Degree MS
Available Programs Accelerated AD/RN to Master's; Accelerated RN to Master's; Master's; Master's for Nurses with Non-Nursing Degrees; RN to Master's.
Concentrations Available Health-care administration; nursing education. *Nurse practitioner programs in:* adult health.
Study Options Full-time and part-time.
Program Entrance Requirements Clinical experience, minimum overall college GPA of 3.25, transcript of college record, written essay, immunizations, interview, 3 letters of recommendation, statistics course. *Application deadline:* Applications may be processed on a rolling basis for some programs. *Application fee:* $25.
Advanced Placement Credit given for nursing courses completed elsewhere dependent upon specific evaluations.
Degree Requirements 30 total credit hours, thesis or project.

POST-MASTER'S PROGRAM

Areas of Study Health-care administration; nursing education. *Nurse practitioner programs in:* adult health.

DOCTORAL DEGREE PROGRAM

Degree DNP
Available Programs Doctorate.
Areas of Study Advanced practice nursing.
Program Entrance Requirements Minimum overall college GPA of 3.25, interview, 3 letters of recommendation, statistics course, vita,

writing sample. *Application deadline:* Applications may be processed on a rolling basis for some programs. *Application fee:* $25.
Degree Requirements 36 total credit hours, dissertation.

Dominican College
Department of Nursing
Orangeburg, New York

Founded in 1952
DEGREES • BSN • M SC N
Nursing Program Faculty 14 (21% with doctorates).
Baccalaureate Enrollment 182 **Women** 87% **Men** 13% **Minority** 44% **International** 40% **Part-time** 43%
Graduate Enrollment 37 **Women** 100% **Minority** 66% **International** 60% **Part-time** 100%
Nursing Student Activities Nursing Honor Society, Sigma Theta Tau, Student Nurses' Association.
Nursing Student Resources Academic advising; academic or career counseling; assistance for students with disabilities; bookstore; campus computer network; career placement assistance; computer lab; computer-assisted instruction; e-mail services; externships; Internet; learning resource lab; library services; nursing audiovisuals; paid internships; remedial services; resume preparation assistance; skills, simulation, or other laboratory; tutoring.
Library Facilities 125,000 volumes (5,650 in health); 450 periodical subscriptions (235 health-care related).

BACCALAUREATE PROGRAMS

Degree BSN
Available Programs Accelerated Baccalaureate for Second Degree; Accelerated LPN to Baccalaureate; Accelerated RN Baccalaureate; Generic Baccalaureate; LPN to Baccalaureate; RN Baccalaureate.
Study Options Full-time and part-time.
Program Entrance Requirements Minimum overall college GPA of 2.7, transcript of college record, CPR certification, health exam, health insurance, high school transcript, immunizations, minimum GPA in nursing prerequisites of 2.0, professional liability insurance/malpractice insurance, prerequisite course work. Transfer students are accepted.
Advanced Placement Credit by examination available. Credit given for nursing courses completed elsewhere dependent upon specific evaluations.
Contact *Telephone:* 845-848-6051. *Fax:* 845-398-4891.

GRADUATE PROGRAMS

Contact *Telephone:* 845-848-6026. *Fax:* 845-398-4891.

MASTER'S DEGREE PROGRAM

Degree M Sc N
Available Programs Master's.
Concentrations Available *Nurse practitioner programs in:* family health.
Study Options Full-time and part-time.
Program Entrance Requirements Clinical experience, minimum overall college GPA of 3.0, transcript of college record, written essay, immunizations, 3 letters of recommendation, nursing research course, physical assessment course, professional liability insurance/malpractice insurance, prerequisite course work, statistics course.
Degree Requirements 42 total credit hours, thesis or project.

D'Youville College
School of Nursing
Buffalo, New York

http://www.dyc.edu/academics/nursing/
Founded in 1908
DEGREES • BSN • MS
Nursing Program Faculty 41 (20% with doctorates).
Baccalaureate Enrollment 492 **Women** 90% **Men** 10% **Minority** 20% **International** 10% **Part-time** 30%
Graduate Enrollment 115 **Women** 96% **Men** 4% **Minority** 10% **International** 35% **Part-time** 40%
Distance Learning Courses Available.

Nursing Student Activities Sigma Theta Tau, Student Nurses' Association.

Nursing Student Resources Academic advising; academic or career counseling; assistance for students with disabilities; bookstore; campus computer network; career placement assistance; computer lab; computer-assisted instruction; e-mail services; externships; interactive nursing skills videos; Internet; learning resource lab; library services; nursing audiovisuals; paid internships; placement services for program completers; remedial services; resume preparation assistance; skills, simulation, or other laboratory; tutoring.

Library Facilities 116,237 volumes (100,000 in health, 17,000 in nursing); 725 periodical subscriptions (171 health-care related).

BACCALAUREATE PROGRAMS

Degree BSN

Available Programs Generic Baccalaureate; RN Baccalaureate.

Site Options Buffalo, NY.

Study Options Full-time and part-time.

Program Entrance Requirements Minimum overall college GPA of 2.5, transcript of college record, health exam, health insurance, high school biology, high school chemistry, 1 year of high school math, 1 year of high school science, high school transcript, immunizations, minimum high school GPA of 2.0, minimum high school rank 50%, minimum GPA in nursing prerequisites of 2.0, professional liability insurance/malpractice insurance, prerequisite course work. Transfer students are accepted.

Advanced Placement Credit given for nursing courses completed elsewhere dependent upon specific evaluations.

Contact *Telephone:* 716-881-7600. *Fax:* 716-515-0679.

GRADUATE PROGRAMS

Contact *Telephone:* 716-881-7744. *Fax:* 716-515-0679.

MASTER'S DEGREE PROGRAM

Degree MS

Available Programs Master's; RN to Master's.

Concentrations Available Nursing education. *Clinical nurse specialist programs in:* community health, palliative care. *Nurse practitioner programs in:* family health.

Study Options Full-time and part-time.

Program Entrance Requirements Clinical experience, computer literacy, minimum overall college GPA of 3.0, transcript of college record, CPR certification, written essay, immunizations, interview, 2 letters of recommendation, nursing research course, physical assessment course, professional liability insurance/malpractice insurance, prerequisite course work, resume, statistics course.

Advanced Placement Credit given for nursing courses completed elsewhere dependent upon specific evaluations.

Degree Requirements 41 total credit hours, thesis or project.

POST-MASTER'S PROGRAM

Areas of Study *Nurse practitioner programs in:* family health.

See display below and full description on page 480.

Elmira College
Program in Nursing Education
Elmira, New York

http://www.elmira.edu/

Founded in 1855

DEGREE • BS

Nursing Program Faculty 22 (1% with doctorates).

Baccalaureate Enrollment 220 **Women** 89% **Men** 11% **Minority** 4% **International** 2% **Part-time** 20%

Nursing Student Activities Sigma Theta Tau, Student Nurses' Association, nursing club.

Nursing Student Resources Academic advising; academic or career counseling; assistance for students with disabilities; bookstore; campus computer network; career placement assistance; computer lab; computer-assisted instruction; e-mail services; housing assistance; interactive nursing skills videos; Internet; learning resource lab; library services; nursing audiovisuals; placement services for program completers; resume preparation assistance; skills, simulation, or other laboratory; tutoring; unpaid internships.

Library Facilities 203,343 volumes (7,461 in health, 5,200 in nursing); 337 periodical subscriptions (72 health-care related).

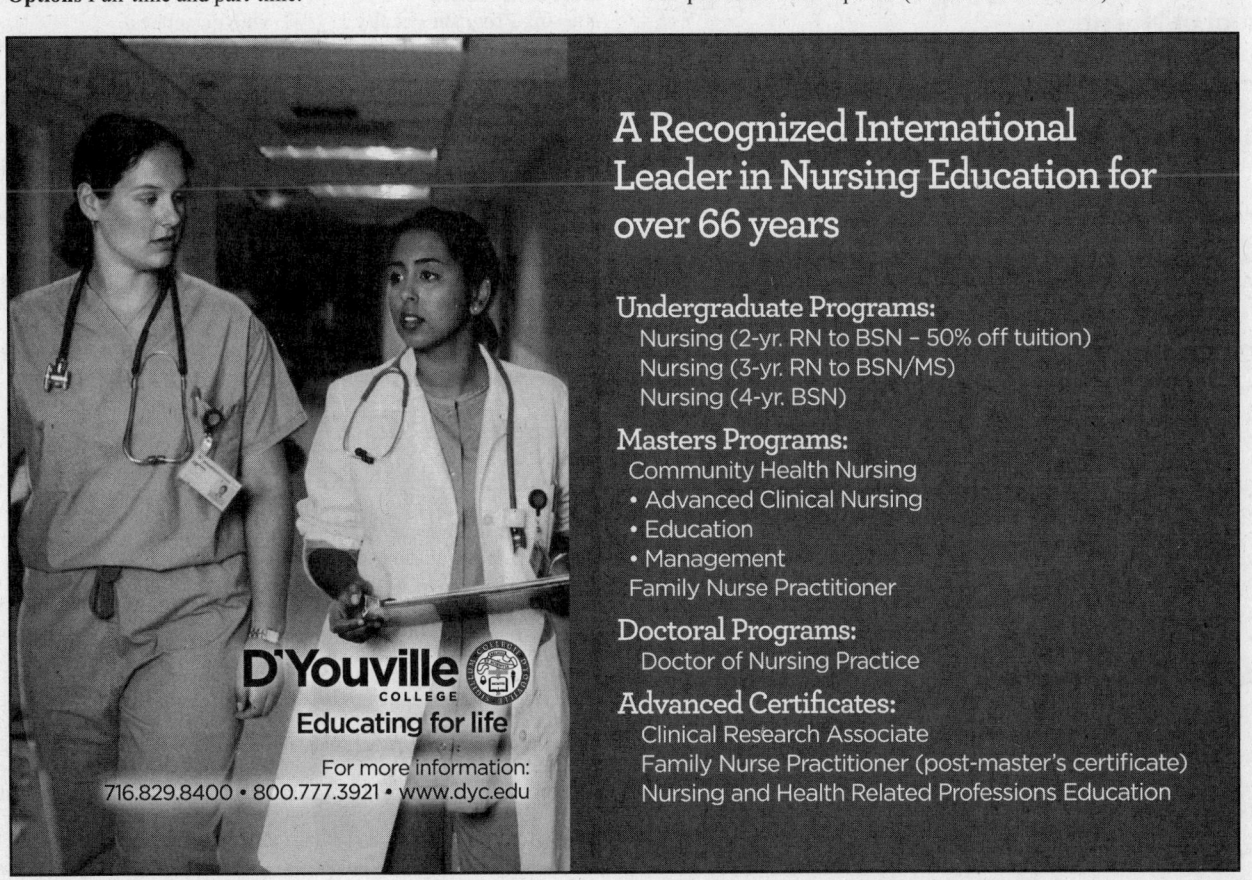

BACCALAUREATE PROGRAMS

Degree BS

Available Programs ADN to Baccalaureate; Generic Baccalaureate; RN Baccalaureate.

Study Options Full-time and part-time.

Program Entrance Requirements Minimum overall college GPA of 2.0, transcript of college record, CPR certification, written essay, health exam, health insurance, high school biology, high school chemistry, 3 years high school math, 3 years high school science, high school transcript, immunizations, 2 letters of recommendation, minimum high school GPA of 2.5. Transfer students are accepted. *Application deadline:* Applications may be processed on a rolling basis for some programs. *Application fee:* $100.

Advanced Placement Credit by examination available. Credit given for nursing courses completed elsewhere dependent upon specific evaluations.

Expenses (2012–13) *Tuition:* full-time $36,600; part-time $325 per credit hour. *International tuition:* $36,600 full-time. *Room and board:* room only: $6300 per academic year. *Required fees:* full-time $500; part-time $50 per term.

Financial Aid 80% of baccalaureate students in nursing programs received some form of financial aid in 2011–12. *Gift aid (need-based):* Federal Pell, FSEOG, state, private, college/university gift aid from institutional funds. *Loans:* Federal Direct (Subsidized and Unsubsidized Stafford PLUS), Perkins, college/university.*Work-study:* Federal Work-Study, part-time campus jobs.*Financial aid application deadline (priority):* 2/1.

Contact Mrs. Julianna Baumann, Dean, Program in Nursing Education, Elmira College, One Park Place, Elmira, NY 14901. *Telephone:* 607-735-1724. *Fax:* 607-735-1718. *E-mail:* admissions@elmira.edu.

CONTINUING EDUCATION PROGRAM

Contact Dr. Lois Schoener, Director of Nurse Education, Program in Nursing Education, Elmira College, One Park Place, Elmira, NY 14901. *Telephone:* 607-735-1890. *Fax:* 607-735-1159. *E-mail:* lschoener@elmira.edu.

Excelsior College

School of Nursing
Albany, New York

Founded in 1970

DEGREES • BS • MS

Distance Learning Courses Available.

Nursing Student Activities Sigma Theta Tau.

Nursing Student Resources Academic advising; academic or career counseling; assistance for students with disabilities; bookstore; computer-assisted instruction; e-mail services; Internet; learning resource lab; library services; nursing audiovisuals; other; resume preparation assistance; skills, simulation, or other laboratory; tutoring.

BACCALAUREATE PROGRAMS

Degree BS

Available Programs RN Baccalaureate.

Study Options Part-time.

Program Entrance Requirements Transcript of college record, high school transcript, RN licensure. Transfer students are accepted. *Application deadline:* Applications may be processed on a rolling basis for some programs.

Advanced Placement Credit by examination available. Credit given for nursing courses completed elsewhere dependent upon specific evaluations.

Contact *Telephone:* 518-464-8500. *Fax:* 518-464-8777.

GRADUATE PROGRAMS

Contact *Telephone:* 518-464-8500. *Fax:* 518-464-8777.

MASTER'S DEGREE PROGRAM

Degree MS

Available Programs Master's; RN to Master's.

Concentrations Available Nursing administration; nursing education; nursing informatics.

Study Options Full-time and part-time.

Online Degree Options Yes (online only).

Program Entrance Requirements Computer literacy, minimum overall college GPA of 3, transcript of college record, written essay, resume. *Application deadline:* Applications may be processed on a rolling basis for some programs.

Advanced Placement Credit given for nursing courses completed elsewhere dependent upon specific evaluations.

Degree Requirements 39 total credit hours, thesis or project.

POST-MASTER'S PROGRAM

Areas of Study Nursing education.

Farmingdale State College

Nursing Department
Farmingdale, New York

Founded in 1912

DEGREE • BS

Library Facilities 125,000 volumes; 800 periodical subscriptions.

BACCALAUREATE PROGRAMS

Degree BS

Available Programs Generic Baccalaureate; RN Baccalaureate.

Contact *Telephone:* 631-420-2229. *Fax:* 631-420-2269.

Hartwick College

Department of Nursing
Oneonta, New York

http://www.hartwick.edu/

Founded in 1797

DEGREE • BS

Nursing Program Faculty 11 (18% with doctorates).

Baccalaureate Enrollment 145 **Women** 93% **Men** 7% **Minority** 9% **International** 1% **Part-time** 12%

Nursing Student Activities Sigma Theta Tau, Student Nurses' Association.

Nursing Student Resources Academic advising; academic or career counseling; assistance for students with disabilities; bookstore; campus computer network; career placement assistance; computer lab; computer-assisted instruction; e-mail services; employment services for current students; externships; housing assistance; interactive nursing skills videos; Internet; learning resource lab; library services; nursing audiovisuals; placement services for program completers; remedial services; resume preparation assistance; skills, simulation, or other laboratory; tutoring; unpaid internships.

Library Facilities 299,336 volumes (5,697 in health, 1,199 in nursing); 12,204 periodical subscriptions (30 health-care related).

BACCALAUREATE PROGRAMS

Degree BS

Available Programs Accelerated Baccalaureate; Accelerated Baccalaureate for Second Degree; Generic Baccalaureate; RN Baccalaureate.

Site Options Cooperstown, NY; Albany, NY.

Study Options Full-time and part-time.

Program Entrance Requirements Minimum overall college GPA of 2.5, transcript of college record, CPR certification, written essay, health exam, high school biology, high school chemistry, high school foreign language, 3 years high school math, 2 years high school science, high school transcript, immunizations, 2 letters of recommendation, minimum GPA in nursing prerequisites of 2.5, professional liability insurance/malpractice insurance. Transfer students are accepted. *Application deadline:* Applications may be processed on a rolling basis for some programs. *Application fee:* $35.

Advanced Placement Credit given for nursing courses completed elsewhere dependent upon specific evaluations.

Contact *Telephone:* 607-431-4780. *Fax:* 607-431-4850.

Hunter College of the City University of New York

Hunter-Bellevue School of Nursing
New York, New York

http://www.hunter.cuny.edu/schoolhp/nursing
Founded in 1870

DEGREES • BSN • DNP • MS • MSN/MPA • MSN/MPH

Nursing Program Faculty 124 (31% with doctorates).

Baccalaureate Enrollment 435 **Women** 83% **Men** 17% **Minority** 62% **International** 2% **Part-time** 38%

Graduate Enrollment 528 **Women** 86% **Men** 14% **Minority** 53% **International** 2% **Part-time** 90%

Nursing Student Activities Sigma Theta Tau, Student Nurses' Association.

Nursing Student Resources Academic advising; academic or career counseling; assistance for students with disabilities; bookstore; campus computer network; computer lab; computer-assisted instruction; e-mail services; interactive nursing skills videos; Internet; learning resource lab; library services; nursing audiovisuals; skills, simulation, or other laboratory.

Library Facilities 548,104 volumes (39,245 in health, 4,295 in nursing); 59,796 periodical subscriptions (375 health-care related).

BACCALAUREATE PROGRAMS

Degree BSN

Available Programs Accelerated Baccalaureate; Generic Baccalaureate; RN Baccalaureate.

Study Options Full-time.

Program Entrance Requirements Minimum overall college GPA of 3.0, transcript of college record, CPR certification, health exam, immunizations, minimum GPA in nursing prerequisites of 3.0, professional liability insurance/malpractice insurance, prerequisite course work. Transfer students are accepted. *Application deadline:* 2/1 (fall). *Application fee:* $75.

Advanced Placement Credit given for nursing courses completed elsewhere dependent upon specific evaluations.

Expenses (2012–13) *Tuition, state resident:* full-time $5430; part-time $340 per credit. *Tuition, nonresident:* full-time $10,640; part-time $720 per credit. *International tuition:* $10,640 full-time. *Room and board:* $11,700; room only: $6000 per academic year. *Required fees:* full-time $399; part-time $60 per term.

Financial Aid 60% of baccalaureate students in nursing programs received some form of financial aid in 2011–12. *Gift aid (need-based):* Federal Pell, FSEOG, state, private, college/university gift aid from institutional funds. *Loans:* Federal Direct (Subsidized and Unsubsidized Stafford PLUS), Perkins. *Work-study:* Federal Work-Study, part-time campus jobs. *Financial aid application deadline (priority):* 4/1.

Contact Ms. Maria Mendoza, Pre-Nursing Adviser, Hunter-Bellevue School of Nursing, Hunter College of the City University of New York, 425 East 25th Street, New York, NY 10010. *Telephone:* 212-481-4473. *Fax:* 212-481-8237. *E-mail:* prenursingadvising@hunter.cuny.edu.

GRADUATE PROGRAMS

Expenses (2012–13) *Tuition, state resident:* full-time $8690; part-time $365 per credit. *Tuition, nonresident:* full-time $16,200; part-time $675 per credit. *International tuition:* $16,200 full-time. *Required fees:* full-time $256; part-time $78 per term.

Financial Aid 50% of graduate students in nursing programs received some form of financial aid in 2011–12. Federal Work-Study, scholarships, traineeships, and tuition waivers (partial) available. Aid available to part-time students. *Financial aid application deadline:* 5/1.

Contact Dr. David Keepnews, Director of Graduate Program, Hunter-Bellevue School of Nursing, Hunter College of the City University of New York, 425 East 25th Street, New York, NY 10010. *Telephone:* 212-481-4465. *Fax:* 212-481-4427. *E-mail:* knokes@hunter.cuny.edu.

MASTER'S DEGREE PROGRAM

Degrees MS; MSN/MPA; MSN/MPH

Available Programs Master's; RN to Master's.

Concentrations Available Clinical nurse leader; nursing administration. *Clinical nurse specialist programs in:* adult health, community health, gerontology, psychiatric/mental health, public health. *Nurse practitioner programs in:* community health, family health, gerontology, psychiatric/mental health.

Study Options Full-time and part-time.

Program Entrance Requirements Clinical experience, minimum overall college GPA of 3.0, transcript of college record, written essay, immunizations, 2 letters of recommendation, resume, statistics course. *Application deadline:* 4/1 (fall), 11/1 (spring). Applications may be processed on a rolling basis for some programs. *Application fee:* $125.

Advanced Placement Credit given for nursing courses completed elsewhere dependent upon specific evaluations.

Degree Requirements 42 total credit hours, thesis or project.

POST-MASTER'S PROGRAM

Areas of Study Nursing education. *Nurse practitioner programs in:* psychiatric/mental health.

DOCTORAL DEGREE PROGRAM

Degree DNP

Available Programs Post-Baccalaureate Doctorate.

Areas of Study Community health, family health, gerontology, neurobehavior.

Program Entrance Requirements Clinical experience, minimum overall college GPA of 3.5, interview, 2 letters of recommendation, statistics course, vita. *Application deadline:* 4/1 (fall), 11/1 (spring). Applications may be processed on a rolling basis for some programs. *Application fee:* $125.

Degree Requirements 90 total credit hours.

CONTINUING EDUCATION PROGRAM

Contact Continuing Education, Hunter-Bellevue School of Nursing, Hunter College of the City University of New York, 695 Park Avenue, East Building, 10th Floor, New York, NY 10021. *Telephone:* 212-650-3850. *Fax:* 212-772-3402. *E-mail:* ce@hunter.cuny.edu.

Keuka College

Division of Nursing
Keuka Park, New York

http://academics.keuka.edu/asap/programs/bs_nursing
Founded in 1890

DEGREE • BS

Nursing Program Faculty 5 (20% with doctorates).

Baccalaureate Enrollment 238 **Women** 94% **Men** 6% **Minority** 4%

Distance Learning Courses Available.

Nursing Student Activities Sigma Theta Tau.

Nursing Student Resources Academic advising; academic or career counseling; assistance for students with disabilities; bookstore; campus computer network; computer lab; computer-assisted instruction; e-mail services; employment services for current students; interactive nursing skills videos; Internet; learning resource lab; library services; nursing audiovisuals; resume preparation assistance; tutoring.

Library Facilities 112,541 volumes (986 in health, 532 in nursing); 384 periodical subscriptions (48 health-care related).

BACCALAUREATE PROGRAMS

Degree BS

Available Programs Accelerated RN Baccalaureate.

Site Options Geneva, NY; Rochester, NY; Canandaigua, NY.

Study Options Full-time and part-time.

Program Entrance Requirements Minimum overall college GPA of 2.5, transcript of college record, CPR certification, health exam, immunizations, minimum GPA in nursing prerequisites of 2.5, prerequisite course work, RN licensure. Transfer students are accepted.

Advanced Placement Credit by examination available. Credit given for nursing courses completed elsewhere dependent upon specific evaluations.

Contact *Telephone:* 315-279-5393. *Fax:* 315-279-5407.

Lehman College of the City University of New York

Department of Nursing
Bronx, New York

http://www.lehman.edu/academics/nursing/
Founded in 1931
DEGREES • BS • DNS • MS
Nursing Program Faculty 43 (35% with doctorates).
Baccalaureate Enrollment 300 **Women** 80% **Men** 20% **Minority** 85%
International 40% **Part-time** 50%
Graduate Enrollment 200 **Women** 90% **Men** 10% **Minority** 75%
International 25% **Part-time** 75%
Distance Learning Courses Available.
Nursing Student Activities Nursing Honor Society, Sigma Theta Tau, Student Nurses' Association, nursing club.
Nursing Student Resources Academic advising; academic or career counseling; assistance for students with disabilities; bookstore; campus computer network; career placement assistance; computer lab; computer-assisted instruction; daycare for children of students; e-mail services; employment services for current students; externships; interactive nursing skills videos; Internet; learning resource lab; library services; nursing audiovisuals; paid internships; placement services for program completers; resume preparation assistance; skills, simulation, or other laboratory; tutoring; unpaid internships.
Library Facilities 660,616 volumes (1,000 in health, 500 in nursing); 9,370 periodical subscriptions (200 health-care related).

BACCALAUREATE PROGRAMS

Degree BS
Available Programs ADN to Baccalaureate; Accelerated Baccalaureate for Second Degree; Accelerated RN Baccalaureate; Baccalaureate for Second Degree; Generic Baccalaureate; International Nurse to Baccalaureate; RN Baccalaureate.
Site Options New York, NY; Queens, NY.
Study Options Full-time.
Online Degree Options Yes.
Program Entrance Requirements Minimum overall college GPA of 2.0, transcript of college record, health exam, high school transcript, immunizations, minimum GPA in nursing prerequisites of 2.75, professional liability insurance/malpractice insurance, prerequisite course work. Transfer students are accepted. *Application deadline:* 3/15 (fall).
Advanced Placement Credit given for nursing courses completed elsewhere dependent upon specific evaluations.
Contact *Telephone:* 718-960-8214. *Fax:* 718-960-8488.

GRADUATE PROGRAMS

Contact *Telephone:* 718-960-8213. *Fax:* 718-960-8488.

MASTER'S DEGREE PROGRAM
Degree MS
Available Programs Master's; Master's for Nurses with Non-Nursing Degrees.
Concentrations Available Nursing administration; nursing education. *Clinical nurse specialist programs in:* adult health, gerontology, parent-child. *Nurse practitioner programs in:* family health, pediatric.
Site Options New York, NY.
Study Options Full-time and part-time.
Program Entrance Requirements Clinical experience, minimum overall college GPA of 3.0, transcript of college record, written essay, immunizations, interview, 2 letters of recommendation, professional liability insurance/malpractice insurance, prerequisite course work. *Application deadline:* 4/1 (fall), 11/1 (spring). Applications may be processed on a rolling basis for some programs. *Application fee:* $125.
Degree Requirements 43 total credit hours.

POST-MASTER'S PROGRAM
Areas of Study *Nurse practitioner programs in:* family health, pediatric.

DOCTORAL DEGREE PROGRAM
Degree DNS
Available Programs Doctorate.
Areas of Study Urban health.
Site Options New York, NY.
Program Entrance Requirements Clinical experience, minimum overall college GPA of 3.5, interview by faculty committee, interview, letters of recommendation, MSN or equivalent, statistics course, vita, writing sample. *Application deadline:* 4/1 (fall).
Degree Requirements 51 total credit hours, dissertation, oral exam, written exam, residency.

CONTINUING EDUCATION PROGRAM

Contact *Telephone:* 718-960-8799.

Le Moyne College

Nursing Programs
Syracuse, New York

http://www.lemoyne.edu/nursing
Founded in 1946
DEGREES • BS • MS
Nursing Program Faculty 8 (50% with doctorates).
Baccalaureate Enrollment 202 **Women** 91% **Men** 9% **Minority** 5%
Part-time 20%
Graduate Enrollment 31 **Women** 100% **Minority** 2% **Part-time** 99%
Distance Learning Courses Available.
Nursing Student Activities Nursing Honor Society.
Nursing Student Resources Academic advising; academic or career counseling; assistance for students with disabilities; bookstore; campus computer network; career placement assistance; computer lab; computer-assisted instruction; e-mail services; employment services for current students; housing assistance; interactive nursing skills videos; Internet; learning resource lab; library services; nursing audiovisuals; placement services for program completers; remedial services; resume preparation assistance; skills, simulation, or other laboratory; tutoring.
Library Facilities 257,672 volumes (2,761 in health, 624 in nursing); 60,686 periodical subscriptions (4,311 health-care related).

BACCALAUREATE PROGRAMS

Degree BS
Available Programs ADN to Baccalaureate; RN Baccalaureate.
Site Options Syracuse, NY.
Study Options Full-time and part-time.
Program Entrance Requirements Minimum overall college GPA of 2.6, transcript of college record, CPR certification, written essay, health exam, health insurance, high school biology, high school chemistry, high school foreign language, 3 years high school math, 3 years high school science, high school transcript, immunizations, 2 letters of recommendation, minimum high school GPA of 3.0, minimum high school rank 85%, minimum GPA in nursing prerequisites of 2.5, RN licensure. Transfer students are accepted. *Application deadline:* 2/1 (fall), 8/1 (spring), 5/1 (summer). Applications may be processed on a rolling basis for some programs. *Application fee:* $35.
Advanced Placement Credit by examination available. Credit given for nursing courses completed elsewhere dependent upon specific evaluations.
Expenses (2012–13) *Tuition:* full-time $28,470; part-time $597 per credit hour. *Room and board:* $11,000; room only: $7180 per academic year. *Required fees:* full-time $990; part-time $25 per term.
Financial Aid 90% of baccalaureate students in nursing programs received some form of financial aid in 2011–12.
Contact Dr. Susan B. Bastable, Chair and Professor, Nursing Programs, Le Moyne College, 1419 Salt Springs Road, Syracuse, NY 13214. *Telephone:* 315-445-5435. *Fax:* 315-445-6024. *E-mail:* bastabsb@lemoyne.edu.

GRADUATE PROGRAMS

Expenses (2012–13) *Tuition:* part-time $622 per credit hour. *Required fees:* part-time $25 per term.
Financial Aid 100% of graduate students in nursing programs received some form of financial aid in 2011–12.
Contact Mrs. Kristen P. Trapasso, Director of Graduate Admissions, Nursing Programs, Le Moyne College, 1419 Salt Springs Road, Syracuse, NY 13214. *Telephone:* 315-445-4265. *Fax:* 315-445-6027. *E-mail:* trapaskp@lemoyne.edu.

MASTER'S DEGREE PROGRAM
Degree MS
Available Programs Master's; Master's for Nurses with Non-Nursing Degrees.
Concentrations Available Nursing administration; nursing education.

Study Options Full-time and part-time.

Program Entrance Requirements Computer literacy, minimum overall college GPA of 3.0, transcript of college record, written essay, immunizations, interview, 2 letters of recommendation, nursing research course, physical assessment course, resume, statistics course. *Application deadline:* 8/1 (fall), 12/15 (spring), 5/1 (summer). Applications may be processed on a rolling basis for some programs. *Application fee:* $50.

Advanced Placement Credit given for nursing courses completed elsewhere dependent upon specific evaluations.

Degree Requirements 39 total credit hours, thesis or project.

POST-MASTER'S PROGRAM

Areas of Study Nursing administration; nursing education.

Long Island University–Brooklyn Campus
School of Nursing
Brooklyn, New York

http://www.liunet.edu/
Founded in 1926
DEGREES • BS • MS
Nursing Program Faculty 85 (30% with doctorates).
Baccalaureate Enrollment 868 **Women** 85% **Men** 15% **Minority** 85% **International** 2% **Part-time** 35%
Graduate Enrollment 240 **Women** 90% **Men** 10% **Minority** 85% **Part-time** 83%
Nursing Student Activities Nursing Honor Society, Student Nurses' Association, nursing club.
Nursing Student Resources Academic advising; academic or career counseling; assistance for students with disabilities; bookstore; campus computer network; career placement assistance; computer lab; computer-assisted instruction; e-mail services; employment services for current students; externships; interactive nursing skills videos; Internet; learning resource lab; library services; nursing audiovisuals; paid internships; remedial services; resume preparation assistance; skills, simulation, or other laboratory; tutoring; unpaid internships.
Library Facilities 314,565 volumes; 329,366 periodical subscriptions.

BACCALAUREATE PROGRAMS

Degree BS
Available Programs ADN to Baccalaureate; Accelerated Baccalaureate for Second Degree; Generic Baccalaureate.
Site Options Brooklyn, NY.
Study Options Full-time and part-time.
Program Entrance Requirements Minimum overall college GPA of 2.75, transcript of college record, CPR certification, health exam, health insurance, high school biology, high school chemistry, 2 years high school math, 2 years high school science, high school transcript, immunizations, interview, minimum high school GPA of 3.0, minimum GPA in nursing prerequisites of 2.75, professional liability insurance/malpractice insurance, prerequisite course work. Transfer students are accepted. *Application deadline:* Applications may be processed on a rolling basis for some programs. *Application fee:* $30.
Advanced Placement Credit given for nursing courses completed elsewhere dependent upon specific evaluations.
Expenses (2012–13) *Tuition:* part-time $974 per credit. *Room and board:* $9920; room only: $5540 per academic year. *Required fees:* part-time $415 per term.
Financial Aid 96% of baccalaureate students in nursing programs received some form of financial aid in 2011–12. *Gift aid (need-based):* Federal Pell, FSEOG, state, private, college/university gift aid from institutional funds, Scholarships for Disadvantaged Students (Nursing and Pharmacy). *Loans:* Federal Direct (Subsidized and Unsubsidized Stafford PLUS), Perkins, alternative loans, Health Professions Student Loans (HPSL). *Work-study:* Federal Work-Study, part-time campus jobs. *Financial aid application deadline:* Continuous.
Contact Miss Keisha King, School of Nursing Secretary, School of Nursing, Long Island University–Brooklyn Campus, 1 University Plaza, Brooklyn, NY 11201. *Telephone:* 718-488-1059. *Fax:* 718-780-4019. *E-mail:* keisha.king@liu.edu.

GRADUATE PROGRAMS

Expenses (2012–13) *Tuition:* part-time $1068 per credit. *Room and board:* $11,799; room only: $7220 per academic year. *Required fees:* part-time $415 per term.
Financial Aid 75% of graduate students in nursing programs received some form of financial aid in 2011–12. Scholarships and unspecified assistantships available. Aid available to part-time students.
Contact Prof. Susanne Flower, Director, School of Nursing, Long Island University–Brooklyn Campus, 1 University Plaza, Brooklyn, NY 11201. *Telephone:* 718-488-1059. *Fax:* 718-780-4019. *E-mail:* susanne.flower@liu.edu.

MASTER'S DEGREE PROGRAM
Degree MS
Available Programs Master's; RN to Master's.
Concentrations Available Health-care administration; nursing administration; nursing education. *Nurse practitioner programs in:* adult health, family health.
Site Options Brooklyn, NY.
Study Options Full-time and part-time.
Program Entrance Requirements Clinical experience, computer literacy, minimum overall college GPA of 3.0, transcript of college record, CPR certification, immunizations, interview, 3 letters of recommendation, nursing research course, physical assessment course, professional liability insurance/malpractice insurance, prerequisite course work, resume, statistics course. *Application deadline:* Applications may be processed on a rolling basis for some programs. *Application fee:* $30.
Advanced Placement Credit given for nursing courses completed elsewhere dependent upon specific evaluations.
Degree Requirements 45 total credit hours.

POST-MASTER'S PROGRAM
Areas of Study Nursing education. *Nurse practitioner programs in:* adult health, family health.

Long Island University–C. W. Post Campus
Department of Nursing
Brookville, New York

http://www.liu.edu/cwpost/nursing
Founded in 1954
DEGREES • BS • MS
Nursing Program Faculty 13 (54% with doctorates).
Baccalaureate Enrollment 65 **Women** 97% **Men** 3% **Minority** 30% **Part-time** 100%
Graduate Enrollment 86 **Women** 94% **Men** 6% **Minority** 30% **Part-time** 100%
Nursing Student Activities Student Nurses' Association.
Nursing Student Resources Academic advising; academic or career counseling; assistance for students with disabilities; bookstore; campus computer network; career placement assistance; computer lab; computer-assisted instruction; e-mail services; employment services for current students; housing assistance; interactive nursing skills videos; Internet; library services; nursing audiovisuals; placement services for program completers; remedial services; resume preparation assistance; skills, simulation, or other laboratory; tutoring.
Library Facilities 177,108 volumes (20,000 in health, 15,000 in nursing); 3,100 periodical subscriptions health-care related.

BACCALAUREATE PROGRAMS
Degree BS
Available Programs RN Baccalaureate.
Site Options Manhasset, NY.
Study Options Part-time.
Program Entrance Requirements Minimum overall college GPA of 3.0, transcript of college record, health exam, health insurance, immunizations, minimum GPA in nursing prerequisites of 3.0, professional liability insurance/malpractice insurance, prerequisite course work, RN licensure. Transfer students are accepted. *Application deadline:* Applications may be processed on a rolling basis for some programs. *Application fee:* $40.
Advanced Placement Credit by examination available. Credit given for nursing courses completed elsewhere dependent upon specific evaluations.

Financial Aid 15% of baccalaureate students in nursing programs received some form of financial aid in 2011–12. *Gift aid (need-based):* Federal Pell, FSEOG, state, private, college/university gift aid from institutional funds. *Loans:* Federal Direct (Subsidized and Unsubsidized Stafford PLUS), Perkins.*Work-study:* Federal Work-Study, part-time campus jobs.*Financial aid application deadline:* 3/1.

Contact Dr. Mary Infantino, Chairperson and Associate Professor, Department of Nursing, Long Island University–C. W. Post Campus, Life Science, Room 270, 720 Northern Boulevard, Brookville, NY 11548-1300. *Telephone:* 516-299-2320. *Fax:* 516-299-2352. *E-mail:* mary.infantino@liu.edu.

GRADUATE PROGRAMS

Expenses (2012–13) *Tuition:* part-time $1068 per credit.

Financial Aid 15% of graduate students in nursing programs received some form of financial aid in 2011–12. Federal Work-Study and unspecified assistantships available. Aid available to part-time students. *Financial aid application deadline:* 5/15.

Contact Dr. Mary Infantino, Chairperson and Associate Professor, Department of Nursing, Long Island University–C. W. Post Campus, Life Science, Room 270, 720 Northern Boulevard, Brookville, NY 11548-1300. *Telephone:* 516-299-2320. *Fax:* 516-299-2352. *E-mail:* mary.infantino@liu.edu.

MASTER'S DEGREE PROGRAM

Degree MS

Available Programs Master's; Master's for Nurses with Non-Nursing Degrees.

Concentrations Available Nursing education. *Clinical nurse specialist programs in:* adult health. *Nurse practitioner programs in:* family health.

Study Options Part-time.

Program Entrance Requirements Clinical experience, minimum overall college GPA of 3.0, transcript of college record, written essay, immunizations, interview, 2 letters of recommendation, physical assessment course, professional liability insurance/malpractice insurance, prerequisite course work. *Application deadline:* Applications may be processed on a rolling basis for some programs. *Application fee:* $40.

Advanced Placement Credit given for nursing courses completed elsewhere dependent upon specific evaluations.

Degree Requirements 46 total credit hours, thesis or project.

POST-MASTER'S PROGRAM

Areas of Study Nursing education. *Nurse practitioner programs in:* family health.

See display below and full description on page 488.

Medgar Evers College of the City University of New York

Department of Nursing
Brooklyn, New York

http://www.mec.cuny.edu/nursing/

Founded in 1969

DEGREE • BSN

Nursing Program Faculty 7 (85% with doctorates).

Baccalaureate Enrollment 60 **Women** 98% **Men** 2% **Minority** 99% **Part-time** 90%

Nursing Student Activities Student Nurses' Association, nursing club.

Nursing Student Resources Academic advising; academic or career counseling; assistance for students with disabilities; bookstore; campus computer network; computer lab; computer-assisted instruction; daycare for children of students; e-mail services; interactive nursing skills videos; Internet; learning resource lab; library services; nursing audiovisuals; remedial services; resume preparation assistance; skills, simulation, or other laboratory; tutoring; unpaid internships.

Library Facilities 120,000 volumes; 24,410 periodical subscriptions.

BACCALAUREATE PROGRAMS

Degree BSN

Available Programs ADN to Baccalaureate; Accelerated RN Baccalaureate.

Study Options Full-time and part-time.

Program Entrance Requirements Minimum overall college GPA of 2.5, transcript of college record, CPR certification, health exam, health insurance, immunizations, professional liability insurance/malpractice insurance, prerequisite course work, RN licensure. Transfer students are accepted.

Advanced Placement Credit given for nursing courses completed elsewhere dependent upon specific evaluations.
Contact *Telephone:* 718-270-6230. *Fax:* 718-270-6235.

Mercy College
Programs in Nursing
Dobbs Ferry, New York

Founded in 1951
DEGREES • BS • MS
Nursing Program Faculty 5 (2% with doctorates).
Baccalaureate Enrollment 333 **Women** 96% **Men** 4% **Minority** 75% **International** 1% **Part-time** 88%
Graduate Enrollment 100 **Women** 99% **Men** 1% **Minority** 50% **International** 10% **Part-time** 75%
Distance Learning Courses Available.
Nursing Student Activities Sigma Theta Tau, Student Nurses' Association.
Nursing Student Resources Academic advising; academic or career counseling; assistance for students with disabilities; bookstore; campus computer network; career placement assistance; computer lab; computer-assisted instruction; e-mail services; employment services for current students; Internet; learning resource lab; library services; nursing audiovisuals; remedial services; resume preparation assistance; skills, simulation, or other laboratory; tutoring.
Library Facilities 249,571 volumes (10,000 in health, 550 in nursing); 736 periodical subscriptions (180 health-care related).

BACCALAUREATE PROGRAMS

Degree BS
Available Programs Accelerated RN Baccalaureate; RN Baccalaureate.
Site Options Dobbs Ferry, NY.
Study Options Full-time and part-time.
Online Degree Options Yes.
Program Entrance Requirements Minimum overall college GPA, transcript of college record, written essay, immunizations, interview, minimum GPA in nursing prerequisites, prerequisite course work, RN licensure. Transfer students are accepted. *Application deadline:* Applications may be processed on a rolling basis for some programs.
Advanced Placement Credit given for nursing courses completed elsewhere dependent upon specific evaluations.
Contact *Telephone:* 914-674-7865. *Fax:* 914-674-7623.

GRADUATE PROGRAMS

Contact *Telephone:* 914-674-7867. *Fax:* 914-674-7623.

MASTER'S DEGREE PROGRAM
Degree MS
Available Programs Accelerated Master's for Non-Nursing College Graduates; Accelerated Master's for Nurses with Non-Nursing Degrees; Accelerated RN to Master's; Master's; Master's for Non-Nursing College Graduates; Master's for Nurses with Non-Nursing Degrees.
Concentrations Available Health-care administration; nursing administration; nursing education.
Site Options Dobbs Ferry, NY.
Study Options Full-time and part-time.
Online Degree Options Yes.
Program Entrance Requirements Clinical experience, minimum overall college GPA of 3.0, transcript of college record, written essay, immunizations, interview, 2 letters of recommendation, professional liability insurance/malpractice insurance, resume. *Application deadline:* Applications may be processed on a rolling basis for some programs.
Advanced Placement Credit given for nursing courses completed elsewhere dependent upon specific evaluations.
Degree Requirements 36 total credit hours, thesis or project.

POST-MASTER'S PROGRAM
Areas of Study Nursing administration; nursing education.

Molloy College
Division of Nursing
Rockville Centre, New York

http://www.molloy.edu/
Founded in 1955
DEGREES • BS • MS • PHD
Nursing Program Faculty 235 (16% with doctorates).
Baccalaureate Enrollment 1,449 **Women** 88% **Men** 12% **Minority** 38% **Part-time** 4%
Graduate Enrollment 471 **Women** 91% **Men** 9% **Minority** 53% **International** 1% **Part-time** 98%
Nursing Student Activities Sigma Theta Tau, Student Nurses' Association.
Nursing Student Resources Academic advising; academic or career counseling; assistance for students with disabilities; bookstore; campus computer network; computer lab; computer-assisted instruction; e-mail services; interactive nursing skills videos; Internet; learning resource lab; library services; nursing audiovisuals; tutoring.
Library Facilities 80,698 volumes; 698 periodical subscriptions.

BACCALAUREATE PROGRAMS

Degree BS
Available Programs ADN to Baccalaureate; Accelerated Baccalaureate for Second Degree; Accelerated RN Baccalaureate; Baccalaureate for Second Degree; Generic Baccalaureate; LPN to Baccalaureate; LPN to RN Baccalaureate; RN Baccalaureate.
Site Options New Hyde Park, NY; Plainview, NY.
Study Options Full-time and part-time.
Program Entrance Requirements Minimum overall college GPA of 3.0, transcript of college record, written essay, health exam, high school biology, high school chemistry, high school foreign language, 3 years high school math, high school transcript, immunizations, minimum high school GPA of 3.0. Transfer students are accepted. *Application deadline:* Applications may be processed on a rolling basis for some programs. *Application fee:* $30.
Advanced Placement Credit given for nursing courses completed elsewhere dependent upon specific evaluations.
Expenses (2012–13) *Tuition:* part-time $735 per credit. *Required fees:* part-time $150 per credit.
Financial Aid 88% of baccalaureate students in nursing programs received some form of financial aid in 2011–12.
Contact Marguerite Lane, Director of Admissions, Division of Nursing, Molloy College, 1000 Hempstead Avenue, PO Box 5002, Rockville Centre, NY 11571-5002. *Telephone:* 516-678-5000 Ext. 6233. *E-mail:* mlane@molloy.edu.

GRADUATE PROGRAMS

Expenses (2012–13) *Tuition:* part-time $895 per credit. *Required fees:* part-time $180 per credit; part-time $260 per term.
Financial Aid 44% of graduate students in nursing programs received some form of financial aid in 2011–12. Research assistantships with partial tuition reimbursements available, teaching assistantships with partial tuition reimbursements available, institutionally sponsored loans, scholarships, and unspecified assistantships available. Aid available to part-time students. *Financial aid application deadline:* 4/1.
Contact Ms. Joanna Forgione, Assistant Director of Admissions, Division of Nursing, Molloy College, 1000 Hempstead Avenue, PO Box 5002, Rockville Centre, NY 11571-5002. *Telephone:* 516-678-5000 Ext. 6322. *E-mail:* jforgione @molloy.edu.

MASTER'S DEGREE PROGRAM
Degree MS
Available Programs Master's.
Concentrations Available Nursing administration; nursing education; nursing informatics. *Clinical nurse specialist programs in:* adult health. *Nurse practitioner programs in:* adult health, family health, pediatric, psychiatric/mental health.
Site Options Farmingdale, NY; New Hyde Park, NY; Plainview, NY.
Study Options Full-time and part-time.
Program Entrance Requirements Clinical experience, minimum overall college GPA of 3.0, transcript of college record, written essay, interview, 3 letters of recommendation, nursing research course, prerequisite course work, statistics course. *Application deadline:* Applications may be processed on a rolling basis for some programs. *Application fee:* $60.

Advanced Placement Credit given for nursing courses completed elsewhere dependent upon specific evaluations.
Degree Requirements 48 total credit hours, thesis or project.

POST-MASTER'S PROGRAM

Areas of Study Nursing administration; nursing education; nursing informatics. *Clinical nurse specialist programs in:* adult health. *Nurse practitioner programs in:* adult health, family health, pediatric, psychiatric/mental health.

DOCTORAL DEGREE PROGRAM

Degree PhD
Available Programs Doctorate.
Areas of Study Health policy, nursing education, nursing research.
Program Entrance Requirements Clinical experience, minimum overall college GPA of 3.5, interview by faculty committee, interview, 3 letters of recommendation, MSN or equivalent, scholarly papers, statistics course, vita, writing sample. *Application deadline:* 2/1 (fall). *Application fee:* $75.
Degree Requirements 45 total credit hours, dissertation.

CONTINUING EDUCATION PROGRAM

Contact Anna Jansson, Associate Director, Continuing Education, Division of Nursing, Molloy College, 1000 Hempstead Avenue, Rockville Centre, NY 11571-5002. *Telephone:* 516-678-5000 Ext. 6106. *Fax:* 516-678-7295. *E-mail:* ajansson@molloy.edu.

See display below and full description on page 494.

Mount Saint Mary College

Division of Nursing
Newburgh, New York

Founded in 1960
DEGREES • BSN • MS
Nursing Program Faculty 36 (50% with doctorates).
Nursing Student Activities Sigma Theta Tau, Student Nurses' Association, nursing club.

Nursing Student Resources Academic advising; academic or career counseling; assistance for students with disabilities; bookstore; campus computer network; career placement assistance; computer lab; computer-assisted instruction; e-mail services; employment services for current students; externships; housing assistance; interactive nursing skills videos; Internet; learning resource lab; library services; nursing audiovisuals; paid internships; remedial services; resume preparation assistance; skills, simulation, or other laboratory; tutoring.
Library Facilities 112,995 volumes (2,443 in health, 1,723 in nursing); 60,280 periodical subscriptions (114 health-care related).

BACCALAUREATE PROGRAMS

Degree BSN
Available Programs Accelerated Baccalaureate; Accelerated RN Baccalaureate; Generic Baccalaureate; RN Baccalaureate.
Study Options Full-time and part-time.
Program Entrance Requirements Minimum overall college GPA of 2.75, transcript of college record, CPR certification, health exam, high school biology, high school chemistry, 3 years high school math, high school transcript, immunizations, interview. Transfer students are accepted.
Advanced Placement Credit by examination available. Credit given for nursing courses completed elsewhere dependent upon specific evaluations.
Contact *Telephone:* 845-569-3248.

GRADUATE PROGRAMS

Contact *Telephone:* 845-569-3248.

MASTER'S DEGREE PROGRAM

Degree MS
Available Programs Master's.
Concentrations Available *Clinical nurse specialist programs in:* adult health. *Nurse practitioner programs in:* adult health.
Study Options Full-time and part-time.
Program Entrance Requirements Clinical experience, computer literacy, minimum overall college GPA of 3.0, transcript of college record, written essay, immunizations, interview, 3 letters of recommendation, nursing research course, physical assessment course, professional liability insurance/malpractice insurance, resume, statistics course.
Degree Requirements 42 total credit hours, thesis or project.

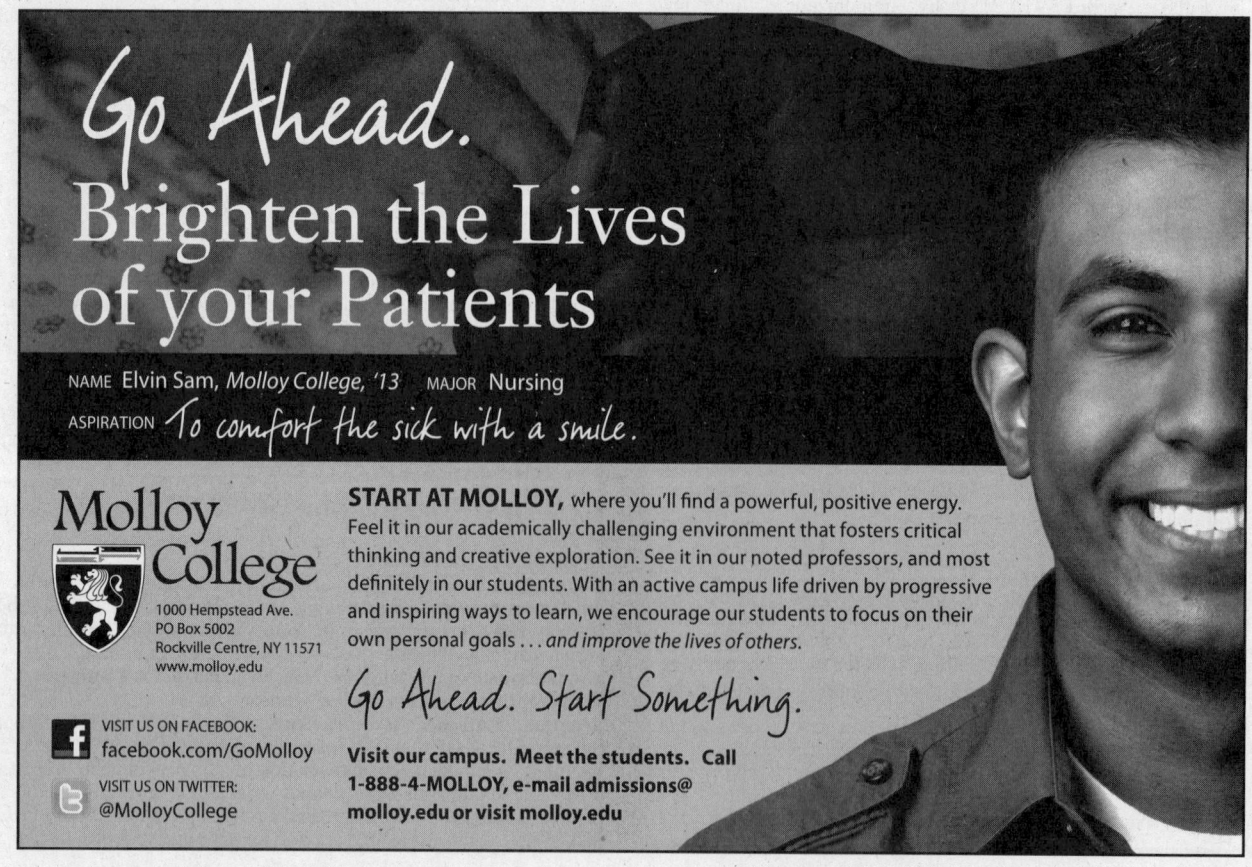

POST-MASTER'S PROGRAM
Areas of Study Nursing administration; nursing education.

Nazareth College of Rochester
Department of Nursing
Rochester, New York

http://www.naz.edu/dept/nursing/
Founded in 1924
DEGREE • BS
Nursing Program Faculty 20 (50% with doctorates).
Baccalaureate Enrollment 20
Distance Learning Courses Available.
Nursing Student Activities Nursing Honor Society, Sigma Theta Tau, Student Nurses' Association, nursing club.
Nursing Student Resources Academic advising; academic or career counseling; assistance for students with disabilities; bookstore; campus computer network; career placement assistance; computer lab; computer-assisted instruction; daycare for children of students; e-mail services; employment services for current students; externships; housing assistance; interactive nursing skills videos; Internet; learning resource lab; library services; nursing audiovisuals; resume preparation assistance; skills, simulation, or other laboratory; tutoring.
Library Facilities 283,248 volumes (267,000 in health, 66,000 in nursing); 16,102 periodical subscriptions (44,000 health-care related).

BACCALAUREATE PROGRAMS

Degree BS
Available Programs Generic Baccalaureate; LPN to Baccalaureate; RN Baccalaureate.
Site Options Rochester, NY.
Study Options Full-time and part-time.
Program Entrance Requirements Minimum overall college GPA of 2.75, transcript of college record, CPR certification, written essay, health exam, high school chemistry, high school transcript, immunizations, minimum high school GPA of 2.75, minimum GPA in nursing prerequisites of 2.5, prerequisite course work. Transfer students are accepted.
Advanced Placement Credit by examination available. Credit given for nursing courses completed elsewhere dependent upon specific evaluations.
Contact Admissions Office, Department of Nursing, Nazareth College of Rochester, 4245 East Avenue, Rochester, NY 14618-3790. *Telephone:* 585-389-2865. *E-mail:* admissions@naz.edu.

New York City College of Technology of the City University of New York
Department of Nursing
Brooklyn, New York

http://nursing.citytech.cuny.edu/
Founded in 1946
DEGREE • BS
Nursing Program Faculty 22
Library Facilities 160,934 volumes; 79,529 periodical subscriptions.

BACCALAUREATE PROGRAMS

Degree BS
Available Programs RN Baccalaureate.
Program Entrance Requirements Minimum overall college GPA of 2.5, immunizations, professional liability insurance/malpractice insurance, RN licensure. Transfer students are accepted.
Contact *Telephone:* 718-260-5660. *Fax:* 718-260-5662.

New York Institute of Technology
Department of Nursing
Old Westbury, New York

Founded in 1955
DEGREE • BSN
Library Facilities 162,222 volumes; 1,245 periodical subscriptions.

BACCALAUREATE PROGRAMS

Degree BSN
Available Programs Generic Baccalaureate.
Contact *Telephone:* 516-686-7516.

New York University
College of Nursing
New York, New York

http://www.nyu.edu/nursing/index.html
Founded in 1831
DEGREES • BS • DNP • MS • MS/MA • MS/MPH • PHD
Nursing Program Faculty 215 (30% with doctorates).
Baccalaureate Enrollment 921 **Women** 87.2% **Men** 12.8% **Minority** 43.1% **International** 1.5% **Part-time** 1.8%
Graduate Enrollment 696 **Women** 89.7% **Men** 10.3% **Minority** 52.4% **International** 1.6% **Part-time** 93%
Distance Learning Courses Available.
Nursing Student Activities Sigma Theta Tau, Student Nurses' Association, nursing club.
Nursing Student Resources Academic advising; academic or career counseling; assistance for students with disabilities; bookstore; campus computer network; career placement assistance; computer lab; computer-assisted instruction; e-mail services; employment services for current students; externships; housing assistance; Internet; learning resource lab; library services; nursing audiovisuals; resume preparation assistance; skills, simulation, or other laboratory; tutoring.
Library Facilities 6 million volumes (102,448 in health, 62,781 in nursing); 170,583 periodical subscriptions (4,658 health-care related).

BACCALAUREATE PROGRAMS

Degree BS
Available Programs Accelerated Baccalaureate for Second Degree; Generic Baccalaureate; RN Baccalaureate.
Study Options Full-time and part-time.
Program Entrance Requirements Minimum overall college GPA of 3.0, transcript of college record, written essay, high school foreign language, 3 years high school math, 4 years high school science, high school transcript, 1 letter of recommendation, minimum GPA in nursing prerequisites of 2.0. Transfer students are accepted. *Application deadline:* 1/1 (fall), 10/1 (spring). *Application fee:* $70.
Advanced Placement Credit given for nursing courses completed elsewhere dependent upon specific evaluations.
Expenses (2012–13) *Tuition:* full-time $20,439; part-time $1204 per credit. *Room and board:* $14,768; room only: $11,768 per academic year. *Required fees:* full-time $1163; part-time $484 per term.
Financial Aid 88% of baccalaureate students in nursing programs received some form of financial aid in 2011–12.
Contact Mr. William Sichel, Assistant Director of Undergraduate Student Affairs and Admissions, College of Nursing, New York University, 726 Broadway, 10th Floor, New York, NY 10003-6677. *Telephone:* 212-998-5336. *Fax:* 212-995-4302. *E-mail:* ws50@nyu.edu.

GRADUATE PROGRAMS

Expenses (2012–13) *Tuition:* part-time $1394 per credit. *Room and board:* room only: $14,326 per academic year. *Required fees:* part-time $497 per term.
Financial Aid 61% of graduate students in nursing programs received some form of financial aid in 2011–12. 2 research assistantships with full and partial tuition reimbursements available (averaging $23,000 per year) were awarded; fellowships with full and partial tuition reimbursements available, career-related internships or fieldwork, institutionally sponsored loans, scholarships, and tuition waivers (partial) also available. Aid available to part-time students. *Financial aid application deadline:* 2/1.
Contact Ms. Elizabeth Ensweiler, Assistant Director of Graduate Student Affairs and Admissions, College of Nursing, New York University, 726

Broadway, 10th Floor, New York, NY 10003-6677. *Telephone:* 212-992-7653. *Fax:* 212-995-4302. *E-mail:* ee39@nyu.edu.

MASTER'S DEGREE PROGRAM

Degrees MS; MS/MA; MS/MPH
Available Programs Master's; RN to Master's.
Concentrations Available Nurse-midwifery; nursing administration; nursing education; nursing informatics. *Nurse practitioner programs in:* acute care, family health, gerontology, pediatric, primary care, psychiatric/mental health.
Study Options Full-time and part-time.
Program Entrance Requirements Clinical experience, minimum overall college GPA of 3.0, transcript of college record, CPR certification, written essay, immunizations, 2 letters of recommendation, nursing research course, resume, statistics course. *Application deadline:* 7/1 (fall), 12/1 (spring). Applications may be processed on a rolling basis for some programs. *Application fee:* $75.
Advanced Placement Credit given for nursing courses completed elsewhere dependent upon specific evaluations.
Degree Requirements 45 total credit hours, thesis or project.

POST-MASTER'S PROGRAM

Areas of Study Nurse-midwifery; nursing administration; nursing education; nursing informatics. *Nurse practitioner programs in:* acute care, family health, gerontology, pediatric, primary care, psychiatric/mental health.

DOCTORAL DEGREE PROGRAM

Degree DNP
Available Programs Doctorate.
Areas of Study Addiction/substance abuse, advanced practice nursing, aging, critical care, family health, gerontology, health promotion/disease prevention, maternity-newborn.
Program Entrance Requirements Minimum overall college GPA of 3.5, clinical experience, graduate level research course (taken no more than 5 years ago), 2 letters of recommendation, Miller Analogies Test (MAT), MSN or equivalent, RN license, vita. *Application deadline:* 3/1 (spring). Applications may be processed on a rolling basis for some programs. *Application fee:* $75.
Degree Requirements 40 total credit hours, Capstone EBP Clinical Project, oral exam.

DOCTORAL DEGREE PROGRAM

Degree PhD
Available Programs Doctorate; Doctorate for Nurses with Non-Nursing Degrees; Post-Baccalaureate Doctorate.
Program Entrance Requirements Minimum overall college GPA of 3.5, interview by faculty committee, interview, 3 letters of recommendation, vita, writing sample, GRE General Test. *Application deadline:* 1/15 (fall). Applications may be processed on a rolling basis for some programs. *Application fee:* $75.
Degree Requirements 45 total credit hours, dissertation, oral exam, residency.

CONTINUING EDUCATION PROGRAM

Contact Dr. Mattia Gilmartin, Continuing Education Director, College of Nursing, New York University, 726 Broadway, 10th Floor, New York, NY 10003-6677. *Telephone:* 212-992-7128. *Fax:* 212-995-3143. *E-mail:* mjg14@nyu.edu.

Niagara University
Department of Nursing
Niagara Falls, Niagara University, New York

http://www.niagara.edu/nursing
Founded in 1856
DEGREE • BS
Nursing Program Faculty 6
Baccalaureate Enrollment 32 **Women** 97% **Men** 3% **Minority** 19% **International** 6% **Part-time** 84%
Distance Learning Courses Available.
Nursing Student Activities Sigma Theta Tau.
Nursing Student Resources Academic advising; academic or career counseling; assistance for students with disabilities; bookstore; campus computer network; computer lab; computer-assisted instruction; e-mail

services; externships; Internet; library services; nursing audiovisuals; tutoring; unpaid internships.
Library Facilities 262,565 volumes; 22,000 periodical subscriptions.

BACCALAUREATE PROGRAMS

Degree BS
Available Programs RN Baccalaureate.
Contact *Telephone:* 716-286-8155. *Fax:* 716-286-8079.

Pace University
Lienhard School of Nursing
New York, New York

http://www.pace.edu/lienhard
Founded in 1906
DEGREES • BS • DNP • MS
Nursing Program Faculty 117 (26% with doctorates).
Baccalaureate Enrollment 469 **Women** 88% **Men** 12% **Minority** 41% **International** .1% **Part-time** 15%
Graduate Enrollment 456 **Women** 92% **Men** 8% **Minority** 47% **International** 1% **Part-time** 95%
Distance Learning Courses Available.
Nursing Student Activities Nursing Honor Society, Sigma Theta Tau, Student Nurses' Association.
Nursing Student Resources Academic advising; academic or career counseling; assistance for students with disabilities; bookstore; campus computer network; career placement assistance; computer lab; computer-assisted instruction; e-mail services; employment services for current students; housing assistance; interactive nursing skills videos; Internet; learning resource lab; library services; nursing audiovisuals; placement services for program completers; resume preparation assistance; skills, simulation, or other laboratory.
Library Facilities 813,367 volumes (17,245 in health, 2,250 in nursing); 135,477 periodical subscriptions (6,819 health-care related).

BACCALAUREATE PROGRAMS

Degree BS
Available Programs Accelerated Baccalaureate for Second Degree; Generic Baccalaureate.
Site Options Pleasantville, NY; New York, NY.
Study Options Full-time and part-time.
Program Entrance Requirements Transcript of college record, CPR certification, written essay, health exam, health insurance, high school biology, high school chemistry, high school foreign language, 4 years high school math, 2 years high school science, high school transcript, immunizations, 2 letters of recommendation, minimum GPA in nursing prerequisites of 2.75. Transfer students are accepted. *Application deadline:* 2/15 (fall). *Application fee:* $50.
Advanced Placement Credit by examination available. Credit given for nursing courses completed elsewhere dependent upon specific evaluations.
Expenses (2012–13) *Tuition:* full-time $35,320; part-time $1013 per credit. *International tuition:* $35,320 full-time. *Room and board:* $14,800 per academic year. *Required fees:* full-time $1294.
Financial Aid 92% of baccalaureate students in nursing programs received some form of financial aid in 2011–12. *Gift aid (need-based):* Federal Pell, FSEOG, state, private, college/university gift aid from institutional funds, Federal Nursing, endowed and restricted scholarships and grants. *Loans:* Federal Nursing Student Loans, Federal Direct (Subsidized and Unsubsidized Stafford PLUS), Perkins.*Work-study:* Federal Work-Study.*Financial aid application deadline (priority):* 2/15.
Contact Dr. Martha Greenberg, Associate Professor and Chairperson, Undergraduate Department, Lienhard School of Nursing, Pace University, 861 Bedford Road, Pleasantville, NY 10570. *Telephone:* 914-773-3325. *Fax:* 914-773-3345. *E-mail:* mgreenberg@pace.edu.

GRADUATE PROGRAMS

Expenses (2012–13) *Tuition:* part-time $898 per credit. *Required fees:* part-time $168 per term.
Financial Aid 43% of graduate students in nursing programs received some form of financial aid in 2011–12. Research assistantships, career-related internships or fieldwork, Federal Work-Study, and tuition waivers (partial) available. Aid available to part-time students.
Contact Dr. Joanne K. Singleton, Chair of the Department of Graduate Studies/Director, Doctor of Nursing Program, Lienhard School of

Nursing, Pace University, 163 William Street, New York, NY 10038. *Telephone:* 212-618-6010. *Fax:* 212-346-1587. *E-mail:* jsingleton@pace.edu.

MASTER'S DEGREE PROGRAM
Degree MS
Available Programs Master's; Master's for Nurses with Non-Nursing Degrees.
Concentrations Available Nursing education. *Nurse practitioner programs in:* family health.
Site Options Pleasantville, NY; New York, NY.
Study Options Full-time and part-time.
Online Degree Options Yes (online only).
Program Entrance Requirements Computer literacy, minimum overall college GPA of 3.0, transcript of college record, CPR certification, immunizations, 2 letters of recommendation, nursing research course, professional liability insurance/malpractice insurance, prerequisite course work, resume, statistics course, GRE General Test or MAT. *Application deadline:* 6/1 (fall), 10/15 (spring). *Application fee:* $70.
Advanced Placement Credit by examination available. Credit given for nursing courses completed elsewhere dependent upon specific evaluations.
Degree Requirements 42 total credit hours, comprehensive exam.

POST-MASTER'S PROGRAM
Areas of Study Nursing education. *Nurse practitioner programs in:* family health.

DOCTORAL DEGREE PROGRAM
Degree DNP
Available Programs Doctorate.
Areas of Study Family health.
Site Options New York, NY.
Program Entrance Requirements Clinical experience, minimum overall college GPA of 3.3, 2 letters of recommendation, MSN or equivalent, vita, writing sample. *Application deadline:* 6/1 (fall). *Application fee:* $70.
Degree Requirements 37 total credit hours, residency.

See display below and full description on page 496.

Roberts Wesleyan College
Division of Nursing
Rochester, New York

http://www.roberts.edu/Nursing/
Founded in 1866
DEGREES • BSCN • M SC N
Nursing Program Faculty 17 (29% with doctorates).
Baccalaureate Enrollment 325 **Women** 94% **Men** 6% **Minority** 16% **International** 3% **Part-time** 7%
Graduate Enrollment 60 **Women** 97% **Men** 3% **Minority** 20% **International** 7%
Distance Learning Courses Available.
Nursing Student Activities Sigma Theta Tau, nursing club.
Nursing Student Resources Academic advising; academic or career counseling; assistance for students with disabilities; bookstore; campus computer network; career placement assistance; computer lab; computer-assisted instruction; e-mail services; employment services for current students; externships; housing assistance; interactive nursing skills videos; Internet; learning resource lab; library services; nursing audiovisuals; placement services for program completers; remedial services; resume preparation assistance; skills, simulation, or other laboratory; tutoring; unpaid internships.
Library Facilities 139,427 volumes (7,669 in health, 6,800 in nursing); 2,148 periodical subscriptions (203 health-care related).

BACCALAUREATE PROGRAMS
Degree BScN
Available Programs Generic Baccalaureate; RN Baccalaureate.
Site Options Dansville, NY; Clifton Springs, NY; Buffalo, NY; Rochester, NY; Weedsport, NY; Rochester, NY.
Study Options Full-time and part-time.
Online Degree Options Yes.
Program Entrance Requirements Minimum overall college GPA of 2.5, transcript of college record, CPR certification, written essay, health exam, health insurance, high school biology, high school chemistry, high school transcript, immunizations, 2 letters of recommendation, minimum GPA in nursing prerequisites of 2.5, prerequisite course work. Transfer

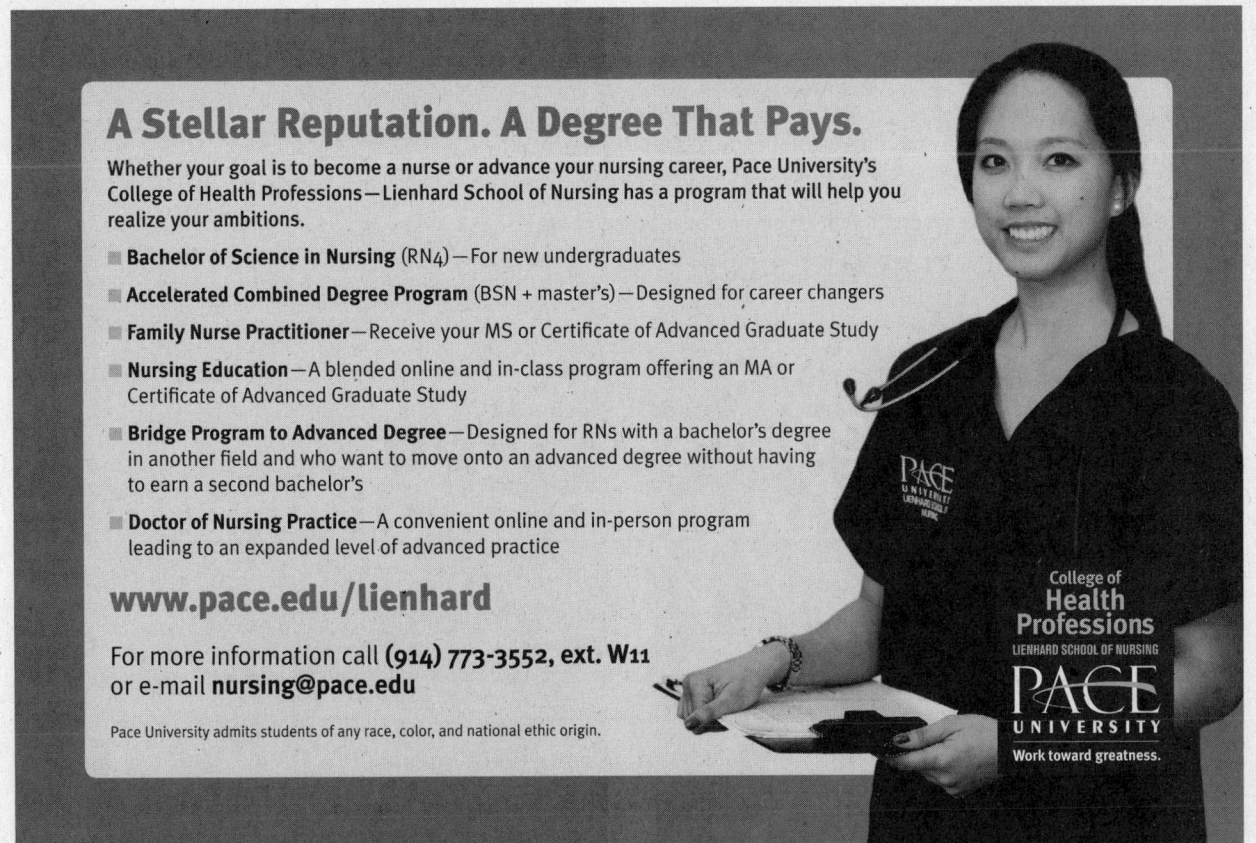

students are accepted. *Application deadline:* 2/1 (fall). Applications may be processed on a rolling basis for some programs. *Application fee:* $35.

Expenses (2012–13) *Tuition:* full-time $25,350; part-time $1056 per credit hour. *International tuition:* $25,350 full-time. *Room and board:* $9264; room only: $5932 per academic year. *Required fees:* full-time $974.

Financial Aid 97% of baccalaureate students in nursing programs received some form of financial aid in 2011–12.

Contact Mr. JP Anderson, Associate Vice President for Undergraduate and Seminary Admissions, Division of Nursing, Roberts Wesleyan College, 2301 Westside Drive, Rochester, NY 14624. *Telephone:* 585-594-6400. *Fax:* 585-549-6371. *E-mail:* admissions@roberts.edu.

GRADUATE PROGRAMS

Expenses (2012–13) *Tuition:* full-time $29,238. *International tuition:* $29,238 full-time. *Required fees:* full-time $300.

Financial Aid 60% of graduate students in nursing programs received some form of financial aid in 2011–12.

Contact Mrs. Brenda Mutton, Graduate Admissions Coordinator, Division of Nursing, Roberts Wesleyan College, 2301 Westside Drive, Rochester, NY 14624-1997. *Telephone:* 585-594-6686. *Fax:* 585-594-6593. *E-mail:* mutton_brenda@roberts.edu.

MASTER'S DEGREE PROGRAM

Degree M Sc N

Available Programs Master's.

Concentrations Available Nursing administration; nursing education.

Study Options Full-time.

Online Degree Options Yes.

Program Entrance Requirements Clinical experience, computer literacy, minimum overall college GPA of 3.0, transcript of college record, written essay, immunizations, interview, 2 letters of recommendation, nursing research course, physical assessment course, prerequisite course work, resume, statistics course. *Application deadline:* Applications may be processed on a rolling basis for some programs. *Application fee:* $35.

Degree Requirements 39 total credit hours, thesis or project.

POST-MASTER'S PROGRAM

Areas of Study Nursing administration; nursing education.

See display below and full description on page 500.

The Sage Colleges
Department of Nursing
Troy, New York

http://www.sage.edu/rsc/academics/programs/nursing/

DEGREES • BS • DNS • MS • MS/MBA

Nursing Program Faculty 20 (40% with doctorates).

Baccalaureate Enrollment 276 **Women** 99% **Men** 1% **Minority** 21% **Part-time** 21%

Graduate Enrollment 210 **Women** 92% **Men** 8% **Minority** 13% **International** 2% **Part-time** 78%

Distance Learning Courses Available.

Nursing Student Activities Nursing Honor Society, Sigma Theta Tau, nursing club.

Nursing Student Resources Academic advising; academic or career counseling; assistance for students with disabilities; bookstore; campus computer network; career placement assistance; computer lab; computer-assisted instruction; e-mail services; employment services for current students; externships; interactive nursing skills videos; Internet; learning resource lab; library services; remedial services; resume preparation assistance; skills, simulation, or other laboratory; tutoring.

Library Facilities 9,000 volumes in health, 6,000 volumes in nursing; 9,000 periodical subscriptions health-care related.

BACCALAUREATE PROGRAMS

Degree BS

Available Programs ADN to Baccalaureate; Accelerated Baccalaureate; Accelerated Baccalaureate for Second Degree; Baccalaureate for Second Degree; Generic Baccalaureate; International Nurse to Baccalaureate; LPN to Baccalaureate; RN Baccalaureate.

Study Options Full-time and part-time.

Program Entrance Requirements Minimum overall college GPA of 2.75, transcript of college record, written essay, health exam, health insurance, high school biology, high school chemistry, 3 years high school math, 3 years high school science, high school transcript, immunizations, interview, 2 letters of recommendation, minimum high school GPA of 2.75, professional liability insurance/malpractice insurance. Transfer students are accepted. *Application deadline:* Applications may be processed on a rolling basis for some programs. *Application fee:* $30.

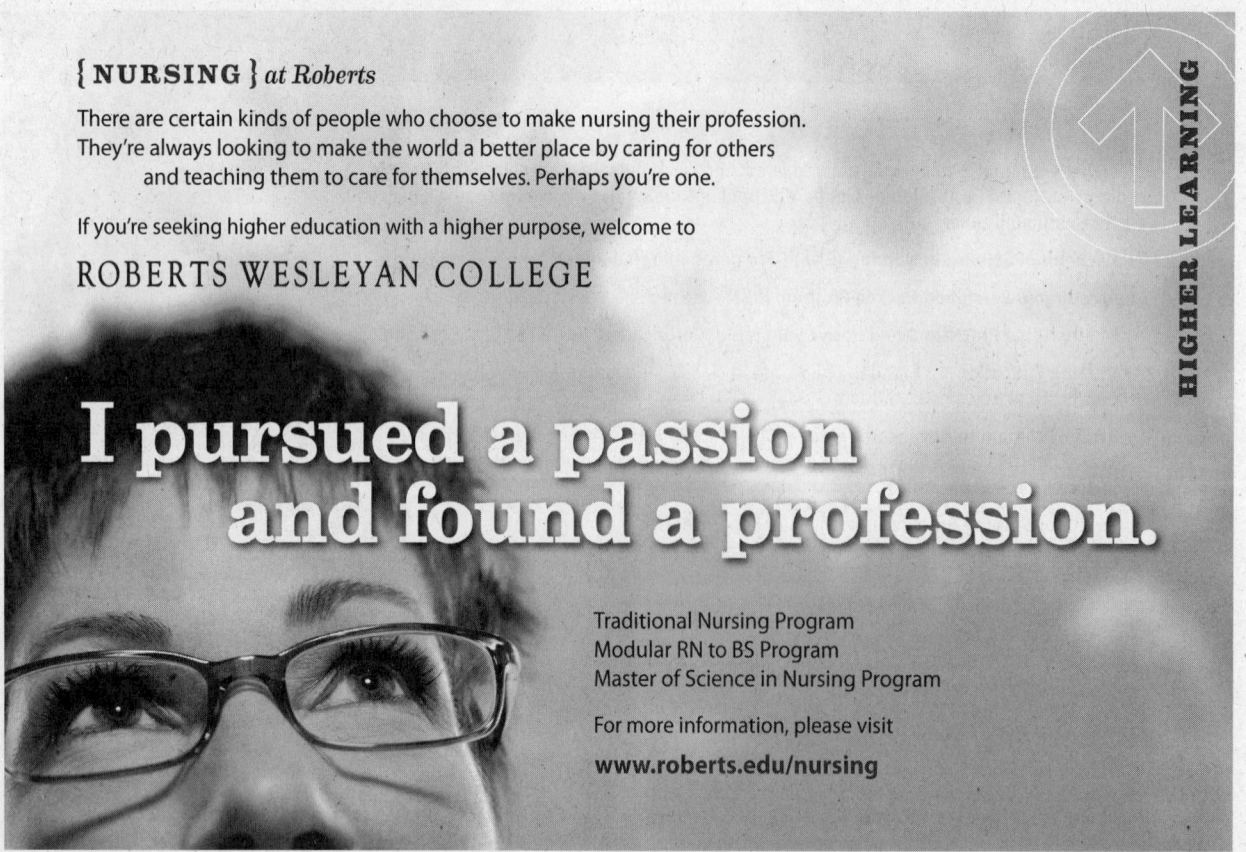

Advanced Placement Credit by examination available. Credit given for nursing courses completed elsewhere dependent upon specific evaluations.

Expenses (2012–13) *Tuition:* full-time $27,000; part-time $900 per credit hour. *International tuition:* $27,000 full-time. *Room and board:* $10,995; room only: $5795 per academic year.

Financial Aid 77% of baccalaureate students in nursing programs received some form of financial aid in 2011–12.

Contact Mary Hayward, MS, Program Contact, Department of Nursing, The Sage Colleges, Troy, NY 12180-4115. *Telephone:* 518-244-2006. *Fax:* 518-244-2009. *E-mail:* nursing@sage.edu.

GRADUATE PROGRAMS

Expenses (2012–13) *Tuition:* full-time $11,880; part-time $660 per credit hour. *International tuition:* $11,880 full-time. *Room and board:* $10,995; room only: $5795 per academic year.

Financial Aid 33% of graduate students in nursing programs received some form of financial aid in 2011–12. Fellowships, research assistantships, Federal Work-Study, scholarships, and unspecified assistantships available. Aid available to part-time students. *Financial aid application deadline:* 3/1.

Contact Dr. Madeline Cafiero, MS Program, Department of Nursing, The Sage Colleges, Troy, NY 12180-4115. *Telephone:* 518-244-4574. *Fax:* 518-244-2009. *E-mail:* nursing@sage.edu.

MASTER'S DEGREE PROGRAM

Degrees MS; MS/MBA

Available Programs Accelerated Master's; Accelerated RN to Master's; Master's.

Concentrations Available Health-care administration; nursing administration; nursing education. *Clinical nurse specialist programs in:* acute care, adult health, cardiovascular, community health, critical care, family health, gerontology, oncology, palliative care, psychiatric/mental health. *Nurse practitioner programs in:* acute care, adult health, community health, family health, gerontology, psychiatric/mental health.

Study Options Full-time and part-time.

Program Entrance Requirements Minimum overall college GPA of 2.75, transcript of college record, CPR certification, written essay, 2 letters of recommendation, physical assessment course, professional liability insurance/malpractice insurance, resume.

Advanced Placement Credit given for nursing courses completed elsewhere dependent upon specific evaluations.

Degree Requirements 42 total credit hours, thesis or project.

POST-MASTER'S PROGRAM

Areas of Study Health-care administration; nursing administration; nursing education. *Clinical nurse specialist programs in:* acute care, adult health, cardiovascular, community health, critical care, family health, gerontology, oncology, palliative care, psychiatric/mental health. *Nurse practitioner programs in:* acute care, adult health, community health, family health, gerontology, psychiatric/mental health.

DOCTORAL DEGREE PROGRAM

Degree DNS

Available Programs Doctorate.

Areas of Study Faculty preparation, health-care systems, nursing administration, nursing education, nursing policy, nursing research, nursing science.

Program Entrance Requirements Minimum overall college GPA of 3.5, interview by faculty committee, 3 letters of recommendation, MSN or equivalent, statistics course, vita, writing sample.

Degree Requirements 42 total credit hours, dissertation.

CONTINUING EDUCATION PROGRAM

Contact Wendy Nelson, Program Contact. *Telephone:* 518-244-3149. *Fax:* 518-244-2009. *E-mail:* nelsow@sage.edu.

St. Francis College
Department of Nursing
Brooklyn Heights, New York

Founded in 1884

DEGREE • BS

Nursing Program Faculty 9

Baccalaureate Enrollment 789

Nursing Student Resources Academic advising; academic or career counseling; assistance for students with disabilities; bookstore; campus computer network; career placement assistance; computer lab; computer-assisted instruction; e-mail services; externships; learning resource lab; library services; nursing audiovisuals; remedial services; resume preparation assistance; skills, simulation, or other laboratory; tutoring; unpaid internships.

Library Facilities 116,716 volumes; 31,391 periodical subscriptions.

BACCALAUREATE PROGRAMS

Degree BS

Available Programs ADN to Baccalaureate; International Nurse to Baccalaureate.

Study Options Full-time and part-time.

Program Entrance Requirements Minimum overall college GPA of 2.0, transcript of college record, written essay, health exam, health insurance, high school transcript, immunizations, interview, 2 letters of recommendation, professional liability insurance/malpractice insurance, prerequisite course work, RN licensure. Transfer students are accepted.

Advanced Placement Credit by examination available. Credit given for nursing courses completed elsewhere dependent upon specific evaluations.

Contact Judy Ashton, Chairperson, Department of Nursing, St. Francis College, 180 Remsen Street, Brooklyn Heights, NY 11201. *Telephone:* 718-489-5267. *Fax:* 718-489-5408. *E-mail:* ssaladino@sfc.edu.

See display on next page and full description on page 504.

St. John Fisher College
Wegmans School of Nursing
Rochester, New York

http://www.sjfc.edu/academics/nursing/about/index.dot

Founded in 1948

DEGREES • BS • DNP • MS

Nursing Program Faculty 53 (30% with doctorates).

Baccalaureate Enrollment 525 **Women** 92% **Men** 8% **Minority** 6% **Part-time** 2%

Graduate Enrollment 111 **Women** 95% **Men** 5% **Minority** 5% **Part-time** 74%

Distance Learning Courses Available.

Nursing Student Activities Sigma Theta Tau, Student Nurses' Association.

Nursing Student Resources Academic advising; academic or career counseling; assistance for students with disabilities; bookstore; campus computer network; career placement assistance; computer lab; computer-assisted instruction; daycare for children of students; e-mail services; employment services for current students; interactive nursing skills videos; Internet; learning resource lab; library services; nursing audiovisuals; resume preparation assistance; skills, simulation, or other laboratory; tutoring.

Library Facilities 229,031 volumes (30,000 in health, 5,000 in nursing); 48,558 periodical subscriptions (200 health-care related).

BACCALAUREATE PROGRAMS

Degree BS

Available Programs ADN to Baccalaureate; Accelerated RN Baccalaureate; Baccalaureate for Second Degree; Generic Baccalaureate; RN Baccalaureate.

Study Options Full-time and part-time.

Program Entrance Requirements Minimum overall college GPA of 2.75, transcript of college record, CPR certification, written essay, health exam, health insurance, high school transcript, immunizations, 2 letters of recommendation, minimum high school GPA of 2.0, minimum GPA in nursing prerequisites of 2.75, prerequisite course work. Transfer students are accepted. *Application deadline:* 3/1 (fall), 10/1 (spring). Applications may be processed on a rolling basis for some programs. *Application fee:* $30.

Advanced Placement Credit given for nursing courses completed elsewhere dependent upon specific evaluations.

Expenses (2012–13) *Tuition:* full-time $26,810; part-time $730 per credit hour. *Room and board:* $10,450; room only: $6950 per academic year. *Required fees:* full-time $1231; part-time $10 per credit.

Financial Aid 95% of baccalaureate students in nursing programs received some form of financial aid in 2011–12. *Gift aid (need-based):* Federal Pell, FSEOG, state, private, college/university gift aid from institutional funds, Federal Nursing. *Loans:* Federal Direct (Subsidized and Unsubsidized Stafford PLUS), Perkins.*Work-study:* Federal Work-Study.*Financial aid application deadline (priority):* 2/15.

Contact Dr. Marilyn Dollinger, Chairperson, Wegmans School of Nursing, St. John Fisher College, 3690 East Avenue, Rochester, NY 14618. *Telephone:* 585-385-8476. *Fax:* 585-385-8466. *E-mail:* mdollinger@sjfc.edu.

GRADUATE PROGRAMS

Expenses (2012–13) *Tuition:* part-time $765 per credit hour. *Required fees:* part-time $10 per credit.

Financial Aid 20% of graduate students in nursing programs received some form of financial aid in 2011–12. Scholarships available.

Contact Dr. Cynthia Ricci McCloskey, Graduate Program Director, Wegmans School of Nursing, St. John Fisher College, 3690 East Avenue, Rochester, NY 14618. *Telephone:* 585-385-8471. *Fax:* 585-385-8466. *E-mail:* cmccloskey@sjfc.eud.

MASTER'S DEGREE PROGRAM

Degree MS

Available Programs Master's; RN to Master's.

Concentrations Available Nursing education. *Clinical nurse specialist programs in:* adult health, gerontology, pediatric, women's health. *Nurse practitioner programs in:* family health.

Study Options Full-time and part-time.

Program Entrance Requirements Computer literacy, minimum overall college GPA of 3.0, transcript of college record, CPR certification, written essay, immunizations, 2 letters of recommendation, nursing research course, physical assessment course, resume, statistics course. *Application deadline:* Applications may be processed on a rolling basis for some programs. *Application fee:* $30.

Advanced Placement Credit given for nursing courses completed elsewhere dependent upon specific evaluations.

Degree Requirements 46 total credit hours, thesis or project, comprehensive exam.

POST-MASTER'S PROGRAM

Areas of Study Nursing education. *Nurse practitioner programs in:* family health.

DOCTORAL DEGREE PROGRAM

Degree DNP

Available Programs Doctorate; Post-Baccalaureate Doctorate.

Areas of Study Advanced practice nursing.

Program Entrance Requirements Clinical experience, minimum overall college GPA of 3.0, interview by faculty committee, letters of recommendation, scholarly papers, vita, writing sample. *Application deadline:* Applications may be processed on a rolling basis for some programs. *Application fee:* $30.

Degree Requirements 48 total credit hours, residency.

St. Joseph's College, New York
Department of Nursing
Brooklyn, New York

http://www.sjcny.edu/
Founded in 1916

DEGREES • BSN • MS

Nursing Program Faculty 18 (61% with doctorates).

Baccalaureate Enrollment 309 **Women** 91% **Men** 9% **Minority** 49% **Part-time** 92%

Graduate Enrollment 58 **Women** 93% **Men** 7% **Minority** 76% **Part-time** 100%

Nursing Student Activities Nursing Honor Society, nursing club.

Nursing Student Resources Academic advising; academic or career counseling; assistance for students with disabilities; bookstore; campus computer network; computer lab; computer-assisted instruction; e-mail services; Internet; learning resource lab; library services; nursing audio-visuals; remedial services; resume preparation assistance; skills, simulation, or other laboratory; tutoring.

Library Facilities 148,315 volumes (14,806 in health, 1,536 in nursing); 21,332 periodical subscriptions (3,321 health-care related).

BACCALAUREATE PROGRAMS

Degree BSN

Available Programs RN Baccalaureate.

Site Options Patchogue, NY.

Study Options Full-time and part-time.

Program Entrance Requirements Minimum overall college GPA of 2.5, transcript of college record, CPR certification, written essay, health exam, health insurance, immunizations, 2 letters of recommendation, minimum GPA in nursing prerequisites of 2.5, professional liability insurance/malpractice insurance, prerequisite course work, RN licensure. Transfer students are accepted. *Application deadline:* 8/31 (fall), 1/15 (spring). Applications may be processed on a rolling basis for some programs. *Application fee:* $25.

Advanced Placement Credit by examination available. Credit given for nursing courses completed elsewhere dependent upon specific evaluations.

Expenses (2012–13) *Tuition:* full-time $19,500; part-time $635 per credit. *International tuition:* $19,500 full-time. *Required fees:* full-time $656; part-time $96 per credit; part-time $187 per term.

Financial Aid 51% of baccalaureate students in nursing programs received some form of financial aid in 2011–12. *Gift aid (need-based):* Federal Pell, FSEOG, state, private, college/university gift aid from institutional funds. *Loans:* Federal Direct (Subsidized and Unsubsidized Stafford PLUS), Perkins, state. *Work-study:* Federal Work-Study, part-time campus jobs. *Financial aid application deadline (priority):* 2/25.

Contact Dr. Barbara L. Sands, Director, Department of Nursing, St. Joseph's College, New York, 245 Clinton Avenue, Brooklyn, NY 11205-3688. *Telephone:* 718-940-5892. *Fax:* 718-638-8839. *E-mail:* bsands@sjcny.edu.

GRADUATE PROGRAMS

Expenses (2012–13) *Tuition:* part-time $715 per credit. *Required fees:* part-time $91 per credit; part-time $175 per term.

Financial Aid 69% of graduate students in nursing programs received some form of financial aid in 2011–12.

Contact Dr. Barbara L. Sands, Director, Department of Nursing, St. Joseph's College, New York, 245 Clinton Avenue, Brooklyn, NY 11205-3688. *Telephone:* 718-940-5892. *Fax:* 718-638-8839. *E-mail:* bsands@sjcny.edu.

MASTER'S DEGREE PROGRAM
Degree MS
Available Programs Master's.
Concentrations Available Nursing education. *Clinical nurse specialist programs in:* adult health.
Site Options Patchogue, NY.
Study Options Part-time.
Program Entrance Requirements Clinical experience, minimum overall college GPA of 3.0, transcript of college record, CPR certification, written essay, immunizations, interview, 2 letters of recommendation, nursing research course, physical assessment course, professional liability insurance/malpractice insurance, prerequisite course work, resume, statistics course. *Application deadline:* 5/15 (fall). Applications may be processed on a rolling basis for some programs. *Application fee:* $25.
Advanced Placement Credit given for nursing courses completed elsewhere dependent upon specific evaluations.
Degree Requirements 38 total credit hours, comprehensive exam.

State University of New York at Plattsburgh
Department of Nursing
Plattsburgh, New York

http://www.plattsburgh.edu/nursing
Founded in 1889
DEGREE • BS
Nursing Program Faculty 20 (20% with doctorates).
Baccalaureate Enrollment 300 Women 90% Men 10% Minority 25% International 4% Part-time 25%
Distance Learning Courses Available.
Nursing Student Activities Nursing Honor Society, Sigma Theta Tau, Student Nurses' Association.
Nursing Student Resources Academic advising; academic or career counseling; assistance for students with disabilities; bookstore; campus computer network; career placement assistance; computer lab; computer-assisted instruction; e-mail services; employment services for current students; interactive nursing skills videos; Internet; learning resource lab; library services; nursing audiovisuals; remedial services; resume preparation assistance; skills, simulation, or other laboratory; tutoring.

Library Facilities 540,476 volumes (19,450 in health, 200 in nursing); 4,902 periodical subscriptions (174 health-care related).

BACCALAUREATE PROGRAMS
Degree BS
Available Programs ADN to Baccalaureate; Generic Baccalaureate; RN Baccalaureate.
Study Options Full-time.
Online Degree Options Yes.
Program Entrance Requirements Minimum overall college GPA of 2.5, transcript of college record, high school biology, high school chemistry, high school foreign language, 3 years high school math, 3 years high school science, high school transcript, minimum GPA in nursing prerequisites of 2.5. Transfer students are accepted. *Application deadline:* Applications may be processed on a rolling basis for some programs.
Expenses (2011–12) *Tuition, state resident:* full-time $5270; part-time $220 per credit. *Tuition, nonresident:* full-time $14,320; part-time $597 per credit. *International tuition:* $14,320 full-time. *Room and board:* $9848; room only: $6198 per academic year. *Required fees:* full-time $1212.
Financial Aid 83% of baccalaureate students in nursing programs received some form of financial aid in 2010–11.
Contact Dr. JoAnn Gleeson-Kreig, Chairperson, Department of Nursing, State University of New York at Plattsburgh, 101 Broad Street, Plattsburgh, NY 12901. *Telephone:* 518-564-3124. *Fax:* 518-564-3100. *E-mail:* joann.gleeson-kreig@plattsburgh.edu.

State University of New York College of Technology at Delhi
Bachelor of Science in Nursing Program
Delhi, New York

Founded in 1913
DEGREE • BSN
Library Facilities 51,821 volumes; 313 periodical subscriptions.

BACCALAUREATE PROGRAMS
Degree BSN
Available Programs RN Baccalaureate.
Study Options Full-time and part-time.
Online Degree Options Yes (online only).
Program Entrance Requirements RN licensure.
Contact *Telephone:* 607-746-4519.

State University of New York Downstate Medical Center
College of Nursing
Brooklyn, New York

http://sls.downstate.edu/admissions/nursing/index.html
Founded in 1858
DEGREES • BS • MS • MS/MPH
Nursing Program Faculty 19 (79% with doctorates).
Baccalaureate Enrollment 133 Women 93% Men 7% Minority 80% International 2% Part-time 77%
Graduate Enrollment 387 Women 90% Men 10% Minority 48% Part-time 40%
Distance Learning Courses Available.
Nursing Student Activities Student Nurses' Association, nursing club.
Nursing Student Resources Academic advising; academic or career counseling; assistance for students with disabilities; bookstore; campus computer network; computer lab; computer-assisted instruction; e-mail services; housing assistance; interactive nursing skills videos; Internet; learning resource lab; library services; nursing audiovisuals; paid internships; skills, simulation, or other laboratory; unpaid internships.
Library Facilities 357,209 volumes in health, 2,679 volumes in nursing; 619 periodical subscriptions health-care related.

BACCALAUREATE PROGRAMS
Degree BS

Available Programs Accelerated Baccalaureate for Second Degree; RN Baccalaureate.

Study Options Full-time.

Program Entrance Requirements Minimum overall college GPA of 3.0, transcript of college record, written essay, health exam, 2 letters of recommendation, professional liability insurance/malpractice insurance, prerequisite course work. Transfer students are accepted. *Application deadline:* 11/1 (fall). Applications may be processed on a rolling basis for some programs. *Application fee:* $40.

Advanced Placement Credit by examination available.

Expenses (2012–13) *Tuition, state resident:* full-time $5570; part-time $232 per credit. *Tuition, nonresident:* full-time $14,820; part-time $618 per credit. *International tuition:* $14,820 full-time. *Room and board:* room only: $4500 per academic year. *Required fees:* full-time $222; part-time $5 per credit.

Financial Aid 33% of baccalaureate students in nursing programs received some form of financial aid in 2011–12.

Contact Dr. Nellie Bailey, Associate Dean, College of Nursing, State University of New York Downstate Medical Center, 450 Clarkson Avenue, Box 22, Brooklyn, NY 11203. *Telephone:* 718-270-7617. *Fax:* 718-270-7641. *E-mail:* nellie.bailey@downstate.edu.

GRADUATE PROGRAMS

Expenses (2012–13) *Tuition, state resident:* full-time $9370; part-time $390 per credit. *Tuition, nonresident:* full-time $16,680; part-time $695 per credit. *International tuition:* $16,680 full-time. *Room and board:* room only: $4500 per academic year. *Required fees:* full-time $222; part-time $5 per credit.

Financial Aid 1% of graduate students in nursing programs received some form of financial aid in 2011–12. Traineeships and health workforce retraining available.

Contact Dr. Laila N. Sedhom, Associate Dean, College of Nursing, State University of New York Downstate Medical Center, 450 Clarkson Avenue, Box 22, Brooklyn, NY 11203-2098. *Telephone:* 718-270-7605. *Fax:* 718-270-7636. *E-mail:* laila.sedhom@downstate.edu.

MASTER'S DEGREE PROGRAM

Degrees MS; MS/MPH

Available Programs Master's.

Concentrations Available Nurse anesthesia; nurse-midwifery. *Clinical nurse specialist programs in:* adult health, maternity-newborn. *Nurse practitioner programs in:* family health, women's health.

Site Options Brooklyn, NY.

Study Options Full-time and part-time.

Program Entrance Requirements Clinical experience, minimum overall college GPA of 3.0, transcript of college record, CPR certification, written essay, interview, 2 letters of recommendation, nursing research course, physical assessment course, professional liability insurance/malpractice insurance, prerequisite course work, resume, statistics course, GRE. *Application deadline:* 11/30 (fall). *Application fee:* $80.

Advanced Placement Credit by examination available. Credit given for nursing courses completed elsewhere dependent upon specific evaluations.

Degree Requirements 44 total credit hours, thesis or project.

POST-MASTER'S PROGRAM

Areas of Study *Nurse practitioner programs in:* family health, women's health.

CONTINUING EDUCATION PROGRAM

Contact Ms. Veronica Arikian, PhD, Director of Continuing Education, College of Nursing, State University of New York Downstate Medical Center, 450 Clarkson Avenue, Box 22, Brooklyn, NY 11203. *Telephone:* 718-270-7488. *Fax:* 718-270-7628. *E-mail:* veronica.arikian@downstate.edu.

State University of New York Empire State College
Bachelor of Science in Nursing Program
Saratoga Springs, New York

http://www.esc.edu/nursing
Founded in 1971
DEGREE • BS
Nursing Program Faculty 6 (33% with doctorates).
Baccalaureate Enrollment 485 **Women** 92.4% **Men** 7.6% **Minority** 17.4% **Part-time** 85.9%
Distance Learning Courses Available.
Nursing Student Resources Academic advising; academic or career counseling; assistance for students with disabilities; bookstore; computer-assisted instruction; e-mail services; interactive nursing skills videos; Internet; library services; nursing audiovisuals; resume preparation assistance; tutoring.
Library Facilities 70,000 volumes; 57,000 periodical subscriptions.

BACCALAUREATE PROGRAMS

Degree BS
Available Programs RN Baccalaureate.
Online Degree Options Yes (online only).
Program Entrance Requirements Minimum overall college GPA of 2.0, transcript of college record, written essay, RN licensure. Transfer students are accepted. *Application deadline:* 6/1 (fall), 10/1 (spring). *Application fee:* $50.
Advanced Placement Credit by examination available. Credit given for nursing courses completed elsewhere dependent upon specific evaluations.
Expenses (2011–12) *Tuition, area resident:* part-time $210 per course.
Financial Aid 27% of baccalaureate students in nursing programs received some form of financial aid in 2010–11.
Contact Ms. Erin White, Coordinator of Student Services, Bachelor of Science in Nursing Program, State University of New York Empire State College, 113 West Avenue, Saratoga Springs, NY 12866. *Telephone:* 518-587-2100 Ext. 2812. *Fax:* 518-587-5126. *E-mail:* erin.white@esc.edu.

State University of New York Institute of Technology
School of Nursing and Health Systems
Utica, New York

http://www.sunyit.edu/
Founded in 1966
DEGREES • BS • MS
Nursing Program Faculty 30 (30% with doctorates).
Baccalaureate Enrollment 200 **Women** 96% **Men** 4% **Minority** 5% **Part-time** 80%
Graduate Enrollment 200 **Women** 90% **Men** 10% **Minority** 10% **Part-time** 70%
Distance Learning Courses Available.
Nursing Student Activities Nursing Honor Society, Sigma Theta Tau, Student Nurses' Association, nursing club.
Nursing Student Resources Academic advising; academic or career counseling; assistance for students with disabilities; bookstore; campus computer network; career placement assistance; computer lab; computer-assisted instruction; e-mail services; employment services for current students; externships; housing assistance; interactive nursing skills videos; Internet; learning resource lab; library services; nursing audiovisuals; other; placement services for program completers; remedial services; resume preparation assistance; skills, simulation, or other laboratory; tutoring; unpaid internships.
Library Facilities 200,730 volumes (14,000 in health, 8,500 in nursing); 372 periodical subscriptions (335 health-care related).

BACCALAUREATE PROGRAMS

Degree BS
Available Programs ADN to Baccalaureate; Accelerated Baccalaureate; Accelerated RN Baccalaureate; RN Baccalaureate.
Study Options Full-time and part-time.

Online Degree Options Yes.

Program Entrance Requirements Minimum overall college GPA of 3.0, transcript of college record, high school biology, high school chemistry, 3 years high school math, 3 years high school science, minimum high school GPA, minimum high school rank 85%, prerequisite course work. Transfer students are accepted. *Application deadline:* 3/15 (fall). *Application fee:* $50.

Advanced Placement Credit by examination available. Credit given for nursing courses completed elsewhere dependent upon specific evaluations.

Expenses (2012–13) *Tuition, state resident:* full-time $5560; part-time $232 per credit hour. *Tuition, nonresident:* full-time $14,820; part-time $618 per credit hour. *Required fees:* full-time $1174; part-time $49 per credit.

Financial Aid 33% of baccalaureate students in nursing programs received some form of financial aid in 2011–12.

Contact Ms. Jennifer Phelan-Ninh, Director of Admissions, School of Nursing and Health Systems, State University of New York Institute of Technology, 100 Seymour Road, Utica, NY 13502. *Telephone:* 315-792-7500. *E-mail:* admissions@sunyit.edu.

GRADUATE PROGRAMS

Expenses (2012–13) *Tuition, state resident:* full-time $9370; part-time $390 per credit hour. *Tuition, nonresident:* full-time $16,680; part-time $695 per credit hour. *Room and board:* $10,500 per academic year. *Required fees:* full-time $1134; part-time $49 per credit.

Financial Aid 60% of graduate students in nursing programs received some form of financial aid in 2011–12. Federal Work-Study, scholarships, traineeships, and unspecified assistantships available.

Contact Ms. Maryrose Raab, Coordinator of Graduate Center, School of Nursing and Health Systems, State University of New York Institute of Technology, 100 Seymour Road, Utica, NY 13502. *Telephone:* 315-792-7297. *Fax:* 315-792-7221. *E-mail:* mb_raab@sunyit.edu.

MASTER'S DEGREE PROGRAM

Degree MS

Available Programs Accelerated AD/RN to Master's; Accelerated RN to Master's; Master's; RN to Master's.

Concentrations Available Nursing education. *Nurse practitioner programs in:* family health.

Study Options Full-time and part-time.

Online Degree Options Yes.

Program Entrance Requirements Clinical experience, computer literacy, minimum overall college GPA of 3.0, transcript of college record, written essay, interview, 2 letters of recommendation, nursing research course, physical assessment course, prerequisite course work, statistics course, GRE General Test (if undergraduate GPA less than 3.3). *Application deadline:* 6/15 (fall), 11/1 (spring). *Application fee:* $50.

Advanced Placement Credit given for nursing courses completed elsewhere dependent upon specific evaluations.

Degree Requirements 45 total credit hours, comprehensive exam.

POST-MASTER'S PROGRAM

Areas of Study Nursing education. *Nurse practitioner programs in:* family health.

CONTINUING EDUCATION PROGRAM

Contact Dr. Deborah Tyksinski, Associate Provost, Sponsored Research and Continuing Education RF Operations Manager, School of Nursing and Health Systems, State University of New York Institute of Technology, 100 Seymour Road, Utica, NY 13502. *Telephone:* 315-792-7151. *Fax:* 315-792-7278. *E-mail:* debtyk@sunyit.edu.

State University of New York Upstate Medical University

College of Nursing
Syracuse, New York

http://www.upstate.edu/con
Founded in 1950
DEGREES • BS • MS
Nursing Program Faculty 21 (40% with doctorates).

Baccalaureate Enrollment 136 **Women** 90% **Men** 10% **Minority** 15% **International** 5% **Part-time** 88%
Graduate Enrollment 277 **Women** 90% **Men** 10% **Minority** 13% **International** 5% **Part-time** 85%
Distance Learning Courses Available.
Nursing Student Activities Sigma Theta Tau, Student Nurses' Association.
Nursing Student Resources Academic advising; academic or career counseling; assistance for students with disabilities; bookstore; campus computer network; career placement assistance; computer lab; computer-assisted instruction; daycare for children of students; e-mail services; Internet; learning resource lab; library services; skills, simulation, or other laboratory; tutoring.
Library Facilities 220,160 volumes (220,382 in health, 1,241 in nursing); 3,200 periodical subscriptions (4,928 health-care related).

BACCALAUREATE PROGRAMS

Degree BS
Available Programs ADN to Baccalaureate.
Site Options Ithaca, NY.
Study Options Full-time and part-time.
Program Entrance Requirements Transcript of college record, CPR certification, written essay, health exam, immunizations, 2 letters of recommendation, prerequisite course work, RN licensure. *Application deadline:* 3/15 (fall), 9/15 (spring). *Application fee:* $50.
Advanced Placement Credit by examination available. Credit given for nursing courses completed elsewhere dependent upon specific evaluations.
Expenses (2011–12) *Tuition, state resident:* full-time $5270; part-time $220 per credit. *Tuition, nonresident:* full-time $14,320; part-time $597 per credit. *Room and board:* room only: $5800 per academic year. *Required fees:* full-time $575.
Financial Aid 35% of baccalaureate students in nursing programs received some form of financial aid in 2010–11.
Contact Mrs. Debora E. Kirsch, Director, Undergraduate Program, College of Nursing, State University of New York Upstate Medical University, 750 East Adams Street, Syracuse, NY 13210. *Telephone:* 315-464-4276. *Fax:* 315-464-5168. *E-mail:* kirschde@upstate.edu.

GRADUATE PROGRAMS

Expenses (2011–12) *Tuition, state resident:* full-time $8870; part-time $370 per credit. *Tuition, nonresident:* full-time $15,160; part-time $632 per credit. *International tuition:* $15,160 full-time. *Room and board:* room only: $5800 per academic year. *Required fees:* full-time $575.
Financial Aid 30% of graduate students in nursing programs received some form of financial aid in 2010–11. Federal Work-Study, institutionally sponsored loans, scholarships, and traineeships available. Aid available to part-time students. *Financial aid application deadline:* 3/1.
Contact Dr. Carol Gavan, Associate Professor/Associate Dean and Director, Graduate Program, College of Nursing, State University of New York Upstate Medical University, 750 East Adams Street, Syracuse, NY 13210. *Telephone:* 315-464-4276. *Fax:* 315-464-5168. *E-mail:* gavanc@upstate.edu.

MASTER'S DEGREE PROGRAM

Degree MS
Available Programs Accelerated RN to Master's; Master's; Master's for Nurses with Non-Nursing Degrees; RN to Master's.
Concentrations Available *Clinical nurse specialist programs in:* medical-surgical. *Nurse practitioner programs in:* adult health, family health, pediatric, psychiatric/mental health.
Site Options Watertown, NY.
Study Options Full-time and part-time.
Program Entrance Requirements Clinical experience, minimum overall college GPA of 3.0, transcript of college record, CPR certification, written essay, immunizations, 3 letters of recommendation, nursing research course, physical assessment course, statistics course. *Application deadline:* 3/15 (fall), 9/15 (spring). *Application fee:* $50.
Advanced Placement Credit by examination available. Credit given for nursing courses completed elsewhere dependent upon specific evaluations.
Degree Requirements 47 total credit hours, thesis or project.

POST-MASTER'S PROGRAM

Areas of Study *Clinical nurse specialist programs in:* medical-surgical. *Nurse practitioner programs in:* adult health, family health, pediatric, psychiatric/mental health.

CONTINUING EDUCATION PROGRAM

Contact Ms. Barbara A. Black, Director, Continuing Nursing Education, College of Nursing, State University of New York Upstate Medical University, 750 East Adams Street, Syracuse, NY 13210. *Telephone:* 315-464-4276. *Fax:* 315-464-5168. *E-mail:* blackb@upstate.edu.

Stony Brook University, State University of New York

School of Nursing
Stony Brook, New York

Founded in 1957

DEGREES • BS • DNP • MS

Nursing Program Faculty 64 (68% with doctorates).
Baccalaureate Enrollment 493 **Women** 83% **Men** 17% **Minority** 46% **International** 12% **Part-time** 71%
Graduate Enrollment 557 **Women** 91% **Men** 9% **Minority** 41% **International** 7% **Part-time** 95%
Distance Learning Courses Available.
Nursing Student Activities Nursing Honor Society, Sigma Theta Tau, Student Nurses' Association, nursing club.
Nursing Student Resources Academic advising; academic or career counseling; assistance for students with disabilities; bookstore; campus computer network; career placement assistance; computer lab; computer-assisted instruction; daycare for children of students; e-mail services; employment services for current students; housing assistance; interactive nursing skills videos; Internet; learning resource lab; library services; nursing audiovisuals; placement services for program completers; resume preparation assistance; skills, simulation, or other laboratory.
Library Facilities 1.5 million volumes (11,022 in health, 5,075 in nursing); 280,000 periodical subscriptions health-care related.

BACCALAUREATE PROGRAMS

Degree BS
Available Programs Accelerated Baccalaureate; Generic Baccalaureate; RN Baccalaureate.
Study Options Full-time and part-time.
Program Entrance Requirements Minimum overall college GPA of 2.5, transcript of college record, CPR certification, written essay, health insurance, immunizations, 3 letters of recommendation, minimum GPA in nursing prerequisites of 2.5, professional liability insurance/malpractice insurance. *Application deadline:* 1/5 (fall), 11/2 (summer). *Application fee:* $40.
Advanced Placement Credit by examination available. Credit given for nursing courses completed elsewhere dependent upon specific evaluations.
Contact *Telephone:* 631-444-3241. *Fax:* 631-444-3136.

GRADUATE PROGRAMS

Contact *Telephone:* 631-444-2644. *Fax:* 631-444-3136.

MASTER'S DEGREE PROGRAM

Degree MS
Available Programs Master's; RN to Master's.
Concentrations Available Nurse-midwifery. *Clinical nurse specialist programs in:* adult health, community health, critical care, parent-child, pediatric, perinatal, psychiatric/mental health, women's health. *Nurse practitioner programs in:* adult health, neonatal health, pediatric, psychiatric/mental health, women's health.
Study Options Full-time and part-time.
Program Entrance Requirements Clinical experience, computer literacy, minimum overall college GPA of 3.0, transcript of college record, CPR certification, written essay, immunizations, interview, 3 letters of recommendation, physical assessment course, professional liability insurance/malpractice insurance, prerequisite course work, resume, statistics course. *Application deadline:* 4/1 (fall), 1/20 (summer). *Application fee:* $40.
Advanced Placement Credit given for nursing courses completed elsewhere dependent upon specific evaluations.
Degree Requirements 45 total credit hours.

POST-MASTER'S PROGRAM

Areas of Study Nurse-midwifery. *Clinical nurse specialist programs in:* adult health, community health, critical care, parent-child, pediatric, perinatal, psychiatric/mental health, women's health. *Nurse practitioner pro-*

grams in: adult health, neonatal health, pediatric, psychiatric/mental health, women's health.

DOCTORAL DEGREE PROGRAM

Degree DNP
Available Programs Doctorate.
Areas of Study Advanced practice nursing, biology of health and illness, clinical practice, ethics, health policy, health promotion/disease prevention, health-care systems, individualized study, nursing policy, nursing research.
Program Entrance Requirements Clinical experience, minimum overall college GPA of 3.0, interview by faculty committee, interview, 3 letters of recommendation, MSN or equivalent, vita, writing sample. *Application deadline:* 12/1 (summer). *Application fee:* $60.
Degree Requirements 42 total credit hours.

CONTINUING EDUCATION PROGRAM

Contact *Telephone:* 631-444-3259. *Fax:* 631-444-3136.

University at Buffalo, the State University of New York

School of Nursing
Buffalo, New York

http://nursing.buffalo.edu/
Founded in 1846

DEGREES • BS • DNP • PHD

Nursing Program Faculty 56 (61% with doctorates).
Baccalaureate Enrollment 216 **Women** 90% **Men** 10% **Minority** 33% **International** 2% **Part-time** 6%
Graduate Enrollment 185 **Women** 80% **Men** 20% **Minority** 31% **International** 8% **Part-time** 54%
Distance Learning Courses Available.
Nursing Student Activities Nursing Honor Society, Sigma Theta Tau, Student Nurses' Association, nursing club.
Nursing Student Resources Academic advising; academic or career counseling; assistance for students with disabilities; bookstore; campus computer network; career placement assistance; computer lab; computer-assisted instruction; daycare for children of students; e-mail services; employment services for current students; externships; housing assistance; interactive nursing skills videos; Internet; learning resource lab; library services; nursing audiovisuals; placement services for program completers; remedial services; resume preparation assistance; skills, simulation, or other laboratory; tutoring; unpaid internships.
Library Facilities 4.1 million volumes (250,000 in health, 25,000 in nursing); 101,268 periodical subscriptions (2,500 health-care related).

BACCALAUREATE PROGRAMS

Degree BS
Available Programs Accelerated Baccalaureate for Second Degree; Generic Baccalaureate; RN Baccalaureate.
Study Options Full-time.
Online Degree Options Yes.
Program Entrance Requirements Minimum overall college GPA of 3.0, transcript of college record, CPR certification, written essay, health exam, health insurance, high school chemistry, immunizations, minimum GPA in nursing prerequisites of 3.0, prerequisite course work. Transfer students are accepted.
Advanced Placement Credit given for nursing courses completed elsewhere dependent upon specific evaluations.
Expenses (2012–13) *Tuition, state resident:* full-time $5570; part-time $232 per credit hour. *Tuition, nonresident:* full-time $16,190; part-time $675 per credit hour. *International tuition:* $16,190 full-time. *Room and board:* $11,496; room only: $6861 per academic year. *Required fees:* full-time $1678; part-time $100 per credit; part-time $468 per term.
Financial Aid 80% of baccalaureate students in nursing programs received some form of financial aid in 2011–12. *Gift aid (need-based):* Federal Pell, FSEOG, state, private, college/university gift aid from institutional funds, Federal Nursing. *Loans:* Federal Nursing Student Loans, Federal Direct (Subsidized and Unsubsidized Stafford PLUS), Perkins, college/university. *Work-study:* Federal Work-Study, part-time campus jobs. *Financial aid application deadline (priority):* 3/1.
Contact Dr. David J. Lang, Director of Student Affairs, School of Nursing, University at Buffalo, the State University of New York, 103

Wende Hall, 3435 Main Street, Buffalo, NY 14214. *Telephone:* 716-829-2537. *Fax:* 716-829-2067. *E-mail:* nursing@buffalo.edu.

GRADUATE PROGRAMS

Expenses (2012–13) *Tuition, state resident:* full-time $9370; part-time $390 per credit hour. *Tuition, nonresident:* full-time $16,680; part-time $695 per credit hour. *International tuition:* $16,680 full-time. *Room and board:* $11,164; room only: $8806 per academic year. *Required fees:* full-time $1239; part-time $135 per credit; part-time $308 per term.

Financial Aid 80% of graduate students in nursing programs received some form of financial aid in 2011–12. 6 fellowships with full tuition reimbursements available (averaging $17,000 per year), 3 research assistantships with full tuition reimbursements available (averaging $10,600 per year), 5 teaching assistantships with full tuition reimbursements available (averaging $10,600 per year) were awarded; scholarships, traineeships, and unspecified assistantships also available. *Financial aid application deadline:* 3/15.

Contact Dr. David J. Lang, Director of Student Affairs, School of Nursing, University at Buffalo, the State University of New York, 103 Wende Hall, 3435 Main Street, Buffalo, NY 14214. *Telephone:* 716-829-2537. *Fax:* 716-829-2067. *E-mail:* nursing@buffalo.edu.

DOCTORAL DEGREE PROGRAM

Degree DNP

Available Programs Doctorate; Post-Baccalaureate Doctorate.

Areas of Study Addiction/substance abuse, advanced practice nursing, aging, clinical practice, critical care, ethics, faculty preparation, family health, gerontology, health policy, health promotion/disease prevention, health-care systems, individualized study, information systems, maternity-newborn, nurse case management, nursing administration, nursing education, nursing policy, nursing research, nursing science, oncology, women's health.

Online Degree Options Yes.

Program Entrance Requirements Clinical experience, minimum overall college GPA of 3.25, interview by faculty committee, interview, 3 letters of recommendation, vita, writing sample, GRE or MAT. *Application deadline:* Applications may be processed on a rolling basis for some programs. *Application fee:* $75.

Degree Requirements 120 total credit hours, dissertation, written exam.

DOCTORAL DEGREE PROGRAM

Degree PhD

Available Programs Doctorate, Post-Baccalaureate Doctorate.

Areas of Study Addiction/substance abuse, advanced practice nursing, aging, clinical practice, critical care, ethics, faculty preparation, family health, gerontology, health policy, health promotion/disease prevention, health-care systems, individualized study, information systems, maternity-newborn, nurse case management, nursing administration, nursing education, nursing policy, nursing research, nursing science, oncology, women's health.

Online Degree Options Yes.

Program Entrance Requirements Minimum overall college GPA of 3.2, interview, interview by faculty member, 3 letters of recommendation, MSN or equivalent, vita, writing sample. *Application deadline:* Applications processed on a rolling basis. *Application fee:* $75.

Degree Requirements 120 total credit hours, dissertation, written exam.

University of Rochester
School of Nursing
Rochester, New York

http://www.son.rochester.edu/
Founded in 1850

DEGREES • BS • DNP • MS • MSN/PHD • PHD
Contact Ms. Elaine M. Andolina, Director of Admissions, School of Nursing, University of Rochester, Box SON, 601 Elmwood Avenue, Rochester NY 14642. *Telephone:* 585-275-2375. *Fax:* 585-756-8299. *E-mail:* son_admissions@urmc.rochester.edu.

Utica College
Department of Nursing
Utica, New York

http://www.utica.edu/
Founded in 1946

DEGREE • BS
Nursing Program Faculty 42 (10% with doctorates).
Baccalaureate Enrollment 523 **Women** 90% **Men** 10% **Minority** 21% **International** .01% **Part-time** 40%
Distance Learning Courses Available.
Nursing Student Activities Sigma Theta Tau, Student Nurses' Association.
Nursing Student Resources Academic advising; academic or career counseling; assistance for students with disabilities; bookstore; campus computer network; career placement assistance; computer lab; computer-assisted instruction; e-mail services; employment services for current students; externships; housing assistance; interactive nursing skills videos; Internet; learning resource lab; library services; nursing audiovisuals; paid internships; placement services for program completers; remedial services; resume preparation assistance; skills, simulation, or other laboratory; tutoring; unpaid internships.
Library Facilities 164,053 volumes (2,652 in health, 1,122 in nursing); 829 periodical subscriptions (118 health-care related).

BACCALAUREATE PROGRAMS

Degree BS

Available Programs Accelerated Baccalaureate for Second Degree; Generic Baccalaureate; RN Baccalaureate.

Study Options Full-time and part-time.

Online Degree Options Yes.

Program Entrance Requirements Minimum overall college GPA of 2.8, transcript of college record, written essay, health exam, health insurance, high school biology, high school chemistry, 3 years high school math, 3 years high school science, high school transcript, immunizations, 3 letters of recommendation, minimum high school GPA of 3.0, minimum high school rank 25%, minimum GPA in nursing prerequisites of 2.8. Transfer students are accepted. *Application deadline:* 1/15 (fall), 10/15 (spring). Applications may be processed on a rolling basis for some programs. *Application fee:* $40.

Advanced Placement Credit by examination available. Credit given for nursing courses completed elsewhere dependent upon specific evaluations.

Expenses (2012–13) *Tuition:* full-time $30,890; part-time $1030 per credit hour. *Room and board:* $11,934 per academic year. *Required fees:* full-time $520; part-time $50 per term.

Financial Aid 97% of baccalaureate students in nursing programs received some form of financial aid in 2011–12.

Contact Mr. Patrick A. Quinn, Vice President for Enrollment Management, Department of Nursing, Utica College, 1600 Burrstone Road, Utica, NY 13502-4892. *Telephone:* 315-792-3006. *Fax:* 315-792-3003. *E-mail:* pquinn@utica.edu.

Wagner College
Department of Nursing
Staten Island, New York

http://www.wagner.edu/departments/nursing/
Founded in 1883

DEGREES • BS • MSN
Nursing Program Faculty 17 (90% with doctorates).
Baccalaureate Enrollment 60 **Women** 82% **Men** 18% **Minority** 20% **International** 10% **Part-time** 5%
Graduate Enrollment 63 **Women** 90% **Men** 10% **Minority** 10% **Part-time** 95%
Nursing Student Activities Nursing Honor Society, Sigma Theta Tau, Student Nurses' Association.
Nursing Student Resources Academic advising; academic or career counseling; assistance for students with disabilities; bookstore; campus computer network; career placement assistance; computer lab; computer-assisted instruction; e-mail services; externships; housing assistance; interactive nursing skills videos; Internet; learning resource lab; library services; nursing audiovisuals; remedial services; skills, simulation, or other laboratory; tutoring; unpaid internships.

Library Facilities 196,140 volumes (4,505 in health, 859 in nursing); 20,196 periodical subscriptions (87 health-care related).

BACCALAUREATE PROGRAMS

Degree BS
Available Programs Baccalaureate for Second Degree; Generic Baccalaureate.
Study Options Full-time.
Program Entrance Requirements Minimum overall college GPA of 3.0, written essay, health exam, health insurance, high school chemistry, high school transcript, immunizations, letters of recommendation, minimum high school GPA of 2.7, minimum GPA in nursing prerequisites of 3.0, prerequisite course work. Transfer students are accepted.
Advanced Placement Credit by examination available. Credit given for nursing courses completed elsewhere dependent upon specific evaluations.
Contact *Telephone:* 718-390-3452. *Fax:* 718-420-4009.

GRADUATE PROGRAMS

Contact *Telephone:* 718-390-3444. *Fax:* 718-420-4009.

MASTER'S DEGREE PROGRAM

Degree MSN
Concentrations Available Nursing education. *Nurse practitioner programs in:* family health.
Study Options Full-time and part-time.
Program Entrance Requirements Clinical experience, minimum overall college GPA of 2.7, transcript of college record, CPR certification, immunizations, interview, 2 letters of recommendation, nursing research course, professional liability insurance/malpractice insurance, resume.
Degree Requirements 44 total credit hours.

POST-MASTER'S PROGRAM

Areas of Study *Nurse practitioner programs in:* family health.

York College of the City University of New York

Program in Nursing
Jamaica, New York

http://www.york.cuny.edu/academics/departments/health-professions/nursing
Founded in 1967

DEGREE • BS
Nursing Program Faculty 9 (20% with doctorates).
Baccalaureate Enrollment 80 **Women** 85% **Men** 15% **Minority** 80% **Part-time** 50%
Nursing Student Activities Nursing club.
Nursing Student Resources Academic advising; academic or career counseling; assistance for students with disabilities; bookstore; campus computer network; career placement assistance; computer lab; computer-assisted instruction; daycare for children of students; e-mail services; employment services for current students; Internet; library services; resume preparation assistance; skills, simulation, or other laboratory; tutoring.
Library Facilities 575,480 volumes (8,714 in health, 567 in nursing); 71,713 periodical subscriptions.

BACCALAUREATE PROGRAMS

Degree BS
Available Programs ADN to Baccalaureate; RN Baccalaureate.
Program Entrance Requirements Minimum overall college GPA of 3.0, transcript of college record, CPR certification, health exam, immunizations, minimum GPA in nursing prerequisites of 3.0, professional liability insurance/malpractice insurance, prerequisite course work, RN licensure. Transfer students are accepted.
Advanced Placement Credit by examination available. Credit given for nursing courses completed elsewhere dependent upon specific evaluations.
Contact *Telephone:* 718-262-2165.

NORTH CAROLINA

Appalachian State University
Department of Nursing
Boone, North Carolina

http://www.nursing.appstate.edu/
Founded in 1899
DEGREE • BSN
Nursing Program Faculty 15 (50% with doctorates).
Baccalaureate Enrollment 146 **Women** 90% **Men** 10% **Minority** 5%
Distance Learning Courses Available.
Nursing Student Activities Nursing Honor Society, Sigma Theta Tau, Student Nurses' Association, nursing club.
Nursing Student Resources Academic advising; academic or career counseling; assistance for students with disabilities; bookstore; campus computer network; career placement assistance; computer lab; computer-assisted instruction; e-mail services; interactive nursing skills videos; Internet; learning resource lab; library services; nursing audiovisuals; remedial services; skills, simulation, or other laboratory; tutoring.
Library Facilities 925,290 volumes (3.2 million in health, 541,000 in nursing); 23,861 periodical subscriptions (6,764 health-care related).

BACCALAUREATE PROGRAMS

Degree BSN
Available Programs Generic Baccalaureate; RN Baccalaureate.
Study Options Full-time.
Online Degree Options Yes.
Program Entrance Requirements Minimum overall college GPA of 3.0, transcript of college record, CPR certification, health exam, immunizations, minimum GPA in nursing prerequisites of 2.5, professional liability insurance/malpractice insurance, prerequisite course work. Transfer students are accepted. *Application deadline:* 1/15 (fall). *Application fee:* $50.
Financial Aid 50% of baccalaureate students in nursing programs received some form of financial aid in 2011–12. *Gift aid (need-based):* Federal Pell, FSEOG, state, private, college/university gift aid from institutional funds. *Loans:* Federal Direct (Subsidized and Unsubsidized Stafford PLUS), Perkins. *Work-study:* Federal Work-Study. *Financial aid application deadline:* Continuous.
Contact Ms. Teri Goodman, Administrative Assistant, Department of Nursing, Appalachian State University, Edwin Duncan Hall, Suite 318, 730 River Street, Boone, NC 28608. *Telephone:* 828-262-8039. *Fax:* 828-262-8066. *E-mail:* goodmantk@appstate.edu.

Barton College
School of Nursing
Wilson, North Carolina

http://www.barton.edu
Founded in 1902
DEGREE • BSN
Nursing Program Faculty 10 (30% with doctorates).
Baccalaureate Enrollment 98 **Women** 94.8% **Men** 5.2% **Minority** 17.9% **International** 2.5% **Part-time** 3.8%
Nursing Student Activities Sigma Theta Tau, Student Nurses' Association, nursing club.
Nursing Student Resources Academic advising; academic or career counseling; assistance for students with disabilities; bookstore; campus computer network; career placement assistance; computer lab; computer-assisted instruction; e-mail services; employment services for current students; externships; interactive nursing skills videos; Internet; learning resource lab; library services; nursing audiovisuals; paid internships; placement services for program completers; remedial services; resume preparation assistance; skills, simulation, or other laboratory; tutoring; unpaid internships.
Library Facilities 3,500 volumes in health, 2,250 volumes in nursing; 100 periodical subscriptions health-care related.

BACCALAUREATE PROGRAMS

Degree BSN

Available Programs ADN to Baccalaureate; Generic Baccalaureate; RN Baccalaureate.

Study Options Full-time and part-time.

Program Entrance Requirements Minimum overall college GPA of 2.5, transcript of college record, CPR certification, health exam, health insurance, high school biology, high school chemistry, high school transcript, immunizations, minimum GPA in nursing prerequisites of 2.7, professional liability insurance/malpractice insurance, prerequisite course work. Transfer students are accepted. *Application deadline:* 11/1 (fall).

Advanced Placement Credit given for nursing courses completed elsewhere dependent upon specific evaluations.

Financial Aid 92% of baccalaureate students in nursing programs received some form of financial aid in 2010–11. *Gift aid (need-based):* Federal Pell, FSEOG, state, private, college/university gift aid from institutional funds. *Loans:* Perkins, alternative loans.*Work-study:* Federal Work-Study, part-time campus jobs.*Financial aid application deadline (priority):* 4/1.

Contact Ms. Joan Taylor, Department Administrator, School of Nursing, Barton College, PO Box 5000, Wilson, NC 27893-7000. *Telephone:* 252-399-6400. *Fax:* 252-399-6416. *E-mail:* jtaylor@barton.edu.

Cabarrus College of Health Sciences
Louise Harkey School of Nursing
Concord, North Carolina

http://www.cabarruscollege.edu/
Founded in 1942
DEGREE • BSN
Nursing Program Faculty 3 (25% with doctorates).
Baccalaureate Enrollment 35 **Women** 90% **Men** 10% **Minority** 10% **Part-time** 50%
Distance Learning Courses Available.
Nursing Student Activities Sigma Theta Tau, Student Nurses' Association, nursing club.
Nursing Student Resources Academic advising; academic or career counseling; assistance for students with disabilities; bookstore; campus computer network; career placement assistance; computer lab; computer-assisted instruction; e-mail services; interactive nursing skills videos; Internet; library services; resume preparation assistance; skills, simulation, or other laboratory.
Library Facilities 500 volumes in health, 300 volumes in nursing; 300 periodical subscriptions health-care related.

BACCALAUREATE PROGRAMS
Degree BSN
Available Programs RN Baccalaureate.
Study Options Full-time and part-time.
Program Entrance Requirements Minimum overall college GPA of 2.5, transcript of college record, CPR certification, written essay, health exam, health insurance, 4 years high school math, immunizations, 2 letters of recommendation, RN licensure. Transfer students are accepted. *Application deadline:* 5/1 (fall), 10/1 (spring). Applications may be processed on a rolling basis for some programs. *Application fee:* $35.
Advanced Placement Credit by examination available.
Contact *Telephone:* 704-403-1756. *Fax:* 704-403-2077.

Duke University
School of Nursing
Durham, North Carolina

http://www.nursing.duke.edu/
Founded in 1838
DEGREES • BSN • MSN • MSN/MBA • PHD
Nursing Program Faculty 81 (94% with doctorates).
Baccalaureate Enrollment 211 **Women** 88% **Men** 12% **Minority** 19% **International** 1%
Graduate Enrollment 606 **Women** 90% **Men** 10% **Minority** 20% **International** 2% **Part-time** 72%
Distance Learning Courses Available.

Nursing Student Activities Sigma Theta Tau, Student Nurses' Association.
Nursing Student Resources Academic advising; academic or career counseling; assistance for students with disabilities; bookstore; campus computer network; career placement assistance; computer lab; computer-assisted instruction; e-mail services; Internet; library services; nursing audiovisuals; resume preparation assistance; skills, simulation, or other laboratory.
Library Facilities 6 million volumes (280,606 in health, 12,366 in nursing); 62,639 periodical subscriptions (3,948 health-care related).

BACCALAUREATE PROGRAMS
Degree BSN
Available Programs Accelerated Baccalaureate for Second Degree.
Site Options Durham, NC.
Study Options Full-time.
Program Entrance Requirements Minimum overall college GPA of 3.0, transcript of college record, CPR certification, written essay, health exam, health insurance, immunizations, interview, 3 letters of recommendation, prerequisite course work. *Application deadline:* 12/1 (fall), 6/1 (spring). *Application fee:* $50.
Financial Aid 97% of baccalaureate students in nursing programs received some form of financial aid in 2011–12. *Gift aid (need-based):* Federal Pell, FSEOG, state, private, college/university gift aid from institutional funds. *Loans:* Federal Direct (Subsidized and Unsubsidized Stafford PLUS), Perkins, college/university, alternative loans.*Work-study:* Federal Work-Study, part-time campus jobs.*Financial aid application deadline:* 3/1.
Contact Mr. Christopher Lambert, Admissions Officer, School of Nursing, Duke University, DUMC 3322 Trent Drive, Durham, NC 27710. *Telephone:* 919-684-9182. *Fax:* 919-668-4693. *E-mail:* christopher.lambert@duke.edu.

GRADUATE PROGRAMS
Financial Aid 64% of graduate students in nursing programs received some form of financial aid in 2011–12. Career-related internships or fieldwork, institutionally sponsored loans, scholarships, traineeships, and tuition waivers (partial) available. Aid available to part-time students. *Financial aid application deadline:* 4/1.
Contact Ms. Mary-Charles Barrett, Admissions Officer, School of Nursing, Duke University, DUMC 3322, Durham, NC 27710. *Telephone:* 919-684-9163. *Fax:* 919-668-4693. *E-mail:* marycharles.barrett@duke.edu.

MASTER'S DEGREE PROGRAM
Degrees MSN; MSN/MBA
Available Programs Master's; RN to Master's.
Concentrations Available Health-care administration; nurse anesthesia; nurse case management; nursing administration; nursing education; nursing informatics. *Nurse practitioner programs in:* acute care, adult health, family health, gerontology, neonatal health, oncology, pediatric, primary care.
Site Options Durham, NC.
Study Options Full-time and part-time.
Online Degree Options Yes.
Program Entrance Requirements Clinical experience, computer literacy, minimum overall college GPA of 3.0, transcript of college record, CPR certification, written essay, immunizations, interview, 3 letters of recommendation, prerequisite course work, resume, statistics course, GRE General Test. *Application deadline:* 12/1 (fall), 6/1 (spring). *Application fee:* $50.
Advanced Placement Credit given for nursing courses completed elsewhere dependent upon specific evaluations.
Degree Requirements 39 total credit hours.

POST-MASTER'S PROGRAM
Areas of Study Health-care administration; nurse anesthesia; nurse case management; nursing administration; nursing education; nursing informatics. *Nurse practitioner programs in:* acute care, adult health, family health, gerontology, neonatal health, oncology, pediatric, primary care.

DOCTORAL DEGREE PROGRAM
Degree PhD
Available Programs Doctorate; Post-Baccalaureate Doctorate.
Areas of Study Health-care systems, illness and transition.
Site Options Durham, NC.
Program Entrance Requirements Minimum overall college GPA of 3.5, interview by faculty committee, interview, 3 letters of recommen-

dation, MSN or equivalent, statistics course, vita. *Application deadline:* 12/15 (fall). *Application fee:* $75.
Degree Requirements 54 total credit hours, dissertation, oral exam.

East Carolina University
College of Nursing
Greenville, North Carolina

http://www.nursing.ecu.edu/
Founded in 1907
DEGREES • BSN • MSN • PHD
Nursing Program Faculty 104 (40% with doctorates).
Baccalaureate Enrollment 628 **Women** 90.6% **Men** 9.4% **Minority** 13.4% **International** .4% **Part-time** 16.2%
Graduate Enrollment 559 **Women** 90.8% **Men** 9.2% **Minority** 14.6% **Part-time** 73.2%
Distance Learning Courses Available.
Nursing Student Activities Nursing Honor Society, Sigma Theta Tau, Student Nurses' Association.
Nursing Student Resources Academic advising; academic or career counseling; assistance for students with disabilities; bookstore; campus computer network; career placement assistance; computer lab; computer-assisted instruction; e-mail services; employment services for current students; externships; housing assistance; interactive nursing skills videos; Internet; learning resource lab; library services; nursing audiovisuals; remedial services; resume preparation assistance; skills, simulation, or other laboratory; tutoring; unpaid internships.
Library Facilities 2.4 million volumes (135,271 in health, 4,000 in nursing); 73,166 periodical subscriptions (16,000 health-care related).

BACCALAUREATE PROGRAMS

Degree BSN
Available Programs ADN to Baccalaureate; Generic Baccalaureate.
Study Options Full-time.
Online Degree Options Yes.
Program Entrance Requirements Minimum overall college GPA of 2.5, transcript of college record, CPR certification, health exam, health insurance, immunizations, professional liability insurance/malpractice insurance, prerequisite course work. Transfer students are accepted. *Application deadline:* 2/1 (fall), 9/1 (spring).
Advanced Placement Credit given for nursing courses completed elsewhere dependent upon specific evaluations.
Contact *Telephone:* 252-744-6477. *Fax:* 252-744-6391.

GRADUATE PROGRAMS

Contact *Telephone:* 252-744-6477. *Fax:* 252-744-6391.

MASTER'S DEGREE PROGRAM
Degree MSN
Available Programs Accelerated Master's for Non-Nursing College Graduates; Accelerated Master's for Nurses with Non-Nursing Degrees; Master's; RN to Master's.
Concentrations Available Nurse anesthesia; nurse-midwifery; nursing administration; nursing education. *Clinical nurse specialist programs in:* adult health. *Nurse practitioner programs in:* adult health, family health, neonatal health.
Study Options Full-time and part-time.
Online Degree Options Yes.
Program Entrance Requirements Clinical experience, computer literacy, minimum overall college GPA of 3.0, transcript of college record, CPR certification, written essay, immunizations, interview, 3 letters of recommendation, nursing research course, professional liability insurance/malpractice insurance, prerequisite course work, statistics course, GRE General Test or MAT. *Application deadline:* Applications may be processed on a rolling basis for some programs.
Advanced Placement Credit given for nursing courses completed elsewhere dependent upon specific evaluations.
Degree Requirements Comprehensive exam.

POST-MASTER'S PROGRAM
Areas of Study Nurse anesthesia; nurse-midwifery; nursing administration; nursing education. *Clinical nurse specialist programs in:* adult health. *Nurse practitioner programs in:* adult health, family health, neonatal health.

DOCTORAL DEGREE PROGRAM
Degree PhD
Available Programs Doctorate; Post-Baccalaureate Doctorate.
Areas of Study Nursing science.
Program Entrance Requirements Minimum overall college GPA of 3.2, interview by faculty committee, interview, 3 letters of recommendation, MSN or equivalent, scholarly papers, statistics course, vita, writing sample. *Application deadline:* 3/1 (fall).
Degree Requirements 54 total credit hours, dissertation, oral exam, written exam.

Fayetteville State University
Program in Nursing
Fayetteville, North Carolina

http://www.uncfsu.edu/nursing/
Founded in 1867
DEGREE • BSN
Library Facilities 333,698 volumes; 4,725 periodical subscriptions.

BACCALAUREATE PROGRAMS

Degree BSN
Available Programs Generic Baccalaureate; RN Baccalaureate.
Program Entrance Requirements Minimum overall college GPA of 2.0, transcript of college record, CPR certification, health exam, health insurance, high school biology, 2.0 years high school math, high school transcript, immunizations, minimum high school GPA of 2.0, minimum GPA in nursing prerequisites of 2.0, professional liability insurance/malpractice insurance, prerequisite course work, RN licensure. Transfer students are accepted.
Contact Ms. Jacinta Williams, Lecturer/Student Coordinator, Program in Nursing, Fayetteville State University, 1200 Murchison Road, Fayetteville, NC 28301-4298. *Telephone:* 910-672-1925. *E-mail:* jwill126@uncfsu.edu.

Gardner-Webb University
School of Nursing
Boiling Springs, North Carolina

http://www.nursing.gardner-webb.edu/index.html
Founded in 1905
DEGREES • BSN • DNP • MSN • MSN/MBA
Nursing Program Faculty 17 (47% with doctorates).
Baccalaureate Enrollment 227 **Women** 92% **Men** 8% **Minority** 19% **Part-time** 57%
Graduate Enrollment 154 **Women** 96% **Men** 4% **Minority** 94% **International** 1% **Part-time** 38%
Distance Learning Courses Available.
Nursing Student Activities Sigma Theta Tau, Student Nurses' Association.
Nursing Student Resources Academic advising; assistance for students with disabilities; bookstore; campus computer network; computer lab; computer-assisted instruction; e-mail services; housing assistance; interactive nursing skills videos; Internet; learning resource lab; library services; nursing audiovisuals; other; paid internships; remedial services; resume preparation assistance; skills, simulation, or other laboratory; tutoring.
Library Facilities 252,450 volumes (6,002 in health, 2,146 in nursing); 109,011 periodical subscriptions (7,808 health-care related).

BACCALAUREATE PROGRAMS

Degree BSN
Available Programs ADN to Baccalaureate; Generic Baccalaureate.
Study Options Full-time and part-time.
Online Degree Options Yes.
Program Entrance Requirements Minimum overall college GPA of 2.5, transcript of college record, CPR certification, high school biology, high school chemistry, high school transcript, immunizations, minimum high school GPA, minimum GPA in nursing prerequisites of 2.5, professional liability insurance/malpractice insurance, prerequisite course work. Transfer students are accepted.

Expenses (2012–13) *Tuition:* full-time $12,125; part-time $387 per credit hour. *Room and board:* $3970; room only: $2040 per academic year. *Required fees:* full-time $535; part-time $250 per term.
Financial Aid 99% of baccalaureate students in nursing programs received some form of financial aid in 2011–12. *Gift aid (need-based):* Federal Pell, FSEOG, state, private, college/university gift aid from institutional funds. *Loans:* Federal Direct (Subsidized and Unsubsidized Stafford PLUS), Perkins, state, alternative loans.*Work-study:* Federal Work-Study, part-time campus jobs.*Financial aid application deadline (priority):* 3/15.
Contact Dr. Mary Alice Hodge, Director, School of Nursing, Gardner-Webb University, PO Box 7268, Boiling Springs, NC 28017. *Telephone:* 704-406-3886. *Fax:* 704-406-3919. *E-mail:* mahodge@gardner-webb.edu.

GRADUATE PROGRAMS

Expenses (2012–13) *Tuition:* full-time $6750; part-time $375 per credit hour. *International tuition:* $6750 full-time. *Room and board:* $3970; room only: $2040 per academic year. *Required fees:* part-time $63 per term.
Financial Aid 58% of graduate students in nursing programs received some form of financial aid in 2011–12.
Contact Dr. Rebecca Beck-Little, Director of MSN Program, School of Nursing, Gardner-Webb University, PO Box 7268, Boiling Springs, NC 28017. *Telephone:* 704-406-4358. *Fax:* 704-406-3919. *E-mail:* rbeck-little@gardner-webb.edu.

MASTER'S DEGREE PROGRAM

Degrees MSN; MSN/MBA
Available Programs Master's; Master's for Non-Nursing College Graduates; RN to Master's.
Concentrations Available Nursing administration; nursing education. *Nurse practitioner programs in:* family health.
Study Options Full-time and part-time.
Online Degree Options Yes (online only).
Program Entrance Requirements Minimum overall college GPA of 2.7, transcript of college record, immunizations, 3 letters of recommendation, statistics course. *Application deadline:* Applications may be processed on a rolling basis for some programs.
Advanced Placement Credit given for nursing courses completed elsewhere dependent upon specific evaluations.
Degree Requirements 36 total credit hours, thesis or project.

DOCTORAL DEGREE PROGRAM

Degree DNP
Available Programs Doctorate.
Areas of Study Ethics, faculty preparation, gerontology, health policy, health promotion/disease prevention, health-care systems, human health and illness, information systems, nurse case management, nursing administration, nursing education, nursing policy, nursing research, nursing science.
Program Entrance Requirements Clinical experience, minimum overall college GPA of 3.2, interview by faculty committee, 3 letters of recommendation, MSN or equivalent, vita, writing sample. *Application deadline:* 1/15 (summer).
Degree Requirements 36 total credit hours, dissertation.

Lees-McRae College
Nursing Program
Banner Elk, North Carolina

http://www.go.lmc.edu/nursing
Founded in 1900
DEGREE • BSN
Nursing Program Faculty 6
Baccalaureate Enrollment 51 **Women** 88% **Men** 12% **Minority** 2% **International** 2%
Distance Learning Courses Available.
Nursing Student Resources Academic advising; academic or career counseling; bookstore; computer lab; computer-assisted instruction; e-mail services; Internet; learning resource lab; library services; nursing audiovisuals; skills, simulation, or other laboratory.
Library Facilities 214,778 volumes; 22,091 periodical subscriptions.

BACCALAUREATE PROGRAMS

Degree BSN

Available Programs ADN to Baccalaureate.
Site Options Spruce Pine, NC.
Study Options Full-time.
Program Entrance Requirements Transcript of college record, immunizations, 2 letters of recommendation, RN licensure. Transfer students are accepted. *Application deadline:* Applications may be processed on a rolling basis for some programs.
Financial Aid 100% of baccalaureate students in nursing programs received some form of financial aid in 2011–12. *Gift aid (need-based):* Federal Pell, FSEOG, state, private, college/university gift aid from institutional funds. *Loans:* Federal Direct (Subsidized and Unsubsidized Stafford PLUS), Perkins, state, college/university.*Work-study:* Federal Work-Study, part-time campus jobs.*Financial aid application deadline:* Continuous.
Contact Ms. Martha P. Hartley, Director of RN to BSN Completion Program, Nursing Program, Lees-McRae College, 375 College Drive, PO Box 128, Banner Elk, NC 28604. *Telephone:* 828-898-8752. *Fax:* 866-774-4280. *E-mail:* hartley@lmc.edu.

Lenoir-Rhyne University
Program in Nursing
Hickory, North Carolina

http://nur.lr.edu/
Founded in 1891
DEGREES • BS • MSN
Nursing Program Faculty 30 (4% with doctorates).
Baccalaureate Enrollment 300 **Women** 90% **Men** 10% **Minority** 11% **International** 2% **Part-time** 4%
Distance Learning Courses Available.
Nursing Student Activities Sigma Theta Tau, Student Nurses' Association.
Nursing Student Resources Academic advising; academic or career counseling; assistance for students with disabilities; bookstore; campus computer network; career placement assistance; computer lab; computer-assisted instruction; e-mail services; employment services for current students; externships; housing assistance; interactive nursing skills videos; Internet; learning resource lab; library services; nursing audiovisuals; placement services for program completers; remedial services; resume preparation assistance; skills, simulation, or other laboratory; tutoring; unpaid internships.
Library Facilities 5,000 volumes in health, 4,200 volumes in nursing; 220 periodical subscriptions health-care related.

BACCALAUREATE PROGRAMS

Degree BS
Available Programs ADN to Baccalaureate; Generic Baccalaureate.
Study Options Full-time and part-time.
Program Entrance Requirements Minimum overall college GPA of 3.0, transcript of college record, CPR certification, written essay, health exam, high school chemistry, high school foreign language, 3 years high school math, high school transcript, immunizations, minimum high school GPA of 3.0, minimum GPA in nursing prerequisites of 2.7, prerequisite course work. Transfer students are accepted. *Application deadline:* 3/1 (fall), 4/1 (summer). Applications may be processed on a rolling basis for some programs. *Application fee:* $35.
Advanced Placement Credit by examination available. Credit given for nursing courses completed elsewhere dependent upon specific evaluations.
Financial Aid 100% of baccalaureate students in nursing programs received some form of financial aid in 2010–11. *Gift aid (need-based):* Federal Pell, FSEOG, state, private, college/university gift aid from institutional funds. *Loans:* Federal Direct (Subsidized and Unsubsidized Stafford PLUS), Perkins, state.*Work-study:* Federal Work-Study, part-time campus jobs.*Financial aid application deadline:* Continuous.
Contact Dr. Kerry C. Thompson, Chair, School of Nursing, Program in Nursing, Lenoir-Rhyne University, PO Box 7292, Hickory, NC 28603. *Telephone:* 828-328-7282. *Fax:* 828-328-7284. *E-mail:* thompsonk@lr.edu.

GRADUATE PROGRAMS

Contact Dr. Kerry C. Thompson, Chair, School of Nursing, Program in Nursing, Lenoir-Rhyne University, Box 7292, Hickory, NC 28601. *Telephone:* 828-328-7282. *E-mail:* thompsonk@lr.edu.

MASTER'S DEGREE PROGRAM

Degree MSN

Available Programs Master's; RN to Master's.

Concentrations Available Health-care administration; nursing education.

Site Options Asheville, NC.

Study Options Full-time and part-time.

Program Entrance Requirements Computer literacy, minimum overall college GPA of 3.0, transcript of college record, CPR certification, written essay, immunizations, interview, letters of recommendation, nursing research course, resume, statistics course. *Application deadline:* Applications may be processed on a rolling basis for some programs. *Application fee:* $35.

Advanced Placement Credit given for nursing courses completed elsewhere dependent upon specific evaluations.

Degree Requirements 36 total credit hours, thesis or project.

North Carolina Agricultural and Technical State University

School of Nursing
Greensboro, North Carolina

http://www.ncat.edu/academics/schools-colleges1/son/index.html
Founded in 1891

DEGREE • BSN

Nursing Program Faculty 29 (15% with doctorates).

Baccalaureate Enrollment 110 **Women** 91% **Men** 9% **Minority** 95%

Nursing Student Activities Sigma Theta Tau, Student Nurses' Association, nursing club.

Nursing Student Resources Academic advising; academic or career counseling; assistance for students with disabilities; bookstore; campus computer network; career placement assistance; computer lab; computer-assisted instruction; e-mail services; housing assistance; interactive nursing skills videos; Internet; learning resource lab; library services; nursing audiovisuals; remedial services; resume preparation assistance; skills, simulation, or other laboratory; tutoring.

Library Facilities 702,159 volumes; 3,205 periodical subscriptions.

BACCALAUREATE PROGRAMS

Degree BSN

Available Programs Accelerated Baccalaureate for Second Degree; Generic Baccalaureate; RN Baccalaureate.

Site Options Greensboro, NC.

Study Options Full-time.

Program Entrance Requirements Minimum overall college GPA of 2.8, transcript of college record, CPR certification, written essay, health exam, health insurance, high school biology, high school foreign language, 3 years high school math, 3 years high school science, high school transcript, immunizations, minimum high school GPA of 3.0, minimum GPA in nursing prerequisites of 2.8, professional liability insurance/malpractice insurance, prerequisite course work. Transfer students are accepted. *Application deadline:* 2/15 (spring). *Application fee:* $45.

Expenses (2012–13) *Tuition, area resident:* full-time $3238. *Tuition, state resident:* full-time $8537. *Room and board:* $3077 per academic year. *Required fees:* full-time $1703.

Contact Mrs. Carliss Jacobs, Student Services Director, School of Nursing, North Carolina Agricultural and Technical State University, Noble Hall, 1601 East Market Street, Greensboro, NC 27411. *Telephone:* 336-334-7750. *Fax:* 336-334-7637. *E-mail:* carlissl@ncat.edu.

North Carolina Central University

Department of Nursing
Durham, North Carolina

http://www.nccu.edu/
Founded in 1910

DEGREE • BSN

Nursing Program Faculty 30 (4% with doctorates).

Nursing Student Activities Sigma Theta Tau.

Nursing Student Resources Academic advising; academic or career counseling; assistance for students with disabilities; bookstore; campus computer network; career placement assistance; computer lab; computer-assisted instruction; e-mail services; employment services for current students; externships; housing assistance; interactive nursing skills videos; Internet; learning resource lab; library services; nursing audiovisuals; paid internships; placement services for program completers; resume preparation assistance; skills, simulation, or other laboratory; tutoring.

Library Facilities 695,876 volumes; 1,952 periodical subscriptions.

BACCALAUREATE PROGRAMS

Degree BSN

Available Programs Generic Baccalaureate.

Study Options Full-time.

Program Entrance Requirements Minimum overall college GPA of 2.0, transcript of college record, health exam, immunizations, minimum GPA in nursing prerequisites of 2.5, professional liability insurance/malpractice insurance, prerequisite course work. Transfer students are accepted.

Advanced Placement Credit given for nursing courses completed elsewhere dependent upon specific evaluations.

Contact *Telephone:* 919-530-5336. *Fax:* 919-530-5343.

Queens University of Charlotte

Presbyterian School of Nursing
Charlotte, North Carolina

http://www.queens.edu/nursing/
Founded in 1857

DEGREES • BSN • MSN • MSN/MBA

Nursing Program Faculty 60 (20% with doctorates).

Baccalaureate Enrollment 260 **Women** 95% **Men** 5% **Minority** 25% **International** 5% **Part-time** 10%

Graduate Enrollment 55 **Women** 95% **Men** 5% **Minority** 25% **International** 5% **Part-time** 50%

Distance Learning Courses Available.

Nursing Student Activities Nursing Honor Society, Sigma Theta Tau, Student Nurses' Association.

Nursing Student Resources Academic advising; academic or career counseling; assistance for students with disabilities; bookstore; campus computer network; career placement assistance; computer lab; computer-assisted instruction; e-mail services; employment services for current students; externships; housing assistance; interactive nursing skills videos; Internet; learning resource lab; library services; nursing audiovisuals; placement services for program completers; remedial services; resume preparation assistance; skills, simulation, or other laboratory; tutoring; unpaid internships.

Library Facilities 126,242 volumes (1,703 in health, 713 in nursing); 592 periodical subscriptions (516 health-care related).

BACCALAUREATE PROGRAMS

Degree BSN

Available Programs ADN to Baccalaureate; Accelerated Baccalaureate; Accelerated Baccalaureate for Second Degree; Baccalaureate for Second Degree; Generic Baccalaureate; RN Baccalaureate.

Site Options Charlotte, NC.

Study Options Full-time.

Online Degree Options Yes.

Program Entrance Requirements Minimum overall college GPA of 2.5, transcript of college record, CPR certification, written essay, health exam, health insurance, high school biology, high school chemistry, 2 years high school math, 1 year of high school science, high school transcript, immunizations, minimum high school GPA of 3.0, minimum GPA in nursing prerequisites of 2.5, prerequisite course work. Transfer students are accepted. *Application deadline:* 3/15 (fall), 9/21 (spring). *Application fee:* $40.

Advanced Placement Credit given for nursing courses completed elsewhere dependent upon specific evaluations.

Contact *Telephone:* 704-688-2780. *Fax:* 704-714-1027.

GRADUATE PROGRAMS

Contact *Telephone:* 704-337-2382. *Fax:* 704-337-2477.

MASTER'S DEGREE PROGRAM

Degrees MSN; MSN/MBA

Available Programs Master's; RN to Master's.

Concentrations Available Clinical nurse leader; nursing administration; nursing education.

Site Options Charlotte, NC.

Study Options Full-time and part-time.

Program Entrance Requirements Minimum overall college GPA of 3.0, transcript of college record, 2 letters of recommendation, professional liability insurance/malpractice insurance, resume. *Application deadline:* Applications may be processed on a rolling basis for some programs. *Application fee:* $40.

Advanced Placement Credit given for nursing courses completed elsewhere dependent upon specific evaluations.

Degree Requirements 36 total credit hours, thesis or project.

CONTINUING EDUCATION PROGRAM

Contact *Telephone:* 704-337-2491.

The University of North Carolina at Chapel Hill
School of Nursing
Chapel Hill, North Carolina

http://nursing.unc.edu/
Founded in 1789
DEGREES • BSN • MSN • PHD

Nursing Program Faculty 141 (70% with doctorates).

Baccalaureate Enrollment 379 **Women** 82.9% **Men** 17.1% **Minority** 28.2% **International** 5% **Part-time** 7.1%

Graduate Enrollment 343 **Women** 90% **Men** 10% **Minority** 28.2% **International** 3.3% **Part-time** 46%

Distance Learning Courses Available.

Nursing Student Activities Sigma Theta Tau, Student Nurses' Association, nursing club.

Nursing Student Resources Academic advising; academic or career counseling; assistance for students with disabilities; bookstore; campus computer network; career placement assistance; computer lab; computer-assisted instruction; daycare for children of students; e-mail services; employment services for current students; housing assistance; interactive nursing skills videos; Internet; learning resource lab; library services; nursing audiovisuals; other; remedial services; resume preparation assistance; skills, simulation, or other laboratory; tutoring.

Library Facilities 7.3 million volumes (347,000 in health, 9,200 in nursing); 92,483 periodical subscriptions (200,000 health-care related).

BACCALAUREATE PROGRAMS

Degree BSN

Available Programs Accelerated Baccalaureate; Accelerated Baccalaureate for Second Degree; Baccalaureate for Second Degree; Generic Baccalaureate.

Study Options Full-time.

Program Entrance Requirements Minimum overall college GPA, transcript of college record, CPR certification, written essay, health exam, health insurance, high school transcript, immunizations, minimum GPA in nursing prerequisites of 2.5, professional liability insurance/malpractice insurance, prerequisite course work. Transfer students are accepted. *Application deadline:* 8/10 (spring), 12/22 (summer). *Application fee:* $80.

Advanced Placement Credit given for nursing courses completed elsewhere dependent upon specific evaluations.

Expenses (2012–13) *Tuition, state resident:* full-time $9580. *Tuition, nonresident:* full-time $34,607. *International tuition:* $34,607 full-time. *Room and board:* $9470; room only: $5520 per academic year. *Required fees:* full-time $1020.

Financial Aid *Gift aid (need-based):* Federal Pell, FSEOG, state, private, college/university gift aid from institutional funds, State Grants. *Loans:* Federal Direct (Subsidized and Unsubsidized Stafford PLUS), Perkins, state, college/university, alternative loans. *Work-study:* Federal Work-Study. *Financial aid application deadline (priority):* 3/1.

Contact Ms. Amy Burdette, Assistant Director for Undergraduate Admissions, School of Nursing, The University of North Carolina at Chapel Hill, CB #7460, Chapel Hill, NC 27599-7460. *Telephone:* 919-966-4260. *Fax:* 919-966-3540. *E-mail:* amy_burdette@unc.edu.

GRADUATE PROGRAMS

Expenses (2012–13) *Tuition, state resident:* full-time $11,134. *Tuition, nonresident:* full-time $27,224. *International tuition:* $27,224 full-time. *Room and board:* $15,364; room only: $11,260 per academic year. *Required fees:* full-time $1850.

Financial Aid 8 fellowships, 6 research assistantships (averaging $8,000 per year), 10 teaching assistantships (averaging $8,000 per year) were awarded; scholarships, traineeships, and unspecified assistantships also available.

Contact Ms. Jennifer Moore, Admissions Counselor for Graduate Program and RN Options, School of Nursing, The University of North Carolina at Chapel Hill, CB #7460, Chapel Hill, NC 27599-7460. *Telephone:* 919-966-4260. *Fax:* 919-966-3540. *E-mail:* jennifer.j.moore@unc.edu.

MASTER'S DEGREE PROGRAM

Degree MSN

Available Programs Master's; RN to Master's.

Concentrations Available Clinical nurse leader; health-care administration; nursing administration; nursing education; nursing informatics. *Nurse practitioner programs in:* adult health, family health, gerontology, oncology, pediatric, primary care, psychiatric/mental health.

Study Options Full-time and part-time.

Program Entrance Requirements Clinical experience, minimum overall college GPA of 3.0, transcript of college record, CPR certification, written essay, immunizations, 3 letters of recommendation, physical assessment course, professional liability insurance/malpractice insurance, resume, statistics course, GRE General Test. *Application deadline:* 1/8 (fall), 10/9 (spring). *Application fee:* $85.

Advanced Placement Credit given for nursing courses completed elsewhere dependent upon specific evaluations.

Degree Requirements 42 total credit hours, thesis or project, comprehensive exam.

POST-MASTER'S PROGRAM

Areas of Study Clinical nurse leader; health-care administration; nursing administration; nursing education; nursing informatics. *Nurse practitioner programs in:* adult health, family health, gerontology, oncology, pediatric, primary care, psychiatric/mental health.

DOCTORAL DEGREE PROGRAM

Degree PhD

Available Programs Doctorate; Post-Baccalaureate Doctorate.

Areas of Study Addiction/substance abuse, advanced practice nursing, aging, bio-behavioral research, biology of health and illness, clinical practice, community health, critical care, ethics, faculty preparation, family health, forensic nursing, gerontology, health policy, health promotion/disease prevention, health-care systems, human health and illness, illness and transition, individualized study, information systems, maternity-newborn, neuro-behavior, nurse case management, nursing administration, nursing education, nursing policy, nursing research, nursing science, oncology, urban health, women's health.

Program Entrance Requirements Minimum overall college GPA of 3.0, interview, 3 letters of recommendation, vita, writing sample, GRE General Test. *Application deadline:* 1/8 (fall), 10/9 (spring). Applications may be processed on a rolling basis for some programs. *Application fee:* $85.

Degree Requirements 54 total credit hours, dissertation, oral exam, written exam, residency.

POSTDOCTORAL PROGRAM

Areas of Study Addiction/substance abuse, adolescent health, aging, cancer care, chronic illness, community health, family health, gerontology, health promotion/disease prevention, individualized study, infection prevention/skin care, information systems, neuro-behavior, nursing informatics, nursing interventions, nursing research, nursing science, outcomes, self-care, vulnerable population, women's health.

Postdoctoral Program Contact Dr. Suzanne Thoyre, Director, PhD and Post-Doctoral Programs, School of Nursing, The University of North Carolina at Chapel Hill, 1002 Carrington Hall, CB #7460, Chapel Hill, NC 27599-7460. *Telephone:* 919-966-8418. *Fax:* 919-843-9969. *E-mail:* thoyre@email.unc.edu.

CONTINUING EDUCATION PROGRAM

Contact Dr. Sonda Oppewal, Director, Center for Lifelong Learning, School of Nursing, The University of North Carolina at Chapel Hill, L400 Carrington Hall, CB #7460, Chapel Hill, NC 27599-7460.

Telephone: 919-966-3638. *Fax:* 919-966-7298. *E-mail:* oppewal@
email.unc.edu.

The University of North Carolina at Charlotte

School of Nursing
Charlotte, North Carolina

http://www.nursing.uncc.edu/
Founded in 1946

DEGREES • BSN • MSN

Nursing Program Faculty 51 (50% with doctorates).

Baccalaureate Enrollment 330 **Women** 92% **Men** 8% **Minority** 8%
Part-time 5%

Graduate Enrollment 200 **Women** 80% **Men** 20% **Minority** 10% **Part-time** 65%

Distance Learning Courses Available.

Nursing Student Activities Sigma Theta Tau, Student Nurses' Association.

Nursing Student Resources Academic advising; academic or career
counseling; assistance for students with disabilities; bookstore; campus
computer network; career placement assistance; computer lab; computer-
assisted instruction; e-mail services; externships; interactive nursing
skills videos; Internet; learning resource lab; library services; nursing
audiovisuals; resume preparation assistance; skills, simulation, or other
laboratory; tutoring.

Library Facilities 1.1 million volumes (39,000 in health, 2,400 in
nursing); 57,471 periodical subscriptions (160 health-care related).

BACCALAUREATE PROGRAMS

Degree BSN

Available Programs ADN to Baccalaureate; Generic Baccalaureate; RN
Baccalaureate.

Study Options Full-time.

Program Entrance Requirements Minimum overall college GPA of
2.5, transcript of college record, CPR certification, written essay, health
exam, health insurance, high school biology, high school chemistry, high
school foreign language, 3 years high school math, 3 years high school
science, high school transcript, immunizations, 3 letters of recommendation, minimum GPA in nursing prerequisites of 2.5, prerequisite course
work. Transfer students are accepted. *Application deadline:* 1/31 (fall),
8/31 (winter).

Contact *Telephone:* 704-687-4676. *Fax:* 704-687-3180.

GRADUATE PROGRAMS

Contact *Telephone:* 704-687-7992. *Fax:* 704-687-6017.

MASTER'S DEGREE PROGRAM

Degree MSN

Available Programs Master's; RN to Master's.

Concentrations Available Nurse anesthesia; nursing administration;
nursing education. *Clinical nurse specialist programs in:* community
health. *Nurse practitioner programs in:* adult health, family health.

Study Options Full-time and part-time.

Online Degree Options Yes.

Program Entrance Requirements Clinical experience, computer literacy, minimum overall college GPA of 3.0, transcript of college record,
CPR certification, written essay, immunizations, interview, 3 letters of
recommendation, nursing research course, professional liability
insurance/malpractice insurance, resume, statistics course.

POST-MASTER'S PROGRAM

Areas of Study Nurse anesthesia; nursing administration; nursing education. *Nurse practitioner programs in:* family health.

The University of North Carolina at Greensboro

School of Nursing
Greensboro, North Carolina

http://www.uncg.edu/nur/
Founded in 1891

DEGREES • BSN • MSN • MSN/MBA • PHD

Nursing Program Faculty 60 (60% with doctorates).

Baccalaureate Enrollment 1,138 **Women** 93% **Men** 7% **Minority** 29%
International 4% **Part-time** 33%

Graduate Enrollment 275 **Women** 80% **Men** 20% **Minority** 18%
International 4% **Part-time** 30%

Nursing Student Activities Nursing Honor Society, Sigma Theta Tau,
Student Nurses' Association.

Nursing Student Resources Academic advising; academic or career
counseling; assistance for students with disabilities; bookstore; campus
computer network; career placement assistance; computer lab; computer-
assisted instruction; e-mail services; externships; Internet; learning
resource lab; library services; nursing audiovisuals; paid internships;
placement services for program completers; remedial services; resume
preparation assistance; skills, simulation, or other laboratory; tutoring;
unpaid internships.

Library Facilities 2 million volumes; 4,648 periodical subscriptions.

BACCALAUREATE PROGRAMS

Degree BSN

Available Programs ADN to Baccalaureate; Baccalaureate for Second
Degree; Generic Baccalaureate; LPN to Baccalaureate; LPN to RN Baccalaureate; RN Baccalaureate.

Site Options Hickory, NC; Greensboro, NC.

Study Options Full-time.

Program Entrance Requirements Minimum overall college GPA of
2.7, transcript of college record, CPR certification, health exam, immunizations, minimum GPA in nursing prerequisites of 3.0, professional liability insurance/malpractice insurance, prerequisite course work. Transfer
students are accepted.

Contact *Telephone:* 336-334-5280. *Fax:* 336-334-3628.

GRADUATE PROGRAMS

Contact *Telephone:* 336-334-5561. *Fax:* 336-334-3628.

MASTER'S DEGREE PROGRAM

Degrees MSN; MSN/MBA

Available Programs Master's.

Concentrations Available Nurse anesthesia; nursing administration;
nursing education. *Nurse practitioner programs in:* adult health, gerontology.

Site Options Hickory, NC.

Study Options Full-time and part-time.

Program Entrance Requirements Clinical experience, minimum
overall college GPA of 3.0, transcript of college record, CPR certification, immunizations, 3 letters of recommendation, physical assessment
course, professional liability insurance/malpractice insurance, prerequisite course work, statistics course, GRE General Test or MAT.

Advanced Placement Credit given for nursing courses completed elsewhere dependent upon specific evaluations.

Degree Requirements 36 total credit hours, thesis or project, comprehensive exam.

POST-MASTER'S PROGRAM

Areas of Study Nurse anesthesia. *Nurse practitioner programs in:* adult
health, gerontology.

DOCTORAL DEGREE PROGRAM

Degree PhD

Available Programs Doctorate.

Areas of Study Aging, faculty preparation, gerontology, health policy,
health promotion/disease prevention, nursing administration, nursing
education, nursing research, nursing science, women's health.

Program Entrance Requirements Minimum overall college GPA of
3.0, interview by faculty committee, interview, 3 letters of recommendation, MSN or equivalent, writing sample.

Degree Requirements 57 total credit hours, dissertation, oral exam,
written exam, residency.

The University of North Carolina at Pembroke

Nursing Program
Pembroke, North Carolina

http://www.uncp.edu/nursing/
Founded in 1887

DEGREE • BSN

Nursing Program Faculty 20 (5% with doctorates).
Baccalaureate Enrollment 139
Distance Learning Courses Available.
Nursing Student Activities Student Nurses' Association.
Nursing Student Resources Academic advising; academic or career counseling; assistance for students with disabilities; bookstore; campus computer network; computer lab; computer-assisted instruction; e-mail services; housing assistance; interactive nursing skills videos; Internet; learning resource lab; library services; nursing audiovisuals; remedial services; resume preparation assistance; skills, simulation, or other laboratory; tutoring.
Library Facilities 376,901 volumes; 54,986 periodical subscriptions.

BACCALAUREATE PROGRAMS

Degree BSN
Available Programs Generic Baccalaureate; RN Baccalaureate.
Site Options Southern Pines, NC; Fayetteville, NC; Hamlet, NC.
Study Options Full-time.
Program Entrance Requirements Minimum overall college GPA, health exam, minimum GPA in nursing prerequisites, prerequisite course work, RN licensure. Transfer students are accepted. *Application deadline:* 1/15 (spring).
Advanced Placement Credit given for nursing courses completed elsewhere dependent upon specific evaluations.
Contact *Telephone:* 910-521-6522. *Fax:* 910-521-6178.

The University of North Carolina Wilmington

School of Nursing
Wilmington, North Carolina

http://www.uncw.edu/son
Founded in 1947

DEGREES • BS • MSN

Nursing Program Faculty 42 (45% with doctorates).
Baccalaureate Enrollment 277 **Women** 92% **Men** 8% **Minority** 9% **Part-time** 7%
Graduate Enrollment 72 **Women** 93% **Men** 7% **Minority** 19% **Part-time** 51%
Distance Learning Courses Available.
Nursing Student Activities Sigma Theta Tau, Student Nurses' Association.
Nursing Student Resources Academic advising; academic or career counseling; assistance for students with disabilities; bookstore; campus computer network; career placement assistance; computer lab; computer-assisted instruction; e-mail services; employment services for current students; externships; housing assistance; interactive nursing skills videos; Internet; learning resource lab; library services; nursing audiovisuals; remedial services; resume preparation assistance; skills, simulation, or other laboratory; tutoring; unpaid internships.
Library Facilities 1 million volumes (18,668 in health, 983 in nursing); 34,029 periodical subscriptions (2,744 health-care related).

BACCALAUREATE PROGRAMS

Degree BS
Available Programs Generic Baccalaureate; RN Baccalaureate.
Site Options Jacksonville, NC.
Study Options Full-time.
Online Degree Options Yes.
Program Entrance Requirements Minimum overall college GPA of 2.7, transcript of college record, CPR certification, written essay, health exam, health insurance, immunizations, minimum GPA in nursing prerequisites of 2.7, professional liability insurance/malpractice insurance,

prerequisite course work. Transfer students are accepted. *Application deadline:* 1/10 (fall), 8/10 (spring).
Advanced Placement Credit given for nursing courses completed elsewhere dependent upon specific evaluations.
Expenses (2012–13) *Tuition, state resident:* full-time $3743; part-time $126 per credit hour. *Tuition, nonresident:* full-time $15,846; part-time $535 per credit hour. *Room and board:* $8338 per academic year. *Required fees:* full-time $2456; part-time $27 per credit.
Financial Aid 72% of baccalaureate students in nursing programs received some form of financial aid in 2011–12.
Contact Mr. Mark Werbeach, Student Service Coordinator, School of Nursing, The University of North Carolina Wilmington, 601 South College Road, Wilmington, NC 28403-5995. *Telephone:* 910-962-7211. *Fax:* 910-962-7656. *E-mail:* werbeachm@uncw.edu.

GRADUATE PROGRAMS

Expenses (2012–13) *Tuition, state resident:* full-time $3880; part-time $190 per credit hour. *Tuition, nonresident:* full-time $15,781; part-time $774 per credit hour. *Room and board:* $10,023 per academic year. *Required fees:* full-time $2456; part-time $39 per credit.
Financial Aid 75% of graduate students in nursing programs received some form of financial aid in 2011–12. 2 teaching assistantships with full and partial tuition reimbursements available (averaging $9,500 per year) were awarded. *Financial aid application deadline:* 3/15.
Contact Dr. Julie S. Taylor, Graduate Coordinator, School of Nursing, The University of North Carolina Wilmington, 601 South College Road, Wilmington, NC 28403-5995. *Telephone:* 910-962-7927. *Fax:* 910-962-4921. *E-mail:* taylorjs@uncw.edu.

MASTER'S DEGREE PROGRAM

Degree MSN
Available Programs Master's.
Concentrations Available Nursing education. *Nurse practitioner programs in:* family health.
Site Options Burgaw, NC; Bolton, NC; Southport, NC; Whiteville, NC; Jacksonville, NC.
Study Options Full-time and part-time.
Program Entrance Requirements Clinical experience, computer literacy, minimum overall college GPA of 3.0, transcript of college record, CPR certification, written essay, immunizations, 3 letters of recommendation, physical assessment course, professional liability insurance/malpractice insurance, prerequisite course work, resume, statistics course, GRE General Test. *Application deadline:* 3/1 (fall). *Application fee:* $60.
Advanced Placement Credit given for nursing courses completed elsewhere dependent upon specific evaluations.
Degree Requirements 47 total credit hours, thesis or project, comprehensive exam.

POST-MASTER'S PROGRAM

Areas of Study Nursing education. *Nurse practitioner programs in:* family health.

Western Carolina University

School of Nursing
Cullowhee, North Carolina

http://www.wcu.edu/
Founded in 1889

DEGREES • BSN • MS

Nursing Program Faculty 31 (50% with doctorates).
Baccalaureate Enrollment 200 **Women** 94% **Men** 6% **Minority** 2%
Graduate Enrollment 122 **Women** 90% **Men** 10% **Minority** 2%
Distance Learning Courses Available.
Nursing Student Activities Sigma Theta Tau, Student Nurses' Association.
Nursing Student Resources Academic advising; academic or career counseling; assistance for students with disabilities; bookstore; campus computer network; career placement assistance; computer lab; computer-assisted instruction; daycare for children of students; e-mail services; externships; housing assistance; interactive nursing skills videos; Internet; learning resource lab; library services; nursing audiovisuals; resume preparation assistance; skills, simulation, or other laboratory; tutoring.
Library Facilities 629,010 volumes (10,000 in health, 900 in nursing); 14,831 periodical subscriptions (70 health-care related).

BACCALAUREATE PROGRAMS

Degree BSN
Available Programs Accelerated Baccalaureate; Generic Baccalaureate; RN Baccalaureate.
Site Options Enka, NC.
Study Options Full-time.
Online Degree Options Yes.
Program Entrance Requirements Minimum overall college GPA of 3.0, transcript of college record, CPR certification, health exam, high school transcript, immunizations, minimum GPA in nursing prerequisites of 2.0, professional liability insurance/malpractice insurance, prerequisite course work. Transfer students are accepted. *Application deadline:* 2/1 (fall), 7/1 (spring). *Application fee:* $45.
Expenses (2011–12) *Tuition, area resident:* full-time $7500. *Tuition, nonresident:* full-time $17,500. *Room and board:* $3200; room only: $2600 per academic year. *Required fees:* full-time $3200.
Financial Aid 75% of baccalaureate students in nursing programs received some form of financial aid in 2010–11. *Gift aid (need-based):* Federal Pell, FSEOG, state, private, college/university gift aid from institutional funds. *Loans:* Federal Direct (Subsidized and Unsubsidized Stafford PLUS), Perkins.*Work-study:* Federal Work-Study.*Financial aid application deadline (priority):* 3/15.
Contact Dr. Judy Neubrander, Director, School of Nursing, Western Carolina University, 209 Moore Building, Cullowhee, NC 28723. *Telephone:* 828-227-7467. *Fax:* 828-227-7052. *E-mail:* jneubrander@wcu.edu.

GRADUATE PROGRAMS

Financial Aid 75% of graduate students in nursing programs received some form of financial aid in 2010–11.
Contact Ms. Jessica Shirley, Director of Student Services, School of Nursing, Western Carolina University, 1459 Sand Hill Road, AB Tech Campus, Suite 33, Enka, NC 28715. *Telephone:* 828-670-8810 Ext. 247. *E-mail:* jshirley@email.wcu.edu.

MASTER'S DEGREE PROGRAM
Degree MS
Available Programs Master's.
Concentrations Available Nurse anesthesia; nursing administration; nursing education. *Nurse practitioner programs in:* family health.
Site Options Enka, NC.
Study Options Full-time and part-time.
Online Degree Options Yes.
Program Entrance Requirements Clinical experience, minimum overall college GPA of 3.0, transcript of college record, CPR certification, written essay, immunizations, interview, 3 letters of recommendation, nursing research course, physical assessment course, professional liability insurance/malpractice insurance, resume, statistics course. *Application deadline:* 4/15 (fall), 10/15 (winter). *Application fee:* $45.
Advanced Placement Credit given for nursing courses completed elsewhere dependent upon specific evaluations.
Degree Requirements Thesis or project, comprehensive exam.

POST-MASTER'S PROGRAM
Areas of Study Nursing administration; nursing education. *Nurse practitioner programs in:* family health.

POSTDOCTORAL PROGRAM
Postdoctoral Program Contact Dr. Sandra Grenwicki, Head, School of Nursing, Western Carolina University, Cullowhee, NC 28723. *Telephone:* 828-227-7467. *Fax:* 828-227-7071. *E-mail:* grenwicki@wcu.edu.

Winston-Salem State University
Department of Nursing
Winston-Salem, North Carolina

http://www.wssu.edu/
Founded in 1892
DEGREES • BSN • MSN
Nursing Program Faculty 34 (13% with doctorates).
Baccalaureate Enrollment 252 **Women** 77% **Men** 23% **Minority** 61%
Graduate Enrollment 15
Nursing Student Activities Nursing Honor Society, Sigma Theta Tau, Student Nurses' Association.
Nursing Student Resources Academic advising; academic or career counseling; assistance for students with disabilities; bookstore; campus computer network; computer lab; interactive nursing skills videos; learning resource lab; nursing audiovisuals; skills, simulation, or other laboratory.
Library Facilities 4,381 volumes in health, 2,691 volumes in nursing; 2,205 periodical subscriptions health-care related.

BACCALAUREATE PROGRAMS

Degree BSN
Available Programs ADN to Baccalaureate; Accelerated RN Baccalaureate; Baccalaureate for Second Degree; Generic Baccalaureate; LPN to Baccalaureate; RN Baccalaureate.
Site Options Wilkesboro, NC; Salisbury, NC; Boone, NC.
Study Options Full-time.
Program Entrance Requirements Minimum overall college GPA of 2.6, transcript of college record, CPR certification, health exam, immunizations, professional liability insurance/malpractice insurance, prerequisite course work. Transfer students are accepted.
Advanced Placement Credit by examination available. Credit given for nursing courses completed elsewhere dependent upon specific evaluations.
Contact *Telephone:* 336-750-2560. *Fax:* 336-750-2599.

GRADUATE PROGRAMS

Contact *Telephone:* 336-750-2275. *Fax:* 336-750-2007.

MASTER'S DEGREE PROGRAM
Degree MSN
Available Programs Master's.
Concentrations Available Nursing education. *Nurse practitioner programs in:* family health, psychiatric/mental health.
Study Options Full-time and part-time.
Program Entrance Requirements Clinical experience, transcript of college record, CPR certification, immunizations, interview, 3 letters of recommendation, nursing research course, physical assessment course, professional liability insurance/malpractice insurance, resume, statistics course.
Advanced Placement Credit given for nursing courses completed elsewhere dependent upon specific evaluations.
Degree Requirements 50 total credit hours, thesis or project.

CONTINUING EDUCATION PROGRAM

Contact *Telephone:* 336-750-2665. *Fax:* 336-750-2599.

NORTH DAKOTA

Dickinson State University
Department of Nursing
Dickinson, North Dakota

http://www.dickinsonstate.edu
Founded in 1918
DEGREE • BSN
Nursing Program Faculty 6 (33% with doctorates).
Baccalaureate Enrollment 32 **Women** 92% **Men** 8% **Minority** 6% **International** 16% **Part-time** 24%
Nursing Student Activities Student Nurses' Association.
Nursing Student Resources Academic advising; academic or career counseling; assistance for students with disabilities; bookstore; campus computer network; career placement assistance; computer lab; computer-assisted instruction; e-mail services; employment services for current students; externships; housing assistance; interactive nursing skills videos; Internet; learning resource lab; library services; nursing audiovisuals; other; placement services for program completers; remedial services; resume preparation assistance; skills, simulation, or other laboratory; tutoring; unpaid internships.
Library Facilities 105,713 volumes (2,319 in health, 912 in nursing); 823 periodical subscriptions (4,540 health-care related).

BACCALAUREATE PROGRAMS

Degree BSN
Available Programs ADN to Baccalaureate; LPN to Baccalaureate; LPN to RN Baccalaureate; RN Baccalaureate.

Study Options Full-time and part-time.
Program Entrance Requirements Minimum overall college GPA of 2.5, transcript of college record, CPR certification, health exam, health insurance, immunizations, minimum GPA in nursing prerequisites of 2.5, prerequisite course work. Transfer students are accepted. *Application deadline:* 2/1 (fall).
Advanced Placement Credit given for nursing courses completed elsewhere dependent upon specific evaluations.
Expenses (2012–13) *Tuition, state resident:* full-time $5718; part-time $189 per credit hour. *Tuition, nonresident:* full-time $7979; part-time $283 per credit hour. *International tuition:* $7979 full-time. *Room and board:* $5197; room only: $1862 per academic year. *Required fees:* full-time $1793; part-time $50 per credit.
Financial Aid 100% of baccalaureate students in nursing programs received some form of financial aid in 2011–12. *Gift aid (need-based):* Federal Pell, FSEOG, state, college/university gift aid from institutional funds, National Guard tuition waivers, staff waivers. *Loans:* Federal Nursing Student Loans, Perkins, state, college/university, Alaska Loans, alternative loans.*Work-study:* Federal Work-Study, part-time campus jobs.*Financial aid application deadline (priority):* 3/15.
Contact Dr. Mary Anne Marsh, Chair, Department of Nursing, Dickinson State University, 291 Campus Drive, Dickinson, ND 58601-4896. *Telephone:* 800-279-4295 Ext. 2133. *Fax:* 701-483-2524. *E-mail:* maryanne.marsh@dickinsonstate.edu.

Jamestown College
Department of Nursing
Jamestown, North Dakota

Founded in 1883
DEGREE • BSN
Nursing Program Faculty 11 (9% with doctorates).
Baccalaureate Enrollment 80
Nursing Student Activities Sigma Theta Tau, Student Nurses' Association.
Nursing Student Resources Academic advising; academic or career counseling; bookstore; campus computer network; computer lab; computer-assisted instruction; e-mail services; externships; interactive nursing skills videos; Internet; learning resource lab; library services; nursing audiovisuals; resume preparation assistance; skills, simulation, or other laboratory; tutoring.
Library Facilities 117,539 volumes (990 in health, 983 in nursing); 21,626 periodical subscriptions (163 health-care related).

BACCALAUREATE PROGRAMS
Degree BSN
Study Options Full-time and part-time.
Program Entrance Requirements Minimum overall college GPA of 3.0, transcript of college record, written essay, high school transcript, immunizations, prerequisite course work. Transfer students are accepted.
Advanced Placement Credit given for nursing courses completed elsewhere dependent upon specific evaluations.
Contact *Telephone:* 701-252-3467 Ext. 2562. *Fax:* 701-253-4318.

Minot State University
Department of Nursing
Minot, North Dakota

http://www.minotstateu.edu/nursing/
Founded in 1913
DEGREE • BSN
Nursing Program Faculty 22 (27% with doctorates).
Baccalaureate Enrollment 179 **Women** 92% **Men** 8% **Minority** 23% **International** 5% **Part-time** 20%
Distance Learning Courses Available.
Nursing Student Activities Sigma Theta Tau, Student Nurses' Association.
Nursing Student Resources Academic advising; academic or career counseling; assistance for students with disabilities; bookstore; campus computer network; career placement assistance; computer lab; computer-assisted instruction; e-mail services; housing assistance; interactive nursing skills videos; Internet; learning resource lab; library services; nursing audiovisuals; paid internships; remedial services; resume prepa-

ration assistance; skills, simulation, or other laboratory; tutoring; unpaid internships.
Library Facilities 419,712 volumes (8,500 in health, 1,750 in nursing); 730 periodical subscriptions (37 health-care related).

BACCALAUREATE PROGRAMS
Degree BSN
Available Programs Generic Baccalaureate; RN Baccalaureate.
Study Options Full-time.
Online Degree Options Yes.
Program Entrance Requirements Minimum overall college GPA of 2.75, transcript of college record, CPR certification, written essay, immunizations, 2 letters of recommendation, minimum GPA in nursing prerequisites of 2.8, prerequisite course work. Transfer students are accepted. *Application deadline:* 9/15 (fall), 2/1 (spring). *Application fee:* $25.
Advanced Placement Credit given for nursing courses completed elsewhere dependent upon specific evaluations.
Expenses (2012–13) *Tuition, state resident:* full-time $6000; part-time $190 per credit. *Tuition, nonresident:* full-time $6000; part-time $190 per credit. *International tuition:* $6000 full-time. *Required fees:* full-time $900.
Financial Aid 70% of baccalaureate students in nursing programs received some form of financial aid in 2011–12. *Gift aid (need-based):* Federal Pell, FSEOG, state, private, college/university gift aid from institutional funds. *Loans:* Federal Nursing Student Loans, Federal Direct (Subsidized and Unsubsidized Stafford PLUS), Perkins.*Work-study:* Federal Work-Study.*Financial aid application deadline (priority):* 3/15.
Contact Ms. Nicola J. Roed, Chair, Department of Nursing, Department of Nursing, Minot State University, 500 University Avenue West, Minot, ND 58707-0002. *Telephone:* 701-858-3526. *Fax:* 701-858-4309. *E-mail:* nicola.roed@minotstateu.edu.

North Dakota State University
Department of Nursing
Fargo, North Dakota

http://www.ndsu.edu/ndsu/nursing/
Founded in 1890
DEGREES • BSN • DNP • MS
Nursing Program Faculty 15 (49% with doctorates).
Baccalaureate Enrollment 195 **Women** 90% **Men** 10% **Minority** 5% **International** 3% **Part-time** 10%
Graduate Enrollment 24 **Women** 95% **Men** 5% **Minority** 1% **Part-time** 45%
Nursing Student Activities Sigma Theta Tau, Student Nurses' Association.
Nursing Student Resources Academic advising; academic or career counseling; assistance for students with disabilities; bookstore; campus computer network; career placement assistance; computer lab; computer-assisted instruction; daycare for children of students; e-mail services; employment services for current students; interactive nursing skills videos; Internet; learning resource lab; library services; nursing audiovisuals; paid internships; placement services for program completers; remedial services; resume preparation assistance; skills, simulation, or other laboratory; tutoring.
Library Facilities 8,631 volumes in health, 1,841 volumes in nursing; 121 periodical subscriptions health-care related.

BACCALAUREATE PROGRAMS
Degree BSN
Available Programs ADN to Baccalaureate; Generic Baccalaureate; LPN to Baccalaureate.
Study Options Full-time.
Program Entrance Requirements Minimum overall college GPA of 3.0, transcript of college record, CPR certification, health exam, health insurance, immunizations, 2 letters of recommendation, minimum GPA in nursing prerequisites of 3.0, prerequisite course work. Transfer students are accepted.
Advanced Placement Credit by examination available. Credit given for nursing courses completed elsewhere dependent upon specific evaluations.
Contact *Telephone:* 701-231-7395. *Fax:* 701-231-7606.

GRADUATE PROGRAMS
Contact *Telephone:* 701-231-8355. *Fax:* 701-231-7606.

MASTER'S DEGREE PROGRAM

Degree MS

Available Programs Master's.

Concentrations Available Nursing education. *Clinical nurse specialist programs in:* adult health. *Nurse practitioner programs in:* family health.

Study Options Full-time and part-time.

Program Entrance Requirements Computer literacy, minimum overall college GPA of 3.0, transcript of college record, CPR certification, immunizations, interview, 3 letters of recommendation, nursing research course, physical assessment course, professional liability insurance/malpractice insurance, resume, statistics course.

Advanced Placement Credit given for nursing courses completed elsewhere dependent upon specific evaluations.

Degree Requirements 58 total credit hours, thesis or project, comprehensive exam.

DOCTORAL DEGREE PROGRAM

Degree DNP

Available Programs Post-Baccalaureate Doctorate.

Areas of Study Advanced practice nursing, family health.

Online Degree Options Yes.

Program Entrance Requirements Clinical experience, minimum overall college GPA of 3.0, interview by faculty committee, 2 letters of recommendation, statistics course, vita, writing sample.

Degree Requirements 86 total credit hours, dissertation, oral exam.

Sanford College of Nursing

Sanford College of Nursing
Bismarck, North Dakota

http://bismarck.sanfordhealth.org/collegeofnursing/
Founded in 1988

DEGREE • BSN

Nursing Program Faculty 15 (7% with doctorates).

Baccalaureate Enrollment 109 **Women** 89% **Men** 11% **Minority** 15%

Nursing Student Activities Sigma Theta Tau, Student Nurses' Association.

Nursing Student Resources Academic advising; bookstore; computer lab; computer-assisted instruction; e-mail services; Internet; library services; nursing audiovisuals; paid internships; placement services for program completers; resume preparation assistance; skills, simulation, or other laboratory; tutoring.

Library Facilities 26,909 volumes (1,485 in health, 1,335 in nursing); 275 periodical subscriptions (655 health-care related).

BACCALAUREATE PROGRAMS

Degree BSN

Available Programs RN Baccalaureate.

Study Options Full-time and part-time.

Program Entrance Requirements Minimum overall college GPA of 2.5, transcript of college record, written essay, health exam, high school transcript, immunizations, interview, minimum GPA in nursing prerequisites of 2.5, prerequisite course work. Transfer students are accepted. *Application deadline:* 11/1 (fall), 2/1 (spring). *Application fee:* $40.

Advanced Placement Credit by examination available. Credit given for nursing courses completed elsewhere dependent upon specific evaluations.

Expenses (2012–13) *Tuition:* full-time $10,312; part-time $430 per credit. *Required fees:* full-time $855.

Financial Aid 98% of baccalaureate students in nursing programs received some form of financial aid in 2011–12. *Gift aid (need-based):* Federal Pell, FSEOG, state, private, college/university gift aid from institutional funds. *Loans:* Federal Nursing Student Loans, Federal Direct (Subsidized and Unsubsidized Stafford PLUS), Perkins, college/university. *Work-study:* Federal Work-Study. *Financial aid application deadline (priority):* 4/15.

Contact Ms. Mary Smith, Director of Student Services, Sanford College of Nursing, 512 North 7th Street, Bismarck, ND 58501. *Telephone:* 701-323-6271. *Fax:* 701-323-6289. *E-mail:* msmith@mocn.edu.

University of Mary

Division of Nursing
Bismarck, North Dakota

http://www.umary.edu/templates/template_degrees.php?degree=Nursing
Founded in 1959

DEGREES • BSN • MSN

Nursing Program Faculty 45 (31% with doctorates).

Baccalaureate Enrollment 123 **Women** 88% **Men** 12% **Minority** 7%

Graduate Enrollment 198 **Women** 98% **Men** 2% **Minority** 14% **Part-time** 23%

Distance Learning Courses Available.

Nursing Student Activities Sigma Theta Tau, Student Nurses' Association.

Nursing Student Resources Academic advising; academic or career counseling; assistance for students with disabilities; bookstore; campus computer network; career placement assistance; computer lab; computer-assisted instruction; e-mail services; employment services for current students; externships; housing assistance; interactive nursing skills videos; Internet; library services; nursing audiovisuals; placement services for program completers; resume preparation assistance; skills, simulation, or other laboratory; unpaid internships.

Library Facilities 64,524 volumes (4,350 in health, 800 in nursing); 210 periodical subscriptions (70 health-care related).

BACCALAUREATE PROGRAMS

Degree BSN

Available Programs Generic Baccalaureate; LPN to Baccalaureate; RN Baccalaureate.

Study Options Full-time and part-time.

Online Degree Options Yes.

Program Entrance Requirements Minimum overall college GPA of 2.75, transcript of college record, CPR certification, written essay, health exam, high school transcript, immunizations, interview, 2 letters of recommendation, minimum GPA in nursing prerequisites of 2.0, professional liability insurance/malpractice insurance, prerequisite course work. Transfer students are accepted.

Advanced Placement Credit by examination available. Credit given for nursing courses completed elsewhere dependent upon specific evaluations.

Expenses (2011–12) *Tuition:* full-time $13,200; part-time $435 per credit. *Room and board:* $5800; room only: $3200 per academic year. *Required fees:* full-time $200.

Financial Aid 100% of baccalaureate students in nursing programs received some form of financial aid in 2010–11.

Contact Admissions Office, Division of Nursing, University of Mary, 7500 University Drive, Bismarck, ND 58504. *Telephone:* 701-255-7500. *Fax:* 701-255-7687.

GRADUATE PROGRAMS

Expenses (2011–12) *Tuition:* part-time $465 per credit.

Financial Aid 95% of graduate students in nursing programs received some form of financial aid in 2010–11. 14 fellowships with partial tuition reimbursements available, 3 teaching assistantships with partial tuition reimbursements available were awarded. *Financial aid application deadline:* 8/1.

Contact Dr. Billie Madler, Graduate Program Director, Division of Nursing, University of Mary, 7500 University Drive, Bismarck, ND 58504. *Telephone:* 701-355-8266. *Fax:* 701-255-7687. *E-mail:* bmadler@umary.edu.

MASTER'S DEGREE PROGRAM

Degree MSN

Available Programs Master's; RN to Master's.

Concentrations Available Nursing administration; nursing education. *Nurse practitioner programs in:* family health.

Site Options Billings, MT; Gillette, WY; Kansas City, MO.

Study Options Full-time and part-time.

Online Degree Options Yes.

Program Entrance Requirements Clinical experience, minimum overall college GPA of 2.75, transcript of college record, CPR certification, written essay, immunizations, interview, 2 letters of recommendation, physical assessment course, prerequisite course work, resume. *Application deadline:* Applications may be processed on a rolling basis for some programs.

Advanced Placement Credit given for nursing courses completed elsewhere dependent upon specific evaluations.
Degree Requirements 45 total credit hours, thesis or project, comprehensive exam.

University of North Dakota
College of Nursing
Grand Forks, North Dakota

http://www.nursing.und.edu/
Founded in 1883
DEGREES • BSN • MS • PHD
Nursing Program Faculty 75 (30% with doctorates).
Baccalaureate Enrollment 304 **Women** 84% **Men** 16% **Minority** 8% **International** 1% **Part-time** 9%
Graduate Enrollment 264 **Women** 88.1% **Men** 11.9% **Minority** 12.8% **International** 1% **Part-time** 52.3%
Distance Learning Courses Available.
Nursing Student Activities Nursing Honor Society, Sigma Theta Tau, Student Nurses' Association.
Nursing Student Resources Academic advising; academic or career counseling; assistance for students with disabilities; bookstore; career placement assistance; computer lab; computer-assisted instruction; daycare for children of students; e-mail services; employment services for current students; externships; housing assistance; interactive nursing skills videos; Internet; learning resource lab; library services; nursing audiovisuals; paid internships; placement services for program completers; remedial services; resume preparation assistance; skills, simulation, or other laboratory; tutoring.
Library Facilities 1.2 million volumes (81,000 in health, 10,200 in nursing); 44,704 periodical subscriptions (30,000 health-care related).

BACCALAUREATE PROGRAMS

Degree BSN
Available Programs ADN to Baccalaureate; Accelerated Baccalaureate for Second Degree; Baccalaureate for Second Degree; Generic Baccalaureate; LPN to Baccalaureate.
Study Options Full-time and part-time.
Program Entrance Requirements Minimum overall college GPA of 2.5, transcript of college record, CPR certification, written essay, health insurance, immunizations, minimum GPA in nursing prerequisites of 2.5, prerequisite course work. Transfer students are accepted. *Application deadline:* 2/1 (fall), 7/1 (spring).
Advanced Placement Credit by examination available. Credit given for nursing courses completed elsewhere dependent upon specific evaluations.
Expenses (2012–13) *Tuition, state resident:* full-time $7254; part-time $302 per credit. *Tuition, nonresident:* full-time $10,223; part-time $426 per credit. *International tuition:* $17,170 full-time. *Room and board:* $6084; room only: $5942 per academic year. *Required fees:* full-time $1000; part-time $45 per credit; part-time $500 per term.
Financial Aid 82% of baccalaureate students in nursing programs received some form of financial aid in 2011–12.
Contact Ms. Lucy Heintz, Director of the Office of Student Services, College of Nursing, University of North Dakota, UND Nursing Building, 430 Oxford Street, Stop 9025, Grand Forks, ND 58202-9025. *Telephone:* 701-777-4534. *Fax:* 701-777-4096. *E-mail:* lucy.heintz@email.und.edu.

GRADUATE PROGRAMS

Expenses (2012–13) *Tuition, state resident:* full-time $7704; part-time $361 per credit. *Tuition, nonresident:* full-time $7704; part-time $361 per credit. *International tuition:* $7704 full-time. *Room and board:* $6084; room only: $3627 per academic year. *Required fees:* full-time $1000; part-time $42 per credit.
Financial Aid 84% of graduate students in nursing programs received some form of financial aid in 2011–12. 3 research assistantships with full and partial tuition reimbursements available (averaging $10,498 per year), 6 teaching assistantships with full and partial tuition reimbursements available (averaging $10,669 per year) were awarded; fellowships with full and partial tuition reimbursements available, Federal Work-Study, institutionally sponsored loans, scholarships, traineeships, and tuition waivers (full and partial) also available. Aid available to part-time students. *Financial aid application deadline:* 3/15.
Contact Dr. Laurel Shepherd, Chair, Graduate Nursing Department, College of Nursing, University of North Dakota, 430 Oxford Street, Stop 9025, Room 361, Grand Forks, ND 58202-9025. *Telephone:* 701-777-4543. *Fax:* 701-777-4096. *E-mail:* laurel.shepherd@und.edu.

MASTER'S DEGREE PROGRAM
Degree MS
Available Programs Master's.
Concentrations Available Nurse anesthesia; nursing education. *Clinical nurse specialist programs in:* gerontology, psychiatric/mental health, public health. *Nurse practitioner programs in:* family health, gerontology, primary care, psychiatric/mental health.
Study Options Full-time and part-time.
Online Degree Options Yes.
Program Entrance Requirements Clinical experience, minimum overall college GPA of 3.0, transcript of college record, CPR certification, written essay, immunizations, interview, 3 letters of recommendation, prerequisite course work, resume, statistics course. *Application deadline:* 1/15 (fall). *Application fee:* $35.
Advanced Placement Credit given for nursing courses completed elsewhere dependent upon specific evaluations.
Degree Requirements 57 total credit hours, thesis or project.

POST-MASTER'S PROGRAM
Areas of Study Nurse anesthesia; nursing education. *Clinical nurse specialist programs in:* gerontology, psychiatric/mental health. *Nurse practitioner programs in:* family health, gerontology, primary care, psychiatric/mental health.

DOCTORAL DEGREE PROGRAM
Degree PhD
Available Programs Doctorate.
Areas of Study Bio-behavioral research, nursing research.
Online Degree Options Yes (online only).
Program Entrance Requirements Minimum overall college GPA of 3.5, interview by faculty committee, 3 letters of recommendation, MSN or equivalent, statistics course, vita, GRE or MAT. *Application deadline:* 2/1 (fall). *Application fee:* $35.
Degree Requirements 90 total credit hours, dissertation, oral exam, written exam.

OHIO

Ashland University
Dwight Schar College of Nursing and Health Sciences
Ashland, Ohio

http://www.ashland.edu/nursing
Founded in 1878
DEGREE • BSN
Nursing Program Faculty 24 (19% with doctorates).
Baccalaureate Enrollment 368 **Women** 84% **Men** 16% **Minority** 6% **Part-time** 3%
Distance Learning Courses Available.
Nursing Student Activities Nursing Honor Society, Sigma Theta Tau, Student Nurses' Association, nursing club.
Nursing Student Resources Academic advising; academic or career counseling; assistance for students with disabilities; bookstore; campus computer network; career placement assistance; computer lab; computer-assisted instruction; e-mail services; employment services for current students; interactive nursing skills videos; Internet; learning resource lab; library services; nursing audiovisuals; remedial services; resume preparation assistance; skills, simulation, or other laboratory; tutoring; unpaid internships.
Library Facilities 205,200 volumes; 1,625 periodical subscriptions.

BACCALAUREATE PROGRAMS

Degree BSN
Available Programs ADN to Baccalaureate; Accelerated Baccalaureate; Accelerated Baccalaureate for Second Degree; Baccalaureate for Second Degree; RN Baccalaureate.
Study Options Full-time and part-time.
Online Degree Options Yes.

Program Entrance Requirements Minimum overall college GPA of 3.0, transcript of college record, CPR certification, health exam, health insurance, high school transcript, immunizations, minimum high school GPA. Transfer students are accepted. *Application deadline:* Applications may be processed on a rolling basis for some programs. *Application fee:* $300.

Expenses (2012–13) *Tuition:* full-time $27,930; part-time $856 per term. *Room and board:* $9400 per academic year. *Required fees:* full-time $1800.

Financial Aid 95% of baccalaureate students in nursing programs received some form of financial aid in 2011–12. *Gift aid (need-based):* Federal Pell, FSEOG, state, private, college/university gift aid from institutional funds. *Loans:* Federal Direct (Subsidized and Unsubsidized Stafford PLUS), Perkins, college/university.*Work-study:* Federal Work-Study.*Financial aid application deadline (priority):* 3/15.

Contact Ms. Jennifer McElwain, Admission Representative, Dwight Schar College of Nursing and Health Sciences, Ashland University, 1020 Trimble Road, Mansfield, OH 44906. *Telephone:* 419-521-6831. *Fax:* 419-521-6826. *E-mail:* jmcelwai@ashland.edu.

Capital University
School of Nursing
Columbus, Ohio

http://www.capital.edu/
Founded in 1830

DEGREES • BSN • MN/MBA • MSN • MSN/JD • MSN/MDIV
Nursing Program Faculty 45 (30% with doctorates).
Baccalaureate Enrollment 464 **Women** 82% **Men** 18% **Minority** 9% **International** 1% **Part-time** 19%
Graduate Enrollment 45 **Women** 87% **Men** 13% **Minority** 31% **International** 2% **Part-time** 98%
Nursing Student Activities Sigma Theta Tau, Student Nurses' Association.
Nursing Student Resources Academic advising; academic or career counseling; assistance for students with disabilities; bookstore; campus computer network; computer lab; computer-assisted instruction; e-mail services; interactive nursing skills videos; Internet; learning resource lab; library services; nursing audiovisuals; remedial services; resume preparation assistance; skills, simulation, or other laboratory; tutoring; unpaid internships.
Library Facilities 220,594 volumes (6,209 in health); 163,236 periodical subscriptions (82 health-care related).

BACCALAUREATE PROGRAMS

Degree BSN
Available Programs ADN to Baccalaureate; Accelerated Baccalaureate for Second Degree; Generic Baccalaureate; RN Baccalaureate.
Study Options Full-time and part-time.
Program Entrance Requirements Minimum overall college GPA of 3.0, transcript of college record, health exam, high school biology, high school chemistry, high school foreign language, 3 years high school math, 3 years high school science, high school transcript, immunizations, minimum high school GPA of 3.0. Transfer students are accepted. *Application deadline:* 5/1 (fall). Applications may be processed on a rolling basis for some programs. *Application fee:* $25.
Advanced Placement Credit by examination available. Credit given for nursing courses completed elsewhere dependent upon specific evaluations.
Financial Aid 100% of baccalaureate students in nursing programs received some form of financial aid in 2011–12.
Contact Dr. Judi Macke, Program Coordinator, School of Nursing, Capital University, 1 College and Main, Columbus, OH 43209-2394. *Telephone:* 614-236-6339. *Fax:* 614-236-6157. *E-mail:* jmacke@capital.edu.

GRADUATE PROGRAMS

Financial Aid 30% of graduate students in nursing programs received some form of financial aid in 2011–12. Career-related internships or fieldwork and traineeships available.
Contact Dr. Sharon Stout-Shaffer, Program Coordinator, School of Nursing, Capital University, 1 College and Main, Columbus, OH 43209-2394. *Telephone:* 614-236-6363. *Fax:* 614-236-6703. *E-mail:* sstoutsh@capital.edu.

MASTER'S DEGREE PROGRAM
Degrees MN/MBA; MSN; MSN/JD; MSN/MDIV
Available Programs Master's; RN to Master's.
Concentrations Available Legal nurse consultant; nursing administration; nursing education. *Clinical nurse specialist programs in:* adult health.
Study Options Full-time and part-time.
Program Entrance Requirements Computer literacy, minimum overall college GPA of 3.0, transcript of college record, CPR certification, written essay, immunizations, 3 letters of recommendation, nursing research course, physical assessment course, professional liability insurance/malpractice insurance, resume, statistics course. *Application deadline:* 8/1 (fall), 12/1 (winter), 12/1 (spring), 5/1 (summer). Applications may be processed on a rolling basis for some programs. *Application fee:* $25.
Advanced Placement Credit given for nursing courses completed elsewhere dependent upon specific evaluations.
Degree Requirements 36 total credit hours, thesis or project, comprehensive exam.

POST-MASTER'S PROGRAM
Areas of Study Legal nurse consultant; nursing education. *Clinical nurse specialist programs in:* adult health.

Case Western Reserve University
Frances Payne Bolton School of Nursing
Cleveland, Ohio

http://fpb.case.edu/
Founded in 1826

DEGREES • BSN • MSN • MSN/MA • MSN/MBA • MSN/MPH • PHD
Nursing Program Faculty 108 (76% with doctorates).
Baccalaureate Enrollment 294 **Women** 89% **Men** 11% **Minority** 13% **International** 1.6% **Part-time** .3%
Graduate Enrollment 523 **Women** 88% **Men** 12% **Minority** 6% **International** 6.3% **Part-time** 42%
Distance Learning Courses Available.
Nursing Student Activities Sigma Theta Tau, Student Nurses' Association.
Nursing Student Resources Academic advising; academic or career counseling; assistance for students with disabilities; bookstore; campus computer network; career placement assistance; computer lab; computer-assisted instruction; e-mail services; employment services for current students; housing assistance; interactive nursing skills videos; Internet; learning resource lab; library services; nursing audiovisuals; other; placement services for program completers; remedial services; resume preparation assistance; skills, simulation, or other laboratory; tutoring.
Library Facilities 2.9 million volumes (475,000 in health); 106,581 periodical subscriptions (2,500 health-care related).

BACCALAUREATE PROGRAMS

Degree BSN
Available Programs Generic Baccalaureate.
Study Options Full-time.
Program Entrance Requirements CPR certification, written essay, health insurance, high school biology, high school chemistry, 2 years high school science, high school transcript, immunizations, 2 letters of recommendation, minimum high school GPA of 3.0. Transfer students are accepted. *Application deadline:* 1/15 (fall). *Application fee:* $35.
Advanced Placement Credit given for nursing courses completed elsewhere dependent upon specific evaluations.
Expenses (2012–13) *Tuition:* full-time $40,120; part-time $1672 per credit hour. *Room and board:* $14,111; room only: $8845 per academic year. *Required fees:* full-time $551.
Financial Aid 100% of baccalaureate students in nursing programs received some form of financial aid in 2011–12. *Gift aid (need-based):* Federal Pell, FSEOG, state, private, college/university gift aid from institutional funds. *Loans:* Federal Nursing Student Loans, Federal Direct (Subsidized and Unsubsidized Stafford PLUS), Perkins, college/university, alternative loans.*Work-study:* Federal Work-Study.*Financial aid application deadline (priority):* 2/15.
Contact Office of Student Services, Frances Payne Bolton School of Nursing, Case Western Reserve University, 10900 Euclid Avenue, Cleveland, OH 44106-4904. *Telephone:* 216-368-2529. *Fax:* 216-368-0124. *E-mail:* admissions@fpb.case.edu.

GRADUATE PROGRAMS

Expenses (2012–13) *Tuition:* full-time $30,240; part-time $1680 per credit hour. *Required fees:* full-time $30.

Financial Aid 90% of graduate students in nursing programs received some form of financial aid in 2011–12. 32 research assistantships (averaging $4,448 per year), 17 teaching assistantships (averaging $12,038 per year) were awarded; fellowships, Federal Work-Study, institutionally sponsored loans, scholarships, and tuition waivers (partial) also available. Aid available to part-time students. *Financial aid application deadline:* 5/15.

Contact Office of Student Services, Frances Payne Bolton School of Nursing, Case Western Reserve University, 10900 Euclid Avenue, Cleveland, OH 44106-4904. *Telephone:* 216-368-2529. *Fax:* 216-368-0124. *E-mail:* admissions@fbp.case.edu.

MASTER'S DEGREE PROGRAM

Degrees MSN; MSN/MA; MSN/MBA; MSN/MPH

Available Programs Accelerated AD/RN to Master's; Master's; Master's for Non-Nursing College Graduates; RN to Master's.

Concentrations Available Nurse anesthesia; nurse-midwifery. *Clinical nurse specialist programs in:* oncology. *Nurse practitioner programs in:* acute care, adult health, family health, gerontology, neonatal health, oncology, pediatric, psychiatric/mental health, women's health.

Study Options Full-time and part-time.

Program Entrance Requirements Minimum overall college GPA of 3.0, transcript of college record, written essay, immunizations, 3 letters of recommendation, resume, statistics course, MAT or GRE General Test. *Application deadline:* 6/1 (fall), 10/1 (spring), 3/1 (summer). Applications may be processed on a rolling basis for some programs. *Application fee:* $75.

Advanced Placement Credit given for nursing courses completed elsewhere dependent upon specific evaluations.

Degree Requirements 40 total credit hours.

POST-MASTER'S PROGRAM

Areas of Study Nurse anesthesia; nurse-midwifery. *Clinical nurse specialist programs in:* oncology. *Nurse practitioner programs in:* acute care, adult health, family health, gerontology, neonatal health, oncology, pediatric, psychiatric/mental health, women's health.

DOCTORAL DEGREE PROGRAM

Degree PhD

Available Programs Doctorate; Doctorate for Nurses with Non-Nursing Degrees; Post-Baccalaureate Doctorate.

Areas of Study Aging, bio-behavioral research, biology of health and illness, community health, critical care, ethics, family health, gerontology, health policy, health promotion/disease prevention, health-care systems, human health and illness, illness and transition, information systems, maternity-newborn, neuro-behavior, nursing administration, nursing education, nursing policy, nursing research, nursing science, oncology, urban health, women's health.

Program Entrance Requirements Minimum overall college GPA of 3.0, interview by faculty committee, 3 letters of recommendation, statistics course, vita, writing sample, GRE General Test, MAT (DNP). *Application deadline:* 1/1 (fall), 10/1 (spring), 3/1 (summer). Applications may be processed on a rolling basis for some programs. *Application fee:* $75.

Degree Requirements 57 total credit hours, dissertation, oral exam, residency.

POSTDOCTORAL PROGRAM

Areas of Study Adolescent health, aging, cancer care, chronic illness, community health, family health, gerontology, health promotion/disease prevention, individualized study, infection prevention/skin care, information systems, neuro-behavior, nursing informatics, nursing interventions, nursing research, nursing science, outcomes, self-care, vulnerable population, women's health.

Postdoctoral Program Contact Dr. Shirley M. Moore, Professor and Associate Dean for Research, Frances Payne Bolton School of Nursing, Case Western Reserve University, 10900 Euclid Avenue, Cleveland, OH 44106-4904. *Telephone:* 216-368-5978. *Fax:* 216-368-3542. *E-mail:* shirley.moore@case.edu.

CONTINUING EDUCATION PROGRAM

Contact Ms. Mary Variath, Instructor in Nursing, Frances Payne Bolton School of Nursing, Case Western Reserve University, 10900 Euclid Avenue, Cleveland, OH 44106-4904. *Telephone:* 216-368-2202. *Fax:* 216-368-5303. *E-mail:* mary.variath@case.edu.

Cedarville University
Department of Nursing
Cedarville, Ohio

http://www.cedarville.edu/academics/nursing
Founded in 1887
DEGREES • BSN • MSN
Nursing Program Faculty 22 (36% with doctorates).
Baccalaureate Enrollment 376 **Women** 91.8% **Men** 8.2% **Minority** 4% **International** .5% **Part-time** .3%
Graduate Enrollment 38 **Women** 90% **Men** 10% **Minority** 18% **International** 16% **Part-time** 47%
Nursing Student Activities Nursing Honor Society, Student Nurses' Association.
Nursing Student Resources Academic advising; academic or career counseling; assistance for students with disabilities; bookstore; campus computer network; career placement assistance; computer lab; computer-assisted instruction; e-mail services; employment services for current students; housing assistance; interactive nursing skills videos; Internet; library services; nursing audiovisuals; paid internships; resume preparation assistance; skills, simulation, or other laboratory; tutoring.
Library Facilities 230,524 volumes (6,386 in health, 1,160 in nursing); 24,519 periodical subscriptions (70 health-care related).

BACCALAUREATE PROGRAMS

Degree BSN

Available Programs RN Baccalaureate.

Study Options Full-time.

Program Entrance Requirements Minimum overall college GPA of 2.8, transcript of college record, CPR certification, written essay, health exam, health insurance, high school biology, high school chemistry, high school foreign language, 4 years high school math, 4 years high school science, high school transcript, immunizations, 1 letter of recommendation, minimum high school GPA of 3.0, minimum high school rank 50%, minimum GPA in nursing prerequisites of 2.8, professional liability insurance/malpractice insurance, prerequisite course work. Transfer students are accepted. *Application deadline:* 5/1 (spring). Applications may be processed on a rolling basis for some programs. *Application fee:* $30.

Advanced Placement Credit given for nursing courses completed elsewhere dependent upon specific evaluations.

Expenses (2012–13) *Tuition:* full-time $25,496; part-time $965 per credit hour. *International tuition:* $25,496 full-time. *Room and board:* $5540; room only: $3140 per academic year.

Financial Aid 96% of baccalaureate students in nursing programs received some form of financial aid in 2011–12. *Gift aid (need-based):* Federal Pell, FSEOG, state, private, college/university gift aid from institutional funds, Federal Nursing. *Loans:* Federal Nursing Student Loans, Federal Direct (Subsidized and Unsubsidized Stafford PLUS), Perkins, college/university. *Work-study:* Federal Work-Study, part-time campus jobs. *Financial aid application deadline (priority):* 3/1.

Contact Ms. Amy Holderby, Director of Admissions, Department of Nursing, Cedarville University, 251 North Main Street, Cedarville, OH 45314-0601. *Telephone:* 800-233-2784. *Fax:* 937-766-7700. *E-mail:* admissions@cedarville.edu.

GRADUATE PROGRAMS

Expenses (2012–13) *Tuition:* full-time $4120; part-time $515 per credit hour. *International tuition:* $4120 full-time.

Financial Aid 73% of graduate students in nursing programs received some form of financial aid in 2011–12.

Contact Ashley Wasserman, MSN Representative, Department of Nursing, Cedarville University, 251 North Main Street, Cedarville, OH 45314. *Telephone:* 937-766-7700. *E-mail:* awasserman@cedarville.edu.

MASTER'S DEGREE PROGRAM

Degree MSN

Available Programs Master's.

Concentrations Available *Clinical nurse specialist programs in:* family health. *Nurse practitioner programs in:* community health.

Study Options Full-time and part-time.

Program Entrance Requirements Clinical experience, computer literacy, minimum overall college GPA of 3.0, transcript of college record, written essay, interview, 3 letters of recommendation, prerequisite course work, resume. *Application deadline:* Applications may be processed on a rolling basis for some programs. *Application fee:* $30.

Degree Requirements 42 total credit hours, thesis or project.

Chamberlain College of Nursing
Chamberlain College of Nursing
Columbus, Ohio

DEGREES • BSN • MSN
Distance Learning Courses Available.

BACCALAUREATE PROGRAMS

Degree BSN
Available Programs Accelerated Baccalaureate; Accelerated Baccalaureate for Second Degree; RN Baccalaureate.
Contact Telephone: 888-556-8226.

GRADUATE PROGRAMS

Contact Telephone: 888-556-8226.

MASTER'S DEGREE PROGRAM
Degree MSN
Available Programs Master's.

Cleveland State University
School of Nursing
Cleveland, Ohio

http://www.csuohio.edu/nursing
Founded in 1964
DEGREES • BSN • MSN • MSN/MBA • PHD
Nursing Program Faculty 66 (18% with doctorates).
Baccalaureate Enrollment 378 Women 81% Men 19% Minority 22%
International 3%
Graduate Enrollment 65 Women 93.8% Men 6.2% Minority 27.6%
Part-time 100%
Distance Learning Courses Available.
Nursing Student Activities Sigma Theta Tau, Student Nurses' Association.
Nursing Student Resources Academic advising; academic or career counseling; assistance for students with disabilities; bookstore; campus computer network; computer lab; computer-assisted instruction; daycare for children of students; e-mail services; employment services for current students; interactive nursing skills videos; Internet; learning resource lab; library services; nursing audiovisuals; remedial services; resume preparation assistance; skills, simulation, or other laboratory; tutoring.
Library Facilities 538,700 volumes (6,000 in health, 300 in nursing); 11,132 periodical subscriptions (70 health-care related).

BACCALAUREATE PROGRAMS

Degree BSN
Available Programs Accelerated Baccalaureate for Second Degree; Generic Baccalaureate; RN Baccalaureate.
Study Options Full-time.
Online Degree Options Yes.
Program Entrance Requirements Minimum overall college GPA of 2.5, transcript of college record, CPR certification, written essay, health exam, health insurance, immunizations, interview, 2 letters of recommendation, minimum GPA in nursing prerequisites of 2.75, prerequisite course work. Transfer students are accepted. Application deadline: 3/1 (fall). Application fee: $25.
Advanced Placement Credit given for nursing courses completed elsewhere dependent upon specific evaluations.
Expenses (2012–13) Tuition, state resident: full-time $9264. Tuition, nonresident: full-time $12,386. International tuition: $12,386 full-time. Room and board: $11,848; room only: $7648 per academic year.
Financial Aid 80% of baccalaureate students in nursing programs received some form of financial aid in 2011–12. Gift aid (need-based): Federal Pell, FSEOG, state, private, college/university gift aid from institutional funds. Loans: Federal Direct (Subsidized and Unsubsidized Stafford PLUS), Perkins, state, alternative loans.Work-study: Federal Work-Study, part-time campus jobs.Financial aid application deadline (priority): 2/15.
Contact Mrs. Mary Leanza Manzuk, Recruiter/Advisor, School of Nursing, Cleveland State University, 2121 Euclid Avenue, JH 238, Cleveland, OH 44115-2214. Telephone: 216-687-3810. Fax: 216-687-3556. E-mail: sonadvising@csuohio.edu.

GRADUATE PROGRAMS

Expenses (2012–13) Tuition, state resident: part-time $511 per credit hour. Tuition, nonresident: part-time $521 per credit hour. Required fees: part-time $25 per credit.
Financial Aid 50% of graduate students in nursing programs received some form of financial aid in 2011–12.
Contact Ms. Carol Ivan, Recruiter/Advisor, School of Nursing, Cleveland State University, 2121 Euclid Avenue, JH 238, Cleveland, OH 44115-2214. Telephone: 216-687-5517. Fax: 216-687-3556. E-mail: sonadvising@csuohio.edu.

MASTER'S DEGREE PROGRAM
Degrees MSN; MSN/MBA
Available Programs Master's.
Concentrations Available Clinical nurse leader; nursing education. Clinical nurse specialist programs in: community health, forensic nursing.
Study Options Part-time.
Online Degree Options Yes (online only).
Program Entrance Requirements Computer literacy, minimum overall college GPA of 3.0, transcript of college record, CPR certification, written essay, immunizations, 2 letters of recommendation, professional liability insurance/malpractice insurance, resume, statistics course. Application deadline: 3/1 (fall). Application fee: $55.
Advanced Placement Credit given for nursing courses completed elsewhere dependent upon specific evaluations.
Degree Requirements 31 total credit hours.

POST-MASTER'S PROGRAM
Areas of Study Nursing education.

DOCTORAL DEGREE PROGRAM
Degree PhD
Available Programs Doctorate.
Areas of Study Nursing education.
Program Entrance Requirements Clinical experience, minimum overall college GPA of 3.25, interview by faculty committee, 2 letters of recommendation, MSN or equivalent, statistics course, vita, writing sample. Application deadline: 2/1 (fall). Application fee: $30.
Degree Requirements 67 total credit hours, dissertation, written exam, residency.

CONTINUING EDUCATION PROGRAM

Contact Noelle Muscatello, Program Assistant, Continuing Education Programs for Health Care Professionals, School of Nursing, Cleveland State University, 2121 Euclid Avenue, Julka Hall, Room 238, Cleveland, OH 44115. Telephone: 216-687-3867. Fax: 216-687-3556. E-mail: j.n.muscatello@csuohio.edu.

College of Mount St. Joseph
Department of Nursing
Cincinnati, Ohio

http://www.msj.edu/
Founded in 1920
DEGREES • BSN • MN
Nursing Program Faculty 32 (4% with doctorates).
Baccalaureate Enrollment 287 Women 97% Men 3% Minority 5%
Part-time 60%
Graduate Enrollment 21 Women 90% Men 10% Minority 5%
Nursing Student Activities Nursing Honor Society, Sigma Theta Tau, Student Nurses' Association.
Nursing Student Resources Academic advising; academic or career counseling; assistance for students with disabilities; bookstore; campus computer network; career placement assistance; computer lab; computer-assisted instruction; daycare for children of students; e-mail services; employment services for current students; externships; housing assistance; interactive nursing skills videos; Internet; learning resource lab; library services; nursing audiovisuals; placement services for program completers; remedial services; resume preparation assistance; skills, simulation, or other laboratory; tutoring.
Library Facilities 96,966 volumes (1,800 in health, 1,200 in nursing); 9,244 periodical subscriptions (300 health-care related).

BACCALAUREATE PROGRAMS

Degree BSN
Available Programs Accelerated RN Baccalaureate; Generic Baccalaureate.
Site Options Cincinnati, OH; Covington, KY.
Study Options Full-time and part-time.
Program Entrance Requirements Minimum overall college GPA of 2.75, transcript of college record, CPR certification, health exam, health insurance, high school chemistry, 2 years high school math, 2 years high school science, high school transcript, immunizations, interview, minimum high school GPA of 2.75, minimum high school rank 60%, minimum GPA in nursing prerequisites of 2.75, professional liability insurance/malpractice insurance, prerequisite course work. Transfer students are accepted. *Application deadline:* Applications may be processed on a rolling basis for some programs. *Application fee:* $25.
Advanced Placement Credit by examination available. Credit given for nursing courses completed elsewhere dependent upon specific evaluations.
Contact *Telephone:* 513-244-4511. *Fax:* 513-451-2547.

GRADUATE PROGRAMS

Contact *Telephone:* 513-244-4503. *Fax:* 513-451-2547.

MASTER'S DEGREE PROGRAM
Degree MN
Available Programs Accelerated Master's for Non-Nursing College Graduates.
Study Options Full-time.
Program Entrance Requirements Minimum overall college GPA of 3.0, transcript of college record, CPR certification, written essay, immunizations, interview, professional liability insurance/malpractice insurance, prerequisite course work, statistics course. *Application deadline:* Applications may be processed on a rolling basis for some programs. *Application fee:* $50.
Advanced Placement Credit by examination available. Credit given for nursing courses completed elsewhere dependent upon specific evaluations.
Degree Requirements 64 total credit hours, thesis or project.

Defiance College
Bachelor's Degree in Nursing
Defiance, Ohio

Founded in 1850
DEGREE • BSN
Library Facilities 175,083 volumes; 38,108 periodical subscriptions.

BACCALAUREATE PROGRAMS

Degree BSN
Available Programs Generic Baccalaureate; RN Baccalaureate.
Program Entrance Requirements Transcript of college record, minimum GPA in nursing prerequisites of 2.75, RN licensure.
Contact *Telephone:* 419-783-2448.

Franciscan University of Steubenville
Department of Nursing
Steubenville, Ohio

Founded in 1946
DEGREES • BSN • MSN
Nursing Program Faculty 15 (20% with doctorates).
Baccalaureate Enrollment 177 **Women** 91% **Men** 9% **Minority** 5% **International** 1% **Part-time** 5%
Graduate Enrollment 23 **Women** 78% **Men** 22% **Minority** 4% **Part-time** 83%
Nursing Student Activities Student Nurses' Association.
Nursing Student Resources Academic advising; academic or career counseling; assistance for students with disabilities; bookstore; campus computer network; computer lab; e-mail services; Internet; learning resource lab; library services; resume preparation assistance; tutoring.

Library Facilities 29,761 volumes in health, 8,946 volumes in nursing; 178 periodical subscriptions health-care related.

BACCALAUREATE PROGRAMS

Degree BSN
Available Programs Generic Baccalaureate; RN Baccalaureate; RPN to Baccalaureate.
Study Options Full-time and part-time.
Program Entrance Requirements Minimum overall college GPA of 2.5, transcript of college record, health exam, health insurance, high school biology, high school chemistry, 2 years high school science, high school transcript, immunizations, 2 letters of recommendation, minimum high school GPA of 2.4, minimum GPA in nursing prerequisites of 2.5, professional liability insurance/malpractice insurance, prerequisite course work. Transfer students are accepted.
Advanced Placement Credit by examination available. Credit given for nursing courses completed elsewhere dependent upon specific evaluations.
Contact *Telephone:* 740-283-6324. *Fax:* 740-283-6449.

GRADUATE PROGRAMS

Contact *Telephone:* 740-284-7245. *Fax:* 740-283-6449.

MASTER'S DEGREE PROGRAM
Degree MSN
Available Programs Master's; RN to Master's.
Concentrations Available Nursing education. *Nurse practitioner programs in:* family health.
Study Options Full-time and part-time.
Program Entrance Requirements Clinical experience, minimum overall college GPA of 3.0, transcript of college record, interview, 2 letters of recommendation, nursing research course, physical assessment course, professional liability insurance/malpractice insurance, prerequisite course work, statistics course.
Advanced Placement Credit given for nursing courses completed elsewhere dependent upon specific evaluations.
Degree Requirements 48 total credit hours, thesis or project.

Hiram College
Nursing Department
Hiram, Ohio

http://www.hiram.edu/nursing
Founded in 1850
DEGREE • BSN
Nursing Program Faculty 18 (20% with doctorates).
Baccalaureate Enrollment 83 **Women** 88% **Men** 12% **Minority** 18% **International** 2% **Part-time** 1%
Nursing Student Activities Sigma Theta Tau, Student Nurses' Association.
Nursing Student Resources Academic advising; academic or career counseling; assistance for students with disabilities; bookstore; campus computer network; career placement assistance; computer lab; computer-assisted instruction; e-mail services; employment services for current students; externships; interactive nursing skills videos; Internet; learning resource lab; library services; nursing audiovisuals; remedial services; resume preparation assistance; skills, simulation, or other laboratory; tutoring.
Library Facilities 506,792 volumes (3,846 in health, 869 in nursing); 8,890 periodical subscriptions (555 health-care related).

BACCALAUREATE PROGRAMS

Degree BSN
Available Programs Generic Baccalaureate.
Study Options Full-time.
Program Entrance Requirements Transcript of college record, written essay, health exam, high school biology, high school chemistry, high school foreign language, high school transcript, immunizations, minimum high school GPA of 2.75. Transfer students are accepted. *Application deadline:* Applications may be processed on a rolling basis for some programs.
Advanced Placement Credit given for nursing courses completed elsewhere dependent upon specific evaluations.

Expenses (2011–12) *Tuition:* full-time $28,000. *International tuition:* $28,000 full-time. *Room and board:* $9460; room only: $4620 per academic year. *Required fees:* full-time $950.
Financial Aid 100% of baccalaureate students in nursing programs received some form of financial aid in 2010–11.
Contact Jennifer LaBenne, Nurse Recruiter, Nursing Department, Hiram College, PO Box 96, Hiram, OH 44234. *Telephone:* 330-569-6104. *Fax:* 330-569-6136. *E-mail:* labenneja@hiram.edu.

Kent State University
College of Nursing
Kent, Ohio

http://www.kent.edu/nursing
Founded in 1910
DEGREES • BSN • MSN • MSN/MBA • MSN/MPA • PHD
Nursing Program Faculty 120 (20% with doctorates).
Baccalaureate Enrollment 1,211 **Women** 83% **Men** 17% **Minority** 27% **International** 2% **Part-time** 16%
Graduate Enrollment 529 **Women** 87% **Men** 13% **Minority** 41% **International** 2% **Part-time** 85%
Distance Learning Courses Available.
Nursing Student Activities Nursing Honor Society, Sigma Theta Tau, Student Nurses' Association.
Nursing Student Resources Academic advising; academic or career counseling; assistance for students with disabilities; bookstore; campus computer network; career placement assistance; computer lab; computer-assisted instruction; e-mail services; employment services for current students; externships; housing assistance; interactive nursing skills videos; Internet; learning resource lab; library services; nursing audiovisuals; other; paid internships; placement services for program completers; remedial services; resume preparation assistance; skills, simulation, or other laboratory; tutoring.
Library Facilities 2.3 million volumes; 12,000 periodical subscriptions (300 health-care related).

BACCALAUREATE PROGRAMS

Degree BSN
Available Programs ADN to Baccalaureate; Accelerated Baccalaureate; Accelerated Baccalaureate for Second Degree; Accelerated RN Baccalaureate; Baccalaureate for Second Degree; Generic Baccalaureate; RN Baccalaureate.
Site Options Canton, OH; Warren, OH; Salem, OH; Burton, OH.
Study Options Full-time and part-time.
Program Entrance Requirements Minimum overall college GPA of 2.75, transcript of college record, CPR certification, written essay, health exam, high school biology, high school transcript, immunizations, 2 letters of recommendation, minimum high school GPA of 2.75, minimum GPA in nursing prerequisites of 2.75, prerequisite course work. Transfer students are accepted. *Application deadline:* 4/15 (fall), 11/30 (spring).
Advanced Placement Credit given for nursing courses completed elsewhere dependent upon specific evaluations.
Expenses (2011–12) *Tuition, state resident:* full-time $9346; part-time $425 per credit hour. *Tuition, nonresident:* full-time $17,306; part-time $787 per credit hour. *Room and board:* room only: $8830 per academic year. *Required fees:* full-time $1514; part-time $69 per credit.
Financial Aid 95% of baccalaureate students in nursing programs received some form of financial aid in 2010–11. *Gift aid (need-based):* Federal Pell, FSEOG, state, private, college/university gift aid from institutional funds. *Loans:* Federal Nursing Student Loans, Federal Direct (Subsidized and Unsubsidized Stafford PLUS), Perkins, state, college/university, alternative loans.*Work-study:* Federal Work-Study.*Financial aid application deadline (priority):* 3/1.
Contact Mr. Curtis Good, Director of Student Services, College of Nursing, Kent State University, Henderson Hall, Kent, OH 44242-0001. *Telephone:* 330-672-9972. *Fax:* 330-672-7911. *E-mail:* cjgood@kent.edu.

GRADUATE PROGRAMS

Expenses (2011–12) *Tuition, state resident:* full-time $8428; part-time $383 per credit hour. *Tuition, nonresident:* full-time $15,944; part-time $725 per credit hour. *International tuition:* $15,944 full-time. *Room and board:* $8830 per academic year. *Required fees:* full-time $1512; part-time $138 per credit.
Financial Aid 85% of graduate students in nursing programs received some form of financial aid in 2010–11. 10 research assistantships with

full tuition reimbursements available, 10 teaching assistantships with full tuition reimbursements available were awarded; Federal Work-Study, institutionally sponsored loans, traineeships, tuition waivers (full), and unspecified assistantships also available. *Financial aid application deadline:* 2/1.
Contact Dr. Gail Bromley, Associate Dean, Academics, College of Nursing, Kent State University, 214 Henderson Hall, PO Box 5190, Kent, OH 44242-0001. *Telephone:* 330-672-8761. *Fax:* 330-672-6387. *E-mail:* gbromley@kent.edu.

MASTER'S DEGREE PROGRAM
Degrees MSN; MSN/MBA; MSN/MPA
Available Programs Accelerated RN to Master's; Master's.
Concentrations Available Health-care administration; nursing education. *Clinical nurse specialist programs in:* adult health, gerontology, pediatric, psychiatric/mental health, women's health. *Nurse practitioner programs in:* acute care, adult health, family health, pediatric, primary care, psychiatric/mental health, women's health.
Study Options Full-time and part-time.
Program Entrance Requirements Clinical experience, computer literacy, minimum overall college GPA of 3.0, transcript of college record, CPR certification, written essay, immunizations, interview, 3 letters of recommendation, professional liability insurance/malpractice insurance, resume, statistics course, GRE (if undergraduate GPA less than 3.0). *Application deadline:* 3/1 (fall), 9/1 (spring). Applications may be processed on a rolling basis for some programs. *Application fee:* $30.
Advanced Placement Credit given for nursing courses completed elsewhere dependent upon specific evaluations.
Degree Requirements 46 total credit hours.

POST-MASTER'S PROGRAM
Areas of Study Health-care administration; nursing education. *Clinical nurse specialist programs in:* adult health, pediatric, psychiatric/mental health. *Nurse practitioner programs in:* acute care, adult health, family health, pediatric, primary care, psychiatric/mental health, women's health.

DOCTORAL DEGREE PROGRAM
Degree PhD
Available Programs Doctorate.
Areas of Study Aging, clinical practice, ethics, gerontology, health policy, health promotion/disease prevention, maternity-newborn, nurse case management, nursing administration, nursing education, nursing research, nursing science, women's health.
Online Degree Options Yes (online only).
Program Entrance Requirements Clinical experience, minimum overall college GPA of 3.0, interview, 2 letters of recommendation, MSN or equivalent, scholarly papers, statistics course, vita, writing sample, GRE. *Application deadline:* 7/15 (fall). Applications may be processed on a rolling basis for some programs. *Application fee:* $30.
Degree Requirements 72 total credit hours, dissertation, written exam.

CONTINUING EDUCATION PROGRAM
Contact Shirley Hemminger, Coordinator of Continuing Nursing Education, College of Nursing, Kent State University, PO Box 5190, Kent, OH 44242-0001. *Telephone:* 330-672-8812. *Fax:* 330-672-2433. *E-mail:* shemming@kent.edu.

Kettering College
Division of Nursing
Kettering, Ohio

http://www.kc.edu/nursing
Founded in 1967
DEGREE • BSN
Nursing Program Faculty 20 (15% with doctorates).
Baccalaureate Enrollment 60 **Women** 95% **Part-time** 100%
Distance Learning Courses Available.
Nursing Student Activities Student Nurses' Association.
Nursing Student Resources Academic advising; academic or career counseling; assistance for students with disabilities; bookstore; campus computer network; computer lab; computer-assisted instruction; e-mail services; externships; interactive nursing skills videos; Internet; learning resource lab; library services; nursing audiovisuals; remedial services; resume preparation assistance; skills, simulation, or other laboratory; tutoring.

Library Facilities 29,390 volumes (4,060 in health, 1,073 in nursing); 266 periodical subscriptions (173 health-care related).

BACCALAUREATE PROGRAMS

Degree BSN
Available Programs Generic Baccalaureate; RN Baccalaureate.
Study Options Full-time and part-time.
Online Degree Options Yes (online only).
Program Entrance Requirements Minimum overall college GPA of 2.5, transcript of college record, CPR certification, health insurance, immunizations, minimum high school GPA of 2.75, minimum GPA in nursing prerequisites of 2.5, prerequisite course work. Transfer students are accepted. *Application deadline:* 5/15 (spring).
Advanced Placement Credit given for nursing courses completed elsewhere dependent upon specific evaluations.
Contact *Telephone:* 937-395-8642. *Fax:* 937-395-8810.

Lourdes University
School of Nursing
Sylvania, Ohio

http://www.lourdes.edu/
Founded in 1958
DEGREES • BSN • MSN
Nursing Program Faculty 28 (30% with doctorates).
Baccalaureate Enrollment 277 Women 86% Men 14% Minority 19% Part-time 39%
Graduate Enrollment 119 Women 89% Men 11% Minority 13%
Nursing Student Activities Nursing Honor Society, Sigma Theta Tau, Student Nurses' Association.
Nursing Student Resources Academic advising; academic or career counseling; assistance for students with disabilities; bookstore; campus computer network; career placement assistance; computer lab; computer-assisted instruction; e-mail services; employment services for current students; housing assistance; interactive nursing skills videos; Internet; learning resource lab; library services; nursing audiovisuals; placement services for program completers; remedial services; resume preparation assistance; skills, simulation, or other laboratory; tutoring.
Library Facilities 180,146 volumes (1,200 in health, 700 in nursing); 68,904 periodical subscriptions (101 health-care related).

BACCALAUREATE PROGRAMS

Degree BSN
Available Programs Generic Baccalaureate; LPN to Baccalaureate; RN Baccalaureate.
Study Options Full-time and part-time.
Program Entrance Requirements Minimum overall college GPA of 2.5, transcript of college record, CPR certification, high school transcript, minimum GPA in nursing prerequisites of 2.5, prerequisite course work. Transfer students are accepted. *Application deadline:* 1/2 (fall), 8/1 (winter).
Advanced Placement Credit by examination available. Credit given for nursing courses completed elsewhere dependent upon specific evaluations.
Expenses (2012–13) *Tuition:* full-time $16,950; part-time $565 per credit. *International tuition:* $16,950 full-time. *Room and board:* $8000; room only: $4400 per academic year. *Required fees:* full-time $1320; part-time $55 per credit.
Financial Aid 98% of baccalaureate students in nursing programs received some form of financial aid in 2011–12. *Gift aid (need-based):* Federal Pell, FSEOG, state, private, college/university gift aid from institutional funds. *Loans:* Federal Direct (Subsidized and Unsubsidized Stafford PLUS), Perkins, state, college/university, alternative loans.*Work-study:* Federal Work-Study, part-time campus jobs.*Financial aid application deadline (priority):* 3/1.
Contact Ms. Kerry Loe, Nursing Advisor/Recruiter, School of Nursing, Lourdes University, 6832 Convent Boulevard, Sylvania, OH 43560. *Telephone:* 419-824-3793. *Fax:* 419-824-3985. *E-mail:* kloe@lourdes.edu.

GRADUATE PROGRAMS

Expenses (2012–13) *Tuition:* full-time $3000; part-time $600 per credit. *International tuition:* $3000 full-time.
Financial Aid 50% of graduate students in nursing programs received some form of financial aid in 2011–12.

Contact Dr. Deborah Vargo, MSN Director, School of Nursing, Lourdes University, 6832 Convent Boulevard, Sylvania, OH 43560. *Telephone:* 419-824-3792. *Fax:* 419-824-3985. *E-mail:* dvargo@lourdes.edu.

MASTER'S DEGREE PROGRAM

Degree MSN
Available Programs Master's; RN to Master's.
Concentrations Available Nurse anesthesia; nursing administration; nursing education.
Study Options Full-time and part-time.
Program Entrance Requirements Transcript of college record, written essay, interview, letters of recommendation, nursing research course. *Application deadline:* 8/1 (fall), 1/2 (winter). Applications may be processed on a rolling basis for some programs.
Degree Requirements 33 total credit hours, thesis or project.

Malone University
School of Nursing
Canton, Ohio

http://www.malone.edu/
Founded in 1892
DEGREES • BSN • MSN
Nursing Program Faculty 45 (33% with doctorates).
Baccalaureate Enrollment 291 Women 82.1% Men 17.9% Minority 7.2% International .7% Part-time 15.1%
Graduate Enrollment 62 Women 83.9% Men 16.1% Minority 4.8% Part-time 100%
Nursing Student Activities Sigma Theta Tau, Student Nurses' Association.
Nursing Student Resources Academic advising; academic or career counseling; assistance for students with disabilities; bookstore; campus computer network; career placement assistance; computer lab; computer-assisted instruction; e-mail services; employment services for current students; interactive nursing skills videos; Internet; learning resource lab; library services; nursing audiovisuals; placement services for program completers; remedial services; resume preparation assistance; skills, simulation, or other laboratory; tutoring.
Library Facilities 272,314 volumes (5,669 in health, 4,825 in nursing); 49,942 periodical subscriptions (316 health-care related).

BACCALAUREATE PROGRAMS

Degree BSN
Available Programs ADN to Baccalaureate; Generic Baccalaureate; RN Baccalaureate.
Study Options Full-time and part-time.
Program Entrance Requirements Minimum overall college GPA of 2.5, transcript of college record, CPR certification, health exam, health insurance, high school biology, high school chemistry, 2 years high school math, 3 years high school science, high school transcript, immunizations, 2 letters of recommendation, minimum high school GPA of 2.5, minimum GPA in nursing prerequisites of 2.0, professional liability insurance/malpractice insurance, prerequisite course work. Transfer students are accepted. *Application deadline:* 8/1 (fall), 12/1 (spring). Applications may be processed on a rolling basis for some programs. *Application fee:* $20.
Advanced Placement Credit given for nursing courses completed elsewhere dependent upon specific evaluations.
Expenses (2011–12) *Tuition:* full-time $22,832; part-time $435 per credit hour. *Room and board:* $8090; room only: $4222 per academic year. *Required fees:* full-time $798.
Financial Aid 97% of baccalaureate students in nursing programs received some form of financial aid in 2010–11.
Contact Vice President for Enrollment Management, School of Nursing, Malone University, 2600 Cleveland Avenue NW, Canton, OH 44709. *Telephone:* 330-471-8145. *Fax:* 330-471-8149. *E-mail:* admissions@malone.edu.

GRADUATE PROGRAMS

Expenses (2011–12) *Tuition:* full-time $16,897; part-time $615 per hour. *Required fees:* full-time $3725.
Financial Aid 87% of graduate students in nursing programs received some form of financial aid in 2010–11.
Contact Ms. Jean Yanok, Administrative Assistant, School of Nursing, Malone University, 2600 Cleveland Avenue NW, Canton, OH 44709.

Telephone: 330-471-8366. *Fax:* 330-471-8607. *E-mail:* jyanok@malone.edu.

MASTER'S DEGREE PROGRAM

Degree MSN

Available Programs Master's.

Concentrations Available *Clinical nurse specialist programs in:* adult health, medical-surgical. *Nurse practitioner programs in:* family health.

Study Options Full-time and part-time.

Program Entrance Requirements Clinical experience, computer literacy, minimum overall college GPA of 3.0, transcript of college record, CPR certification, written essay, immunizations, interview, 2 letters of recommendation, nursing research course, physical assessment course, professional liability insurance/malpractice insurance, resume, statistics course. *Application deadline:* Applications may be processed on a rolling basis for some programs.

Advanced Placement Credit given for nursing courses completed elsewhere dependent upon specific evaluations.

Degree Requirements 56 total credit hours, thesis or project.

Mercy College of Ohio
Division of Nursing
Toledo, Ohio

http://www.mercycollege.edu/
Founded in 1993

DEGREE • BSN

Nursing Program Faculty 75 (15% with doctorates).

Baccalaureate Enrollment 297 **Women** 86% **Men** 14% **Minority** 13% **Part-time** 42%

Distance Learning Courses Available.

Nursing Student Activities Sigma Theta Tau, Student Nurses' Association.

Nursing Student Resources Academic advising; academic or career counseling; assistance for students with disabilities; campus computer network; career placement assistance; computer lab; computer-assisted instruction; e-mail services; employment services for current students; housing assistance; Internet; learning resource lab; library services; nursing audiovisuals; placement services for program completers; remedial services; resume preparation assistance; skills, simulation, or other laboratory; tutoring.

Library Facilities 6,000 volumes (3,580 in health, 800 in nursing); 128 periodical subscriptions (325 health-care related).

BACCALAUREATE PROGRAMS

Degree BSN

Available Programs Generic Baccalaureate; RN Baccalaureate.

Study Options Full-time and part-time.

Online Degree Options Yes.

Program Entrance Requirements Minimum overall college GPA of 2.7, transcript of college record, CPR certification, health exam, high school biology, high school chemistry, 2 years high school math, high school transcript, immunizations, minimum high school GPA of 2.7. Transfer students are accepted. *Application deadline:* 8/1 (fall). *Application fee:* $25.

Advanced Placement Credit by examination available.

Expenses (2012–13) *Tuition:* full-time $9780; part-time $377 per credit hour. *Required fees:* full-time $660; part-time $22 per credit; part-time $660 per term.

Financial Aid 85% of baccalaureate students in nursing programs received some form of financial aid in 2011–12.

Contact Ms. Aimee Bishop-Stuart, Director of Admissions, Division of Nursing, Mercy College of Ohio, 2221 Madison Avenue, Toledo, OH 43604. *Telephone:* 888-806-3729. *Fax:* 419-251-1462. *E-mail:* aimee.bishop-stuart@mercycollege.edu.

Miami University
Department of Nursing
Hamilton, Ohio

http://www.eas.muohio.edu/nsg
Founded in 1809

DEGREE • BSN

Nursing Program Faculty 13 (23% with doctorates).

Baccalaureate Enrollment 106 **Women** 98% **Men** 2% **Minority** 7% **Part-time** 56%

Distance Learning Courses Available.

Nursing Student Activities Sigma Theta Tau, Student Nurses' Association.

Nursing Student Resources Academic advising; academic or career counseling; assistance for students with disabilities; bookstore; campus computer network; computer lab; daycare for children of students; e-mail services; interactive nursing skills videos; Internet; learning resource lab; library services; nursing audiovisuals; resume preparation assistance; tutoring.

Library Facilities 4.1 million volumes (29,000 in nursing); 106,179 periodical subscriptions (852 health-care related).

BACCALAUREATE PROGRAMS

Degree BSN

Available Programs ADN to Baccalaureate; Generic Baccalaureate; RN Baccalaureate.

Site Options Hamilton, OH; Middletown, OH.

Study Options Full-time and part-time.

Program Entrance Requirements Minimum overall college GPA of 2.5, transcript of college record, health exam, health insurance, high school chemistry, 2 years high school math, 1 year of high school science, high school transcript, immunizations, minimum high school GPA of 3.0, minimum GPA in nursing prerequisites of 2.5, professional liability insurance/malpractice insurance. Transfer students are accepted.

Advanced Placement Credit given for nursing courses completed elsewhere dependent upon specific evaluations.

Contact *Telephone:* 513-785-7751. *Fax:* 513-785-7767.

Miami University Hamilton
Bachelor of Science in Nursing Program
Hamilton, Ohio

Founded in 1968

DEGREE • BSN

Nursing Program Faculty 27 (15% with doctorates).

Baccalaureate Enrollment 116

Distance Learning Courses Available.

Nursing Student Activities Sigma Theta Tau, Student Nurses' Association.

Nursing Student Resources Academic advising; academic or career counseling; assistance for students with disabilities; bookstore; campus computer network; career placement assistance; computer lab; computer-assisted instruction; daycare for children of students; e-mail services; employment services for current students; interactive nursing skills videos; Internet; learning resource lab; library services; nursing audiovisuals; placement services for program completers; remedial services; resume preparation assistance; skills, simulation, or other laboratory; tutoring.

Library Facilities 68,000 volumes; 400 periodical subscriptions.

BACCALAUREATE PROGRAMS

Degree BSN

Available Programs Generic Baccalaureate; RN Baccalaureate.

Site Options West Chester, OH; Middletown, OH.

Contact *Telephone:* 513-785-7772. *Fax:* 513-785-7767.

Mount Carmel College of Nursing
Nursing Programs
Columbus, Ohio

http://www.mccn.edu/
Founded in 1903
DEGREES • BSN • MS
Nursing Program Faculty 115 (20% with doctorates).
Baccalaureate Enrollment 886 **Women** 90% **Men** 10% **Minority** 10% **Part-time** 28%
Graduate Enrollment 170 **Women** 95% **Men** 5% **Minority** 21% **Part-time** 45%
Distance Learning Courses Available.
Nursing Student Activities Sigma Theta Tau, Student Nurses' Association.
Nursing Student Resources Academic advising; academic or career counseling; assistance for students with disabilities; bookstore; campus computer network; computer lab; computer-assisted instruction; e-mail services; housing assistance; interactive nursing skills videos; Internet; learning resource lab; library services; nursing audiovisuals; resume preparation assistance; skills, simulation, or other laboratory; tutoring.
Library Facilities 35,004 volumes (4,666 in health, 2,252 in nursing); 386 periodical subscriptions (5,178 health-care related).

BACCALAUREATE PROGRAMS

Degree BSN
Available Programs Accelerated Baccalaureate for Second Degree; Generic Baccalaureate; RN Baccalaureate.
Site Options Lancaster, OH.
Study Options Full-time and part-time.
Online Degree Options Yes.
Program Entrance Requirements Minimum overall college GPA of 2.8, transcript of college record, written essay, health exam, high school biology, high school chemistry, high school foreign language, 3 years high school math, 3 years high school science, high school transcript, immunizations, minimum high school GPA of 3.0. Transfer students are accepted. *Application deadline:* 4/1 (fall), 11/1 (winter). Applications may be processed on a rolling basis for some programs. *Application fee:* $30.
Advanced Placement Credit given for nursing courses completed elsewhere dependent upon specific evaluations.
Expenses (2012–13) *Tuition:* full-time $16,403; part-time $513 per credit. *Room and board:* room only: $5000 per academic year. *Required fees:* full-time $851.
Financial Aid 81% of baccalaureate students in nursing programs received some form of financial aid in 2011–12. *Gift aid (need-based):* Federal Pell, FSEOG, state, private, college/university gift aid from institutional funds. *Loans:* Federal Nursing Student Loans, Perkins, state, college/university. *Work-study:* part-time campus jobs. *Financial aid application deadline:* Continuous.
Contact Kim M. Campbell, Director, Admissions and Recruitment, Nursing Programs, Mount Carmel College of Nursing, 127 South Davis Avenue, Columbus, OH 43222-1504. *Telephone:* 614-234-5144. *Fax:* 614-234-2875. *E-mail:* kcampbell@mccn.edu.

GRADUATE PROGRAMS

Expenses (2012–13) *Tuition:* full-time $8093; part-time $415 per credit. *Room and board:* room only: $5000 per academic year. *Required fees:* full-time $98.
Financial Aid 83% of graduate students in nursing programs received some form of financial aid in 2011–12.
Contact Kip Sexton, MS Program Coordinator, Nursing Programs, Mount Carmel College of Nursing, 127 South Davis Avenue, Columbus, OH 43222-1504. *Telephone:* 614-234-5169. *Fax:* 614-234-2875. *E-mail:* ksexton@mccn.edu.

MASTER'S DEGREE PROGRAM
Degree MS
Available Programs Master's.
Concentrations Available Nursing administration; nursing education. *Clinical nurse specialist programs in:* adult health. *Nurse practitioner programs in:* family health, gerontology.

Study Options Full-time and part-time.
Program Entrance Requirements Minimum overall college GPA of 3.0, transcript of college record, CPR certification, written essay, 3 letters of recommendation, professional liability insurance/malpractice insurance, resume. *Application deadline:* 7/1 (fall), 11/1 (spring), 4/1 (summer). Applications may be processed on a rolling basis for some programs. *Application fee:* $30.
Degree Requirements 33 total credit hours, thesis or project.

POST-MASTER'S PROGRAM
Areas of Study Nursing education. *Nurse practitioner programs in:* family health.

Mount Vernon Nazarene University
School of Nursing and Health Sciences
Mount Vernon, Ohio

http://www.mvnu.edu/
Founded in 1964
DEGREE • BS
Nursing Program Faculty 12 (8% with doctorates).
Baccalaureate Enrollment 89 **Women** 85.4% **Men** 14.6% **Minority** 8.9% **International** 1%
Nursing Student Activities Sigma Theta Tau, nursing club.
Nursing Student Resources Academic advising; academic or career counseling; assistance for students with disabilities; bookstore; campus computer network; career placement assistance; computer lab; computer-assisted instruction; e-mail services; employment services for current students; interactive nursing skills videos; Internet; learning resource lab; library services; nursing audiovisuals; remedial services; resume preparation assistance; skills, simulation, or other laboratory; tutoring.
Library Facilities 170,871 volumes; 9,538 periodical subscriptions.

BACCALAUREATE PROGRAMS

Degree BS
Available Programs Generic Baccalaureate.
Study Options Full-time and part-time.
Program Entrance Requirements Transcript of college record, CPR certification, health exam, health insurance, immunizations, minimum GPA in nursing prerequisites of 2.0, prerequisite course work. Transfer students are accepted. *Application deadline:* Applications may be processed on a rolling basis for some programs.
Financial Aid *Gift aid (need-based):* Federal Pell, FSEOG, state, private, college/university gift aid from institutional funds. *Loans:* Federal Nursing Student Loans, Federal Direct (Subsidized and Unsubsidized Stafford PLUS), Perkins, state, Schell Loans. *Work-study:* Federal Work-Study, part-time campus jobs. *Financial aid application deadline (priority):* 3/15.
Contact Nursing Program, School of Nursing and Health Sciences, Mount Vernon Nazarene University, 800 Martinsburg Road, Mount Vernon, OH 43050. *Telephone:* 740-392-6868.

Muskingum University
Department of Nursing
New Concord, Ohio

Founded in 1837
DEGREE • BSN
Library Facilities 233,000 volumes; 900 periodical subscriptions.

BACCALAUREATE PROGRAMS

Degree BSN
Available Programs Generic Baccalaureate.
Contact *Telephone:* 740-826-6151.

Notre Dame College

Nursing Department
South Euclid, Ohio

Founded in 1922
DEGREE • BSN

BACCALAUREATE PROGRAMS

Degree BSN
Available Programs Generic Baccalaureate; RN Baccalaureate.
Contact *Telephone:* 216-373-5183.

Ohio Northern University

Nursing Program
Ada, Ohio

Founded in 1871
DEGREE • BSN

BACCALAUREATE PROGRAMS

Degree BSN
Available Programs RN Baccalaureate.
Contact *Telephone:* 419-772-2000.

The Ohio State University

College of Nursing
Columbus, Ohio

http://www.nursing.osu.edu/
Founded in 1870
DEGREES • BSN • MS • MS/MPH • PHD
Nursing Program Faculty 100 (20% with doctorates).
Baccalaureate Enrollment 674 **Women** 85% **Men** 15% **Minority** 13%
International 2% **Part-time** 20%
Graduate Enrollment 517 **Women** 83% **Men** 17% **Minority** 13%
International 2% **Part-time** 43%
Distance Learning Courses Available.
Nursing Student Activities Nursing Honor Society, Sigma Theta Tau, Student Nurses' Association, nursing club.
Nursing Student Resources Academic advising; academic or career counseling; assistance for students with disabilities; bookstore; campus computer network; career placement assistance; computer lab; computer-assisted instruction; daycare for children of students; e-mail services; employment services for current students; externships; housing assistance; interactive nursing skills videos; Internet; learning resource lab; library services; nursing audiovisuals; other; paid internships; placement services for program completers; remedial services; resume preparation assistance; skills, simulation, or other laboratory; tutoring; unpaid internships.
Library Facilities 6.2 million volumes (188,602 in health, 4,198 in nursing); 75,963 periodical subscriptions (5,060 health-care related).

BACCALAUREATE PROGRAMS

Degree BSN
Available Programs Generic Baccalaureate; RN Baccalaureate.
Study Options Full-time.
Online Degree Options Yes.
Program Entrance Requirements Minimum overall college GPA of 3.2, transcript of college record, CPR certification, written essay, health insurance, high school biology, high school chemistry, high school foreign language, 3 years high school math, 2 years high school science, high school transcript, immunizations, minimum GPA in nursing prerequisites of 3.2, professional liability insurance/malpractice insurance, prerequisite course work. *Application deadline:* 1/15 (fall). *Application fee:* $60.
Advanced Placement Credit by examination available. Credit given for nursing courses completed elsewhere dependent upon specific evaluations.
Expenses (2012–13) *Tuition, state resident:* full-time $9168; part-time $382 per credit hour. *Tuition, nonresident:* full-time $15,408; part-time $642 per credit hour. *International tuition:* $26,445 full-time. *Room and*

board: $10,392 per academic year. *Required fees:* full-time $1327; part-time $92 per credit; part-time $623 per term.
Financial Aid 80% of baccalaureate students in nursing programs received some form of financial aid in 2011–12. *Gift aid (need-based):* Federal Pell, FSEOG, state, private, college/university gift aid from institutional funds. *Loans:* Federal Nursing Student Loans, Federal Direct (Subsidized and Unsubsidized Stafford PLUS), Perkins, college/university.*Work-study:* Federal Work-Study, part-time campus jobs.*Financial aid application deadline (priority):* 2/15.
Contact Ms. Jennifer Marinello, Associate Director, College of Nursing, The Ohio State University, Graduate and Professional Admissions, 105 Student Academic Services Building, Columbus, OH 43210. *Telephone:* 614-292-9444. *Fax:* 614-292-3895. *E-mail:* marinello.1@osu.edu.

GRADUATE PROGRAMS

Expenses (2012–13) *Tuition, state resident:* full-time $11,336; part-time $709 per credit hour. *Tuition, nonresident:* full-time $17,312; part-time $1082 per credit hour. *International tuition:* $32,000 full-time. *Room and board:* room only: $9240 per academic year. *Required fees:* full-time $1174; part-time $109 per credit; part-time $554 per term.
Financial Aid 90% of graduate students in nursing programs received some form of financial aid in 2011–12. Fellowships, research assistantships, teaching assistantships, Federal Work-Study, institutionally sponsored loans, and unspecified assistantships available. Aid available to part-time students.
Contact Ms. Jackie Min, Graduate Outreach Coordinator, College of Nursing, The Ohio State University, 1585 Neil Avenue, 212 Newton Hall, Columbus, OH 43210-1289. *Telephone:* 614-688-8145. *Fax:* 614-292-9399. *E-mail:* min.37@osu.edu.

MASTER'S DEGREE PROGRAM

Degrees MS; MS/MPH
Available Programs Accelerated Master's for Non-Nursing College Graduates; Accelerated Master's for Nurses with Non-Nursing Degrees; Accelerated RN to Master's; Master's; Master's for Non-Nursing College Graduates; Master's for Nurses with Non-Nursing Degrees.
Concentrations Available Clinical nurse leader; health-care administration; nurse-midwifery; nursing administration. *Clinical nurse specialist programs in:* adult health, cardiovascular, community health, oncology, psychiatric/mental health, public health. *Nurse practitioner programs in:* acute care, adult health, community health, family health, gerontology, neonatal health, pediatric, primary care, psychiatric/mental health, women's health.
Study Options Full-time and part-time.
Online Degree Options Yes (online only).
Program Entrance Requirements Minimum overall college GPA of 3.5, transcript of college record, CPR certification, written essay, immunizations, 3 letters of recommendation, nursing research course, physical assessment course, prerequisite course work, resume, statistics course. *Application deadline:* 4/2 (fall), 9/12 (spring), 10/12 (summer). *Application fee:* $40.
Advanced Placement Credit given for nursing courses completed elsewhere dependent upon specific evaluations.
Degree Requirements 30 total credit hours, thesis or project, comprehensive exam.

POST-MASTER'S PROGRAM

Areas of Study Clinical nurse leader; health-care administration; nurse-midwifery; nursing administration. *Clinical nurse specialist programs in:* adult health, cardiovascular, community health, oncology, psychiatric/mental health, public health. *Nurse practitioner programs in:* acute care, adult health, community health, family health, gerontology, neonatal health, pediatric, primary care, psychiatric/mental health, women's health.

DOCTORAL DEGREE PROGRAM

Degree PhD
Available Programs Doctorate; Doctorate for Nurses with Non-Nursing Degrees; Post-Baccalaureate Doctorate.
Areas of Study Addiction/substance abuse, advanced practice nursing, aging, bio-behavioral research, biology of health and illness, clinical practice, community health, critical care, ethics, faculty preparation, family health, gerontology, health policy, health promotion/disease prevention, health-care systems, human health and illness, illness and transition, individualized study, information systems, maternity-newborn, neuro-behavior, nurse case management, nursing administration, nursing policy, nursing research, nursing science, oncology, urban health, women's health.

Program Entrance Requirements Clinical experience, minimum overall college GPA of 3.5, interview, 3 letters of recommendation, MSN or equivalent, statistics course, vita, writing sample. *Application deadline:* 4/2 (fall). *Application fee:* $40.
Degree Requirements 54 total credit hours, dissertation, oral exam, written exam, residency.

CONTINUING EDUCATION PROGRAM

Contact Ms. Jackie Loversidge, Director of Continuing Education, College of Nursing, The Ohio State University, 1585 Neil Avenue, Columbus, OH 43210-1289. *Telephone:* 614-292-6379. *Fax:* 614-292-7976. *E-mail:* loversidge.1@osu.edu.

Ohio University
School of Nursing
Athens, Ohio

http://www.ohio.edu/chsp/nrse/
Founded in 1804
DEGREES • BSN • MSN
Nursing Program Faculty 9 (89% with doctorates).
Nursing Student Activities Nursing Honor Society, Sigma Theta Tau.
Nursing Student Resources Academic or career counseling; career placement assistance; computer lab; e-mail services; Internet; library services.
Library Facilities 3 million volumes; 57,813 periodical subscriptions.

BACCALAUREATE PROGRAMS

Degree BSN
Available Programs Generic Baccalaureate; RN Baccalaureate.
Online Degree Options Yes.
Program Entrance Requirements Transfer students are accepted.
Contact *Telephone:* 740-593-4494. *Fax:* 740-593-0286.

GRADUATE PROGRAMS

Contact *Telephone:* 740-593-4494. *Fax:* 740-593-0144.

MASTER'S DEGREE PROGRAM
Degree MSN
Available Programs Master's.
Concentrations Available Nursing administration; nursing education. *Nurse practitioner programs in:* family health.
Study Options Full-time and part-time.
Program Entrance Requirements Minimum overall college GPA of 3.0, transcript of college record, written essay, 3 letters of recommendation, resume, statistics course.
Advanced Placement Credit given for nursing courses completed elsewhere dependent upon specific evaluations.
Degree Requirements 55 total credit hours.

Otterbein University
Department of Nursing
Westerville, Ohio

http://www.otterbein.edu
Founded in 1847
DEGREES • BSN • MSN
Nursing Student Activities Nursing Honor Society, Sigma Theta Tau.
Library Facilities 182,629 volumes; 1,012 periodical subscriptions.

BACCALAUREATE PROGRAMS

Degree BSN
Available Programs Accelerated RN Baccalaureate; Generic Baccalaureate; LPN to Baccalaureate; RN Baccalaureate.
Program Entrance Requirements Transfer students are accepted.
Advanced Placement Credit by examination available. Credit given for nursing courses completed elsewhere dependent upon specific evaluations.
Contact *Telephone:* 614-823-1614. *Fax:* 614-823-3131.

GRADUATE PROGRAMS

Contact *Telephone:* 614-823-1614.

MASTER'S DEGREE PROGRAM
Degree MSN
Available Programs Master's.
Concentrations Available Nursing administration; nursing education. *Clinical nurse specialist programs in:* adult health. *Nurse practitioner programs in:* adult health, family health.
Study Options Part-time.

POST-MASTER'S PROGRAM
Areas of Study Nursing education. *Nurse practitioner programs in:* adult health, family health.

CONTINUING EDUCATION PROGRAM

Contact *Telephone:* 614-823-1614.

Shawnee State University
Department of Nursing
Portsmouth, Ohio

http://www.shawnee.edu/acad/hs/nursing/index.html
Founded in 1986
DEGREE • BSN
Nursing Program Faculty 9
Nursing Student Activities Student Nurses' Association.
Nursing Student Resources Academic advising; academic or career counseling; assistance for students with disabilities; bookstore; campus computer network; career placement assistance; computer lab; computer-assisted instruction; daycare for children of students; e-mail services; employment services for current students; housing assistance; interactive nursing skills videos; Internet; learning resource lab; library services; nursing audiovisuals; other; placement services for program completers; remedial services; resume preparation assistance; skills, simulation, or other laboratory; tutoring.
Library Facilities 138,059 volumes (8,273 in health, 870 in nursing); 64,694 periodical subscriptions (1,798 health-care related).

BACCALAUREATE PROGRAMS

Degree BSN
Available Programs ADN to Baccalaureate; RN Baccalaureate.
Study Options Full-time and part-time.
Program Entrance Requirements Minimum overall college GPA of 2.5, transcript of college record, CPR certification, health exam, health insurance, high school transcript, immunizations, professional liability insurance/malpractice insurance, prerequisite course work, RN licensure. Transfer students are accepted.
Advanced Placement Credit given for nursing courses completed elsewhere dependent upon specific evaluations.
Contact *Telephone:* 740-351-3378. *Fax:* 740-351-3354.

CONTINUING EDUCATION PROGRAM

Contact *Telephone:* 740-351-3281.

The University of Akron
College of Nursing
Akron, Ohio

http://www.uakron.edu/nursing/
Founded in 1870
DEGREES • BSN • MSN • PHD
Nursing Program Faculty 98 (25% with doctorates).
Baccalaureate Enrollment 551 **Women** 78% **Men** 22% **Minority** 10% **Part-time** 1%
Graduate Enrollment 329 **Women** 87% **Men** 13% **Minority** 9% **Part-time** 74%
Distance Learning Courses Available.
Nursing Student Activities Sigma Theta Tau, Student Nurses' Association, nursing club.
Nursing Student Resources Academic advising; academic or career counseling; assistance for students with disabilities; bookstore; campus computer network; career placement assistance; computer lab; computer-assisted instruction; daycare for children of students; e-mail services; employment services for current students; interactive nursing skills

videos; Internet; learning resource lab; library services; nursing audiovisuals; remedial services; resume preparation assistance; skills, simulation, or other laboratory; tutoring.
Library Facilities 1.3 million volumes (36,800 in health, 10,258 in nursing); 481,872 periodical subscriptions (7,804 health-care related).

BACCALAUREATE PROGRAMS

Degree BSN
Available Programs ADN to Baccalaureate; Accelerated Baccalaureate for Second Degree; Accelerated RN Baccalaureate; Generic Baccalaureate; LPN to Baccalaureate; LPN to RN Baccalaureate.
Site Options Lorain, OH; Orville, OH; Medina, OH; Lakewood (UA Lakewood), OH; Kirtland (Lakeland Community College), OH.
Study Options Full-time and part-time.
Online Degree Options Yes.
Program Entrance Requirements Transcript of college record, CPR certification, health exam, immunizations, minimum GPA in nursing prerequisites of 2.75, prerequisite course work. Transfer students are accepted. *Application deadline:* Applications may be processed on a rolling basis for some programs. *Application fee:* $40.
Advanced Placement Credit given for nursing courses completed elsewhere dependent upon specific evaluations.
Expenses (2012–13) *Tuition, state resident:* full-time $9552; part-time $345 per credit hour. *Tuition, nonresident:* full-time $17,753; part-time $687 per credit hour. *International tuition:* $17,753 full-time. *Room and board:* $11,878; room only: $6306 per academic year. *Required fees:* full-time $634; part-time $53 per credit; part-time $317 per term.
Financial Aid 80% of baccalaureate students in nursing programs received some form of financial aid in 2011–12. *Gift aid (need-based):* Federal Pell, FSEOG, state, college/university gift aid from institutional funds. *Loans:* Federal Nursing Student Loans, Federal Direct (Subsidized and Unsubsidized Stafford PLUS), Perkins, college/university.*Work-study:* Federal Work-Study, part-time campus jobs.*Financial aid application deadline (priority):* 2/1.
Contact School of Nursing, College of Nursing, The University of Akron, Mary Gladwin Hall, 209 Carroll Street, Akron, OH 44325-3701. *Telephone:* 330-972-7551. *Fax:* 330-972-5737.

GRADUATE PROGRAMS

Expenses (2012–13) *Tuition, state resident:* full-time $7285; part-time $405 per credit hour. *Tuition, nonresident:* full-time $12,473; part-time $693 per credit hour. *Room and board:* $11,878; room only: $6306 per academic year. *Required fees:* full-time $613; part-time $34 per credit; part-time $306 per term.
Financial Aid 80% of graduate students in nursing programs received some form of financial aid in 2011–12. 10 teaching assistantships with full tuition reimbursements available were awarded; career-related internships or fieldwork and Federal Work-Study also available.
Contact Dr. Marlene S. Huff, Coordinator, Educational Progression and Graduate Programs, College of Nursing, The University of Akron, Akron, OH 44325-3701. *Telephone:* 330-972-5930. *Fax:* 330-972-5737. *E-mail:* mhuff@uakron.edu.

MASTER'S DEGREE PROGRAM
Degree MSN
Available Programs Master's; RN to Master's.
Concentrations Available Nurse anesthesia; nursing administration. *Clinical nurse specialist programs in:* adult health, gerontology, pediatric, psychiatric/mental health. *Nurse practitioner programs in:* acute care, adult health, gerontology, pediatric, primary care, psychiatric/mental health.
Site Options Lorain, OH; Orville, OH.
Study Options Full-time and part-time.
Program Entrance Requirements Clinical experience, computer literacy, minimum overall college GPA of 3.0, transcript of college record, CPR certification, written essay, immunizations, interview, 3 letters of recommendation, physical assessment course, professional liability insurance/malpractice insurance, prerequisite course work, resume, statistics course. *Application deadline:* Applications may be processed on a rolling basis for some programs. *Application fee:* $40.
Advanced Placement Credit given for nursing courses completed elsewhere dependent upon specific evaluations.
Degree Requirements 53 total credit hours.

POST-MASTER'S PROGRAM
Areas of Study Nurse anesthesia. *Clinical nurse specialist programs in:* adult health, gerontology, pediatric, psychiatric/mental health. *Nurse practitioner programs in:* acute care, adult health, family health, gerontology, pediatric, primary care, psychiatric/mental health.

DOCTORAL DEGREE PROGRAM
Degree PhD
Available Programs Doctorate.
Areas of Study Advanced practice nursing, aging, clinical practice, community health, critical care, ethics, family health, gerontology, health policy, health promotion/disease prevention, health-care systems, human health and illness, illness and transition, individualized study, maternity-newborn, nursing administration, nursing policy, nursing research, nursing science, women's health.
Program Entrance Requirements Minimum overall college GPA of 3.0, interview by faculty committee, interview, 3 letters of recommendation, MSN or equivalent, vita, writing sample, GRE. *Application deadline:* Applications may be processed on a rolling basis for some programs. *Application fee:* $40.
Degree Requirements 72 total credit hours, dissertation, oral exam, written exam, residency.

CONTINUING EDUCATION PROGRAM

Contact Dr. Marlene S. Huff, Coordinator, Educational Progression and Graduate Programs, College of Nursing, The University of Akron, Akron, OH 44325-3701. *Telephone:* 330-972-5930. *Fax:* 330-972-5737. *E-mail:* mhuff@uakron.edu.

See display on next page and full description on page 506.

University of Cincinnati
College of Nursing
Cincinnati, Ohio

http://www.nursing.uc.edu/
Founded in 1819
DEGREES • BSN • MSN • MSN/MBA • MSN/PHD • PHD
Nursing Program Faculty 143 (31% with doctorates).
Baccalaureate Enrollment 631 **Women** 90% **Men** 10% **Minority** 14% **Part-time** 13%
Graduate Enrollment 360 **Women** 86% **Men** 14% **Minority** 14% **International** 2%
Distance Learning Courses Available.
Nursing Student Activities Sigma Theta Tau, Student Nurses' Association.
Nursing Student Resources Academic advising; academic or career counseling; assistance for students with disabilities; bookstore; campus computer network; computer lab; computer-assisted instruction; e-mail services; employment services for current students; externships; housing assistance; interactive nursing skills videos; Internet; learning resource lab; library services; nursing audiovisuals; paid internships; remedial services; resume preparation assistance; skills, simulation, or other laboratory; tutoring; unpaid internships.
Library Facilities 3.7 million volumes (221,630 in health, 21,306 in nursing); 103,066 periodical subscriptions (2,384 health-care related).

BACCALAUREATE PROGRAMS

Degree BSN
Available Programs ADN to Baccalaureate; Accelerated Baccalaureate for Second Degree; Generic Baccalaureate; RN Baccalaureate.
Site Options Cincinnati, OH.
Study Options Full-time.
Program Entrance Requirements Minimum overall college GPA of 2.5, transcript of college record, CPR certification, health insurance, high school biology, high school chemistry, 3 years high school math, high school transcript, immunizations, prerequisite course work. Transfer students are accepted. *Application deadline:* 6/30 (fall).
Advanced Placement Credit by examination available. Credit given for nursing courses completed elsewhere dependent upon specific evaluations.
Contact *Telephone:* 513-558-5070. *Fax:* 513-558-7523.

GRADUATE PROGRAMS

Contact *Telephone:* 513-558-5072. *Fax:* 513-558-7523.

MASTER'S DEGREE PROGRAM
Degrees MSN; MSN/MBA; MSN/PhD
Available Programs Accelerated Master's for Non-Nursing College Graduates; Master's.

Nursing

At The University of Akron, we prepare nurses to deal with the reality of today's high-tech health care environment while embracing the human element of patient and family care.

Whether earning a BSN, MSN, PhD or DNP degree, you will graduate as an ethical, honest and compassionate caregiver who can and does transform lives.

Call us for more information on how The University of Akron can transform you.

330-972-5103

www.uakron.edu/nursing

Concentrations Available Nurse anesthesia; nurse-midwifery; nursing administration. *Clinical nurse specialist programs in:* adult health, critical care, gerontology, medical-surgical, occupational health, public health. *Nurse practitioner programs in:* adult health, family health, neonatal health, occupational health, pediatric, women's health.
Site Options Cincinnati, OH.
Study Options Full-time and part-time.
Online Degree Options Yes.
Program Entrance Requirements Clinical experience, computer literacy, transcript of college record, CPR certification, written essay, immunizations, interview, 3 letters of recommendation, physical assessment course, professional liability insurance/malpractice insurance, resume, statistics course, GRE General Test. *Application deadline:* 10/1 (fall), 9/1 (winter), 1/1 (spring), 3/1 (summer). Applications may be processed on a rolling basis for some programs. *Application fee:* $40.
Advanced Placement Credit given for nursing courses completed elsewhere dependent upon specific evaluations.
Degree Requirements 65 total credit hours, thesis or project.

POST-MASTER'S PROGRAM
Areas of Study Nursing education. *Nurse practitioner programs in:* adult health, family health, neonatal health, occupational health, pediatric, psychiatric/mental health, women's health.

DOCTORAL DEGREE PROGRAM
Degree PhD
Available Programs Doctorate; Post-Baccalaureate Doctorate.
Areas of Study Addiction/substance abuse, community health, critical care, ethics, faculty preparation, family health, health promotion/disease prevention, health-care systems, human health and illness, illness and transition, individualized study, maternity-newborn, nursing administration, nursing research, nursing science, oncology, women's health.
Site Options Cincinnati, OH.
Program Entrance Requirements Minimum overall college GPA of 3.0, interview by faculty committee, interview, 3 letters of recommendation, statistics course, vita, writing sample, GRE General Test. *Application deadline:* 8/15 (fall). Applications may be processed on a rolling basis for some programs. *Application fee:* $40.
Degree Requirements 135 total credit hours, dissertation, oral exam, written exam, residency.

CONTINUING EDUCATION PROGRAM
Contact *Telephone:* 513-558-5311. *Fax:* 513-558-5054.

University of Phoenix–Cleveland Campus
College of Nursing
Independence, Ohio

Founded in 2000
DEGREES • BSN • MSN
Nursing Program Faculty 10 (20% with doctorates).
Baccalaureate Enrollment 17 **Women** 82.4% **Men** 17.6% **Minority** 11.8%
Graduate Enrollment 4 **Women** 100%
Nursing Student Activities Sigma Theta Tau.
Nursing Student Resources Academic advising; academic or career counseling; assistance for students with disabilities; bookstore; campus computer network; computer lab; computer-assisted instruction; e-mail services; interactive nursing skills videos; Internet; learning resource lab; library services; nursing audiovisuals; remedial services; skills, simulation, or other laboratory; tutoring.
Library Facilities 16,781 periodical subscriptions (1,300 health-care related).

BACCALAUREATE PROGRAMS
Degree BSN
Available Programs Accelerated Baccalaureate.
Site Options Beachwood, OH.
Study Options Full-time.
Program Entrance Requirements Transcript of college record, CPR certification, immunizations, 1 letter of recommendation, RN licensure. Transfer students are accepted. *Application deadline:* Applications may be processed on a rolling basis for some programs.

Advanced Placement Credit by examination available. Credit given for nursing courses completed elsewhere dependent upon specific evaluations.

Contact *Telephone:* 216-447-8807.

GRADUATE PROGRAMS

Contact *Telephone:* 216-447-8807.

MASTER'S DEGREE PROGRAM
Degree MSN
Available Programs Master's.
Concentrations Available Nursing administration.
Site Options Beachwood, OH.
Study Options Full-time.
Program Entrance Requirements Clinical experience, computer literacy, minimum overall college GPA of 2.5, transcript of college record. *Application deadline:* Applications may be processed on a rolling basis for some programs. *Application fee:* $45.
Advanced Placement Credit given for nursing courses completed elsewhere dependent upon specific evaluations.
Degree Requirements 39 total credit hours, thesis or project.

University of Rio Grande
Holzer School of Nursing
Rio Grande, Ohio

Founded in 1876
DEGREE • BSN
Nursing Program Faculty 9
Library Facilities 96,731 volumes; 850 periodical subscriptions.

BACCALAUREATE PROGRAMS

Degree BSN
Available Programs RN Baccalaureate.
Study Options Full-time and part-time.
Contact *Telephone:* 800-282-7201 Ext. 7308. *Fax:* 740-245-7177.

The University of Toledo
College of Nursing
Toledo, Ohio

http://www.utoledo.edu/nursing
Founded in 1872
DEGREES • BSN • DNP • MSN
Nursing Program Faculty 51 (50% with doctorates).
Baccalaureate Enrollment 459 **Women** 85% **Men** 15% **Minority** 12% **International** 3% **Part-time** 17%
Graduate Enrollment 280 **Women** 91% **Men** 9% **Minority** 5% **Part-time** 71%
Distance Learning Courses Available.
Nursing Student Activities Sigma Theta Tau, Student Nurses' Association, nursing club.
Nursing Student Resources Academic advising; academic or career counseling; assistance for students with disabilities; bookstore; campus computer network; computer lab; computer-assisted instruction; daycare for children of students; e-mail services; employment services for current students; interactive nursing skills videos; Internet; learning resource lab; library services; nursing audiovisuals; paid internships; resume preparation assistance; skills, simulation, or other laboratory; tutoring.
Library Facilities 2.1 million volumes (33,000 in health, 4,000 in nursing); 1,841 periodical subscriptions (2,400 health-care related).

BACCALAUREATE PROGRAMS

Degree BSN
Available Programs ADN to Baccalaureate; Generic Baccalaureate; RN Baccalaureate.
Study Options Full-time and part-time.
Online Degree Options Yes.
Program Entrance Requirements Minimum overall college GPA of 3.0, transcript of college record, CPR certification, health exam, health insurance, high school biology, high school chemistry, high school foreign language, 3 years high school math, 3 years high school science, high school transcript, immunizations, minimum high school GPA of 3.0, professional liability insurance/malpractice insurance, prerequisite course work. Transfer students are accepted. *Application deadline:* 5/1 (fall), 9/1 (spring), 1/15 (summer). *Application fee:* $45.
Advanced Placement Credit given for nursing courses completed elsewhere dependent upon specific evaluations.
Expenses (2012–13) *Tuition, state resident:* full-time $7864; part-time $328 per credit hour. *Tuition, nonresident:* full-time $16,984; part-time $708 per credit hour. *International tuition:* $17,004 full-time. *Room and board:* $12,468 per academic year. *Required fees:* full-time $1798; part-time $50 per credit.
Financial Aid 91% of baccalaureate students in nursing programs received some form of financial aid in 2011–12. *Gift aid (need-based):* Federal Pell, FSEOG, state, private, college/university gift aid from institutional funds, Academic Competitiveness Grants, National SMART Grants, TEACH Grants. *Loans:* Federal Direct (Subsidized and Unsubsidized Stafford PLUS), Perkins, alternative loans.*Work-study:* Federal Work-Study.*Financial aid application deadline (priority):* 4/1.
Contact Ms. Kathleen Mitchell, Assistant Dean for Student Services, College of Nursing, The University of Toledo, Mail Stop #1026, 3000 Arlington Avenue, Toledo, OH 43614-2598. *Telephone:* 419-383-5839. *Fax:* 419-383-5894. *E-mail:* kathleen.mitchell@utoledo.edu.

GRADUATE PROGRAMS

Expenses (2012–13) *Tuition, state resident:* full-time $12,595; part-time $525 per credit hour. *Tuition, nonresident:* full-time $22,828; part-time $951 per credit hour. *International tuition:* $22,848 full-time. *Room and board:* $12,468 per academic year. *Required fees:* full-time $1798; part-time $50 per credit.
Financial Aid 70% of graduate students in nursing programs received some form of financial aid in 2011–12. Federal Work-Study, institutionally sponsored loans, scholarships, traineeships, and tuition waivers (full and partial) available.
Contact Ms. Kathleen Mitchell, Graduate Nursing Advisor, College of Nursing, The University of Toledo, Mail Stop #1026, 3000 Arlington Avenue, Toledo, OH 43614-2598. *Telephone:* 419-383-5841. *Fax:* 419-383-5894. *E-mail:* kathleen.mitchell@utoledo.edu.

MASTER'S DEGREE PROGRAM
Degree MSN
Available Programs Master's; Master's for Non-Nursing College Graduates; Master's for Nurses with Non-Nursing Degrees.
Concentrations Available Clinical nurse leader; nursing education. *Nurse practitioner programs in:* family health, pediatric.
Study Options Full-time and part-time.
Program Entrance Requirements Computer literacy, minimum overall college GPA of 3.0, transcript of college record, CPR certification, written essay, immunizations, 2 letters of recommendation, resume, GRE. *Application deadline:* 12/15 (fall), 9/1 (spring). *Application fee:* $110.
Advanced Placement Credit given for nursing courses completed elsewhere dependent upon specific evaluations.
Degree Requirements 55 total credit hours, thesis or project, comprehensive exam.

POST-MASTER'S PROGRAM
Areas of Study Nursing education. *Nurse practitioner programs in:* family health, pediatric.

DOCTORAL DEGREE PROGRAM
Degree DNP
Available Programs Doctorate; Post-Baccalaureate Doctorate.
Areas of Study Advanced practice nursing, nursing administration.
Online Degree Options Yes.
Program Entrance Requirements Clinical experience, minimum overall college GPA of 3.0, interview by faculty committee, interview, 3 letters of recommendation, MSN or equivalent, statistics course, vita, writing sample. *Application deadline:* 12/15 (fall). *Application fee:* $110.

CONTINUING EDUCATION PROGRAM
Contact Ms. Deborah Mattin, Director, Continuing Nursing Education, College of Nursing, The University of Toledo, Mail Stop #1026, 3000 Arlington Avenue, Toledo, OH 43614-2598. *Telephone:* 419-383-5812. *Fax:* 419-383-5894. *E-mail:* deborah.mattin@utoledo.edu.

Urbana University
College of Nursing and Allied Health
Urbana, Ohio

http://www.urbana.edu/academics/college-of-nursing-and-allied-health/
Founded in 1850
DEGREES • BSN • MSN
Nursing Program Faculty 4 (100% with doctorates).
Baccalaureate Enrollment 50 **Women** 98% **Men** 2% **Minority** 2% **Part-time** 100%
Graduate Enrollment 100 **Women** 100% **Minority** 10% **Part-time** 100%
Distance Learning Courses Available.
Nursing Student Activities Nursing Honor Society.
Nursing Student Resources Academic advising; academic or career counseling; assistance for students with disabilities; bookstore; campus computer network; career placement assistance; computer lab; e-mail services; Internet; learning resource lab; library services; nursing audiovisuals; placement services for program completers; remedial services; resume preparation assistance; tutoring.
Library Facilities 61,600 volumes (320 in health, 250 in nursing); 800 periodical subscriptions (1,000 health-care related).

BACCALAUREATE PROGRAMS

Degree BSN
Available Programs ADN to Baccalaureate.
Site Options Dayton, OH; Springfield, OH.
Study Options Full-time and part-time.
Program Entrance Requirements Transcript of college record, CPR certification, health exam, health insurance, immunizations, letters of recommendation, professional liability insurance/malpractice insurance, RN licensure. Transfer students are accepted. *Application deadline:* Applications may be processed on a rolling basis for some programs. *Application fee:* $25.
Advanced Placement Credit given for nursing courses completed elsewhere dependent upon specific evaluations.
Expenses (2012–13) *Tuition:* part-time $450 per credit hour. *Required fees:* part-time $165 per term.
Financial Aid 10% of baccalaureate students in nursing programs received some form of financial aid in 2011–12.
Contact Dr. Sue Z. Green, BSN Program Chair, College of Nursing and Allied Health, Urbana University, Losch Hall, Suite #6, 579 College Way, Urbana, OH 43078. *Telephone:* 937-652-6734. *E-mail:* sgreen@urbana.edu.

GRADUATE PROGRAMS

Expenses (2012–13) *Tuition:* part-time $510 per credit hour. *Required fees:* part-time $165 per term.
Financial Aid 10% of graduate students in nursing programs received some form of financial aid in 2011–12.
Contact Dr. Barbara Miville, MSN Program Chair, College of Nursing and Allied Health, Urbana University, Losch Hall, Suite #6, 579 College Way, Urbana, OH 43078. *Telephone:* 937-652-6735. *E-mail:* bmiville@urbana.edu.

MASTER'S DEGREE PROGRAM
Degree MSN
Available Programs Master's; Master's for Nurses with Non-Nursing Degrees; RN to Master's.
Concentrations Available Nursing administration; nursing education.
Site Options Dayton, OH; Springfield, OH.
Study Options Full-time and part-time.
Program Entrance Requirements Computer literacy, minimum overall college GPA of 3.0, transcript of college record, CPR certification, written essay, immunizations, interview, 3 letters of recommendation, professional liability insurance/malpractice insurance, resume. *Application deadline:* 8/1 (fall), 12/1 (spring), 5/1 (summer). Applications may be processed on a rolling basis for some programs. *Application fee:* $25.
Advanced Placement Credit given for nursing courses completed elsewhere dependent upon specific evaluations.
Degree Requirements 47 total credit hours, thesis or project.

CONTINUING EDUCATION PROGRAM

Contact Ms. Terry Pope, Director, The Center for Leadership Excellence, College of Nursing and Allied Health, Urbana University, 579 College Way, Urbana, OH 43078. *Telephone:* 937-484-1239. *E-mail:* tpope@urbana.edu.

Ursuline College
The Breen School of Nursing
Pepper Pike, Ohio

Founded in 1871
DEGREES • BSN • DNP • MSN
Nursing Program Faculty 25 (35% with doctorates).
Baccalaureate Enrollment 350
Graduate Enrollment 270 **Women** 90% **Men** 10% **Minority** 28% **International** 2% **Part-time** 75%
Nursing Student Activities Nursing Honor Society, Sigma Theta Tau, Student Nurses' Association.
Nursing Student Resources Academic advising; academic or career counseling; assistance for students with disabilities; bookstore; campus computer network; career placement assistance; computer lab; computer-assisted instruction; e-mail services; employment services for current students; externships; interactive nursing skills videos; Internet; learning resource lab; library services; nursing audiovisuals; placement services for program completers; remedial services; resume preparation assistance; skills, simulation, or other laboratory; tutoring.
Library Facilities 202,253 volumes; 45,818 periodical subscriptions.

BACCALAUREATE PROGRAMS

Degree BSN
Available Programs ADN to Baccalaureate; Accelerated Baccalaureate for Second Degree; Accelerated RN Baccalaureate; Generic Baccalaureate.
Study Options Full-time.
Program Entrance Requirements Minimum overall college GPA of 2.5, transcript of college record, written essay, health exam, health insurance, high school biology, high school chemistry, 2 years high school math, 2 years high school science, high school transcript, immunizations, 1 letter of recommendation, minimum high school GPA of 2.75, minimum GPA in nursing prerequisites of 2.75. Transfer students are accepted. *Application deadline:* Applications may be processed on a rolling basis for some programs.
Advanced Placement Credit given for nursing courses completed elsewhere dependent upon specific evaluations.
Financial Aid *Gift aid (need-based):* Federal Pell, FSEOG, state, private, college/university gift aid from institutional funds, United Negro College Fund. *Loans:* Federal Direct (Subsidized and Unsubsidized Stafford PLUS), Perkins, state, college/university. *Work-study:* Federal Work-Study. *Financial aid application deadline:* Continuous.
Contact Elizabeth Beach, Coordinator, BSN Enrollment, The Breen School of Nursing, Ursuline College, 2550 Lander Road, Pepper Pike, OH 44124-4398. *Telephone:* 440-449-4200. *Fax:* 440-449-4267.

GRADUATE PROGRAMS

Contact Dr. Janet R. Baker, Director, Graduate Program, The Breen School of Nursing, Ursuline College, 2550 Lander Road, Pepper Pike, OH 44124-4398. *Telephone:* 440-449-4200 Ext. 8172. *Fax:* 440-684-6053. *E-mail:* jbaker@ursuline.edu.

MASTER'S DEGREE PROGRAM
Degree MSN
Available Programs Accelerated Master's; Master's.
Concentrations Available Nurse case management; nursing education; nursing informatics. *Clinical nurse specialist programs in:* adult health, palliative care. *Nurse practitioner programs in:* adult health, family health.
Study Options Full-time and part-time.
Program Entrance Requirements Clinical experience, minimum overall college GPA of 3.0, transcript of college record, CPR certification, written essay, immunizations, 3 letters of recommendation, resume. *Application deadline:* 6/15 (fall), 12/15 (spring). Applications may be processed on a rolling basis for some programs.
Advanced Placement Credit given for nursing courses completed elsewhere dependent upon specific evaluations.
Degree Requirements 43 total credit hours, thesis or project.

POST-MASTER'S PROGRAM

Areas of Study Nurse case management; nursing education; nursing informatics. *Clinical nurse specialist programs in:* adult health, palliative care. *Nurse practitioner programs in:* adult health, family health.

DOCTORAL DEGREE PROGRAM

Degree DNP

Available Programs Doctorate.

Program Entrance Requirements Clinical experience, minimum overall college GPA of 3.0, 2 letters of recommendation, MSN or equivalent, vita, writing sample. *Application deadline:* 5/15 (fall). *Application fee:* $25.

Degree Requirements 38 total credit hours, dissertation.

See display on this page and full description on page 512.

Walsh University
Department of Nursing
North Canton, Ohio

http://www.walsh.edu/
Founded in 1958

DEGREES • BSN • DNP • MSN

Nursing Program Faculty 18 (40% with doctorates).
Baccalaureate Enrollment 271 **Women** 77% **Men** 23% **Minority** 5% **International** 1% **Part-time** 10%
Graduate Enrollment 32 **Women** 100% **Part-time** 80%
Distance Learning Courses Available.
Nursing Student Activities Sigma Theta Tau, Student Nurses' Association.
Nursing Student Resources Academic advising; academic or career counseling; assistance for students with disabilities; bookstore; campus computer network; career placement assistance; computer lab; computer-assisted instruction; e-mail services; employment services for current students; housing assistance; interactive nursing skills videos; Internet; learning resource lab; library services; nursing audiovisuals; placement services for program completers; remedial services; resume preparation assistance; skills, simulation, or other laboratory; tutoring.
Library Facilities 252,014 volumes (4,000 in health, 2,000 in nursing); 61,193 periodical subscriptions (114 health-care related).

BACCALAUREATE PROGRAMS

Degree BSN

Available Programs Accelerated Baccalaureate; Accelerated Baccalaureate for Second Degree; Generic Baccalaureate; RN Baccalaureate.
Site Options Akron, OH; Canton, OH.
Study Options Full-time and part-time.
Program Entrance Requirements Transcript of college record, CPR certification, health exam, health insurance, high school chemistry, high school foreign language, 3 years high school math, 3 years high school science, high school transcript, immunizations, minimum high school GPA of 2.3, minimum GPA in nursing prerequisites of 2.75, professional liability insurance/malpractice insurance, prerequisite course work. Transfer students are accepted. *Application deadline:* 8/15 (fall), 12/31 (spring), 4/15 (summer). Applications may be processed on a rolling basis for some programs. *Application fee:* $25.
Advanced Placement Credit by examination available. Credit given for nursing courses completed elsewhere dependent upon specific evaluations.
Expenses (2012–13) *Tuition:* full-time $23,550; part-time $785 per credit. *International tuition:* $23,550 full-time. *Room and board:* $10,200; room only: $6000 per academic year. *Required fees:* full-time $1140; part-time $38 per credit.
Financial Aid 94% of baccalaureate students in nursing programs received some form of financial aid in 2011–12.
Contact Dr. Linda G. Linc, Professor and Chair, Department of Nursing, Walsh University, 2020 East Maple Street, North Canton, OH 44720-3336. *Telephone:* 330-490-7251. *Fax:* 330-490-7206. *E-mail:* llinc@walsh.edu.

GRADUATE PROGRAMS

Expenses (2012–13) *Tuition:* full-time $5265; part-time $585 per credit. *International tuition:* $5265 full-time. *Room and board:* $10,200; room only: $6000 per academic year.

Financial Aid 40% of graduate students in nursing programs received some form of financial aid in 2011–12.
Contact Dr. Karen Gehrling, Director, Graduate Programs, Department of Nursing, Walsh University, 2020 East Maple Street, North Canton, OH 44720. *Telephone:* 330-490-7251. *Fax:* 330-490-7206. *E-mail:* kgehrling@walsh.edu.

MASTER'S DEGREE PROGRAM
Degree MSN
Available Programs Accelerated AD/RN to Master's; Master's.
Concentrations Available Clinical nurse leader; nursing education.
Study Options Full-time and part-time.
Online Degree Options Yes (online only).
Program Entrance Requirements Minimum overall college GPA of 3.0, transcript of college record, written essay, interview, statistics course. *Application deadline:* Applications may be processed on a rolling basis for some programs. *Application fee:* $25.
Advanced Placement Credit given for nursing courses completed elsewhere dependent upon specific evaluations.
Degree Requirements 36 total credit hours, thesis or project.

DOCTORAL DEGREE PROGRAM
Degree DNP
Available Programs Post-Baccalaureate Doctorate.
Areas of Study Ethics, health policy, health promotion/disease prevention, health-care systems, information systems, nurse case management, nursing administration, nursing policy, nursing research, nursing science.
Online Degree Options Yes (online only).
Program Entrance Requirements Minimum overall college GPA of 3.0, interview by faculty committee, interview, 2 letters of recommendation, MSN or equivalent, statistics course, writing sample. *Application deadline:* Applications may be processed on a rolling basis for some programs. *Application fee:* $25.
Degree Requirements 38 total credit hours, residency.

Wright State University
College of Nursing and Health
Dayton, Ohio

http://nursing.wright.edu/
Founded in 1964
DEGREES • BSN • DNP • MS • MS/MBA
Nursing Program Faculty 68 (33% with doctorates).
Baccalaureate Enrollment 787 **Women** 84% **Men** 16% **Minority** 16% **International** 1% **Part-time** 35%
Graduate Enrollment 257 **Women** 94% **Men** 6% **Minority** 14% **Part-time** 86%
Distance Learning Courses Available.
Nursing Student Activities Nursing Honor Society, Sigma Theta Tau, Student Nurses' Association, nursing club.
Nursing Student Resources Academic advising; academic or career counseling; assistance for students with disabilities; bookstore; campus computer network; career placement assistance; computer lab; computer-assisted instruction; daycare for children of students; e-mail services; employment services for current students; externships; housing assistance; interactive nursing skills videos; Internet; learning resource lab; library services; nursing audiovisuals; remedial services; resume preparation assistance; skills, simulation, or other laboratory; tutoring.
Library Facilities 910,287 volumes (111,826 in health, 7,646 in nursing); 36,138 periodical subscriptions (1,279 health-care related).

BACCALAUREATE PROGRAMS
Degree BSN
Available Programs Accelerated Baccalaureate for Second Degree; Baccalaureate for Second Degree; Generic Baccalaureate; RN Baccalaureate.
Site Options Dayton, OH; Chillicothe, OH; Celina, OH.
Study Options Full-time and part-time.
Program Entrance Requirements Minimum overall college GPA of 2.5, transcript of college record, written essay, high school transcript, minimum GPA in nursing prerequisites of 2.5, prerequisite course work. Transfer students are accepted. *Application deadline:* 6/30 (fall), 12/30 (spring).

Advanced Placement Credit by examination available. Credit given for nursing courses completed elsewhere dependent upon specific evaluations.
Contact *Telephone:* 937-775-3132. *Fax:* 937-775-4571.

GRADUATE PROGRAMS
Contact *Telephone:* 937-775-3577. *Fax:* 937-775-4571.

MASTER'S DEGREE PROGRAM
Degrees MS; MS/MBA
Available Programs Master's; Master's for Nurses with Non-Nursing Degrees.
Concentrations Available Clinical nurse leader; health-care administration; nursing administration. *Clinical nurse specialist programs in:* adult health, community health, pediatric, public health, school health. *Nurse practitioner programs in:* acute care, family health, pediatric.
Study Options Full-time and part-time.
Online Degree Options Yes.
Program Entrance Requirements Clinical experience, computer literacy, minimum overall college GPA of 3.0, transcript of college record, written essay, interview, physical assessment course, statistics course, GRE General Test. *Application deadline:* Applications may be processed on a rolling basis for some programs. *Application fee:* $30.
Advanced Placement Credit given for nursing courses completed elsewhere dependent upon specific evaluations.
Degree Requirements 48 total credit hours, thesis or project.

POST-MASTER'S PROGRAM
Areas of Study *Clinical nurse specialist programs in:* school health. *Nurse practitioner programs in:* acute care, family health, pediatric.

DOCTORAL DEGREE PROGRAM
Degree DNP
Available Programs Doctorate.
Areas of Study Advanced practice nursing, biology of health and illness, clinical practice, community health, family health, health policy, health promotion/disease prevention, health-care systems, information systems, nursing administration, nursing policy, nursing science.
Online Degree Options Yes (online only).
Program Entrance Requirements Clinical experience, minimum overall college GPA of 3.3, interview by faculty committee, 3 letters of recommendation, MSN or equivalent, statistics course, vita, writing sample.
Degree Requirements 54 total credit hours, dissertation.

CONTINUING EDUCATION PROGRAM
Contact *Telephone:* 937-775-3577. *Fax:* 937-775-4571.

Xavier University
School of Nursing
Cincinnati, Ohio

Founded in 1831
DEGREES • BSN • MSN • MSN/ED D • MSN/MBA
Nursing Program Faculty 72 (11% with doctorates).
Baccalaureate Enrollment 317 **Women** 90% **Men** 10% **Minority** 10% **Part-time** 18%
Graduate Enrollment 235 **Women** 96% **Men** 4% **Minority** 10% **Part-time** 72%
Nursing Student Activities Sigma Theta Tau, nursing club.
Nursing Student Resources Academic advising; academic or career counseling; assistance for students with disabilities; bookstore; campus computer network; career placement assistance; computer lab; computer-assisted instruction; e-mail services; employment services for current students; externships; housing assistance; interactive nursing skills videos; Internet; learning resource lab; library services; nursing audiovisuals; remedial services; resume preparation assistance; skills, simulation, or other laboratory; tutoring.
Library Facilities 470,438 volumes (8,900 in health, 1,160 in nursing); 62,558 periodical subscriptions (200 health-care related).

BACCALAUREATE PROGRAMS
Degree BSN
Available Programs Generic Baccalaureate.
Study Options Full-time and part-time.

Program Entrance Requirements Minimum overall college GPA of 2.7, transcript of college record, written essay, high school chemistry, high school foreign language, 3 years high school math, 2 years high school science, high school transcript, minimum high school GPA of 3.0. Transfer students are accepted. *Application deadline:* Applications may be processed on a rolling basis for some programs. *Application fee:* $35.
Advanced Placement Credit given for nursing courses completed elsewhere dependent upon specific evaluations.
Expenses (2012–13) *Room and board:* $10,000; room only: $5600 per academic year.
Financial Aid 90% of baccalaureate students in nursing programs received some form of financial aid in 2011–12. *Gift aid (need-based):* Federal Pell, FSEOG, state, private, college/university gift aid from institutional funds. *Loans:* Federal Direct (Subsidized and Unsubsidized Stafford PLUS), Perkins.*Work-study:* Federal Work-Study, part-time campus jobs.*Financial aid application deadline (priority):* 2/15.
Contact Ms. Marilyn Volk Gomez, Director of Nursing Student Services, School of Nursing, Xavier University, 3800 Victory Parkway, Cincinnati, OH 45207-7351. *Telephone:* 513-745-4392. *Fax:* 513-745-1087. *E-mail:* gomez@xavier.edu.

GRADUATE PROGRAMS

Expenses (2012–13) *Tuition:* part-time $588 per credit hour.
Financial Aid 30% of graduate students in nursing programs received some form of financial aid in 2011–12.
Contact Ms. Marilyn Volk Gomez, Director of Nursing Student Services, School of Nursing, Xavier University, 3800 Victory Parkway, Cincinnati, OH 45207-7351. *Telephone:* 513-745-4392. *Fax:* 513-745-1087. *E-mail:* gomez@xavier.edu.

MASTER'S DEGREE PROGRAM

Degrees MSN; MSN/Ed D; MSN/MBA
Available Programs Accelerated Master's for Non-Nursing College Graduates; Master's; Master's for Nurses with Non-Nursing Degrees; RN to Master's.
Concentrations Available Clinical nurse leader; nursing administration; nursing education; nursing informatics. *Clinical nurse specialist programs in:* forensic nursing, school health.
Study Options Full-time and part-time.
Program Entrance Requirements Minimum overall college GPA of 2.8, transcript of college record, written essay, 3 letters of recommendation, statistics course, GRE. *Application deadline:* Applications may be processed on a rolling basis for some programs.
Degree Requirements 36 total credit hours, thesis or project.

Youngstown State University

Department of Nursing
Youngstown, Ohio

Founded in 1908
DEGREES • BSN • MSN
Nursing Program Faculty 22 (18% with doctorates).
Baccalaureate Enrollment 22
Graduate Enrollment 24 **Women** 75% **Men** 25% **Minority** 13%
Nursing Student Activities Sigma Theta Tau, Student Nurses' Association.
Nursing Student Resources Academic advising; academic or career counseling; assistance for students with disabilities; bookstore; campus computer network; career placement assistance; computer lab; computer-assisted instruction; e-mail services; housing assistance; interactive nursing skills videos; Internet; learning resource lab; library services; nursing audiovisuals; placement services for program completers; resume preparation assistance; skills, simulation, or other laboratory; tutoring.
Library Facilities 853,993 volumes; 44,678 periodical subscriptions.

BACCALAUREATE PROGRAMS

Degree BSN
Site Options Boardman, OH.
Study Options Full-time.
Program Entrance Requirements Minimum overall college GPA of 2.0, transcript of college record, CPR certification, health exam, health insurance, high school biology, high school chemistry, high school foreign language, 3 years high school math, 3 years high school science, high school transcript, immunizations, minimum high school GPA, minimum high school rank, minimum GPA in nursing prerequisites of 2.5, prerequisite course work. Transfer students are accepted.

Advanced Placement Credit by examination available. Credit given for nursing courses completed elsewhere dependent upon specific evaluations.
Contact *Telephone:* 330-941-2328. *Fax:* 330-941-2309.

GRADUATE PROGRAMS

Contact *Telephone:* 330-941-1796. *Fax:* 330-941-2309.

MASTER'S DEGREE PROGRAM

Degree MSN
Concentrations Available Nurse anesthesia; nursing education.
Study Options Full-time and part-time.
Program Entrance Requirements Clinical experience, computer literacy, transcript of college record, CPR certification, written essay, immunizations, nursing research course, physical assessment course, prerequisite course work, resume, GRE General Test.
Advanced Placement Credit given for nursing courses completed elsewhere dependent upon specific evaluations.
Degree Requirements Thesis or project.

OKLAHOMA

Bacone College
Department of Nursing
Muskogee, Oklahoma

Founded in 1880
DEGREE • BSN
Nursing Program Faculty 8
Baccalaureate Enrollment 16 **Women** 100% **Minority** 65%
Nursing Student Activities Student Nurses' Association, nursing club.
Nursing Student Resources Academic advising; bookstore; campus computer network; computer lab; computer-assisted instruction; interactive nursing skills videos; Internet; learning resource lab; library services; nursing audiovisuals; remedial services; skills, simulation, or other laboratory.
Library Facilities 34,564 volumes; 121 periodical subscriptions.

BACCALAUREATE PROGRAMS

Degree BSN
Available Programs Accelerated RN Baccalaureate.
Program Entrance Requirements Transcript of college record, CPR certification, health exam, health insurance, immunizations, 2 letters of recommendation, minimum GPA in nursing prerequisites of 2.5, prerequisite course work, RN licensure.
Contact *Telephone:* 888-682-5514.

East Central University
Department of Nursing
Ada, Oklahoma

http://www.ecok.edu/colleges/health_sciences/nursing/index.htm
Founded in 1909
DEGREE • BS
Nursing Program Faculty 17 (31% with doctorates).
Baccalaureate Enrollment 495 **Women** 86% **Men** 14% **Minority** 44%
International 1% **Part-time** 14%
Distance Learning Courses Available.
Nursing Student Activities Student Nurses' Association.
Nursing Student Resources Academic advising; academic or career counseling; assistance for students with disabilities; bookstore; campus computer network; career placement assistance; computer lab; computer-assisted instruction; daycare for children of students; e-mail services; employment services for current students; externships; housing assistance; interactive nursing skills videos; Internet; learning resource lab; library services; nursing audiovisuals; other; placement services for program completers; resume preparation assistance; skills, simulation, or other laboratory; tutoring.

Library Facilities 268,734 volumes (2,236 in health, 893 in nursing); 47,935 periodical subscriptions (266 health-care related).

BACCALAUREATE PROGRAMS

Degree BS
Available Programs ADN to Baccalaureate; Generic Baccalaureate.
Site Options Ardmore, OK; McAlester, OK; Durant, OK.
Study Options Full-time and part-time.
Program Entrance Requirements Minimum overall college GPA of 2.5, transcript of college record, CPR certification, health exam, immunizations, minimum GPA in nursing prerequisites of 2.5, professional liability insurance/malpractice insurance, prerequisite course work. Transfer students are accepted. *Application deadline:* 9/17 (spring).
Advanced Placement Credit given for nursing courses completed elsewhere dependent upon specific evaluations.
Contact *Telephone:* 580-310-5434. *Fax:* 580-310-5785.

Langston University
School of Nursing and Health Professions
Langston, Oklahoma

http://www.langston.edu/academics/nursing_health_professions.aspx
Founded in 1897

DEGREE • BSN
Nursing Program Faculty 16 (13% with doctorates).
Nursing Student Activities Student Nurses' Association, nursing club.
Nursing Student Resources Academic advising; academic or career counseling; assistance for students with disabilities; bookstore; campus computer network; career placement assistance; computer lab; computer-assisted instruction; daycare for children of students; e-mail services; housing assistance; interactive nursing skills videos; Internet; learning resource lab; library services; nursing audiovisuals; remedial services; resume preparation assistance; skills, simulation, or other laboratory; tutoring.
Library Facilities 97,565 volumes (35,397 in health, 2,664 in nursing); 1,235 periodical subscriptions (978 health-care related).

BACCALAUREATE PROGRAMS

Degree BSN
Available Programs Generic Baccalaureate; LPN to Baccalaureate; RN Baccalaureate.
Site Options Tulsa, OK.
Study Options Full-time and part-time.
Program Entrance Requirements Minimum overall college GPA of 2.5, transcript of college record, written essay, health exam, immunizations, minimum GPA in nursing prerequisites of 2.5, professional liability insurance/malpractice insurance, prerequisite course work. Transfer students are accepted.
Advanced Placement Credit by examination available. Credit given for nursing courses completed elsewhere dependent upon specific evaluations.
Contact *Telephone:* 405-466-3411. *Fax:* 405-466-2195.

Northeastern State University
Department of Nursing
Tahlequah, Oklahoma

http://academics.nsuok.edu/Default.aspx?alias=academics.nsuok.edu/healthprofessions
Founded in 1846

DEGREES • BSN • MSN
Nursing Program Faculty 6 (33% with doctorates).
Baccalaureate Enrollment 120 Women 92% Men 8% Minority 29% Part-time 94%
Graduate Enrollment 15 Women 93% Men 7% Minority 27% Part-time 100%
Distance Learning Courses Available.
Nursing Student Activities Sigma Theta Tau, Student Nurses' Association.
Nursing Student Resources Academic advising; academic or career counseling; assistance for students with disabilities; bookstore; campus computer network; career placement assistance; computer lab; computer-assisted instruction; e-mail services; employment services for current students; housing assistance; Internet; library services; nursing audiovisuals; placement services for program completers; resume preparation assistance; tutoring.
Library Facilities 429,808 volumes (21,000 in health, 15,500 in nursing); 5,758 periodical subscriptions (1,000 health-care related).

BACCALAUREATE PROGRAMS

Degree BSN
Available Programs Accelerated RN Baccalaureate; RN Baccalaureate.
Site Options Broken Arrow, OK; Miami, OK; Muskogee, OK.
Online Degree Options Yes (online only).
Program Entrance Requirements Minimum overall college GPA of 2.0, transcript of college record, CPR certification, health exam, immunizations, 3 letters of recommendation, minimum GPA in nursing prerequisites of 2.0, professional liability insurance/malpractice insurance, prerequisite course work, RN licensure. Transfer students are accepted.
Expenses (2011–12) *Tuition, state resident:* full-time $3495; part-time $117 per credit hour. *Tuition, nonresident:* full-time $10,020; part-time $334 per credit hour. *International tuition:* $10,060 full-time. *Room and board:* $6550 per academic year. *Required fees:* full-time $1107; part-time $37 per credit.
Financial Aid 80% of baccalaureate students in nursing programs received some form of financial aid in 2010–11.
Contact Dr. Joyce A. Van Nostrand, Chair, Nursing Program and Department of Health Professions, Department of Nursing, Northeastern State University, PO Box 549, Muskogee, OK 74402-0549. *Telephone:* 918-781-5410. *Fax:* 918-781-5411. *E-mail:* vannostr@nsuok.edu.

GRADUATE PROGRAMS

Expenses (2011–12) *Tuition, state resident:* full-time $4530; part-time $151 per credit hour. *Tuition, nonresident:* full-time $11,940; part-time $398 per credit hour. *International tuition:* $11,980 full-time. *Room and board:* $6525 per academic year. *Required fees:* full-time $1107; part-time $37 per credit.
Financial Aid 80% of graduate students in nursing programs received some form of financial aid in 2010–11.
Contact Dr. Joyce A. Van Nostrand, Chair, Nursing Program and Department of Health Professions, Department of Nursing, Northeastern State University, PO Box 549, Muskogee, OK 74402-0549. *Telephone:* 918-781-5410. *Fax:* 918-781-5411. *E-mail:* vannostr@nsuok.edu.

MASTER'S DEGREE PROGRAM
Degree MSN
Available Programs Master's.
Concentrations Available Nursing education.
Site Options Broken Arrow, OK; Miami, OK; Muskogee, OK.
Study Options Full-time and part-time.
Online Degree Options Yes (online only).
Program Entrance Requirements Minimum overall college GPA of 3.0, transcript of college record, CPR certification, immunizations, 3 letters of recommendation, nursing research course, professional liability insurance/malpractice insurance, statistics course. *Application deadline:* 8/1 (fall), 1/2 (spring).
Advanced Placement Credit given for nursing courses completed elsewhere dependent upon specific evaluations.
Degree Requirements 32 total credit hours, thesis or project.

Northwestern Oklahoma State University
Division of Nursing
Alva, Oklahoma

http://www.nwosu.edu/nursing
Founded in 1897

DEGREE • BSN
Nursing Program Faculty 15 (.02% with doctorates).
Baccalaureate Enrollment 60 Women 98% Men 2% Minority 2% International 2% Part-time 1%
Distance Learning Courses Available.
Nursing Student Activities Nursing Honor Society, Student Nurses' Association.
Nursing Student Resources Academic advising; academic or career counseling; assistance for students with disabilities; bookstore; campus

computer network; career placement assistance; computer lab; computer-assisted instruction; e-mail services; housing assistance; interactive nursing skills videos; Internet; learning resource lab; library services; nursing audiovisuals; remedial services; skills, simulation, or other laboratory; tutoring.
Library Facilities 233,792 volumes; 17,100 periodical subscriptions (59 health-care related).

BACCALAUREATE PROGRAMS

Degree BSN
Available Programs ADN to Baccalaureate; Accelerated Baccalaureate; Accelerated LPN to Baccalaureate; Accelerated RN Baccalaureate; Baccalaureate for Second Degree; Generic Baccalaureate; LPN to Baccalaureate; LPN to RN Baccalaureate; RN Baccalaureate.
Site Options Enid, OK; Woodward, OK; Alva, OK.
Study Options Full-time and part-time.
Program Entrance Requirements Minimum overall college GPA of 2.5, transcript of college record, CPR certification, health exam, high school transcript, immunizations, 3 letters of recommendation, minimum high school GPA of 2.5, minimum GPA in nursing prerequisites of 2.5, professional liability insurance/malpractice insurance, prerequisite course work. Transfer students are accepted. *Application deadline:* 2/2 (spring).
Advanced Placement Credit by examination available. Credit given for nursing courses completed elsewhere dependent upon specific evaluations.
Expenses (2011–12) *Tuition, state resident:* full-time $3968; part-time $132 per credit hour. *Tuition, nonresident:* full-time $9518; part-time $317 per credit hour. *Room and board:* $3700 per academic year. *Required fees:* full-time $623.
Financial Aid 74% of baccalaureate students in nursing programs received some form of financial aid in 2010–11. *Gift aid (need-based):* Federal Pell, FSEOG, state, private, college/university gift aid from institutional funds. *Loans:* Federal Direct (Subsidized and Unsubsidized Stafford PLUS).*Work-study:* Federal Work-Study, part-time campus jobs.*Financial aid application deadline:* Continuous.
Contact Dr. Carole McKenzie, Division Chair, Division of Nursing, Northwestern Oklahoma State University, 709 Oklahoma Boulevard, Alva, OK 73717-2799. *Telephone:* 580-327-8489. *Fax:* 580-327-8434. *E-mail:* camckenzie@nwosu.edu.

Oklahoma Baptist University
School of Nursing
Shawnee, Oklahoma

http://www.okbu.edu/
Founded in 1910
DEGREES • BSN • MSN
Nursing Program Faculty 24 (28% with doctorates).
Baccalaureate Enrollment 203 **Women** 95% **Men** 5% **Minority** 8% **International** 1% **Part-time** 4%
Graduate Enrollment 34 **Women** 94% **Men** 6% **Minority** 8% **International** 6%
Nursing Student Activities Sigma Theta Tau, Student Nurses' Association.
Nursing Student Resources Academic advising; academic or career counseling; assistance for students with disabilities; bookstore; campus computer network; computer lab; computer-assisted instruction; e-mail services; externships; Internet; learning resource lab; library services; nursing audiovisuals; remedial services; resume preparation assistance; skills, simulation, or other laboratory; tutoring; unpaid internships.
Library Facilities 230,000 volumes (10,000 in health, 5,500 in nursing); 1,800 periodical subscriptions (65 health-care related).

BACCALAUREATE PROGRAMS

Degree BSN
Available Programs ADN to Baccalaureate; Baccalaureate for Second Degree; Generic Baccalaureate; LPN to RN Baccalaureate; RN Baccalaureate.
Study Options Full-time and part-time.
Program Entrance Requirements Minimum overall college GPA of 2.25, transcript of college record, CPR certification, health exam, high school transcript, immunizations, minimum GPA in nursing prerequisites of 2.3, prerequisite course work. Transfer students are accepted. *Application deadline:* 4/1 (fall), 4/1 (winter), 4/1 (spring), 7/15 (summer).
Expenses (2011–12) *Tuition:* full-time $17,220; part-time $560 per credit hour. *International tuition:* $17,295 full-time. *Room and board:* $2815;

room only: $686 per academic year. *Required fees:* full-time $560; part-time $20 per credit.
Financial Aid 93% of baccalaureate students in nursing programs received some form of financial aid in 2010–11.
Contact Dr. Lana Bolhouse, Dean, School of Nursing, Oklahoma Baptist University, 500 West University, Shawnee, OK 74804. *Telephone:* 405-878-2081. *Fax:* 405-878-2083. *E-mail:* lana.bolhouse@okbu.edu.

GRADUATE PROGRAMS

Expenses (2011–12) *Tuition:* full-time $16,575; part-time $425 per credit hour.
Financial Aid 100% of graduate students in nursing programs received some form of financial aid in 2010–11.
Contact Mrs. Lana Melton, Administrative Assistant, School of Nursing, Oklahoma Baptist University, 111 Harrison, Oklahoma City, OK 73104. *Telephone:* 405-319-8470. *E-mail:* Lana.Melton@okbu.edu.

MASTER'S DEGREE PROGRAM
Degree MSN
Available Programs Master's.
Concentrations Available Nursing education.
Site Options Oklahoma City, OK.
Study Options Full-time.
Program Entrance Requirements Clinical experience, minimum overall college GPA of 3.0, transcript of college record, written essay, resume, statistics course. *Application deadline:* 7/30 (fall), 12/20 (winter), 7/30 (spring), 7/30 (summer). Applications may be processed on a rolling basis for some programs.
Degree Requirements 39 total credit hours, thesis or project.

Oklahoma Christian University
Nursing Program
Oklahoma City, Oklahoma

Founded in 1950
DEGREE • BSN
Library Facilities 141,980 volumes; 30,835 periodical subscriptions.

BACCALAUREATE PROGRAMS

Degree BSN
Available Programs Generic Baccalaureate.
Program Entrance Requirements Minimum overall college GPA of 2.75, 3 letters of recommendation.
Contact *Telephone:* 405-425-1921.

Oklahoma City University
Kramer School of Nursing
Oklahoma City, Oklahoma

http://www.okcu.edu/nursing
Founded in 1904
DEGREES • BSN • DNP • MSN • MSN/MBA • PHD
Nursing Program Faculty 49 (31% with doctorates).
Baccalaureate Enrollment 457 **Women** 80% **Men** 20% **Minority** 40% **International** 20% **Part-time** 10%
Graduate Enrollment 73 **Women** 85% **Men** 15% **Minority** 15% **International** 4% **Part-time** 65%
Nursing Student Activities Sigma Theta Tau, Student Nurses' Association.
Nursing Student Resources Academic advising; academic or career counseling; assistance for students with disabilities; bookstore; campus computer network; career placement assistance; computer lab; computer-assisted instruction; e-mail services; employment services for current students; housing assistance; interactive nursing skills videos; Internet; learning resource lab; library services; nursing audiovisuals; placement services for program completers; remedial services; resume preparation assistance; skills, simulation, or other laboratory; tutoring.
Library Facilities 520,953 volumes (2,714 in health, 590 in nursing); 14,000 periodical subscriptions (234 health-care related).

BACCALAUREATE PROGRAMS

Degree BSN

Available Programs ADN to Baccalaureate; Accelerated Baccalaureate; Accelerated Baccalaureate for Second Degree; Baccalaureate for Second Degree; Generic Baccalaureate; International Nurse to Baccalaureate; RN Baccalaureate.

Site Options Lawton, OK; Ardmore , OK.

Study Options Full-time and part-time.

Program Entrance Requirements Minimum overall college GPA of 3.0, transcript of college record, CPR certification, written essay, health insurance, high school transcript, immunizations, minimum GPA in nursing prerequisites of 3.0, prerequisite course work. Transfer students are accepted. *Application deadline:* 8/1 (fall), 12/1 (spring), 4/1 (summer). Applications may be processed on a rolling basis for some programs. *Application fee:* $50.

Advanced Placement Credit by examination available. Credit given for nursing courses completed elsewhere dependent upon specific evaluations.

Expenses (2012–13) *Tuition:* full-time $24,740; part-time $840 per credit hour. *International tuition:* $24,740 full-time. *Room and board:* $9210 per academic year. *Required fees:* full-time $6720; part-time $210 per credit.

Financial Aid 85% of baccalaureate students in nursing programs received some form of financial aid in 2011–12. *Gift aid (need-based):* Federal Pell, FSEOG, state, private, college/university gift aid from institutional funds, United Negro College Fund, Federal Nursing, Native American Grants. *Loans:* Federal Nursing Student Loans, Federal Direct (Subsidized and Unsubsidized Stafford PLUS), Perkins. *Work-study:* Federal Work-Study, part-time campus jobs. *Financial aid application deadline (priority):* 3/1.

Contact Ms. Debbie Taber, Intake Specialist, Kramer School of Nursing, Oklahoma City University, 2501 North Blackwelder Avenue, Oklahoma City, OK 73106-1493. *Telephone:* 405-208-5924. *Fax:* 405-208-5914. *E-mail:* djtaber@okcu.edu.

GRADUATE PROGRAMS

Expenses (2012–13) *Tuition:* full-time $11,232; part-time $936 per credit hour. *International tuition:* $11,232 full-time. *Room and board:* $9210 per academic year. *Required fees:* full-time $2520; part-time $210 per credit.

Financial Aid 92% of graduate students in nursing programs received some form of financial aid in 2011–12.

Contact Mrs. Nicole Allison-Catalfu, Graduate Specialist, Kramer School of Nursing, Oklahoma City University, 2501 North Blackwelder Avenue, Oklahoma City, OK 73106-1493. *Telephone:* 405-208-5960. *Fax:* 405-208-5914. *E-mail:* neallisoncatalfu@okcu.edu.

MASTER'S DEGREE PROGRAM

Degrees MSN; MSN/MBA

Available Programs Accelerated AD/RN to Master's; Accelerated Master's; Accelerated Master's for Nurses with Non-Nursing Degrees; Accelerated RN to Master's; Master's; Master's for Nurses with Non-Nursing Degrees; RN to Master's.

Concentrations Available Nursing administration; nursing education.

Study Options Full-time and part-time.

Program Entrance Requirements Minimum overall college GPA of 3.0, transcript of college record, written essay, nursing research course, physical assessment course, statistics course. *Application deadline:* 8/1 (fall), 12/1 (spring), 4/1 (summer). Applications may be processed on a rolling basis for some programs. *Application fee:* $50.

Advanced Placement Credit given for nursing courses completed elsewhere dependent upon specific evaluations.

Degree Requirements 33 total credit hours, thesis or project.

POST-MASTER'S PROGRAM

Areas of Study *Nurse practitioner programs in:* family health.

DOCTORAL DEGREE PROGRAM

Degree DNP

Available Programs Doctorate, Doctorate for Nurses with Non-Nursing Degrees, Post-Baccalaureate Doctorate.

Areas of Study Clinical practice, nursing administration, nursing education.

Program Entrance Requirements Minimum overall college GPA of 3.5, clinical experience, interview by faculty committee, MSN or equivalent, statistics course, vita, writing sample. *Application deadline:* 4/1 (fall). *Application fee:* $50.

Degree Requirements 90 total credit hours, dissertation, oral exam, residency, written exam.

DOCTORAL DEGREE PROGRAM

Degree PhD

Available Programs Doctorate; Doctorate for Nurses with Non-Nursing Degrees; Post-Baccalaureate Doctorate.

Areas of Study Nursing administration, nursing education.

Program Entrance Requirements Clinical experience, minimum overall college GPA of 3.5, interview by faculty committee, MSN or equivalent, statistics course, vita, writing sample. *Application deadline:* 4/1 (fall). *Application fee:* $50.

Degree Requirements 90 total credit hours, dissertation, oral exam, written exam, residency.

CONTINUING EDUCATION PROGRAM

Contact Mr. Christopher Black, Director of Communications and Outreach, Kramer School of Nursing, Oklahoma City University, 2501 North Blackwelder Avenue, Oklahoma City, OK 73106-1493. *Telephone:* 405-208-5832. *Fax:* 405-208-5914. *E-mail:* cblack@okcu.edu.

Oklahoma Panhandle State University
Bachelor of Science in Nursing Program
Goodwell, Oklahoma

http://www.opsu.edu/
Founded in 1909

DEGREE • BSN

Nursing Program Faculty 4

Baccalaureate Enrollment 57 **Women** 90% **Men** 10% **Minority** 19% **Part-time** 73%

Distance Learning Courses Available.

Nursing Student Activities Student Nurses' Association.

Nursing Student Resources Academic advising; academic or career counseling; assistance for students with disabilities; bookstore; campus computer network; computer-assisted instruction; e-mail services; Internet; library services.

Library Facilities 1,019 volumes in health, 380 volumes in nursing; 2,032 periodical subscriptions health-care related.

BACCALAUREATE PROGRAMS

Degree BSN

Available Programs ADN to Baccalaureate.

Study Options Full-time and part-time.

Online Degree Options Yes (online only).

Program Entrance Requirements Minimum overall college GPA of 2.0, transcript of college record, CPR certification, immunizations, minimum GPA in nursing prerequisites of 2.0, RN licensure. Transfer students are accepted. *Application deadline:* 8/1 (fall), 1/10 (spring), 5/20 (summer).

Advanced Placement Credit given for nursing courses completed elsewhere dependent upon specific evaluations.

Contact *Telephone:* 580-349-1520. *Fax:* 580-349-1529.

Oklahoma Wesleyan University
School of Nursing
Bartlesville, Oklahoma

http://www.okwu.edu/
Founded in 1909

DEGREE • BSN

Nursing Program Faculty 31 (35% with doctorates).

Baccalaureate Enrollment 140 **Women** 96% **Men** 4% **Minority** 23%

Nursing Student Resources Academic advising; academic or career counseling; assistance for students with disabilities; bookstore; campus computer network; computer lab; computer-assisted instruction; interactive nursing skills videos; Internet; learning resource lab; library services; nursing audiovisuals; skills, simulation, or other laboratory.

Library Facilities 108,717 volumes (946 in health, 483 in nursing); 82 periodical subscriptions (40 health-care related).

BACCALAUREATE PROGRAMS

Degree BSN

Available Programs ADN to Baccalaureate; Accelerated RN Baccalaureate; Baccalaureate for Second Degree; Generic Baccalaureate; International Nurse to Baccalaureate; LPN to Baccalaureate; RN Baccalaureate.
Study Options Full-time.
Program Entrance Requirements Minimum overall college GPA of 2.3, transcript of college record, CPR certification, health exam, health insurance, immunizations, 2 letters of recommendation, minimum GPA in nursing prerequisites of 2.75, professional liability insurance/malpractice insurance, prerequisite course work, RN licensure. Transfer students are accepted.
Advanced Placement Credit by examination available. Credit given for nursing courses completed elsewhere dependent upon specific evaluations.
Contact *Telephone:* 918-335-6254. *Fax:* 918-335-6204.

Oral Roberts University

Anna Vaughn School of Nursing
Tulsa, Oklahoma

http://www.oru.edu/
Founded in 1963
DEGREE • BSN
Nursing Program Faculty 28 (11% with doctorates).
Baccalaureate Enrollment 104 **Women** 89% **Men** 11% **Minority** 24%
International 5% **Part-time** 4%
Nursing Student Activities Student Nurses' Association.
Nursing Student Resources Academic advising; academic or career counseling; assistance for students with disabilities; bookstore; campus computer network; computer lab; computer-assisted instruction; e-mail services; employment services for current students; housing assistance; interactive nursing skills videos; Internet; learning resource lab; library services; nursing audiovisuals; remedial services; resume preparation assistance; skills, simulation, or other laboratory; tutoring.
Library Facilities 7,964 volumes in health, 2,558 volumes in nursing; 54 periodical subscriptions health-care related.

BACCALAUREATE PROGRAMS

Degree BSN
Available Programs ADN to Baccalaureate; Generic Baccalaureate; RN Baccalaureate.
Study Options Full-time and part-time.
Program Entrance Requirements Minimum overall college GPA of 3.3, transcript of college record, CPR certification, health exam, health insurance, high school biology, high school chemistry, 2 years high school math, 2 years high school science, high school transcript, immunizations, minimum high school GPA of 2.5, minimum GPA in nursing prerequisites of 2.5. Transfer students are accepted. *Application deadline:* 8/1 (fall), 12/1 (spring). *Application fee:* $35.
Advanced Placement Credit given for nursing courses completed elsewhere dependent upon specific evaluations.
Expenses (2012–13) *Tuition:* full-time $20,862; part-time $872 per credit hour. *International tuition:* $20,862 full-time. *Room and board:* $8938; room only: $4578 per academic year. *Required fees:* full-time $1064; part-time $1064 per credit.
Financial Aid 98% of baccalaureate students in nursing programs received some form of financial aid in 2011–12.
Contact Dr. Kenda Jezek, Dean, Anna Vaughn School of Nursing, Oral Roberts University, 7777 South Lewis Avenue, Tulsa, OK 74171. *Telephone:* 918-495-6198. *Fax:* 918-495-6020. *E-mail:* kjezek@oru.edu.

Rogers State University

Nursing Program
Claremore, Oklahoma

Founded in 1909
DEGREE • BSN
Baccalaureate Enrollment 18 **Women** 94% **Men** 6% **Minority** 38%
International 11%
Distance Learning Courses Available.
Nursing Student Activities Student Nurses' Association.
Nursing Student Resources Academic advising; academic or career counseling; assistance for students with disabilities; bookstore; campus computer network; career placement assistance; computer lab; computer-

assisted instruction; daycare for children of students; e-mail services; housing assistance; interactive nursing skills videos; Internet; learning resource lab; library services; nursing audiovisuals; placement services for program completers; remedial services; resume preparation assistance; skills, simulation, or other laboratory.
Library Facilities 86,664 volumes; 40,178 periodical subscriptions.

BACCALAUREATE PROGRAMS

Degree BSN
Available Programs ADN to Baccalaureate.
Site Options Bartlesville, OK.
Program Entrance Requirements Minimum overall college GPA, CPR certification, health exam, health insurance, immunizations, minimum GPA in nursing prerequisites, RN licensure. Transfer students are accepted.
Contact *Telephone:* 918-343-7885. *Fax:* 918-343-7628.

Southern Nazarene University

School of Nursing
Bethany, Oklahoma

http://www.snu.edu/
Founded in 1899
DEGREES • BS • MS
Nursing Program Faculty 35 (40% with doctorates).
Baccalaureate Enrollment 101 **Women** 90% **Men** 10% **Minority** 35%
International 2% **Part-time** 10%
Graduate Enrollment 34 **Women** 90% **Men** 10% **Minority** 10%
Distance Learning Courses Available.
Nursing Student Activities Sigma Theta Tau, Student Nurses' Association.
Nursing Student Resources Academic advising; academic or career counseling; assistance for students with disabilities; bookstore; campus computer network; career placement assistance; computer lab; computer-assisted instruction; e-mail services; employment services for current students; externships; housing assistance; interactive nursing skills videos; Internet; learning resource lab; library services; nursing audiovisuals; paid internships; remedial services; skills, simulation, or other laboratory; tutoring.
Library Facilities 101,117 volumes; 41,048 periodical subscriptions.

BACCALAUREATE PROGRAMS

Degree BS
Available Programs ADN to Baccalaureate; Baccalaureate for Second Degree; Generic Baccalaureate; LPN to Baccalaureate.
Study Options Full-time.
Program Entrance Requirements Minimum overall college GPA of 2.75, transcript of college record, CPR certification, health exam, health insurance, immunizations, minimum GPA in nursing prerequisites of 2.75, professional liability insurance/malpractice insurance, prerequisite course work. Transfer students are accepted. *Application deadline:* 12/5 (fall). Applications may be processed on a rolling basis for some programs.
Advanced Placement Credit by examination available. Credit given for nursing courses completed elsewhere dependent upon specific evaluations.
Contact *Telephone:* 405-717-6217. *Fax:* 405-717-6264.

GRADUATE PROGRAMS

Contact *Telephone:* 405-717-6217. *Fax:* 405-717-6264.

MASTER'S DEGREE PROGRAM
Degree MS
Available Programs Accelerated Master's; Accelerated Master's for Nurses with Non-Nursing Degrees.
Concentrations Available Nursing administration; nursing education.
Site Options Tulsa, OK.
Study Options Full-time.
Program Entrance Requirements Clinical experience, computer literacy, minimum overall college GPA of 3.0, transcript of college record, immunizations, interview, 3 letters of recommendation, nursing research course, physical assessment course, resume, statistics course. *Application deadline:* Applications may be processed on a rolling basis for some programs.

Advanced Placement Credit given for nursing courses completed elsewhere dependent upon specific evaluations.
Degree Requirements 39 total credit hours, thesis or project.

Southwestern Oklahoma State University
School of Nursing
Weatherford, Oklahoma

http://www.swosu.edu/academics/nursing/index.asp
Founded in 1901
DEGREE • BSN
Nursing Program Faculty 9 (15% with doctorates).
Baccalaureate Enrollment 80 Women 90% Men 10% Minority 12% International 1%
Distance Learning Courses Available.
Nursing Student Activities Sigma Theta Tau, Student Nurses' Association, nursing club.
Nursing Student Resources Academic advising; academic or career counseling; assistance for students with disabilities; bookstore; campus computer network; computer lab; computer-assisted instruction; e-mail services; externships; housing assistance; interactive nursing skills videos; Internet; learning resource lab; library services; nursing audiovisuals; remedial services; skills, simulation, or other laboratory; tutoring.
Library Facilities 284 periodical subscriptions health-care related.

BACCALAUREATE PROGRAMS
Degree BSN
Available Programs ADN to Baccalaureate; Generic Baccalaureate; RN Baccalaureate.
Site Options Oklahoma City, OK; Weatherford, OK; Elk City, OK.
Study Options Full-time.
Online Degree Options Yes.
Program Entrance Requirements Minimum overall college GPA of 2.25, transcript of college record, CPR certification, immunizations, 2 letters of recommendation, minimum GPA in nursing prerequisites of 2.25, professional liability insurance/malpractice insurance, prerequisite course work. Transfer students are accepted. *Application deadline:* 2/1 (fall).
Advanced Placement Credit given for nursing courses completed elsewhere dependent upon specific evaluations.
Financial Aid 70% of baccalaureate students in nursing programs received some form of financial aid in 2010–11. *Gift aid (need-based):* Federal Pell, FSEOG, state, private, college/university gift aid from institutional funds. *Loans:* Federal Direct (Subsidized and Unsubsidized Stafford PLUS).*Work-study:* Federal Work-Study.*Financial aid application deadline:* 3/1.
Contact Ms. Pam Colvard, Administrative Assistant, School of Nursing, Southwestern Oklahoma State University, 100 Campus Drive, Weatherford, OK 73096-3098. *Telephone:* 580-774-3261. *Fax:* 580-774-7075. *E-mail:* pam.colvard@swosu.edu.

University of Central Oklahoma
Department of Nursing
Edmond, Oklahoma

http://www.uco.edu/cms/nursing
Founded in 1890
DEGREE • BSN
Nursing Program Faculty 44 (13% with doctorates).
Baccalaureate Enrollment 264 Women 90% Men 10% Minority 19% International 5% Part-time 1%
Nursing Student Activities Nursing Honor Society, Sigma Theta Tau, Student Nurses' Association.
Nursing Student Resources Academic advising; academic or career counseling; assistance for students with disabilities; bookstore; campus computer network; career placement assistance; computer lab; computer-assisted instruction; e-mail services; externships; interactive nursing skills videos; Internet; library services; nursing audiovisuals; skills, simulation, or other laboratory; tutoring.
Library Facilities 3,000 volumes in health, 1,661 volumes in nursing.

BACCALAUREATE PROGRAMS
Degree BSN
Available Programs Generic Baccalaureate; LPN to Baccalaureate; RN Baccalaureate.
Site Options Midwest City, OK; Oklahoma City, OK.
Study Options Full-time and part-time.
Program Entrance Requirements Minimum overall college GPA of 2.5, transcript of college record, CPR certification, immunizations, 3 letters of recommendation, professional liability insurance/malpractice insurance, prerequisite course work. Transfer students are accepted. *Application deadline:* 9/14 (fall), 1/25 (spring). *Application fee:* $25.
Advanced Placement Credit given for nursing courses completed elsewhere dependent upon specific evaluations.
Expenses (2012–13) *Tuition, area resident:* full-time $6487; part-time $232 per hour. *International tuition:* $13,651 full-time. *Room and board:* $6708; room only: $3248 per academic year. *Required fees:* full-time $1736.
Financial Aid 35% of baccalaureate students in nursing programs received some form of financial aid in 2011–12.
Contact Vicki Addison, Administrative Secretary, Department of Nursing, University of Central Oklahoma, 100 North University Drive, Edmond, OK 73034-5209. *Telephone:* 405-974-5000. *E-mail:* vaddison@ucok.edu.

University of Oklahoma Health Sciences Center
College of Nursing
Oklahoma City, Oklahoma

http://nursing.ouhsc.edu/
Founded in 1890
DEGREES • BSN • MS • PHD
Nursing Program Faculty 185 (16% with doctorates).
Baccalaureate Enrollment 892 Women 85% Men 15% Minority 37% International 1% Part-time 4%
Graduate Enrollment 256 Women 93% Men 7% Minority 26% International 1% Part-time 71%
Distance Learning Courses Available.
Nursing Student Activities Sigma Theta Tau, Student Nurses' Association.
Nursing Student Resources Academic advising; academic or career counseling; assistance for students with disabilities; bookstore; campus computer network; computer lab; computer-assisted instruction; e-mail services; employment services for current students; housing assistance; Internet; learning resource lab; library services; nursing audiovisuals; skills, simulation, or other laboratory; tutoring.
Library Facilities 334,976 volumes; 4,941 periodical subscriptions.

BACCALAUREATE PROGRAMS
Degree BSN
Available Programs ADN to Baccalaureate; Accelerated Baccalaureate for Second Degree; Generic Baccalaureate; LPN to RN Baccalaureate.
Site Options Lawton, OK; Tulsa, OK.
Study Options Full-time.
Program Entrance Requirements Minimum overall college GPA of 2.5, transcript of college record, high school transcript, minimum GPA in nursing prerequisites of 2.5, prerequisite course work. Transfer students are accepted. *Application deadline:* 1/15 (fall). *Application fee:* $65.
Advanced Placement Credit by examination available. Credit given for nursing courses completed elsewhere dependent upon specific evaluations.
Contact *Telephone:* 405-271-2128. *Fax:* 405-271-7341.

GRADUATE PROGRAMS
Contact *Telephone:* 405-271-2128. *Fax:* 405-271-7341.

MASTER'S DEGREE PROGRAM
Degree MS
Available Programs Master's; Master's for Non-Nursing College Graduates.
Concentrations Available Clinical nurse leader; health-care administration; nursing education. *Clinical nurse specialist programs in:* acute care. *Nurse practitioner programs in:* adult health, family health, neonatal health, pediatric.

Site Options Lawton, OK; Tulsa, OK.

Study Options Full-time and part-time.

Online Degree Options Yes.

Program Entrance Requirements Computer literacy, minimum overall college GPA of 3.0, transcript of college record, 3 letters of recommendation, nursing research course, professional liability insurance/malpractice insurance, prerequisite course work, statistics course. *Application deadline:* 3/1 (fall), 8/1 (spring), 1/15 (summer). *Application fee:* $65.

Advanced Placement Credit given for nursing courses completed elsewhere dependent upon specific evaluations.

Degree Requirements 38 total credit hours, thesis or project, comprehensive exam.

POST-MASTER'S PROGRAM

Areas of Study Clinical nurse leader; health-care administration; nursing education. *Nurse practitioner programs in:* adult health, family health, neonatal health, pediatric.

DOCTORAL DEGREE PROGRAM

Degree PhD

Available Programs Doctorate.

Areas of Study Nursing education.

Program Entrance Requirements Minimum overall college GPA of 3.5, interview by faculty committee, 3 letters of recommendation, scholarly papers, statistics course, vita, writing sample. *Application deadline:* 4/14 (fall). *Application fee:* $65.

Degree Requirements 90 total credit hours, dissertation, oral exam, written exam.

CONTINUING EDUCATION PROGRAM

Contact *Telephone:* 405-271-2428. *Fax:* 405-271-7341.

University of Phoenix–Oklahoma City Campus

College of Health and Human Services
Oklahoma City, Oklahoma

Founded in 1976

Nursing Program Faculty 1

Nursing Student Activities Sigma Theta Tau.

Nursing Student Resources Academic advising; academic or career counseling; assistance for students with disabilities; bookstore; campus computer network; computer lab; computer-assisted instruction; e-mail services; interactive nursing skills videos; Internet; learning resource lab; library services; nursing audiovisuals; skills, simulation, or other laboratory; tutoring.

Library Facilities 16,781 periodical subscriptions (1,300 health-care related).

University of Phoenix–Tulsa Campus

College of Health and Human Services
Tulsa, Oklahoma

Founded in 1998

Nursing Student Activities Sigma Theta Tau.

Nursing Student Resources Academic advising; academic or career counseling; assistance for students with disabilities; bookstore; campus computer network; computer lab; computer-assisted instruction; e-mail services; interactive nursing skills videos; Internet; learning resource lab; library services; nursing audiovisuals; remedial services; skills, simulation, or other laboratory; tutoring.

Library Facilities 16,781 periodical subscriptions (1,300 health-care related).

University of Tulsa

School of Nursing
Tulsa, Oklahoma

http://www.utulsa.edu/nursing

Founded in 1894

DEGREE • BSN

Nursing Program Faculty 13 (33% with doctorates).

Baccalaureate Enrollment 80 **Women** 88% **Men** 12% **Minority** 20% **International** 1% **Part-time** 2%

Nursing Student Activities Sigma Theta Tau, Student Nurses' Association.

Nursing Student Resources Academic advising; academic or career counseling; assistance for students with disabilities; bookstore; campus computer network; career placement assistance; computer lab; computer-assisted instruction; daycare for children of students; e-mail services; employment services for current students; externships; housing assistance; interactive nursing skills videos; Internet; learning resource lab; library services; nursing audiovisuals; placement services for program completers; remedial services; resume preparation assistance; skills, simulation, or other laboratory; tutoring.

Library Facilities 1.2 million volumes (4,300 in nursing); 51,790 periodical subscriptions (118 health-care related).

BACCALAUREATE PROGRAMS

Degree BSN

Available Programs Generic Baccalaureate; LPN to RN Baccalaureate; RN Baccalaureate.

Study Options Full-time.

Program Entrance Requirements Minimum overall college GPA of 2.5, transcript of college record, CPR certification, written essay, health exam, immunizations, minimum GPA in nursing prerequisites. Transfer students are accepted. *Application deadline:* 2/1 (fall). Applications may be processed on a rolling basis for some programs.

Advanced Placement Credit by examination available. Credit given for nursing courses completed elsewhere dependent upon specific evaluations.

Expenses (2012–13) *Tuition:* full-time $32,410; part-time $1035 per credit hour. *International tuition:* $32,410 full-time. *Room and board:* $9934; room only: $5524 per academic year. *Required fees:* full-time $400.

Financial Aid 90% of baccalaureate students in nursing programs received some form of financial aid in 2011–12. *Gift aid (need-based):* Federal Pell, FSEOG, state, private, college/university gift aid from institutional funds. *Loans:* Federal Direct (Subsidized and Unsubsidized Stafford PLUS), Perkins. *Work-study:* Federal Work-Study, part-time campus jobs. *Financial aid application deadline (priority):* 3/1.

Contact Dr. Susan Kathleen Gaston, Director, School of Nursing, University of Tulsa, 800 South Tucker Drive, Tulsa, OK 74104-9700. *Telephone:* 918-631-3116. *Fax:* 918-631-2068. *E-mail:* susan-gaston@utulsa.edu.

OREGON

George Fox University

Nursing Department
Newberg, Oregon

http://www.georgefox.edu/academics/undergrad/departments/nursing/index.html

Founded in 1891

DEGREE • BSN

Nursing Program Faculty 15 (20% with doctorates).

Baccalaureate Enrollment 110 **Women** 91% **Men** 9% **Minority** 8%

Nursing Student Activities Nursing club.

Nursing Student Resources Academic advising; academic or career counseling; assistance for students with disabilities; bookstore; campus computer network; career placement assistance; computer lab; computer-assisted instruction; e-mail services; employment services for current students; housing assistance; interactive nursing skills videos; Internet; learning resource lab; library services; nursing audiovisuals; remedial

services; resume preparation assistance; skills, simulation, or other laboratory; tutoring.
Library Facilities 219,143 volumes (490 in health, 100 in nursing); 6,129 periodical subscriptions (5,600 health-care related).

BACCALAUREATE PROGRAMS

Degree BSN
Available Programs Generic Baccalaureate.
Study Options Full-time.
Program Entrance Requirements Minimum overall college GPA of 2.8, transcript of college record, CPR certification, written essay, immunizations, 2 letters of recommendation, minimum GPA in nursing prerequisites of 2.8, prerequisite course work. Transfer students are accepted. *Application deadline:* 10/2 (fall). *Application fee:* $50.
Contact *Telephone:* 503-554-2950. *Fax:* 503-554-3900.

Linfield College
School of Nursing
McMinnville, Oregon

http://www.linfield.edu/portland
Founded in 1849
DEGREE • BSN
Nursing Program Faculty 64 (22% with doctorates).
Baccalaureate Enrollment 314 **Women** 85.4% **Men** 14.6% **Minority** 17.8% **International** .3% **Part-time** 3.5%
Nursing Student Activities Sigma Theta Tau, Student Nurses' Association, nursing club.
Nursing Student Resources Academic advising; academic or career counseling; bookstore; campus computer network; computer lab; e-mail services; Internet; learning resource lab; library services; nursing audiovisuals; resume preparation assistance; skills, simulation, or other laboratory.
Library Facilities 186,725 volumes (7,201 in health, 1,482 in nursing); 961 periodical subscriptions (249 health-care related).

BACCALAUREATE PROGRAMS

Degree BSN
Available Programs ADN to Baccalaureate; Accelerated Baccalaureate for Second Degree; Baccalaureate for Second Degree; Generic Baccalaureate.
Site Options Portland, OR.
Study Options Full-time.
Program Entrance Requirements Minimum overall college GPA of 2.9, transcript of college record, CPR certification, written essay, health exam, health insurance, immunizations, 1 letter of recommendation, minimum GPA in nursing prerequisites of 2.75, professional liability insurance/malpractice insurance, prerequisite course work. Transfer students are accepted.
Advanced Placement Credit given for nursing courses completed elsewhere dependent upon specific evaluations.
Contact *Telephone:* 503-413-8481. *Fax:* 503-413-6283.

CONTINUING EDUCATION PROGRAM

Contact *Telephone:* 503-413-7163. *Fax:* 503-413-6846.

Oregon Health & Science University
School of Nursing
Portland, Oregon

http://www.ohsu.edu/xd/education/schools/school-of-nursing/
Founded in 1974
DEGREES • BS • MN/MPH • MS • PHD
Nursing Program Faculty 138 (40% with doctorates).
Baccalaureate Enrollment 573 **Women** 83% **Men** 17% **Minority** 7% **International** 1% **Part-time** 68%
Graduate Enrollment 219 **Women** 74% **Men** 26% **Minority** 4% **International** 2% **Part-time** 56%
Distance Learning Courses Available.

Nursing Student Activities Nursing Honor Society, Sigma Theta Tau, Student Nurses' Association, nursing club.
Nursing Student Resources Academic advising; assistance for students with disabilities; bookstore; campus computer network; computer lab; e-mail services; externships; interactive nursing skills videos; Internet; learning resource lab; library services; nursing audiovisuals; resume preparation assistance; skills, simulation, or other laboratory.
Library Facilities 286,950 volumes (227,344 in health, 7,666 in nursing); 13,811 periodical subscriptions (2,357 health-care related).

BACCALAUREATE PROGRAMS

Degree BS
Available Programs Accelerated Baccalaureate; Generic Baccalaureate; RN Baccalaureate.
Site Options Klamath Falls, OR; Ashland, OR; La Grande, OR.
Study Options Full-time.
Program Entrance Requirements Transcript of college record, written essay, minimum GPA in nursing prerequisites of 3.0, prerequisite course work. Transfer students are accepted. *Application deadline:* 2/15 (fall). *Application fee:* $120.
Advanced Placement Credit given for nursing courses completed elsewhere dependent upon specific evaluations.
Contact *Telephone:* 503-494-7725. *Fax:* 503-494-6433.

GRADUATE PROGRAMS

Contact *Telephone:* 503-494-7725. *Fax:* 503-494-4350.

MASTER'S DEGREE PROGRAM
Degrees MN/MPH; MS
Available Programs Accelerated Master's for Non-Nursing College Graduates; Master's.
Concentrations Available Nurse anesthesia; nurse-midwifery; nursing education. *Nurse practitioner programs in:* family health, psychiatric/mental health.
Site Options Klamath Falls, OR; Ashland, OR; La Grande, OR.
Study Options Full-time and part-time.
Program Entrance Requirements Clinical experience, computer literacy, minimum overall college GPA of 3.0, transcript of college record, CPR certification, written essay, immunizations, interview, 3 letters of recommendation, resume, statistics course, GRE General Test. *Application deadline:* 12/1 (fall). Applications may be processed on a rolling basis for some programs. *Application fee:* $120.
Advanced Placement Credit given for nursing courses completed elsewhere dependent upon specific evaluations.
Degree Requirements 45 total credit hours, comprehensive exam.

POST-MASTER'S PROGRAM
Areas of Study Nurse-midwifery; nursing education. *Nurse practitioner programs in:* family health, gerontology, psychiatric/mental health.

DOCTORAL DEGREE PROGRAM
Degree PhD
Available Programs Doctorate; Post-Baccalaureate Doctorate.
Areas of Study Advanced practice nursing, aging, clinical practice, ethics, faculty preparation, family health, gerontology, health policy, health promotion/disease prevention, health-care systems, human health and illness, illness and transition, nursing policy, nursing research, nursing science, women's health.
Program Entrance Requirements Clinical experience, minimum overall college GPA of 3.0, interview by faculty committee, 3 letters of recommendation, MSN or equivalent, scholarly papers, statistics course, vita, writing sample, GRE General Test. *Application deadline:* 12/1 (fall). Applications may be processed on a rolling basis for some programs. *Application fee:* $120.
Degree Requirements 90 total credit hours, dissertation, oral exam, written exam, residency.

POSTDOCTORAL PROGRAM
Areas of Study Adolescent health, aging, chronic illness, family health, gerontology, health promotion/disease prevention, nursing interventions, nursing research, nursing science, outcomes, self-care, vulnerable population, women's health.
Postdoctoral Program Contact*Telephone:* 503-494-7725. *Fax:* 503-494-4350.

CONTINUING EDUCATION PROGRAM

Contact *Telephone:* 503-494-6772. *Fax:* 503-494-4350.

University of Portland
School of Nursing
Portland, Oregon

http://nursing.up.edu/
Founded in 1901

DEGREES • BSN • DNP • MS
Nursing Program Faculty 48 (38% with doctorates).
Baccalaureate Enrollment 567 **Women** 90% **Men** 10% **Minority** 25% **International** 4%
Graduate Enrollment 83 **Women** 86% **Men** 14% **Minority** 13% **International** 1%
Distance Learning Courses Available.
Nursing Student Activities Sigma Theta Tau, Student Nurses' Association, nursing club.
Nursing Student Resources Academic advising; academic or career counseling; assistance for students with disabilities; bookstore; campus computer network; career placement assistance; computer lab; computer-assisted instruction; daycare for children of students; e-mail services; employment services for current students; housing assistance; interactive nursing skills videos; Internet; learning resource lab; library services; nursing audiovisuals; remedial services; resume preparation assistance; skills, simulation, or other laboratory; tutoring.
Library Facilities 228,138 volumes (5,545 in health, 1,024 in nursing); 6,977 periodical subscriptions (504 health-care related).

BACCALAUREATE PROGRAMS

Degree BSN
Available Programs Generic Baccalaureate.
Study Options Full-time.
Program Entrance Requirements Minimum overall college GPA of 2.7, transcript of college record, CPR certification, written essay, health exam, health insurance, high school chemistry, high school transcript, immunizations, 1 letter of recommendation, minimum high school GPA of 2.7, minimum GPA in nursing prerequisites of 2.7, prerequisite course work. Transfer students are accepted. *Application deadline:* 1/15 (fall), 1/15 (spring). *Application fee:* $50.
Advanced Placement Credit by examination available. Credit given for nursing courses completed elsewhere dependent upon specific evaluations.
Expenses (2012–13) *Tuition:* full-time $41,390. *Room and board:* $10,040 per academic year. *Required fees:* full-time $2260.
Financial Aid 95% of baccalaureate students in nursing programs received some form of financial aid in 2011–12.
Contact Mr. Jason McDonald, Dean of Admissions, School of Nursing, University of Portland, 5000 North Willamette Boulevard, Portland, OR 97203-5798. *Telephone:* 503-943-7147. *E-mail:* mcdonaja@up.edu.

GRADUATE PROGRAMS

Expenses (2012–13) *Tuition:* part-time $980 per credit. *Room and board:* $12,090 per academic year. *Required fees:* part-time $50 per credit.
Financial Aid 84% of graduate students in nursing programs received some form of financial aid in 2011–12. Fellowships, research assistantships, Federal Work-Study and scholarships available. Aid available to part-time students. *Financial aid application deadline:* 3/1.
Contact Mrs. Stacey Boatright, Nursing Program Counselor and Grant Manager, School of Nursing, University of Portland, 5000 North Willamette Boulevard, MSC-153, Portland, OR 97203-5798. *Telephone:* 503-943-7423. *Fax:* 503-943-7729. *E-mail:* boatrigh@up.edu.

MASTER'S DEGREE PROGRAM
Degree MS
Available Programs Master's.
Concentrations Available Clinical nurse leader; nursing education.
Study Options Part-time.
Program Entrance Requirements Computer literacy, minimum overall college GPA of 3.0, transcript of college record, written essay, interview, 2 letters of recommendation, resume, statistics course, GRE General Test or MAT. *Application deadline:* 1/15 (summer). Applications may be processed on a rolling basis for some programs. *Application fee:* $50.
Advanced Placement Credit given for nursing courses completed elsewhere dependent upon specific evaluations.
Degree Requirements 42 total credit hours, thesis or project.

DOCTORAL DEGREE PROGRAM
Degree DNP
Available Programs Doctorate; Post-Baccalaureate Doctorate.

Areas of Study Advanced practice nursing.
Program Entrance Requirements Minimum overall college GPA of 3.0, interview by faculty committee, 3 letters of recommendation, statistics course, vita, writing sample, GRE General Test or MAT. *Application deadline:* 1/15 (summer). Applications may be processed on a rolling basis for some programs. *Application fee:* $50.
Degree Requirements 83 total credit hours, residency.

PENNSYLVANIA

Alvernia University
Nursing
Reading, Pennsylvania

http://www.alvernia.edu/
Founded in 1958

DEGREE • BSN
Nursing Program Faculty 9 (2% with doctorates).
Baccalaureate Enrollment 203 **Women** 98% **Men** 2% **Minority** 10% **International** 3% **Part-time** 20%
Nursing Student Activities Nursing Honor Society, Sigma Theta Tau, Student Nurses' Association.
Nursing Student Resources Academic advising; academic or career counseling; bookstore; campus computer network; computer lab; computer-assisted instruction; e-mail services; employment services for current students; externships; interactive nursing skills videos; Internet; learning resource lab; library services; nursing audiovisuals; remedial services; skills, simulation, or other laboratory; tutoring.
Library Facilities 2,931 volumes in health, 995 volumes in nursing; 89 periodical subscriptions health-care related.

BACCALAUREATE PROGRAMS

Degree BSN
Available Programs Generic Baccalaureate; LPN to Baccalaureate; LPN to RN Baccalaureate; RN Baccalaureate.
Site Options Reading, PA; Pottsville, PA; Ashland, PA.
Study Options Full-time.
Program Entrance Requirements Minimum overall college GPA of 2.7, transcript of college record, CPR certification, written essay, health exam, health insurance, high school biology, high school chemistry, 2 years high school math, 2 years high school science, high school transcript, immunizations, 2 letters of recommendation, minimum high school GPA of 2.7, minimum GPA in nursing prerequisites of 2.7. Transfer students are accepted.
Advanced Placement Credit by examination available. Credit given for nursing courses completed elsewhere dependent upon specific evaluations.
Contact *Telephone:* 610-796-8460. *Fax:* 610-796-8464.

CONTINUING EDUCATION PROGRAM

Contact *Telephone:* 610-796-5611. *Fax:* 610-796-8464.

Bloomsburg University of Pennsylvania
Department of Nursing
Bloomsburg, Pennsylvania

http://www.bloomu.edu/
Founded in 1839

DEGREES • BSN • MSN • MSN/MBA
Nursing Program Faculty 36 (36% with doctorates).
Baccalaureate Enrollment 306 **Women** 86% **Men** 14% **Minority** 5% **Part-time** 8%
Graduate Enrollment 96 **Women** 89% **Men** 11% **Minority** 10% **Part-time** 73%
Distance Learning Courses Available.
Nursing Student Activities Sigma Theta Tau, Student Nurses' Association, nursing club.

Nursing Student Resources Academic advising; academic or career counseling; assistance for students with disabilities; bookstore; campus computer network; career placement assistance; computer lab; computer-assisted instruction; daycare for children of students; e-mail services; employment services for current students; externships; housing assistance; interactive nursing skills videos; Internet; learning resource lab; library services; nursing audiovisuals; paid internships; placement services for program completers; remedial services; resume preparation assistance; skills, simulation, or other laboratory; tutoring; unpaid internships.

Library Facilities 496,203 volumes (6,082 in health, 3,612 in nursing); 68,400 periodical subscriptions (7,564 health-care related).

BACCALAUREATE PROGRAMS

Degree BSN

Available Programs ADN to Baccalaureate; Baccalaureate for Second Degree; Generic Baccalaureate; LPN to RN Baccalaureate; RN Baccalaureate.

Study Options Full-time.

Program Entrance Requirements Minimum overall college GPA of 2.5, transcript of college record, health exam, health insurance, high school biology, high school chemistry, 2 years high school math, 3 years high school science, high school transcript, immunizations, 3 letters of recommendation, minimum high school GPA of 3.0, minimum high school rank 80%, minimum GPA in nursing prerequisites of 2.5, prerequisite course work. Transfer students are accepted. *Application deadline:* 11/15 (fall). *Application fee:* $35.

Advanced Placement Credit by examination available. Credit given for nursing courses completed elsewhere dependent upon specific evaluations.

Expenses (2012–13) *Tuition, state resident:* full-time $6428; part-time $268 per credit. *Tuition, nonresident:* full-time $16,070; part-time $670 per credit. *International tuition:* $16,070 full-time. *Room and board:* $7498; room only: $4598 per academic year. *Required fees:* full-time $1915.

Financial Aid 61% of baccalaureate students in nursing programs received some form of financial aid in 2011–12. *Gift aid (need-based):* Federal Pell, FSEOG, state, private, college/university gift aid from institutional funds. *Loans:* Federal Direct (Subsidized and Unsubsidized Stafford PLUS), Perkins, state, alternative loans. *Work-study:* Federal Work-Study, part-time campus jobs. *Financial aid application deadline (priority):* 3/15.

Contact Dr. Michelle Ficca, Department Chairperson, Department of Nursing, Bloomsburg University of Pennsylvania, 400 East 2nd Street, Room 3109, MCHS, Bloomsburg, PA 17815. *Telephone:* 570-389-4615. *Fax:* 570-389-5008. *E-mail:* mficca@bloomu.edu.

GRADUATE PROGRAMS

Expenses (2012–13) *Tuition, state resident:* full-time $8580; part-time $429 per credit. *Tuition, nonresident:* full-time $12,880; part-time $644 per credit. *International tuition:* $12,880 full-time. *Room and board:* $7498; room only: $4598 per academic year. *Required fees:* full-time $1988.

Financial Aid 35% of graduate students in nursing programs received some form of financial aid in 2011–12. Unspecified assistantships available.

Contact Dr. Michelle Ficca, Coordinator of Graduate Program, Department of Nursing, Bloomsburg University of Pennsylvania, 400 East Second Street, Room 3136, MCHS, Bloomsburg, PA 17815. *Telephone:* 570-389-4615. *Fax:* 570-389-5008. *E-mail:* mficca@bloomu.edu.

MASTER'S DEGREE PROGRAM

Degrees MSN; MSN/MBA

Available Programs Master's; Master's for Nurses with Non-Nursing Degrees; RN to Master's.

Concentrations Available Nurse anesthesia; nursing administration. *Nurse practitioner programs in:* adult health.

Site Options Danville, PA.

Study Options Full-time and part-time.

Program Entrance Requirements Clinical experience, minimum overall college GPA of 3.0, transcript of college record, CPR certification, written essay, immunizations, interview, 3 letters of recommendation, nursing research course, physical assessment course, professional liability insurance/malpractice insurance, resume, statistics course. *Application deadline:* Applications may be processed on a rolling basis for some programs. *Application fee:* $35.

Advanced Placement Credit by examination available. Credit given for nursing courses completed elsewhere dependent upon specific evaluations.

Degree Requirements 39–66 total credit hours, comprehensive exam.

POST-MASTER'S PROGRAM

Areas of Study Nursing administration. *Clinical nurse specialist programs in:* school health. *Nurse practitioner programs in:* adult health, family health.

CONTINUING EDUCATION PROGRAM

Contact Dr. Michelle Ficca, Department Chairperson, Department of Nursing, Bloomsburg University of Pennsylvania, 400 East 2nd Street, Room 3109, MCHS, Bloomsburg, PA 17815. *Telephone:* 570-389-4615. *Fax:* 570-389-5008. *E-mail:* mficca@bloomu.edu.

California University of Pennsylvania
Department of Nursing
California, Pennsylvania

http://www.calu.edu/academics/colleges/eberly/nursing/index.htm
Founded in 1852

DEGREE • BSN
Nursing Program Faculty 5 (60% with doctorates).
Baccalaureate Enrollment 145 **Women** 83% **Men** 17% **Minority** 3% **Part-time** 92%
Nursing Student Activities Sigma Theta Tau.
Nursing Student Resources Academic advising; academic or career counseling; assistance for students with disabilities; bookstore; campus computer network; career placement assistance; computer lab; computer-assisted instruction; daycare for children of students; e-mail services; employment services for current students; Internet; library services; nursing audiovisuals; placement services for program completers; remedial services; resume preparation assistance; tutoring.
Library Facilities 3,840 volumes in health, 2,010 volumes in nursing; 80 periodical subscriptions health-care related.

BACCALAUREATE PROGRAMS

Degree BSN
Available Programs RN Baccalaureate.
Site Options West Mifflin, PA.
Study Options Full-time and part-time.
Program Entrance Requirements Minimum overall college GPA of 2.0, transcript of college record, CPR certification, health exam, health insurance, immunizations, 2 letters of recommendation, professional liability insurance/malpractice insurance, prerequisite course work, RN licensure. Transfer students are accepted.
Advanced Placement Credit by examination available. Credit given for nursing courses completed elsewhere dependent upon specific evaluations.
Contact *Telephone:* 724-938-5739. *Fax:* 724-938-1612.

Carlow University
School of Nursing
Pittsburgh, Pennsylvania

http://www.carlow.edu/academics/schools/sch-nurs/index.html
Founded in 1929

DEGREES • BSN • MSN
Nursing Program Faculty 31 (23% with doctorates).
Baccalaureate Enrollment 333 **Women** 99% **Men** 1% **Minority** 13% **Part-time** 21%
Graduate Enrollment 54 **Women** 94% **Men** 6% **Minority** 11% **Part-time** 94%
Nursing Student Activities Nursing Honor Society, Sigma Theta Tau, Student Nurses' Association.
Nursing Student Resources Academic advising; academic or career counseling; assistance for students with disabilities; bookstore; campus computer network; career placement assistance; computer lab; computer-assisted instruction; daycare for children of students; e-mail services;

employment services for current students; externships; housing assistance; Internet; learning resource lab; library services; nursing audiovisuals; other; paid internships; placement services for program completers; remedial services; resume preparation assistance; skills, simulation, or other laboratory; tutoring; unpaid internships.
Library Facilities 136,177 volumes (14,100 in health, 5,450 in nursing); 15,804 periodical subscriptions (60 health-care related).

BACCALAUREATE PROGRAMS

Degree BSN
Available Programs Accelerated RN Baccalaureate; Baccalaureate for Second Degree; Generic Baccalaureate.
Site Options Cranberry Township, PA; Greensburg, PA.
Study Options Full-time and part-time.
Program Entrance Requirements Minimum overall college GPA of 3.0, transcript of college record, CPR certification, health exam, health insurance, high school biology, high school chemistry, 2 years high school math, 2 years high school science, high school transcript, immunizations, interview, minimum high school GPA of 3.0, minimum GPA in nursing prerequisites of 2.0, professional liability insurance/malpractice insurance, prerequisite course work. Transfer students are accepted.
Advanced Placement Credit by examination available. Credit given for nursing courses completed elsewhere dependent upon specific evaluations.
Contact *Telephone:* 412-578-6059. *Fax:* 412-578-6668.

GRADUATE PROGRAMS

Contact *Telephone:* 412-578-8764. *Fax:* 412-578-6321.

MASTER'S DEGREE PROGRAM

Degree MSN
Available Programs Accelerated Master's; Master's; RN to Master's.
Concentrations Available Nurse case management; nursing administration; nursing education. *Clinical nurse specialist programs in:* home health care. *Nurse practitioner programs in:* family health.
Site Options Cranberry Township, PA; Greensburg, PA.
Study Options Full-time and part-time.
Program Entrance Requirements Clinical experience, computer literacy, minimum overall college GPA of 3.0, transcript of college record, CPR certification, written essay, immunizations, interview, 3 letters of recommendation, professional liability insurance/malpractice insurance, prerequisite course work, resume, statistics course.
Advanced Placement Credit by examination available. Credit given for nursing courses completed elsewhere dependent upon specific evaluations.
Degree Requirements 56 total credit hours, thesis or project, comprehensive exam.

POST-MASTER'S PROGRAM

Areas of Study *Clinical nurse specialist programs in:* home health care. *Nurse practitioner programs in:* family health.

CONTINUING EDUCATION PROGRAM

Contact *Telephone:* 412-578-8764. *Fax:* 412-578-6321.

Cedar Crest College
Department of Nursing
Allentown, Pennsylvania

http://www.cedarcrest.edu/
Founded in 1867
DEGREES • BS • MSN
Nursing Program Faculty 21 (24% with doctorates).
Baccalaureate Enrollment 287 **Women** 96% **Men** 4% **Minority** 23% **International** 8% **Part-time** 68%
Graduate Enrollment 23 **Women** 96% **Men** 4% **Minority** 4% **Part-time** 100%
Nursing Student Activities Nursing Honor Society, Sigma Theta Tau, Student Nurses' Association.
Nursing Student Resources Academic advising; academic or career counseling; assistance for students with disabilities; bookstore; campus computer network; career placement assistance; computer lab; computer-assisted instruction; e-mail services; interactive nursing skills videos; Internet; learning resource lab; library services; nursing audiovisuals; remedial services; skills, simulation, or other laboratory; tutoring.

Library Facilities 149,853 volumes; 28,278 periodical subscriptions.

BACCALAUREATE PROGRAMS

Degree BS
Available Programs Baccalaureate for Second Degree; Generic Baccalaureate; LPN to Baccalaureate; RN Baccalaureate.
Study Options Full-time and part-time.
Program Entrance Requirements Minimum overall college GPA of 2.5, CPR certification, written essay, health exam, health insurance, high school biology, high school chemistry, 3 years high school math, 2 years high school science, high school transcript, immunizations, minimum GPA in nursing prerequisites of 2.7, prerequisite course work. Transfer students are accepted. *Application deadline:* Applications may be processed on a rolling basis for some programs.
Advanced Placement Credit given for nursing courses completed elsewhere dependent upon specific evaluations.
Contact *Telephone:* 610-740-3780. *Fax:* 610-606-4647.

GRADUATE PROGRAMS

Contact *Telephone:* 610-606-4666 Ext. 3480.

MASTER'S DEGREE PROGRAM

Degree MSN
Available Programs Master's.
Study Options Part-time.
Program Entrance Requirements Clinical experience, minimum overall college GPA of 3.0, transcript of college record, CPR certification, immunizations, interview, 3 letters of recommendation, nursing research course, physical assessment course, resume, statistics course. *Application deadline:* Applications may be processed on a rolling basis for some programs. *Application fee:* $30.
Advanced Placement Credit given for nursing courses completed elsewhere dependent upon specific evaluations.
Degree Requirements 38 total credit hours, thesis or project.

Chatham University
Nursing Programs
Pittsburgh, Pennsylvania

http://www.chatham.edu/
Founded in 1869
DEGREES • BSN • DNP • MSN
Nursing Program Faculty 27 (80% with doctorates).
Baccalaureate Enrollment 99 **Women** 83% **Men** 17% **Minority** 5% **Part-time** 80%
Graduate Enrollment 116 **Women** 86% **Men** 14% **Minority** 28% **Part-time** 63%
Distance Learning Courses Available.
Nursing Student Activities Nursing Honor Society, Sigma Theta Tau.
Nursing Student Resources Academic advising; academic or career counseling; assistance for students with disabilities; bookstore; campus computer network; career placement assistance; computer lab; e-mail services; employment services for current students; housing assistance; Internet; library services; other; placement services for program completers; remedial services; resume preparation assistance; tutoring.
Library Facilities 115,775 volumes (1,747 in health, 1,732 in nursing); 29,961 periodical subscriptions (967 health-care related).

BACCALAUREATE PROGRAMS

Degree BSN
Available Programs RN Baccalaureate; RPN to Baccalaureate.
Study Options Full-time and part-time.
Program Entrance Requirements Written essay, health insurance, high school transcript, immunizations, 2 letters of recommendation. Transfer students are accepted. *Application deadline:* 4/15 (fall), 11/1 (spring). Applications may be processed on a rolling basis for some programs.
Advanced Placement Credit by examination available. Credit given for nursing courses completed elsewhere dependent upon specific evaluations.
Expenses (2012–13) *Tuition:* part-time $737 per credit.
Contact Ms. Brittani Uberti, Admission Counselor, Nursing Programs, Chatham University, Berry Hall, Woodland Road, Pittsburgh, PA 15232. *Telephone:* 412-365-1107. *Fax:* 412-365-1609. *E-mail:* buberti@chatham.edu.

GRADUATE PROGRAMS

Expenses (2012–13) *Tuition:* part-time $802 per credit. *Required fees:* part-time $21 per credit.
Financial Aid 75% of graduate students in nursing programs received some form of financial aid in 2011–12.
Contact Mr. David A. Vey, Assistant Director of Online Admission, Nursing Programs, Chatham University, Admission Office, Woodland Road, Pittsburgh, PA 15232. *Telephone:* 412-365-1498. *Fax:* 412-365-1609. *E-mail:* dvey@chatham.edu.

MASTER'S DEGREE PROGRAM
Degree MSN
Available Programs Master's.
Concentrations Available Nursing administration; nursing education; nursing informatics.
Study Options Full-time.
Online Degree Options Yes (online only).
Program Entrance Requirements Minimum overall college GPA of 3.0, transcript of college record, written essay, resume. *Application deadline:* 8/15 (fall). Applications may be processed on a rolling basis for some programs.
Advanced Placement Credit given for nursing courses completed elsewhere dependent upon specific evaluations.
Degree Requirements 36 total credit hours, thesis or project.

DOCTORAL DEGREE PROGRAM
Degree DNP
Available Programs Doctorate.
Online Degree Options Yes (online only).
Program Entrance Requirements Clinical experience, minimum overall college GPA of 3.0, 2 letters of recommendation, MSN or equivalent, vita, writing sample. *Application deadline:* 4/15 (fall), 9/15 (spring).
Degree Requirements 27 total credit hours, residency.

Clarion University of Pennsylvania
School of Nursing
Oil City, Pennsylvania

http://www.clarion.edu/
Founded in 1867
DEGREES • BSN • MSN
Nursing Program Faculty 20 (25% with doctorates).
Baccalaureate Enrollment 105 **Women** 90% **Men** 10% **Minority** 2% **International** 1% **Part-time** 88%
Graduate Enrollment 82 **Women** 98% **Men** 2% **Minority** 3% **Part-time** 80%
Distance Learning Courses Available.
Nursing Student Activities Sigma Theta Tau, nursing club.
Nursing Student Resources Academic advising; academic or career counseling; assistance for students with disabilities; bookstore; campus computer network; career placement assistance; computer lab; computer-assisted instruction; daycare for children of students; e-mail services; employment services for current students; externships; housing assistance; interactive nursing skills videos; Internet; learning resource lab; library services; nursing audiovisuals; placement services for program completers; remedial services; resume preparation assistance; skills, simulation, or other laboratory; tutoring.
Library Facilities 474,723 volumes (12,000 in health, 7,000 in nursing); 33,515 periodical subscriptions (300 health-care related).

BACCALAUREATE PROGRAMS

Degree BSN
Available Programs ADN to Baccalaureate; RN Baccalaureate.
Study Options Full-time and part-time.
Online Degree Options Yes (online only).
Program Entrance Requirements Minimum overall college GPA of 2.5, transcript of college record, CPR certification, health exam, health insurance, high school transcript, immunizations, minimum GPA in nursing prerequisites of 2.0, professional liability insurance/malpractice insurance, RN licensure. Transfer students are accepted. *Application deadline:* 8/1 (fall), 12/1 (winter). Applications may be processed on a rolling basis for some programs. *Application fee:* $30.
Contact *Telephone:* 814-393-1258. *Fax:* 814-676-0251.

GRADUATE PROGRAMS

Contact *Telephone:* 412-578-7277.

MASTER'S DEGREE PROGRAM
Degree MSN
Available Programs Master's; RN to Master's.
Concentrations Available Nursing education: *Nurse practitioner programs in:* family health.
Site Options Edinboro, PA; Pittsburgh, PA.
Study Options Full-time and part-time.
Program Entrance Requirements Clinical experience, computer literacy, minimum overall college GPA of 3.0, transcript of college record, CPR certification, written essay, immunizations, interview, 3 letters of recommendation, professional liability insurance/malpractice insurance, statistics course. *Application deadline:* 4/1 (fall), 11/1 (winter), 11/1 (spring), 4/1 (summer). *Application fee:* $50.
Advanced Placement Credit given for nursing courses completed elsewhere dependent upon specific evaluations.
Degree Requirements 45 total credit hours, thesis or project, comprehensive exam.

POST-MASTER'S PROGRAM
Areas of Study Nursing education. *Nurse practitioner programs in:* family health.

DeSales University
Department of Nursing and Health
Center Valley, Pennsylvania

http://www.desales.edu/
Founded in 1964
DEGREES • BSN • MSN • MSN/MBA
Nursing Program Faculty 74 (23% with doctorates).
Baccalaureate Enrollment 193 **Women** 88% **Men** 12% **Minority** 4% **International** 2% **Part-time** 23%
Graduate Enrollment 85 **Women** 93% **Men** 7% **Minority** 2% **Part-time** 95%
Nursing Student Activities Nursing Honor Society, Sigma Theta Tau, Student Nurses' Association.
Nursing Student Resources Academic advising; academic or career counseling; bookstore; campus computer network; career placement assistance; computer lab; computer-assisted instruction; e-mail services; employment services for current students; externships; interactive nursing skills videos; Internet; learning resource lab; library services; nursing audiovisuals; paid internships; placement services for program completers; remedial services; resume preparation assistance; skills, simulation, or other laboratory; tutoring; unpaid internships.
Library Facilities 174,563 volumes (1,215 in health, 100 in nursing); 12,733 periodical subscriptions (100 health-care related).

BACCALAUREATE PROGRAMS

Degree BSN
Available Programs ADN to Baccalaureate; Accelerated Baccalaureate; Accelerated RN Baccalaureate; Baccalaureate for Second Degree; Generic Baccalaureate; RN Baccalaureate.
Study Options Full-time and part-time.
Program Entrance Requirements Minimum overall college GPA of 2.5, transcript of college record, written essay, high school biology, high school chemistry, high school foreign language, 2 years high school math, 3 years high school science, high school transcript, 2 letters of recommendation, minimum high school GPA of 2.5, minimum high school rank 33%, minimum GPA in nursing prerequisites of 2.0. Transfer students are accepted. *Application deadline:* Applications may be processed on a rolling basis for some programs. *Application fee:* $30.
Advanced Placement Credit by examination available. Credit given for nursing courses completed elsewhere dependent upon specific evaluations.
Contact *Telephone:* 610-282-1100 Ext. 1285. *Fax:* 610-282-2091.

GRADUATE PROGRAMS

Contact *Telephone:* 610-282-1100 Ext. 1664. *Fax:* 610-282-2091.

MASTER'S DEGREE PROGRAM
Degrees MSN; MSN/MBA

Available Programs Accelerated AD/RN to Master's; Master's; RN to Master's.

Concentrations Available Nursing administration; nursing education. *Clinical nurse specialist programs in:* adult health. *Nurse practitioner programs in:* family health.

Study Options Full-time and part-time.

Program Entrance Requirements Minimum overall college GPA of 3.0, transcript of college record, written essay, interview, 3 letters of recommendation, prerequisite course work, statistics course. *Application deadline:* Applications may be processed on a rolling basis for some programs. *Application fee:* $35.

Advanced Placement Credit given for nursing courses completed elsewhere dependent upon specific evaluations.

Degree Requirements 47 total credit hours.

POST-MASTER'S PROGRAM

Areas of Study Nursing education. *Clinical nurse specialist programs in:* adult health. *Nurse practitioner programs in:* family health.

CONTINUING EDUCATION PROGRAM

Contact *Telephone:* 610-282-1100 Ext. 1271. *Fax:* 610-282-2091.

Drexel University
College of Nursing and Health Professions
Philadelphia, Pennsylvania

http://www.drexel.edu/cnhp
Founded in 1891
DEGREES • BSN • DR NP • MSN
Nursing Program Faculty 73 (52% with doctorates).
Baccalaureate Enrollment 1,696 **Women** 87% **Men** 13% **Minority** 21% **International** 1% **Part-time** 46%
Graduate Enrollment 1,010 **Women** 89% **Men** 11% **Minority** 19% **International** 2% **Part-time** 96%
Distance Learning Courses Available.
Nursing Student Activities Nursing Honor Society, Sigma Theta Tau, Student Nurses' Association, nursing club.
Nursing Student Resources Academic advising; academic or career counseling; assistance for students with disabilities; bookstore; campus computer network; career placement assistance; computer lab; computer-assisted instruction; e-mail services; housing assistance; interactive nursing skills videos; Internet; learning resource lab; library services; nursing audiovisuals; paid internships; placement services for program completers; remedial services; resume preparation assistance; skills, simulation, or other laboratory; tutoring.
Library Facilities 643,869 volumes (51,000 in health, 5,015 in nursing); 27,399 periodical subscriptions (63,000 health-care related).

BACCALAUREATE PROGRAMS

Degree BSN
Available Programs Accelerated Baccalaureate; Accelerated Baccalaureate for Second Degree; Generic Baccalaureate; RN Baccalaureate.
Site Options Philadelphia, PA.
Study Options Full-time.
Program Entrance Requirements CPR certification, written essay, health insurance, high school biology, high school chemistry, 3 years high school math, 2 years high school science, high school transcript, immunizations, 2 letters of recommendation. Transfer students are accepted. *Application deadline:* 1/15 (fall). *Application fee:* $75.
Expenses (2012–13) *Tuition:* full-time $33,800; part-time $930 per credit. *International tuition:* $33,800 full-time. *Room and board:* $11,200; room only: $5625 per academic year. *Required fees:* full-time $3170; part-time $145 per term.
Financial Aid 66% of baccalaureate students in nursing programs received some form of financial aid in 2011–12.
Contact Ms. Vanessa Thomas, Director of Undergraduate Admissions, College of Nursing and Health Professions, Drexel University, 3141 Chestnut Street, Enrollment Management, Philadelphia, PA 19104. *Telephone:* 215-895-6732. *Fax:* 215-895-5939. *E-mail:* VMT26@drexel.edu.

GRADUATE PROGRAMS

Expenses (2012–13) *Tuition:* part-time $800 per credit.
Financial Aid 44% of graduate students in nursing programs received some form of financial aid in 2011–12. Fellowships, research assistant-ships, teaching assistantships, career-related internships or fieldwork, Federal Work-Study, institutionally sponsored loans, and tuition waivers (partial) available. Aid available to part-time students. *Financial aid application deadline:* 5/1.
Contact Mr. Redian Furxhui, Academic Advisor, MSN Programs, College of Nursing and Health Professions, Drexel University, 1505 Race Street, Mail Stop 501, Philadelphia, PA 19102-1192. *Telephone:* 215-762-3999. *Fax:* 215-762-1259. *E-mail:* rf53@drexel.edu.

MASTER'S DEGREE PROGRAM

Degree MSN
Available Programs Master's; RN to Master's.
Concentrations Available Clinical nurse leader; nurse anesthesia; nursing administration; nursing education. *Clinical nurse specialist programs in:* women's health. *Nurse practitioner programs in:* acute care, adult health, family health, pediatric, psychiatric/mental health, women's health.
Site Options Philadelphia, PA.
Study Options Full-time and part-time.
Online Degree Options Yes.
Program Entrance Requirements Clinical experience, computer literacy, minimum overall college GPA of 3.0, transcript of college record, CPR certification, written essay, immunizations, 2 letters of recommendation, resume. *Application deadline:* 1/1 (fall). Applications may be processed on a rolling basis for some programs. *Application fee:* $75.
Advanced Placement Credit given for nursing courses completed elsewhere dependent upon specific evaluations.
Degree Requirements 55 total credit hours, thesis or project, comprehensive exam.

POST-MASTER'S PROGRAM

Areas of Study Nursing administration; nursing education. *Nurse practitioner programs in:* family health, pediatric.

DOCTORAL DEGREE PROGRAM

Degree Dr NP
Available Programs Doctorate.
Areas of Study Clinical practice, faculty preparation, nursing administration, nursing education, nursing research, nursing science.
Site Options Philadelphia, PA.
Online Degree Options Yes (online only).
Program Entrance Requirements Clinical experience, minimum overall college GPA of 3.25, interview by faculty committee, interview, 2 letters of recommendation, vita, writing sample, GRE General Test. *Application deadline:* 6/1 (fall).
Degree Requirements 48 total credit hours, dissertation, oral exam, written exam, residency.

CONTINUING EDUCATION PROGRAM

Contact Mr. Wayne Miller, Director of Continuing Nursing Education, College of Nursing and Health Professions, Drexel University, 245 North 15th Street, Mail Stop #501, Philadelphia, PA 19102. *Telephone:* 215-762-8521. *Fax:* 215-762-7778. *E-mail:* wdm22@drexel.edu.

Duquesne University
School of Nursing
Pittsburgh, Pennsylvania

http://www.duq.edu/nursing
Founded in 1878
DEGREES • BSN • MSN • PHD
Nursing Program Faculty 83 (78% with doctorates).
Baccalaureate Enrollment 471 **Women** 89% **Men** 11% **Minority** 11%
Graduate Enrollment 233 **Women** 95% **Men** 5% **Minority** 18% **International** 1% **Part-time** 37%
Distance Learning Courses Available.
Nursing Student Activities Nursing Honor Society, Sigma Theta Tau, Student Nurses' Association, nursing club.
Nursing Student Resources Academic advising; academic or career counseling; assistance for students with disabilities; bookstore; campus computer network; career placement assistance; computer lab; computer-assisted instruction; daycare for children of students; e-mail services; employment services for current students; externships; housing assistance; interactive nursing skills videos; Internet; learning resource lab; library services; nursing audiovisuals; paid internships; placement services for program completers; remedial services; resume preparation

assistance; skills, simulation, or other laboratory; tutoring; unpaid internships.
Library Facilities 728,587 volumes (27,613 in health, 1,951 in nursing); 78,125 periodical subscriptions (1,779 health-care related).

BACCALAUREATE PROGRAMS

Degree BSN
Available Programs Accelerated Baccalaureate for Second Degree; Generic Baccalaureate.
Study Options Full-time and part-time.
Program Entrance Requirements Minimum overall college GPA of 3.0, transcript of college record, written essay, high school biology, high school chemistry, high school foreign language, 2 years high school math, 3 years high school science, high school transcript, 2 letters of recommendation, minimum high school GPA of 3.0, minimum high school rank 40%. Transfer students are accepted. *Application deadline:* 5/1 (fall), 11/1 (spring). Applications may be processed on a rolling basis for some programs. *Application fee:* $50.
Advanced Placement Credit by examination available.
Expenses (2012–13) *Tuition:* full-time $27,668; part-time $902 per credit. *International tuition:* $27,668 full-time. *Room and board:* $10,198 per academic year. *Required fees:* full-time $2366; part-time $92 per credit.
Financial Aid 89% of baccalaureate students in nursing programs received some form of financial aid in 2011–12.
Contact Ms. Susan Hardner, Nursing Recruiter, School of Nursing, Duquesne University, 600 Forbes Avenue, Pittsburgh, PA 15282-1760. *Telephone:* 412-396-4945. *Fax:* 412-396-6346. *E-mail:* hardnersue@ duq.edu.

GRADUATE PROGRAMS

Expenses (2012–13) *Tuition:* part-time $991 per credit. *Required fees:* part-time $92 per credit.
Financial Aid 48% of graduate students in nursing programs received some form of financial aid in 2011–12. 17 research assistantships with partial tuition reimbursements available (averaging $1,170 per year), 8 teaching assistantships with partial tuition reimbursements available (averaging $1,170 per year) were awarded; institutionally sponsored loans, scholarships, traineeships, tuition waivers (partial), and unspecified assistantships also available. Aid available to part-time students. *Financial aid application deadline:* 7/1.
Contact Ms. Susan Hardner, Nursing Recruiter, School of Nursing, Duquesne University, 600 Forbes Avenue, Pittsburgh, PA 15282-1760. *Telephone:* 412-396-4945. *Fax:* 412-396-6346. *E-mail:* hardnersue@ duq.edu.

MASTER'S DEGREE PROGRAM
Degree MSN
Available Programs Master's.
Concentrations Available Nursing education. *Clinical nurse specialist programs in:* forensic nursing. *Nurse practitioner programs in:* family health.
Study Options Full-time and part-time.
Online Degree Options Yes (online only).
Program Entrance Requirements Clinical experience, computer literacy, minimum overall college GPA of 3.0, transcript of college record, written essay, interview, 2 letters of recommendation, nursing research course, physical assessment course, prerequisite course work, resume, statistics course. *Application deadline:* 3/1 (summer).
Advanced Placement Credit given for nursing courses completed elsewhere dependent upon specific evaluations.
Degree Requirements 47 total credit hours, thesis or project.

POST-MASTER'S PROGRAM
Areas of Study *Clinical nurse specialist programs in:* forensic nursing. *Nurse practitioner programs in:* family health.

DOCTORAL DEGREE PROGRAM
Degree PhD
Available Programs Doctorate.
Areas of Study Nursing research.
Online Degree Options Yes (online only).
Program Entrance Requirements Minimum overall college GPA of 3.5, interview by faculty committee, 3 letters of recommendation, MSN or equivalent, scholarly papers, statistics course, vita, writing sample. *Application deadline:* 1/15 (summer).
Degree Requirements 58 total credit hours, dissertation, oral exam, written exam, residency.

CONTINUING EDUCATION PROGRAM

Contact Miss Alyssa Kramer, Administrative Assistant, School of Nursing, Duquesne University, 600 Forbes Avenue, Pittsburgh, PA 15282-1760. *Telephone:* 412-396-5203. *Fax:* 412-396-6346. *E-mail:* kramera@duq.edu.

See display on next page and full description on page 478.

Eastern University
Program in Nursing
St. Davids, Pennsylvania

http://www.eastern.edu/academic/ccgps/nursing/index.html
Founded in 1952
DEGREE • BSN
Nursing Program Faculty 7 (43% with doctorates).
Baccalaureate Enrollment 100 **Women** 92% **Men** 8% **Minority** 25% **International** 32%
Distance Learning Courses Available.
Nursing Student Activities Sigma Theta Tau, Student Nurses' Association.
Nursing Student Resources Academic advising; academic or career counseling; assistance for students with disabilities; bookstore; campus computer network; career placement assistance; computer lab; computer-assisted instruction; e-mail services; employment services for current students; Internet; learning resource lab; library services; nursing audiovisuals; placement services for program completers; remedial services; resume preparation assistance; skills, simulation, or other laboratory; tutoring; unpaid internships.
Library Facilities 5,858 volumes in health, 3,000 volumes in nursing; 821 periodical subscriptions health-care related.

BACCALAUREATE PROGRAMS

Degree BSN
Available Programs Accelerated RN Baccalaureate; Baccalaureate for Second Degree; Generic Baccalaureate; International Nurse to Baccalaureate.
Site Options Wynnewood, PA; West Chester, PA; Harrisburg, PA.
Study Options Full-time.
Program Entrance Requirements Minimum overall college GPA of 3.0, transcript of college record, CPR certification, written essay, health exam, health insurance, high school chemistry, high school transcript, immunizations, interview, 2 letters of recommendation, minimum GPA in nursing prerequisites of 3.0, professional liability insurance/malpractice insurance, prerequisite course work, RN licensure. Transfer students are accepted. *Application deadline:* Applications may be processed on a rolling basis for some programs. *Application fee:* $40.
Contact *Telephone:* 800-732-7669. *Fax:* 610-341-1468.

East Stroudsburg University of Pennsylvania
Department of Nursing
East Stroudsburg, Pennsylvania

http://www4.esu.edu/academics/departments/nursing/index. cfm
Founded in 1893
DEGREE • BS
Nursing Program Faculty 14 (77% with doctorates).
Baccalaureate Enrollment 166 **Women** 75% **Men** 25%
Nursing Student Activities Nursing Honor Society, Sigma Theta Tau, Student Nurses' Association, nursing club.
Nursing Student Resources Academic advising; academic or career counseling; assistance for students with disabilities; bookstore; campus computer network; career placement assistance; computer lab; computer-assisted instruction; daycare for children of students; e-mail services; employment services for current students; externships; housing assistance; interactive nursing skills videos; Internet; learning resource lab; library services; nursing audiovisuals; other; placement services for program completers; remedial services; resume preparation assistance; skills, simulation, or other laboratory; tutoring; unpaid internships.

Library Facilities 569,096 volumes (16,810 in health, 2,035 in nursing); 3,900 periodical subscriptions (495 health-care related).

BACCALAUREATE PROGRAMS

Degree BS

Available Programs Generic Baccalaureate; RN Baccalaureate.

Study Options Full-time.

Program Entrance Requirements Minimum overall college GPA of 2.75, transcript of college record, health exam, 2 years high school math, 2 years high school science, high school transcript, immunizations, minimum high school GPA of 3.0, minimum high school rank 75%, minimum GPA in nursing prerequisites of 2.75. Transfer students are accepted. *Application deadline:* 5/1 (fall), 1/1 (winter), 1/1 (spring). Applications may be processed on a rolling basis for some programs. *Application fee:* $100.

Advanced Placement Credit by examination available. Credit given for nursing courses completed elsewhere dependent upon specific evaluations.

Contact *Telephone:* 570-422-3569. *Fax:* 570-422-3848.

Edinboro University of Pennsylvania

Department of Nursing
Edinboro, Pennsylvania

http://www.edinboro.edu/

Founded in 1857

DEGREE • BS

Nursing Program Faculty 23 (52% with doctorates).

Baccalaureate Enrollment 295 **Women** 86.2% **Men** 13.8% **Minority** 10.6% **International** 7.2% **Part-time** .4%

Nursing Student Activities Sigma Theta Tau, Student Nurses' Association, nursing club.

Nursing Student Resources Academic advising; academic or career counseling; assistance for students with disabilities; bookstore; campus computer network; career placement assistance; computer lab; computer-assisted instruction; e-mail services; employment services for current students; housing assistance; interactive nursing skills videos; Internet; learning resource lab; library services; nursing audiovisuals; remedial services; resume preparation assistance; skills, simulation, or other laboratory; tutoring.

Library Facilities 503,349 volumes (500,000 in health, 100 in nursing); 1,170 periodical subscriptions (105 health-care related).

BACCALAUREATE PROGRAMS

Degree BS

Available Programs ADN to Baccalaureate; Accelerated Baccalaureate; Accelerated Baccalaureate for Second Degree; Baccalaureate for Second Degree; Generic Baccalaureate; International Nurse to Baccalaureate.

Site Options Erie, PA.

Study Options Full-time and part-time.

Program Entrance Requirements Minimum overall college GPA of 2.75, CPR certification, health exam, high school biology, high school chemistry, 2 years high school math, 2 years high school science, high school transcript, immunizations, minimum high school rank 40%, minimum GPA in nursing prerequisites of 2.75, professional liability insurance/malpractice insurance. *Application deadline:* Applications may be processed on a rolling basis for some programs. *Application fee:* $25.

Advanced Placement Credit by examination available.

Expenses (2012–13) *Tuition, state resident:* full-time $6428; part-time $268 per credit. *Tuition, nonresident:* full-time $9642; part-time $402 per credit. *International tuition:* $9642 full-time. *Room and board:* $10,368; room only: $7400 per academic year. *Required fees:* full-time $1075.

Financial Aid 75% of baccalaureate students in nursing programs received some form of financial aid in 2011–12.

Contact Dr. Thomas R. White, Chairperson, Department of Nursing, Department of Nursing, Edinboro University of Pennsylvania, Human Services Building #125, 215 Scotland Road, Edinboro, PA 16444. *Telephone:* 814-732-2900. *Fax:* 814-732-2536. *E-mail:* twhite@edinboro.edu.

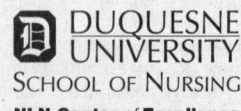

Gannon University
Villa Maria School of Nursing
Erie, Pennsylvania

http://www.gannon.edu/Academic-Offerings/Health-Professions-and-Sciences/Villa-Maria-School-of-Nursing/
Founded in 1925
DEGREES • BSN • DNP • MSN
Nursing Program Faculty 16 (20% with doctorates).
Baccalaureate Enrollment 350 **Women** 88% **Men** 12% **Minority** 4%
International 3% **Part-time** 5%
Graduate Enrollment 97 **Women** 68% **Men** 32% **Minority** 6% **Part-time** 38%
Distance Learning Courses Available.
Nursing Student Activities Nursing Honor Society, Sigma Theta Tau.
Nursing Student Resources Academic advising; academic or career counseling; assistance for students with disabilities; bookstore; campus computer network; career placement assistance; computer lab; computer-assisted instruction; e-mail services; employment services for current students; externships; housing assistance; interactive nursing skills videos; Internet; learning resource lab; library services; nursing audiovisuals; other; paid internships; placement services for program completers; remedial services; resume preparation assistance; skills, simulation, or other laboratory; tutoring; unpaid internships.
Library Facilities 266,136 volumes (140,000 in health, 20,000 in nursing); 58,039 periodical subscriptions (3,000 health-care related).

BACCALAUREATE PROGRAMS

Degree BSN
Available Programs ADN to Baccalaureate; Baccalaureate for Second Degree; Generic Baccalaureate; International Nurse to Baccalaureate; RN Baccalaureate.
Study Options Full-time and part-time.
Online Degree Options Yes.
Program Entrance Requirements Minimum overall college GPA of 2.7, transcript of college record, CPR certification, written essay, health exam, health insurance, high school biology, high school chemistry, 4 years high school math, 2 years high school science, high school transcript, immunizations, 1 letter of recommendation, minimum high school GPA of 2.5, minimum high school rank 40%, minimum GPA in nursing prerequisites of 2.7. Transfer students are accepted. *Application deadline:* Applications may be processed on a rolling basis for some programs. *Application fee:* $25.
Expenses (2012–13) *Tuition:* full-time $27,550; part-time $675 per credit. *Room and board:* $9600; room only: $7000 per academic year. *Required fees:* full-time $700; part-time $18 per credit.
Financial Aid 40% of baccalaureate students in nursing programs received some form of financial aid in 2011–12. *Gift aid (need-based):* Federal Pell, FSEOG, state, private, college/university gift aid from institutional funds. *Loans:* Federal Nursing Student Loans, Federal Direct (Subsidized and Unsubsidized Stafford PLUS), Perkins. *Work-study:* Federal Work-Study, part-time campus jobs. *Financial aid application deadline (priority):* 3/15.
Contact Ms. Patricia Ann Marshall, Director, Undergraduate Programs in Nursing, Villa Maria School of Nursing, Gannon University, 109 University Square, Morosky Academic Center, Erie, PA 16541-0001. *Telephone:* 814-871-5470. *Fax:* 814-871-5662. *E-mail:* marshall001@gannon.edu.

GRADUATE PROGRAMS

Expenses (2012–13) *Tuition:* part-time $850 per credit. *Required fees:* part-time $18 per credit.
Financial Aid Scholarships available.
Contact Dr. Kathleen Patterson, School and Graduate Program Director, Villa Maria School of Nursing, Gannon University, 109 University Square, Erie, PA 16541-0001. *Telephone:* 814-871-5547. *Fax:* 814-871-5662. *E-mail:* patterso018@gannon.edu.

MASTER'S DEGREE PROGRAM
Degree MSN
Available Programs Accelerated AD/RN to Master's; Accelerated RN to Master's; Master's; RN to Master's.
Concentrations Available Nurse anesthesia; nursing administration. *Nurse practitioner programs in:* family health.
Study Options Full-time and part-time.
Program Entrance Requirements Clinical experience, computer literacy, minimum overall college GPA of 3.0, transcript of college record,

CPR certification, written essay, immunizations, interview, 3 letters of recommendation, nursing research course, professional liability insurance/malpractice insurance, prerequisite course work, statistics course, GRE General Test. *Application deadline:* Applications may be processed on a rolling basis for some programs. *Application fee:* $50.
Advanced Placement Credit given for nursing courses completed elsewhere dependent upon specific evaluations.
Degree Requirements 46 total credit hours, thesis or project.

POST-MASTER'S PROGRAM
Areas of Study Nurse anesthesia; nursing administration. *Nurse practitioner programs in:* family health.

DOCTORAL DEGREE PROGRAM
Degree DNP
Available Programs Doctorate.
Areas of Study Clinical practice, family health.
Program Entrance Requirements Clinical experience, minimum overall college GPA of 3.0, interview by faculty committee, 3 letters of recommendation, MSN or equivalent, statistics course, vita, writing sample. *Application deadline:* Applications may be processed on a rolling basis for some programs. *Application fee:* $50.
Degree Requirements 42 total credit hours, dissertation, residency.

See display on next page and full description on page 484.

Gwynedd-Mercy College
School of Nursing
Gwynedd Valley, Pennsylvania

Founded in 1948
DEGREES • BSN • MSN
Nursing Program Faculty 21 (43% with doctorates).
Baccalaureate Enrollment 85 **Women** 95% **Men** 5% **Minority** 5% **Part-time** 28%
Graduate Enrollment 40 **Women** 85% **Men** 15% **Minority** 10% **International** 5% **Part-time** 80%
Nursing Student Activities Sigma Theta Tau, Student Nurses' Association.
Nursing Student Resources Academic advising; bookstore; campus computer network; computer lab; computer-assisted instruction; daycare for children of students; e-mail services; interactive nursing skills videos; learning resource lab; library services; nursing audiovisuals; resume preparation assistance; skills, simulation, or other laboratory; tutoring.
Library Facilities 105,070 volumes; 667 periodical subscriptions.

BACCALAUREATE PROGRAMS

Degree BSN
Available Programs ADN to Baccalaureate; Accelerated RN Baccalaureate; RN Baccalaureate.
Site Options Fort Washington, PA.
Study Options Full-time and part-time.
Program Entrance Requirements Minimum overall college GPA of 2.8, transcript of college record, CPR certification, health exam, health insurance, high school biology, high school chemistry, 2 years high school math, high school transcript, immunizations, letters of recommendation, minimum high school rank 33%, minimum GPA in nursing prerequisites, professional liability insurance/malpractice insurance, RN licensure. Transfer students are accepted.
Advanced Placement Credit by examination available. Credit given for nursing courses completed elsewhere dependent upon specific evaluations.
Contact *Telephone:* 215-646-7300 Ext. 425. *Fax:* 215-641-5556 Ext. 528.

GRADUATE PROGRAMS

Contact *Telephone:* 215-646-7300 Ext. 407. *Fax:* 215-542-5789.

MASTER'S DEGREE PROGRAM
Degree MSN
Available Programs Master's; RN to Master's.
Concentrations Available *Clinical nurse specialist programs in:* gerontology, oncology, pediatric. *Nurse practitioner programs in:* adult health, pediatric.
Study Options Full-time and part-time.

Program Entrance Requirements Clinical experience, minimum overall college GPA of 3.0, transcript of college record, written essay, immunizations, interview, 2 letters of recommendation, physical assessment course, professional liability insurance/malpractice insurance, statistics course, GRE General Test or MAT.

Advanced Placement Credit by examination available. Credit given for nursing courses completed elsewhere dependent upon specific evaluations.

Degree Requirements 43 total credit hours.

POST-MASTER'S PROGRAM
Areas of Study *Nurse practitioner programs in:* adult health, pediatric.

Holy Family University
School of Nursing and Allied Health Professions
Philadelphia, Pennsylvania

http://www.holyfamily.edu/sn/index.shtml
Founded in 1954

DEGREES • BSN • MSN
Nursing Program Faculty 80 (28% with doctorates).
Baccalaureate Enrollment 700 **Women** 90% **Men** 10% **Minority** 40% **International** 5% **Part-time** 14%
Graduate Enrollment 60 **Women** 97% **Men** 3% **Minority** 27% **Part-time** 100%
Distance Learning Courses Available.
Nursing Student Activities Nursing Honor Society, Sigma Theta Tau, Student Nurses' Association, nursing club.
Nursing Student Resources Academic advising; academic or career counseling; assistance for students with disabilities; bookstore; campus computer network; career placement assistance; computer lab; computer-assisted instruction; daycare for children of students; e-mail services; employment services for current students; externships; housing assistance; interactive nursing skills videos; Internet; learning resource lab; library services; nursing audiovisuals; other; remedial services; resume preparation assistance; skills, simulation, or other laboratory; tutoring; unpaid internships.
Library Facilities 145,700 volumes (8,159 in health, 2,177 in nursing); 14,250 periodical subscriptions (279 health-care related).

BACCALAUREATE PROGRAMS
Degree BSN
Available Programs ADN to Baccalaureate; Accelerated RN Baccalaureate; Generic Baccalaureate; International Nurse to Baccalaureate.
Site Options Bensalem, PA; Meadowbrook, PA; Philadelphia, PA.
Study Options Full-time.
Program Entrance Requirements Transcript of college record, CPR certification, health exam, health insurance, high school biology, high school chemistry, high school foreign language, 3 years high school math, 3 years high school science, high school transcript, immunizations, 2 letters of recommendation, minimum high school GPA of 3.0, minimum high school rank 60%, minimum GPA in nursing prerequisites of 3.0, prerequisite course work. Transfer students are accepted. *Application deadline:* 8/1 (fall), 1/5 (spring), 5/10 (summer). Applications may be processed on a rolling basis for some programs. *Application fee:* $25.
Expenses (2012–13) *Tuition:* full-time $25,000; part-time $535 per credit. *International tuition:* $25,000 full-time. *Room and board:* $5700; room only: $3500 per academic year. *Required fees:* full-time $900; part-time $60 per term.
Financial Aid 85% of baccalaureate students in nursing programs received some form of financial aid in 2011–12. *Gift aid (need-based):* Federal Pell, FSEOG, state, private, college/university gift aid from institutional funds. *Loans:* Federal Nursing Student Loans, Federal Direct (Subsidized and Unsubsidized Stafford PLUS), Perkins. *Work-study:* Federal Work-Study. *Financial aid application deadline (priority):* 3/1.
Contact Lauren A. Campbell, Director of Undergraduate Admissions, School of Nursing and Allied Health Professions, Holy Family University, 9801 Frankford Avenue, Philadelphia, PA 19114-2094. *Telephone:* 215-637-3050. *Fax:* 215-281-1022. *E-mail:* admissions@holyfamily.edu.

GRADUATE PROGRAMS
Expenses (2012–13) *Tuition:* part-time $655 per credit hour. *International tuition:* $655 full-time. *Required fees:* part-time $85 per term.
Financial Aid 85% of graduate students in nursing programs received some form of financial aid in 2011–12.
Contact Gidget Montelibano, Graduate Admissions, School of Nursing and Allied Health Professions, Holy Family University, 9701 Frankford Avenue, Philadelphia, PA 19114-2094. *Telephone:* 267-341-3358. *E-mail:* gmontelibano@holyfamily.edu.

MASTER'S DEGREE PROGRAM

Degree MSN

Available Programs Master's; Master's for Nurses with Non-Nursing Degrees.

Concentrations Available Nursing education.

Study Options Part-time.

Program Entrance Requirements Minimum overall college GPA of 3.0, transcript of college record, written essay, immunizations, 2 letters of recommendation, nursing research course, professional liability insurance/malpractice insurance, prerequisite course work, resume, statistics course. *Application deadline:* 8/1 (fall), 1/10 (spring), 5/10 (summer). Applications may be processed on a rolling basis for some programs. *Application fee:* $25.

Advanced Placement Credit by examination available. Credit given for nursing courses completed elsewhere dependent upon specific evaluations.

Degree Requirements 39 total credit hours, comprehensive exam.

POST-MASTER'S PROGRAM

Areas of Study Health-care administration; nursing education. *Nurse practitioner programs in:* community health.

CONTINUING EDUCATION PROGRAM

Contact Dr. Mary Maria Wombwell, School of Nursing and Allied Health Professions, Holy Family University, 9801 Frankford Avenue, Philadelphia, PA 19114. *Telephone:* 267-341-3300. *Fax:* 215-637-6598. *E-mail:* mwombwell@holyfamily.edu.

Immaculata University
Department of Nursing
Immaculata, Pennsylvania

http://www.immaculata.edu/nursing/
Founded in 1920

DEGREES • BSN • MSN

Nursing Program Faculty 80 (50% with doctorates).

Baccalaureate Enrollment 1,125 **Women** 92% **Men** 8% **Minority** 13% **International** 2% **Part-time** 90%

Graduate Enrollment 105 **Women** 97% **Men** 3% **Minority** 15% **Part-time** 100%

Nursing Student Activities Sigma Theta Tau, nursing club.

Nursing Student Resources Academic advising; academic or career counseling; assistance for students with disabilities; bookstore; campus computer network; career placement assistance; computer lab; computer-assisted instruction; e-mail services; employment services for current students; externships; interactive nursing skills videos; Internet; learning resource lab; library services; nursing audiovisuals; placement services for program completers; resume preparation assistance; skills, simulation, or other laboratory; tutoring.

Library Facilities 1,500 volumes in health, 1,500 volumes in nursing; 115 periodical subscriptions health-care related.

BACCALAUREATE PROGRAMS

Degree BSN

Available Programs Accelerated RN Baccalaureate; Generic Baccalaureate; RN Baccalaureate.

Site Options Philadelphia, PA; Abington, PA; Christiana, DE.

Study Options Full-time.

Program Entrance Requirements Transcript of college record, CPR certification, written essay, health exam, high school chemistry, high school foreign language, 2 years high school math, 3 years high school science, high school transcript, immunizations, interview, 2 letters of recommendation, minimum high school GPA of 3.0, prerequisite course work. Transfer students are accepted. *Application deadline:* 1/31 (fall). *Application fee:* $35.

Advanced Placement Credit by examination available.

Expenses (2012–13) *Tuition:* full-time $29,000; part-time $470 per credit. *International tuition:* $29,000 full-time. *Room and board:* $8000; room only: $5500 per academic year. *Required fees:* full-time $500; part-time $50 per term.

Financial Aid 75% of baccalaureate students in nursing programs received some form of financial aid in 2011–12.

Contact Mr. Chris Mayerski, Admissions Counselor, Department of Nursing, Immaculata University, 1145 King Road, Immaculata, PA 19345. *Telephone:* 610-647-4400 Ext. 3044. *Fax:* 610-640-0836. *E-mail:* cmayerski@immaculata.edu.

GRADUATE PROGRAMS

Expenses (2012–13) *Tuition:* part-time $620 per credit. *International tuition:* $620 full-time. *Required fees:* part-time $150 per credit.

Financial Aid 25% of graduate students in nursing programs received some form of financial aid in 2011–12.

Contact Dr. Jane Tang, Coordinator, MSN Program, Department of Nursing, Immaculata University, 1145 King Road, Immaculata, PA 19345-0691. *Telephone:* 610-647-4400 Ext. 3309. *Fax:* 610-640-0286. *E-mail:* jtang@immaculata.edu.

MASTER'S DEGREE PROGRAM

Degree MSN

Available Programs Master's; Master's for Non-Nursing College Graduates.

Concentrations Available Nursing administration; nursing education.

Site Options Abington, PA; Christiana, DE.

Study Options Part-time.

Program Entrance Requirements Minimum overall college GPA of 3.0, transcript of college record, written essay, interview, 3 letters of recommendation, physical assessment course, statistics course. *Application deadline:* Applications may be processed on a rolling basis for some programs. *Application fee:* $50.

Advanced Placement Credit given for nursing courses completed elsewhere dependent upon specific evaluations.

Degree Requirements 39 total credit hours, thesis or project.

Indiana University of Pennsylvania
Department of Nursing and Allied Health
Indiana, Pennsylvania

http://www.iup.edu/rn-alliedhealth/default.aspx
Founded in 1875

DEGREES • BSN • MS • PHD

Nursing Program Faculty 39 (54% with doctorates).

Baccalaureate Enrollment 112 **Women** 87.57% **Men** 12.43% **Minority** 4.02% **International** 4.39%

Graduate Enrollment 44 **Women** 93.18% **Men** 6.82% **Minority** 2.27% **Part-time** 100%

Distance Learning Courses Available.

Nursing Student Activities Nursing Honor Society, Sigma Theta Tau, Student Nurses' Association, nursing club.

Nursing Student Resources Academic advising; academic or career counseling; assistance for students with disabilities; bookstore; campus computer network; career placement assistance; computer lab; computer-assisted instruction; e-mail services; employment services for current students; housing assistance; interactive nursing skills videos; Internet; learning resource lab; library services; nursing audiovisuals; remedial services; resume preparation assistance; skills, simulation, or other laboratory; tutoring.

Library Facilities 884,379 volumes (5,758 in health, 3,395 in nursing); 33,549 periodical subscriptions (225 health-care related).

BACCALAUREATE PROGRAMS

Degree BSN

Available Programs Baccalaureate for Second Degree; Generic Baccalaureate; LPN to Baccalaureate.

Study Options Full-time and part-time.

Program Entrance Requirements Minimum overall college GPA of 3.0, transcript of college record, high school chemistry, 3 years high school math, high school transcript, minimum high school GPA of 3.0, prerequisite course work. Transfer students are accepted. *Application deadline:* Applications may be processed on a rolling basis for some programs. *Application fee:* $50.

Expenses (2012–13) *Tuition, state resident:* full-time $6428; part-time $268 per credit. *Tuition, nonresident:* full-time $16,070; part-time $670 per credit. *International tuition:* $16,070 full-time. *Room and board:* $10,466; room only: $7740 per academic year. *Required fees:* full-time $2244; part-time $52 per credit; part-time $203 per term.

Financial Aid 85% of baccalaureate students in nursing programs received some form of financial aid in 2011–12.

Contact Mr. Chris Kitas, Associate Director of Institutional Research, Planning and Assessment, Department of Nursing and Allied Health, Indiana University of Pennsylvania, Institutional Research Planning and

Assessment, 404 Sutton Hall, Indiana, PA 15705. *Telephone:* 724-357-5562. *Fax:* 724-357-3833. *E-mail:* Chris.Kitas@iup.edu.

GRADUATE PROGRAMS

Expenses (2012–13) *Tuition, state resident:* full-time $8136; part-time $452 per credit. *Tuition, nonresident:* full-time $12,204; part-time $678 per credit. *International tuition:* $12,204 full-time. *Room and board:* $10,466; room only: $7740 per academic year. *Required fees:* full-time $2232.

Financial Aid 68% of graduate students in nursing programs received some form of financial aid in 2011–12. 5 fellowships (averaging $5,179 per year), 4 research assistantships with full and partial tuition reimbursements available (averaging $3,599 per year) were awarded; teaching assistantships, Federal Work-Study also available. Aid available to part-time students. *Financial aid application deadline:* 4/15.

Contact Dr. Elizabeth A. Palmer, Department Chair, Department of Nursing and Allied Health, Indiana University of Pennsylvania, 1010 Oakland Avenue, Indiana, PA 15705-1087. *Telephone:* 724-357-2557. *Fax:* 724-357-3267. *E-mail:* lpalmer@iup.edu.

MASTER'S DEGREE PROGRAM

Degree MS

Available Programs Master's; Master's for Nurses with Non-Nursing Degrees.

Concentrations Available Nursing administration; nursing education.

Site Options Monroeville, PA.

Study Options Part-time.

Program Entrance Requirements Clinical experience, minimum overall college GPA of 3.0, transcript of college record, written essay, 2 letters of recommendation, nursing research course, resume, statistics course. *Application deadline:* Applications may be processed on a rolling basis for some programs. *Application fee:* $50.

Advanced Placement Credit given for nursing courses completed elsewhere dependent upon specific evaluations.

Degree Requirements 36 total credit hours.

DOCTORAL DEGREE PROGRAM

Degree PhD

Available Programs Doctorate.

Areas of Study Nursing education.

Program Entrance Requirements Minimum overall college GPA of 3.5, interview by faculty committee, 2 letters of recommendation, MSN or equivalent, statistics course, vita, writing sample. *Application deadline:* Applications may be processed on a rolling basis for some programs. *Application fee:* $50.

Degree Requirements 60 total credit hours, dissertation, oral exam, written exam, residency.

Lancaster General College of Nursing & Health Sciences

Bachelor of Science in Nursing Program

Lancaster, Pennsylvania

Founded in 1903

DEGREE • BSN

BACCALAUREATE PROGRAMS

Degree BSN

Available Programs RN Baccalaureate.

Program Entrance Requirements Minimum overall college GPA of 2.0, RN licensure.

Expenses (2012–13) *Tuition:* part-time $425 per credit hour.

Contact Program Chair, Bachelor of Science in Nursing Program, Lancaster General College of Nursing & Health Sciences, 410 North Lime Street, Lancaster, PA 17602. *Telephone:* 800-622-5443. *E-mail:* jlhershe@lancastergeneralcollege.edu.

La Roche College

Department of Nursing and Nursing Management

Pittsburgh, Pennsylvania

http://www.laroche.edu/

Founded in 1963

DEGREES • BSN • MSN

Nursing Program Faculty 11 (90% with doctorates).

Baccalaureate Enrollment 77 **Women** 85% **Men** 15% **International** 5% **Part-time** 75%

Graduate Enrollment 30 **Women** 83% **Men** 17% **International** 5% **Part-time** 94%

Distance Learning Courses Available.

Nursing Student Activities Sigma Theta Tau.

Nursing Student Resources Academic advising; academic or career counseling; assistance for students with disabilities; bookstore; campus computer network; computer lab; e-mail services; externships; Internet; library services; resume preparation assistance; tutoring.

Library Facilities 133,556 volumes; 582 periodical subscriptions (850 health-care related).

BACCALAUREATE PROGRAMS

Degree BSN

Available Programs Accelerated RN Baccalaureate; LPN to RN Baccalaureate; RN Baccalaureate.

Study Options Full-time and part-time.

Online Degree Options Yes (online only).

Program Entrance Requirements Minimum overall college GPA of 3.0, transcript of college record, CPR certification, written essay, health exam, health insurance, high school transcript, immunizations, interview, 2 letters of recommendation, minimum high school GPA of 3.0, professional liability insurance/malpractice insurance, RN licensure. Transfer students are accepted. *Application deadline:* Applications may be processed on a rolling basis for some programs. *Application fee:* $50.

Advanced Placement Credit by examination available. Credit given for nursing courses completed elsewhere dependent upon specific evaluations.

Expenses (2012–13) *Tuition:* full-time $23,000; part-time $595 per credit hour. *Room and board:* $3200; room only: $2900 per academic year. *Required fees:* full-time $200.

Financial Aid 87% of baccalaureate students in nursing programs received some form of financial aid in 2011–12. *Gift aid (need-based):* Federal Pell, FSEOG, state, private, college/university gift aid from institutional funds. *Loans:* Federal Direct (Subsidized and Unsubsidized Stafford PLUS), Perkins, state. *Work-study:* Federal Work-Study. *Financial aid application deadline (priority):* 5/1.

Contact Ms. Hope A. Schiffgens, Director, Graduate Studies and Adult Education, Department of Nursing and Nursing Management, La Roche College, 9000 Babcock Boulevard, Pittsburgh, PA 15237. *Telephone:* 412-536-1266. *Fax:* 412-536-1283. *E-mail:* hope.schiffgens@laroche.edu.

GRADUATE PROGRAMS

Expenses (2012–13) *Tuition:* part-time $625 per credit hour. *Room and board:* $3500; room only: $2500 per academic year.

Financial Aid 85% of graduate students in nursing programs received some form of financial aid in 2011–12.

Contact Ms. Hope A. Schiffgens, Director, Graduate Studies and Adult Education, Department of Nursing and Nursing Management, La Roche College, 9000 Babcock Boulevard, Pittsburgh, PA 15237. *Telephone:* 412-536-1262. *Fax:* 412-536-1283. *E-mail:* hope.schiffgens@laroche.edu.

MASTER'S DEGREE PROGRAM

Degree MSN

Available Programs Master's; RN to Master's.

Concentrations Available Nursing administration; nursing education.

Study Options Full-time and part-time.

Online Degree Options Yes (online only).

Program Entrance Requirements Clinical experience, minimum overall college GPA of 3.0, transcript of college record, immunizations, interview, 2 letters of recommendation, professional liability insurance/malpractice insurance, resume. *Application deadline:* Applications may be processed on a rolling basis for some programs. *Application fee:* $50.

Advanced Placement Credit given for nursing courses completed elsewhere dependent upon specific evaluations.
Degree Requirements 41 total credit hours.

CONTINUING EDUCATION PROGRAM

Contact Ms. Hope A. Schiffgens, Director, Graduate Studies and Adult Education, Department of Nursing and Nursing Management, La Roche College, 9000 Babcock Boulevard, Pittsburgh, PA 15237. *Telephone:* 412-536-1260. *Fax:* 412-536-1283. *E-mail:* hope.schiffgens@ laroche.edu.

La Salle University
School of Nursing and Health Sciences
Philadelphia, Pennsylvania

http://www.lasalle.edu/schools/snhs/
Founded in 1863
DEGREES • BSN • MSN • MSN/MBA
Nursing Program Faculty 45 (32% with doctorates).
Nursing Student Activities Sigma Theta Tau, Student Nurses' Association, nursing club.
Nursing Student Resources Academic advising; academic or career counseling; assistance for students with disabilities; bookstore; campus computer network; career placement assistance; computer lab; computer-assisted instruction; e-mail services; employment services for current students; externships; housing assistance; interactive nursing skills videos; Internet; learning resource lab; library services; nursing audiovisuals; placement services for program completers; remedial services; resume preparation assistance; skills, simulation, or other laboratory; tutoring.
Library Facilities 420,000 volumes (8,350 in nursing); 60,705 periodical subscriptions (310 health-care related).

BACCALAUREATE PROGRAMS

Degree BSN
Available Programs Baccalaureate for Second Degree; Generic Baccalaureate; LPN to Baccalaureate; RN Baccalaureate.
Site Options Newtown, PA.
Study Options Full-time and part-time.
Program Entrance Requirements Minimum overall college GPA of 2.75, transcript of college record, CPR certification, written essay, health exam, health insurance, high school biology, high school chemistry, 3 years high school math, 3 years high school science, high school transcript, immunizations, interview, 2 letters of recommendation, minimum high school GPA of 3.0, minimum high school rank 25%, minimum GPA in nursing prerequisites of 2.75, professional liability insurance/malpractice insurance, prerequisite course work. Transfer students are accepted.
Advanced Placement Credit by examination available. Credit given for nursing courses completed elsewhere dependent upon specific evaluations.
Contact *Telephone:* 215-951-1430. *Fax:* 215-951-1896.

GRADUATE PROGRAMS

Contact *Telephone:* 215-951-1413. *Fax:* 215-951-1896.

MASTER'S DEGREE PROGRAM
Degrees MSN; MSN/MBA
Available Programs Master's; RN to Master's.
Concentrations Available Nurse anesthesia; nursing administration. *Clinical nurse specialist programs in:* adult health, public health. *Nurse practitioner programs in:* adult health, family health.
Site Options Newtown, PA.
Study Options Full-time and part-time.
Program Entrance Requirements Clinical experience, minimum overall college GPA of 3.0, transcript of college record, CPR certification, written essay, immunizations, interview, 2 letters of recommendation, nursing research course, physical assessment course, professional liability insurance/malpractice insurance, resume, statistics course.
Advanced Placement Credit given for nursing courses completed elsewhere dependent upon specific evaluations.
Degree Requirements 41 total credit hours.

POST-MASTER'S PROGRAM
Areas of Study Nurse anesthesia; nursing administration; nursing education. *Clinical nurse specialist programs in:* adult health, public health. *Nurse practitioner programs in:* adult health, family health.

CONTINUING EDUCATION PROGRAM

Contact *Telephone:* 215-951-1432. *Fax:* 215-951-1896.

Mansfield University of Pennsylvania
Department of Health Sciences–Nursing
Mansfield, Pennsylvania

http://www.mansfield.edu/
Founded in 1857
DEGREES • BSN • MSN
Nursing Program Faculty 12 (50% with doctorates).
Baccalaureate Enrollment 186 **Women** 95% **Men** 5% **Minority** 4% **International** 1% **Part-time** 5%
Graduate Enrollment 52 **Women** 98% **Men** 2% **Minority** 1% **Part-time** 100%
Distance Learning Courses Available.
Nursing Student Activities Nursing Honor Society, Student Nurses' Association, nursing club.
Nursing Student Resources Academic advising; academic or career counseling; assistance for students with disabilities; bookstore; campus computer network; career placement assistance; computer lab; daycare for children of students; e-mail services; employment services for current students; housing assistance; Internet; learning resource lab; library services; nursing audiovisuals; remedial services; resume preparation assistance; skills, simulation, or other laboratory; tutoring.
Library Facilities 1,300 volumes in health, 500 volumes in nursing; 550 periodical subscriptions health-care related.

BACCALAUREATE PROGRAMS

Degree BSN
Available Programs Generic Baccalaureate; RN Baccalaureate.
Site Options Sayre, PA.
Study Options Full-time and part-time.
Program Entrance Requirements Minimum overall college GPA of 2.7, transcript of college record, CPR certification, health exam, health insurance, high school biology, high school chemistry, 2 years high school math, 2 years high school science, high school transcript, immunizations, minimum high school GPA of 2.7, minimum high school rank 60%, professional liability insurance/malpractice insurance. Transfer students are accepted. *Application deadline:* Applications may be processed on a rolling basis for some programs. *Application fee:* $25.
Advanced Placement Credit by examination available. Credit given for nursing courses completed elsewhere dependent upon specific evaluations.
Expenses (2012–13) *Tuition, area resident:* full-time $6428; part-time $268 per credit. *Tuition, state resident:* full-time $10,608; part-time $429 per credit. *Tuition, nonresident:* full-time $16,070; part-time $429 per credit. *Room and board:* $9974 per academic year. *Required fees:* full-time $2498.
Financial Aid 90% of baccalaureate students in nursing programs received some form of financial aid in 2011–12.
Contact Admissions Office, Department of Health Sciences–Nursing, Mansfield University of Pennsylvania, Alumni Hall, Mansfield, PA 16933. *Telephone:* 570-662-4243. *Fax:* 570-662-4121. *E-mail:* admissions@mansfield.edu.

GRADUATE PROGRAMS

Expenses (2012–13) *Tuition, area resident:* part-time $429 per credit. *Tuition, state resident:* part-time $644 per credit. *Tuition, nonresident:* part-time $644 per credit. *Required fees:* part-time $84 per credit.
Financial Aid 50% of graduate students in nursing programs received some form of financial aid in 2011–12.
Contact Dr. Janeen Bartlett Sheehe, Department Chair and Nursing Program Director, Department of Health Sciences–Nursing, Mansfield University of Pennsylvania, 212C Elliott Hall, Mansfield, PA 16933. *Telephone:* 570-662-4522. *Fax:* 570-662-4137. *E-mail:* jsheehe@ mansfield.edu.

MASTER'S DEGREE PROGRAM

Degree MSN

Available Programs Master's.

Concentrations Available Nursing administration; nursing education.

Study Options Part-time.

Online Degree Options Yes (online only).

Program Entrance Requirements Minimum overall college GPA of 3.0, transcript of college record, 1 letter of recommendation, nursing research course, prerequisite course work. *Application deadline:* Applications may be processed on a rolling basis for some programs. *Application fee:* $25.

Advanced Placement Credit given for nursing courses completed elsewhere dependent upon specific evaluations.

Degree Requirements 33 total credit hours, thesis or project.

Marywood University

Department of Nursing
Scranton, Pennsylvania

http://www.marywood.edu/nursing/index.html
Founded in 1915

DEGREES • BSN • MSN • MSN/MPH

Nursing Program Faculty 16 (50% with doctorates).

Baccalaureate Enrollment 117 **Women** 90% **Men** 10% **Minority** 5% **International** 3% **Part-time** 5%

Graduate Enrollment 17 **Women** 100% **Part-time** 90%

Distance Learning Courses Available.

Nursing Student Activities Sigma Theta Tau, Student Nurses' Association.

Nursing Student Resources Academic advising; academic or career counseling; assistance for students with disabilities; bookstore; campus computer network; computer lab; daycare for children of students; e-mail services; employment services for current students; interactive nursing skills videos; Internet; learning resource lab; library services; nursing audiovisuals; skills, simulation, or other laboratory; tutoring.

Library Facilities 224,294 volumes (7,400 in health, 3,006 in nursing); 29,756 periodical subscriptions (750 health-care related).

BACCALAUREATE PROGRAMS

Degree BSN

Available Programs ADN to Baccalaureate; Generic Baccalaureate; International Nurse to Baccalaureate; LPN to Baccalaureate; RN Baccalaureate.

Study Options Full-time and part-time.

Program Entrance Requirements Transcript of college record, high school biology, high school chemistry, 1 year of high school math, high school transcript, 1 letter of recommendation. Transfer students are accepted.

Advanced Placement Credit given for nursing courses completed elsewhere dependent upon specific evaluations.

Contact *Telephone:* 570-348-6211 Ext. 2374. *Fax:* 570-961-4761.

GRADUATE PROGRAMS

Contact *Telephone:* 570-348-6211 Ext. 2475. *Fax:* 570-961-4761.

MASTER'S DEGREE PROGRAM

Degrees MSN; MSN/MPH

Available Programs Master's.

Concentrations Available Nursing administration.

Study Options Full-time and part-time.

Program Entrance Requirements Clinical experience, minimum overall college GPA of 3.0, transcript of college record, written essay, 2 letters of recommendation, nursing research course, physical assessment course, statistics course.

Degree Requirements 39 total credit hours, thesis or project.

CONTINUING EDUCATION PROGRAM

Contact *Telephone:* 570-340-6060. *Fax:* 570-961-4776.

Messiah College

Department of Nursing
Mechanicsburg, Pennsylvania

http://www.messiah.edu/
Founded in 1909

DEGREE • BSN

Nursing Program Faculty 25 (28% with doctorates).

Baccalaureate Enrollment 232 **Women** 91% **Men** 9% **Minority** 8% **International** .4% **Part-time** 2%

Nursing Student Activities Nursing Honor Society, Sigma Theta Tau, Student Nurses' Association, nursing club.

Nursing Student Resources Academic advising; academic or career counseling; assistance for students with disabilities; bookstore; campus computer network; career placement assistance; computer lab; computer-assisted instruction; e-mail services; employment services for current students; interactive nursing skills videos; Internet; learning resource lab; library services; nursing audiovisuals; remedial services; resume preparation assistance; skills, simulation, or other laboratory; tutoring.

Library Facilities 282,358 volumes (9,021 in health, 1,631 in nursing); 54,706 periodical subscriptions (6,649 health-care related).

BACCALAUREATE PROGRAMS

Degree BSN

Available Programs Generic Baccalaureate.

Study Options Full-time and part-time.

Program Entrance Requirements Minimum overall college GPA of 3.0, transcript of college record, CPR certification, health exam, health insurance, high school foreign language, 2 years high school math, 2 years high school science, high school transcript, immunizations, minimum GPA in nursing prerequisites of 2.7, prerequisite course work. Transfer students are accepted. *Application deadline:* Applications may be processed on a rolling basis for some programs. *Application fee:* $30.

Advanced Placement Credit given for nursing courses completed elsewhere dependent upon specific evaluations.

Expenses (2012–13) *Tuition:* full-time $28,640; part-time $1196 per credit hour. *International tuition:* $28,640 full-time. *Room and board:* $8760; room only: $4640 per academic year. *Required fees:* full-time $2200.

Financial Aid 100% of baccalaureate students in nursing programs received some form of financial aid in 2011–12. *Gift aid (need-based):* Federal Pell, FSEOG, state, private, college/university gift aid from institutional funds. *Loans:* Federal Nursing Student Loans, Federal Direct (Subsidized and Unsubsidized Stafford PLUS), Perkins. *Work-study:* Federal Work-Study, part-time campus jobs. *Financial aid application deadline (priority):* 4/1.

Contact Dana Britton, Director of Admissions, Department of Nursing, Messiah College, Suite 3005, One College Avenue, Mechanicsburg, PA 17055. *Telephone:* 800-233-4220. *Fax:* 717-796-5374. *E-mail:* admiss@messiah.edu.

Millersville University of Pennsylvania

Department of Nursing
Millersville, Pennsylvania

http://www.millersville.edu/nursing/
Founded in 1855

DEGREES • BSN • MSN

Nursing Program Faculty 10 (60% with doctorates).

Baccalaureate Enrollment 101 **Women** 95% **Men** 5% **Minority** 18% **Part-time** 90%

Graduate Enrollment 110 **Women** 86% **Men** 14% **Minority** 3% **Part-time** 100%

Nursing Student Activities Sigma Theta Tau.

Nursing Student Resources Academic advising; academic or career counseling; assistance for students with disabilities; bookstore; computer lab; e-mail services; interactive nursing skills videos; Internet; library services; nursing audiovisuals; resume preparation assistance.

Library Facilities 363,250 volumes; 77,665 periodical subscriptions (82 health-care related).

BACCALAUREATE PROGRAMS

Degree BSN

Available Programs RN Baccalaureate.

Site Options Harrisburg, PA.

Study Options Full-time and part-time.

Program Entrance Requirements Minimum overall college GPA of 2.0, transcript of college record, RN licensure. Transfer students are accepted. *Application deadline:* Applications may be processed on a rolling basis for some programs. *Application fee:* $40.

Expenses (2012–13) *Tuition, state resident:* part-time $358 per credit. *Tuition, nonresident:* part-time $768 per credit.

Financial Aid 50% of baccalaureate students in nursing programs received some form of financial aid in 2011–12.

Contact Dr. Barbara Zimmerman, Chairperson, Department of Nursing, Millersville University of Pennsylvania, Caputo Hall, PO Box 1002, Millersville, PA 17551-0302. *Telephone:* 717-872-3376. *Fax:* 717-871-4877. *E-mail:* barbara.zimmerman@millersville.edu.

GRADUATE PROGRAMS

Expenses (2012–13) *Tuition, state resident:* part-time $548 per credit. *Tuition, nonresident:* part-time $773 per credit.

Financial Aid 50% of graduate students in nursing programs received some form of financial aid in 2011–12. 2 research assistantships with partial tuition reimbursements available (averaging $1,871 per year) were awarded; institutionally sponsored loans and unspecified assistantships also available. Aid available to part-time students. *Financial aid application deadline:* 3/15.

Contact Dr. Deborah Castellucci, Graduate Program Coordinator, Department of Nursing, Millersville University of Pennsylvania, Caputo Hall, PO Box 1002, Millersville, PA 17551-0302. *Telephone:* 717-871-5341. *Fax:* 717-871-4887. *E-mail:* deborah.castellucci@millersville.edu.

MASTER'S DEGREE PROGRAM

Degree MSN

Available Programs Master's.

Concentrations Available Nursing education. *Nurse practitioner programs in:* family health.

Study Options Part-time.

Program Entrance Requirements Clinical experience, minimum overall college GPA of 3.0, transcript of college record, interview, 3 letters of recommendation, nursing research course, physical assessment course, resume, statistics course. *Application deadline:* 1/15 (spring). *Application fee:* $40.

Degree Requirements Thesis or project.

POST-MASTER'S PROGRAM

Areas of Study Nursing education. *Nurse practitioner programs in:* family health.

Misericordia University

Department of Nursing
Dallas, Pennsylvania

http://www.misericordia.edu/nursing
Founded in 1924

DEGREES • BSN • MSN

Nursing Program Faculty 34 (5% with doctorates).

Baccalaureate Enrollment 196 **Women** 87% **Men** 13% **Minority** 3% **Part-time** 25%

Graduate Enrollment 63 **Women** 93% **Men** 7% **Part-time** 100%

Distance Learning Courses Available.

Nursing Student Activities Nursing Honor Society, Sigma Theta Tau, Student Nurses' Association, nursing club.

Nursing Student Resources Academic advising; academic or career counseling; assistance for students with disabilities; bookstore; campus computer network; career placement assistance; computer lab; computer-assisted instruction; e-mail services; employment services for current students; externships; housing assistance; interactive nursing skills videos; Internet; learning resource lab; library services; nursing audiovisuals; placement services for program completers; remedial services; resume preparation assistance; skills, simulation, or other laboratory; tutoring.

Library Facilities 80,417 volumes (5 in health, 5 in nursing); 43,545 periodical subscriptions (15 health-care related).

BACCALAUREATE PROGRAMS

Degree BSN

Available Programs Accelerated RN Baccalaureate; Baccalaureate for Second Degree; Generic Baccalaureate; RN Baccalaureate.

Study Options Full-time and part-time. ·

Program Entrance Requirements Minimum overall college GPA of 3.0, transcript of college record, CPR certification, health exam, health insurance, high school biology, high school chemistry, 1 year of high school math, high school transcript, immunizations, letters of recommendation, minimum high school GPA of 2.5, minimum high school rank, minimum GPA in nursing prerequisites of 3.0, professional liability insurance/malpractice insurance. Transfer students are accepted. *Application deadline:* 8/1 (fall), 8/1 (winter), 12/1 (spring), 4/1 (summer). Applications may be processed on a rolling basis for some programs. *Application fee:* $200.

Advanced Placement Credit by examination available. Credit given for nursing courses completed elsewhere dependent upon specific evaluations.

Expenses (2012–13) *Tuition:* full-time $12,940; part-time $495 per credit. *Room and board:* $5800; room only: $3300 per academic year. *Required fees:* full-time $450; part-time $225 per term.

Financial Aid 75% of baccalaureate students in nursing programs received some form of financial aid in 2011–12. *Gift aid (need-based):* Federal Pell, FSEOG, state, private, college/university gift aid from institutional funds, Federal Nursing. *Loans:* Federal Nursing Student Loans, Perkins, state. *Work-study:* Federal Work-Study. *Financial aid application deadline (priority):* 3/1.

Contact Mr. Glenn Bozinski, Admissions, Department of Nursing, Misericordia University, 301 Lake Street, Dallas, PA 18612. *Telephone:* 570-674-6434. *E-mail:* gbozinsk@misericordia.edu.

GRADUATE PROGRAMS

Expenses (2012–13) *Tuition:* part-time $625 per credit. *Required fees:* part-time $250 per term.

Financial Aid 90% of graduate students in nursing programs received some form of financial aid in 2011–12. Teaching assistantships, career-related internships or fieldwork, scholarships, traineeships, tuition waivers (partial), and unspecified assistantships available. Aid available to part-time students. *Financial aid application deadline:* 6/30.

Contact Miss Larree Brown, Adult Education Counselor, Graduate Programs, Department of Nursing, Misericordia University, 301 Lake Street, Dallas, PA 18612. *Telephone:* 570-674-6451. *Fax:* 570-674-8902. *E-mail:* lbrown@misericordia.edu.

MASTER'S DEGREE PROGRAM

Degree MSN

Available Programs Master's; RN to Master's.

Concentrations Available Nursing education. *Clinical nurse specialist programs in:* family health. *Nurse practitioner programs in:* family health.

Study Options Part-time.

Program Entrance Requirements Clinical experience, computer literacy, minimum overall college GPA of 3.0, transcript of college record, written essay, 3 letters of recommendation, nursing research course, physical assessment course, professional liability insurance/malpractice insurance, statistics course. *Application deadline:* 7/18 (fall), 7/18 (winter), 12/1 (spring), 4/1 (summer). Applications may be processed on a rolling basis for some programs. *Application fee:* $200.

Advanced Placement Credit given for nursing courses completed elsewhere dependent upon specific evaluations.

Degree Requirements 45 total credit hours, thesis or project.

POST-MASTER'S PROGRAM

Areas of Study Nursing education. *Clinical nurse specialist programs in:* family health. *Nurse practitioner programs in:* family health.

Moravian College

St. Luke's School of Nursing
Bethlehem, Pennsylvania

http://www.moravian.edu/
Founded in 1742

DEGREES • BS • MS

Nursing Program Faculty 32 (38% with doctorates).

Baccalaureate Enrollment 216 **Women** 94% **Men** 6% **Minority** 5% **International** 1% **Part-time** 38%

Graduate Enrollment 55 **Women** 95% **Men** 5% **Minority** 5% **International** 2% **Part-time** 100%

Nursing Student Activities Sigma Theta Tau, Student Nurses' Association.

Nursing Student Resources Academic advising; academic or career counseling; assistance for students with disabilities; bookstore; campus computer network; career placement assistance; computer lab; computer-assisted instruction; e-mail services; employment services for current students; externships; housing assistance; interactive nursing skills videos; Internet; learning resource lab; library services; nursing audiovisuals; placement services for program completers; remedial services; resume preparation assistance; skills, simulation, or other laboratory; tutoring.

Library Facilities 323,790 volumes (4,600 in health, 1,900 in nursing); 46,210 periodical subscriptions (275 health-care related).

BACCALAUREATE PROGRAMS

Degree BS

Available Programs Generic Baccalaureate; RN Baccalaureate.

Study Options Full-time.

Program Entrance Requirements CPR certification, written essay, health exam, health insurance, high school biology, high school foreign language, 3 years high school math, 3 years high school science, high school transcript, immunizations, minimum GPA in nursing prerequisites of 2.7, prerequisite course work. Transfer students are accepted. *Application deadline:* 3/1 (fall). *Application fee:* $40.

Advanced Placement Credit by examination available. Credit given for nursing courses completed elsewhere dependent upon specific evaluations.

Expenses (2012–13) *Tuition:* full-time $33,919. *Room and board:* $10,330; room only: $5860 per academic year.

Financial Aid 90% of baccalaureate students in nursing programs received some form of financial aid in 2011–12. *Gift aid (need-based):* Federal Pell, FSEOG, state, private, college/university gift aid from institutional funds. *Loans:* Federal Direct (Subsidized and Unsubsidized Stafford PLUS), Perkins. *Work-study:* Federal Work-Study, part-time campus jobs. *Financial aid application deadline (priority):* 2/14.

Contact Ms. Erika E. Mondok, Interim Director of Enrollment, St. Luke's School of Nursing, Moravian College, 1200 Main Street, Bethlehem, PA 18018. *Telephone:* 800-441-3191. *E-mail:* erikamondok@moravian.edu.

GRADUATE PROGRAMS

Expenses (2012–13) *Tuition:* part-time $2145 per course. *Required fees:* part-time $90 per term.

Contact Dr. Lori Hoffman, RN, MS Program Coordinator, St. Luke's School of Nursing, Moravian College, 1200 Main Street, Bethlehem, PA 18018. *Telephone:* 610-625-7769. *Fax:* 610-625-7861. *E-mail:* lorihoffman@moravian.edu.

MASTER'S DEGREE PROGRAM

Degree MS

Available Programs Master's; Master's for Nurses with Non-Nursing Degrees.

Concentrations Available Clinical nurse leader; nursing administration; nursing education.

Study Options Part-time.

Program Entrance Requirements Computer literacy, minimum overall college GPA of 3.0, transcript of college record, written essay, 2 letters of recommendation, prerequisite course work, resume, statistics course. *Application deadline:* Applications may be processed on a rolling basis for some programs. *Application fee:* $35.

Advanced Placement Credit given for nursing courses completed elsewhere dependent upon specific evaluations.

Degree Requirements 36 total credit hours, thesis or project.

CONTINUING EDUCATION PROGRAM

Contact Ms. Dawn Goodolf, RN, RN-to-BS Program Coordinator, St. Luke's School of Nursing, Moravian College, 1200 Main Street, Bethlehem, PA 18018. *Telephone:* 610-625-7764. *Fax:* 610-625-7861. *E-mail:* medmg01@moravian.edu.

Mount Aloysius College
Division of Nursing
Cresson, Pennsylvania

http://www.mtaloy.edu/
Founded in 1939

DEGREE • BSN

Nursing Program Faculty 8 (25% with doctorates).

Baccalaureate Enrollment 72 **Women** 88% **Men** 12% **Minority** 1% **Part-time** 89%

Distance Learning Courses Available.

Nursing Student Activities Student Nurses' Association.

Nursing Student Resources Academic advising; academic or career counseling; assistance for students with disabilities; bookstore; campus computer network; computer lab; computer-assisted instruction; daycare for children of students; e-mail services; interactive nursing skills videos; Internet; learning resource lab; library services; nursing audiovisuals; remedial services; resume preparation assistance; skills, simulation, or other laboratory; tutoring.

Library Facilities 90,750 volumes (6,000 in health, 900 in nursing); 164 periodical subscriptions (42 health-care related).

BACCALAUREATE PROGRAMS

Degree BSN

Available Programs ADN to Baccalaureate; Accelerated RN Baccalaureate.

Site Options Johnstown, PA; Altoona, PA.

Study Options Full-time.

Online Degree Options Yes.

Program Entrance Requirements Transcript of college record, health exam, high school transcript, immunizations, RN licensure. Transfer students are accepted. *Application deadline:* Applications may be processed on a rolling basis for some programs. *Application fee:* $30.

Advanced Placement Credit by examination available. Credit given for nursing courses completed elsewhere dependent upon specific evaluations.

Expenses (2011–12) *Tuition:* full-time $20,180; part-time $560 per credit. *Room and board:* $8950 per academic year. *Required fees:* part-time $30 per term.

Financial Aid 35% of baccalaureate students in nursing programs received some form of financial aid in 2010–11.

Contact Dr. Jacqueline Beck, Chairperson, RN-BSN Department, Division of Nursing, Mount Aloysius College, 7373 Admiral Peary Highway, Cresson, PA 16630. *Telephone:* 814-886-6401. *Fax:* 814-886-6374. *E-mail:* jbeck@mtaloy.edu.

CONTINUING EDUCATION PROGRAM

Contact Ms. Roxane Hogue, Director of Graduate and Continuing Education, Division of Nursing, Mount Aloysius College, 7373 Admiral Peary Highway, Cresson, PA 16630. *Telephone:* 814-886-6403. *Fax:* 814-886-2978. *E-mail:* rhogue@mtaloy.edu.

Neumann University
Program in Nursing and Health Sciences
Aston, Pennsylvania

http://www.neumann.edu/
Founded in 1965

DEGREES • BS • MS

Nursing Program Faculty 37 (14% with doctorates).

Baccalaureate Enrollment 585 **Women** 87.9% **Men** 12.1% **Minority** 23.8% **International** .3% **Part-time** 40.2%

Graduate Enrollment 34 **Women** 100% **Minority** 23.5% **Part-time** 100%

Nursing Student Activities Nursing Honor Society, Sigma Theta Tau, Student Nurses' Association.

Nursing Student Resources Academic advising; academic or career counseling; assistance for students with disabilities; bookstore; campus computer network; career placement assistance; computer lab; computer-assisted instruction; e-mail services; employment services for current students; externships; housing assistance; interactive nursing skills videos; Internet; learning resource lab; library services; nursing audiovisuals; paid internships; remedial services; resume preparation assistance; skills, simulation, or other laboratory; tutoring; unpaid internships.

Library Facilities 60,750 volumes (600 in health, 540 in nursing); 166 periodical subscriptions (6,500 health-care related).

BACCALAUREATE PROGRAMS

Degree BS

Available Programs ADN to Baccalaureate; Accelerated RN Baccalaureate; Baccalaureate for Second Degree; Generic Baccalaureate; International Nurse to Baccalaureate; LPN to Baccalaureate; LPN to RN Baccalaureate.

Study Options Full-time and part-time.

Program Entrance Requirements Minimum overall college GPA of 2.5, transcript of college record, health exam, health insurance, high school biology, high school chemistry, high school foreign language, 2 years high school math, 4 years high school science, high school transcript, immunizations, minimum high school GPA of 2.5, minimum GPA in nursing prerequisites of 2.5, prerequisite course work. Transfer students are accepted. *Application deadline:* Applications may be processed on a rolling basis for some programs.

Advanced Placement Credit by examination available. Credit given for nursing courses completed elsewhere dependent upon specific evaluations.

Expenses (2012–13) *Tuition:* full-time $23,262; part-time $531 per credit. *International tuition:* $23,262 full-time. *Room and board:* $11,070 per academic year. *Required fees:* full-time $810; part-time $100 per credit.

Financial Aid 95% of baccalaureate students in nursing programs received some form of financial aid in 2011–12.

Contact Ms. Rachael Sokolovich, Admissions Counselor, Program in Nursing and Health Sciences, Neumann University, One Neumann Drive, Aston, PA 19014-1298. *Telephone:* 800-963-8626 Ext. 5531. *Fax:* 610-558-5652. *E-mail:* sokolovr@neumann.edu.

GRADUATE PROGRAMS

Expenses (2012–13) *Tuition:* part-time $631 per credit hour.

Financial Aid 50% of graduate students in nursing programs received some form of financial aid in 2011–12. Available to part-time students. *Application deadline:* 3/15.

Contact Ms. Kittie Pain, Associate Director, Admissions, Program in Nursing and Health Sciences, Neumann University, One Neumann Drive, Aston, PA 19014-1298. *Telephone:* 800-963-8626 Ext. 5613. *Fax:* 610-558-5652. *E-mail:* nursediv@neumann.edu.

MASTER'S DEGREE PROGRAM

Degree MS

Available Programs Master's.

Concentrations Available Nursing education. *Nurse practitioner programs in:* adult health.

Study Options Full-time and part-time.

Program Entrance Requirements Computer literacy, minimum overall college GPA of 3.0, transcript of college record, CPR certification, immunizations, interview, 2 letters of recommendation, nursing research course, physical assessment course, professional liability insurance/malpractice insurance, prerequisite course work, statistics course, GRE or MAT. *Application deadline:* Applications may be processed on a rolling basis for some programs.

Advanced Placement Credit given for nursing courses completed elsewhere dependent upon specific evaluations.

Degree Requirements 43 total credit hours, thesis or project.

POST-MASTER'S PROGRAM

Areas of Study Nursing education. *Nurse practitioner programs in:* adult health.

Penn State University Park
School of Nursing
State College, University Park, Pennsylvania

http://www.nursing.psu.edu/
Founded in 1855

DEGREES • BS • MS • MSN/PHD • PHD

Nursing Program Faculty 110 (20% with doctorates).

Baccalaureate Enrollment 824 **Women** 95% **Men** 5% **Minority** 7% **Part-time** 43%

Graduate Enrollment 61 **Women** 92% **Men** 8% **Minority** 10% **Part-time** 59%

Distance Learning Courses Available.

Nursing Student Activities Sigma Theta Tau, Student Nurses' Association.

Nursing Student Resources Academic advising; academic or career counseling; assistance for students with disabilities; bookstore; campus computer network; career placement assistance; computer lab; computer-assisted instruction; daycare for children of students; e-mail services; employment services for current students; externships; housing assistance; interactive nursing skills videos; Internet; learning resource lab; library services; nursing audiovisuals; paid internships; remedial services; resume preparation assistance; skills, simulation, or other laboratory; tutoring.

Library Facilities 5.8 million volumes (244,000 in health); 102,865 periodical subscriptions (3,500 health-care related).

BACCALAUREATE PROGRAMS

Degree BS

Available Programs ADN to Baccalaureate; Generic Baccalaureate; RN Baccalaureate.

Site Options Uniontown, PA; New Kensington, PA; Harrisburg, PA; Hershey, PA; University Park, PA; Altoona, PA; Mont Alto, PA; Sharon, PA: Scranton, PA.

Study Options Full-time.

Online Degree Options Yes.

Program Entrance Requirements Transcript of college record, 3 years high school math, 3 years high school science, high school transcript. Transfer students are accepted. *Application deadline:* 11/30 (fall). *Application fee:* $50.

Advanced Placement Credit given for nursing courses completed elsewhere dependent upon specific evaluations.

Contact *Telephone:* 814-863-8185. *Fax:* 814-863-2925.

GRADUATE PROGRAMS

Contact *Telephone:* 814-863-2211. *Fax:* 814-865-2925.

MASTER'S DEGREE PROGRAM

Degrees MS; MSN/PhD

Available Programs Master's.

Concentrations Available Nursing administration. *Clinical nurse specialist programs in:* adult health, community health, gerontology. *Nurse practitioner programs in:* adult health, family health.

Site Options Hershey, PA; University Park, PA.

Study Options Full-time and part-time.

Online Degree Options Yes.

Program Entrance Requirements Computer literacy, minimum overall college GPA of 3.0, transcript of college record, CPR certification, written essay, immunizations, 2 letters of recommendation, professional liability insurance/malpractice insurance. *Application deadline:* Applications may be processed on a rolling basis for some programs. *Application fee:* $65.

Advanced Placement Credit given for nursing courses completed elsewhere dependent upon specific evaluations.

Degree Requirements 43 total credit hours, thesis or project.

POST-MASTER'S PROGRAM

Areas of Study *Nurse practitioner programs in:* family health.

DOCTORAL DEGREE PROGRAM

Degree PhD

Available Programs Doctorate.

Areas of Study Bio-behavioral research, faculty preparation, gerontology, human health and illness, illness and transition, individualized study, nursing research, nursing science.

Site Options Hershey, PA; University Park, PA.

Program Entrance Requirements Minimum overall college GPA of 3.5, interview, 3 letters of recommendation, MSN or equivalent, writing sample. *Application deadline:* Applications may be processed on a rolling basis for some programs. *Application fee:* $65.

Degree Requirements 58 total credit hours, dissertation, oral exam, written exam, residency.

POSTDOCTORAL PROGRAM

Areas of Study Gerontology.

Postdoctoral Program Contact *Telephone:* 814-865-9337. *Fax:* 814-865-2925.

CONTINUING EDUCATION PROGRAM

Contact *Telephone:* 814-865-8469. *Fax:* 814-865-3779.

Pennsylvania College of Technology
School of Health Sciences
Williamsport, Pennsylvania

Founded in 1965

DEGREE • BSN

Nursing Program Faculty 37 (5% with doctorates).
Baccalaureate Enrollment 12 **Women** 100% **International** 1% **Part-time** 92%
Nursing Student Activities Student Nurses' Association.
Nursing Student Resources Academic advising; academic or career counseling; assistance for students with disabilities; bookstore; campus computer network; career placement assistance; computer lab; computer-assisted instruction; daycare for children of students; e-mail services; employment services for current students; externships; housing assistance; interactive nursing skills videos; Internet; learning resource lab; library services; nursing audiovisuals; placement services for program completers; remedial services; resume preparation assistance; skills, simulation, or other laboratory; tutoring.
Library Facilities 147,200 volumes; 32,086 periodical subscriptions.

BACCALAUREATE PROGRAMS

Degree BSN
Available Programs RN Baccalaureate.
Program Entrance Requirements Transfer students are accepted.
Contact *Telephone:* 800-367-9222 Ext. 4525.

Robert Morris University
School of Nursing and Health Sciences
Moon Township, Pennsylvania

http://www.rmu.edu/web/cms/schools/snhs/nursing/Pages/default.aspx
Founded in 1921

DEGREES • BSN • DNP • MSN

Nursing Program Faculty 30 (50% with doctorates).
Baccalaureate Enrollment 429 **Women** 85% **Men** 15% **Minority** 7% **Part-time** 20%
Graduate Enrollment 149 **Women** 88% **Men** 12% **Minority** 13% **International** 1% **Part-time** 100%
Distance Learning Courses Available.
Nursing Student Activities Nursing Honor Society, Sigma Theta Tau, Student Nurses' Association.
Nursing Student Resources Academic advising; academic or career counseling; assistance for students with disabilities; bookstore; campus computer network; career placement assistance; computer lab; computer-assisted instruction; e-mail services; employment services for current students; externships; housing assistance; interactive nursing skills videos; Internet; learning resource lab; library services; nursing audiovisuals; paid internships; placement services for program completers; remedial services; resume preparation assistance; skills, simulation, or other laboratory; tutoring; unpaid internships.
Library Facilities 115,350 volumes; 19,143 periodical subscriptions.

BACCALAUREATE PROGRAMS

Degree BSN
Available Programs Baccalaureate for Second Degree; Generic Baccalaureate.
Study Options Full-time and part-time.
Online Degree Options Yes.
Program Entrance Requirements Minimum overall college GPA of 3.0, transcript of college record, written essay, health exam, health insurance, high school biology, high school chemistry, 2 years high school math, 2 years high school science, high school transcript, immunizations, 2 letters of recommendation, minimum high school GPA of 3.0, minimum GPA in nursing prerequisites of 2.0, prerequisite course work. Transfer students are accepted. *Application deadline:* 5/1 (fall), 11/1 (spring). Applications may be processed on a rolling basis for some programs. *Application fee:* $30.
Advanced Placement Credit given for nursing courses completed elsewhere dependent upon specific evaluations.

Expenses (2012–13) *Tuition:* full-time $25,750; part-time $835 per credit. *Room and board:* $11,360; room only: $5370 per academic year. *Required fees:* full-time $654; part-time $30 per credit.
Financial Aid 90% of baccalaureate students in nursing programs received some form of financial aid in 2011–12.
Contact Enrollment Services, School of Nursing and Health Sciences, Robert Morris University, 6001 University Boulevard, Moon Township, PA 15108-1189. *Telephone:* 412-397-5200. *Fax:* 412-397-2425. *E-mail:* admissionsoffice@rmu.edu.

GRADUATE PROGRAMS

Expenses (2012–13) *Tuition:* part-time $820 per credit. *Required fees:* part-time $15 per credit.
Financial Aid 80% of graduate students in nursing programs received some form of financial aid in 2011–12. Federal Work-Study, institutionally sponsored loans, and unspecified assistantships available. *Financial aid application deadline:* 5/1.
Contact Enrollment Services, School of Nursing and Health Sciences, Robert Morris University, 6001 University Boulevard, Moon Township, PA 15108-1189. *Telephone:* 412-397-5200. *Fax:* 412-397-2425. *E-mail:* GraduateAdmissions@rmu.edu.

MASTER'S DEGREE PROGRAM

Degree MSN
Available Programs Master's.
Concentrations Available Nursing education.
Site Options Cranberry, PA.
Study Options Part-time.
Program Entrance Requirements Clinical experience, minimum overall college GPA of 3.25, transcript of college record, CPR certification, written essay, interview, 2 letters of recommendation, statistics course. *Application deadline:* Applications may be processed on a rolling basis for some programs. *Application fee:* $35.
Degree Requirements 36 total credit hours, thesis or project.

DOCTORAL DEGREE PROGRAM

Degree DNP
Available Programs Doctorate; Post-Baccalaureate Doctorate.
Areas of Study Advanced practice nursing.
Program Entrance Requirements Clinical experience, minimum overall college GPA of 3.25, interview by faculty committee, 2 letters of recommendation, vita, writing sample. *Application deadline:* Applications may be processed on a rolling basis for some programs. *Application fee:* $35.

Saint Francis University
Department of Nursing
Loretto, Pennsylvania

http://francis.edu/nursing/
Founded in 1847

DEGREE • BSN

Nursing Program Faculty 7 (1% with doctorates).
Baccalaureate Enrollment 85 **Women** 90% **Men** 10% **Minority** 2%
Nursing Student Activities Student Nurses' Association, nursing club.
Nursing Student Resources Academic advising; academic or career counseling; assistance for students with disabilities; bookstore; campus computer network; career placement assistance; computer lab; computer-assisted instruction; e-mail services; employment services for current students; externships; interactive nursing skills videos; Internet; learning resource lab; library services; nursing audiovisuals; resume preparation assistance; skills, simulation, or other laboratory; tutoring.
Library Facilities 152,712 volumes (150,000 in health, 120,000 in nursing); 30,029 periodical subscriptions (25 health-care related).

BACCALAUREATE PROGRAMS

Degree BSN
Available Programs Generic Baccalaureate.
Study Options Full-time and part-time.
Program Entrance Requirements Transcript of college record, high school biology, high school chemistry, 2 years high school math, 2 years high school science, high school transcript, minimum high school GPA of 3.0, minimum high school rank 50%, minimum GPA in nursing prerequisites of 2.7, prerequisite course work. Transfer students are accepted. *Application deadline:* Applications may be processed on a rolling basis for some programs. *Application fee:* $30.

Advanced Placement Credit by examination available. Credit given for nursing courses completed elsewhere dependent upon specific evaluations.

Expenses (2011–12) *Room and board:* $2392 per academic year.

Financial Aid 100% of baccalaureate students in nursing programs received some form of financial aid in 2010–11. *Gift aid (need-based):* Federal Pell, FSEOG, state, private, college/university gift aid from institutional funds. *Loans:* Federal Direct (Subsidized and Unsubsidized Stafford PLUS), Perkins, private loans. *Work-study:* Federal Work-Study, part-time campus jobs. *Financial aid application deadline (priority):* 5/1.

Contact Dr. Rita M. Trofino, Chairperson, Department of Nursing, Saint Francis University, PO Box 600, 117 Evergreen Drive, 103 Schwab Hall, Loretto, PA 15940-0600. *Telephone:* 814-472-3027. *Fax:* 814-472-3849. *E-mail:* rtrofino@francis.edu.

Slippery Rock University of Pennsylvania
Department of Nursing
Slippery Rock, Pennsylvania

http://www.sru.edu/academics/colleges/ches/nursing/Pages/ Welcome.aspx
Founded in 1889

DEGREE • BSN

Nursing Program Faculty 7 (100% with doctorates).
Baccalaureate Enrollment 230 **Women** 95% **Men** 5% **Minority** 1% **Part-time** 97%
Distance Learning Courses Available.
Nursing Student Activities Sigma Theta Tau.
Nursing Student Resources Academic advising; academic or career counseling; assistance for students with disabilities; bookstore; campus computer network; career placement assistance; computer lab; computer-assisted instruction; daycare for children of students; e-mail services; employment services for current students; housing assistance; Internet; library services; nursing audiovisuals; placement services for program completers; resume preparation assistance; tutoring.
Library Facilities 621,761 volumes (7,214 in health, 925 in nursing); 343 periodical subscriptions (1,299 health-care related).

BACCALAUREATE PROGRAMS

Degree BSN
Available Programs ADN to Baccalaureate; RN Baccalaureate.
Study Options Full-time and part-time.
Online Degree Options Yes (online only).
Program Entrance Requirements Minimum overall college GPA of 2.5, transcript of college record, minimum GPA in nursing prerequisites of 2.5, professional liability insurance/malpractice insurance, RN licensure. Transfer students are accepted. *Application deadline:* Applications may be processed on a rolling basis for some programs. *Application fee:* $30.
Advanced Placement Credit by examination available. Credit given for nursing courses completed elsewhere dependent upon specific evaluations.
Contact *Telephone:* 724-738-4921. *Fax:* 724-738-2509.

Temple University
Department of Nursing
Philadelphia, Pennsylvania

http://www.temple.edu/nursing
Founded in 1884

DEGREES • BSN • DNP • MSN

Nursing Program Faculty 37 (50% with doctorates).
Baccalaureate Enrollment 400 **Women** 85% **Men** 15% **Minority** 49% **Part-time** 62%
Graduate Enrollment 120 **Women** 95% **Men** 5% **Minority** 16% **Part-time** 100%
Distance Learning Courses Available.
Nursing Student Activities Nursing Honor Society, Sigma Theta Tau, Student Nurses' Association, nursing club.

Nursing Student Resources Academic advising; academic or career counseling; assistance for students with disabilities; bookstore; campus computer network; career placement assistance; computer lab; computer-assisted instruction; e-mail services; externships; housing assistance; interactive nursing skills videos; Internet; learning resource lab; library services; nursing audiovisuals; remedial services; resume preparation assistance; skills, simulation, or other laboratory; tutoring.
Library Facilities 60,374 volumes in health, 1,350 volumes in nursing; 62,173 periodical subscriptions (1,350 health-care related).

BACCALAUREATE PROGRAMS

Degree BSN
Available Programs Generic Baccalaureate; RN Baccalaureate.
Study Options Full-time.
Program Entrance Requirements Minimum overall college GPA of 3.0, transcript of college record, CPR certification, written essay, health exam, health insurance, high school biology, high school chemistry, high school foreign language, 3 years high school math, 3 years high school science, high school transcript, immunizations, interview, minimum high school GPA of 3.0, minimum GPA in nursing prerequisites of 3.0, prerequisite course work. Transfer students are accepted. *Application deadline:* 2/15 (fall). *Application fee:* $50.
Advanced Placement Credit given for nursing courses completed elsewhere dependent upon specific evaluations.
Contact *Telephone:* 215-707-4618. *Fax:* 215-707-1599.

GRADUATE PROGRAMS

Contact *Telephone:* 215-707-3789. *Fax:* 215-707-1599.

MASTER'S DEGREE PROGRAM

Degree MSN
Available Programs Master's.
Concentrations Available Nursing education. *Clinical nurse specialist programs in:* psychiatric/mental health. *Nurse practitioner programs in:* adult health, family health, pediatric.
Study Options Full-time and part-time.
Program Entrance Requirements Clinical experience, minimum overall college GPA of 3.0, transcript of college record, CPR certification, written essay, immunizations, interview, 2 letters of recommendation, nursing research course, physical assessment course, professional liability insurance/malpractice insurance, statistics course, GRE General Test.
Advanced Placement Credit given for nursing courses completed elsewhere dependent upon specific evaluations.
Degree Requirements 36 total credit hours.

POST-MASTER'S PROGRAM

Areas of Study Nursing education. *Clinical nurse specialist programs in:* psychiatric/mental health. *Nurse practitioner programs in:* adult health, family health, pediatric.

DOCTORAL DEGREE PROGRAM

Degree DNP
Available Programs Doctorate.

Thomas Jefferson University
Department of Nursing
Philadelphia, Pennsylvania

http://www.tju.edu/
Founded in 1824

DEGREES • BSN • DNP • MSN

Nursing Program Faculty 38 (42% with doctorates).
Nursing Student Activities Nursing Honor Society, Sigma Theta Tau, Student Nurses' Association.
Nursing Student Resources Academic advising; academic or career counseling; assistance for students with disabilities; bookstore; campus computer network; career placement assistance; computer lab; computer-assisted instruction; e-mail services; interactive nursing skills videos; Internet; learning resource lab; library services; nursing audiovisuals; paid internships; placement services for program completers; remedial services; resume preparation assistance; skills, simulation, or other laboratory; tutoring.
Library Facilities 146,000 volumes in health, 4,700 volumes in nursing; 2,100 periodical subscriptions health-care related.

BACCALAUREATE PROGRAMS

Degree BSN

Available Programs ADN to Baccalaureate; Accelerated Baccalaureate; Accelerated Baccalaureate for Second Degree; Accelerated RN Baccalaureate; Baccalaureate for Second Degree; Generic Baccalaureate; RN Baccalaureate.

Site Options Atlantic City, NJ; Philadelphia, PA.

Study Options Full-time and part-time.

Program Entrance Requirements Minimum overall college GPA of 2.9, transcript of college record, CPR certification, written essay, health exam, health insurance, high school transcript, immunizations, 2 letters of recommendation, prerequisite course work. Transfer students are accepted.

Advanced Placement Credit by examination available. Credit given for nursing courses completed elsewhere dependent upon specific evaluations.

Contact *Telephone:* 215-503-8104. *Fax:* 215-503-0376.

GRADUATE PROGRAMS

Contact *Telephone:* 215-503-8057. *Fax:* 215-932-1468.

MASTER'S DEGREE PROGRAM

Degree MSN

Available Programs Accelerated Master's; Accelerated RN to Master's; Master's; Master's for Non-Nursing College Graduates; Master's for Nurses with Non-Nursing Degrees; RN to Master's.

Concentrations Available Nurse anesthesia; nursing education; nursing informatics. *Clinical nurse specialist programs in:* acute care, adult health, community health, critical care, home health care, medical-surgical, oncology, pediatric, public health. *Nurse practitioner programs in:* acute care, adult health, family health, neonatal health, oncology, pediatric.

Site Options Philadelphia, PA.

Study Options Full-time and part-time.

Program Entrance Requirements Clinical experience, computer literacy, minimum overall college GPA of 3.0, transcript of college record, CPR certification, written essay, interview, 3 letters of recommendation, nursing research course, physical assessment course, professional liability insurance/malpractice insurance, resume, statistics course.

Advanced Placement Credit given for nursing courses completed elsewhere dependent upon specific evaluations.

Degree Requirements 36 total credit hours.

POST-MASTER'S PROGRAM

Areas of Study Nursing education; nursing informatics. *Nurse practitioner programs in:* acute care, adult health, family health, neonatal health, oncology, pediatric.

DOCTORAL DEGREE PROGRAM

Degree DNP

Available Programs Doctorate.

Areas of Study Advanced practice nursing, clinical practice, individualized study.

Program Entrance Requirements Clinical experience, minimum overall college GPA of 3.2, interview by faculty committee, interview, 3 letters of recommendation, MSN or equivalent, scholarly papers, statistics course, vita, writing sample.

Degree Requirements 36 total credit hours, written exam, residency.

CONTINUING EDUCATION PROGRAM

Contact *Telephone:* 215-503-8057. *Fax:* 215-503-0376.

University of Pennsylvania
School of Nursing
Philadelphia, Pennsylvania

http://www.nursing.upenn.edu/
Founded in 1740

DEGREES · BSN · MSN · MSN/MBA · MSN/MPH · MSN/PHD · PHD

Nursing Program Faculty 337 (16% with doctorates).
Baccalaureate Enrollment 554 **Women** 89% **Men** 11% **Minority** 37.4% **International** 2.3% **Part-time** 1.3%
Graduate Enrollment 503 **Women** 91.6% **Men** 8.4% **Minority** 23.3% **International** 3.4% **Part-time** 60.6%

Nursing Student Activities Nursing Honor Society, Sigma Theta Tau, Student Nurses' Association.

Nursing Student Resources Academic advising; academic or career counseling; assistance for students with disabilities; bookstore; campus computer network; career placement assistance; computer lab; computer-assisted instruction; daycare for children of students; e-mail services; employment services for current students; externships; housing assistance; interactive nursing skills videos; Internet; learning resource lab; library services; nursing audiovisuals; other; paid internships; placement services for program completers; remedial services; resume preparation assistance; skills, simulation, or other laboratory; tutoring; unpaid internships.

Library Facilities 6 million volumes; 105,721 periodical subscriptions.

BACCALAUREATE PROGRAMS

Degree BSN

Available Programs ADN to Baccalaureate; Accelerated Baccalaureate; Accelerated Baccalaureate for Second Degree; Accelerated RN Baccalaureate; Baccalaureate for Second Degree; Generic Baccalaureate; RN Baccalaureate.

Study Options Full-time and part-time.

Program Entrance Requirements Minimum overall college GPA of 3.0, transcript of college record, written essay, health exam, health insurance, high school biology, high school chemistry, high school foreign language, 4 years high school math, 4 years high school science, high school transcript, immunizations, interview, 2 letters of recommendation, minimum high school GPA of 3.0, minimum high school rank 10%. Transfer students are accepted. *Application deadline:* 1/1 (fall). *Application fee:* $75.

Advanced Placement Credit given for nursing courses completed elsewhere dependent upon specific evaluations.

Financial Aid 96% of baccalaureate students in nursing programs received some form of financial aid in 2011–12.

Contact Office of Enrollment Management, School of Nursing, University of Pennsylvania, 418 Curie Boulevard, Philadelphia, PA 19104-4217. *Telephone:* 215-898-4271. *Fax:* 215-573-8439. *E-mail:* admissions@nursing.upenn.edu.

GRADUATE PROGRAMS

Financial Aid 94% of graduate students in nursing programs received some form of financial aid in 2011–12. Fellowships, research assistantships, teaching assistantships, institutionally sponsored loans, scholarships, traineeships, and unspecified assistantships available. *Financial aid application deadline:* 12/15.

Contact Carol Ladden, Assistant Dean of Admissions and Financial Aid, School of Nursing, University of Pennsylvania, 418 Curie Boulevard, Philadelphia, PA 19104-4217. *Telephone:* 215-898-4271. *Fax:* 215-573-8439. *E-mail:* admissions@nursing.upenn.edu.

MASTER'S DEGREE PROGRAM

Degrees MSN; MSN/MBA; MSN/MPH; MSN/PhD

Available Programs Accelerated Master's for Non-Nursing College Graduates; Accelerated RN to Master's; Master's.

Concentrations Available Health-care administration; nurse anesthesia; nurse-midwifery; nursing administration. *Clinical nurse specialist programs in:* acute care, adult health, maternity-newborn, pediatric. *Nurse practitioner programs in:* acute care, adult health, family health, gerontology, neonatal health, pediatric, primary care, psychiatric/mental health, women's health.

Study Options Full-time and part-time.

Program Entrance Requirements Clinical experience, computer literacy, minimum overall college GPA of 3.0, transcript of college record, CPR certification, written essay, immunizations, interview, 3 letters of recommendation, prerequisite course work, resume, statistics course, GRE General Test. *Application deadline:* 7/1 (fall), 11/1 (winter), 11/1 (spring), 4/1 (summer). Applications may be processed on a rolling basis for some programs. *Application fee:* $80.

Advanced Placement Credit given for nursing courses completed elsewhere dependent upon specific evaluations.

Degree Requirements 36 total credit hours.

POST-MASTER'S PROGRAM

Areas of Study Health-care administration; nurse anesthesia; nurse-midwifery; nursing administration; nursing education. *Clinical nurse specialist programs in:* acute care, adult health, maternity-newborn, medical-surgical, pediatric. *Nurse practitioner programs in:* acute care, adult health, family health, gerontology, neonatal health, oncology, pediatric, primary care, psychiatric/mental health, women's health.

DOCTORAL DEGREE PROGRAM

Degree PhD
Available Programs Doctorate; Post-Baccalaureate Doctorate.
Areas of Study Addiction/substance abuse, aging, bio-behavioral research, biology of health and illness, clinical practice, community health, critical care, ethics, faculty preparation, family health, gerontology, health policy, health promotion/disease prevention, health-care systems, human health and illness, illness and transition, individualized study, information systems, maternity-newborn, neuro-behavior, nursing administration, nursing policy, nursing research, nursing science, oncology, urban health, women's health.
Program Entrance Requirements Minimum overall college GPA of 3.5, interview by faculty committee, interview, 3 letters of recommendation, MSN or equivalent, statistics course, vita, writing sample, GRE General Test. *Application deadline:* 11/1 (fall). *Application fee:* $80.
Degree Requirements 39 total credit hours, dissertation, oral exam, written exam, residency.

POSTDOCTORAL PROGRAM

Areas of Study Adolescent health, aging, cancer care, chronic illness, community health, family health, gerontology, health promotion/disease prevention, individualized study, nursing informatics, nursing interventions, nursing research, nursing science, outcomes, self-care, vulnerable population, women's health.
Postdoctoral Program Contact Dr. Yvonne Paterson, Associate Dean for Nursing Research, School of Nursing, University of Pennsylvania, 418 Curie Boulevard, Claire M. Fagin Hall, 4th Floor, Philadelphia, PA 19104-4271. *Telephone:* 215-898-3151. *E-mail:* research@nursing.upenn.edu.

CONTINUING EDUCATION PROGRAM

Contact Janet L. Tomcavage, Program Management, School of Nursing, University of Pennsylvania, 418 Curie Boulevard, Philadelphia, PA 19104-4271. *Telephone:* 215-898-5422. *E-mail:* tomcavag@nursing.upenn.edu.

University of Pittsburgh

School of Nursing
Pittsburgh, Pennsylvania

http://www.nursing.pitt.edu/
Founded in 1787
DEGREES • BSN • MSN • PHD
Nursing Program Faculty 114 (75% with doctorates).
Baccalaureate Enrollment 624 **Women** 88% **Men** 12% **Minority** 11% **International** .5% **Part-time** 2%
Graduate Enrollment 432 **Women** 84% **Men** 16% **Minority** 12% **International** 3% **Part-time** 54%
Distance Learning Courses Available.
Nursing Student Activities Nursing Honor Society, Sigma Theta Tau, Student Nurses' Association.
Nursing Student Resources Academic advising; academic or career counseling; assistance for students with disabilities; bookstore; campus computer network; career placement assistance; computer lab; computer-assisted instruction; daycare for children of students; e-mail services; employment services for current students; externships; housing assistance; interactive nursing skills videos; Internet; learning resource lab; library services; nursing audiovisuals; other; paid internships; placement services for program completers; remedial services; resume preparation assistance; skills, simulation, or other laboratory; tutoring.
Library Facilities 6.4 million volumes (338,365 in health, 8,941 in nursing); 130,107 periodical subscriptions (4,469 health-care related).

BACCALAUREATE PROGRAMS

Degree BSN
Available Programs Accelerated Baccalaureate for Second Degree; Generic Baccalaureate; RN Baccalaureate.
Study Options Full-time.
Program Entrance Requirements Minimum overall college GPA of 3.0, transcript of college record, written essay, health exam, health insurance, high school biology, high school chemistry, 4 years high school math, 3 years high school science, high school transcript, immunizations, 1 letter of recommendation, minimum high school GPA of 3.3, minimum GPA in nursing prerequisites of 3.0. Transfer students are accepted. *Application deadline:* Applications may be processed on a rolling basis for some programs. *Application fee:* $45.

Advanced Placement Credit by examination available.
Expenses (2012–13) *Tuition, state resident:* full-time $19,802; part-time $825 per credit. *Tuition, nonresident:* full-time $32,308; part-time $1346 per credit. *International tuition:* $32,308 full-time. *Room and board:* $5700; room only: $2950 per academic year. *Required fees:* full-time $884; part-time $226 per term.
Financial Aid 76% of baccalaureate students in nursing programs received some form of financial aid in 2011–12.
Contact Mrs. Suzanne Brody, Associate Director of Student Services Recruitment, School of Nursing, University of Pittsburgh, 239 Victoria Building, 3500 Victoria Street, Pittsburgh, PA 15261. *Telephone:* 412-624-1291. *Fax:* 412-624-2409. *E-mail:* brodys@pitt.edu.

GRADUATE PROGRAMS

Expenses (2012–13) *Tuition, state resident:* full-time $22,672; part-time $925 per credit. *Tuition, nonresident:* full-time $26,148; part-time $1069 per credit. *International tuition:* $26,148 full-time. *Required fees:* full-time $764; part-time $212 per term.
Financial Aid 78% of graduate students in nursing programs received some form of financial aid in 2011–12. 13 fellowships with full and partial tuition reimbursements available (averaging $20,997 per year), 16 research assistantships with full and partial tuition reimbursements available (averaging $13,807 per year), 7 teaching assistantships with full and partial tuition reimbursements available (averaging $17,688 per year) were awarded; scholarships, traineeships, and unspecified assistantships also available. Aid available to part-time students. *Financial aid application deadline:* 7/1.
Contact Mrs. Suzanne Brody, Associate Director of Student Services Recruitment, School of Nursing, University of Pittsburgh, 239 Victoria Building, 3500 Victoria Street, Pittsburgh, PA 15261. *Telephone:* 412-624-1291. *Fax:* 412-624-2409. *E-mail:* brodys@pitt.edu.

MASTER'S DEGREE PROGRAM

Degree MSN
Available Programs Master's; RN to Master's.
Concentrations Available Clinical nurse leader; nurse anesthesia; nursing administration; nursing informatics.
Site Options Johnstown, PA; Greensburg, PA; Bradford, PA.
Study Options Full-time and part-time.
Online Degree Options Yes.
Program Entrance Requirements Clinical experience, minimum overall college GPA of 3.0, transcript of college record, CPR certification, written essay, immunizations, interview, 3 letters of recommendation, professional liability insurance/malpractice insurance, resume, statistics course, GRE or MAT. *Application deadline:* Applications may be processed on a rolling basis for some programs. *Application fee:* $50.
Advanced Placement Credit by examination available. Credit given for nursing courses completed elsewhere dependent upon specific evaluations.
Degree Requirements 52 total credit hours, comprehensive exam.

POST-MASTER'S PROGRAM

Areas of Study Nurse case management; nursing education; nursing informatics. *Nurse practitioner programs in:* acute care, gerontology, neonatal health, psychiatric/mental health.

DOCTORAL DEGREE PROGRAM

Degree PhD
Available Programs Doctorate; Post-Baccalaureate Doctorate.
Areas of Study Nursing research, nursing science.
Program Entrance Requirements Minimum overall college GPA of 3.5, interview by faculty committee, interview, 3 letters of recommendation, MSN or equivalent, statistics course, vita, writing sample, GRE. *Application deadline:* Applications may be processed on a rolling basis for some programs. *Application fee:* $50.
Degree Requirements 64 total credit hours, dissertation.

POSTDOCTORAL PROGRAM

Areas of Study Nursing research, nursing science.
Postdoctoral Program Contact Dr. Judith A. Erlen, PhD Program Coordinator/Associate Director of Center for Research in Chronic Disorders, School of Nursing, University of Pittsburgh, 3500 Victoria Street, Pittsburgh, PA 15261. *Telephone:* 412-624-1905. *Fax:* 412-624-8521. *E-mail:* jae001@pitt.edu.

CONTINUING EDUCATION PROGRAM

Contact Mrs. Mary Rodgers Schubert, Interim Director of Continuing Education Program, School of Nursing, University of Pittsburgh, 226

Victoria Building, 3500 Victoria Street, Pittsburgh, PA 15261. *Telephone:* 412-624-3156. *E-mail:* mschuber@pitt.edu.

University of Pittsburgh at Bradford
Department of Nursing
Bradford, Pennsylvania

http://www.upb.pitt.edu
Founded in 1963
DEGREE • BSN
Nursing Program Faculty 9 (33% with doctorates).
Baccalaureate Enrollment 8 **Women** 87% **Men** 13% **Part-time** 25%
Distance Learning Courses Available.
Nursing Student Activities Nursing club.
Nursing Student Resources Academic advising; academic or career counseling; assistance for students with disabilities; bookstore; campus computer network; career placement assistance; computer lab; computer-assisted instruction; e-mail services; employment services for current students; externships; housing assistance; Internet; learning resource lab; library services; nursing audiovisuals; remedial services; resume preparation assistance; skills, simulation, or other laboratory; tutoring; unpaid internships.
Library Facilities 97,963 volumes (356 in health, 223 in nursing); 245 periodical subscriptions (13 health-care related).

BACCALAUREATE PROGRAMS
Degree BSN
Available Programs Generic Baccalaureate; RN Baccalaureate.
Site Options St. Marys, PA.
Study Options Full-time and part-time.
Program Entrance Requirements Transcript of college record, CPR certification, health exam, health insurance, high school transcript, immunizations, minimum high school GPA of 2.5, minimum GPA in nursing prerequisites of 2.5, professional liability insurance/malpractice insurance, prerequisite course work, RN licensure. Transfer students are accepted. *Application deadline:* Applications may be processed on a rolling basis for some programs. *Application fee:* $45.
Advanced Placement Credit by examination available. Credit given for nursing courses completed elsewhere dependent upon specific evaluations.
Expenses (2012–13) *Tuition, state resident:* full-time $15,334; part-time $638 per credit. *Tuition, nonresident:* full-time $28,523; part-time $1188 per credit. *International tuition:* $28,523 full-time. *Room and board:* $7960; room only: $4920 per academic year. *Required fees:* full-time $852; part-time $156 per term.
Financial Aid 88% of baccalaureate students in nursing programs received some form of financial aid in 2011–12.
Contact Mr. Alexander Nazemetz, Nursing Admissions, Department of Nursing, University of Pittsburgh at Bradford, 300 Campus Drive, Bradford, PA 16701. *Telephone:* 800-872-1787. *Fax:* 814-362-5150. *E-mail:* nazemetz@pitt.edu.

The University of Scranton
Department of Nursing
Scranton, Pennsylvania

http://www.scranton.edu/academics/pcps/nursing/index.shtml
Founded in 1888
DEGREES • BS • MSN
Nursing Program Faculty 50 (85% with doctorates).
Baccalaureate Enrollment 265 **Women** 92% **Men** 8% **Minority** 7% **Part-time** 8%
Graduate Enrollment 95 **Women** 70% **Men** 30% **Minority** 6% **Part-time** 50%
Nursing Student Activities Nursing Honor Society, Sigma Theta Tau, Student Nurses' Association, nursing club.
Nursing Student Resources Academic advising; academic or career counseling; bookstore; campus computer network; career placement assistance; computer lab; computer-assisted instruction; e-mail services; employment services for current students; interactive nursing skills videos; Internet; learning resource lab; library services; nursing audiovisuals; placement services for program completers; remedial services; resume preparation assistance; skills, simulation, or other laboratory; tutoring.
Library Facilities 405,128 volumes (28,400 in health, 8,484 in nursing); 41,297 periodical subscriptions (106 health-care related).

BACCALAUREATE PROGRAMS
Degree BS
Available Programs Baccalaureate for Second Degree; Generic Baccalaureate; LPN to RN Baccalaureate; RN Baccalaureate.
Study Options Full-time and part-time.
Program Entrance Requirements Minimum overall college GPA of 2.5, transcript of college record, written essay, health exam, health insurance, high school biology, high school chemistry, high school foreign language, 3 years high school math, 3 years high school science, high school transcript, immunizations, minimum high school rank 30%, minimum GPA in nursing prerequisites. Transfer students are accepted. *Application deadline:* 3/1 (fall). Applications may be processed on a rolling basis for some programs.
Advanced Placement Credit by examination available. Credit given for nursing courses completed elsewhere dependent upon specific evaluations.
Financial Aid 80% of baccalaureate students in nursing programs received some form of financial aid in 2011–12.
Contact Dr. Patricia Harrington, Chairperson, Department of Nursing, The University of Scranton, 800 Linden Street, McGurrin Hall, Scranton, PA 18510-4595. *Telephone:* 570-941-7673. *Fax:* 570-941-7903. *E-mail:* harringtonp1@scranton.edu.

GRADUATE PROGRAMS
Financial Aid 90% of graduate students in nursing programs received some form of financial aid in 2011–12. 7 teaching assistantships with full and partial tuition reimbursements available (averaging $6,914 per year) were awarded; career-related internships or fieldwork, Federal Work-Study, and unspecified assistantships also available. Aid available to part-time students. *Financial aid application deadline:* 3/1.
Contact Dr. Mary Jane Hanson, Director, Graduate Nursing Program, Department of Nursing, The University of Scranton, 800 Linden Street, McGurrin Hall, Scranton, PA 18510-4595. *Telephone:* 570-941-4060. *Fax:* 570-941-7903. *E-mail:* hansonm2@scranton.edu.

MASTER'S DEGREE PROGRAM
Degree MSN
Available Programs Accelerated AD/RN to Master's; Accelerated RN to Master's; Master's; RN to Master's.
Concentrations Available Nurse anesthesia; nursing education. *Clinical nurse specialist programs in:* adult health. *Nurse practitioner programs in:* family health.
Site Options Wilkes-Barre, PA.
Study Options Full-time and part-time.
Program Entrance Requirements Clinical experience, minimum overall college GPA of 3.0, transcript of college record, CPR certification, written essay, immunizations, interview, 3 letters of recommendation, nursing research course, physical assessment course, professional liability insurance/malpractice insurance, prerequisite course work, statistics course. *Application deadline:* Applications may be processed on a rolling basis for some programs. *Application fee:* $50.
Advanced Placement Credit given for nursing courses completed elsewhere dependent upon specific evaluations.
Degree Requirements 46 total credit hours, comprehensive exam.

POST-MASTER'S PROGRAM
Areas of Study Nurse anesthesia; nursing education. *Clinical nurse specialist programs in:* adult health. *Nurse practitioner programs in:* family health.

Villanova University
College of Nursing
Villanova, Pennsylvania

http://www.nursing.villanova.edu/
Founded in 1842
DEGREES • BSN • MSN • PHD
Nursing Program Faculty 81 (47% with doctorates).

Baccalaureate Enrollment 544 **Women** 94% **Men** 6% **Minority** 20% **International** 1.3% **Part-time** 2%
Graduate Enrollment 233 **Women** 91% **Men** 9% **Minority** 10% **International** 6% **Part-time** 88%
Distance Learning Courses Available.
Nursing Student Activities Nursing Honor Society, Sigma Theta Tau, Student Nurses' Association, nursing club.
Nursing Student Resources Academic advising; academic or career counseling; assistance for students with disabilities; bookstore; campus computer network; career placement assistance; computer lab; computer-assisted instruction; e-mail services; employment services for current students; housing assistance; interactive nursing skills videos; Internet; learning resource lab; library services; nursing audiovisuals; remedial services; resume preparation assistance; skills, simulation, or other laboratory; tutoring.
Library Facilities 755,000 volumes (14,147 in health, 1,592 in nursing); 12,000 periodical subscriptions (113 health-care related).

BACCALAUREATE PROGRAMS

Degree BSN
Available Programs ADN to Baccalaureate; Accelerated Baccalaureate for Second Degree; Baccalaureate for Second Degree; Generic Baccalaureate; International Nurse to Baccalaureate; RN Baccalaureate.
Study Options Full-time.
Program Entrance Requirements Minimum overall college GPA of 2.75, transcript of college record, CPR certification, written essay, health exam, health insurance, high school biology, high school chemistry, high school foreign language, 3 years high school math, 3 years high school science, high school transcript, immunizations, 2 letters of recommendation, minimum high school GPA of 3.0, minimum GPA in nursing prerequisites. Transfer students are accepted. *Application deadline:* 11/1 (fall), 1/7 (winter). *Application fee:* $80.
Advanced Placement Credit given for nursing courses completed elsewhere dependent upon specific evaluations.
Expenses (2012–13) *Tuition:* full-time $42,150; part-time $1760 per credit. *Room and board:* $11,800; room only: $6460 per academic year. *Required fees:* full-time $590; part-time $30 per credit; part-time $60 per term.
Financial Aid 65% of baccalaureate students in nursing programs received some form of financial aid in 2011–12. *Gift aid (need-based):* Federal Pell, FSEOG, state, private, college/university gift aid from institutional funds, endowed and restricted scholarships and grants. *Loans:* Federal Nursing Student Loans, Federal Direct (Subsidized and Unsubsidized Stafford PLUS), Perkins. *Work-study:* Federal Work-Study, part-time campus jobs. *Financial aid application deadline:* 2/7 (priority: 2/7).
Contact Dr. Angelina A. Arcamone, Assistant Dean and Director, Undergraduate Program, College of Nursing, Villanova University, Driscoll Hall, 800 Lancaster Avenue, Villanova, PA 19085-1690. *Telephone:* 610-519-4926. *Fax:* 610-519-7650. *E-mail:* angelina.arcamone@villanova.edu.

GRADUATE PROGRAMS

Expenses (2012–13) *Tuition:* full-time $6795; part-time $755 per credit. *International tuition:* $6795 full-time. *Required fees:* full-time $60.
Financial Aid 46% of graduate students in nursing programs received some form of financial aid in 2011–12. 5 teaching assistantships with full tuition reimbursements available (averaging $13,100 per year) were awarded; institutionally sponsored loans, scholarships, traineeships, tuition waivers (full), and unspecified assistantships also available. *Financial aid application deadline:* 7/1.
Contact Dr. Marguerite K. Schlag, Assistant Dean and Director, Graduate Program, College of Nursing, Villanova University, Driscoll Hall, 800 Lancaster Avenue, Villanova, PA 19085-1690. *Telephone:* 610-519-4934. *Fax:* 610-519-7997. *E-mail:* marguerite.schlag@villanova.edu.

MASTER'S DEGREE PROGRAM

Degree MSN
Available Programs Master's.
Concentrations Available Health-care administration; nurse anesthesia; nursing education. *Nurse practitioner programs in:* adult health, family health, pediatric.
Site Options Philadelphia, PA.
Study Options Full-time and part-time.
Program Entrance Requirements Clinical experience, computer literacy, minimum overall college GPA of 3.0, transcript of college record, written essay, immunizations, 3 letters of recommendation, nursing research course, physical assessment course, professional liability insurance/malpractice insurance, resume, statistics course, GRE or MAT.

Application deadline: 7/1 (fall), 11/1 (spring), 4/1 (summer). Applications may be processed on a rolling basis for some programs. *Application fee:* $50.
Advanced Placement Credit given for nursing courses completed elsewhere dependent upon specific evaluations.
Degree Requirements 45 total credit hours, thesis or project.

POST-MASTER'S PROGRAM

Areas of Study Health-care administration; nurse anesthesia; nursing education. *Nurse practitioner programs in:* adult health, family health, pediatric.

DOCTORAL DEGREE PROGRAM

Degree PhD
Available Programs Doctorate.
Areas of Study Faculty preparation, nursing education, nursing research.
Program Entrance Requirements Clinical experience, minimum overall college GPA of 3.5, interview, 3 letters of recommendation, MSN or equivalent, scholarly papers, vita, writing sample, GRE. *Application deadline:* 12/1 (fall), 12/1 (summer). *Application fee:* $70.
Degree Requirements 51 total credit hours, dissertation, oral exam, written exam.

CONTINUING EDUCATION PROGRAM

Contact Dr. Lynore DeSilets, Assistant Dean and Director, Continuing Education, College of Nursing, Villanova University, Driscoll Hall, 800 Lancaster Avenue, Villanova, PA 19085-1690. *Telephone:* 610-519-4931. *Fax:* 610-519-6780. *E-mail:* lyn.desilets@villanova.edu.

Waynesburg University
Department of Nursing
Waynesburg, Pennsylvania

http://www.waynesburg.edu/
Founded in 1849
DEGREES • BSN • DNP • MSN • MSN/MBA
Nursing Program Faculty 48 (39% with doctorates).
Baccalaureate Enrollment 337 **Women** 91% **Men** 9% **Minority** 1%
Graduate Enrollment 240 **Women** 95% **Men** 5% **Minority** 1% **Part-time** 95%
Nursing Student Activities Sigma Theta Tau, Student Nurses' Association.
Nursing Student Resources Academic advising; academic or career counseling; assistance for students with disabilities; bookstore; campus computer network; career placement assistance; computer lab; computer-assisted instruction; e-mail services; employment services for current students; externships; Internet; learning resource lab; library services; nursing audiovisuals; paid internships; placement services for program completers; remedial services; resume preparation assistance; skills, simulation, or other laboratory; tutoring.
Library Facilities 100,000 volumes (4,500 in nursing); 1,206 periodical subscriptions (46 health-care related).

BACCALAUREATE PROGRAMS

Degree BSN
Available Programs Accelerated Baccalaureate; Accelerated Baccalaureate for Second Degree; Generic Baccalaureate; LPN to Baccalaureate.
Site Options Canonsburg, PA; Wexford, PA; Monroeville, PA.
Study Options Full-time.
Program Entrance Requirements Minimum overall college GPA of 3.0, transcript of college record, CPR certification, health exam, high school biology, high school chemistry, 2 years high school math, 2 years high school science, high school transcript, immunizations, minimum high school GPA of 3.0, minimum GPA in nursing prerequisites of 3.0, professional liability insurance/malpractice insurance, prerequisite course work. Transfer students are accepted. *Application deadline:* Applications may be processed on a rolling basis for some programs. *Application fee:* $75.
Advanced Placement Credit by examination available.
Expenses (2012–13) *Tuition:* full-time $19,450. *Room and board:* $8250; room only: $4170 per academic year. *Required fees:* full-time $380.
Financial Aid 90% of baccalaureate students in nursing programs received some form of financial aid in 2011–12.
Contact Dr. Nancy R. Mosser, Director/Chairperson, Department of Nursing, Waynesburg University, 51 West College Street, Waynesburg,

PA 15370-1222. *Telephone:* 724-852-3356. *Fax:* 724-852-3220. *E-mail:* nmosser@waynesburg.edu.

GRADUATE PROGRAMS

Expenses (2012–13) *Tuition:* part-time $580 per contact hour.
Financial Aid 50% of graduate students in nursing programs received some form of financial aid in 2011–12.
Contact Dr. Kimberly Stephens, Co-Chair of Graduate and Professional Studies Program, Department of Nursing, Waynesburg University, Monroeville Center, Penn Center, Building 3, Pittsburgh, PA 15235. *Telephone:* 412-824-3700. *E-mail:* kpstephe@waynesburg.edu.

MASTER'S DEGREE PROGRAM

Degrees MSN; MSN/MBA
Available Programs Accelerated Master's; Accelerated Master's for Nurses with Non-Nursing Degrees; Accelerated RN to Master's.
Concentrations Available Nursing administration; nursing education.
Site Options Canonsburg, PA; Wexford, PA; Monroeville, PA.
Study Options Part-time.
Program Entrance Requirements Clinical experience, computer literacy, minimum overall college GPA of 3.0, transcript of college record, 2 letters of recommendation, resume. *Application deadline:* Applications may be processed on a rolling basis for some programs. *Application fee:* $75.
Degree Requirements 36 total credit hours, thesis or project.

DOCTORAL DEGREE PROGRAM

Degree DNP
Available Programs Doctorate; Post-Baccalaureate Doctorate.
Areas of Study Advanced practice nursing, health-care systems, nursing administration.
Site Options Monroeville, PA.
Program Entrance Requirements Minimum overall college GPA of 3.0, interview by faculty committee, interview, letters of recommendation, MSN or equivalent, statistics course, vita, writing sample. *Application deadline:* Applications may be processed on a rolling basis for some programs.
Degree Requirements 80 total credit hours, oral exam, written exam, residency.

West Chester University of Pennsylvania

Department of Nursing
West Chester, Pennsylvania

http://www.wcupa.edu/_academics/Healthsciences/nursing/
Founded in 1871

DEGREES • BSN • MSN

Nursing Program Faculty 40 (28% with doctorates).
Baccalaureate Enrollment 384 **Women** 88% **Men** 12% **Minority** 11% **International** .5% **Part-time** 28%
Graduate Enrollment 42 **Women** 93% **Men** 7% **Minority** 19% **International** 1% **Part-time** 81%.
Distance Learning Courses Available.
Nursing Student Activities Nursing Honor Society, Sigma Theta Tau, Student Nurses' Association.
Nursing Student Resources Academic advising; academic or career counseling; assistance for students with disabilities; bookstore; campus computer network; career placement assistance; computer lab; computer-assisted instruction; e-mail services; employment services for current students; externships; housing assistance; interactive nursing skills videos; Internet; learning resource lab; library services; nursing audiovisuals; remedial services; resume preparation assistance; skills, simulation, or other laboratory; tutoring.
Library Facilities 1.4 million volumes (88 in nursing); 19,636 periodical subscriptions (173 health-care related).

BACCALAUREATE PROGRAMS

Degree BSN
Available Programs Accelerated Baccalaureate for Second Degree; Generic Baccalaureate; RN Baccalaureate.
Study Options Full-time and part-time.
Program Entrance Requirements Written essay, health exam, health insurance, high school biology, high school chemistry, 3 years high school math, 3 years high school science, high school transcript,

minimum high school GPA, minimum high school rank. *Application deadline:* Applications may be processed on a rolling basis for some programs. *Application fee:* $45.
Advanced Placement Credit given for nursing courses completed elsewhere dependent upon specific evaluations.
Expenses (2012–13) *Tuition, state resident:* full-time $6428; part-time $268 per credit. *Tuition, nonresident:* full-time $16,070; part-time $670 per credit. *International tuition:* $16,070 full-time. *Room and board:* $7784; room only: $4848 per academic year. *Required fees:* full-time $2192; part-time $91 per credit.
Financial Aid 85% of baccalaureate students in nursing programs received some form of financial aid in 2011–12.
Contact Dr. Cheryl Monturo, Interim Chairperson, Department of Nursing, West Chester University of Pennsylvania, 855 South New Street, West Chester, PA 19383. *Telephone:* 610-436-2693. *Fax:* 610-436-3083. *E-mail:* cmonturo@wcupa.edu.

GRADUATE PROGRAMS

Expenses (2012–13) *Tuition, state resident:* full-time $8494; part-time $429 per credit. *Tuition, nonresident:* full-time $12,750; part-time $644 per credit. *International tuition:* $12,750 full-time. *Required fees:* part-time $105 per credit; part-time $865 per term.
Financial Aid 60% of graduate students in nursing programs received some form of financial aid in 2011–12. Unspecified assistantships available. Aid available to part-time students. *Financial aid application deadline:* 2/15.
Contact Dr. Ann C. Stowe, Graduate Program Coordinator, Department of Nursing, West Chester University of Pennsylvania, 855 South New Street, Sturzebecker Health Sciences Center, West Chester, PA 19383. *Telephone:* 610-436-2331. *Fax:* 610-436-3083. *E-mail:* astowe@wcupa.edu.

MASTER'S DEGREE PROGRAM

Degree MSN
Available Programs Master's.
Concentrations Available Nursing administration; nursing education. *Clinical nurse specialist programs in:* public health.
Study Options Full-time and part-time.
Program Entrance Requirements Clinical experience, minimum overall college GPA of 2.8, transcript of college record, written essay, interview, 2 letters of recommendation, physical assessment course, resume, statistics course. *Application deadline:* Applications may be processed on a rolling basis for some programs. *Application fee:* $45.
Advanced Placement Credit given for nursing courses completed elsewhere dependent upon specific evaluations.
Degree Requirements 39 total credit hours, comprehensive exam.

Widener University

School of Nursing
Chester, Pennsylvania

http://www.widener.edu/
Founded in 1821

DEGREES • BSN • MSN • MSN/PHD • PHD

Nursing Program Faculty 93 (31% with doctorates).
Baccalaureate Enrollment 578 **Women** 90% **Men** 10% **Minority** 23% **International** 1% **Part-time** 1%.
Graduate Enrollment 267 **Women** 94% **Men** 6% **Minority** 15% **Part-time** 88%
Distance Learning Courses Available.
Nursing Student Activities Nursing Honor Society, Sigma Theta Tau, Student Nurses' Association.
Nursing Student Resources Academic advising; academic or career counseling; assistance for students with disabilities; bookstore; campus computer network; career placement assistance; computer lab; computer-assisted instruction; e-mail services; employment services for current students; housing assistance; interactive nursing skills videos; Internet; learning resource lab; library services; nursing audiovisuals; placement services for program completers; remedial services; resume preparation assistance; skills, simulation, or other laboratory; tutoring.
Library Facilities 208,847 volumes (14,890 in health, 2,639 in nursing); 2,695 periodical subscriptions (451 health-care related).

BACCALAUREATE PROGRAMS

Degree BSN

Available Programs ADN to Baccalaureate; Generic Baccalaureate; RN Baccalaureate.

Study Options Full-time.

Program Entrance Requirements Transcript of college record, health exam, health insurance, high school biology, high school chemistry, high school foreign language, 3 years high school math, 3 years high school science, high school transcript, immunizations, minimum high school GPA of 2.85, minimum GPA in nursing prerequisites of 3.0. Transfer students are accepted. *Application deadline:* Applications may be processed on a rolling basis for some programs.

Advanced Placement Credit by examination available. Credit given for nursing courses completed elsewhere dependent upon specific evaluations.

Expenses (2012–13) *Tuition:* full-time $35,764; part-time $1190 per credit. *International tuition:* $35,764 full-time. *Room and board:* $11,300; room only: $6300 per academic year. *Required fees:* full-time $795; part-time $349 per term.

Financial Aid 98% of baccalaureate students in nursing programs received some form of financial aid in 2011–12. *Gift aid (need-based):* Federal Pell, FSEOG, state, private, college/university gift aid from institutional funds, Federal Nursing. *Loans:* Federal Direct (Subsidized and Unsubsidized Stafford PLUS), Perkins. *Work-study:* Federal Work-Study, part-time campus jobs. *Financial aid application deadline (priority):* 2/15.

Contact Dr. Rose Schwartz, RN, Director, Prelicensure BSN, School of Nursing, Widener University, One University Place, Chester, PA 19013-5892. *Telephone:* 610-499-4211. *Fax:* 610-499-4216. *E-mail:* raschwartz@widener.edu.

GRADUATE PROGRAMS

Expenses (2012–13) *Tuition:* part-time $840 per credit. *Required fees:* part-time $111 per credit.

Financial Aid 49% of graduate students in nursing programs received some form of financial aid in 2011–12. Career-related internships or fieldwork, Federal Work-Study, and traineeships available. Aid available to part-time students. *Financial aid application deadline:* 4/1.

Contact Mrs. Betty Boyles, Administrative Assistant for Graduate Programs, School of Nursing, Widener University, One University Place, Chester, PA 19013-5892. *Telephone:* 610-499-4208. *Fax:* 610-499-4216. *E-mail:* eaboyles@widener.edu.

MASTER'S DEGREE PROGRAM

Degrees MSN; MSN/PhD

Available Programs Master's; Master's for Nurses with Non-Nursing Degrees.

Concentrations Available Nursing education. *Clinical nurse specialist programs in:* acute care, adult health, critical care, gerontology. *Nurse practitioner programs in:* family health.

Site Options Harrisburg, PA.

Study Options Full-time and part-time.

Program Entrance Requirements Clinical experience, computer literacy, minimum overall college GPA of 3.0, transcript of college record, immunizations, interview, 2 letters of recommendation, nursing research course, resume, statistics course, GRE General Test. *Application deadline:* 7/15 (fall), 11/15 (spring), 3/16 (summer). Applications may be processed on a rolling basis for some programs.

Advanced Placement Credit given for nursing courses completed elsewhere dependent upon specific evaluations.

Degree Requirements 42 total credit hours.

POST-MASTER'S PROGRAM

Areas of Study Nursing education. *Clinical nurse specialist programs in:* acute care, adult health, critical care, gerontology. *Nurse practitioner programs in:* family health.

DOCTORAL DEGREE PROGRAM

Degree PhD

Available Programs Doctorate.

Areas of Study Faculty preparation, nursing education, nursing research, nursing science.

Program Entrance Requirements Minimum overall college GPA of 3.5, interview, 2 letters of recommendation, MSN or equivalent, statistics course, vita, writing sample, GRE General Test. *Application deadline:* 7/15 (fall), 11/15 (spring), 3/17 (summer). Applications may be processed on a rolling basis for some programs.

Degree Requirements 63 total credit hours, dissertation, written exam.

CONTINUING EDUCATION PROGRAM

Contact Ms. Marcia Bowers, Director for Community Relations and Continuing Education, School of Nursing, Widener University, One University Place, Chester, PA 19013. *Telephone:* 610-499-1327. *Fax:* 610-499-4216. *E-mail:* mdbowers@widener.edu.

Wilkes University
Department of Nursing
Wilkes-Barre, Pennsylvania

http://www.wilkes.edu/
Founded in 1933

DEGREES • BS • MS

Nursing Program Faculty 25 (20% with doctorates).

Baccalaureate Enrollment 300 **Women** 90% **Men** 10% **Minority** 5% **Part-time** 15%

Graduate Enrollment 65 **Women** 85% **Men** 15% **Minority** 5% **Part-time** 75%

Distance Learning Courses Available.

Nursing Student Activities Sigma Theta Tau, Student Nurses' Association, nursing club.

Nursing Student Resources Academic advising; academic or career counseling; assistance for students with disabilities; bookstore; campus computer network; career placement assistance; computer lab; computer-assisted instruction; daycare for children of students; e-mail services; employment services for current students; externships; housing assistance; interactive nursing skills videos; Internet; learning resource lab; library services; nursing audiovisuals; paid internships; placement services for program completers; remedial services; resume preparation assistance; skills, simulation, or other laboratory; tutoring; unpaid internships.

Library Facilities 13,450 volumes in health, 13,000 volumes in nursing; 70 periodical subscriptions health-care related.

BACCALAUREATE PROGRAMS

Degree BS

Available Programs ADN to Baccalaureate; Accelerated Baccalaureate for Second Degree; Accelerated LPN to Baccalaureate; Accelerated RN Baccalaureate; Generic Baccalaureate; LPN to RN Baccalaureate; RN Baccalaureate.

Study Options Full-time and part-time.

Program Entrance Requirements Minimum overall college GPA of 2.0, transcript of college record, CPR certification, health exam, health insurance, high school biology, high school chemistry, 2 years high school math, 3 years high school science, high school transcript, immunizations, minimum high school GPA, professional liability insurance/malpractice insurance. Transfer students are accepted.

Advanced Placement Credit by examination available. Credit given for nursing courses completed elsewhere dependent upon specific evaluations.

Contact *Telephone:* 570-408-4074. *Fax:* 570-408-7807.

GRADUATE PROGRAMS

Contact *Telephone:* 570-408-4078. *Fax:* 570-408-7807.

MASTER'S DEGREE PROGRAM

Degree MS

Available Programs Accelerated AD/RN to Master's; Accelerated RN to Master's; Master's; Master's for Non-Nursing College Graduates; RN to Master's.

Concentrations Available Nursing administration; nursing education. *Clinical nurse specialist programs in:* gerontology, psychiatric/mental health.

Study Options Full-time and part-time.

Program Entrance Requirements Clinical experience, minimum overall college GPA of 3.0, transcript of college record, CPR certification, immunizations, interview, 3 letters of recommendation, nursing research course, physical assessment course, professional liability insurance/malpractice insurance, statistics course.

Advanced Placement Credit given for nursing courses completed elsewhere dependent upon specific evaluations.

Degree Requirements 37 total credit hours, thesis or project.

POST-MASTER'S PROGRAM

Areas of Study Nursing administration; nursing education. *Clinical nurse specialist programs in:* gerontology, psychiatric/mental health.

CONTINUING EDUCATION PROGRAM

Contact *Telephone:* 570-408-4462.

York College of Pennsylvania
Department of Nursing
York, Pennsylvania

http://www.ycp.edu/academics/academic-departments/nursing/
Founded in 1787

DEGREES • BS • DNP • MS
Nursing Program Faculty 74 (26% with doctorates).
Baccalaureate Enrollment 614 **Women** 94% **Men** 6% **Minority** 4% **Part-time** 6%
Graduate Enrollment 94 **Women** 92% **Men** 8% **Minority** 6% **International** 1% **Part-time** 47%
Distance Learning Courses Available.
Nursing Student Activities Sigma Theta Tau, Student Nurses' Association, nursing club.
Nursing Student Resources Academic advising; academic or career counseling; assistance for students with disabilities; bookstore; campus computer network; career placement assistance; computer lab; computer-assisted instruction; e-mail services; employment services for current students; externships; housing assistance; interactive nursing skills videos; Internet; learning resource lab; library services; nursing audiovisuals; paid internships; placement services for program completers; remedial services; resume preparation assistance; skills, simulation, or other laboratory; tutoring.
Library Facilities 403,800 volumes (6,681 in health, 1,226 in nursing); 42,568 periodical subscriptions (83 health-care related).

BACCALAUREATE PROGRAMS

Degree BS
Available Programs ADN to Baccalaureate; Generic Baccalaureate; LPN to Baccalaureate; RN Baccalaureate.
Study Options Full-time and part-time.
Program Entrance Requirements Minimum overall college GPA of 2.8, transcript of college record, CPR certification, health exam, health insurance, high school biology, high school chemistry, 1 year of high school math, 3 years high school science, high school transcript, immunizations, 2 letters of recommendation, minimum high school GPA of 3.4, minimum high school rank 40%, minimum GPA in nursing prerequisites of 2.8, professional liability insurance/malpractice insurance, prerequisite course work. *Application deadline:* Applications may be processed on a rolling basis for some programs.
Advanced Placement Credit by examination available. Credit given for nursing courses completed elsewhere dependent upon specific evaluations.
Expenses (2012–13) *Tuition:* full-time $14,900. *Room and board:* $9300; room only: $5220 per academic year. *Required fees:* full-time $1620.
Financial Aid 90% of baccalaureate students in nursing programs received some form of financial aid in 2011–12.
Contact Karen S. March, Chairperson and Professor, Department of Nursing, York College of Pennsylvania, 441 Country Club Road, York, PA 17405-7199. *Telephone:* 717-815-1243. *Fax:* 717-849-1651. *E-mail:* kmarch@ycp.edu.

GRADUATE PROGRAMS

Expenses (2012–13) *Tuition:* part-time $670 per credit. *Required fees:* part-time $340 per term.
Financial Aid 8% of graduate students in nursing programs received some form of financial aid in 2011–12.
Contact Dr. Linda Coniff Pugh, Director, Department of Nursing, York College of Pennsylvania, York, PA 17405-7199. *Telephone:* 717-815-6592. *Fax:* 717-849-1659. *E-mail:* lpugh@ycp.edu.

MASTER'S DEGREE PROGRAM
Degree MS

Available Programs Master's; RN to Master's.
Concentrations Available Nurse anesthesia; nursing education. *Clinical nurse specialist programs in:* adult health. *Nurse practitioner programs in:* adult health.
Study Options Part-time.
Program Entrance Requirements Clinical experience, computer literacy, minimum overall college GPA of 3.0, transcript of college record, CPR certification, written essay, immunizations, interview, 2 letters of recommendation, nursing research course, physical assessment course, professional liability insurance/malpractice insurance, resume, statistics course. *Application deadline:* 6/30 (fall). Applications may be processed on a rolling basis for some programs. *Application fee:* $50.
Advanced Placement Credit given for nursing courses completed elsewhere dependent upon specific evaluations.
Degree Requirements 41 total credit hours, thesis or project.

POST-MASTER'S PROGRAM
Areas of Study *Nurse practitioner programs in:* adult health.

DOCTORAL DEGREE PROGRAM
Degree DNP
Available Programs Doctorate.
Areas of Study Advanced practice nursing, clinical practice, health policy, health-care systems, individualized study, information systems, nursing policy, nursing science.
Program Entrance Requirements Clinical experience, minimum overall college GPA of 3.5, interview by faculty committee, 2 letters of recommendation, MSN or equivalent, statistics course, vita, writing sample. *Application deadline:* 3/1 (fall). Applications may be processed on a rolling basis for some programs. *Application fee:* $50.
Degree Requirements 37 total credit hours, residency.

PUERTO RICO

Inter American University of Puerto Rico, Aguadilla Campus
Nursing Program
Aguadilla, Puerto Rico

Founded in 1957
DEGREE • BSN
Library Facilities 61,359 volumes; 277 periodical subscriptions.

BACCALAUREATE PROGRAMS

Degree BSN
Available Programs RN Baccalaureate.
Contact Admissions, Nursing Program, Inter American University of Puerto Rico, Aguadilla Campus, PO Box 20000, Aguadilla, PR 00605. *Telephone:* 787-891-0925. *E-mail:* dperez@aguadilla.inter.edu.

Inter American University of Puerto Rico, Arecibo Campus
Nursing Program
Arecibo, Puerto Rico

Founded in 1957
DEGREE • BS
Library Facilities 73,642 volumes; 640 periodical subscriptions.

BACCALAUREATE PROGRAMS

Degree BS
Available Programs Generic Baccalaureate.
Contact *Telephone:* 787-878-5475.

Inter American University of Puerto Rico, Metropolitan Campus
Carmen Torres de Tiburcio School of Nursing
San Juan, Puerto Rico

http://www.metro.inter.edu/index.asp
Founded in 1960
DEGREE • BSN
Nursing Program Faculty 26 (27% with doctorates).
Baccalaureate Enrollment 312 **Women** 57% **Men** 43%
Nursing Student Activities Student Nurses' Association.
Nursing Student Resources Academic advising; academic or career counseling; assistance for students with disabilities; bookstore; campus computer network; career placement assistance; computer lab; computer-assisted instruction; daycare for children of students; e-mail services; employment services for current students; externships; interactive nursing skills videos; Internet; learning resource lab; library services; nursing audiovisuals; paid internships; placement services for program completers; remedial services; skills, simulation, or other laboratory; tutoring.
Library Facilities 171,173 volumes (36,000 in health, 21,759 in nursing); 41,660 periodical subscriptions (2,090 health-care related).

BACCALAUREATE PROGRAMS

Degree BSN
Available Programs ADN to Baccalaureate; Accelerated Baccalaureate; Generic Baccalaureate.
Study Options Full-time and part-time.
Program Entrance Requirements Minimum overall college GPA of 2.0, transcript of college record, CPR certification, health exam, health insurance, high school transcript, immunizations, 2 letters of recommendation, minimum high school rank 4%, minimum GPA in nursing prerequisites of 2. Transfer students are accepted.
Advanced Placement Credit by examination available. Credit given for nursing courses completed elsewhere dependent upon specific evaluations.
Contact *Telephone:* 787-763-3066. *Fax:* 787-250-1242 Ext. 2159.

Pontifical Catholic University of Puerto Rico
Department of Nursing
Ponce, Puerto Rico

http://www.pucpr.edu/catalogo/espanol/ciencias/dep_enf.htm
Founded in 1948
DEGREE • BSN
Library Facilities 1,499 volumes in nursing.

BACCALAUREATE PROGRAMS

Degree BSN
Available Programs Generic Baccalaureate.
Program Entrance Requirements Minimum overall college GPA of 2.0, CPR certification, health exam, health insurance, immunizations, interview, letters of recommendation, minimum high school GPA of 2.5, prerequisite course work.
Contact *Telephone:* 787-841-2000 Ext. 1604.

Universidad Adventista de las Antillas
Department of Nursing
Mayagüez, Puerto Rico

Founded in 1957
DEGREE • BSN
Nursing Program Faculty 11 (18% with doctorates).

Baccalaureate Enrollment 257 **Women** 69% **Men** 31% **Minority** 100% **International** 13% **Part-time** 1%
Nursing Student Activities Nursing club.
Nursing Student Resources Academic advising; academic or career counseling; assistance for students with disabilities; campus computer network; computer lab; computer-assisted instruction; e-mail services; employment services for current students; housing assistance; interactive nursing skills videos; Internet; learning resource lab; library services; nursing audiovisuals; remedial services; resume preparation assistance; skills, simulation, or other laboratory; tutoring; unpaid internships.
Library Facilities 2,488 volumes in health, 1,556 volumes in nursing; 29 periodical subscriptions health-care related.

BACCALAUREATE PROGRAMS

Degree BSN
Available Programs Generic Baccalaureate; RN Baccalaureate.
Study Options Full-time.
Program Entrance Requirements Minimum overall college GPA of 2.3, transcript of college record, health exam, health insurance, high school transcript, immunizations, interview, 2 letters of recommendation, minimum high school GPA of 2.5. Transfer students are accepted.
Advanced Placement Credit given for nursing courses completed elsewhere dependent upon specific evaluations.
Contact *Telephone:* 787-834-9595 Ext. 2209. *Fax:* 787-834-9597.

CONTINUING EDUCATION PROGRAM

Contact *Telephone:* 787-834-9595 Ext. 2284. *Fax:* 787-834-9597.

Universidad del Turabo
Nursing Program
Gurabo, Puerto Rico

Founded in 1972
DEGREE • BS

BACCALAUREATE PROGRAMS

Degree BS
Available Programs Generic Baccalaureate.
Contact *Telephone:* 787-743-7979.

Universidad Metropolitana
Department of Nursing
San Juan, Puerto Rico

http://www.suagm.edu/umet/oa_pe_cs_programas.asp?cn_id=686
Founded in 1980
DEGREE • BSN
Library Facilities 5,438 volumes in health; 110 periodical subscriptions health-care related.

BACCALAUREATE PROGRAMS

Degree BSN
Contact *Telephone:* 787-766-1717 Ext. 6422. *Fax:* 787-769-7663.

University of Puerto Rico at Arecibo
Department of Nursing
Arecibo, Puerto Rico

http://www.upra.edu/
Founded in 1967
DEGREE • BSN
Nursing Program Faculty 21
Library Facilities 65,000 volumes; 3,660 periodical subscriptions.

BACCALAUREATE PROGRAMS

Degree BSN

Available Programs Generic Baccalaureate.
Contact *Telephone:* 787-878-2830. *Fax:* 787-880-4972.

University of Puerto Rico at Humacao

Department of Nursing
Humacao, Puerto Rico

http://www1.uprh.edu/enfe/
Founded in 1962

DEGREE • BS

Nursing Program Faculty 16 (12% with doctorates).
Nursing Student Activities Student Nurses' Association.
Nursing Student Resources Skills, simulation, or other laboratory.
Library Facilities 75,518 volumes; 57,383 periodical subscriptions.

BACCALAUREATE PROGRAMS

Degree BS
Available Programs Generic Baccalaureate.
Study Options Full-time and part-time.
Program Entrance Requirements Minimum overall college GPA, transcript of college record, health exam, health insurance, high school transcript, immunizations, minimum high school GPA of 2.0, minimum GPA in nursing prerequisites of 2.5. Transfer students are accepted.
Advanced Placement Credit by examination available. Credit given for nursing courses completed elsewhere dependent upon specific evaluations.
Contact *Telephone:* 787-850-9346. *Fax:* 787-850-9411.

University of Puerto Rico, Mayagüez Campus

Department of Nursing
Mayagüez, Puerto Rico

http://www.uprm.edu/enfe/
Founded in 1911

DEGREE • BSN

Nursing Program Faculty 21 (10% with doctorates).
Nursing Student Activities Nursing Honor Society, Sigma Theta Tau, Student Nurses' Association.
Nursing Student Resources Academic advising; academic or career counseling; assistance for students with disabilities; bookstore; campus computer network; career placement assistance; computer lab; computer-assisted instruction; e-mail services; employment services for current students; interactive nursing skills videos; Internet; learning resource lab; library services; nursing audiovisuals; paid internships; placement services for program completers; remedial services; resume preparation assistance; skills, simulation, or other laboratory; tutoring.
Library Facilities 68 periodical subscriptions health-care related.

BACCALAUREATE PROGRAMS

Degree BSN
Available Programs Generic Baccalaureate.
Study Options Full-time.
Program Entrance Requirements High school transcript, immunizations. Transfer students are accepted.
Advanced Placement Credit by examination available.
Contact *Telephone:* 787-263-3482. *Fax:* 787-832-3875.

CONTINUING EDUCATION PROGRAM

Contact *Telephone:* 787-265-3842. *Fax:* 787-832-3875.

University of Puerto Rico, Medical Sciences Campus

School of Nursing
San Juan, Puerto Rico

http://enfermeria.rcm.upr.edu/doctorado.html
Founded in 1950

DEGREES • BSN • MSN

Nursing Program Faculty 37 (25% with doctorates).
Baccalaureate Enrollment 241 **Women** 85% **Men** 15% **Part-time** 12%
Graduate Enrollment 158 **Women** 79% **Men** 21% **Part-time** 6%
Nursing Student Activities Sigma Theta Tau, Student Nurses' Association.
Nursing Student Resources Academic advising; academic or career counseling; assistance for students with disabilities; computer lab; computer-assisted instruction; e-mail services; employment services for current students; interactive nursing skills videos; Internet; library services; nursing audiovisuals; skills, simulation, or other laboratory; tutoring.
Library Facilities 7,830 volumes in health, 1,143 volumes in nursing; 1,215 periodical subscriptions health-care related.

BACCALAUREATE PROGRAMS

Degree BSN
Available Programs ADN to Baccalaureate; Generic Baccalaureate.
Study Options Full-time and part-time.
Program Entrance Requirements Minimum overall college GPA of 2.0, transcript of college record, health exam, immunizations, interview, minimum high school GPA of 2.0, prerequisite course work. Transfer students are accepted.
Contact *Telephone:* 787-758-2525 Ext. 1984. *Fax:* 787-281-0721.

GRADUATE PROGRAMS

Contact *Telephone:* 787-758-2525 Ext. 3105. *Fax:* 787-281-0721.

MASTER'S DEGREE PROGRAM
Degree MSN
Available Programs Master's.
Concentrations Available Nurse anesthesia; nursing administration; nursing education. *Clinical nurse specialist programs in:* adult health, community health, critical care, gerontology, maternity-newborn, pediatric, psychiatric/mental health.
Site Options Mayaguez, PR.
Study Options Full-time and part-time.
Program Entrance Requirements Clinical experience, minimum overall college GPA of 2.5, transcript of college record, immunizations, interview, resume, statistics course, GRE or EXADEP.
Degree Requirements 48 total credit hours, thesis or project.

CONTINUING EDUCATION PROGRAM

Contact *Telephone:* 787-758-2525 Ext. 2102. *Fax:* 787-281-0721.

University of the Sacred Heart

Program in Nursing
San Juan, Puerto Rico

Founded in 1935
DEGREES • BSN • MSN
Nursing Student Resources Skills, simulation, or other laboratory.

BACCALAUREATE PROGRAMS

Degree BSN
Available Programs Generic Baccalaureate.
Contact *Telephone:* 787-728-1515. *Fax:* 787-727-1250.

GRADUATE PROGRAMS

Contact *Telephone:* 787-728-1515 Ext. 2427. *Fax:* 787-727-1250.

MASTER'S DEGREE PROGRAM
Degree MSN
Available Programs Master's.

Concentrations Available *Nurse practitioner programs in:* occupational health.
Degree Requirements 37 total credit hours.

RHODE ISLAND

Rhode Island College
Department of Nursing
Providence, Rhode Island

http://www.ric.edu/nursing
Founded in 1854
DEGREES • BSN • MSN
Nursing Program Faculty 49 (39% with doctorates).
Baccalaureate Enrollment 415 **Women** 89% **Men** 11% **Minority** 36%
Part-time 38%
Graduate Enrollment 43 **Women** 98% **Men** 2% **Minority** 19% **Part-time** 98%
Distance Learning Courses Available.
Nursing Student Activities Sigma Theta Tau, Student Nurses' Association, nursing club.
Nursing Student Resources Academic advising; academic or career counseling; assistance for students with disabilities; bookstore; campus computer network; career placement assistance; computer lab; computer-assisted instruction; daycare for children of students; e-mail services; employment services for current students; housing assistance; interactive nursing skills videos; Internet; learning resource lab; library services; nursing audiovisuals; paid internships; placement services for program completers; remedial services; resume preparation assistance; skills, simulation, or other laboratory; tutoring.
Library Facilities 749,979 volumes (574 in nursing); 1.4 million periodical subscriptions (63 health-care related).

BACCALAUREATE PROGRAMS

Degree BSN
Available Programs Baccalaureate for Second Degree; Generic Baccalaureate; RN Baccalaureate.
Site Options Providence, RI.
Study Options Full-time and part-time.
Program Entrance Requirements Minimum overall college GPA of 2.7, CPR certification, health exam, health insurance, high school biology, high school chemistry, high school foreign language, 4 years high school math, 2 years high school science, high school transcript, immunizations, letters of recommendation, minimum GPA in nursing prerequisites of 3.0, prerequisite course work. Transfer students are accepted. *Application deadline:* 10/15 (fall), 4/15 (spring).
Advanced Placement Credit given for nursing courses completed elsewhere dependent upon specific evaluations.
Contact *Telephone:* 401-456-8014. *Fax:* 401-456-8206.

GRADUATE PROGRAMS

Contact *Telephone:* 401-456-9720. *Fax:* 401-456-8206.

MASTER'S DEGREE PROGRAM
Degree MSN
Available Programs Master's.
Concentrations Available *Clinical nurse specialist programs in:* acute care, adult health, community health. *Nurse practitioner programs in:* acute care, adult health.
Site Options Providence, RI.
Study Options Full-time and part-time.
Program Entrance Requirements Minimum overall college GPA of 3.0, transcript of college record, written essay, letters of recommendation, resume, statistics course. *Application deadline:* 2/15 (fall). *Application fee:* $50.
Advanced Placement Credit given for nursing courses completed elsewhere dependent upon specific evaluations.
Degree Requirements 45 total credit hours, thesis or project.

Salve Regina University
Department of Nursing
Newport, Rhode Island

http://www.salve.edu/academics/departments/nur/
Founded in 1934
DEGREE • BS
Nursing Program Faculty 23 (18% with doctorates).
Baccalaureate Enrollment 314 **Women** 91% **Men** 9% **Minority** 10%
International 1% Part-time 15%
Nursing Student Activities Sigma Theta Tau, Student Nurses' Association, nursing club.
Nursing Student Resources Academic advising; academic or career counseling; assistance for students with disabilities; bookstore; campus computer network; career placement assistance; computer lab; computer-assisted instruction; e-mail services; housing assistance; interactive nursing skills videos; Internet; learning resource lab; library services; nursing audiovisuals; paid internships; resume preparation assistance; skills, simulation, or other laboratory; tutoring; unpaid internships.
Library Facilities 6,882 volumes in health, 1,081 volumes in nursing; 76 periodical subscriptions health-care related.

BACCALAUREATE PROGRAMS

Degree BS
Available Programs Generic Baccalaureate; RN Baccalaureate.
Site Options Warwick, RI.
Study Options Full-time and part-time.
Program Entrance Requirements Minimum overall college GPA of 2.7, transcript of college record, written essay, high school biology, high school chemistry, high school foreign language, 3 years high school math, 3 years high school science, high school transcript, 2 letters of recommendation, minimum GPA in nursing prerequisites of 2.0, prerequisite course work. Transfer students are accepted. *Application deadline:* 2/1 (fall). Applications may be processed on a rolling basis for some programs. *Application fee:* $50.
Advanced Placement Credit by examination available. Credit given for nursing courses completed elsewhere dependent upon specific evaluations.
Expenses (2012–13) *Tuition:* full-time $33,450; part-time $1115 per credit. *International tuition:* $33,450 full-time. *Room and board:* $11,950; room only: $7000 per academic year. *Required fees:* full-time $500; part-time $40 per term.
Financial Aid 85% of baccalaureate students in nursing programs received some form of financial aid in 2011–12. *Gift aid (need-based):* Federal Pell, FSEOG, state, private, college/university gift aid from institutional funds. *Loans:* Federal Nursing Student Loans, Federal Direct (Subsidized and Unsubsidized Stafford PLUS), Perkins, college/university, alternative loans.*Work-study:* Federal Work-Study, part-time campus jobs.*Financial aid application deadline (priority):* 3/1.
Contact Mrs. Colleen Emerson, Dean of Undergraduate Admissions, Department of Nursing, Salve Regina University, 100 Ochre Point Avenue, Newport, RI 02840-4192. *Telephone:* 888-467-2583. *Fax:* 401-848-2823. *E-mail:* sruadmis@salve.edu.

CONTINUING EDUCATION PROGRAM

Contact Ms. Kelly Alverson, Director of Continuing Education and Graduate Enrollment, Department of Nursing, Salve Regina University, Graduate Studies and Continuing Education Office, Newport, RI 02840-4192. *Telephone:* 800-637-0002. *Fax:* 401-341-2973. *E-mail:* kelly.alverson@salve.edu.

University of Rhode Island
College of Nursing
Kingston, Rhode Island

http://www.uri.edu/nursing
Founded in 1892
DEGREES • BS • MS • PHD
Nursing Program Faculty 47 (50% with doctorates).
Baccalaureate Enrollment 851 **Women** 87% **Men** 13% **Minority** 24%
International 1% Part-time 10%
Graduate Enrollment 110 **Women** 95% **Men** 5% **Minority** 5% **International** 6% **Part-time** 75%

Nursing Student Activities Sigma Theta Tau, Student Nurses' Association.

Nursing Student Resources Academic advising; academic or career counseling; assistance for students with disabilities; bookstore; campus computer network; career placement assistance; computer lab; computer-assisted instruction; e-mail services; externships; housing assistance; interactive nursing skills videos; Internet; learning resource lab; library services; nursing audiovisuals; remedial services; resume preparation assistance; skills, simulation, or other laboratory; tutoring.

Library Facilities 1.5 million volumes; 25,309 periodical subscriptions.

BACCALAUREATE PROGRAMS

Degree BS

Available Programs ADN to Baccalaureate; Generic Baccalaureate; RN Baccalaureate.

Site Options Providence, RI.

Study Options Full-time and part-time.

Program Entrance Requirements Minimum overall college GPA of 2.5, transcript of college record, CPR certification, written essay, health exam, health insurance, high school foreign language, 3 years high school math, 2 years high school science, high school transcript, immunizations, 2 letters of recommendation, minimum high school rank 30%, minimum GPA in nursing prerequisites of 2.2. Transfer students are accepted.

Advanced Placement Credit given for nursing courses completed elsewhere dependent upon specific evaluations.

Contact *Telephone:* 401-874-7100.

GRADUATE PROGRAMS

Contact *Telephone:* 401-874-2766. *Fax:* 401-874-2061.

MASTER'S DEGREE PROGRAM

Degree MS

Available Programs Master's; RN to Master's.

Concentrations Available Clinical nurse leader; nursing administration; nursing education. *Clinical nurse specialist programs in:* gerontology, psychiatric/mental health. *Nurse practitioner programs in:* family health, gerontology.

Site Options Providence, RI.

Study Options Full-time and part-time.

Program Entrance Requirements Clinical experience, minimum overall college GPA of 3.0, transcript of college record, written essay, immunizations, 3 letters of recommendation, nursing research course, professional liability insurance/malpractice insurance, resume, statistics course, GRE or MAT.

Degree Requirements 41 total credit hours, thesis or project, comprehensive exam.

POST-MASTER'S PROGRAM

Areas of Study Nursing administration; nursing education. *Clinical nurse specialist programs in:* gerontology, psychiatric/mental health. *Nurse practitioner programs in:* family health, gerontology.

DOCTORAL DEGREE PROGRAM

Degree PhD

Available Programs Doctorate.

Areas of Study Nursing research, nursing science.

Program Entrance Requirements Clinical experience, minimum overall college GPA of 3.0, interview by faculty committee, 3 letters of recommendation, MSN or equivalent, scholarly papers, statistics course, vita, writing sample, GRE.

Degree Requirements 61 total credit hours, dissertation, oral exam, written exam, residency.

SOUTH CAROLINA

Charleston Southern University
Wingo School of Nursing
Charleston, South Carolina

http://www.csuniv.edu/
Founded in 1964

DEGREES • BSN • MSN
Nursing Program Faculty 18 (22% with doctorates).
Baccalaureate Enrollment 111 **Women** 90% **Men** 10% **Minority** 25%
Graduate Enrollment 16 **Women** 99% **Men** 1% **Minority** 10%
Distance Learning Courses Available.
Nursing Student Activities Sigma Theta Tau, Student Nurses' Association.
Nursing Student Resources Academic advising; academic or career counseling; assistance for students with disabilities; bookstore; campus computer network; career placement assistance; computer lab; computer-assisted instruction; e-mail services; externships; interactive nursing skills videos; Internet; learning resource lab; library services; nursing audiovisuals; remedial services; resume preparation assistance; skills, simulation, or other laboratory; tutoring.
Library Facilities 192,600 volumes (2,400 in health, 250 in nursing); 1,111 periodical subscriptions (55 health-care related).

BACCALAUREATE PROGRAMS

Degree BSN
Available Programs ADN to Baccalaureate; Generic Baccalaureate; RN Baccalaureate.
Study Options Full-time.
Online Degree Options Yes.
Program Entrance Requirements Minimum overall college GPA of 2.75, transcript of college record, CPR certification, written essay, health exam, health insurance, immunizations, minimum GPA in nursing prerequisites of 3.0, professional liability insurance/malpractice insurance, prerequisite course work. Transfer students are accepted. *Application deadline:* 3/15 (fall).
Advanced Placement Credit given for nursing courses completed elsewhere dependent upon specific evaluations.
Expenses (2011–12) *Tuition:* full-time $20,600; part-time $450 per credit. *Room and board:* $8000 per academic year. *Required fees:* full-time $1600.
Financial Aid 90% of baccalaureate students in nursing programs received some form of financial aid in 2010–11.
Contact Dr. Tara Hulsey, Dean of Nursing, Wingo School of Nursing, Charleston Southern University, 9200 University Boulevard, PO Box 118087, Charleston, SC 29423-8087. *Telephone:* 843-863-7075. *Fax:* 843-863-7540. *E-mail:* thulsey@csuniv.edu.

GRADUATE PROGRAMS

Financial Aid 95% of graduate students in nursing programs received some form of financial aid in 2010–11.
Contact Dr. Tara Hulsey, Dean, Wingo School of Nursing, Charleston Southern University, 9200 University Boulevard, PO Box 118087, Charleston, SC 29423. *Telephone:* 843-863-7075. *Fax:* 843-863-7540. *E-mail:* thulsey@csuniv.edu.

MASTER'S DEGREE PROGRAM

Degree MSN
Available Programs Master's; RN to Master's.
Concentrations Available Nursing education.
Study Options Full-time.
Online Degree Options Yes (online only).
Program Entrance Requirements Clinical experience, minimum overall college GPA of 3.0, transcript of college record, written essay, 3 letters of recommendation, resume. *Application deadline:* 6/31 (fall). *Application fee:* $20.
Advanced Placement Credit given for nursing courses completed elsewhere dependent upon specific evaluations.
Degree Requirements 39 total credit hours, thesis or project.

Clemson University
School of Nursing
Clemson, South Carolina

http://www.clemson.edu/hehd/departments/nursing/
Founded in 1889
DEGREES • BS • MS
Nursing Program Faculty 22 (71% with doctorates).
Baccalaureate Enrollment 402 **Women** 99% **Men** 1% **Minority** 11%
Graduate Enrollment 82 **Women** 90% **Men** 10% **Minority** 8% **Part-time** 54%
Distance Learning Courses Available.
Nursing Student Activities Nursing Honor Society, Sigma Theta Tau, Student Nurses' Association.
Nursing Student Resources Academic advising; academic or career counseling; assistance for students with disabilities; bookstore; campus computer network; career placement assistance; computer lab; computer-assisted instruction; e-mail services; employment services for current students; externships; housing assistance; interactive nursing skills videos; Internet; learning resource lab; library services; nursing audiovisuals; other; remedial services; resume preparation assistance; skills, simulation, or other laboratory; tutoring; unpaid internships.
Library Facilities 1.2 million volumes (29,800 in health, 5,548 in nursing); 5,587 periodical subscriptions (877 health-care related).

BACCALAUREATE PROGRAMS

Degree BS
Available Programs Accelerated Baccalaureate; Generic Baccalaureate; RN Baccalaureate.
Site Options Greenville, SC.
Study Options Full-time and part-time.
Program Entrance Requirements Minimum overall college GPA of 2.5, transcript of college record, CPR certification, health insurance, high school biology, high school chemistry, 3 years high school math, 3 years high school science, high school transcript, immunizations, minimum high school GPA of 2.5, professional liability insurance/malpractice insurance, prerequisite course work. Transfer students are accepted.
Advanced Placement Credit by examination available. Credit given for nursing courses completed elsewhere dependent upon specific evaluations.
Financial Aid 90% of baccalaureate students in nursing programs received some form of financial aid in 2011–12. *Gift aid (need-based):* Federal Pell, FSEOG, state, private, college/university gift aid from institutional funds. *Loans:* Federal Direct (Subsidized and Unsubsidized Stafford PLUS), Perkins, state, college/university, private loans.*Work-study:* Federal Work-Study, part-time campus jobs.*Financial aid application deadline (priority):* 4/1.
Contact Mr. Robert S. Barkley, Director of Admissions, School of Nursing, Clemson University, 106 Sikes Hall, Clemson, SC 29634. *Telephone:* 864-656-5463. *Fax:* 864-656-2464. *E-mail:* rbrtbkl@clemson.edu.

GRADUATE PROGRAMS

Financial Aid 75% of graduate students in nursing programs received some form of financial aid in 2011–12. 2 research assistantships with partial tuition reimbursements available (averaging $2,000 per year), teaching assistantships with partial tuition reimbursements available (averaging $5,122 per year) were awarded; fellowships with full and partial tuition reimbursements available, career-related internships or fieldwork, institutionally sponsored loans, scholarships, and unspecified assistantships also available. Aid available to part-time students.
Contact Mr. Patrick R. Harris, Student Services Program Coordinator, School of Nursing, Clemson University, 225 South Pleasantburg Drive, Greenville, SC 29606. *Telephone:* 864-250-8881. *Fax:* 864-250-6711. *E-mail:* pharri4@clemson.edu.

MASTER'S DEGREE PROGRAM
Degree MS
Available Programs Master's.
Concentrations Available Nursing administration; nursing education. *Nurse practitioner programs in:* adult health, family health, gerontology.
Site Options Greenville, SC.
Study Options Full-time and part-time.
Program Entrance Requirements Clinical experience, computer literacy, minimum overall college GPA of 3.0, transcript of college record, CPR certification, written essay, immunizations, 2 letters of recommendation, nursing research course, physical assessment course, professional liability insurance/malpractice insurance, prerequisite course work, resume, statistics course, GRE General Test. *Application deadline:* 4/1 (fall), 10/1 (spring).
Advanced Placement Credit given for nursing courses completed elsewhere dependent upon specific evaluations.
Degree Requirements 45 total credit hours, thesis or project, comprehensive exam.

POST-MASTER'S PROGRAM
Areas of Study Nursing administration; nursing education. *Nurse practitioner programs in:* adult health, family health, gerontology.

Coastal Carolina University
Nursing Completion Program
Conway, South Carolina

Founded in 1954
DEGREE • BSN
Library Facilities 216,564 volumes; 30,812 periodical subscriptions.

BACCALAUREATE PROGRAMS

Degree BSN
Available Programs RN Baccalaureate.
Program Entrance Requirements Immunizations, professional liability insurance/malpractice insurance, prerequisite course work, RN licensure.
Contact Director of the Nursing Completion Program, Nursing Completion Program, Coastal Carolina University, PO Box 261954, Conway, SC 29528-6054. *Telephone:* 843-349-4112. *E-mail:* pbohanna@coastal.edu.

Francis Marion University
Department of Nursing
Florence, South Carolina

http://www.fmarion.edu/
Founded in 1970
DEGREE • BSN
Nursing Program Faculty 13 (38% with doctorates).
Baccalaureate Enrollment 213 **Women** 86% **Men** 14% **Minority** 26%
Distance Learning Courses Available.
Nursing Student Activities Nursing Honor Society, Sigma Theta Tau, Student Nurses' Association.
Nursing Student Resources Academic advising; academic or career counseling; assistance for students with disabilities; bookstore; campus computer network; career placement assistance; computer lab; computer-assisted instruction; daycare for children of students; e-mail services; externships; housing assistance; interactive nursing skills videos; Internet; learning resource lab; library services; nursing audiovisuals; paid internships; placement services for program completers; remedial services; resume preparation assistance; skills, simulation, or other laboratory; tutoring; unpaid internships.
Library Facilities 412,000 volumes; 1,110 periodical subscriptions.

BACCALAUREATE PROGRAMS

Degree BSN
Available Programs ADN to Baccalaureate; Generic Baccalaureate.
Study Options Full-time.
Online Degree Options Yes.
Program Entrance Requirements Transcript of college record, CPR certification, written essay, health insurance, immunizations, 3 letters of recommendation, minimum GPA in nursing prerequisites of 3.0, prerequisite course work. Transfer students are accepted. *Application deadline:* 3/1 (fall), 10/1 (spring). *Application fee:* $78.
Expenses (2011–12) *Tuition, area resident:* full-time $13,220; part-time $1322 per credit hour. *Tuition, nonresident:* full-time $26,440; part-time $2644 per credit hour. *Room and board:* $3310 per academic year. *Required fees:* full-time $348.
Financial Aid 90% of baccalaureate students in nursing programs received some form of financial aid in 2010–11. *Gift aid (need-based):* Federal Pell, FSEOG, state, private, Academic Competitiveness Grants, National SMART Grants. *Loans:* Federal Direct (Subsidized and Unsubsidized Stafford PLUS), state.*Work-study:* Federal Work-Study, part-time campus jobs.*Financial aid application deadline:* 6/30(priority: 3/1).

Contact Miss Devin V. Cribb, Coordinator of Student Services, Department of Nursing, Francis Marion University, PO Box 100547, Florence, SC 29502-0547. *Telephone:* 843-661-1226. *Fax:* 843-661-1696. *E-mail:* dcribb@fmarion.edu.

Lander University
School of Nursing
Greenwood, South Carolina

http://www.lander.edu/nursing/
Founded in 1872

DEGREE • BSN
Nursing Program Faculty 21 (10% with doctorates).
Baccalaureate Enrollment 273 **Women** 92% **Men** 8% **Minority** 21% **Part-time** 16%
Distance Learning Courses Available.
Nursing Student Activities Sigma Theta Tau, Student Nurses' Association.
Nursing Student Resources Academic advising; academic or career counseling; assistance for students with disabilities; bookstore; campus computer network; career placement assistance; computer lab; computer-assisted instruction; e-mail services; externships; housing assistance; interactive nursing skills videos; Internet; learning resource lab; library services; nursing audiovisuals; resume preparation assistance; skills, simulation, or other laboratory.
Library Facilities 186,690 volumes (6,209 in health, 1,145 in nursing); 657 periodical subscriptions (36 health-care related).

BACCALAUREATE PROGRAMS
Degree BSN
Available Programs Accelerated Baccalaureate; Accelerated Baccalaureate for Second Degree; Accelerated RN Baccalaureate; Baccalaureate for Second Degree; Generic Baccalaureate; RN Baccalaureate.
Site Options Greenwood, SC.
Study Options Full-time and part-time.
Online Degree Options Yes.
Program Entrance Requirements Minimum overall college GPA of 2.6, transcript of college record, CPR certification, health exam, health insurance, immunizations, professional liability insurance/malpractice insurance, prerequisite course work. Transfer students are accepted. *Application deadline:* Applications may be processed on a rolling basis for some programs. *Application fee:* $35.
Advanced Placement Credit given for nursing courses completed elsewhere dependent upon specific evaluations.
Contact *Telephone:* 864-388-8307. *Fax:* 864-388-8125.

Medical University of South Carolina
College of Nursing
Charleston, South Carolina

http://www.musc.edu/nursing
Founded in 1824

DEGREES • BSN • MSN • PHD
Nursing Program Faculty 38 (80% with doctorates).
Baccalaureate Enrollment 183 **Women** 82% **Men** 18% **Minority** 31% **Part-time** 1%
Graduate Enrollment 202 **Women** 95% **Men** 5% **Minority** 16% **Part-time** 28%
Distance Learning Courses Available.
Nursing Student Activities Sigma Theta Tau, Student Nurses' Association.
Nursing Student Resources Academic advising; bookstore; campus computer network; computer lab; computer-assisted instruction; e-mail services; housing assistance; interactive nursing skills videos; Internet; learning resource lab; library services; nursing audiovisuals; other; resume preparation assistance; skills, simulation, or other laboratory; tutoring.
Library Facilities 151,763 volumes (40,000 in health, 1,500 in nursing); 20,173 periodical subscriptions (19,000 health-care related).

BACCALAUREATE PROGRAMS
Degree BSN
Available Programs Accelerated Baccalaureate; Accelerated Baccalaureate for Second Degree.
Site Options Charleston, SC.
Study Options Full-time.
Program Entrance Requirements Minimum overall college GPA of 3.0, transcript of college record, CPR certification, written essay, health exam, health insurance, immunizations, 3 letters of recommendation, minimum GPA in nursing prerequisites of 3.0, prerequisite course work. Transfer students are accepted. *Application deadline:* 1/15 (fall), 9/15 (spring). *Application fee:* $95.
Advanced Placement Credit by examination available. Credit given for nursing courses completed elsewhere dependent upon specific evaluations.
Expenses (2012–13) *Tuition, state resident:* full-time $21,447; part-time $647 per credit hour. *Tuition, nonresident:* full-time $36,450; part-time $1124 per credit hour. *Required fees:* full-time $1410; part-time $193 per term.
Financial Aid 85% of baccalaureate students in nursing programs received some form of financial aid in 2011–12.
Contact Mrs. Mardi Long, Program Coordinator, College of Nursing, Medical University of South Carolina, 99 Jonathan Lucas Street, MSC 160, Charleston, SC 29425-1600. *Telephone:* 843-792-6683. *Fax:* 843-792-9258. *E-mail:* longm@musc.edu.

GRADUATE PROGRAMS
Expenses (2012–13) *Tuition, state resident:* full-time $23,175; part-time $795 per credit hour. *Tuition, nonresident:* full-time $25,659; part-time $985 per credit hour. *Required fees:* full-time $1355; part-time $510 per credit; part-time $845 per term.
Financial Aid 83% of graduate students in nursing programs received some form of financial aid in 2011–12. Federal Work-Study, scholarships, and traineeships available. Aid available to part-time students. *Financial aid application deadline:* 3/10.
Contact Dr. Robin L. Bissinger, Director of Graduate Programs, College of Nursing, Medical University of South Carolina, 99 Jonathan Lucas Street, Room 209, MSC 160, Charleston, SC 29425-1600. *Telephone:* 843-792-0531. *Fax:* 843-792-1741. *E-mail:* bissinrl@musc.edu.

MASTER'S DEGREE PROGRAM
Degree MSN
Available Programs Master's.
Concentrations Available *Nurse practitioner programs in:* adult health, family health, pediatric.
Site Options Charleston, SC.
Study Options Full-time and part-time.
Online Degree Options Yes (online only).
Program Entrance Requirements Minimum overall college GPA of 3.0, transcript of college record, CPR certification, written essay, immunizations, 3 letters of recommendation, prerequisite course work, resume, statistics course. *Application deadline:* 3/1 (fall). *Application fee:* $95.
Advanced Placement Credit given for nursing courses completed elsewhere dependent upon specific evaluations.
Degree Requirements 60 total credit hours.

DOCTORAL DEGREE PROGRAM
Degree PhD
Available Programs Doctorate; Post-Baccalaureate Doctorate.
Areas of Study Community health, family health, nursing administration, nursing education, nursing policy, nursing research.
Site Options Charleston, SC.
Online Degree Options Yes (online only).
Program Entrance Requirements Minimum overall college GPA of 3.5, interview by faculty committee, interview, 3 letters of recommendation, MSN or equivalent, statistics course, vita, writing sample. *Application deadline:* 3/1 (fall). Applications may be processed on a rolling basis for some programs. *Application fee:* $95.
Degree Requirements 62 total credit hours, dissertation, oral exam, written exam.

POSTDOCTORAL PROGRAM
Areas of Study Gerontology, nursing interventions, nursing research, vulnerable population.
Postdoctoral Program Contact Dr. William Basco, Program Director, College of Nursing, Medical University of South Carolina, Rutledge Towers, MSC 106, Charleston, SC 29425. *Telephone:* 843-876-6512. *Fax:* 843-876-8709. *E-mail:* bascob@musc.edu.

Newberry College

Department of Nursing
Newberry, South Carolina

Founded in 1856

DEGREE • BSN

Library Facilities 85,473 volumes; 105 periodical subscriptions.

BACCALAUREATE PROGRAMS

Degree BSN

Available Programs RN Baccalaureate.

Program Entrance Requirements Minimum overall college GPA of 2.75, prerequisite course work.

Contact Department Chair, Department of Nursing, Newberry College, 2100 College Street, Newberry, SC 29108. *Telephone:* 800-845-4955. *E-mail:* mcdowell@newberry.edu.

South Carolina State University

Department of Nursing
Orangeburg, South Carolina

Founded in 1896

DEGREE • BSN

Library Facilities 313,329 volumes; 3,031 periodical subscriptions.

BACCALAUREATE PROGRAMS

Degree BSN

Available Programs Generic Baccalaureate; RN Baccalaureate.

Program Entrance Requirements Minimum overall college GPA of 2.8, immunizations, minimum high school GPA of 2.8.

Contact *Telephone:* 803-536-7063. *Fax:* 803-536-8593.

University of South Carolina

College of Nursing
Columbia, South Carolina

http://www.sc.edu/nursing

Founded in 1801

DEGREES • BSN • MSN • PHD

Nursing Program Faculty 102 (25% with doctorates).

Baccalaureate Enrollment 1,038 **Women** 93% **Men** 7% **Minority** 17% **International** .2% **Part-time** 4%

Graduate Enrollment 223 **Women** 90% **Men** 10% **Minority** 15% **Part-time** 62%

Distance Learning Courses Available.

Nursing Student Activities Sigma Theta Tau, Student Nurses' Association, nursing club.

Nursing Student Resources Academic advising; academic or career counseling; assistance for students with disabilities; bookstore; campus computer network; career placement assistance; computer lab; computer-assisted instruction; daycare for children of students; e-mail services; housing assistance; interactive nursing skills videos; Internet; learning resource lab; library services; nursing audiovisuals; remedial services; resume preparation assistance; skills, simulation, or other laboratory; tutoring.

Library Facilities 4 million volumes (98,901 in health, 10,716 in nursing); 67,016 periodical subscriptions (285 health-care related).

BACCALAUREATE PROGRAMS

Degree BSN

Available Programs Generic Baccalaureate.

Site Options Allendale, SC; Lancaster, SC; Walterboro, SC.

Study Options Full-time and part-time.

Program Entrance Requirements Minimum overall college GPA of 3.0, transcript of college record, high school biology, high school chemistry, high school foreign language, 1.5 years high school math, 1.5 years high school science, high school transcript, immunizations, minimum GPA in nursing prerequisites of 3.0. Transfer students are accepted. *Application deadline:* 12/1 (fall), 11/1 (spring), 12/1 (summer). *Application fee:* $50.

Advanced Placement Credit by examination available. Credit given for nursing courses completed elsewhere dependent upon specific evaluations.

Expenses (2011–12) *Tuition, state resident:* full-time $11,068; part-time $492 per credit hour. *Tuition, nonresident:* full-time $28,352; part-time $1232 per credit hour. *Room and board:* $8192; room only: $5440 per academic year. *Required fees:* full-time $2880.

Financial Aid 91% of baccalaureate students in nursing programs received some form of financial aid in 2010–11. *Gift aid (need-based):* Federal Pell, FSEOG, state, private, college/university gift aid from institutional funds, United Negro College Fund, Federal Nursing. *Loans:* Federal Nursing Student Loans, Federal Direct (Subsidized and Unsubsidized Stafford PLUS), Perkins.*Work-study:* Federal Work-Study, part-time campus jobs.*Financial aid application deadline (priority):* 4/1.

Contact Mrs. Gail S. Vereen, Student Services Manager, College of Nursing, University of South Carolina, 1601 Greene Street, Columbia, SC 29208. *Telephone:* 803-777-7412. *Fax:* 803-777-0616. *E-mail:* gsveree@mailbox.sc.edu.

GRADUATE PROGRAMS

Expenses (2011–12) *Tuition, state resident:* full-time $12,416; part-time $555 per credit hour. *Tuition, nonresident:* full-time $25,444; part-time $1077 per credit hour. *International tuition:* $25,444 full-time. *Room and board:* room only: $835 per academic year. *Required fees:* full-time $2680; part-time $204 per credit; part-time $169 per term.

Financial Aid 67% of graduate students in nursing programs received some form of financial aid in 2010–11. 1 fellowship (averaging $1,200 per year), 3 research assistantships with partial tuition reimbursements available (averaging $2,790 per year), 11 teaching assistantships (averaging $5,533 per year) were awarded; scholarships, traineeships, and unspecified assistantships also available. *Financial aid application deadline:* 4/1.

Contact Ms. Cheryl Nelson, Student Services Coordinator, Graduate Programs, College of Nursing, University of South Carolina, 1601 Greene Street, Columbia, SC 29208. *Telephone:* 803-777-3780. *Fax:* 803-777-2305. *E-mail:* cyjackso@mailbox.sc.edu.

MASTER'S DEGREE PROGRAM

Degree MSN

Available Programs Master's.

Concentrations Available *Nurse practitioner programs in:* acute care, family health.

Study Options Full-time and part-time.

Program Entrance Requirements Minimum overall college GPA of 3.0, transcript of college record, written essay, immunizations, 2 letters of recommendation, resume, GRE General Test, MAT. *Application deadline:* 5/1 (fall). *Application fee:* $50.

Advanced Placement Credit given for nursing courses completed elsewhere dependent upon specific evaluations.

Degree Requirements 45 total credit hours, comprehensive exam.

POST-MASTER'S PROGRAM

Areas of Study *Nurse practitioner programs in:* acute care, family health.

DOCTORAL DEGREE PROGRAM

Degree PhD

Available Programs Doctorate; Post-Baccalaureate Doctorate.

Areas of Study Health promotion/disease prevention, health-care systems, individualized study, nursing science.

Program Entrance Requirements Minimum overall college GPA of 3.0, interview by faculty committee, 3 letters of recommendation, scholarly papers, vita, writing sample, GRE General Test. *Application deadline:* 5/1 (fall). *Application fee:* $50.

Degree Requirements 60 total credit hours, dissertation, written exam, residency.

CONTINUING EDUCATION PROGRAM

Contact Dr. Eileen Shake, Director, Center for Nursing Leadership, College of Nursing, University of South Carolina, 1601 Greene Street, Columbia, SC 29208. *Telephone:* 803-777-5881. *Fax:* 803-777-6800. *E-mail:* shakee@mailbox.sc.edu.

University of South Carolina Aiken

School of Nursing
Aiken, South Carolina

http://www.usca.edu/nursing/
Founded in 1961

DEGREE • BSN

Nursing Program Faculty 16 (50% with doctorates).
Baccalaureate Enrollment 250 Women 90% Men 10% Minority 30% International 1% Part-time 3%
Distance Learning Courses Available.
Nursing Student Activities Sigma Theta Tau, Student Nurses' Association.
Nursing Student Resources Academic advising; academic or career counseling; assistance for students with disabilities; bookstore; campus computer network; career placement assistance; computer lab; computer-assisted instruction; daycare for children of students; e-mail services; employment services for current students; housing assistance; interactive nursing skills videos; Internet; learning resource lab; library services; nursing audiovisuals; placement services for program completers; resume preparation assistance; skills, simulation, or other laboratory; tutoring.
Library Facilities 212,758 volumes (200 in health, 100 in nursing); 656 periodical subscriptions (100 health-care related).

BACCALAUREATE PROGRAMS

Degree BSN
Available Programs ADN to Baccalaureate; Generic Baccalaureate; International Nurse to Baccalaureate; LPN to Baccalaureate; RN Baccalaureate.
Study Options Full-time and part-time.
Online Degree Options Yes.
Program Entrance Requirements CPR certification, written essay, health exam, immunizations, 2 letters of recommendation, minimum GPA in nursing prerequisites of 2.75, prerequisite course work. Transfer students are accepted. *Application deadline:* 3/15 (fall), 10/15 (spring).
Advanced Placement Credit by examination available. Credit given for nursing courses completed elsewhere dependent upon specific evaluations.
Contact *Telephone:* 803-648-3392. *Fax:* 803-641-3725.

University of South Carolina Beaufort

Nursing Program
Bluffton, South Carolina

http://www.uscb.edu/academics/undergraduate/Nursing/index/index.php
Founded in 1959

DEGREE • BSN

Nursing Program Faculty 9 (43% with doctorates).
Baccalaureate Enrollment 84 Women 91% Men 9% Minority 6% Part-time 10%
Distance Learning Courses Available.
Nursing Student Activities Student Nurses' Association.
Nursing Student Resources Academic advising; academic or career counseling; assistance for students with disabilities; bookstore; campus computer network; career placement assistance; computer lab; computer-assisted instruction; e-mail services; employment services for current students; externships; housing assistance; interactive nursing skills videos; Internet; learning resource lab; library services; nursing audiovisuals; paid internships; remedial services; resume preparation assistance; skills, simulation, or other laboratory; tutoring; unpaid internships.
Library Facilities 84,865 volumes (2,273 in health, 173 in nursing); 146 periodical subscriptions (23 health-care related).

BACCALAUREATE PROGRAMS

Degree BSN
Available Programs Generic Baccalaureate; RN Baccalaureate.
Study Options Full-time.
Program Entrance Requirements Minimum overall college GPA of 2.75, transcript of college record, CPR certification, written essay, health

exam, health insurance, immunizations, interview, 2 letters of recommendation, minimum GPA in nursing prerequisites of 2.75, prerequisite course work. Transfer students are accepted. *Application deadline:* 9/1 (spring).
Advanced Placement Credit by examination available. Credit given for nursing courses completed elsewhere dependent upon specific evaluations.
Expenses (2012–13) *Tuition, state resident:* full-time $8172; part-time $344 per credit. *Tuition, nonresident:* full-time $17,570; part-time $734 per credit. *International tuition:* $17,570 full-time. *Room and board:* $8540 per academic year. *Required fees:* full-time $1300.
Financial Aid 90% of baccalaureate students in nursing programs received some form of financial aid in 2011–12. *Gift aid (need-based):* Federal Pell, FSEOG, state, private, college/university gift aid from institutional funds. *Loans:* Federal Direct (Subsidized and Unsubsidized Stafford PLUS).*Work-study:* Federal Work-Study, part-time campus jobs.*Financial aid application deadline (priority):* 3/1.
Contact Dr. Rose Kearney-Nunnery, Professor and Chair, Department of Nursing, Nursing Program, University of South Carolina Beaufort, 1 University Boulevard, Bluffton, SC 29909. *Telephone:* 843-208-8124. *E-mail:* nursing@uscb.edu.

University of South Carolina Upstate

Mary Black School of Nursing
Spartanburg, South Carolina

https://www.uscupstate.edu/academics/nursing/default.aspx?id=2287
Founded in 1967

DEGREE • BSN

Nursing Program Faculty 80 (15% with doctorates).
Baccalaureate Enrollment 448 Women 90% Men 10% Minority 28% International 2% Part-time 6%
Distance Learning Courses Available.
Nursing Student Activities Nursing Honor Society, Sigma Theta Tau, Student Nurses' Association.
Nursing Student Resources Academic advising; academic or career counseling; assistance for students with disabilities; bookstore; campus computer network; career placement assistance; computer lab; computer-assisted instruction; daycare for children of students; e-mail services; employment services for current students; externships; housing assistance; interactive nursing skills videos; Internet; learning resource lab; library services; nursing audiovisuals; paid internships; resume preparation assistance; skills, simulation, or other laboratory; tutoring; unpaid internships.
Library Facilities 300,892 volumes (214,998 in health, 23,359 in nursing); 31,024 periodical subscriptions.

BACCALAUREATE PROGRAMS

Degree BSN
Available Programs Generic Baccalaureate; RN Baccalaureate.
Site Options Greenville, SC.
Study Options Full-time and part-time.
Online Degree Options Yes.
Program Entrance Requirements Transcript of college record, CPR certification, health exam, health insurance, immunizations, minimum GPA in nursing prerequisites of 2.75, professional liability insurance/malpractice insurance, prerequisite course work. Transfer students are accepted. *Application deadline:* 1/15 (fall), 5/1 (spring).
Advanced Placement Credit by examination available. Credit given for nursing courses completed elsewhere dependent upon specific evaluations.
Expenses (2011–12) *Tuition, state resident:* full-time $4573; part-time $390 per credit hour. *Tuition, nonresident:* full-time $9286; part-time $789 per credit hour. *International tuition:* $9286 full-time. *Room and board:* $3986; room only: $2650 per academic year. *Required fees:* full-time $2000; part-time $54 per credit.
Financial Aid 85% of baccalaureate students in nursing programs received some form of financial aid in 2010–11.
Contact Dr. Katharine M. Gibb, Interim Dean, Mary Black School of Nursing, University of South Carolina Upstate, 800 University Way, Spartanburg, SC 29303. *Telephone:* 864-503-5444. *Fax:* 864-503-5405. *E-mail:* kgibb@uscupstate.edu.

SOUTH DAKOTA

Augustana College
Department of Nursing
Sioux Falls, South Dakota

http://www.augie.edu/
Founded in 1860
DEGREE • BA
Nursing Program Faculty 15 (27% with doctorates).
Baccalaureate Enrollment 207 **Women** 87% **Men** 13% **Minority** 6% **Part-time** 2%
Distance Learning Courses Available.
Nursing Student Activities Sigma Theta Tau, Student Nurses' Association.
Nursing Student Resources Academic advising; academic or career counseling; assistance for students with disabilities; bookstore; campus computer network; career placement assistance; computer lab; computer-assisted instruction; daycare for children of students; e-mail services; employment services for current students; housing assistance; interactive nursing skills videos; Internet; learning resource lab; library services; nursing audiovisuals; remedial services; resume preparation assistance; skills, simulation, or other laboratory; tutoring; unpaid internships.
Library Facilities 271,973 volumes; 8,815 periodical subscriptions.

BACCALAUREATE PROGRAMS
Degree BA
Available Programs Generic Baccalaureate.
Study Options Full-time.
Program Entrance Requirements Minimum overall college GPA of 2.7, transcript of college record, CPR certification, written essay, health exam, health insurance, high school transcript, immunizations, 2 letters of recommendation, minimum high school GPA of 3.5, minimum GPA in nursing prerequisites of 2.7, prerequisite course work. Transfer students are accepted. *Application deadline:* 2/15 (fall). Applications may be processed on a rolling basis for some programs.
Advanced Placement Credit given for nursing courses completed elsewhere dependent upon specific evaluations.
Expenses (2012–13) *Tuition:* full-time $27,380. *Room and board:* $6626 per academic year. *Required fees:* full-time $640.
Financial Aid 98% of baccalaureate students in nursing programs received some form of financial aid in 2011–12.
Contact Debbie Anderson, Office Assistant, Department of Nursing, Augustana College, 2001 South Summit Avenue, Sioux Falls, SD 57197. *Telephone:* 605-274-4721. *Fax:* 605-274-4723. *E-mail:* debbie.anderson@augie.edu.

Mount Marty College
Nursing Program
Yankton, South Dakota

http://www.mtmc.edu/
Founded in 1936
DEGREE • BSN
Nursing Program Faculty 13 (15% with doctorates).
Baccalaureate Enrollment 89 **Women** 89% **Men** 11% **Minority** 7% **Part-time** 2%
Nursing Student Activities Sigma Theta Tau, Student Nurses' Association, nursing club.
Nursing Student Resources Academic advising; academic or career counseling; assistance for students with disabilities; bookstore; campus computer network; career placement assistance; computer lab; computer-assisted instruction; daycare for children of students; e-mail services; employment services for current students; externships; housing assistance; interactive nursing skills videos; Internet; learning resource lab; library services; nursing audiovisuals; paid internships; placement services for program completers; remedial services; resume preparation assistance; skills, simulation, or other laboratory; tutoring; unpaid internships.
Library Facilities 79,076 volumes (8,750 in health, 5,350 in nursing); 307 periodical subscriptions (85 health-care related).

BACCALAUREATE PROGRAMS
Degree BSN
Available Programs ADN to Baccalaureate; Accelerated LPN to Baccalaureate; Generic Baccalaureate; International Nurse to Baccalaureate; LPN to Baccalaureate; LPN to RN Baccalaureate; RN Baccalaureate.
Site Options Watertown, SD.
Study Options Full-time and part-time.
Program Entrance Requirements Minimum overall college GPA of 2.7, transcript of college record, CPR certification, health exam, health insurance, high school transcript, immunizations, minimum GPA in nursing prerequisites of 2.0, prerequisite course work. Transfer students are accepted. *Application deadline:* Applications may be processed on a rolling basis for some programs.
Advanced Placement Credit given for nursing courses completed elsewhere dependent upon specific evaluations.
Contact *Telephone:* 605-668-1594. *Fax:* 605-668-1607.

National American University
School of Nursing
Rapid City, South Dakota

Founded in 1941
DEGREE • BSN
Library Facilities 31,018 volumes; 268 periodical subscriptions.

BACCALAUREATE PROGRAMS
Degree BSN
Available Programs Generic Baccalaureate.
Contact *Telephone:* 303-876-7181. *Fax:* 303-876-7105.

Presentation College
Department of Nursing
Aberdeen, South Dakota

http://www.presentation.edu/
Founded in 1951
DEGREE • BSN
Nursing Program Faculty 21 (9% with doctorates).
Baccalaureate Enrollment 185 **Women** 95% **Men** 5% **Minority** 4% **Part-time** 24%
Distance Learning Courses Available.
Nursing Student Activities Nursing Honor Society, Sigma Theta Tau, Student Nurses' Association, nursing club.
Nursing Student Resources Academic advising; academic or career counseling; assistance for students with disabilities; bookstore; campus computer network; career placement assistance; computer lab; computer-assisted instruction; e-mail services; employment services for current students; externships; interactive nursing skills videos; Internet; learning resource lab; library services; nursing audiovisuals; placement services for program completers; remedial services; resume preparation assistance; skills, simulation, or other laboratory; tutoring; unpaid internships.
Library Facilities 89,703 volumes (378 in health, 353 in nursing); 48,740 periodical subscriptions (2,172 health-care related).

BACCALAUREATE PROGRAMS
Degree BSN
Available Programs ADN to Baccalaureate; Baccalaureate for Second Degree; Generic Baccalaureate; LPN to RN Baccalaureate; RN Baccalaureate.
Site Options Fargo , ND; Fairmont, MN.
Study Options Full-time and part-time.
Online Degree Options Yes.
Program Entrance Requirements Minimum overall college GPA of 2.5, transcript of college record, CPR certification, written essay, health exam, high school biology, high school chemistry, 2 years high school math, high school transcript, immunizations, 2 letters of recommendation, minimum high school GPA of 2.7, minimum GPA in nursing prerequisites of 2.5, prerequisite course work. Transfer students are accepted. *Application deadline:* 3/1 (fall).

Advanced Placement Credit by examination available. Credit given for nursing courses completed elsewhere dependent upon specific evaluations.
Contact *Telephone:* 605-229-8492. *Fax:* 605-229-8489.

South Dakota State University
College of Nursing
Brookings, South Dakota

http://www.sdstate.edu/nurs/
Founded in 1881
DEGREES • BS • MS • PHD
Nursing Program Faculty 127 (22% with doctorates).
Baccalaureate Enrollment 553 **Women** 82% **Men** 18% **Minority** 4%
Graduate Enrollment 166 **Women** 96% **Men** 4% **Minority** 2% **Part-time** 100%
Distance Learning Courses Available.
Nursing Student Activities Sigma Theta Tau, Student Nurses' Association, nursing club.
Nursing Student Resources Academic advising; academic or career counseling; assistance for students with disabilities; bookstore; campus computer network; career placement assistance; computer lab; computer-assisted instruction; e-mail services; employment services for current students; externships; interactive nursing skills videos; Internet; learning resource lab; library services; nursing audiovisuals; paid internships; placement services for program completers; remedial services; resume preparation assistance; skills, simulation, or other laboratory; tutoring.
Library Facilities 777,287 volumes (20,000 in health, 5,700 in nursing); 31,512 periodical subscriptions (4,402 health-care related).

BACCALAUREATE PROGRAMS

Degree BS
Available Programs Accelerated Baccalaureate; Generic Baccalaureate; RN Baccalaureate.
Site Options Rapid City, SD; Sioux Falls, SD.
Study Options Full-time.
Online Degree Options Yes.
Program Entrance Requirements Minimum overall college GPA of 2.7, transcript of college record, CPR certification, health exam, health insurance, immunizations, interview, minimum GPA in nursing prerequisites of 2.7, professional liability insurance/malpractice insurance, prerequisite course work. Transfer students are accepted. *Application deadline:* 1/25 (fall), 9/25 (spring).
Advanced Placement Credit given for nursing courses completed elsewhere dependent upon specific evaluations.
Contact *Telephone:* 605-688-6153. *Fax:* 605-688-6523.

GRADUATE PROGRAMS

Contact *Telephone:* 605-688-4114. *Fax:* 605-688-5827.

MASTER'S DEGREE PROGRAM
Degree MS
Available Programs Master's; RN to Master's.
Concentrations Available Clinical nurse leader; nursing administration; nursing education. *Nurse practitioner programs in:* family health, neonatal health, psychiatric/mental health.
Site Options Rapid City, SD; Sioux Falls, SD.
Study Options Full-time and part-time.
Online Degree Options Yes.
Program Entrance Requirements Clinical experience, minimum overall college GPA of 3.0, transcript of college record, CPR certification, written essay, immunizations, 3 letters of recommendation, professional liability insurance/malpractice insurance, statistics course. *Application deadline:* 3/1 (fall). *Application fee:* $200.
Advanced Placement Credit given for nursing courses completed elsewhere dependent upon specific evaluations.
Degree Requirements 48 total credit hours, thesis or project, comprehensive exam.

POST-MASTER'S PROGRAM
Areas of Study Nursing education. *Nurse practitioner programs in:* family health.

DOCTORAL DEGREE PROGRAM
Degree PhD
Available Programs Doctorate.

Areas of Study Nursing research.
Site Options Sioux Falls, SD.
Program Entrance Requirements Minimum overall college GPA of 3.3, interview by faculty committee, 4 letters of recommendation, MSN or equivalent, scholarly papers, vita, writing sample. *Application deadline:* 3/1 (fall).
Degree Requirements 60 total credit hours, dissertation, oral exam, written exam.

CONTINUING EDUCATION PROGRAM

Contact *Telephone:* 605-688-5178. *Fax:* 605-688-5745.

University of Sioux Falls
School of Nursing
Sioux Falls, South Dakota

http://www.usiouxfalls.edu/nursing
Founded in 1883
DEGREE • BSN
Nursing Program Faculty 5 (20% with doctorates).
Baccalaureate Enrollment 169
Distance Learning Courses Available.
Nursing Student Activities Nursing Honor Society, Sigma Theta Tau, Student Nurses' Association.
Nursing Student Resources Academic advising; academic or career counseling; assistance for students with disabilities; bookstore; campus computer network; career placement assistance; computer lab; computer-assisted instruction; e-mail services; employment services for current students; interactive nursing skills videos; Internet; learning resource lab; library services; nursing audiovisuals; other; placement services for program completers; remedial services; resume preparation assistance; skills, simulation, or other laboratory; tutoring.
Library Facilities 85,713 volumes; 378 periodical subscriptions.

BACCALAUREATE PROGRAMS

Degree BSN
Available Programs Accelerated Baccalaureate; Generic Baccalaureate; RN Baccalaureate.
Online Degree Options Yes.
Program Entrance Requirements Minimum overall college GPA of 2.75, written essay, letters of recommendation, minimum high school GPA of 2.75, prerequisite course work, RN licensure.
Contact School of Nursing, School of Nursing, University of Sioux Falls, 1101 West 22nd Street, Sioux Falls, SD 57105. *Telephone:* 605-331-6697. *E-mail:* Nursing@usiouxfalls.edu.

TENNESSEE

Aquinas College
School of Nursing
Nashville, Tennessee

http://www.aquinas.edu/nursing/
Founded in 1961
DEGREES • BSN • MSN
Nursing Program Faculty 6 (33% with doctorates).
Baccalaureate Enrollment 24 **Women** 92% **Men** 8% **Minority** 12% **International** 1% **Part-time** 100%
Graduate Enrollment 11 **Women** 100% **Part-time** 11%
Nursing Student Activities Nursing Honor Society, nursing club.
Nursing Student Resources Academic advising; academic or career counseling; assistance for students with disabilities; bookstore; campus computer network; career placement assistance; computer lab; computer-assisted instruction; e-mail services; employment services for current students; interactive nursing skills videos; Internet; learning resource lab; library services; nursing audiovisuals; remedial services; resume preparation assistance; skills, simulation, or other laboratory; tutoring.
Library Facilities 2,290 volumes in health, 1,220 volumes in nursing; 85 periodical subscriptions health-care related.

BACCALAUREATE PROGRAMS

Degree BSN
Available Programs Accelerated RN Baccalaureate.
Study Options Part-time.
Program Entrance Requirements Transfer students are accepted. *Application deadline:* Applications may be processed on a rolling basis for some programs. *Application fee:* $25.
Advanced Placement Credit by examination available. Credit given for nursing courses completed elsewhere dependent upon specific evaluations.
Expenses (2012–13) *Tuition:* full-time $19,200; part-time $640 per credit. *International tuition:* $19,200 full-time. *Required fees:* full-time $600.
Contact Br. Ignatius Perkins, OP, RN to BSN Program Director, School of Nursing, Aquinas College, 4210 Harding Pike, Nashville, TN 37205. *Telephone:* 615-297-2008. *Fax:* 615-783-0562. *E-mail:* perkinsi@aquinascollege.edu.

GRADUATE PROGRAMS

Expenses (2012–13) *Tuition:* part-time $665 per credit. *Required fees:* part-time $110 per credit.
Contact Br. Ignatius Perkins, OP, Dean, School of Nursing/Director, MSN Program, School of Nursing, Aquinas College, 4210 Harding Pike, Nashville, TN 37205. *Telephone:* 615-297-2008. *Fax:* 615-783-0562. *E-mail:* perkinsi@aquinascollege.edu.

MASTER'S DEGREE PROGRAM

Degree MSN
Available Programs Master's.
Concentrations Available Nursing education.
Study Options Part-time.
Program Entrance Requirements Computer literacy, minimum overall college GPA of 3.0, transcript of college record, CPR certification, written essay, immunizations, interview, professional liability insurance/malpractice insurance, resume. *Application deadline:* Applications may be processed on a rolling basis for some programs. *Application fee:* $25.
Advanced Placement Credit by examination available. Credit given for nursing courses completed elsewhere dependent upon specific evaluations.
Degree Requirements 40 total credit hours, thesis or project.

POST-MASTER'S PROGRAM
Areas of Study Nursing education.

Austin Peay State University
School of Nursing
Clarksville, Tennessee

http://www.apsu.edu/nursing01
Founded in 1927
DEGREES • BSN • MSN
Nursing Program Faculty 39 (26% with doctorates).
Baccalaureate Enrollment 258 **Women** 89.53% **Men** 10.47% **Minority** 23.64% **International** .1% **Part-time** 5.4%
Graduate Enrollment 146 **Women** 89.53% **Men** 10.47% **Minority** 23.64% **Part-time** 73.3%
Nursing Student Activities Nursing Honor Society, Sigma Theta Tau, Student Nurses' Association.
Nursing Student Resources Academic advising; computer lab; computer-assisted instruction; interactive nursing skills videos; Internet; nursing audiovisuals; skills, simulation, or other laboratory.
Library Facilities 366,955 volumes (4,700 in health, 800 in nursing); 34,899 periodical subscriptions (80 health-care related).

BACCALAUREATE PROGRAMS

Degree BSN
Available Programs ADN to Baccalaureate; Baccalaureate for Second Degree; Generic Baccalaureate; RN Baccalaureate.
Study Options Full-time.
Program Entrance Requirements Minimum overall college GPA of 3.0, transcript of college record, immunizations, minimum GPA in nursing prerequisites of 3.0, prerequisite course work. Transfer students are accepted. *Application deadline:* 5/1 (fall), 9/1 (spring).

Expenses (2012–13) *Tuition, state resident:* full-time $6648. *Tuition, nonresident:* full-time $20,736. *International tuition:* $20,736 full-time. *Room and board:* $8380; room only: $5600 per academic year. *Required fees:* full-time $3212.
Financial Aid 64% of baccalaureate students in nursing programs received some form of financial aid in 2011–12.
Contact Ms. Debbie Cochener, Administrative Specialist/Pre-Nursing Advisor, School of Nursing, Austin Peay State University, PO Box 4658, Clarksville, TN 37044. *Telephone:* 931-221-7708. *Fax:* 931-221-7595. *E-mail:* cochenerd@apsu.edu.

GRADUATE PROGRAMS

Expenses (2012–13) *Tuition, state resident:* part-time $364 per credit hour. *Tuition, nonresident:* part-time $364 per credit hour. *Required fees:* part-time $115 per credit.
Financial Aid 63% of graduate students in nursing programs received some form of financial aid in 2011–12.
Contact Dr. Doris Davenport, Coordinator of the MSN RODP, School of Nursing, Austin Peay State University, PO Box 4685, Clarksville, TN 37044. *Telephone:* 931-221-9467. *Fax:* 931-221-7595. *E-mail:* davenportd@apsu.edu.

MASTER'S DEGREE PROGRAM

Degree MSN
Available Programs Master's.
Concentrations Available Nursing administration; nursing education; nursing informatics. *Nurse practitioner programs in:* family health.
Study Options Full-time and part-time.
Online Degree Options Yes (online only).
Program Entrance Requirements Minimum overall college GPA of 3.0, transcript of college record, statistics course. *Application deadline:* 7/1 (fall), 12/1 (spring), 4/1 (summer). Applications may be processed on a rolling basis for some programs. *Application fee:* $25.
Advanced Placement Credit given for nursing courses completed elsewhere dependent upon specific evaluations.
Degree Requirements 46 total credit hours.

POST-MASTER'S PROGRAM
Areas of Study Nursing administration; nursing education; nursing informatics. *Nurse practitioner programs in:* family health.

Baptist College of Health Sciences
Nursing Division
Memphis, Tennessee

http://www.bchs.edu/
Founded in 1994
DEGREE • BSN
Nursing Program Faculty 40 (20% with doctorates).
Baccalaureate Enrollment 731 **Women** 89% **Men** 11% **Minority** 43% **Part-time** 45%
Distance Learning Courses Available.
Nursing Student Activities Sigma Theta Tau, Student Nurses' Association.
Nursing Student Resources Academic advising; academic or career counseling; assistance for students with disabilities; bookstore; campus computer network; computer lab; computer-assisted instruction; e-mail services; employment services for current students; externships; housing assistance; interactive nursing skills videos; Internet; learning resource lab; library services; nursing audiovisuals; paid internships; placement services for program completers; resume preparation assistance; skills, simulation, or other laboratory; tutoring.
Library Facilities 14,547 volumes (2,573 in health, 1,790 in nursing); 260 periodical subscriptions (213 health-care related).

BACCALAUREATE PROGRAMS

Degree BSN
Available Programs Generic Baccalaureate; LPN to Baccalaureate; RN Baccalaureate.
Study Options Full-time and part-time.
Program Entrance Requirements Minimum overall college GPA of 2.5, CPR certification, health exam, health insurance, 2 years high school math, 2 years high school science, high school transcript, immunizations, 3 letters of recommendation, minimum high school GPA of 2.75.

Transfer students are accepted. *Application deadline:* 6/1 (fall), 11/1 (spring). *Application fee:* $25.
Contact *Telephone:* 901-572-2441. *Fax:* 901-572-2461.

Belmont University
School of Nursing
Nashville, Tennessee

http://www.belmont.edu/nursing
Founded in 1951
DEGREES • BSN • MSN
Nursing Program Faculty 65 (19% with doctorates).
Baccalaureate Enrollment 406 **Women** 84% **Men** 16% **Minority** 6% **International** 3% **Part-time** 8%
Graduate Enrollment 43 **Women** 98% **Men** 2% **Minority** 12% **International** 2% **Part-time** 63%
Nursing Student Activities Nursing Honor Society, Sigma Theta Tau, Student Nurses' Association.
Nursing Student Resources Academic advising; academic or career counseling; assistance for students with disabilities; bookstore; campus computer network; career placement assistance; computer lab; computer-assisted instruction; e-mail services; employment services for current students; externships; housing assistance; interactive nursing skills videos; Internet; learning resource lab; library services; nursing audiovisuals; placement services for program completers; remedial services; resume preparation assistance; skills, simulation, or other laboratory; tutoring.
Library Facilities 228,427 volumes (6,000 in health, 800 in nursing); 1,084 periodical subscriptions (7,500 health-care related).

BACCALAUREATE PROGRAMS

Degree BSN
Available Programs ADN to Baccalaureate; Accelerated Baccalaureate; Accelerated Baccalaureate for Second Degree; Baccalaureate for Second Degree; Generic Baccalaureate; LPN to RN Baccalaureate; RN Baccalaureate.
Study Options Full-time and part-time.
Program Entrance Requirements Minimum overall college GPA of 2.5, transcript of college record, CPR certification, written essay, health exam, health insurance, high school biology, high school chemistry, 3 years high school math, 3 years high school science, high school transcript, immunizations, 1 letter of recommendation, minimum high school GPA of 2.5, minimum GPA in nursing prerequisites of 3.0. Transfer students are accepted. *Application deadline:* Applications may be processed on a rolling basis for some programs. *Application fee:* $50.
Advanced Placement Credit by examination available. Credit given for nursing courses completed elsewhere dependent upon specific evaluations.
Contact *Telephone:* 615-460-6120. *Fax:* 615-460-6125.

GRADUATE PROGRAMS

Contact *Telephone:* 615-460-6027. *Fax:* 615-460-6125.

MASTER'S DEGREE PROGRAM
Degree MSN
Available Programs Master's.
Concentrations Available Nursing education. *Nurse practitioner programs in:* family health.
Study Options Full-time and part-time.
Program Entrance Requirements Clinical experience, minimum overall college GPA of 3.0, transcript of college record, CPR certification, written essay, immunizations, interview, 2 letters of recommendation, resume, GRE. *Application fee:* $50.
Advanced Placement Credit given for nursing courses completed elsewhere dependent upon specific evaluations.
Degree Requirements 41 total credit hours, comprehensive exam.

POST-MASTER'S PROGRAM
Areas of Study Nursing education. *Nurse practitioner programs in:* family health.

Bethel University
Nursing Program
McKenzie, Tennessee

http://www.bethelu.edu/
Founded in 1842
DEGREE • BSN
Nursing Program Faculty 7
Baccalaureate Enrollment 46 **Women** 83% **Men** 17% **Minority** 17% **International** 4%
Distance Learning Courses Available.
Nursing Student Activities Student Nurses' Association.
Nursing Student Resources Academic advising; academic or career counseling; assistance for students with disabilities; bookstore; campus computer network; career placement assistance; computer lab; computer-assisted instruction; e-mail services; housing assistance; interactive nursing skills videos; Internet; learning resource lab; library services; nursing audiovisuals; remedial services; resume preparation assistance; skills, simulation, or other laboratory; tutoring.
Library Facilities 45,000 volumes (1,146 in nursing); 111,700 periodical subscriptions (99 health-care related).

BACCALAUREATE PROGRAMS

Degree BSN
Available Programs ADN to Baccalaureate; Generic Baccalaureate.
Study Options Full-time.
Program Entrance Requirements Minimum overall college GPA of 2.75, transcript of college record, CPR certification, health exam, health insurance, immunizations, minimum GPA in nursing prerequisites of 2.0, professional liability insurance/malpractice insurance, prerequisite course work. Transfer students are accepted. *Application deadline:* 3/1 (spring). *Application fee:* $25.
Advanced Placement Credit given for nursing courses completed elsewhere dependent upon specific evaluations.
Expenses (2012–13) *Tuition:* full-time $12,900; part-time $398 per credit. *Required fees:* full-time $1070; part-time $535 per term.
Financial Aid 80% of baccalaureate students in nursing programs received some form of financial aid in 2011–12.
Contact Ms. Mary Bess Griffith, Director, Nursing Program, Bethel University, 325 Cherry Avenue, McKenzie, TN 38201. *Telephone:* 731-352-6768. *Fax:* 731-352-2771. *E-mail:* griffithmb@bethelu.edu.

Carson-Newman University
Department of Nursing
Jefferson City, Tennessee

http://www.cn.edu/
Founded in 1851
DEGREES • BSN • MSN
Nursing Program Faculty 12 (58% with doctorates).
Baccalaureate Enrollment 102 **Women** 89% **Men** 11% **Minority** 13% **International** 1%
Graduate Enrollment 60 **Women** 77% **Men** 23% **Minority** 2% **Part-time** 87%
Distance Learning Courses Available.
Nursing Student Activities Sigma Theta Tau, Student Nurses' Association.
Nursing Student Resources Academic advising; academic or career counseling; assistance for students with disabilities; bookstore; campus computer network; career placement assistance; computer lab; computer-assisted instruction; e-mail services; employment services for current students; housing assistance; interactive nursing skills videos; Internet; learning resource lab; library services; nursing audiovisuals; placement services for program completers; remedial services; resume preparation assistance; skills, simulation, or other laboratory; tutoring.
Library Facilities 218,371 volumes (6,515 in health, 4,781 in nursing); 3,966 periodical subscriptions (10,824 health-care related).

BACCALAUREATE PROGRAMS

Degree BSN
Available Programs Accelerated Baccalaureate; Accelerated Baccalaureate for Second Degree; Generic Baccalaureate; LPN to Baccalaureate; LPN to RN Baccalaureate; RN Baccalaureate.
Study Options Full-time.

Online Degree Options Yes.

Program Entrance Requirements Minimum overall college GPA of 2.75, transcript of college record, health exam, health insurance, high school transcript, immunizations, minimum GPA in nursing prerequisites of 2.75, prerequisite course work. Transfer students are accepted. *Application deadline:* 3/1 (fall), 9/1 (spring), 3/1 (summer). Applications may be processed on a rolling basis for some programs.

Advanced Placement Credit by examination available. Credit given for nursing courses completed elsewhere dependent upon specific evaluations.

Expenses (2012–13) *Tuition:* full-time $21,660; part-time $902 per credit hour. *International tuition:* $21,660 full-time. *Room and board:* $8256; room only: $4416 per academic year. *Required fees:* full-time $1603; part-time $328 per term.

Financial Aid 95% of baccalaureate students in nursing programs received some form of financial aid in 2011–12. *Gift aid (need-based):* Federal Pell, FSEOG, state, private, college/university gift aid from institutional funds. *Loans:* Perkins, state, college/university, alternative loans. *Work-study:* Federal Work-Study, part-time campus jobs. *Financial aid application deadline (priority):* 4/1.

Contact Dr. Gregory A. Casalenuovo, Chair, Department of Nursing and Behavioral Health, Department of Nursing, Carson-Newman University, 1646 Russell Avenue, C-N Box 71883, Jefferson City, TN 37760. *Telephone:* 865-471-3425. *Fax:* 865-471-4574. *E-mail:* gcasalenuovo@cn.edu.

GRADUATE PROGRAMS

Expenses (2012–13) *Tuition:* full-time $4626; part-time $514 per credit hour. *International tuition:* $4626 full-time. *Room and board:* $8256; room only: $4416 per academic year. *Required fees:* full-time $242; part-time $162 per term.

Financial Aid 95% of graduate students in nursing programs received some form of financial aid in 2011–12.

Contact Dr. Kimberly S. Bolton, Graduate Program Director, Graduate Studies in Nursing, Department of Nursing, Carson-Newman University, 1646 Russell Avenue, C-N Box 71883, Jefferson City, TN 37760. *Telephone:* 865-471-4056. *Fax:* 865-471-4574. *E-mail:* kbolton@cn.edu.

MASTER'S DEGREE PROGRAM

Degree MSN

Available Programs Accelerated AD/RN to Master's; Master's.

Concentrations Available Nursing education. *Nurse practitioner programs in:* family health.

Study Options Full-time and part-time.

Program Entrance Requirements Minimum overall college GPA of 3.0, transcript of college record, written essay, interview, 3 letters of recommendation. *Application deadline:* 4/15 (fall), 10/15 (spring), 3/15 (summer). Applications may be processed on a rolling basis for some programs. *Application fee:* $50.

Advanced Placement Credit given for nursing courses completed elsewhere dependent upon specific evaluations.

Degree Requirements 45 total credit hours, thesis or project, comprehensive exam.

POST-MASTER'S PROGRAM

Areas of Study Nursing education. *Nurse practitioner programs in:* family health.

Cumberland University
Rudy School of Nursing and Health Professions
Lebanon, Tennessee

http://www.cumberland.edu/Nursing/
Founded in 1842

DEGREE • BSN

Nursing Program Faculty 20 (20% with doctorates).

Baccalaureate Enrollment 321 **Women** 84% **Men** 16% **Minority** 11% **Part-time** .5%

Distance Learning Courses Available.

Nursing Student Activities Sigma Theta Tau, Student Nurses' Association.

Nursing Student Resources Academic advising; academic or career counseling; assistance for students with disabilities; bookstore; campus computer network; career placement assistance; computer lab; computer-assisted instruction; e-mail services; externships; housing assistance; interactive nursing skills videos; Internet; learning resource lab; library

services; nursing audiovisuals; remedial services; resume preparation assistance; skills, simulation, or other laboratory; tutoring.

Library Facilities 112,112 volumes (125 in health, 66 in nursing); 232 periodical subscriptions (25 health-care related).

BACCALAUREATE PROGRAMS

Degree BSN

Available Programs ADN to Baccalaureate; Accelerated Baccalaureate; Accelerated Baccalaureate for Second Degree; Accelerated RN Baccalaureate; Baccalaureate for Second Degree; Generic Baccalaureate; RN Baccalaureate.

Site Options Mt. Juliet, TN.

Study Options Full-time and part-time.

Online Degree Options Yes.

Program Entrance Requirements Minimum overall college GPA of 3.0, transcript of college record, CPR certification, written essay, health exam, health insurance, high school transcript, immunizations, minimum high school GPA of 2.75, minimum GPA in nursing prerequisites of 3.0, professional liability insurance/malpractice insurance, prerequisite course work. Transfer students are accepted. *Application deadline:* 6/1 (fall), 10/1 (spring), 2/1 (summer). Applications may be processed on a rolling basis for some programs. *Application fee:* $25.

Advanced Placement Credit by examination available. Credit given for nursing courses completed elsewhere dependent upon specific evaluations.

Expenses (2012–13) *Tuition:* full-time $19,200; part-time $800 per credit. *International tuition:* $19,350 full-time. *Room and board:* $6800 per academic year. *Required fees:* full-time $1550; part-time $50 per credit; part-time $600 per term.

Financial Aid 95% of baccalaureate students in nursing programs received some form of financial aid in 2011–12.

Contact Dr. Carole Ann Bach, Professor and Dean, Rudy School of Nursing and Health Professions, Cumberland University, One Cumberland Square, McFarland Campus, Lebanon, TN 37087-3554. *Telephone:* 615-547-1200. *Fax:* 615-449-1368. *E-mail:* cbach@cumberland.edu.

East Tennessee State University
College of Nursing
Johnson City, Tennessee

http://www.etsu.edu/nursing
Founded in 1911

DEGREES • BSN • DNP • MSN • PHD

Nursing Program Faculty 70 (36% with doctorates).

Baccalaureate Enrollment 768 **Women** 82% **Men** 18% **Minority** 7% **Part-time** 11%

Graduate Enrollment 289 **Women** 94% **Men** 6% **Minority** 2% **International** 1% **Part-time** 49%

Distance Learning Courses Available.

Nursing Student Activities Nursing Honor Society, Sigma Theta Tau, Student Nurses' Association.

Nursing Student Resources Academic advising; academic or career counseling; assistance for students with disabilities; bookstore; campus computer network; career placement assistance; computer lab; computer-assisted instruction; daycare for children of students; e-mail services; employment services for current students; externships; housing assistance; interactive nursing skills videos; Internet; learning resource lab; library services; nursing audiovisuals; remedial services; resume preparation assistance; skills, simulation, or other laboratory; tutoring.

Library Facilities 1.1 million volumes; 3,714 periodical subscriptions.

BACCALAUREATE PROGRAMS

Degree BSN

Available Programs ADN to Baccalaureate; Accelerated Baccalaureate for Second Degree; Accelerated RN Baccalaureate; Generic Baccalaureate; LPN to Baccalaureate; RN Baccalaureate.

Site Options Cleveland, TN; Kingsport, TN; Pellissippi, TN; Sevierville, TN.

Study Options Full-time and part-time.

Online Degree Options Yes.

Program Entrance Requirements Minimum overall college GPA of 2.6, transcript of college record, minimum GPA in nursing prerequisites of 2.6, prerequisite course work. Transfer students are accepted. *Application deadline:* 10/1 (fall), 2/1 (spring).

Advanced Placement Credit given for nursing courses completed elsewhere dependent upon specific evaluations.

Expenses (2012–13) *Tuition, state resident:* full-time $2961; part-time $2350 per semester. *Tuition, nonresident:* full-time $7686; part-time $6100 per semester. *Required fees:* full-time $538.

Financial Aid 95% of baccalaureate students in nursing programs received some form of financial aid in 2011–12. *Gift aid (need-based):* Federal Pell, FSEOG, state, private, college/university gift aid from institutional funds, Federal Nursing. *Loans:* Federal Nursing Student Loans, Federal Direct (Subsidized and Unsubsidized Stafford PLUS), Perkins, state, college/university.*Work-study:* Federal Work-Study, part-time campus jobs.*Financial aid application deadline (priority):* 4/15.

Contact Mr. Scott Vaughn, Director, Student Services, College of Nursing, East Tennessee State University, PO Box 70664, Office of Student Services, Johnson City, TN 37614. *Telephone:* 423-439-4578. *Fax:* 423-439-4522. *E-mail:* nursing@etsu.edu.

GRADUATE PROGRAMS

Expenses (2012–13) *Tuition, state resident:* full-time $17,000; part-time $472 per credit. *Tuition, nonresident:* full-time $24,000; part-time $661 per credit. *Required fees:* full-time $1100; part-time $25 per credit; part-time $300 per term.

Financial Aid 90% of graduate students in nursing programs received some form of financial aid in 2011–12. 3 research assistantships with full and partial tuition reimbursements available (averaging $4,000 per year) were awarded; career-related internships or fieldwork, institutionally sponsored loans, scholarships, and unspecified assistantships also available. *Financial aid application deadline:* 7/1.

Contact Ms. Amy Bower, Coordinator, College of Nursing, East Tennessee State University, PO Box 70664, Office of Student Services, Johnson City, TN 37614. *Telephone:* 423-439-4578. *Fax:* 423-439-4522. *E-mail:* bowera@etsu.edu.

MASTER'S DEGREE PROGRAM

Degree MSN

Available Programs Master's; Master's for Nurses with Non-Nursing Degrees.

Concentrations Available Clinical nurse leader; nursing administration; nursing education; nursing informatics. *Nurse practitioner programs in:* family health.

Study Options Full-time and part-time.

Online Degree Options Yes.

Program Entrance Requirements Minimum overall college GPA of 3.0, transcript of college record, written essay, 3 letters of recommendation, resume, statistics course. *Application deadline:* 2/1 (fall), 7/1 (spring), 12/1 (summer). *Application fee:* $35.

Advanced Placement Credit given for nursing courses completed elsewhere dependent upon specific evaluations.

Degree Requirements 46 total credit hours, comprehensive exam.

POST-MASTER'S PROGRAM

Areas of Study Nursing administration; nursing education; nursing informatics. *Nurse practitioner programs in:* family health.

DOCTORAL DEGREE PROGRAM

Degree DNP

Available Programs Doctorate, Doctorate for Nurses with Non-Nursing Degrees, Post-Baccalaureate Doctorate.

Areas of Study Advanced practice nursing, nursing administration.

Program Entrance Requirements Minimum overall college GPA of 3.0, clinical experience, interview by faculty committee, letters of recommendation, MSN or equivalent, vita, writing sample. *Application deadline:* 2/1 (fall), 10/1 (spring). *Application fee:* $35.

Degree Requirements 79-85 total credit hours, residency.

DOCTORAL DEGREE PROGRAM

Degree PhD

Available Programs Doctorate.

Areas of Study Individualized study.

Program Entrance Requirements Clinical experience, minimum overall college GPA of 3.0, interview by faculty committee, 3 letters of recommendation, MSN or equivalent, statistics course, vita, writing sample, GRE General Test. *Application deadline:* 2/1 (spring). *Application fee:* $35.

Degree Requirements 62 total credit hours, dissertation, written exam, residency.

CONTINUING EDUCATION PROGRAM

Contact Ms. Lisa Davenport, Assistant Professor and Coordinator, Continuing Education, College of Nursing, East Tennessee State University, PO Box 70629, 807 University Parkway, Johnson City, TN 37614-1709. *Telephone:* 423-439-4052. *E-mail:* davenpol@etsu.edu.

King College
School of Nursing
Bristol, Tennessee

http://www.king.edu/
Founded in 1867

DEGREES • BSN • MSN • MSN/MBA

Nursing Program Faculty 31 (26% with doctorates).

Baccalaureate Enrollment 366 **Women** 96% **Men** 4% **Minority** 1% **International** 1%

Graduate Enrollment 35 **Women** 99% **Men** 1% **Minority** 1%

Distance Learning Courses Available.

Nursing Student Activities Student Nurses' Association.

Nursing Student Resources Academic advising; academic or career counseling; assistance for students with disabilities; bookstore; campus computer network; career placement assistance; computer lab; computer-assisted instruction; e-mail services; employment services for current students; externships; interactive nursing skills videos; Internet; learning resource lab; library services; nursing audiovisuals; paid internships; remedial services; resume preparation assistance; skills, simulation, or other laboratory; tutoring.

Library Facilities 97,836 volumes (929 in health, 158 in nursing); 352 periodical subscriptions (87 health-care related).

BACCALAUREATE PROGRAMS

Degree BSN

Available Programs Accelerated RN Baccalaureate; Generic Baccalaureate.

Site Options Kingsport, TN.

Study Options Full-time.

Program Entrance Requirements Minimum overall college GPA of 2.0, transcript of college record, CPR certification, written essay, health exam, health insurance, high school biology, high school chemistry, high school foreign language, 2 years high school math, 2 years high school science, high school transcript, immunizations, minimum high school GPA of 2.6, minimum high school rank 25%, minimum GPA in nursing prerequisites of 2.75. Transfer students are accepted. *Application deadline:* 6/1 (fall). *Application fee:* $100.

Contact *Telephone:* 423-652-4841. *Fax:* 423-652-4833.

GRADUATE PROGRAMS

Contact *Telephone:* 423-652-4841. *Fax:* 423-652-4833.

MASTER'S DEGREE PROGRAM

Degrees MSN; MSN/MBA

Available Programs Accelerated RN to Master's; Master's.

Concentrations Available *Clinical nurse specialist programs in:* acute care, adult health, oncology.

Study Options Full-time.

Program Entrance Requirements Clinical experience, computer literacy, minimum overall college GPA of 3.0, transcript of college record, CPR certification, written essay, immunizations, 2 letters of recommendation, nursing research course, physical assessment course, resume, statistics course. *Application deadline:* 4/15 (fall). *Application fee:* $100.

Degree Requirements 39 total credit hours, thesis or project.

Lincoln Memorial University
Caylor School of Nursing
Harrogate, Tennessee

http://www.lmunet.edu/academics/nursing/index2.shtml
Founded in 1897

DEGREES • BSN • MSN

Nursing Program Faculty 50 (57% with doctorates).

Baccalaureate Enrollment 70 **Women** 80% **Men** 20% **Minority** 3% **International** 3%

Graduate Enrollment 65

Nursing Student Activities Student Nurses' Association.

Nursing Student Resources Academic advising; academic or career counseling; bookstore; campus computer network; career placement assistance; computer lab; e-mail services; externships; interactive nursing skills videos; Internet; learning resource lab; library services; nursing audiovisuals; other; placement services for program completers; skills, simulation, or other laboratory; tutoring.

Library Facilities 323,046 volumes (1,230 in health, 630 in nursing); 334 periodical subscriptions (36 health-care related).

BACCALAUREATE PROGRAMS

Degree BSN

Available Programs ADN to Baccalaureate; Accelerated Baccalaureate; Generic Baccalaureate; RN Baccalaureate.

Site Options Knoxville, TN.

Study Options Full-time.

Program Entrance Requirements Minimum overall college GPA of 2.75, transcript of college record, CPR certification, immunizations, professional liability insurance/malpractice insurance, prerequisite course work, RN licensure. Transfer students are accepted. *Application deadline:* Applications may be processed on a rolling basis for some programs.

Expenses (2011–12) *Tuition:* full-time $17,520; part-time $730 per credit hour.

Financial Aid 80% of baccalaureate students in nursing programs received some form of financial aid in 2010–11.

Contact Admissions, Caylor School of Nursing, Lincoln Memorial University, Cumberland Gap Parkway, Harrogate, TN 37752. *Telephone:* 423-869-3611. *Fax:* 423-869-6444. *E-mail:* admissions@lmunet.edu.

GRADUATE PROGRAMS

Contact Sherry M. Pearman, Director of Nursing Recruitment and Advising, Caylor School of Nursing, Lincoln Memorial University, 6965 Cumberland Gap Parkway, Harrogate, TN 37752. *Telephone:* 423-869-6283. *Fax:* 423-869-6244. *E-mail:* sherry.pearman@lmuent.edu.

MASTER'S DEGREE PROGRAM

Degree MSN

Available Programs Master's.

Concentrations Available Nurse anesthesia. *Nurse practitioner programs in:* family health, psychiatric/mental health.

Site Options Knoxville, TN.

Study Options Full-time and part-time.

Program Entrance Requirements Clinical experience, computer literacy, transcript of college record, CPR certification, written essay, immunizations, interview, 3 letters of recommendation, professional liability insurance/malpractice insurance, prerequisite course work, statistics course. *Application deadline:* Applications may be processed on a rolling basis for some programs.

POST-MASTER'S PROGRAM

Areas of Study *Nurse practitioner programs in:* family health, psychiatric/mental health.

Lipscomb University

Department of Nursing
Nashville, Tennessee

Founded in 1891

DEGREE • BSN

Library Facilities 227,885 volumes; 719 periodical subscriptions.

BACCALAUREATE PROGRAMS

Degree BSN

Available Programs Generic Baccalaureate.

Contact *Telephone:* 615-996-6650.

Martin Methodist College

Division of Nursing
Pulaski, Tennessee

http://martinmethodist.edu/

Founded in 1870

DEGREE • BSN

Nursing Program Faculty 7 (43% with doctorates).

Baccalaureate Enrollment 71 Women 96% Men 4% Minority 2%

Distance Learning Courses Available.

Nursing Student Activities Student Nurses' Association.

Nursing Student Resources Academic advising; academic or career counseling; bookstore; campus computer network; career placement assistance; computer lab; computer-assisted instruction; e-mail services; employment services for current students; housing assistance; interactive nursing skills videos; Internet; learning resource lab; library services; nursing audiovisuals; placement services for program completers; remedial services; resume preparation assistance; skills, simulation, or other laboratory; tutoring; unpaid internships.

Library Facilities 84,000 volumes (875 in nursing); 664 periodical subscriptions (400 health-care related).

BACCALAUREATE PROGRAMS

Degree BSN

Available Programs Generic Baccalaureate.

Study Options Full-time.

Program Entrance Requirements Transcript of college record, CPR certification, health insurance, immunizations, minimum GPA in nursing prerequisites, prerequisite course work. Transfer students are accepted. *Application deadline:* 2/1 (fall), 2/1 (winter). *Application fee:* $30.

Expenses (2012–13) *Tuition:* full-time $20,000. *Room and board:* $10,000; room only: $7000 per academic year. *Required fees:* full-time $700; part-time $350 per term.

Financial Aid 100% of baccalaureate students in nursing programs received some form of financial aid in 2011–12.

Contact Dr. Kenneth R. Burns, Professor and Chair, Division of Nursing, Martin Methodist College, 433 West Madison Street, Pulaski, TN 38478. *Telephone:* 931-424-7395. *Fax:* 931-363-9891. *E-mail:* kburns@martinmethodist.edu.

Middle Tennessee State University

School of Nursing
Murfreesboro, Tennessee

http://www.mtsu.edu/

Founded in 1911

DEGREES • BSN • MSN

Nursing Program Faculty 45 (65% with doctorates).

Baccalaureate Enrollment 300 Women 85% Men 15% Minority 15%

Graduate Enrollment 100 Women 80% Men 20% Minority 15% Part-time 50%

Distance Learning Courses Available.

Nursing Student Activities Sigma Theta Tau, Student Nurses' Association.

Nursing Student Resources Academic advising; academic or career counseling; assistance for students with disabilities; bookstore; campus computer network; career placement assistance; computer lab; computer-assisted instruction; e-mail services; interactive nursing skills videos; Internet; learning resource lab; library services; nursing audiovisuals; remedial services; resume preparation assistance; skills, simulation, or other laboratory; tutoring.

Library Facilities 100 volumes in health, 45 volumes in nursing; 100 periodical subscriptions health-care related.

BACCALAUREATE PROGRAMS

Degree BSN

Available Programs Generic Baccalaureate; LPN to RN Baccalaureate; RN Baccalaureate.

Study Options Full-time.

Online Degree Options Yes.

Program Entrance Requirements Minimum overall college GPA of 2.8, transcript of college record, CPR certification, health exam, health

insurance, immunizations, interview, minimum GPA in nursing prerequisites of 2.75, professional liability insurance/malpractice insurance, prerequisite course work. Transfer students are accepted. *Application deadline:* 2/1 (fall), 10/1 (spring).
Advanced Placement Credit by examination available. Credit given for nursing courses completed elsewhere dependent upon specific evaluations.
Financial Aid *Gift aid (need-based):* Federal Pell, FSEOG, state, private, college/university gift aid from institutional funds. *Loans:* Federal Direct (Subsidized and Unsubsidized Stafford PLUS), Perkins, college/university.*Work-study:* Federal Work-Study.*Financial aid application deadline (priority):* 3/1.
Contact Dr. Karen S. Ward, Interim Director, School of Nursing, Middle Tennessee State University, PO Box 81, 1301 East Main Street, Murfreesboro, TN 37132-0001. *Telephone:* 615-898-2437. *Fax:* 615-898-5441. *E-mail:* karen.ward@mtsu.edu.

GRADUATE PROGRAMS

Contact Dr. Karen S. Ward, Interim Director, School of Nursing, Middle Tennessee State University, PO Box 81, 1301 East Main Street, Murfreesboro, TN 37132-0001. *Telephone:* 615-898-2437. *Fax:* 615-898-5441. *E-mail:* karen.ward@mtsu.edu.

MASTER'S DEGREE PROGRAM
Degree MSN
Available Programs Accelerated AD/RN to Master's; Master's.
Concentrations Available Nursing administration; nursing education; nursing informatics. *Nurse practitioner programs in:* family health.
Site Options multiple cities.
Study Options Full-time and part-time.
Online Degree Options Yes.
Program Entrance Requirements Minimum overall college GPA of 3.0, transcript of college record, 3 letters of recommendation, prerequisite course work, resume. *Application deadline:* Applications may be processed on a rolling basis for some programs.
Degree Requirements 43 total credit hours, thesis or project.

POST-MASTER'S PROGRAM
Areas of Study *Nurse practitioner programs in:* family health.

Milligan College
Department of Nursing
Milligan College, Tennessee

http://www.milligan.edu/BSN/
Founded in 1866
DEGREE • BSN
Nursing Program Faculty 10 (25% with doctorates).
Baccalaureate Enrollment 195 **Women** 90% **Men** 10% **Minority** 2%
Nursing Student Activities Nursing Honor Society, Student Nurses' Association.
Nursing Student Resources Academic advising; academic or career counseling; assistance for students with disabilities; bookstore; campus computer network; career placement assistance; computer lab; computer-assisted instruction; e-mail services; employment services for current students; externships; interactive nursing skills videos; Internet; learning resource lab; library services; nursing audiovisuals; placement services for program completers; remedial services; resume preparation assistance; skills, simulation, or other laboratory; tutoring; unpaid internships.
Library Facilities 145,605 volumes (2,430 in health, 184 in nursing); 11,097 periodical subscriptions (340 health-care related).

BACCALAUREATE PROGRAMS
Degree BSN
Available Programs ADN to Baccalaureate; Baccalaureate for Second Degree; Generic Baccalaureate; LPN to Baccalaureate; LPN to RN Baccalaureate; RN Baccalaureate.
Study Options Full-time and part-time.
Program Entrance Requirements Minimum overall college GPA of 2.5, transcript of college record, CPR certification, written essay, health exam, immunizations, letters of recommendation, minimum GPA in nursing prerequisites of 2.5, professional liability insurance/malpractice insurance, prerequisite course work. Transfer students are accepted. *Application deadline:* Applications may be processed on a rolling basis for some programs. *Application fee:* $30.

Advanced Placement Credit given for nursing courses completed elsewhere dependent upon specific evaluations.
Expenses (2011–12) *Tuition:* full-time $24,360; part-time $400 per credit hour. *International tuition:* $24,360 full-time. *Room and board:* $5650; room only: $2650 per academic year. *Required fees:* full-time $900; part-time $524 per term.
Financial Aid 94% of baccalaureate students in nursing programs received some form of financial aid in 2010–11.
Contact Dr. Melinda K. Collins, Area Chair and Director of Nursing, Department of Nursing, Milligan College, Wilson Way, Suite 302, Milligan College, TN 37682. *Telephone:* 423-461-8655. *Fax:* 423-461-8982. *E-mail:* mcollins@milligan.edu.

South College
Department of Nursing
Knoxville, Tennessee

Founded in 1882
DEGREE • BSN

BACCALAUREATE PROGRAMS
Degree BSN
Available Programs Generic Baccalaureate.
Program Entrance Requirements Immunizations, minimum high school GPA of 2.5. Transfer students are accepted.
Contact *Telephone:* 865-251-1800.

Southern Adventist University
School of Nursing
Collegedale, Tennessee

http://www.southern.edu/nursing
Founded in 1892
DEGREES • BS • DNP • MSN • MSN/MBA
Nursing Program Faculty 21 (28% with doctorates).
Baccalaureate Enrollment 144 **Women** 80% **Men** 20% **Minority** 29% **International** 15% **Part-time** 38%
Graduate Enrollment 205 **Women** 85% **Men** 15% **Minority** 7% **International** 1% **Part-time** 45%
Distance Learning Courses Available.
Nursing Student Activities Sigma Theta Tau, nursing club.
Nursing Student Resources Academic advising; academic or career counseling; assistance for students with disabilities; bookstore; campus computer network; career placement assistance; computer lab; computer-assisted instruction; e-mail services; employment services for current students; housing assistance; interactive nursing skills videos; Internet; learning resource lab; library services; nursing audiovisuals; remedial services; resume preparation assistance; skills, simulation, or other laboratory; tutoring.
Library Facilities 170,176 volumes (7,795 in health, 974 in nursing); 56,047 periodical subscriptions (86 health-care related).

BACCALAUREATE PROGRAMS
Degree BS
Available Programs ADN to Baccalaureate.
Site Options Chattanooga, TN.
Study Options Full-time and part-time.
Online Degree Options Yes.
Program Entrance Requirements Minimum overall college GPA of 2.5, transcript of college record, CPR certification, health exam, high school transcript, immunizations, 2 letters of recommendation, minimum GPA in nursing prerequisites of 2.0, prerequisite course work, RN licensure. Transfer students are accepted. *Application deadline:* 2/1 (fall), 9/1 (winter). Applications may be processed on a rolling basis for some programs.
Advanced Placement Credit given for nursing courses completed elsewhere dependent upon specific evaluations.
Expenses (2012–13) *Tuition:* full-time $18,324; part-time $774 per credit hour. *International tuition:* $18,324 full-time. *Room and board:* $5584; room only: $3484 per academic year. *Required fees:* full-time $1280.
Financial Aid 80% of baccalaureate students in nursing programs received some form of financial aid in 2011–12. *Gift aid (need-based):*

Federal Pell, FSEOG, state, private, college/university gift aid from institutional funds. *Loans:* Federal Nursing Student Loans, Federal Direct (Subsidized and Unsubsidized Stafford PLUS), Perkins, college/university.*Work-study:* Federal Work-Study, part-time campus jobs.*Financial aid application deadline (priority):* 3/1.

Contact Mrs. Linda Marlowe, Admissions and Progression Coordinator, School of Nursing, Southern Adventist University, PO Box 370, Collegedale, TN 37315-0370. *Telephone:* 423-236-2941. *Fax:* 423-236-1940. *E-mail:* lmarlowe@southern.edu.

GRADUATE PROGRAMS

Expenses (2012–13) *Tuition:* full-time $9900; part-time $550 per credit hour. *International tuition:* $9900 full-time. *Room and board:* $8000; room only: $6000 per academic year.

Financial Aid 50% of graduate students in nursing programs received some form of financial aid in 2011–12.

Contact Mrs. Diane Proffitt, Applications Manager, School of Nursing, Southern Adventist University, PO Box 370, Collegedale, TN 37315-0370. *Telephone:* 423-236-2957. *Fax:* 423-236-1940. *E-mail:* dproffit@southern.edu.

MASTER'S DEGREE PROGRAM

Degrees MSN; MSN/MBA

Available Programs Accelerated RN to Master's; Master's.

Concentrations Available Nursing education. *Nurse practitioner programs in:* acute care, adult health, family health.

Study Options Full-time and part-time.

Program Entrance Requirements Clinical experience, minimum overall college GPA of 3.0, transcript of college record, CPR certification, written essay, immunizations, interview, 2 letters of recommendation, prerequisite course work, statistics course. *Application deadline:* 7/1 (fall), 11/1 (winter). *Application fee:* $25.

Advanced Placement Credit given for nursing courses completed elsewhere dependent upon specific evaluations.

Degree Requirements 46 total credit hours, thesis or project.

DOCTORAL DEGREE PROGRAM

Degree DNP

Available Programs Doctorate.

Online Degree Options Yes (online only).

Program Entrance Requirements Clinical experience, minimum overall college GPA of 3.0, interview by faculty committee, letters of recommendation, MSN or equivalent, scholarly papers, statistics course, vita, writing sample. *Application fee:* $25.

Degree Requirements 42 total credit hours.

CONTINUING EDUCATION PROGRAM

Contact Mrs. Linda Marlowe, Admissions and Progression Coordinator, School of Nursing, Southern Adventist University, PO Box 370, Collegedale, TN 37315-0370. *Telephone:* 423-236-2941. *Fax:* 423-236-1940. *E-mail:* lmarlowe@southern.edu.

Tennessee State University

School of Nursing
Nashville, Tennessee

http://www.tnstate.edu/nursing/

Founded in 1912

DEGREES • BSN • MSN

Nursing Program Faculty 47 (34% with doctorates).

Baccalaureate Enrollment 107 **Women** 81% **Men** 19% **Minority** 66% **Part-time** 21%

Graduate Enrollment 301 **Women** 93% **Men** 7% **Minority** 40% **International** 6% **Part-time** 86%

Distance Learning Courses Available.

Nursing Student Activities Sigma Theta Tau.

Nursing Student Resources Academic advising; academic or career counseling; assistance for students with disabilities; bookstore; campus computer network; computer lab; e-mail services; interactive nursing skills videos; Internet; learning resource lab; library services; nursing audiovisuals; skills, simulation, or other laboratory; tutoring.

Library Facilities 630,890 volumes (50,000 in health, 25,000 in nursing); 300 periodical subscriptions health-care related.

BACCALAUREATE PROGRAMS

Degree BSN

Available Programs Generic Baccalaureate; RN Baccalaureate.

Site Options Nashville, TN.

Study Options Full-time.

Program Entrance Requirements Minimum overall college GPA of 2.8, transcript of college record, CPR certification, health exam, immunizations, minimum high school GPA of 2.8, minimum GPA in nursing prerequisites of 2.8, professional liability insurance/malpractice insurance, prerequisite course work. Transfer students are accepted. *Application deadline:* 3/1 (fall).

Expenses (2012–13) *Tuition, state resident:* full-time $6426; part-time $287 per credit hour. *Tuition, nonresident:* full-time $18,954; part-time $809 per credit hour. *Room and board:* $8240; room only: $5520 per academic year. *Required fees:* full-time $1700.

Financial Aid 80% of baccalaureate students in nursing programs received some form of financial aid in 2011–12. *Gift aid (need-based):* Federal Pell, FSEOG, state, private, college/university gift aid from institutional funds. *Loans:* Federal Direct (Subsidized and Unsubsidized Stafford PLUS), Perkins.*Work-study:* Federal Work-Study.*Financial aid application deadline (priority):* 4/1.

Contact Dr. Pamela D. Ark, BSN Program Director, School of Nursing, Tennessee State University, 3500 John A. Merritt Boulevard, Box 9590, Nashville, TN 37209-1561. *Telephone:* 615-963-7615. *Fax:* 615-963-5593. *E-mail:* park@tnstate.edu.

GRADUATE PROGRAMS

Expenses (2012–13) *Tuition, state resident:* full-time $8310; part-time $427 per credit hour. *Tuition, nonresident:* full-time $19,790; part-time $1001 per credit hour. *Required fees:* full-time $1500; part-time $25 per credit.

Financial Aid 80% of graduate students in nursing programs received some form of financial aid in 2011–12. Research assistantships (averaging $6,500 per year), 3 teaching assistantships (averaging $6,500 per year) were awarded.

Contact Dr. Jane C. Norman, MSN Program Director, School of Nursing, Tennessee State University, 3500 John A. Merritt Boulevard, Box 9590, Nashville, TN 37209-1561. *Telephone:* 615-963-5255. *Fax:* 615-963-7614. *E-mail:* jnorman@tnstate.edu.

MASTER'S DEGREE PROGRAM

Degree MSN

Available Programs RN to Master's.

Concentrations Available Nursing administration; nursing education; nursing informatics. *Nurse practitioner programs in:* family health.

Site Options Nashville, TN.

Study Options Full-time and part-time.

Online Degree Options Yes.

Program Entrance Requirements Computer literacy, minimum overall college GPA of 3.0, transcript of college record, CPR certification, written essay, immunizations, 3 letters of recommendation, resume, GRE General Test or MAT. *Application deadline:* 7/15 (fall), 11/15 (spring), 3/15 (summer). Applications may be processed on a rolling basis for some programs. *Application fee:* $25.

Advanced Placement Credit given for nursing courses completed elsewhere dependent upon specific evaluations.

Degree Requirements 45 total credit hours, thesis or project, comprehensive exam.

POST-MASTER'S PROGRAM

Areas of Study Nursing administration; nursing education; nursing informatics. *Nurse practitioner programs in:* family health.

CONTINUING EDUCATION PROGRAM

Contact Dr. Kathy L. Martin, Associate Dean, Health Sciences/Executive Director, Nursing, School of Nursing, Tennessee State University, 3500 John A. Merritt Boulevard, Box 9590, Nashville, TN 37209-1561. *Telephone:* 615-963-5251. *Fax:* 615-963-5049. *E-mail:* kmartin3@tnstate.edu.

Tennessee Technological University

Whitson-Hester School of Nursing
Cookeville, Tennessee

http://www.tntech.edu/nursing
Founded in 1915
DEGREES • BSN • M SC N • MSN
Nursing Program Faculty 21 (19% with doctorates).
Baccalaureate Enrollment 187 **Women** 91% **Men** 9% **Minority** 3% **Part-time** 1%
Graduate Enrollment 47 **Women** 89% **Men** 11% **Minority** 4% **Part-time** 94%
Distance Learning Courses Available.
Nursing Student Activities Sigma Theta Tau, Student Nurses' Association.
Nursing Student Resources Academic advising; academic or career counseling; assistance for students with disabilities; bookstore; campus computer network; career placement assistance; computer lab; computer-assisted instruction; daycare for children of students; e-mail services; employment services for current students; externships; housing assistance; Internet; learning resource lab; library services; nursing audiovisuals; paid internships; placement services for program completers; remedial services; resume preparation assistance; skills, simulation, or other laboratory; tutoring; unpaid internships.
Library Facilities 704,377 volumes (312,892 in health, 11,893 in nursing); 1,636 periodical subscriptions (96 health-care related).

BACCALAUREATE PROGRAMS

Degree BSN
Available Programs ADN to Baccalaureate; Baccalaureate for Second Degree; Generic Baccalaureate; RN Baccalaureate.
Study Options Full-time.
Program Entrance Requirements Minimum overall college GPA of 2.5, transcript of college record, CPR certification, written essay, health exam, high school biology, high school foreign language, 4 years high school math, 2 years high school science, high school transcript, immunizations, minimum high school GPA of 3.0, minimum GPA in nursing prerequisites of 2.5, professional liability insurance/malpractice insurance, prerequisite course work. Transfer students are accepted. *Application deadline:* 2/1 (fall), 6/1 (spring).
Advanced Placement Credit given for nursing courses completed elsewhere dependent upon specific evaluations.
Expenses (2011–12) *Tuition, state resident:* full-time $6702; part-time $296 per credit hour. *Tuition, nonresident:* full-time $21,012; part-time $864 per credit hour. *Room and board:* $7384; room only: $3830 per academic year. *Required fees:* full-time $750; part-time $25 per credit.
Financial Aid 85% of baccalaureate students in nursing programs received some form of financial aid in 2010–11. *Gift aid (need-based):* Federal Pell, FSEOG, state, private, college/university gift aid from institutional funds, United Negro College Fund. *Loans:* Federal Direct (Subsidized and Unsubsidized Stafford PLUS, Perkins, college/university. *Work-study:* Federal Work-Study, part-time campus jobs. *Financial aid application deadline (priority):* 3/15.
Contact Ms. Kristi L. Burris, Academic Advisor, Whitson-Hester School of Nursing, Tennessee Technological University, Box 5001, Cookeville, TN 38505-0001. *Telephone:* 931-372-3229. *Fax:* 931-372-6244. *E-mail:* KLLoftis@tntech.edu.

GRADUATE PROGRAMS

Expenses (2011–12) *Tuition, state resident:* part-time $441 per credit hour. *Tuition, nonresident:* part-time $1065 per credit hour.
Financial Aid 5% of graduate students in nursing programs received some form of financial aid in 2010–11.
Contact Ms. Kristi L. Burris, Academic Advisor, Whitson-Hester School of Nursing, Tennessee Technological University, Box 5001, Cookeville, TN 38505-0001. *Telephone:* 931-372-3229. *Fax:* 931-372-6244. *E-mail:* KLLoftis@tntech.edu.

MASTER'S DEGREE PROGRAM

Degrees M Sc N; MSN
Available Programs Master's; Master's for Nurses with Non-Nursing Degrees.
Concentrations Available Nursing administration; nursing education; nursing informatics. *Nurse practitioner programs in:* family health.
Study Options Full-time and part-time.

Online Degree Options Yes (online only).
Program Entrance Requirements Computer literacy, minimum overall college GPA of 3.0, transcript of college record, CPR certification, written essay, immunizations, 3 letters of recommendation, nursing research course, professional liability insurance/malpractice insurance, resume. *Application deadline:* 8/1 (fall), 12/1 (spring), 5/1 (summer). Applications may be processed on a rolling basis for some programs. *Application fee:* $25.
Advanced Placement Credit given for nursing courses completed elsewhere dependent upon specific evaluations.
Degree Requirements 46 total credit hours, thesis or project.

Tennessee Wesleyan College

Fort Sanders Nursing Department
Knoxville, Tennessee

http://www.twcnet.edu/admissions/nursing-program/
Founded in 1857
DEGREE • BSN
Nursing Program Faculty 18 (6% with doctorates).
Baccalaureate Enrollment 128 **Women** 89% **Men** 11% **Minority** 3% **International** 2% **Part-time** 3%
Distance Learning Courses Available.
Nursing Student Activities Nursing Honor Society, Sigma Theta Tau, Student Nurses' Association.
Nursing Student Resources Academic advising; assistance for students with disabilities; bookstore; campus computer network; computer lab; e-mail services; Internet; library services; nursing audiovisuals; other; skills, simulation, or other laboratory.
Library Facilities 5,000 volumes in health, 4,000 volumes in nursing; 135 periodical subscriptions health-care related.

BACCALAUREATE PROGRAMS

Degree BSN
Available Programs ADN to Baccalaureate; Generic Baccalaureate; RN Baccalaureate.
Site Options Knoxville, TN.
Study Options Full-time.
Program Entrance Requirements Minimum overall college GPA of 2.7, transcript of college record, CPR certification, written essay, health exam, high school transcript, immunizations, interview, minimum GPA in nursing prerequisites of 2.7, prerequisite course work. Transfer students are accepted. *Application deadline:* 1/15 (fall). *Application fee:* $25.
Advanced Placement Credit given for nursing courses completed elsewhere dependent upon specific evaluations.
Expenses (2011–12) *Tuition:* full-time $20,900; part-time $792 per credit hour. *Room and board:* $6480 per academic year. *Required fees:* full-time $1900; part-time $79 per credit.
Financial Aid 97% of baccalaureate students in nursing programs received some form of financial aid in 2010–11. *Gift aid (need-based):* Federal Pell, FSEOG, state, private, college/university gift aid from institutional funds. *Loans:* Federal Direct (Subsidized and Unsubsidized Stafford PLUS). *Work-study:* Federal Work-Study, part-time campus jobs. *Financial aid application deadline:* Continuous.
Contact Nursing Contact, Fort Sanders Nursing Department, Tennessee Wesleyan College, 9845 Cogdill Road, Knoxville, TN 37932. *Telephone:* 865-777-5100. *Fax:* 865-777-5114.

Union University

School of Nursing
Jackson, Tennessee

http://www.uu.edu/academics/son/
Founded in 1823
DEGREES • BSN • MSN
Nursing Program Faculty 28 (36% with doctorates).
Baccalaureate Enrollment 285 **Women** 93% **Men** 7% **Minority** 27% **International** 2% **Part-time** 56%
Graduate Enrollment 55 **Women** 80% **Men** 20% **Minority** 25% **Part-time** 4%
Nursing Student Activities Nursing Honor Society, Sigma Theta Tau, Student Nurses' Association.

Nursing Student Resources Academic advising; academic or career counseling; assistance for students with disabilities; bookstore; campus computer network; career placement assistance; computer lab; computer-assisted instruction; e-mail services; employment services for current students; housing assistance; Internet; learning resource lab; library services; nursing audiovisuals; resume preparation assistance; skills, simulation, or other laboratory; tutoring.
Library Facilities 155,500 volumes (6,005 in nursing); 20,324 periodical subscriptions (1,284 health-care related).

BACCALAUREATE PROGRAMS

Degree BSN
Available Programs Accelerated Baccalaureate for Second Degree; Generic Baccalaureate; LPN to Baccalaureate; RN Baccalaureate.
Site Options Germantown, TN.
Study Options Full-time.
Program Entrance Requirements Minimum overall college GPA of 2.8, transcript of college record, CPR certification, health exam, immunizations, minimum GPA in nursing prerequisites of 2.8, prerequisite course work. Transfer students are accepted.
Advanced Placement Credit by examination available. Credit given for nursing courses completed elsewhere dependent upon specific evaluations.
Contact *Telephone:* 731-661-5538. *Fax:* 731-661-5504.

GRADUATE PROGRAMS

Contact *Telephone:* 731-661-5538. *Fax:* 901-661-5504.

MASTER'S DEGREE PROGRAM
Degree MSN
Available Programs Master's.
Concentrations Available Nurse anesthesia; nursing administration; nursing education. *Clinical nurse specialist programs in:* adult health, pediatric. *Nurse practitioner programs in:* family health.
Site Options Germantown, TN.
Study Options Full-time and part-time.
Program Entrance Requirements Minimum overall college GPA of 3.0, transcript of college record, CPR certification, written essay, immunizations, interview, 3 letters of recommendation, professional liability insurance/malpractice insurance, GRE.
Advanced Placement Credit given for nursing courses completed elsewhere dependent upon specific evaluations.
Degree Requirements 46 total credit hours.

POST-MASTER'S PROGRAM
Areas of Study Nursing administration; nursing education. *Clinical nurse specialist programs in:* adult health, pediatric. *Nurse practitioner programs in:* family health.

CONTINUING EDUCATION PROGRAM

Contact *Telephone:* 731-661-5152. *Fax:* 731-661-5504.

University of Memphis
Loewenberg School of Nursing
Memphis, Tennessee

http://nursing.memphis.edu/
Founded in 1912
DEGREES • BSN • MSN
Nursing Program Faculty 65 (22% with doctorates).
Baccalaureate Enrollment 441 **Women** 91% **Men** 9% **Minority** 23% **Part-time** 15%
Graduate Enrollment 124 **Women** 92% **Men** 8% **Minority** 30% **Part-time** 75%
Distance Learning Courses Available.
Nursing Student Activities Sigma Theta Tau, Student Nurses' Association.
Nursing Student Resources Academic advising; academic or career counseling; assistance for students with disabilities; bookstore; campus computer network; career placement assistance; computer lab; computer-assisted instruction; daycare for children of students; e-mail services; externships; housing assistance; interactive nursing skills videos; Internet; learning resource lab; library services; nursing audiovisuals; paid internships; remedial services; resume preparation assistance; skills, simulation, or other laboratory; tutoring.

Library Facilities 1.5 million volumes (74,513 in health); 6,771 periodical subscriptions (878 health-care related).

BACCALAUREATE PROGRAMS

Degree BSN
Available Programs ADN to Baccalaureate; Accelerated Baccalaureate; Accelerated Baccalaureate for Second Degree; Accelerated RN Baccalaureate; Baccalaureate for Second Degree; Generic Baccalaureate; RN Baccalaureate.
Site Options Jackson, TN.
Study Options Full-time.
Program Entrance Requirements Minimum overall college GPA of 2.7, transcript of college record, CPR certification, health exam, high school biology, high school chemistry, high school foreign language, 3 years high school math, 2 years high school science, high school transcript, immunizations, minimum high school GPA of 3.0, minimum GPA in nursing prerequisites of 2.4, prerequisite course work. Transfer students are accepted.
Advanced Placement Credit by examination available. Credit given for nursing courses completed elsewhere dependent upon specific evaluations.
Contact *Telephone:* 901-678-2003. *Fax:* 901-678-4906.

GRADUATE PROGRAMS

Contact *Telephone:* 901-678-2003. *Fax:* 901-678-4906.

MASTER'S DEGREE PROGRAM
Degree MSN
Available Programs Accelerated Master's for Nurses with Non-Nursing Degrees; Master's; Master's for Non-Nursing College Graduates; Master's for Nurses with Non-Nursing Degrees.
Concentrations Available Nursing administration; nursing education. *Nurse practitioner programs in:* family health.
Site Options Jackson, TN.
Study Options Full-time and part-time.
Online Degree Options Yes.
Program Entrance Requirements Minimum overall college GPA of 2.8, CPR certification, immunizations, 3 letters of recommendation, professional liability insurance/malpractice insurance.
Advanced Placement Credit given for nursing courses completed elsewhere dependent upon specific evaluations.
Degree Requirements 45 total credit hours, comprehensive exam.

POST-MASTER'S PROGRAM
Areas of Study *Nurse practitioner programs in:* family health.

The University of Tennessee
College of Nursing
Knoxville, Tennessee

http://nightingale.con.utk.edu/
Founded in 1794
DEGREES • BSN • MSN • PHD
Nursing Program Faculty 54 (54% with doctorates).
Baccalaureate Enrollment 215 **Women** 91% **Men** 9% **Minority** 5.6% **International** 3.3% **Part-time** 7.4%
Graduate Enrollment 139 **Women** 89.3% **Men** 10.7% **Minority** 3.5% **International** 1.4% **Part-time** 32%
Distance Learning Courses Available.
Nursing Student Activities Sigma Theta Tau, Student Nurses' Association.
Nursing Student Resources Academic advising; academic or career counseling; assistance for students with disabilities; bookstore; campus computer network; computer lab; computer-assisted instruction; e-mail services; employment services for current students; externships; interactive nursing skills videos; Internet; learning resource lab; library services; nursing audiovisuals; remedial services; skills, simulation, or other laboratory; tutoring.
Library Facilities 3.1 million volumes (59,214 in health, 3,711 in nursing); 66,447 periodical subscriptions (572 health-care related).

BACCALAUREATE PROGRAMS

Degree BSN
Available Programs Accelerated Baccalaureate; Accelerated RN Baccalaureate; Generic Baccalaureate.

Study Options Full-time and part-time.

Program Entrance Requirements Transcript of college record, CPR certification, written essay, health exam, health insurance, high school biology, high school chemistry, 3 years high school math, 2 years high school science, high school transcript, immunizations, interview, minimum high school GPA of 3.2, minimum GPA in nursing prerequisites of 3.2, professional liability insurance/malpractice insurance, prerequisite course work. Transfer students are accepted. *Application deadline:* 12/1 (fall), 12/1 (summer). *Application fee:* $30.

Advanced Placement Credit given for nursing courses completed elsewhere dependent upon specific evaluations.

Contact *Telephone:* 865-974-7606. *Fax:* 865-974-3569.

GRADUATE PROGRAMS

Contact *Telephone:* 865-974-4151. *Fax:* 865-974-3569.

MASTER'S DEGREE PROGRAM

Degree MSN

Available Programs Accelerated Master's for Nurses with Non-Nursing Degrees; Accelerated RN to Master's; Master's; Master's for Non-Nursing College Graduates; Master's for Nurses with Non-Nursing Degrees; RN to Master's.

Concentrations Available Nurse anesthesia; nursing administration. *Clinical nurse specialist programs in:* adult health, pediatric, psychiatric/mental health. *Nurse practitioner programs in:* adult health, family health, pediatric, psychiatric/mental health.

Study Options Full-time.

Program Entrance Requirements Minimum overall college GPA of 3.0, transcript of college record, CPR certification, written essay, immunizations, 3 letters of recommendation, physical assessment course, professional liability insurance/malpractice insurance, prerequisite course work, statistics course, GRE General Test. *Application deadline:* 2/1 (fall), 10/1 (spring), 10/1 (summer). *Application fee:* $30.

Advanced Placement Credit by examination available. Credit given for nursing courses completed elsewhere dependent upon specific evaluations.

Degree Requirements 41 total credit hours, comprehensive exam.

POST-MASTER'S PROGRAM

Areas of Study Nurse anesthesia; nursing administration; nursing education. *Clinical nurse specialist programs in:* adult health, pediatric, psychiatric/mental health. *Nurse practitioner programs in:* adult health, family health, pediatric, psychiatric/mental health.

DOCTORAL DEGREE PROGRAM

Degree PhD

Available Programs Doctorate; Post-Baccalaureate Doctorate.

Areas of Study Bio-behavioral research, biology of health and illness, faculty preparation, family health, gerontology, health policy, health promotion/disease prevention, human health and illness, individualized study, neuro-behavior, nursing administration, nursing education, nursing research, nursing science, women's health.

Online Degree Options Yes (online only).

Program Entrance Requirements Minimum overall college GPA of 3.0, interview by faculty committee, interview, 3 letters of recommendation, writing sample, GRE General Test. *Application deadline:* 10/1 (summer). *Application fee:* $30.

Degree Requirements 67 total credit hours, dissertation, oral exam, written exam, residency.

CONTINUING EDUCATION PROGRAM

Contact *Telephone:* 865-974-7598. *Fax:* 865-974-3569.

The University of Tennessee at Chattanooga
School of Nursing
Chattanooga, Tennessee

http://www.utc.edu/Academic/Nursing
Founded in 1886

DEGREES • BSN • DNP • MSN

Nursing Program Faculty 27 (48% with doctorates).
Baccalaureate Enrollment 172 **Women** 90% **Men** 10% **Minority** 8%
Graduate Enrollment 107 **Women** 70% **Men** 30% **Minority** 15% **Part-time** 32%

Distance Learning Courses Available.

Nursing Student Activities Sigma Theta Tau, Student Nurses' Association.

Nursing Student Resources Academic advising; academic or career counseling; assistance for students with disabilities; bookstore; campus computer network; career placement assistance; computer lab; computer-assisted instruction; daycare for children of students; e-mail services; employment services for current students; interactive nursing skills videos; Internet; learning resource lab; library services; nursing audiovisuals; skills, simulation, or other laboratory; tutoring.

Library Facilities 510,890 volumes (19,370 in health, 3,100 in nursing); 2,335 periodical subscriptions (200 health-care related).

BACCALAUREATE PROGRAMS

Degree BSN

Available Programs ADN to Baccalaureate; Baccalaureate for Second Degree; Generic Baccalaureate.

Study Options Full-time.

Online Degree Options Yes (online only).

Program Entrance Requirements Minimum overall college GPA of 2.75, transcript of college record, CPR certification, health exam, health insurance, high school foreign language, 3 years high school math, high school transcript, immunizations, 2 letters of recommendation, minimum high school GPA of 2.0, minimum GPA in nursing prerequisites of 2.75, professional liability insurance/malpractice insurance, prerequisite course work. Transfer students are accepted. *Application deadline:* 3/1 (fall).

Advanced Placement Credit given for nursing courses completed elsewhere dependent upon specific evaluations.

Expenses (2011–12) *Tuition, state resident:* full-time $3359; part-time $385 per credit hour. *Tuition, nonresident:* full-time $10,126; part-time $949 per credit hour.

Financial Aid 60% of baccalaureate students in nursing programs received some form of financial aid in 2010–11. *Gift aid (need-based):* Federal Pell, FSEOG, state, private, college/university gift aid from institutional funds, United Negro College Fund, Federal Nursing. *Loans:* Federal Direct (Subsidized and Unsubsidized Stafford PLUS), Perkins. *Work-study:* Federal Work-Study, part-time campus jobs. *Financial aid application deadline (priority):* 5/1.

Contact Dr. Katherine S. Lindgren, Director, School of Nursing, The University of Tennessee at Chattanooga, 615 McCallie Avenue, Department 1051, Chattanooga, TN 37403-2598. *Telephone:* 423-425-4750. *Fax:* 423-425-4668. *E-mail:* kay-lindgren@utc.edu.

GRADUATE PROGRAMS

Expenses (2011–12) *Tuition, state resident:* full-time $3896; part-time $519 per credit hour. *Tuition, nonresident:* full-time $10,663; part-time $1271 per credit hour. *International tuition:* $10,663 full-time. *Required fees:* full-time $38.

Financial Aid 70% of graduate students in nursing programs received some form of financial aid in 2010–11. Career-related internships or fieldwork and scholarships available. Aid available to part-time students.

Contact Dr. Katherine S. Lindgren, Director, School of Nursing, The University of Tennessee at Chattanooga, 615 McCallie Avenue, Department 1051, Chattanooga, TN 37403-2598. *Telephone:* 423-425-4750. *Fax:* 423-425-4668. *E-mail:* kay-lindgren@utc.edu.

MASTER'S DEGREE PROGRAM

Degree MSN

Available Programs Master's.

Concentrations Available Nurse anesthesia. *Nurse practitioner programs in:* family health.

Site Options Tupelo, MS.

Study Options Full-time and part-time.

Program Entrance Requirements Clinical experience, computer literacy, minimum overall college GPA of 3.0, transcript of college record, CPR certification, written essay, immunizations, interview, 3 letters of recommendation, nursing research course, physical assessment course, professional liability insurance/malpractice insurance, resume, statistics course, GRE General Test, MAT. *Application deadline:* 1/31 (winter), 8/1 (summer). *Application fee:* $30.

Advanced Placement Credit given for nursing courses completed elsewhere dependent upon specific evaluations.

Degree Requirements 48 total credit hours, comprehensive exam.

POST-MASTER'S PROGRAM

Areas of Study Nurse anesthesia. *Nurse practitioner programs in:* family health.

DOCTORAL DEGREE PROGRAM

Degree DNP

Available Programs Doctorate.

Online Degree Options Yes (online only).

Program Entrance Requirements Clinical experience, minimum overall college GPA of 3.0, interview by faculty committee, 3.0 letters of recommendation, MSN or equivalent, vita. *Application deadline:* 9/1 (winter). *Application fee:* $30.

Degree Requirements 36 total credit hours.

The University of Tennessee at Martin

Department of Nursing
Martin, Tennessee

http://www.utm.edu/
Founded in 1900

DEGREE • BSN

Nursing Program Faculty 15 (20% with doctorates).

Baccalaureate Enrollment 198 **Women** 88% **Men** 12% **Minority** 6% **Part-time** 27%

Distance Learning Courses Available.

Nursing Student Activities Nursing Honor Society, Sigma Theta Tau, Student Nurses' Association, nursing club.

Nursing Student Resources Academic advising; academic or career counseling; assistance for students with disabilities; bookstore; campus computer network; career placement assistance; computer lab; computer-assisted instruction; daycare for children of students; e-mail services; employment services for current students; housing assistance; interactive nursing skills videos; Internet; learning resource lab; library services; nursing audiovisuals; remedial services; resume preparation assistance; skills, simulation, or other laboratory; tutoring.

Library Facilities 525,603 volumes (1,772 in health, 1,645 in nursing); 1,031 periodical subscriptions (10,803 health-care related).

BACCALAUREATE PROGRAMS

Degree BSN

Available Programs ADN to Baccalaureate; Generic Baccalaureate; LPN to RN Baccalaureate.

Site Options Ripley, TN; Selmer, TN; Parsons, TN.

Study Options Full-time.

Program Entrance Requirements Minimum overall college GPA of 2.0, transcript of college record, CPR certification, written essay, health exam, health insurance, high school biology, high school chemistry, high school foreign language, 3 years high school math, 2 years high school science, high school transcript, immunizations, interview, minimum high school GPA of 3.0, minimum GPA in nursing prerequisites of 2.0, professional liability insurance/malpractice insurance, prerequisite course work. Transfer students are accepted. *Application deadline:* 2/1 (fall).

Advanced Placement Credit by examination available. Credit given for nursing courses completed elsewhere dependent upon specific evaluations.

Expenses (2011–12) *Tuition, state resident:* full-time $6718; part-time $281 per credit hour. *Tuition, nonresident:* full-time $19,128; part-time $799 per credit hour. *International tuition:* $19,128 full-time. *Required fees:* full-time $1500; part-time $750 per term.

Financial Aid 96% of baccalaureate students in nursing programs received some form of financial aid in 2010–11. *Gift aid (need-based):* Federal Pell, FSEOG, state, private, college/university gift aid from institutional funds. *Loans:* Perkins. *Work-study:* Federal Work-Study. *Financial aid application deadline (priority):* 2/15.

Contact Mrs. Brenda W. Campbell, Program Resource Specialist, Department of Nursing, The University of Tennessee at Martin, Gooch Hall 136J, Martin, TN 38238. *Telephone:* 731-881-7138. *Fax:* 731-881-7939. *E-mail:* brendac@utm.edu.

The University of Tennessee Health Science Center

College of Nursing
Memphis, Tennessee

http://www.uthsc.edu/
Founded in 1911

DEGREES • DNP • MSN

Nursing Program Faculty 51 (87% with doctorates).

Graduate Enrollment 227 **Women** 85% **Men** 15% **Minority** 22%

Distance Learning Courses Available.

Nursing Student Activities Sigma Theta Tau, Student Nurses' Association.

Nursing Student Resources Academic advising; academic or career counseling; assistance for students with disabilities; bookstore; campus computer network; computer lab; computer-assisted instruction; e-mail services; housing assistance; interactive nursing skills videos; Internet; learning resource lab; library services; nursing audiovisuals; paid internships; remedial services; skills, simulation, or other laboratory; tutoring.

Library Facilities 165,200 volumes (198,936 in health, 8,061 in nursing); 1,784 periodical subscriptions (3,800 health-care related).

GRADUATE PROGRAMS

Contact *Telephone:* 901-448-6139. *Fax:* 901-448-4121.

MASTER'S DEGREE PROGRAM

Degree MSN

Available Programs Accelerated Master's for Non-Nursing College Graduates.

Concentrations Available Clinical nurse leader.

Study Options Full-time.

Program Entrance Requirements Computer literacy, minimum overall college GPA of 3.0, transcript of college record, CPR certification, written essay, immunizations, interview, 3 letters of recommendation, prerequisite course work, statistics course, GRE General Test. *Application deadline:* 1/15 (summer).

Degree Requirements 80 total credit hours.

POST-MASTER'S PROGRAM

Areas of Study Nurse anesthesia. *Clinical nurse specialist programs in:* acute care, critical care, family health, psychiatric/mental health, public health. *Nurse practitioner programs in:* acute care, family health, neonatal health, pediatric, primary care, psychiatric/mental health.

DOCTORAL DEGREE PROGRAM

Degree DNP

Available Programs Doctorate; Post-Baccalaureate Doctorate.

Areas of Study Addiction/substance abuse, advanced practice nursing, clinical practice, community health, critical care, family health, forensic nursing, gerontology, women's health.

Online Degree Options Yes (online only).

Program Entrance Requirements Minimum overall college GPA of 3.0, interview by faculty committee, interview, 3 letters of recommendation, writing sample. *Application deadline:* 2/1 (fall).

Degree Requirements Residency.

Vanderbilt University

Vanderbilt University School of Nursing
Nashville, Tennessee

http://www.nursing.vanderbilt.edu/
Founded in 1873

DEGREES • DNP • MSN • MSN/MDIV • MSN/MTS • PHD

Nursing Program Faculty 168 (50% with doctorates).

Graduate Enrollment 909 **Women** 90% **Men** 10% **Minority** 13.5% **International** 1% **Part-time** 46.5%

Distance Learning Courses Available.

Nursing Student Activities Nursing Honor Society, Sigma Theta Tau.

Nursing Student Resources Academic advising; academic or career counseling; assistance for students with disabilities; bookstore; campus computer network; career placement assistance; computer lab; computer-assisted instruction; e-mail services; housing assistance; interactive nursing skills videos; Internet; learning resource lab; library services;

nursing audiovisuals; remedial services; resume preparation assistance; skills, simulation, or other laboratory; tutoring.

Library Facilities 2.6 million volumes (213,202 in health); 78,041 periodical subscriptions (3,816 health-care related).

GRADUATE PROGRAMS

Expenses (2012–13) *Tuition:* full-time $43,914; part-time $1126 per credit hour. *Required fees:* full-time $3703.

Financial Aid 85% of graduate students in nursing programs received some form of financial aid in 2011–12. Scholarships available. Aid available to part-time students. *Financial aid application deadline:* 3/15.

Contact Patricia Peerman, Assistant Dean of Enrollment Management, Vanderbilt University School of Nursing, Vanderbilt University, 207 Godchaux Hall, Nashville, TN 37240. *Telephone:* 615-322-3800. *Fax:* 615-343-0333. *E-mail:* paddy.peerman@vanderbilt.edu.

MASTER'S DEGREE PROGRAM

Degrees MSN; MSN/MDIV; MSN/MTS

Available Programs Master's; Master's for Non-Nursing College Graduates; RN to Master's.

Concentrations Available Health-care administration; nurse-midwifery; nursing administration; nursing informatics. *Nurse practitioner programs in:* acute care, adult health, family health, gerontology, neonatal health, pediatric, psychiatric/mental health, women's health.

Study Options Full-time and part-time.

Online Degree Options Yes (online only).

Program Entrance Requirements Computer literacy, minimum overall college GPA of 3.0, transcript of college record, CPR certification, written essay, immunizations, 3 letters of recommendation, prerequisite course work, statistics course, GRE General Test (within the past 5 years). *Application deadline:* 12/1 (fall). Applications may be processed on a rolling basis for some programs. *Application fee:* $50.

Advanced Placement Credit by examination available. Credit given for nursing courses completed elsewhere dependent upon specific evaluations.

Degree Requirements 39 total credit hours.

POST-MASTER'S PROGRAM

Areas of Study Health-care administration; nurse-midwifery; nursing administration; nursing informatics. *Nurse practitioner programs in:* acute care, adult health, family health, gerontology, neonatal health, pediatric, psychiatric/mental health, women's health.

DOCTORAL DEGREE PROGRAM

Degree DNP

Available Programs Doctorate.

Areas of Study Biology of health and illness, clinical practice, community health, critical care, family health, gerontology, health policy, health promotion/disease prevention, health-care systems, human health and illness, information systems, maternity-newborn, nursing administration, nursing policy, women's health.

Program Entrance Requirements Minimum overall college GPA of 3.5, interview by faculty committee, 3 letters of recommendation, MSN or equivalent, statistics course, vita, writing sample, GRE General Test. *Application deadline:* 1/15 (fall). Applications may be processed on a rolling basis for some programs. *Application fee:* $50.

Degree Requirements 74 total credit hours, oral exam.

DOCTORAL DEGREE PROGRAM

Degree PhD

Available Programs Doctorate.

Areas of Study Nursing research.

Program Entrance Requirements Minimum overall college GPA of 3.5, interview by faculty committee, 3 letters of recommendation, MSN or equivalent, statistics course, vita, writing sample. *Application deadline:* 1/15 (fall).

Degree Requirements 72 semester credit hours, dissertation, oral exam.

POSTDOCTORAL PROGRAM

Areas of Study Individualized study.

Postdoctoral Program Contact Dr. Ann Minnick, Director, Vanderbilt University School of Nursing, Vanderbilt University, 415 Godchaux Hall, Nashville, TN 37240. *Telephone:* 615-343-2998. *Fax:* 615-343-5898. *E-mail:* ann.minnick@vanderbilt.edu.

TEXAS

Abilene Christian University
Patty Hanks Shelton School of Nursing
Abilene, Texas

See description of programs under Patty Hanks Shelton School of Nursing (Abilene, Texas)

Angelo State University
Department of Nursing and Rehabilitation Sciences
San Angelo, Texas

http://www.angelo.edu/dept/nursing
Founded in 1928
DEGREES • BSN • MSN
Nursing Program Faculty 35 (34% with doctorates).
Baccalaureate Enrollment 231 **Women** 85% **Men** 15% **Minority** 24% **Part-time** 69%
Graduate Enrollment 117 **Women** 85% **Men** 15% **Minority** 22% **Part-time** 84%
Distance Learning Courses Available.
Nursing Student Activities Nursing Honor Society, Student Nurses' Association.
Nursing Student Resources Academic advising; academic or career counseling; bookstore; campus computer network; computer lab; computer-assisted instruction; e-mail services; housing assistance; interactive nursing skills videos; Internet; learning resource lab; library services; nursing audiovisuals; skills, simulation, or other laboratory; tutoring.
Library Facilities 709,223 volumes (7,830 in health, 5,224 in nursing); 46,684 periodical subscriptions (170 health-care related).

BACCALAUREATE PROGRAMS

Degree BSN
Available Programs Generic Baccalaureate; RN Baccalaureate.
Study Options Full-time.
Online Degree Options Yes.
Program Entrance Requirements Minimum overall college GPA of 2.5, transcript of college record, CPR certification, health insurance, immunizations, 2 letters of recommendation, prerequisite course work. Transfer students are accepted. *Application deadline:* 2/15 (fall), 10/1 (spring).
Expenses (2012–13) *Tuition, state resident:* full-time $9478; part-time $698 per credit hour. *Tuition, nonresident:* full-time $21,658; part-time $1050 per credit hour. *Room and board:* $7484; room only: $4659 per academic year. *Required fees:* full-time $1800.
Financial Aid 36% of baccalaureate students in nursing programs received some form of financial aid in 2011–12.
Contact Ms. Crystal M. Schobel, Academic College Advisor, Department of Nursing and Rehabilitation Sciences, Angelo State University, ASU Station #10911, San Angelo, TX 76909. *Telephone:* 325-942-2630. *Fax:* 325-942-2631. *E-mail:* chhs@angelo.edu.

GRADUATE PROGRAMS

Expenses (2012–13) *Tuition, state resident:* full-time $10,986; part-time $718 per credit hour. *Tuition, nonresident:* full-time $23,166; part-time $1069 per credit hour. *Room and board:* $7484; room only: $4659 per academic year. *Required fees:* full-time $1800.
Financial Aid 75% of graduate students in nursing programs received some form of financial aid in 2011–12. Career-related internships or fieldwork, Federal Work-Study, and scholarships available. Aid available to part-time students. *Financial aid application deadline:* 3/1.
Contact Dr. Molly Walker, Graduate Adviser, MSN Program, Department of Nursing and Rehabilitation Sciences, Angelo State University, ASU Station #10902, San Angelo, TX 76909. *Telephone:* 325-942-2224. *Fax:* 325-942-2236. *E-mail:* molly.walker@angelo.edu.

MASTER'S DEGREE PROGRAM

Degree MSN
Available Programs Master's; Master's for Non-Nursing College Graduates; RN to Master's.

Concentrations Available Nursing education. *Clinical nurse specialist programs in:* adult health, medical-surgical. *Nurse practitioner programs in:* family health.
Study Options Full-time and part-time.
Online Degree Options Yes (online only).
Program Entrance Requirements Computer literacy, minimum overall college GPA of 3.0, transcript of college record, CPR certification, written essay, immunizations, 3 letters of recommendation, physical assessment course, prerequisite course work, statistics course. *Application deadline:* 4/1 (fall), 9/1 (spring).
Advanced Placement Credit given for nursing courses completed elsewhere dependent upon specific evaluations.
Degree Requirements 34 total credit hours, comprehensive exam.

Baylor University
Louise Herrington School of Nursing
Waco, Texas

http://www.baylor.edu/nursing
Founded in 1845
DEGREES • BSN • DNP • MSN
Nursing Program Faculty 68 (27% with doctorates).
Baccalaureate Enrollment 327 **Women** 90% **Men** 10% **Minority** 36% **International** 1.5% **Part-time** 5%
Graduate Enrollment 81 **Women** 91% **Men** 9% **Minority** 23.5% **International** 4% **Part-time** 53%
Distance Learning Courses Available.
Nursing Student Activities Sigma Theta Tau, Student Nurses' Association.
Nursing Student Resources Academic advising; academic or career counseling; assistance for students with disabilities; campus computer network; career placement assistance; computer lab; e-mail services; housing assistance; interactive nursing skills videos; Internet; learning resource lab; library services; nursing audiovisuals; resume preparation assistance; skills, simulation, or other laboratory; tutoring.
Library Facilities 2.9 million volumes (4,800 in health, 4,800 in nursing); 73,204 periodical subscriptions (101 health-care related).

BACCALAUREATE PROGRAMS

Degree BSN
Available Programs Accelerated Baccalaureate for Second Degree; Generic Baccalaureate.
Study Options Full-time.
Program Entrance Requirements Transcript of college record, CPR certification, health exam, health insurance, immunizations, minimum GPA in nursing prerequisites of 3.0, prerequisite course work. Transfer students are accepted. *Application deadline:* 1/15 (fall), 5/31 (spring), 1/5 (summer).
Advanced Placement Credit by examination available. Credit given for nursing courses completed elsewhere dependent upon specific evaluations.
Expenses (2012–13) *Tuition:* full-time $32,574; part-time $1274 per hour. *International tuition:* $32,574 full-time. *Room and board:* room only: $5000 per academic year. *Required fees:* full-time $3598; part-time $131 per credit.
Financial Aid 92% of baccalaureate students in nursing programs received some form of financial aid in 2011–12. *Gift aid (need-based):* Federal Pell, FSEOG, state, college/university gift aid from institutional funds. *Loans:* Federal Nursing Student Loans, Federal Direct (Subsidized and Unsubsidized Stafford PLUS), Perkins, state, private loans. *Work-study:* Federal Work-Study, part-time campus jobs. *Financial aid application deadline (priority):* 3/1.
Contact Recruiter, Louise Herrington School of Nursing, Baylor University, 3700 Worth Street, Dallas, TX 75246. *Telephone:* 214-820-3361. *Fax:* 214-820-3835. *E-mail:* BU_Nursing@baylor.edu.

GRADUATE PROGRAMS

Expenses (2012–13) *Tuition:* part-time $1274 per hour. *Room and board:* room only: $5000 per academic year. *Required fees:* part-time $131 per credit.
Financial Aid 100% of graduate students in nursing programs received some form of financial aid in 2011–12.
Contact Dr. Barbara Camune, Director, Graduate Program, Louise Herrington School of Nursing, Baylor University, 3700 Worth Street, Dallas, TX 75246. *Telephone:* 214-820-3361. *Fax:* 214-820-4770. *E-mail:* barvara_camune@baylor.edu.

MASTER'S DEGREE PROGRAM
Degree MSN
Available Programs Master's.
Concentrations Available *Nurse practitioner programs in:* family health, neonatal health.
Study Options Full-time and part-time.
Online Degree Options Yes.
Program Entrance Requirements Clinical experience, minimum overall college GPA of 3.0, transcript of college record, CPR certification, written essay, immunizations, interview, 3 letters of recommendation, prerequisite course work, statistics course, GRE General Test or MAT. *Application deadline:* 4/15 (fall). *Application fee:* $40.
Advanced Placement Credit given for nursing courses completed elsewhere dependent upon specific evaluations.
Degree Requirements 39 total credit hours.

POST-MASTER'S PROGRAM
Areas of Study *Nurse practitioner programs in:* family health, neonatal health.

DOCTORAL DEGREE PROGRAM
Degree DNP
Available Programs Doctorate.
Areas of Study Maternity-newborn.
Program Entrance Requirements Minimum overall college GPA of 3.0, interview by faculty committee, interview, 3 letters of recommendation, MSN or equivalent, statistics course, writing sample, GRE General Test. *Application deadline:* 4/15 (fall). *Application fee:* $40.
Degree Requirements 75 total credit hours, residency.

See display on next page and full description on page 476.

East Texas Baptist University
Department of Nursing
Marshall, Texas

http://www.etbu.edu/academicPrograms/School_of_Nursing/
Founded in 1912
DEGREE • BSN
Nursing Program Faculty 8 (25% with doctorates).
Baccalaureate Enrollment 43 **Women** 95% **Men** 5% **Minority** 10%
Nursing Student Activities Student Nurses' Association.
Nursing Student Resources Academic advising; academic or career counseling; assistance for students with disabilities; bookstore; campus computer network; computer lab; computer-assisted instruction; e-mail services; employment services for current students; housing assistance; interactive nursing skills videos; Internet; learning resource lab; library services; nursing audiovisuals; remedial services; resume preparation assistance; skills, simulation, or other laboratory; tutoring.
Library Facilities 2.2 million volumes (568 in health, 291 in nursing); 25,000 periodical subscriptions (2,100 health-care related).

BACCALAUREATE PROGRAMS

Degree BSN
Available Programs Generic Baccalaureate.
Study Options Full-time.
Program Entrance Requirements Transcript of college record, CPR certification, written essay, health insurance, immunizations, 2 letters of recommendation, minimum GPA in nursing prerequisites of 2.8, prerequisite course work. Transfer students are accepted. *Application deadline:* 3/1 (fall).
Advanced Placement Credit given for nursing courses completed elsewhere dependent upon specific evaluations.
Expenses (2011–12) *Tuition:* full-time $18,368; part-time $656 per contact hour. *Room and board:* $5666; room only: $2440 per academic year. *Required fees:* full-time $1250.
Financial Aid 99% of baccalaureate students in nursing programs received some form of financial aid in 2010–11. *Gift aid (need-based):* Federal Pell, FSEOG, state, private, college/university gift aid from institutional funds, Federal Nursing. *Loans:* Federal Direct (Subsidized and Unsubsidized Stafford PLUS), Perkins, state. *Work-study:* Federal Work-Study, part-time campus jobs. *Financial aid application deadline (priority):* 6/1.
Contact Julie Warbington, Administrative Assistant and Interim Admissions Counselor, Department of Nursing, East Texas Baptist

University, One Tiger Drive, Marshall, TX 75670-1498. *Telephone:* 903-923-2210. *Fax:* 903-938-9225. *E-mail:* jwarbington@etbu.edu.

Hardin-Simmons University
Patty Hanks Shelton School of Nursing
Abilene, Texas

See description of programs under Patty Hanks Shelton School of Nursing (Abilene, Texas).

Houston Baptist University
School of Nursing and Allied Health
Houston, Texas

Founded in 1960
DEGREE • BSN
Nursing Program Faculty 19 (3% with doctorates).
Baccalaureate Enrollment 165 **Women** 95% **Men** 5% **Minority** 78% **International** 2%
Nursing Student Activities Nursing Honor Society, Sigma Theta Tau, Student Nurses' Association.
Nursing Student Resources Academic advising; academic or career counseling; assistance for students with disabilities; bookstore; career placement assistance; computer lab; e-mail services; employment services for current students; externships; housing assistance; interactive nursing skills videos; Internet; learning resource lab; library services; nursing audiovisuals; paid internships; placement services for program completers; remedial services; resume preparation assistance; skills, simulation, or other laboratory; tutoring; unpaid internships.
Library Facilities 306,834 volumes (4,276 in health, 1,200 in nursing); 74,168 periodical subscriptions (117 health-care related).

BACCALAUREATE PROGRAMS
Degree BSN
Available Programs RN Baccalaureate.

Site Options Houston, TX.
Study Options Full-time.
Program Entrance Requirements Minimum overall college GPA of 3.0, transcript of college record, CPR certification, health exam, health insurance, immunizations, minimum GPA in nursing prerequisites of 3.0, prerequisite course work. Transfer students are accepted. *Application deadline:* 3/1 (fall), 10/1 (spring).
Advanced Placement Credit by examination available.
Expenses (2012–13) *Tuition:* full-time $24,000; part-time $1000 per credit hour.
Financial Aid 80% of baccalaureate students in nursing programs received some form of financial aid in 2011–12. *Gift aid (need-based):* Federal Pell, FSEOG, state, private, college/university gift aid from institutional funds. *Loans:* Federal Direct (Subsidized and Unsubsidized Stafford PLUS).*Work-study:* Federal Work-Study, part-time campus jobs.*Financial aid application deadline:* 4/15(priority: 3/1).
Contact Dr. Nancy Yuill, Dean, School of Nursing and Allied Health, Houston Baptist University, 7502 Fondren Street, Houston, TX 77074. *Telephone:* 281-649-3300. *Fax:* 281-649-3340. *E-mail:* nyuill@hbu.edu.

Lamar University
Department of Nursing
Beaumont, Texas

http://dept.lamar.edu/nursing/
Founded in 1923
DEGREES • BSN • MSN • MSN/MBA
Nursing Program Faculty 42 (31% with doctorates).
Baccalaureate Enrollment 260 **Women** 80% **Men** 20% **Minority** 10%
Graduate Enrollment 60 **Women** 95% **Men** 5% **Minority** 25% **Part-time** 92%
Distance Learning Courses Available.
Nursing Student Activities Sigma Theta Tau, Student Nurses' Association.
Nursing Student Resources Academic advising; academic or career counseling; assistance for students with disabilities; bookstore; campus computer network; career placement assistance; computer lab; computer-assisted instruction; e-mail services; employment services for current stu-

dents; housing assistance; interactive nursing skills videos; Internet; learning resource lab; library services; nursing audiovisuals; placement services for program completers; remedial services; resume preparation assistance; skills, simulation, or other laboratory; tutoring.

Library Facilities 526,180 volumes (6,825 in health, 3,160 in nursing); 26,618 periodical subscriptions (166 health-care related).

BACCALAUREATE PROGRAMS

Degree BSN

Available Programs ADN to Baccalaureate; Generic Baccalaureate; RN Baccalaureate.

Study Options Full-time.

Online Degree Options Yes.

Program Entrance Requirements Minimum overall college GPA of 2.5, transcript of college record, CPR certification, health exam, immunizations, minimum GPA in nursing prerequisites of 2.5, professional liability insurance/malpractice insurance, prerequisite course work. Transfer students are accepted. *Application deadline:* 3/1 (fall), 10/1 (spring). *Application fee:* $25.

Advanced Placement Credit given for nursing courses completed elsewhere dependent upon specific evaluations.

Expenses (2012–13) *Tuition, state resident:* part-time $208 per credit hour. *Tuition, nonresident:* part-time $451 per credit hour. *Room and board:* $7966; room only: $5098 per academic year. *Required fees:* part-time $150 per term.

Financial Aid 80% of baccalaureate students in nursing programs received some form of financial aid in 2011–12.

Contact Ms. Melissa I. Chandler, Academic Advisor, Department of Nursing, Lamar University, PO Box 10081, Beaumont, TX 77710. *Telephone:* 409-880-8868. *Fax:* 409-880-7736. *E-mail:* nursing@lamar.edu.

GRADUATE PROGRAMS

Expenses (2012–13) *Tuition, state resident:* part-time $308 per credit hour. *Tuition, nonresident:* part-time $551 per credit hour. *Room and board:* $7966; room only: $5098 per academic year. *Required fees:* part-time $150 per term.

Financial Aid 48% of graduate students in nursing programs received some form of financial aid in 2011–12.

Contact Dr. Nancy Bume, Director of Graduate Nursing Studies, Department of Nursing, Lamar University, PO Box 10081, Beaumont, TX 77710. *Telephone:* 409-880-7720. *Fax:* 409-880-8698. *E-mail:* nancy.blume@lamar.edu.

MASTER'S DEGREE PROGRAM

Degrees MSN; MSN/MBA

Available Programs Master's.

Concentrations Available Nursing administration; nursing education.

Study Options Full-time and part-time.

Online Degree Options Yes (online only).

Program Entrance Requirements Computer literacy, minimum overall college GPA of 3.0, transcript of college record, CPR certification, immunizations, professional liability insurance/malpractice insurance, prerequisite course work, statistics course. *Application deadline:* Applications may be processed on a rolling basis for some programs. *Application fee:* $25.

Advanced Placement Credit given for nursing courses completed elsewhere dependent upon specific evaluations.

Degree Requirements 37 total credit hours, thesis or project, comprehensive exam.

POST-MASTER'S PROGRAM

Areas of Study Nursing administration; nursing education.

CONTINUING EDUCATION PROGRAM

Contact Dr. Cindy Stinson, Coordinator of Continuing Education, Department of Nursing, Lamar University, PO Box 10081, Beaumont, TX 77710. *Telephone:* 409-880-8833. *Fax:* 409-880-1865. *E-mail:* cynthia.stinson@lamar.edu.

Lubbock Christian University
Department of Nursing
Lubbock, Texas

Founded in 1957

DEGREE • BSN
Nursing Program Faculty 5 (40% with doctorates).
Library Facilities 128,090 volumes; 452 periodical subscriptions.

BACCALAUREATE PROGRAMS

Degree BSN
Available Programs RN Baccalaureate.
Study Options Part-time.
Program Entrance Requirements Minimum overall college GPA of 2.5, transcript of college record, CPR certification, health exam, immunizations, interview, 2 letters of recommendation, minimum high school GPA, minimum GPA in nursing prerequisites of 2.5, professional liability insurance/malpractice insurance, prerequisite course work, RN licensure. Transfer students are accepted.

McMurry University
Patty Hanks Shelton School of Nursing
Abilene, Texas

See description of programs under Patty Hanks Shelton School of Nursing (Abilene, Texas).

Midwestern State University
Nursing Program
Wichita Falls, Texas

http://hs2.mwsu.edu/nursing/
Founded in 1922

DEGREES • BSN • MSN
Nursing Program Faculty 20 (35% with doctorates).
Baccalaureate Enrollment 482 **Women** 83% **Men** 17% **Minority** 54% **International** 6% **Part-time** 23%
Graduate Enrollment 122 **Women** 82% **Men** 18% **Minority** 30% **International** 3% **Part-time** 34%
Distance Learning Courses Available.
Nursing Student Activities Nursing Honor Society, Sigma Theta Tau, Student Nurses' Association.
Nursing Student Resources Academic advising; academic or career counseling; assistance for students with disabilities; bookstore; campus computer network; career placement assistance; computer lab; computer-assisted instruction; e-mail services; employment services for current students; externships; housing assistance; interactive nursing skills videos; Internet; learning resource lab; library services; nursing audiovisuals; other; placement services for program completers; remedial services; resume preparation assistance; skills, simulation, or other laboratory; tutoring.
Library Facilities 462,657 volumes (10,000 in health, 5,000 in nursing); 884 periodical subscriptions (6,000 health-care related).

BACCALAUREATE PROGRAMS

Degree BSN
Available Programs ADN to Baccalaureate; Generic Baccalaureate.
Study Options Full-time and part-time.
Program Entrance Requirements Transcript of college record, CPR certification, health exam, health insurance, immunizations, minimum GPA in nursing prerequisites of 3.0, professional liability insurance/malpractice insurance, prerequisite course work. Transfer students are accepted. *Application deadline:* 3/15 (fall), 9/30 (spring). *Application fee:* $25.
Advanced Placement Credit given for nursing courses completed elsewhere dependent upon specific evaluations.
Expenses (2011–12) *Tuition, state resident:* full-time $3470. *Tuition, nonresident:* full-time $3920. *International tuition:* $10,400 full-time. *Room and board:* $3820; room only: $3190 per academic year. *Required fees:* part-time $55 per credit.

Financial Aid 80% of baccalaureate students in nursing programs received some form of financial aid in 2010–11.

Contact Dr. Karen J. Polvado, Chair, Wilson School of Nursing, Nursing Program, Midwestern State University, 3410 Taft Boulevard, Bridwell Hall 308H, Wichita Falls, TX 76308. *Telephone:* 940-397-3254. *Fax:* 940-397-4911. *E-mail:* karen.polvado@mwsu.edu.

GRADUATE PROGRAMS

Expenses (2011–12) *Tuition, state resident:* full-time $2200; part-time $90 per credit hour. *Tuition, nonresident:* part-time $360 per credit hour. *International tuition:* $15,500 full-time. *Room and board:* $5870; room only: $3190 per academic year. *Required fees:* part-time $55 per credit.

Financial Aid 50% of graduate students in nursing programs received some form of financial aid in 2010–11. Teaching assistantships with partial tuition reimbursements available, career-related internships or fieldwork, Federal Work-Study, institutionally sponsored loans, scholarships, tuition waivers (partial), and unspecified assistantships available. Aid available to part-time students. *Financial aid application deadline:* 3/1.

Contact Dr. Debra G. Walker, Graduate Coordinator, Nursing Program, Midwestern State University, 3410 Taft Boulevard, Bridwell Hall 308C, Wichita Falls, TX 76308. *Telephone:* 940-397-4600. *Fax:* 940-397-4911. *E-mail:* debra.walker@mwsu.edu.

MASTER'S DEGREE PROGRAM

Degree MSN

Available Programs Master's; RN to Master's.

Concentrations Available Nursing education. *Nurse practitioner programs in:* family health, psychiatric/mental health.

Study Options Full-time and part-time.

Online Degree Options Yes.

Program Entrance Requirements Clinical experience, minimum overall college GPA of 3.0, transcript of college record, CPR certification, immunizations, interview, professional liability insurance/malpractice insurance, statistics course, GRE General Test or MAT. *Application deadline:* 7/1 (fall), 11/1 (spring), 4/15 (summer). Applications may be processed on a rolling basis for some programs. *Application fee:* $35.

Advanced Placement Credit by examination available. Credit given for nursing courses completed elsewhere dependent upon specific evaluations.

Degree Requirements 40 total credit hours, thesis or project.

POST-MASTER'S PROGRAM

Areas of Study Nursing education. *Nurse practitioner programs in:* family health, psychiatric/mental health.

CONTINUING EDUCATION PROGRAM

Contact Dr. Betty Bowles, Coordinator, Professional Outreach Center, Nursing Program, Midwestern State University, 3410 Taft Boulevard, Wichita Falls, TX 76308. *Telephone:* 940-397-4048. *Fax:* 940-397-4513. *E-mail:* betty.bowles@mwsu.edu.

Patty Hanks Shelton School of Nursing

Patty Hanks Shelton School of Nursing
Abilene, Texas

http://www.phssn.edu/

DEGREES • BSN • MSN

Nursing Program Faculty 17 (30% with doctorates).

Baccalaureate Enrollment 131 **Women** 89% **Men** 11% **Minority** 25% **International** 2% **Part-time** 9%

Graduate Enrollment 18 **Women** 73% **Men** 27% **Minority** 17%

Distance Learning Courses Available.

Nursing Student Activities Nursing Honor Society, Sigma Theta Tau, Student Nurses' Association.

Nursing Student Resources Academic advising; academic or career counseling; assistance for students with disabilities; bookstore; campus computer network; career placement assistance; computer lab; computer-assisted instruction; e-mail services; employment services for current students; externships; interactive nursing skills videos; Internet; learning resource lab; library services; nursing audiovisuals; remedial services; resume preparation assistance; skills, simulation, or other laboratory; tutoring.

Library Facilities 9,200 volumes in health, 1,300 volumes in nursing; 140 periodical subscriptions health-care related.

BACCALAUREATE PROGRAMS

Degree BSN

Available Programs Generic Baccalaureate; RN Baccalaureate.

Study Options Full-time.

Program Entrance Requirements Minimum overall college GPA of 3.0, transcript of college record, CPR certification, health exam, health insurance, immunizations, 2 letters of recommendation, minimum GPA in nursing prerequisites of 3.0, professional liability insurance/malpractice insurance, prerequisite course work. Transfer students are accepted. *Application deadline:* 6/13 (fall), 10/13 (spring).

Advanced Placement Credit by examination available. Credit given for nursing courses completed elsewhere dependent upon specific evaluations.

Financial Aid 80% of baccalaureate students in nursing programs received some form of financial aid in 2011–12.

Contact Mrs. Sharon Eichhorst, Director of Student Development, Patty Hanks Shelton School of Nursing, 2149 Hickory Street, Abilene, TX 79601. *Telephone:* 325-671-2353. *Fax:* 325-671-2386. *E-mail:* seichhorst@phssn.edu.

GRADUATE PROGRAMS

Expenses (2012–13) *Tuition:* part-time $725 per credit hour.

Financial Aid 50% of graduate students in nursing programs received some form of financial aid in 2011–12.

Contact Dr. Indira Tyler, Associate Dean, Patty Hanks Shelton School of Nursing, 2149 Hickory Street, Abilene, TX 79601. *Telephone:* 325-671-2367. *Fax:* 325-671-2386. *E-mail:* Indira.D. Tyler@phssn.edu.

MASTER'S DEGREE PROGRAM

Degree MSN

Available Programs Master's.

Concentrations Available Nursing education. *Nurse practitioner programs in:* family health.

Study Options Full-time and part-time.

Program Entrance Requirements Clinical experience, minimum overall college GPA of 3.5, transcript of college record, CPR certification, written essay, immunizations, interview, 3 letters of recommendation, physical assessment course, professional liability insurance/malpractice insurance, resume, statistics course. *Application deadline:* 8/12 (fall).

Advanced Placement Credit given for nursing courses completed elsewhere dependent upon specific evaluations.

Degree Requirements 49 total credit hours.

POST-MASTER'S PROGRAM

Areas of Study *Nurse practitioner programs in:* family health.

CONTINUING EDUCATION PROGRAM

Contact Dr. Nina Ouimette, Dean and Professor, Patty Hanks Shelton School of Nursing, 2149 Hickory Street, Abilene, TX 79601. *Telephone:* 325-671-2399. *Fax:* 325-671-2386. *E-mail:* nouimette@phssn.edu.

Prairie View A&M University

College of Nursing
Houston, Texas

http://www.pvamu.edu/nursing
Founded in 1878

DEGREES • BSN • MSN

Nursing Program Faculty 66 (26% with doctorates).

Baccalaureate Enrollment 447 **Women** 85% **Men** 15% **Minority** 38% **International** 2% **Part-time** 19%

Graduate Enrollment 103 **Women** 95% **Men** 5% **Minority** 25% **International** 2% **Part-time** 78%

Distance Learning Courses Available.

Nursing Student Activities Nursing Honor Society, Sigma Theta Tau, Student Nurses' Association, nursing club.

Nursing Student Resources Academic advising; academic or career counseling; assistance for students with disabilities; bookstore; campus computer network; career placement assistance; computer lab; computer-assisted instruction; e-mail services; employment services for current students; interactive nursing skills videos; Internet; learning resource lab;

library services; nursing audiovisuals; placement services for program completers; resume preparation assistance; skills, simulation, or other laboratory; tutoring.
Library Facilities 1.2 million volumes (355,707 in health, 7,899 in nursing); 42,660 periodical subscriptions (9,283 health-care related).

BACCALAUREATE PROGRAMS

Degree BSN
Available Programs Generic Baccalaureate; LPN to Baccalaureate; RN Baccalaureate.
Site Options Woodlands, TX; College Station, TX.
Study Options Full-time and part-time.
Program Entrance Requirements Minimum overall college GPA of 2.5, transcript of college record, CPR certification, health exam, immunizations, minimum GPA in nursing prerequisites of 2.0, professional liability insurance/malpractice insurance, prerequisite course work. Transfer students are accepted. *Application deadline:* 3/1 (fall), 10/1 (spring). *Application fee:* $25.
Advanced Placement Credit given for nursing courses completed elsewhere dependent upon specific evaluations.
Contact *Telephone:* 713-797-7031. *Fax:* 713-797-7092.

GRADUATE PROGRAMS

Contact *Telephone:* 713-797-7015. *Fax:* 713-797-7011.

MASTER'S DEGREE PROGRAM

Degree MSN
Available Programs Master's.
Concentrations Available Nursing administration; nursing education. *Nurse practitioner programs in:* family health.
Study Options Full-time and part-time.
Program Entrance Requirements Clinical experience, minimum overall college GPA of 2.75, transcript of college record, CPR certification, immunizations, interview, 3 letters of recommendation, physical assessment course, prerequisite course work, resume, statistics course, MAT or GRE. *Application deadline:* 6/1 (fall), 10/1 (spring), 4/1 (summer). *Application fee:* $25.
Advanced Placement Credit by examination available. Credit given for nursing courses completed elsewhere dependent upon specific evaluations.
Degree Requirements 53 total credit hours, thesis or project.

POST-MASTER'S PROGRAM

Areas of Study Nursing administration; nursing education. *Nurse practitioner programs in:* family health.

Southwestern Adventist University
Department of Nursing
Keene, Texas

http://www.swau.edu/
Founded in 1894
DEGREE • BS
Nursing Program Faculty 17 (40% with doctorates).
Baccalaureate Enrollment 101 **Women** 84% **Men** 16% **Minority** 72% **International** 5% **Part-time** 6%
Nursing Student Activities Student Nurses' Association.
Nursing Student Resources Academic advising; academic or career counseling; assistance for students with disabilities; bookstore; campus computer network; computer lab; computer-assisted instruction; e-mail services; externships; interactive nursing skills videos; Internet; learning resource lab; library services; nursing audiovisuals; remedial services; resume preparation assistance; skills, simulation, or other laboratory; tutoring.
Library Facilities 135,774 volumes (1,791 in health, 847 in nursing); 4,500 periodical subscriptions (5,168 health-care related).

BACCALAUREATE PROGRAMS

Degree BS
Available Programs Generic Baccalaureate; LPN to RN Baccalaureate; RN Baccalaureate.
Study Options Full-time and part-time.
Program Entrance Requirements Transcript of college record, CPR certification, written essay, health exam, health insurance, immuniza-

tions, 3 letters of recommendation, minimum GPA in nursing prerequisites of 2.75, prerequisite course work. *Application deadline:* 8/10 (spring). *Application fee:* $100.
Advanced Placement Credit by examination available.
Expenses (2012–13) *Tuition:* full-time $17,400; part-time $725 per credit hour. *International tuition:* $17,400 full-time. *Room and board:* $7032; room only: $3420 per academic year. *Required fees:* full-time $800.
Financial Aid 65% of baccalaureate students in nursing programs received some form of financial aid in 2011–12.
Contact Dr. Lenora D. Follett, Chair, Department of Nursing, Department of Nursing, Southwestern Adventist University, 300 West Magnolia, PO Box 567, Keene, TX 76059. *Telephone:* 817-202-6670. *Fax:* 817-202-6713. *E-mail:* lenora.follett@swau.edu.

Stephen F. Austin State University
Richard and Lucille Dewitt School of Nursing
Nacogdoches, Texas

http://www.fp.sfasu.edu/nursing/
Founded in 1923
DEGREE • BSN
Nursing Program Faculty 29 (34% with doctorates).
Baccalaureate Enrollment 267
Distance Learning Courses Available.
Nursing Student Activities Sigma Theta Tau, Student Nurses' Association.
Nursing Student Resources Academic advising; academic or career counseling; assistance for students with disabilities; bookstore; campus computer network; computer lab; computer-assisted instruction; e-mail services; employment services for current students; housing assistance; interactive nursing skills videos; Internet; library services; nursing audiovisuals; skills, simulation, or other laboratory; tutoring.
Library Facilities 745,137 volumes; 1,153 periodical subscriptions.

BACCALAUREATE PROGRAMS

Degree BSN
Available Programs RN Baccalaureate.
Site Options Nacogdoches, TX.
Study Options Full-time.
Program Entrance Requirements Minimum overall college GPA of 2.75, transcript of college record, CPR certification, health insurance, high school transcript, immunizations, minimum GPA in nursing prerequisites of 2.5, professional liability insurance/malpractice insurance, prerequisite course work. Transfer students are accepted. *Application deadline:* 2/1 (fall), 9/12 (spring).
Advanced Placement Credit given for nursing courses completed elsewhere dependent upon specific evaluations.
Contact Dr. Glenda C. Walker, Director, Richard and Lucille Dewitt School of Nursing, Stephen F. Austin State University, SFA Box 6156, Nacogdoches, TX 75962. *Telephone:* 936-468-7700. *Fax:* 936-468-7752.

Tarleton State University
Department of Nursing
Stephenville, Texas

http://www.tarleton.edu/~nursing
Founded in 1899
DEGREE • BSN
Nursing Program Faculty 19 (14% with doctorates).
Baccalaureate Enrollment 230 **Women** 95% **Men** 5% **Minority** 15% **International** 2% **Part-time** 25%
Nursing Student Activities Sigma Theta Tau, Student Nurses' Association.
Nursing Student Resources Academic advising; academic or career counseling; assistance for students with disabilities; bookstore; computer lab; computer-assisted instruction; daycare for children of students; e-mail services; employment services for current students; externships; learning resource lab; library services; nursing audiovisuals; remedial services; resume preparation assistance; skills, simulation, or other laboratory; tutoring; unpaid internships.

Library Facilities 400,000 volumes; 25,800 periodical subscriptions.

BACCALAUREATE PROGRAMS

Degree BSN

Available Programs ADN to Baccalaureate; Generic Baccalaureate; LPN to Baccalaureate.

Study Options Full-time and part-time.

Program Entrance Requirements Transcript of college record, CPR certification, written essay, health exam, high school transcript, immunizations, 3 letters of recommendation, minimum GPA in nursing prerequisites of 2.75, professional liability insurance/malpractice insurance, prerequisite course work. Transfer students are accepted.

Advanced Placement Credit by examination available. Credit given for nursing courses completed elsewhere dependent upon specific evaluations.

Contact *Telephone:* 254-968-9139. *Fax:* 254-968-9716.

CONTINUING EDUCATION PROGRAM

Contact *Telephone:* 325-649-8058. *Fax:* 325-649-8959.

Texas A&M Health Science Center

College of Nursing
College Station, Texas

http://www.tamhsc.edu
Founded in 1999

DEGREE • BSN

Nursing Program Faculty 28 (33% with doctorates).

Baccalaureate Enrollment 145 **Women** 89% **Men** 11% **Minority** 7% **Part-time** 2%

Distance Learning Courses Available.

Nursing Student Activities Sigma Theta Tau, Student Nurses' Association, nursing club.

Nursing Student Resources Academic advising; assistance for students with disabilities; bookstore; campus computer network; career placement assistance; computer lab; computer-assisted instruction; e-mail services; externships; interactive nursing skills videos; Internet; learning resource lab; library services; nursing audiovisuals; remedial services; resume preparation assistance; skills, simulation, or other laboratory; tutoring.

BACCALAUREATE PROGRAMS

Degree BSN

Available Programs ADN to Baccalaureate; Accelerated Baccalaureate for Second Degree; Generic Baccalaureate; RN Baccalaureate.

Site Options Round Rock, TX.

Study Options Full-time.

Online Degree Options Yes.

Program Entrance Requirements Minimum overall college GPA of 3.0, transcript of college record, CPR certification, written essay, health exam, health insurance, high school foreign language, immunizations, 1 letter of recommendation, minimum GPA in nursing prerequisites of 2.75, professional liability insurance/malpractice insurance, prerequisite course work. Transfer students are accepted. *Application deadline:* 8/1 (winter), 2/1 (summer). *Application fee:* $50.

Advanced Placement Credit by examination available. Credit given for nursing courses completed elsewhere dependent upon specific evaluations.

Financial Aid 89% of baccalaureate students in nursing programs received some form of financial aid in 2011–12.

Contact Kathryn Willis Cochran, Associate Dean for Student Affairs, College of Nursing, Texas A&M Health Science Center, 8447 State Highway 47, Bryan, TX 77807-3260. *Telephone:* 979-436-0110. *Fax:* 979-436-0098. *E-mail:* cochran@tamhsc.edu.

Texas A&M International University

Canseco School of Nursing
Laredo, Texas

Founded in 1969

DEGREES • BSN • MSN

Nursing Program Faculty 21 (19% with doctorates).

Baccalaureate Enrollment 171 **Women** 70% **Men** 30% **Minority** 98% **International** 1% **Part-time** 25%

Graduate Enrollment 29 **Women** 75% **Men** 25% **Minority** 90% **Part-time** 100%

Distance Learning Courses Available.

Nursing Student Activities Nursing Honor Society, Student Nurses' Association.

Nursing Student Resources Academic advising; academic or career counseling; assistance for students with disabilities; bookstore; campus computer network; career placement assistance; computer lab; computer-assisted instruction; daycare for children of students; e-mail services; employment services for current students; externships; housing assistance; interactive nursing skills videos; Internet; learning resource lab; library services; nursing audiovisuals; paid internships; placement services for program completers; remedial services; resume preparation assistance; skills, simulation, or other laboratory; tutoring.

Library Facilities 332,163 volumes (273,643 in health, 8,500 in nursing); 33,587 periodical subscriptions (80 health-care related).

BACCALAUREATE PROGRAMS

Degree BSN

Available Programs Generic Baccalaureate; RN Baccalaureate.

Study Options Full-time.

Program Entrance Requirements Minimum overall college GPA of 2.5, transcript of college record, CPR certification, written essay, health exam, immunizations, 2 letters of recommendation, minimum high school GPA of 2.5, minimum GPA in nursing prerequisites of 2.5, prerequisite course work. Transfer students are accepted. *Application deadline:* 6/1 (fall). *Application fee:* $25.

Advanced Placement Credit given for nursing courses completed elsewhere dependent upon specific evaluations.

Expenses (2011–12) *Tuition, state resident:* full-time $5417; part-time $373 per credit hour. *Tuition, nonresident:* full-time $13,757; part-time $687 per credit hour. *Room and board:* $6750 per academic year.

Financial Aid 85% of baccalaureate students in nursing programs received some form of financial aid in 2010–11. *Gift aid (need-based):* Federal Pell, FSEOG, state, college/university gift aid from institutional funds, Federal Nursing. *Loans:* Federal Direct (Subsidized and Unsubsidized Stafford PLUS), state, college/university, Hinson-Hazelwood Loan Program. *Work-study:* Federal Work-Study, part-time campus jobs. *Financial aid application deadline:* 8/1 (priority: 3/15).

Contact Dr. Regina C. Aune, Dean, Canseco School of Nursing, Texas A&M International University, 5201 University Boulevard, Laredo, TX 78041-1900. *Telephone:* 956-326-2450. *Fax:* 956-326-2449. *E-mail:* regina.aune@tamiu.edu.

GRADUATE PROGRAMS

Expenses (2011–12) *Tuition, area resident:* full-time $4208; part-time $396 per credit hour. *Tuition, nonresident:* full-time $9768; part-time $709 per credit hour. *International tuition:* $9768 full-time. *Room and board:* $6750 per academic year.

Financial Aid 85% of graduate students in nursing programs received some form of financial aid in 2010–11.

Contact Dr. Regina C. Aune, Dean, Canseco School of Nursing, Texas A&M International University, 5201 University Boulevard, Laredo, TX 78041-1900. *Telephone:* 956-326-2450. *Fax:* 956-326-2449. *E-mail:* sbaker@tamiu.edu.

MASTER'S DEGREE PROGRAM

Degree MSN

Available Programs Master's.

Concentrations Available *Nurse practitioner programs in:* family health.

Study Options Full-time and part-time.

Program Entrance Requirements Clinical experience, minimum overall college GPA of 3.0, transcript of college record, CPR certification, written essay, immunizations, interview, 2 letters of recommen-

dation, nursing research course. *Application deadline:* 6/1 (fall). *Application fee:* $25.
Advanced Placement Credit given for nursing courses completed elsewhere dependent upon specific evaluations.
Degree Requirements 45 total credit hours.

Texas A&M University–Corpus Christi
College of Nursing and Health Sciences
Corpus Christi, Texas

http://conhs.tamucc.edu/
Founded in 1947
DEGREES • BSN • MSN
Nursing Program Faculty 64 (45% with doctorates).
Baccalaureate Enrollment 451 **Women** 79% **Men** 21% **Minority** 55% **International** .01% **Part-time** 13%
Graduate Enrollment 338 **Women** 84% **Men** 16% **Minority** 44% **Part-time** 99%
Distance Learning Courses Available.
Nursing Student Activities Nursing Honor Society, Sigma Theta Tau, Student Nurses' Association.
Nursing Student Resources Academic advising; academic or career counseling; assistance for students with disabilities; bookstore; campus computer network; career placement assistance; computer lab; computer-assisted instruction; e-mail services; employment services for current students; housing assistance; interactive nursing skills videos; Internet; learning resource lab; library services; nursing audiovisuals; placement services for program completers; remedial services; resume preparation assistance; skills, simulation, or other laboratory; tutoring.
Library Facilities 731,586 volumes (500 in health, 350 in nursing); 1,901 periodical subscriptions (100 health-care related).

BACCALAUREATE PROGRAMS
Degree BSN
Available Programs ADN to Baccalaureate; Accelerated Baccalaureate for Second Degree; Baccalaureate for Second Degree; Generic Baccalaureate; RN Baccalaureate.
Study Options Full-time and part-time.
Online Degree Options Yes.
Program Entrance Requirements Minimum overall college GPA of 3.0, transcript of college record, CPR certification, immunizations, professional liability insurance/malpractice insurance, prerequisite course work. Transfer students are accepted. *Application deadline:* 11/15 (fall), 6/1 (spring), 10/1 (summer). *Application fee:* $45.
Advanced Placement Credit by examination available. Credit given for nursing courses completed elsewhere dependent upon specific evaluations.
Expenses (2012–13) *Tuition, state resident:* full-time $5317; part-time $168 per credit hour. *Tuition, nonresident:* full-time $14,522; part-time $519 per credit hour. *International tuition:* $14,522 full-time. *Required fees:* full-time $2634; part-time $268 per credit; part-time $1285 per term.
Financial Aid 78% of baccalaureate students in nursing programs received some form of financial aid in 2011–12.
Contact Dr. Cynthia O'Neal, Undergraduate Chair, College of Nursing and Health Sciences, Texas A&M University–Corpus Christi, 6300 Ocean Drive, Unit 5805, Corpus Christi, TX 78412-5503. *Telephone:* 361-825-2244. *Fax:* 361-825-2484. *E-mail:* Cynthia.O'Neal@tamucc.edu.

GRADUATE PROGRAMS
Expenses (2012–13) *Tuition, state resident:* part-time $197 per credit hour. *Tuition, nonresident:* part-time $547 per credit hour. *Required fees:* part-time $292 per credit; part-time $689 per term.
Financial Aid 20% of graduate students in nursing programs received some form of financial aid in 2011–12.
Contact Dr. Chris Bray, Interim Graduate Chair, College of Nursing and Health Sciences, Texas A&M University–Corpus Christi, 6300 Ocean Drive, Unit 5805, Corpus Christi, TX 78412. *Telephone:* 361-825-2798. *Fax:* 936-462-7662. *E-mail:* chris.bray@tamucc.edu.

MASTER'S DEGREE PROGRAM
Degree MSN

Available Programs Master's; RN to Master's.
Concentrations Available Nursing administration; nursing education. *Nurse practitioner programs in:* family health.
Study Options Part-time.
Online Degree Options Yes (online only).
Program Entrance Requirements Minimum overall college GPA of 3.0, transcript of college record, CPR certification, written essay, immunizations, 3 letters of recommendation, resume, statistics course. *Application deadline:* 4/15 (fall), 11/15 (spring), 4/15 (summer). *Application fee:* $40.
Advanced Placement Credit given for nursing courses completed elsewhere dependent upon specific evaluations.
Degree Requirements 49 total credit hours, thesis or project.

POST-MASTER'S PROGRAM
Areas of Study Nursing administration; nursing education. *Nurse practitioner programs in:* family health.

CONTINUING EDUCATION PROGRAM
Contact Ms. Petra Martinez, Chair of Continuing Education Committee, College of Nursing and Health Sciences, Texas A&M University–Corpus Christi, 6300 Ocean Drive, ST 316, Corpus Christi, TX 78412-5503. *Telephone:* 361-825-2353. *Fax:* 361-825-3491. *E-mail:* petra.martinez@tamucc.edu.

Texas A&M University–Texarkana
Nursing Department
Texarkana, Texas

http://www.tamut.edu/nursing/index.php?pageid=13
Founded in 1971
DEGREES • BSN • MSN
Nursing Program Faculty 5 (60% with doctorates).
Baccalaureate Enrollment 31 **Women** 87% **Men** 13% **Minority** 23% **Part-time** 94%
Graduate Enrollment 26 **Women** 96% **Men** 4% **Minority** 15% **Part-time** 100%
Nursing Student Activities Nursing club.
Nursing Student Resources Academic advising; academic or career counseling; assistance for students with disabilities; bookstore; campus computer network; career placement assistance; computer lab; computer-assisted instruction; e-mail services; Internet; library services; nursing audiovisuals; resume preparation assistance.
Library Facilities 8,743 volumes in health, 2,558 volumes in nursing; 80 periodical subscriptions health-care related.

BACCALAUREATE PROGRAMS
Degree BSN
Available Programs ADN to Baccalaureate.
Study Options Full-time and part-time.
Program Entrance Requirements Minimum overall college GPA of 2.0, transcript of college record, CPR certification, health exam, health insurance, immunizations, letters of recommendation, professional liability insurance/malpractice insurance, prerequisite course work, RN licensure. Transfer students are accepted. *Application deadline:* 7/15 (fall), 12/1 (spring), 4/1 (summer).
Advanced Placement Credit given for nursing courses completed elsewhere dependent upon specific evaluations.
Contact *Telephone:* 903-223-3175. *Fax:* 903-223-3107.

GRADUATE PROGRAMS
Contact *Telephone:* 903-223-3175.

MASTER'S DEGREE PROGRAM
Degree MSN
Available Programs Master's.
Concentrations Available Nursing administration; nursing education.
Study Options Full-time and part-time.
Program Entrance Requirements Minimum overall college GPA of 3.0, transcript of college record, written essay, 3 letters of recommendation, resume. *Application deadline:* 7/15 (fall), 12/1 (spring), 4/1 (summer).
Degree Requirements 36 total credit hours.

Texas Christian University
Harris College of Nursing
Fort Worth, Texas

http://www.nursing.tcu.edu/
Founded in 1873
DEGREES • BSN • DNP • MSN
Nursing Program Faculty 52 (67% with doctorates).
Baccalaureate Enrollment 675 **Women** 91% **Men** 9% **Minority** 21% **International** 1%
Graduate Enrollment 274 **Women** 49% **Men** 51% **Minority** 19% **Part-time** 15%
Distance Learning Courses Available.
Nursing Student Activities Sigma Theta Tau, Student Nurses' Association.
Nursing Student Resources Academic advising; academic or career counseling; assistance for students with disabilities; bookstore; campus computer network; career placement assistance; computer lab; computer-assisted instruction; e-mail services; employment services for current students; externships; interactive nursing skills videos; Internet; learning resource lab; library services; nursing audiovisuals; other; remedial services; resume preparation assistance; skills, simulation, or other laboratory; tutoring; unpaid internships.
Library Facilities 1.4 million volumes (26,500 in health, 2,200 in nursing); 79,353 periodical subscriptions (180 health-care related).

BACCALAUREATE PROGRAMS

Degree BSN
Available Programs Accelerated Baccalaureate for Second Degree; Generic Baccalaureate.
Study Options Full-time and part-time.
Program Entrance Requirements Minimum overall college GPA of 2.5, transcript of college record, CPR certification, written essay, high school foreign language, 2 years high school math, 4 years high school science, high school transcript, immunizations, minimum high school GPA of 3.0, minimum GPA in nursing prerequisites of 2.5, prerequisite course work. Transfer students are accepted. *Application deadline:* 2/1 (fall), 10/1 (spring), 11/15 (summer). *Application fee:* $40.
Advanced Placement Credit by examination available. Credit given for nursing courses completed elsewhere dependent upon specific evaluations.
Expenses (2012–13) *Tuition:* full-time $34,500. *Room and board:* $10,650 per academic year. *Required fees:* full-time $390.
Financial Aid 80% of baccalaureate students in nursing programs received some form of financial aid in 2011–12. *Gift aid (need-based):* Federal Pell, FSEOG, state, private, college/university gift aid from institutional funds. *Loans:* Federal Nursing Student Loans, Federal Direct (Subsidized and Unsubsidized Stafford PLUS), Perkins, state. *Work-study:* Federal Work-Study, part-time campus jobs. *Financial aid application deadline:* 5/1 (priority: 5/1).
Contact Ms. Marinda Allender, Director of Nursing Undergraduate Programs, Harris College of Nursing, Texas Christian University, TCU Box 298620, Fort Worth, TX 76129. *Telephone:* 817-257-7650. *Fax:* 817-257-7944. *E-mail:* m.allender@tcu.edu.

GRADUATE PROGRAMS

Expenses (2012–13) *Tuition:* full-time $21,150; part-time $10,575 per term. *Required fees:* full-time $300; part-time $150 per term.
Financial Aid 100% of graduate students in nursing programs received some form of financial aid in 2011–12.
Contact Ms. Mary Jane Allred, Assistant to Dean of Graduate Studies, Harris College of Nursing, Texas Christian University, TCU Box 298627, Fort Worth, TX 76129. *Telephone:* 817-257-6726. *Fax:* 817-257-8383. *E-mail:* m.allred@tcu.edu.

MASTER'S DEGREE PROGRAM
Degree MSN
Available Programs Master's.
Concentrations Available Clinical nurse leader; nursing education. *Clinical nurse specialist programs in:* gerontology, pediatric.
Study Options Full-time and part-time.
Online Degree Options Yes (online only).
Program Entrance Requirements Clinical experience, computer literacy, minimum overall college GPA of 3.0, transcript of college record, CPR certification, written essay, immunizations, 3 letters of recommendation, professional liability insurance/malpractice insurance, prerequ-

isite course work, resume. *Application deadline:* 11/15 (summer). *Application fee:* $50.
Advanced Placement Credit given for nursing courses completed elsewhere dependent upon specific evaluations.
Degree Requirements 40 total credit hours, thesis or project.

POST-MASTER'S PROGRAM
Areas of Study Clinical nurse leader; nursing education. *Clinical nurse specialist programs in:* gerontology, pediatric.

DOCTORAL DEGREE PROGRAM
Degree DNP
Available Programs Doctorate.
Areas of Study Advanced practice nursing, nursing administration.
Program Entrance Requirements Clinical experience, minimum overall college GPA of 3.0, interview, 3 letters of recommendation, MSN or equivalent, vita, writing sample. *Application deadline:* 11/15 (fall). *Application fee:* $100.
Degree Requirements 30 total credit hours, oral exam, written exam.

CONTINUING EDUCATION PROGRAM

Contact Ms. Barbara Patten, Program Planning and Continuing Nursing Education Coordinator, Harris College of Nursing, Texas Christian University, TCU Box 298620, Fort Worth, TX 76129. *Telephone:* 817-257-7368. *Fax:* 817-257-7944. *E-mail:* bapatten@tcu.edu.

Texas State University–San Marcos
St. David's School of Nursing
San Marcos, Texas

Founded in 1899
DEGREES • BSN • MSN
Library Facilities 1.6 million volumes; 14,764 periodical subscriptions.

BACCALAUREATE PROGRAMS

Degree BSN
Available Programs Baccalaureate for Second Degree; Generic Baccalaureate.
Program Entrance Requirements Health insurance, minimum GPA in nursing prerequisites of 3.0.
Contact School of Nursing, St. David's School of Nursing, Texas State University–San Marcos, 1555 University Drive, Round Rock, TX 78665. *Telephone:* 512-716-2900. *Fax:* 512-716-2949.

GRADUATE PROGRAMS

Contact School of Nursing, St. David's School of Nursing, Texas State University–San Marcos, 1555 University Drive, Round Rock, TX 78665. *Telephone:* 512-716-2900. *Fax:* 512-716-2911.

MASTER'S DEGREE PROGRAM
Degree MSN
Available Programs Master's.
Program Entrance Requirements Transcript of college record, written essay, 3 letters of recommendation, resume.

Texas Tech University Health Sciences Center
School of Nursing
Lubbock, Texas

http://www.ttuhsc.edu/son
Founded in 1969
DEGREES • BSN • DNP • MSN
Nursing Program Faculty 88 (48% with doctorates).
Baccalaureate Enrollment 878 **Women** 80% **Men** 20% **Minority** 45% **International** 20% **Part-time** 2%
Graduate Enrollment 489 **Women** 85% **Men** 15% **Minority** 34% **Part-time** 86%
Distance Learning Courses Available.

Nursing Student Activities Sigma Theta Tau, Student Nurses' Association.

Nursing Student Resources Academic advising; academic or career counseling; assistance for students with disabilities; bookstore; campus computer network; career placement assistance; computer lab; e-mail services; Internet; learning resource lab; library services; nursing audiovisuals; other; skills, simulation, or other laboratory; tutoring.

Library Facilities 320,818 volumes in health, 6,583 volumes in nursing; 28,960 periodical subscriptions health-care related.

BACCALAUREATE PROGRAMS

Degree BSN

Available Programs Accelerated Baccalaureate for Second Degree; Generic Baccalaureate; RN Baccalaureate.

Site Options Odessa, TX; Abilene, TX.

Study Options Full-time.

Online Degree Options Yes (online only).

Program Entrance Requirements Transcript of college record, written essay, immunizations, minimum GPA in nursing prerequisites of 2.5, prerequisite course work, RN licensure. *Application deadline:* 12/15 (fall). *Application fee:* $40.

Advanced Placement Credit given for nursing courses completed elsewhere dependent upon specific evaluations.

Expenses (2012–13) *Tuition, state resident:* full-time $2625. *Tuition, nonresident:* full-time $7890. *International tuition:* $7890 full-time.

Financial Aid 86% of baccalaureate students in nursing programs received some form of financial aid in 2011–12.

Contact Dr. Kathy Sridaromont, Department Chair of Traditional Undergraduate Studies, School of Nursing, Texas Tech University Health Sciences Center, 3601 4th Street, MS 6264, Lubbock, TX 79430. *Telephone:* 806-743-2730. *Fax:* 806-743-1648. *E-mail:* kathy.sridaromont@ttuhsc.edu.

GRADUATE PROGRAMS

Expenses (2012–13) *Tuition, state resident:* full-time $2025; part-time $1350 per semester. *Tuition, nonresident:* full-time $5184; part-time $3456 per semester. *International tuition:* $5184 full-time. *Required fees:* part-time $2016 per term.

Financial Aid 80% of graduate students in nursing programs received some form of financial aid in 2011–12. Institutionally sponsored loans, scholarships, and traineeships available. Aid available to part-time students. *Financial aid application deadline:* 12/1.

Contact Ms. Georgina Barrera, Graduate Program Student Affairs Coordinator, School of Nursing, Texas Tech University Health Sciences Center, 3601 4th Street, MS 6264, Lubbock, TX 79430. *Telephone:* 806-743-2762. *Fax:* 806-743-2324. *E-mail:* georgina.barrera@ttuhsc.edu.

MASTER'S DEGREE PROGRAM

Degree MSN

Available Programs Master's.

Concentrations Available Nurse-midwifery; nursing administration; nursing education. *Nurse practitioner programs in:* acute care, family health, gerontology, pediatric.

Study Options Full-time and part-time.

Online Degree Options Yes (online only).

Program Entrance Requirements Clinical experience, computer literacy, minimum overall college GPA of 3.0, transcript of college record, CPR certification, written essay, immunizations, 3 letters of recommendation, nursing research course, statistics course. *Application deadline:* 5/1 (fall), 9/1 (spring). *Application fee:* $40.

Advanced Placement Credit given for nursing courses completed elsewhere dependent upon specific evaluations.

Degree Requirements 48 total credit hours, thesis or project, comprehensive exam.

POST-MASTER'S PROGRAM

Areas of Study *Nurse practitioner programs in:* acute care, family health, gerontology, pediatric.

DOCTORAL DEGREE PROGRAM

Degree DNP

Available Programs Doctorate.

Areas of Study Nursing administration, nursing education.

Program Entrance Requirements Clinical experience, minimum overall college GPA of 3.0, interview by faculty committee, interview, 3 letters of recommendation, MSN or equivalent, statistics course, vita, writing sample. *Application deadline:* 9/1 (summer).

Degree Requirements 48 total credit hours.

Texas Woman's University
College of Nursing
Denton, Texas

http://www.twu.edu/nursing
Founded in 1901
DEGREES • BS • MS • MSN/MHA • PHD
Nursing Program Faculty 258 (35% with doctorates).
Baccalaureate Enrollment 988 **Women** 90% **Men** 10% **Minority** 51% **International** 4% **Part-time** 14%
Graduate Enrollment 919 **Women** 94% **Men** 6% **Minority** 40% **International** 1% **Part-time** 85%
Distance Learning Courses Available.
Nursing Student Activities Nursing Honor Society, Sigma Theta Tau, Student Nurses' Association, nursing club.
Nursing Student Resources Academic advising; academic or career counseling; assistance for students with disabilities; bookstore; campus computer network; career placement assistance; computer lab; computer-assisted instruction; e-mail services; employment services for current students; interactive nursing skills videos; Internet; learning resource lab; library services; nursing audiovisuals; placement services for program completers; remedial services; resume preparation assistance; skills, simulation, or other laboratory; tutoring; unpaid internships.
Library Facilities 580,832 volumes (250,000 in health, 26,463 in nursing); 55,756 periodical subscriptions (2,644 health-care related).

BACCALAUREATE PROGRAMS

Degree BS

Available Programs Baccalaureate for Second Degree; Generic Baccalaureate; RN Baccalaureate.

Site Options Houston, TX; Dallas, TX.

Study Options Full-time and part-time.

Online Degree Options Yes.

Program Entrance Requirements Transcript of college record, CPR certification, high school transcript, immunizations, minimum GPA in nursing prerequisites of 3.0, professional liability insurance/malpractice insurance, prerequisite course work. Transfer students are accepted. *Application deadline:* 2/1 (fall), 9/1 (spring). *Application fee:* $30.

Advanced Placement Credit given for nursing courses completed elsewhere dependent upon specific evaluations.

Expenses (2012–13) *Tuition, state resident:* full-time $5156; part-time $437 per credit hour. *Tuition, nonresident:* full-time $11,468; part-time $788 per credit hour. *Room and board:* $6930 per academic year. *Required fees:* full-time $2269.

Financial Aid *Gift aid (need-based):* Federal Pell, FSEOG, state, private, college/university gift aid from institutional funds. *Loans:* Federal Nursing Student Loans, Federal Direct (Subsidized and Unsubsidized Stafford PLUS), Perkins, state, college/university, alternative loans. *Work-study:* Federal Work-Study, part-time campus jobs. *Financial aid application deadline (priority):* 4/1.

Contact Heather Close, Nursing Admissions Coordinator, College of Nursing, Texas Woman's University, PO Box 425498, Denton, TX 76204. *Telephone:* 940-898-2401. *Fax:* 940-898-2437. *E-mail:* nursing@twu.edu.

GRADUATE PROGRAMS

Expenses (2012–13) *Tuition, state resident:* full-time $5400; part-time $330 per credit hour. *Tuition, nonresident:* full-time $11,650; part-time $681 per credit hour. *Required fees:* full-time $450.

Financial Aid 30% of graduate students in nursing programs received some form of financial aid in 2011–12. 10 research assistantships (averaging $12,942 per year), 1 teaching assistantship (averaging $12,942 per year) were awarded; career-related internships or fieldwork, Federal Work-Study, institutionally sponsored loans, scholarships, traineeships, and unspecified assistantships also available. Aid available to part-time students. *Financial aid application deadline:* 3/1.

Contact Dr. Ruth Johnson, Associate Dean of the Graduate School, College of Nursing, Texas Woman's University, PO Box 425649, Denton, TX 76204. *Telephone:* 940-898-3415. *E-mail:* rjohnson@twu.edu.

MASTER'S DEGREE PROGRAM

Degrees MS; MSN/MHA

Available Programs Master's; RN to Master's.

Concentrations Available Clinical nurse leader; health-care administration; nursing administration; nursing education. *Nurse practitioner programs in:* acute care, adult health, family health, pediatric, women's health.

Site Options Houston, TX; Dallas, TX.
Study Options Full-time and part-time.
Online Degree Options Yes.
Program Entrance Requirements Clinical experience, minimum overall college GPA of 3.0, transcript of college record, CPR certification, immunizations, professional liability insurance/malpractice insurance, statistics course, GRE or MAT. *Application deadline:* 2/1 (fall), 9/1 (spring).
Advanced Placement Credit given for nursing courses completed elsewhere dependent upon specific evaluations.
Degree Requirements 48 total credit hours, thesis or project.

POST-MASTER'S PROGRAM
Areas of Study *Nurse practitioner programs in:* acute care, adult health, family health, pediatric, women's health.

DOCTORAL DEGREE PROGRAM
Degree PhD
Available Programs Doctorate.
Areas of Study Nursing research, nursing science, women's health.
Site Options Houston, TX; Dallas, TX.
Program Entrance Requirements Minimum overall college GPA of 3.5, 2 letters of recommendation, MSN or equivalent, statistics course, vita, GRE (preferred minimum score 153 [500 old version] Verbal, 144 [500 old version] Quantitative, 4 Analytical).
Degree Requirements 60 total credit hours, dissertation, oral exam, written exam.

University of Houston–Victoria
School of Nursing
Victoria, Texas

Founded in 1973
DEGREES • BSN • MSN

BACCALAUREATE PROGRAMS
Degree BSN
Available Programs Accelerated Baccalaureate for Second Degree; RN Baccalaureate.
Contact *Telephone:* 361-570-4848.

GRADUATE PROGRAMS
Contact *Telephone:* 361-570-4848.

MASTER'S DEGREE PROGRAM
Degree MSN
Available Programs Master's; RN to Master's.
Concentrations Available Nursing administration; nursing education.
Program Entrance Requirements GRE or MAT.

University of Mary Hardin-Baylor
College of Nursing
Belton, Texas

http://www.umhb.edu/
Founded in 1845
DEGREES • BSN • MSN
Nursing Program Faculty 48 (22% with doctorates).
Baccalaureate Enrollment 483 **Women** 88% **Men** 12% **Minority** 35% **International** 4%
Graduate Enrollment 38 **Women** 95% **Men** 5% **Minority** 24% **Part-time** 10%
Distance Learning Courses Available.
Nursing Student Activities Nursing Honor Society, Sigma Theta Tau, Student Nurses' Association.
Nursing Student Resources Academic advising; academic or career counseling; assistance for students with disabilities; bookstore; campus computer network; career placement assistance; computer lab; e-mail services; employment services for current students; housing assistance; Internet; learning resource lab; library services; nursing audiovisuals; placement services for program completers; remedial services; resume preparation assistance; skills, simulation, or other laboratory; tutoring.

Library Facilities 8,116 volumes in health, 6,924 volumes in nursing; 132 periodical subscriptions health-care related.

BACCALAUREATE PROGRAMS
Degree BSN
Available Programs ADN to Baccalaureate; Generic Baccalaureate.
Study Options Full-time and part-time.
Program Entrance Requirements Minimum overall college GPA of 3.0, transcript of college record, CPR certification, written essay, health exam, health insurance, high school transcript, immunizations, minimum GPA in nursing prerequisites of 3.0, prerequisite course work. Transfer students are accepted. *Application deadline:* 3/1 (fall), 10/1 (spring). Applications may be processed on a rolling basis for some programs.
Advanced Placement Credit given for nursing courses completed elsewhere dependent upon specific evaluations.
Expenses (2012–13) *Tuition:* full-time $21,900; part-time $730 per credit hour. *International tuition:* $21,900 full-time. *Room and board:* $5970; room only: $4685 per academic year. *Required fees:* full-time $2380.
Financial Aid 95% of baccalaureate students in nursing programs received some form of financial aid in 2011–12.
Contact Dr. Sharon Souter, Dean and Professor, College of Nursing, University of Mary Hardin-Baylor, Box 8015, 900 College Street, Belton, TX 76513-2599. *Telephone:* 254-295-4665. *Fax:* 254-295-4141. *E-mail:* lpehl@umhb.edu.

GRADUATE PROGRAMS
Expenses (2012–13) *Tuition:* part-time $750 per credit hour.
Financial Aid 40% of graduate students in nursing programs received some form of financial aid in 2011–12.
Contact Dr. Carrie Johnson, Director and Associate Professor, College of Nursing, University of Mary Hardin-Baylor, Box 8015, 900 College Street, Belton, TX 76513-2599. *Telephone:* 254-295-4178. *Fax:* 254-295-4141. *E-mail:* cjohnson@umhb.edu.

MASTER'S DEGREE PROGRAM
Degree MSN
Available Programs Master's.
Concentrations Available Clinical nurse leader; nursing education. *Nurse practitioner programs in:* family health.
Study Options Full-time and part-time.
Program Entrance Requirements Clinical experience, computer literacy, minimum overall college GPA of 3.0, transcript of college record, CPR certification, written essay, immunizations, interview, 2 letters of recommendation, nursing research course, physical assessment course, professional liability insurance/malpractice insurance, prerequisite course work, statistics course. *Application deadline:* 4/1 (fall). Applications may be processed on a rolling basis for some programs.
Advanced Placement Credit given for nursing courses completed elsewhere dependent upon specific evaluations.
Degree Requirements 36 total credit hours, comprehensive exam.

POST-MASTER'S PROGRAM
Areas of Study Clinical nurse leader; nursing education. *Nurse practitioner programs in:* family health.

The University of Texas at Arlington
College of Nursing
Arlington, Texas

http://www.uta.edu/nursing
Founded in 1895
DEGREES • BSN • MSN • MSN/MBA • MSN/MHA • MSN/MPH • PHD
Nursing Program Faculty 126 (34% with doctorates).
Baccalaureate Enrollment 2,243 **Women** 89% **Men** 11% **Minority** 40% **International** 10% **Part-time** 8%
Graduate Enrollment 542 **Women** 91% **Men** 9% **Minority** 22% **Part-time** 70%
Distance Learning Courses Available.
Nursing Student Activities Nursing Honor Society, Sigma Theta Tau, Student Nurses' Association, nursing club.
Nursing Student Resources Academic advising; campus computer network; computer lab; e-mail services; externships; interactive nursing

skills videos; Internet; learning resource lab; nursing audiovisuals; skills, simulation, or other laboratory; tutoring.
Library Facilities 1.5 million volumes (36,000 in health, 23,300 in nursing); 73,846 periodical subscriptions (530 health-care related).

BACCALAUREATE PROGRAMS

Degree BSN
Available Programs Accelerated Baccalaureate; Accelerated Baccalaureate for Second Degree; Accelerated RN Baccalaureate; Baccalaureate for Second Degree; Generic Baccalaureate; RN Baccalaureate.
Site Options Fort Worth, TX; Dallas, TX; Waco, Grayson, Paris, Kaufman, TX.
Study Options Full-time and part-time.
Program Entrance Requirements Minimum overall college GPA of 2.5, transcript of college record, CPR certification, health insurance, immunizations, minimum high school GPA of 2.5, minimum GPA in nursing prerequisites of 2.5, professional liability insurance/malpractice insurance, prerequisite course work. Transfer students are accepted. *Application deadline:* 1/5 (fall), 6/1 (spring).
Advanced Placement Credit given for nursing courses completed elsewhere dependent upon specific evaluations.
Contact *Telephone:* 817-272-2776. *Fax:* 817-272-5006.

GRADUATE PROGRAMS

Contact *Telephone:* 817-272-2776. *Fax:* 817-272-5006.

MASTER'S DEGREE PROGRAM
Degrees MSN; MSN/MBA; MSN/MHA; MSN/MPH
Available Programs Master's.
Concentrations Available Health-care administration; nursing administration; nursing education. *Nurse practitioner programs in:* acute care, adult health, family health, gerontology, neonatal health, pediatric, psychiatric/mental health.
Site Options Fort Worth, TX; Dallas, TX.
Study Options Full-time and part-time.
Online Degree Options Yes.
Program Entrance Requirements Clinical experience, computer literacy, minimum overall college GPA of 3.0, transcript of college record, CPR certification, written essay, immunizations, physical assessment course, statistics course, GRE General Test if GPA less than 3.0. *Application deadline:* 6/1 (fall), 10/15 (spring). *Application fee:* $70.
Advanced Placement Credit given for nursing courses completed elsewhere dependent upon specific evaluations.
Degree Requirements 48 total credit hours.

POST-MASTER'S PROGRAM
Areas of Study *Nurse practitioner programs in:* acute care, adult health, family health, gerontology, neonatal health, pediatric, psychiatric/mental health.

DOCTORAL DEGREE PROGRAM
Degree PhD
Available Programs Doctorate; Post-Baccalaureate Doctorate.
Areas of Study Faculty preparation, nursing education, nursing research.
Program Entrance Requirements Clinical experience, minimum overall college GPA of 3.0, interview by faculty committee, interview, 3 letters of recommendation, statistics course, GRE General Test (waived for MSN-to-PhD applicants). *Application deadline:* 4/2 (fall). *Application fee:* $70.
Degree Requirements 54 total credit hours, dissertation, residency.

CONTINUING EDUCATION PROGRAM

Contact *Telephone:* 817-272-0720. *Fax:* 817-272-5371.

The University of Texas at Austin
School of Nursing
Austin, Texas

http://www.utexas.edu/nursing
Founded in 1883
DEGREES • BSN • MSN • MSN/MBA • PHD
Nursing Program Faculty 73 (62% with doctorates).
Baccalaureate Enrollment 791 **Women** 90.5% **Men** 9.5% **Minority** 33% **International** 1% **Part-time** 13%

Graduate Enrollment 323 **Women** 88% **Men** 12% **Minority** 27% **International** 9% **Part-time** 24%
Distance Learning Courses Available.
Nursing Student Activities Nursing Honor Society, Sigma Theta Tau, Student Nurses' Association, nursing club.
Nursing Student Resources Academic advising; academic or career counseling; assistance for students with disabilities; bookstore; campus computer network; career placement assistance; computer lab; computer-assisted instruction; daycare for children of students; e-mail services; employment services for current students; externships; housing assistance; interactive nursing skills videos; Internet; learning resource lab; library services; nursing audiovisuals; other; paid internships; placement services for program completers; remedial services; resume preparation assistance; skills, simulation, or other laboratory; tutoring; unpaid internships.
Library Facilities 10.8 million volumes (100,000 in health, 80,000 in nursing); 107,456 periodical subscriptions (504 health-care related).

BACCALAUREATE PROGRAMS

Degree BSN
Available Programs Generic Baccalaureate; RN Baccalaureate.
Study Options Full-time.
Program Entrance Requirements Minimum overall college GPA of 2.75, transcript of college record, CPR certification, written essay, 3 years high school math, 2 years high school science, high school transcript, 3 letters of recommendation, minimum GPA in nursing prerequisites of 2.75, professional liability insurance/malpractice insurance, prerequisite course work. Transfer students are accepted. *Application deadline:* 9/15 (fall), 2/15 (spring). *Application fee:* $50.
Advanced Placement Credit by examination available. Credit given for nursing courses completed elsewhere dependent upon specific evaluations.
Expenses (2012–13) *Tuition, state resident:* full-time $5181; part-time $3369 per semester. *Tuition, nonresident:* full-time $17,852; part-time $11,606 per semester. *International tuition:* $17,852 full-time. *Required fees:* full-time $1000; part-time $450 per credit.
Financial Aid 54% of baccalaureate students in nursing programs received some form of financial aid in 2011–12. *Gift aid (need-based):* Federal Pell, FSEOG, state, private, college/university gift aid from institutional funds. *Loans:* Federal Direct (Subsidized and Unsubsidized Stafford PLUS), Perkins, state. *Work-study:* Federal Work-Study, part-time campus jobs. *Financial aid application deadline:* Continuous.
Contact Christina Jarvis, Student Affairs Office, School of Nursing, The University of Texas at Austin, 1710 Red River Street, Austin, TX 78701-1412. *Telephone:* 512-232-4780. *Fax:* 512-232-4777. *E-mail:* sar@mail.nur.utexas.edu.

GRADUATE PROGRAMS

Expenses (2012–13) *Tuition, state resident:* full-time $9482; part-time $3461 per semester. *Tuition, nonresident:* full-time $17,520; part-time $5733 per semester. *International tuition:* $17,520 full-time. *Room and board:* $9246 per academic year.
Financial Aid 35% of graduate students in nursing programs received some form of financial aid in 2011–12. Fellowships, research assistantships, teaching assistantships, scholarships and traineeships available. *Financial aid application deadline:* 2/1.
Contact Mr. Rudy Ortiz, Graduate Student Affairs, School of Nursing, The University of Texas at Austin, 1700 Red River Street, Graduate Student Affairs, Austin, TX 78701-1499. *Telephone:* 512-232-4701. *Fax:* 512-232-4777. *E-mail:* nugrad@uts.cc.utexas.edu.

MASTER'S DEGREE PROGRAM
Degrees MSN; MSN/MBA
Available Programs Master's; Master's for Non-Nursing College Graduates; Master's for Nurses with Non-Nursing Degrees.
Concentrations Available Nursing administration. *Clinical nurse specialist programs in:* adult health. *Nurse practitioner programs in:* family health, pediatric, psychiatric/mental health.
Study Options Full-time and part-time.
Program Entrance Requirements Minimum overall college GPA of 3.0, transcript of college record, written essay, interview, 3 letters of recommendation, prerequisite course work, resume, statistics course, GRE General Test. *Application deadline:* 12/1 (fall), 11/1 (summer). *Application fee:* $65.
Advanced Placement Credit given for nursing courses completed elsewhere dependent upon specific evaluations.
Degree Requirements 39 total credit hours.

POST-MASTER'S PROGRAM

Areas of Study *Clinical nurse specialist programs in:* adult health. *Nurse practitioner programs in:* family health, pediatric, psychiatric/mental health.

DOCTORAL DEGREE PROGRAM

Degree PhD
Available Programs Doctorate; Doctorate for Nurses with Non-Nursing Degrees; Post-Baccalaureate Doctorate.
Areas of Study Addiction/substance abuse, aging, bio-behavioral research, clinical practice, community health, ethics, family health, gerontology, health promotion/disease prevention, health-care systems, human health and illness, illness and transition, individualized study, information systems, maternity-newborn, nursing administration, nursing research, nursing science, oncology, women's health.
Program Entrance Requirements Minimum overall college GPA of 3.0, interview, 3 letters of recommendation, MSN or equivalent, statistics course, vita, writing sample, GRE General Test. *Application deadline:* 12/1 (fall), 11/1 (summer). *Application fee:* $65.
Degree Requirements 57 total credit hours, dissertation, oral exam.

POSTDOCTORAL PROGRAM

Postdoctoral Program Contact Dr. Lorraine Walker, Professor, School of Nursing, The University of Texas at Austin, 1700 Red River Street, Austin, TX 78701. *Telephone:* 512-232-4751. *Fax:* 512-232-4777. *E-mail:* lwalker@mail.nur.utexas.edu.

The University of Texas at Brownsville

Department of Nursing
Brownsville, Texas

http://www.utb.edu/vpaa/nursing/pages/default.aspx
Founded in 1973
DEGREES • BSN • MSN
Nursing Program Faculty 13 (62% with doctorates).
Baccalaureate Enrollment 91 **Women** 74% **Men** 26% **Minority** 90% **International** 2% **Part-time** 82%
Graduate Enrollment 53 **Women** 77% **Men** 23% **Minority** 87% **International** 4% **Part-time** 47%
Distance Learning Courses Available.
Nursing Student Activities Nursing club.
Nursing Student Resources Academic advising; academic or career counseling; assistance for students with disabilities; bookstore; campus computer network; career placement assistance; computer lab; computer-assisted instruction; daycare for children of students; e-mail services; employment services for current students; housing assistance; interactive nursing skills videos; Internet; learning resource lab; library services; nursing audiovisuals; remedial services; resume preparation assistance; skills, simulation, or other laboratory; tutoring.
Library Facilities 174,660 volumes; 4,447 periodical subscriptions.

BACCALAUREATE PROGRAMS

Degree BSN
Available Programs ADN to Baccalaureate.
Study Options Full-time and part-time.
Online Degree Options Yes (online only).
Program Entrance Requirements Minimum overall college GPA of 2.5, transcript of college record, CPR certification, immunizations, minimum GPA in nursing prerequisites of 2.5, professional liability insurance/malpractice insurance, prerequisite course work, RN licensure. Transfer students are accepted. *Application deadline:* 3/1 (fall), 11/1 (spring).
Advanced Placement Credit by examination available.
Financial Aid *Gift aid (need-based):* Federal Pell, FSEOG, state, private, college/university gift aid from institutional funds. *Loans:* Federal Direct (Subsidized and Unsubsidized Stafford PLUS), state, college/university. *Work-study:* Federal Work-Study, part-time campus jobs. *Financial aid application deadline (priority):* 3/1.
Contact Dr. Anne R. Rentfro, Associate Dean, College of Nursing, Department of Nursing, The University of Texas at Brownsville, 80 Fort Brown, Brownsville, TX 78520. *Telephone:* 956-882-5071. *Fax:* 956-882-5100. *E-mail:* anne.rentfro@utb.edu.

GRADUATE PROGRAMS

Contact Dr. Eloisa G. Tamez, Director of Masters Program, Department of Nursing, The University of Texas at Brownsville, 80 Fort Brown, Brownsville, TX 78520. *Telephone:* 956-882-5079. *Fax:* 956-882-5100. *E-mail:* eloisa.tamez@utb.edu.

MASTER'S DEGREE PROGRAM

Degree MSN
Available Programs Master's; Master's for Nurses with Non-Nursing Degrees.
Concentrations Available Nursing administration; nursing education. *Clinical nurse specialist programs in:* public health.
Study Options Full-time and part-time.
Online Degree Options Yes (online only).
Program Entrance Requirements Computer literacy, minimum overall college GPA of 3.0, transcript of college record, CPR certification, written essay, immunizations, interview, professional liability insurance/malpractice insurance, resume, statistics course. *Application deadline:* 4/1 (fall), 10/1 (spring). *Application fee:* $25.
Advanced Placement Credit given for nursing courses completed elsewhere dependent upon specific evaluations.
Degree Requirements 37 total credit hours, thesis or project.

CONTINUING EDUCATION PROGRAM

Contact Dr. Anne Rentfro, Interim Associate Dean College of Nursing, Department of Nursing, The University of Texas at Brownsville, 80 Fort Brown, Brownsville, TX 78520. *Telephone:* 956-882-5084. *Fax:* 956-882-5100. *E-mail:* anne.rentfro@utb.edu.

The University of Texas at El Paso

School of Nursing
El Paso, Texas

http://www.utep.edu/
Founded in 1913
DEGREES • BSN • MSN
Nursing Program Faculty 64 (27% with doctorates).
Baccalaureate Enrollment 514 **Women** 76.5% **Men** 23.5% **Minority** 80.4% **International** 2.7% **Part-time** 58.8%
Graduate Enrollment 153 **Women** 81% **Men** 19% **Minority** 61.4% **International** 3.3% **Part-time** 78.4%
Distance Learning Courses Available.
Nursing Student Activities Nursing Honor Society, Sigma Theta Tau, Student Nurses' Association.
Nursing Student Resources Academic advising; academic or career counseling; assistance for students with disabilities; bookstore; campus computer network; career placement assistance; computer lab; computer-assisted instruction; e-mail services; employment services for current students; interactive nursing skills videos; Internet; learning resource lab; library services; nursing audiovisuals; remedial services; skills, simulation, or other laboratory; tutoring.
Library Facilities 1.3 million volumes (71,389 in health, 13,043 in nursing); 3,065 periodical subscriptions (314 health-care related).

BACCALAUREATE PROGRAMS

Degree BSN
Available Programs Accelerated Baccalaureate; Generic Baccalaureate; RN Baccalaureate.
Site Options El Paso, TX.
Study Options Full-time and part-time.
Program Entrance Requirements Minimum overall college GPA of 2.0, transcript of college record, CPR certification, health exam, high school biology, high school math, high school science, high school transcript, immunizations, minimum GPA in nursing prerequisites of 2.5, professional liability insurance/malpractice insurance, prerequisite course work. Transfer students are accepted. *Application deadline:* 2/28 (fall), 9/30 (spring), 2/28 (summer).
Advanced Placement Credit by examination available. Credit given for nursing courses completed elsewhere dependent upon specific evaluations.
Contact *Telephone:* 915-747-7267. *Fax:* 915-747-8266.

GRADUATE PROGRAMS

Contact *Telephone:* 915-747-7226. *Fax:* 915-747-8266.

MASTER'S DEGREE PROGRAM

Degree MSN
Available Programs Master's; RN to Master's.
Concentrations Available Nursing administration; nursing education. *Nurse practitioner programs in:* family health.
Site Options El Paso, TX.
Study Options Full-time and part-time.
Online Degree Options Yes (online only).
Program Entrance Requirements Clinical experience, minimum overall college GPA of 3.0, transcript of college record, CPR certification, written essay, immunizations, interview, nursing research course, professional liability insurance/malpractice insurance, resume, statistics course, GRE. *Application deadline:* 9/1 (fall), 2/1 (spring). Applications may be processed on a rolling basis for some programs. *Application fee:* $45.
Advanced Placement Credit given for nursing courses completed elsewhere dependent upon specific evaluations.
Degree Requirements 33 total credit hours, thesis or project, comprehensive exam.

POST-MASTER'S PROGRAM

Areas of Study Nursing administration; nursing education. *Nurse practitioner programs in:* family health.

The University of Texas at Tyler
Program in Nursing
Tyler, Texas

http://www.uttyler.edu/nursing
Founded in 1971
DEGREES • BSN • MSN • MSN/MBA • PHD
Nursing Program Faculty 65 (25% with doctorates).
Baccalaureate Enrollment 650 **Women** 70% **Men** 30% **Minority** 10% **International** 1% **Part-time** 15%
Graduate Enrollment 175 **Women** 88% **Men** 12% **Minority** 11% **Part-time** 88%
Nursing Student Activities Nursing Honor Society, Sigma Theta Tau, Student Nurses' Association, nursing club.
Nursing Student Resources Academic advising; academic or career counseling; assistance for students with disabilities; bookstore; campus computer network; career placement assistance; computer lab; computer-assisted instruction; e-mail services; employment services for current students; externships; interactive nursing skills videos; Internet; learning resource lab; library services; nursing audiovisuals; resume preparation assistance; skills, simulation, or other laboratory; tutoring.
Library Facilities 11,000 volumes in health, 5,500 volumes in nursing; 150 periodical subscriptions health-care related.

BACCALAUREATE PROGRAMS

Degree BSN
Available Programs ADN to Baccalaureate; Accelerated RN Baccalaureate; Generic Baccalaureate; International Nurse to Baccalaureate; LPN to Baccalaureate; LPN to RN Baccalaureate; RN Baccalaureate.
Site Options Longview, TX; Palestine, TX.
Study Options Full-time and part-time.
Online Degree Options Yes (online only).
Program Entrance Requirements Minimum overall college GPA of 2.75, transcript of college record, CPR certification, immunizations, minimum GPA in nursing prerequisites of 2.75, professional liability insurance/malpractice insurance, prerequisite course work. Transfer students are accepted. *Application deadline:* 2/15 (fall), 9/15 (spring).
Advanced Placement Credit given for nursing courses completed elsewhere dependent upon specific evaluations.
Expenses (2012–13) *Tuition, state resident:* full-time $7300. *Tuition, nonresident:* full-time $18,000.
Financial Aid 70% of baccalaureate students in nursing programs received some form of financial aid in 2011–12.
Contact Ms. Renee Lampkin, Director of Marketing/Advising, Program in Nursing, The University of Texas at Tyler, 3900 University Boulevard, Tyler, TX 75799. *Telephone:* 903-565-5534. *Fax:* 903-565-5533. *E-mail:* rlampkin@uttyler.edu.

GRADUATE PROGRAMS

Financial Aid 60% of graduate students in nursing programs received some form of financial aid in 2011–12. 1 fellowship (averaging $10,000 per year), 3 research assistantships (averaging $2,200 per year) were awarded; institutionally sponsored loans and scholarships also available. *Financial aid application deadline:* 7/1.
Contact Ms. RaeJean Griffin, Administrative Assistant II, Program in Nursing, The University of Texas at Tyler, 3900 University Boulevard, Tyler, TX 75799. *Telephone:* 903-566-7128. *Fax:* 903-565-5901. *E-mail:* rgriffin@uttyler.edu.

MASTER'S DEGREE PROGRAM

Degrees MSN; MSN/MBA
Available Programs Accelerated AD/RN to Master's; Accelerated RN to Master's; Master's; RN to Master's.
Concentrations Available Nursing administration; nursing education. *Nurse practitioner programs in:* family health, pediatric.
Study Options Full-time and part-time.
Online Degree Options Yes (online only).
Program Entrance Requirements Computer literacy, minimum overall college GPA of 3.0, transcript of college record, CPR certification, written essay, immunizations, 4 letters of recommendation, nursing research course, prerequisite course work, resume, statistics course, GRE General Test or MAT, GMAT. *Application deadline:* 3/15 (fall), 10/15 (spring).
Advanced Placement Credit given for nursing courses completed elsewhere dependent upon specific evaluations.
Degree Requirements 36 total credit hours, thesis or project, comprehensive exam.

POST-MASTER'S PROGRAM

Areas of Study Nursing administration; nursing education. *Nurse practitioner programs in:* family health, pediatric.

DOCTORAL DEGREE PROGRAM

Degree PhD
Available Programs Doctorate.
Areas of Study Nursing science.
Program Entrance Requirements Minimum overall college GPA of 3.0, interview by faculty committee, 3 letters of recommendation, MSN or equivalent, scholarly papers, statistics course, vita, writing sample.
Degree Requirements 65 total credit hours, dissertation, written exam.

The University of Texas Health Science Center at Houston
School of Nursing
Houston, Texas

http://son.uth.tmc.edu/
Founded in 1972
DEGREES • BSN • MSN • MSN/MPH • PHD
Nursing Program Faculty 112 (54% with doctorates).
Baccalaureate Enrollment 497 **Women** 86% **Men** 14% **Minority** 45% **International** 1% **Part-time** 20%
Graduate Enrollment 350 **Women** 87% **Men** 13% **Minority** 35% **International** 12% **Part-time** 60%
Distance Learning Courses Available.
Nursing Student Activities Sigma Theta Tau, Student Nurses' Association.
Nursing Student Resources Academic advising; academic or career counseling; assistance for students with disabilities; bookstore; campus computer network; computer lab; computer-assisted instruction; e-mail services; employment services for current students; housing assistance; interactive nursing skills videos; Internet; learning resource lab; library services; nursing audiovisuals; paid internships; remedial services; skills, simulation, or other laboratory; tutoring.

BACCALAUREATE PROGRAMS

Degree BSN
Available Programs ADN to Baccalaureate; Accelerated Baccalaureate for Second Degree; Generic Baccalaureate.
Site Options Houston, TX.
Study Options Full-time.
Program Entrance Requirements Transcript of college record, CPR certification, written essay, health exam, immunizations, interview, minimum GPA in nursing prerequisites of 2.75, prerequisite course work. Transfer students are accepted. *Application deadline:* 1/15 (fall), 9/1 (spring), 12/1 (summer). *Application fee:* $30.

Advanced Placement Credit given for nursing courses completed elsewhere dependent upon specific evaluations.
Contact *Telephone:* 713-500-2101. *Fax:* 713-500-2107.

GRADUATE PROGRAMS

Contact *Telephone:* 713-500-2101. *Fax:* 713-500-2107.

MASTER'S DEGREE PROGRAM
Degrees MSN; MSN/MPH
Available Programs Master's.
Concentrations Available Nurse anesthesia; nursing administration; nursing education. *Clinical nurse specialist programs in:* acute care, adult health, critical care, gerontology. *Nurse practitioner programs in:* acute care, adult health, family health, gerontology, pediatric, psychiatric/mental health, women's health.
Study Options Full-time and part-time.
Program Entrance Requirements Clinical experience, minimum overall college GPA of 3.0, transcript of college record, CPR certification, immunizations, interview, 3 letters of recommendation, prerequisite course work, resume, statistics course, GRE or MAT. *Application deadline:* 4/15 (fall), 2/15 (summer). *Application fee:* $30.
Advanced Placement Credit given for nursing courses completed elsewhere dependent upon specific evaluations.
Degree Requirements 48 total credit hours, thesis or project.

POST-MASTER'S PROGRAM
Areas of Study Nursing administration; nursing education. *Clinical nurse specialist programs in:* acute care, adult health, critical care, gerontology, oncology. *Nurse practitioner programs in:* acute care, adult health, family health, gerontology, oncology, pediatric, psychiatric/mental health, women's health.

DOCTORAL DEGREE PROGRAM
Degree PhD
Available Programs Doctorate.
Areas of Study Addiction/substance abuse, advanced practice nursing, aging, bio-behavioral research, biology of health and illness, clinical practice, community health, critical care, ethics, faculty preparation, family health, gerontology, health policy, health promotion/disease prevention, health-care systems, human health and illness, illness and transition, individualized study, information systems, maternity-newborn, neuro-behavior, nurse case management, nursing administration, nursing education, nursing policy, nursing research, nursing science, oncology, urban health, women's health.
Program Entrance Requirements Minimum overall college GPA of 3.0, interview by faculty committee, 3 letters of recommendation, MSN or equivalent, vita, writing sample, GRE. *Application deadline:* 4/1 (fall). *Application fee:* $30.
Degree Requirements 66 total credit hours, dissertation.

CONTINUING EDUCATION PROGRAM

Contact *Telephone:* 713-500-2116. *Fax:* 713-500-2026.

The University of Texas Health Science Center at San Antonio
School of Nursing
San Antonio, Texas

http://www.nursing.uthscsa.edu/
Founded in 1976
DEGREES • BSN • MSN • PHD
Nursing Program Faculty 122 (63% with doctorates).
Baccalaureate Enrollment 558 **Women** 84.59% **Men** 15.41% **Minority** 53.23% **International** 1.79% **Part-time** 2.15%
Graduate Enrollment 258 **Women** 16% **Men** 84% **Minority** 54% **International** 2% **Part-time** 41%
Distance Learning Courses Available.
Nursing Student Activities Nursing Honor Society, Sigma Theta Tau, Student Nurses' Association, nursing club.
Nursing Student Resources Academic advising; academic or career counseling; assistance for students with disabilities; bookstore; campus computer network; career placement assistance; computer lab; computer-assisted instruction; e-mail services; employment services for current students; housing assistance; interactive nursing skills videos; Internet; learning resource lab; library services; nursing audiovisuals; placement services for program completers; remedial services; resume preparation assistance; skills, simulation, or other laboratory; tutoring.
Library Facilities 4,793 volumes in health, 4,091 volumes in nursing; 4,367 periodical subscriptions health-care related.

BACCALAUREATE PROGRAMS

Degree BSN
Available Programs Accelerated Baccalaureate for Second Degree; Generic Baccalaureate.
Study Options Full-time.
Program Entrance Requirements Minimum overall college GPA of 2.5, transcript of college record, CPR certification, written essay, health insurance, immunizations, minimum GPA in nursing prerequisites of 3.0, professional liability insurance/malpractice insurance, prerequisite course work. Transfer students are accepted. *Application deadline:* 1/10 (fall), 7/1 (spring), 11/1 (summer). *Application fee:* $45.
Advanced Placement Credit given for nursing courses completed elsewhere dependent upon specific evaluations.
Expenses (2012–13) *Tuition, state resident:* full-time $19,009. *Tuition, nonresident:* full-time $42,169. *International tuition:* $42,169 full-time.
Financial Aid 84% of baccalaureate students in nursing programs received some form of financial aid in 2011–12.
Contact Dr. Ilene M. Decker, Associate Dean for Undergraduate Studies, School of Nursing, The University of Texas Health Science Center at San Antonio, 7703 Floyd Curl Drive, MC 7945, San Antonio, TX 78229-3900. *Telephone:* 210-567-5810. *Fax:* 210-567-3813. *E-mail:* deckerI@uthscsa.edu.

GRADUATE PROGRAMS

Expenses (2012–13) *Tuition, state resident:* full-time $15,960. *Tuition, nonresident:* full-time $36,499. *International tuition:* $36,499 full-time.
Financial Aid 76% of graduate students in nursing programs received some form of financial aid in 2011–12. 3 fellowships with full tuition reimbursements available (averaging $30,000 per year) were awarded; research assistantships, teaching assistantships, institutionally sponsored loans and scholarships also available. *Financial aid application deadline:* 6/30.
Contact Dr. Ilene M. Decker, Associate Dean, School of Nursing, The University of Texas Health Science Center at San Antonio, 7703 Floyd Curl Drive, MC 7945, San Antonio, TX 78229-3900. *Telephone:* 210-567-5810. *Fax:* 210-567-3813. *E-mail:* DeckerI@uthscsa.edu.

MASTER'S DEGREE PROGRAM
Degree MSN
Available Programs Master's; RN to Master's.
Concentrations Available Clinical nurse leader; nursing administration. *Nurse practitioner programs in:* family health, gerontology, pediatric, psychiatric/mental health.
Study Options Full-time and part-time.
Program Entrance Requirements Computer literacy, minimum overall college GPA of 3.0, transcript of college record, CPR certification, written essay, immunizations, 3 letters of recommendation, professional liability insurance/malpractice insurance, statistics course. *Application deadline:* 1/10 (fall), 7/1 (spring). *Application fee:* $65.
Advanced Placement Credit given for nursing courses completed elsewhere dependent upon specific evaluations.
Degree Requirements 50 total credit hours, thesis or project.

POST-MASTER'S PROGRAM
Areas of Study *Nurse practitioner programs in:* family health, pediatric, psychiatric/mental health.

DOCTORAL DEGREE PROGRAM
Degree PhD
Available Programs Doctorate; Post-Baccalaureate Doctorate.
Areas of Study Nursing research.
Program Entrance Requirements Clinical experience, minimum overall college GPA of 3.0, interview, 3 letters of recommendation, MSN or equivalent, statistics course, vita, writing sample, GRE, MAT. *Application deadline:* 2/1 (fall). *Application fee:* $65.
Degree Requirements 80 total credit hours.

CONTINUING EDUCATION PROGRAM

Contact Laura Alvarado, Director of Nursing Continuing Education, School of Nursing, The University of Texas Health Science Center at San Antonio, 7703 Floyd Curl Drive, San Antonio, TX 78229-3900. *Telephone:* 210-567-0170. *Fax:* 210-567-5909. *E-mail:* AlvaradoLV@uthsca.edu.

The University of Texas Medical Branch
School of Nursing
Galveston, Texas

http://www.son.utmb.edu/
Founded in 1891
DEGREES • BSN • MSN • PHD
Nursing Program Faculty 60 (57% with doctorates).
Baccalaureate Enrollment 476 **Women** 82% **Men** 18% **Minority** 30%
International 1% **Part-time** 14%
Graduate Enrollment 442 **Women** 86% **Men** 14% **Minority** 26%
International .27% **Part-time** 79.9%
Distance Learning Courses Available.
Nursing Student Activities Nursing Honor Society, Sigma Theta Tau, Student Nurses' Association.
Nursing Student Resources Academic advising; academic or career counseling; assistance for students with disabilities; bookstore; campus computer network; career placement assistance; computer lab; computer-assisted instruction; e-mail services; employment services for current students; housing assistance; interactive nursing skills videos; Internet; learning resource lab; library services; nursing audiovisuals; resume preparation assistance; skills, simulation, or other laboratory; tutoring.
Library Facilities 287,463 volumes in health, 7,304 volumes in nursing; 11,237 periodical subscriptions health-care related.

BACCALAUREATE PROGRAMS

Degree BSN
Available Programs Accelerated Baccalaureate for Second Degree; Generic Baccalaureate; RN Baccalaureate.
Study Options Full-time.
Program Entrance Requirements Minimum overall college GPA of 2.75, transcript of college record, CPR certification, written essay, health insurance, immunizations, interview, minimum GPA in nursing prerequisites of 2.75, professional liability insurance/malpractice insurance, prerequisite course work. Transfer students are accepted. *Application deadline:* 1/15 (fall), 6/15 (spring). *Application fee:* $25.
Advanced Placement Credit by examination available. Credit given for nursing courses completed elsewhere dependent upon specific evaluations.
Expenses (2012–13) *Tuition, state resident:* full-time $8427; part-time $187 per credit hour. *Tuition, nonresident:* full-time $24,292; part-time $540 per credit hour. *International tuition:* $24,292 full-time. *Room and board:* $14,736; room only: $10,352 per academic year. *Required fees:* full-time $4815.
Financial Aid 95% of baccalaureate students in nursing programs received some form of financial aid in 2011–12.
Contact Dr. Charlotte Wisnewski, Associate Professor and Director of Baccalaureate Programs, School of Nursing, The University of Texas Medical Branch, 301 University Boulevard, Galveston, TX 77555-1132. *Telephone:* 409-772-8235. *Fax:* 409-772-3770. *E-mail:* cwisnews@utmb.edu.

GRADUATE PROGRAMS

Expenses (2012–13) *Tuition, state resident:* full-time $7302; part-time $228 per credit hour. *Tuition, nonresident:* full-time $18,534; part-time $579 per credit hour. *International tuition:* $18,534 full-time. *Room and board:* $14,736; room only: $10,352 per academic year. *Required fees:* full-time $5495.
Financial Aid 42% of graduate students in nursing programs received some form of financial aid in 2011–12.
Contact Dr. Bruce Leonard, Associate Professor and Masters Program Director, School of Nursing, The University of Texas Medical Branch, 301 University Boulevard, Galveston, TX 77555-1029. *Telephone:* 409-772-8225. *Fax:* 409-772-8323. *E-mail:* brleonar@utmb.edu.

MASTER'S DEGREE PROGRAM
Degree MSN
Available Programs Master's.
Concentrations Available Clinical nurse leader; nursing administration; nursing education. *Nurse practitioner programs in:* family health, gerontology, neonatal health.
Study Options Full-time and part-time.
Online Degree Options Yes (online only).
Program Entrance Requirements Clinical experience, computer literacy, minimum overall college GPA of 3.0, transcript of college record, CPR certification, immunizations, interview, 3 letters of recommendation, professional liability insurance/malpractice insurance, prerequisite course work, statistics course. *Application deadline:* 3/1 (fall). *Application fee:* $60.
Advanced Placement Credit given for nursing courses completed elsewhere dependent upon specific evaluations.
Degree Requirements 46 total credit hours.

POST-MASTER'S PROGRAM
Areas of Study Clinical nurse leader; nursing administration; nursing education. *Nurse practitioner programs in:* family health, gerontology, neonatal health.

DOCTORAL DEGREE PROGRAM
Degree PhD
Available Programs Doctorate; Post-Baccalaureate Doctorate.
Areas of Study Health promotion/disease prevention.
Online Degree Options Yes (online only).
Program Entrance Requirements Clinical experience, minimum overall college GPA of 3.5, interview by faculty committee, interview, 3 letters of recommendation, MSN or equivalent, statistics course, vita, writing sample. *Application deadline:* 3/1 (fall). *Application fee:* $50.
Degree Requirements 63 total credit hours, dissertation, oral exam, written exam, residency.

The University of Texas–Pan American
Department of Nursing
Edinburg, Texas

http://www.utpa.edu/
Founded in 1927
DEGREES • BSN • MSN
Nursing Program Faculty 23 (45% with doctorates).
Baccalaureate Enrollment 170 **Women** 78% **Men** 22% **Minority** 90%
Graduate Enrollment 65 **Women** 88% **Men** 12% **Minority** 88% **Part-time** 75%
Nursing Student Activities Sigma Theta Tau, Student Nurses' Association.
Nursing Student Resources Academic advising; academic or career counseling; assistance for students with disabilities; bookstore; campus computer network; career placement assistance; computer lab; computer-assisted instruction; daycare for children of students; e-mail services; employment services for current students; housing assistance; interactive nursing skills videos; Internet; learning resource lab; library services; nursing audiovisuals; remedial services; skills, simulation, or other laboratory; tutoring.
Library Facilities 230 volumes in health, 200 volumes in nursing; 300 periodical subscriptions health-care related.

BACCALAUREATE PROGRAMS

Degree BSN
Available Programs ADN to Baccalaureate; Generic Baccalaureate; RN Baccalaureate.
Study Options Full-time.
Program Entrance Requirements Transcript of college record, CPR certification, immunizations, minimum GPA in nursing prerequisites of 2.5, professional liability insurance/malpractice insurance, prerequisite course work. Transfer students are accepted. *Application deadline:* 10/1 (fall), 10/1 (spring).
Contact *Telephone:* 956-381-3491. *Fax:* 956-381-2875.

GRADUATE PROGRAMS

Contact *Telephone:* 956-381-3491. *Fax:* 956-381-2875.

MASTER'S DEGREE PROGRAM
Degree MSN
Available Programs Master's.
Concentrations Available *Clinical nurse specialist programs in:* adult health. *Nurse practitioner programs in:* family health, pediatric.
Study Options Full-time and part-time.
Program Entrance Requirements Minimum overall college GPA of 2.75, transcript of college record, written essay, immunizations, 3 letters of recommendation, resume, statistics course. *Application deadline:* 7/1 (fall), 10/1 (winter), 4/1 (spring), 4/1 (summer).

Advanced Placement Credit given for nursing courses completed elsewhere dependent upon specific evaluations.

Degree Requirements 48 total credit hours, thesis or project.

POST-MASTER'S PROGRAM

Areas of Study *Clinical nurse specialist programs in:* adult health. *Nurse practitioner programs in:* family health, pediatric.

University of the Incarnate Word

Ila Faye Miller School of Nursing and Health Professions
San Antonio, Texas

http://www.uiw.edu/snhp
Founded in 1881

DEGREES • BSN • DNP • MSN

Nursing Program Faculty 39 (41% with doctorates).

Baccalaureate Enrollment 251 **Women** 87% **Men** 13% **Minority** 70% **International** 2%

Graduate Enrollment 66 **Women** 76% **Men** 24% **Minority** 39% **International** 10% **Part-time** 91%

Distance Learning Courses Available.

Nursing Student Activities Sigma Theta Tau, Student Nurses' Association.

Nursing Student Resources Academic advising; academic or career counseling; assistance for students with disabilities; bookstore; campus computer network; career placement assistance; computer lab; computer-assisted instruction; e-mail services; employment services for current students; externships; housing assistance; interactive nursing skills videos; Internet; learning resource lab; library services; nursing audiovisuals; paid internships; placement services for program completers; remedial services; resume preparation assistance; skills, simulation, or other laboratory; tutoring; unpaid internships.

Library Facilities 273,468 volumes (6,000 in health, 6,000 in nursing); 70,017 periodical subscriptions (3,048 health-care related).

BACCALAUREATE PROGRAMS

Degree BSN

Available Programs ADN to Baccalaureate; Baccalaureate for Second Degree; Generic Baccalaureate.

Study Options Full-time.

Online Degree Options Yes.

Program Entrance Requirements Minimum overall college GPA of 2.5, transcript of college record, CPR certification, health exam, health insurance, immunizations, minimum GPA in nursing prerequisites of 2.5, professional liability insurance/malpractice insurance, prerequisite course work. Transfer students are accepted. *Application deadline:* 2/1 (fall), 9/1 (spring). *Application fee:* $20.

Advanced Placement Credit given for nursing courses completed elsewhere dependent upon specific evaluations.

Expenses (2012–13) *Tuition:* full-time $22,800; part-time $755 per credit hour. *Room and board:* $10,094 per academic year. *Required fees:* full-time $1990.

Financial Aid 90% of baccalaureate students in nursing programs received some form of financial aid in 2011–12. *Gift aid (need-based):* Federal Pell, FSEOG, state, private, college/university gift aid from institutional funds, United Negro College Fund, Federal Nursing. *Loans:* Federal Nursing Student Loans, Federal Direct (Subsidized and Unsubsidized Stafford PLUS), Perkins, state, alternative loans. *Work-study:* Federal Work-Study, part-time campus jobs. *Financial aid application deadline (priority):* 4/1.

Contact Ms. Heather Rodriguez, Office of Admissions, Ila Faye Miller School of Nursing and Health Professions, University of the Incarnate Word, 4301 Broadway, San Antonio, TX 78209. *Telephone:* 210-829-6005. *E-mail:* admis@uiwtx.edu.

GRADUATE PROGRAMS

Expenses (2012–13) *Tuition:* full-time $18,840; part-time $785 per credit. *International tuition:* $18,840 full-time. *Required fees:* full-time $2352; part-time $98 per credit.

Financial Aid 75% of graduate students in nursing programs received some form of financial aid in 2011–12. Federal Work-Study, scholarships, and traineeships available. Aid available to part-time students.

Contact Dr. Holly B. Cassells, Director of Graduate Nursing Programs, Ila Faye Miller School of Nursing and Health Professions, University of the Incarnate Word, 4301 Broadway, San Antonio, TX 78209. *Telephone:* 210-829-3977. *Fax:* 210-829-3174. *E-mail:* cassells@uiwtx.edu.

MASTER'S DEGREE PROGRAM

Degree MSN

Available Programs Accelerated AD/RN to Master's; Master's.

Concentrations Available Clinical nurse leader. *Clinical nurse specialist programs in:* adult health.

Study Options Full-time and part-time.

Program Entrance Requirements Clinical experience, minimum overall college GPA of 3.0, transcript of college record, CPR certification, immunizations, 3 letters of recommendation, physical assessment course, professional liability insurance/malpractice insurance, statistics course. *Application deadline:* Applications may be processed on a rolling basis for some programs. *Application fee:* $20.

Advanced Placement Credit given for nursing courses completed elsewhere dependent upon specific evaluations.

Degree Requirements 42 total credit hours.

POST-MASTER'S PROGRAM

Areas of Study Clinical nurse leader. *Clinical nurse specialist programs in:* adult health.

DOCTORAL DEGREE PROGRAM

Degree DNP

Available Programs Doctorate.

Areas of Study Advanced practice nursing.

Online Degree Options Yes (online only).

Program Entrance Requirements Minimum overall college GPA of 3.0, interview, 3 letters of recommendation, MSN or equivalent, statistics course. *Application deadline:* Applications may be processed on a rolling basis for some programs. *Application fee:* $20.

Degree Requirements 33 total credit hours.

Wayland Baptist University

Bachelor of Science in Nursing Program
Plainview, Texas

Founded in 1908

DEGREE • BSN

Library Facilities 129,646 volumes; 779 periodical subscriptions.

BACCALAUREATE PROGRAMS

Degree BSN

Available Programs RN Baccalaureate.

Contact *Telephone:* 210-826-7595 Ext. 228.

West Texas A&M University

Department of Nursing
Canyon, Texas

http://www.wtamu.edu/nursing
Founded in 1909

DEGREES • BSN • MSN

Nursing Program Faculty 30 (23% with doctorates).

Baccalaureate Enrollment 380 **Women** 84% **Men** 16% **Minority** 27% **International** 1% **Part-time** 35%

Graduate Enrollment 54 **Women** 85% **Men** 15% **Minority** 9% **Part-time** 52%

Nursing Student Activities Sigma Theta Tau, Student Nurses' Association.

Nursing Student Resources Academic advising; academic or career counseling; assistance for students with disabilities; bookstore; campus computer network; career placement assistance; computer lab; computer-assisted instruction; daycare for children of students; e-mail services; employment services for current students; housing assistance; interactive nursing skills videos; Internet; learning resource lab; library services; nursing audiovisuals; placement services for program completers; remedial services; resume preparation assistance; skills, simulation, or other laboratory; tutoring.

Library Facilities 1.1 million volumes (17,000 in health, 10,000 in nursing); 19,022 periodical subscriptions (75 health-care related).

BACCALAUREATE PROGRAMS

Degree BSN
Available Programs ADN to Baccalaureate; Generic Baccalaureate; LPN to Baccalaureate.
Study Options Full-time and part-time.
Program Entrance Requirements Minimum overall college GPA of 2.5, transcript of college record, CPR certification, immunizations, minimum GPA in nursing prerequisites of 2.0, prerequisite course work. Transfer students are accepted.
Advanced Placement Credit given for nursing courses completed elsewhere dependent upon specific evaluations.
Contact *Telephone:* 806-651-2661. *Fax:* 806-651-2632.

GRADUATE PROGRAMS

Contact *Telephone:* 806-651-2637. *Fax:* 806-651-2632.

MASTER'S DEGREE PROGRAM

Degree MSN
Available Programs Master's; RN to Master's.
Concentrations Available Nursing administration; nursing education. *Nurse practitioner programs in:* family health.
Study Options Full-time and part-time.
Program Entrance Requirements Clinical experience, computer literacy, minimum overall college GPA of 3.0, transcript of college record, CPR certification, immunizations, nursing research course, prerequisite course work, statistics course, GRE General Test.
Advanced Placement Credit given for nursing courses completed elsewhere dependent upon specific evaluations.
Degree Requirements 39 total credit hours, thesis or project.

POST-MASTER'S PROGRAM

Areas of Study *Nurse practitioner programs in:* family health.

UTAH

Brigham Young University
College of Nursing
Provo, Utah

http://nursing.byu.edu/
Founded in 1875
DEGREES • BS • MS
Nursing Program Faculty 46 (43% with doctorates).
Baccalaureate Enrollment 370 **Women** 93.5% **Men** 6.5% **Minority** 5.4% **International** 2%
Graduate Enrollment 26 **Women** 69% **Men** 31% **Minority** 3%
Nursing Student Activities Nursing Honor Society, Sigma Theta Tau, Student Nurses' Association.
Nursing Student Resources Academic advising; academic or career counseling; assistance for students with disabilities; bookstore; campus computer network; career placement assistance; computer lab; computer-assisted instruction; e-mail services; employment services for current students; housing assistance; interactive nursing skills videos; Internet; learning resource lab; library services; nursing audiovisuals; other; paid internships; resume preparation assistance; skills, simulation, or other laboratory; tutoring.
Library Facilities 72,332 volumes in health, 5,217 volumes in nursing; 10,500 periodical subscriptions health-care related.

BACCALAUREATE PROGRAMS

Degree BS
Available Programs RN Baccalaureate.
Study Options Full-time.
Program Entrance Requirements Minimum overall college GPA, transcript of college record, CPR certification, written essay, 2 letters of recommendation, minimum GPA in nursing prerequisites of 3.0, prerequisite course work. Transfer students are accepted. *Application deadline:* 5/31 (fall), 9/30 (winter).
Advanced Placement Credit given for nursing courses completed elsewhere dependent upon specific evaluations.

Expenses (2012–13) *Tuition:* full-time $4710; part-time $242 per credit hour. *Room and board:* $3215; room only: $2215 per academic year. *Required fees:* full-time $100.
Financial Aid 30% of baccalaureate students in nursing programs received some form of financial aid in 2011–12.
Contact Dr. Mark E. White, Advisement Center Supervisor, College of Nursing, Brigham Young University, 550 SWKT, Provo, UT 84602-5532. *Telephone:* 801-422-7211. *Fax:* 801-422-0536. *E-mail:* mark_white@byu.edu.

GRADUATE PROGRAMS

Expenses (2012–13) *Tuition:* full-time $5950; part-time $331 per credit hour.
Financial Aid 100% of graduate students in nursing programs received some form of financial aid in 2011–12. 2 research assistantships with full and partial tuition reimbursements available (averaging $10,000 per year), 3 teaching assistantships with full and partial tuition reimbursements available (averaging $10,000 per year) were awarded; institutionally sponsored loans, scholarships, tuition waivers (full), and unspecified assistantships also available. Aid available to part-time students. *Financial aid application deadline:* 2/1.
Contact Ms. Stephanie Von Forell, Research Center and Graduate Program Secretary, College of Nursing, Brigham Young University, 400 SWKT, Provo, UT 84602-5532. *Telephone:* 801-422-4142. *Fax:* 801-422-0536. *E-mail:* nursing_graduate@byu.edu.

MASTER'S DEGREE PROGRAM

Degree MS
Available Programs Master's.
Concentrations Available *Nurse practitioner programs in:* family health.
Study Options Full-time and part-time.
Program Entrance Requirements Clinical experience, minimum overall college GPA of 3.0, transcript of college record, CPR certification, written essay, immunizations, interview, 3 letters of recommendation, prerequisite course work, resume, statistics course, GRE. *Application deadline:* 12/1 (spring). *Application fee:* $50.
Advanced Placement Credit given for nursing courses completed elsewhere dependent upon specific evaluations.
Degree Requirements 56 total credit hours, thesis or project.

POST-MASTER'S PROGRAM

Areas of Study *Nurse practitioner programs in:* family health.

Dixie State College of Utah
Nursing Department
St. George, Utah

Founded in 1911
DEGREE • BSN
Library Facilities 166,120 volumes; 190 periodical subscriptions.

BACCALAUREATE PROGRAMS

Degree BSN
Available Programs RN Baccalaureate.
Program Entrance Requirements Written essay, immunizations, RN licensure. *Application deadline:* 3/15 (fall), 9/15 (spring).
Contact *Telephone:* 435-879-4802.

Southern Utah University
Department of Nursing
Cedar City, Utah

http://www.suu.edu/cose/nursing/
Founded in 1897
DEGREE • BSN
Nursing Program Faculty 9 (2% with doctorates).
Baccalaureate Enrollment 96 **Women** 70% **Men** 30% **Minority** 5% **International** 1%
Nursing Student Activities Nursing Honor Society, Student Nurses' Association, nursing club.
Nursing Student Resources Academic advising; academic or career counseling; assistance for students with disabilities; bookstore; campus

computer network; career placement assistance; computer lab; computer-assisted instruction; daycare for children of students; e-mail services; employment services for current students; externships; housing assistance; interactive nursing skills videos; Internet; learning resource lab; library services; nursing audiovisuals; remedial services; resume preparation assistance; skills, simulation, or other laboratory; tutoring.
Library Facilities 241,996 volumes (1,000 in health, 1,000 in nursing); 5,000 periodical subscriptions health-care related.

BACCALAUREATE PROGRAMS

Degree BSN
Available Programs Generic Baccalaureate; RN Baccalaureate.
Study Options Full-time.
Program Entrance Requirements Minimum overall college GPA of 3.0, transcript of college record, written essay, health insurance, immunizations, 3 letters of recommendation, minimum GPA in nursing prerequisites of 3.0, prerequisite course work. Transfer students are accepted. *Application deadline:* 2/8 (fall), 9/12 (spring). *Application fee:* $20.
Advanced Placement Credit given for nursing courses completed elsewhere dependent upon specific evaluations.
Expenses (2012–13) *Tuition, state resident:* full-time $4100. *Tuition, nonresident:* full-time $14,500. *Room and board:* $7100; room only: $3600 per academic year. *Required fees:* full-time $540.
Financial Aid 80% of baccalaureate students in nursing programs received some form of financial aid in 2011–12.
Contact Vikki Robertson, Department Secretary, Department of Nursing, Southern Utah University, 351 West University Boulevard, GC 005, Cedar City, UT 84720. *Telephone:* 435-586-1906. *Fax:* 435-586-1984. *E-mail:* robertsonv@suu.edu.

University of Phoenix–Utah Campus
College of Health and Human Services
Salt Lake City, Utah

Founded in 1984
Nursing Program Faculty 2
Nursing Student Activities Sigma Theta Tau.
Nursing Student Resources Academic advising; academic or career counseling; assistance for students with disabilities; bookstore; campus computer network; computer lab; computer-assisted instruction; e-mail services; interactive nursing skills videos; Internet; learning resource lab; library services; nursing audiovisuals; remedial services; skills, simulation, or other laboratory; tutoring.
Library Facilities 16,871 periodical subscriptions (1,300 health-care related).

University of Utah
College of Nursing
Salt Lake City, Utah

http://www.nursing.utah.edu/
Founded in 1850
DEGREES • BS • MS • PHD
Nursing Program Faculty 101 (55% with doctorates).
Baccalaureate Enrollment 307 **Women** 80% **Men** 20% **Minority** 9% **International** 3% **Part-time** 19%
Graduate Enrollment 345 **Women** 83% **Men** 17% **Minority** 12% **International** 3% **Part-time** 29%
Distance Learning Courses Available.
Nursing Student Activities Sigma Theta Tau, Student Nurses' Association.
Nursing Student Resources Academic advising; academic or career counseling; assistance for students with disabilities; bookstore; campus computer network; career placement assistance; computer lab; computer-assisted instruction; e-mail services; employment services for current students; interactive nursing skills videos; Internet; learning resource lab; library services; nursing audiovisuals; remedial services; resume preparation assistance; skills, simulation, or other laboratory.
Library Facilities 4.2 million volumes (212,579 in health, 6,603 in nursing); 68,225 periodical subscriptions (5,201 health-care related).

BACCALAUREATE PROGRAMS

Degree BS
Available Programs Accelerated Baccalaureate; Generic Baccalaureate; RN Baccalaureate.
Study Options Full-time.
Program Entrance Requirements Minimum overall college GPA of 2.8, transcript of college record, CPR certification, written essay, health exam, immunizations, interview, 3 letters of recommendation, minimum GPA in nursing prerequisites of 3.0, prerequisite course work. Transfer students are accepted. *Application deadline:* 1/15 (fall), 1/15 (summer).
Advanced Placement Credit by examination available. Credit given for nursing courses completed elsewhere dependent upon specific evaluations.
Expenses (2012–13) *Tuition, state resident:* full-time $8926; part-time $2246 per semester. *Tuition, nonresident:* full-time $23,688; part-time $9321 per semester. *International tuition:* $23,688 full-time. *Room and board:* $7705; room only: $3719 per academic year. *Required fees:* full-time $1771; part-time $57 per credit.
Financial Aid 64% of baccalaureate students in nursing programs received some form of financial aid in 2011–12. *Gift aid (need-based):* Federal Pell, FSEOG, state, private, college/university gift aid from institutional funds, Federal Nursing, Academic Competitiveness Grants, National SMART Grants, TEACH Grants. *Loans:* Federal Nursing Student Loans, Federal Direct (Subsidized and Unsubsidized Stafford PLUS), Perkins, college/university, private loans. *Work-study:* Federal Work-Study. *Financial aid application deadline (priority):* 4/1.
Contact Ms. Cynthia Weatbrook, Undergraduate Academic Advisor, College of Nursing, University of Utah, 10 South 2000 East, Salt Lake City, UT 84112-5880. *Telephone:* 801-581-3414. *Fax:* 801-585-9705. *E-mail:* cynthia.weatbrook@nurs.utah.edu.

GRADUATE PROGRAMS

Expenses (2012–13) *Tuition, state resident:* full-time $11,473. *Tuition, nonresident:* full-time $28,423. *Required fees:* full-time $868.
Financial Aid 41% of graduate students in nursing programs received some form of financial aid in 2011–12. 105 fellowships with full and partial tuition reimbursements available (averaging $6,060 per year), 6 research assistantships with full tuition reimbursements available (averaging $6,500 per year), 13 teaching assistantships with partial tuition reimbursements available (averaging $4,025 per year) were awarded; scholarships, traineeships, and unspecified assistantships also available. Aid available to part-time students. *Financial aid application deadline:* 3/15.
Contact Jennifer Bangerter, PhD, Co-Director, Academic Programs and Student Services, College of Nursing, University of Utah, 10 South 2000 East, Salt Lake City, UT 84112-5880. *Telephone:* 801-585-6658. *Fax:* 801-585-9705. *E-mail:* j.aoyagi.bangerter@nurs.utah.edu.

MASTER'S DEGREE PROGRAM
Degree MS
Available Programs Master's; RN to Master's.
Concentrations Available Nursing education; nursing informatics. *Nurse practitioner programs in:* gerontology, psychiatric/mental health.
Site Options St. George, UT.
Study Options Full-time.
Program Entrance Requirements Clinical experience, computer literacy, minimum overall college GPA of 3.0, transcript of college record, CPR certification, written essay, immunizations, interview, 3 letters of recommendation, professional liability insurance/malpractice insurance, resume, statistics course, GRE General Test (if cumulative GPA less than 3.2). *Application deadline:* 1/15 (fall). *Application fee:* $55.
Advanced Placement Credit given for nursing courses completed elsewhere dependent upon specific evaluations.
Degree Requirements 40 total credit hours, thesis or project, comprehensive exam.

POST-MASTER'S PROGRAM
Areas of Study Nurse-midwifery; nursing education; nursing informatics. *Nurse practitioner programs in:* acute care, adult health, family health, gerontology, pediatric, psychiatric/mental health, women's health.

DOCTORAL DEGREE PROGRAM
Degree PhD
Available Programs Doctorate; Doctorate for Nurses with Non-Nursing Degrees; Post-Baccalaureate Doctorate.
Areas of Study Aging, bio-behavioral research, community health, critical care, ethics, faculty preparation, family health, gerontology, health policy, health promotion/disease prevention, health-care systems, human health and illness, illness and transition, individualized study,

information systems, maternity-newborn, nursing administration, nursing education, nursing policy, nursing research, nursing science, oncology, women's health.

Program Entrance Requirements Clinical experience, minimum overall college GPA of 3.3, interview by faculty committee, interview, 3 letters of recommendation, statistics course, vita, writing sample, GRE General Test. *Application deadline:* 1/15 (fall).

Degree Requirements 62 total credit hours, dissertation, oral exam, written exam, residency.

POSTDOCTORAL PROGRAM

Areas of Study Aging, cancer care, chronic illness, gerontology, information systems, nursing informatics, nursing interventions, nursing research, nursing science, women's health.

Postdoctoral Program Contact Dr. Ginette A. Pepper, Associate Dean for Research and PhD Programs, College of Nursing, University of Utah, 10 South 2000 East, Salt Lake City, UT 84112-5880. *Telephone:* 801-585-7872. *Fax:* 801-581-4642. *E-mail:* ginny.pepper@nurs.utah.edu.

Utah Valley University
Department of Nursing
Orem, Utah

http://www.uvu.edu/
Founded in 1941

DEGREE • BSN

Nursing Program Faculty 22 (25% with doctorates).
Baccalaureate Enrollment 100 **Women** 60% **Men** 40% **Part-time** 99%
Nursing Student Activities Student Nurses' Association.
Nursing Student Resources Academic advising; academic or career counseling; assistance for students with disabilities; bookstore; campus computer network; career placement assistance; computer lab; computer-assisted instruction; daycare for children of students; e-mail services; employment services for current students; interactive nursing skills videos; Internet; learning resource lab; library services; nursing audiovisuals; resume preparation assistance; skills, simulation, or other laboratory; tutoring; unpaid internships.
Library Facilities 228,000 volumes (4,640 in health, 361 in nursing); 568 periodical subscriptions (200 health-care related).

BACCALAUREATE PROGRAMS

Degree BSN
Available Programs ADN to Baccalaureate.
Study Options Part-time.
Program Entrance Requirements CPR certification, health exam, health insurance, immunizations, minimum GPA in nursing prerequisites of 2.5, prerequisite course work, RN licensure. Transfer students are accepted.
Advanced Placement Credit by examination available.
Contact *Telephone:* 801-863-8199. *Fax:* 801-863-6093.

Weber State University
Program in Nursing
Ogden, Utah

http://weber.edu/nursing
Founded in 1889

DEGREES • BSN • MSN

Nursing Program Faculty 42 (5% with doctorates).
Baccalaureate Enrollment 334 **Women** 86% **Men** 14% **Minority** 3% **International** 1% **Part-time** 4%
Graduate Enrollment 43 **Women** 85% **Men** 15% **Minority** 1%
Distance Learning Courses Available.
Nursing Student Activities Sigma Theta Tau, Student Nurses' Association.
Nursing Student Resources Academic advising; academic or career counseling; assistance for students with disabilities; bookstore; campus computer network; career placement assistance; computer lab; computer-assisted instruction; daycare for children of students; e-mail services; employment services for current students; housing assistance; interactive nursing skills videos; Internet; learning resource lab; library services; nursing audiovisuals; placement services for program completers; resume preparation assistance; skills, simulation, or other laboratory; tutoring; unpaid internships.
Library Facilities 694,095 volumes (800 in health, 800 in nursing); 769 periodical subscriptions (120 health-care related).

BACCALAUREATE PROGRAMS

Degree BSN
Available Programs ADN to Baccalaureate.
Site Options Layton, UT.
Study Options Full-time and part-time.
Program Entrance Requirements Minimum overall college GPA of 3.0, transcript of college record, CPR certification, health insurance, immunizations, minimum GPA in nursing prerequisites of 3.0, prerequisite course work, RN licensure. Transfer students are accepted. *Application deadline:* 3/10 (fall), 10/10 (spring). *Application fee:* $25.
Expenses (2011–12) *Tuition, state resident:* full-time $3800. *Tuition, nonresident:* full-time $11,500. *Required fees:* full-time $800.
Financial Aid 30% of baccalaureate students in nursing programs received some form of financial aid in 2010–11.
Contact Mr. Doug Watson, Academic Admissions Advisor, Program in Nursing, Weber State University, 3907 University Circle, Ogden, UT 84408-3907. *Telephone:* 801-626-6128. *Fax:* 801-626-6382. *E-mail:* dwatson@weber.edu.

GRADUATE PROGRAMS

Expenses (2011–12) *Tuition, state resident:* full-time $6000. *Tuition, nonresident:* full-time $60,000. *Required fees:* full-time $800.
Financial Aid 20% of graduate students in nursing programs received some form of financial aid in 2010–11.
Contact Mr. Robert W. Holt, Enrollment Director, Program in Nursing, Weber State University, 3903 University Circle, Ogden, UT 84408-3903. *Telephone:* 801-626-7774. *Fax:* 801-626-6397. *E-mail:* rholt@weber.edu.

MASTER'S DEGREE PROGRAM

Degree MSN
Available Programs Master's.
Concentrations Available Nursing administration; nursing education.
Study Options Full-time.
Program Entrance Requirements Clinical experience, minimum overall college GPA of 3.0, transcript of college record, CPR certification, written essay, immunizations, interview, 2 letters of recommendation, nursing research course, professional liability insurance/malpractice insurance, prerequisite course work, resume, statistics course. *Application deadline:* 3/1 (fall). *Application fee:* $100.
Degree Requirements 40 total credit hours, thesis or project.

Western Governors University
Online College of Health Professions
Salt Lake City, Utah

Founded in 1998

DEGREES • BS • MS

Baccalaureate Enrollment 3,281 **Women** 88% **Men** 12% **Minority** 33%
Graduate Enrollment 2,423 **Women** 89% **Men** 11% **Minority** 26%
Distance Learning Courses Available.
Nursing Student Resources Academic advising; academic or career counseling; assistance for students with disabilities; campus computer network; computer lab; computer-assisted instruction; e-mail services; employment services for current students; interactive nursing skills videos; Internet; learning resource lab; library services; nursing audiovisuals; resume preparation assistance; skills, simulation, or other laboratory; tutoring.

BACCALAUREATE PROGRAMS

Degree BS
Available Programs Accelerated Baccalaureate; Accelerated RN Baccalaureate; Generic Baccalaureate; LPN to RN Baccalaureate; RN Baccalaureate.
Site Options Indianapolis, IN; Los Angeles, CA; Houston, TX.
Study Options Full-time.
Online Degree Options Yes (online only).
Program Entrance Requirements Transfer students are accepted. *Application deadline:* Applications may be processed on a rolling basis for some programs. *Application fee:* $65.

Advanced Placement Credit by examination available.
Expenses (2012–13) *Tuition:* full-time $6500. *Required fees:* full-time $700.
Contact Admissions, Online College of Health Professions, Western Governors University, 4001 South 700 East, Suite 700, Salt Lake City, UT 84107-2533. *Telephone:* 801-274-3280. *Fax:* 801-274-3305.

GRADUATE PROGRAMS

Expenses (2012–13) *Tuition:* full-time $6500. *Required fees:* full-time $700.
Contact Admissions, Online College of Health Professions, Western Governors University, 4001 South 700 East, Suite 700, Salt Lake City, UT 84107-2533. *Telephone:* 801-274-3280. *Fax:* 801-274-3305.

MASTER'S DEGREE PROGRAM

Degree MS
Available Programs Accelerated Master's; Accelerated RN to Master's; Master's; RN to Master's.
Concentrations Available Clinical nurse leader; health-care administration; nursing administration; nursing education.
Study Options Full-time.
Online Degree Options Yes (online only).
Program Entrance Requirements Computer literacy, transcript of college record, interview. *Application deadline:* Applications may be processed on a rolling basis for some programs. *Application fee:* $65.
Advanced Placement Credit by examination available.
Degree Requirements 30 total credit hours, thesis or project.

Westminster College

School of Nursing and Health Sciences
Salt Lake City, Utah

http://www.westminstercollege.edu/nursing/
Founded in 1875
DEGREES • BSN • MSN
Nursing Student Activities Sigma Theta Tau, Student Nurses' Association, nursing club.
Nursing Student Resources Academic advising; academic or career counseling; assistance for students with disabilities; bookstore; campus computer network; career placement assistance; computer lab; computer-assisted instruction; e-mail services; employment services for current students; housing assistance; interactive nursing skills videos; Internet; learning resource lab; library services; nursing audiovisuals; placement services for program completers; remedial services; resume preparation assistance; skills, simulation, or other laboratory; tutoring.
Library Facilities 123,552 volumes; 20,117 periodical subscriptions.

BACCALAUREATE PROGRAMS

Degree BSN
Available Programs Baccalaureate for Second Degree; Generic Baccalaureate; RN Baccalaureate.
Study Options Full-time.
Program Entrance Requirements Transcript of college record, written essay, 3 letters of recommendation, minimum GPA in nursing prerequisites of 2.5, prerequisite course work. Transfer students are accepted.
Contact *Telephone:* 801-832-2150. *Fax:* 801-832-3110.

GRADUATE PROGRAMS

Contact *Telephone:* 801-832-2150. *Fax:* 801-832-3110.

MASTER'S DEGREE PROGRAM

Degree MSN
Available Programs Master's.
Concentrations Available Nursing education. *Nurse practitioner programs in:* family health.
Program Entrance Requirements Transcript of college record, written essay, 3 letters of recommendation, resume, GRE.
Advanced Placement Credit given for nursing courses completed elsewhere dependent upon specific evaluations.
Degree Requirements 42 total credit hours, thesis or project.

POST-MASTER'S PROGRAM

Areas of Study *Nurse practitioner programs in:* family health.

VERMONT

Norwich University
Department of Nursing
Northfield, Vermont

http://programs.norwich.edu/mathscience/nursing/
Founded in 1819
DEGREE • BSN
Nursing Program Faculty 8 (10% with doctorates).
Baccalaureate Enrollment 90 **Women** 90% **Men** 10% **Minority** 10% **Part-time** 20%
Nursing Student Activities Student Nurses' Association, nursing club.
Nursing Student Resources Academic advising; academic or career counseling; assistance for students with disabilities; bookstore; campus computer network; career placement assistance; computer lab; e-mail services; employment services for current students; externships; housing assistance; interactive nursing skills videos; Internet; learning resource lab; library services; nursing audiovisuals; placement services for program completers; remedial services; resume preparation assistance; skills, simulation, or other laboratory; tutoring; unpaid internships.
Library Facilities 280,000 volumes; 904 periodical subscriptions.

BACCALAUREATE PROGRAMS

Degree BSN
Available Programs ADN to Baccalaureate; Generic Baccalaureate; RN Baccalaureate.
Site Options Rutland, VT.
Study Options Full-time and part-time.
Program Entrance Requirements Minimum overall college GPA of 2.5, transcript of college record, CPR certification, written essay, health exam, health insurance, high school biology, high school chemistry, 2 years high school math, 2 years high school science, high school transcript, immunizations, interview, 2 letters of recommendation, minimum GPA in nursing prerequisites of 2.5. Transfer students are accepted.
Advanced Placement Credit given for nursing courses completed elsewhere dependent upon specific evaluations.
Contact *Telephone:* 802-485-2008. *Fax:* 802-485-2032.

Southern Vermont College
Department of Nursing
Bennington, Vermont

http://www.svc.edu/academics/divisions/nursing.html
Founded in 1926
DEGREE • BSN
Nursing Program Faculty 16 (13% with doctorates).
Baccalaureate Enrollment 41 **Women** 76% **Men** 24% **Part-time** 75%
Distance Learning Courses Available.
Nursing Student Activities Student Nurses' Association.
Nursing Student Resources Academic advising; academic or career counseling; assistance for students with disabilities; bookstore; career placement assistance; computer lab; e-mail services; employment services for current students; Internet; library services; resume preparation assistance; skills, simulation, or other laboratory; tutoring.
Library Facilities 20,270 volumes; 33,000 periodical subscriptions.

BACCALAUREATE PROGRAMS

Degree BSN
Available Programs ADN to Baccalaureate; RN Baccalaureate.
Study Options Full-time and part-time.
Program Entrance Requirements CPR certification, written essay, health exam, immunizations, interview, 2 letters of recommendation, RN licensure. Transfer students are accepted. *Application deadline:* Applications may be processed on a rolling basis for some programs. *Application fee:* $30.
Advanced Placement Credit by examination available.
Financial Aid *Gift aid (need-based):* Federal Pell, FSEOG, state, private, college/university gift aid from institutional funds. *Loans:* Federal Direct (Subsidized and Unsubsidized Stafford PLUS).*Work-study:* Federal Work-Study.*Financial aid application deadline (priority):* 3/1.

Contact Dr. Karen Clement-O'Brien, Chair, Division of Nursing, Department of Nursing, Southern Vermont College, 982 Mansion Drive, Bennington, VT 05201. *Telephone:* 802-447-6347. *E-mail:* kcob@svc.edu.

University of Vermont
Department of Nursing
Burlington, Vermont

http://www.uvm.edu/~cnhs/nursing
Founded in 1791
DEGREES • BS • MS
Nursing Program Faculty 37 (14% with doctorates).
Baccalaureate Enrollment 282 **Women** 95% **Men** 5% **Minority** 9%
Graduate Enrollment 78 **Women** 90% **Men** 10% **Minority** 9% **Part-time** 23%
Distance Learning Courses Available.
Nursing Student Activities Nursing Honor Society, Sigma Theta Tau, Student Nurses' Association.
Nursing Student Resources Academic advising; academic or career counseling; assistance for students with disabilities; bookstore; campus computer network; career placement assistance; computer lab; computer-assisted instruction; e-mail services; employment services for current students; interactive nursing skills videos; Internet; learning resource lab; library services; nursing audiovisuals; remedial services; resume preparation assistance; skills, simulation, or other laboratory; tutoring.
Library Facilities 2.6 million volumes (126,689 in health, 1,437 in nursing); 30,000 periodical subscriptions (5,084 health-care related).

BACCALAUREATE PROGRAMS
Degree BS
Available Programs ADN to Baccalaureate; Generic Baccalaureate.
Study Options Full-time and part-time.
Program Entrance Requirements Minimum overall college GPA of 3.0, transcript of college record, written essay, health insurance, high school biology, high school chemistry, high school foreign language, 3 years high school math, 2 years high school science, high school transcript, immunizations, letters of recommendation, minimum GPA in nursing prerequisites of 2.0. Transfer students are accepted. *Application deadline:* 1/15 (fall). *Application fee:* $55.
Advanced Placement Credit by examination available. Credit given for nursing courses completed elsewhere dependent upon specific evaluations.
Contact *Telephone:* 802-656-0968.

GRADUATE PROGRAMS
Contact *Telephone:* 802-656-2018. *Fax:* 802-656-8306.

MASTER'S DEGREE PROGRAM
Degree MS
Available Programs Master's; Master's for Non-Nursing College Graduates; Master's for Nurses with Non-Nursing Degrees; RN to Master's.
Concentrations Available Nursing administration. *Nurse practitioner programs in:* adult health, family health, psychiatric/mental health.
Study Options Full-time and part-time.
Program Entrance Requirements Minimum overall college GPA of 3.0, transcript of college record, written essay, 3 letters of recommendation, physical assessment course, statistics course, GRE General Test. *Application deadline:* Applications may be processed on a rolling basis for some programs. *Application fee:* $40.
Advanced Placement Credit by examination available. Credit given for nursing courses completed elsewhere dependent upon specific evaluations.
Degree Requirements 57 total credit hours, thesis or project, comprehensive exam.

POST-MASTER'S PROGRAM
Areas of Study *Nurse practitioner programs in:* adult health, family health, psychiatric/mental health.

VIRGIN ISLANDS

University of the Virgin Islands
Division of Nursing
Saint Thomas, Virgin Islands

http://www.uvi.edu/
Founded in 1962
DEGREE • BSN
Nursing Program Faculty 8 (15% with doctorates).
Baccalaureate Enrollment 51 **Women** 98% **Men** 2% **Minority** 11% **International** 12% **Part-time** 20%
Nursing Student Activities Student Nurses' Association.
Nursing Student Resources Academic advising; academic or career counseling; assistance for students with disabilities; bookstore; campus computer network; career placement assistance; computer lab; computer-assisted instruction; e-mail services; employment services for current students; externships; housing assistance; interactive nursing skills videos; Internet; learning resource lab; library services; nursing audiovisuals; paid internships; remedial services; resume preparation assistance; skills, simulation, or other laboratory; tutoring.
Library Facilities 104,062 volumes (95,000 in health, 600 in nursing); 370 periodical subscriptions (15 health-care related).

BACCALAUREATE PROGRAMS
Degree BSN
Available Programs ADN to Baccalaureate; Generic Baccalaureate; LPN to Baccalaureate; RN Baccalaureate.
Site Options St. Croix, VI.
Study Options Full-time and part-time.
Program Entrance Requirements Minimum overall college GPA of 2.5, transcript of college record, CPR certification, health exam, 2 years high school math, high school transcript, immunizations, minimum GPA in nursing prerequisites of 2.5, professional liability insurance/malpractice insurance, prerequisite course work. Transfer students are accepted. *Application deadline:* 10/15 (fall). Applications may be processed on a rolling basis for some programs. *Application fee:* $25.
Advanced Placement Credit by examination available. Credit given for nursing courses completed elsewhere dependent upon specific evaluations.
Expenses (2012–13) *Tuition, state resident:* full-time $1995; part-time $133 per credit. *Tuition, nonresident:* full-time $5985; part-time $400 per credit. *International tuition:* $5985 full-time. *Room and board:* $5690; room only: $2800 per academic year. *Required fees:* full-time $484; part-time $373 per term.
Financial Aid 99% of baccalaureate students in nursing programs received some form of financial aid in 2011–12.
Contact Dr. Cheryl P. Franklin, Dean, Division of Nursing, University of the Virgin Islands, RR1, Box 10000, Kingshill, St. Croix, VI 00850-9781. *Telephone:* 340-778-1620 Ext. 4117. *Fax:* 340-693-1285. *E-mail:* cfrankl@uvi.edu.

VIRGINIA

Bon Secours Memorial College of Nursing
Bon Secours Memorial College of Nursing
Richmond, Virginia

DEGREE • BSN

BACCALAUREATE PROGRAMS
Degree BSN
Available Programs Generic Baccalaureate; RN Baccalaureate.
Online Degree Options Yes.
Program Entrance Requirements Minimum overall college GPA of 2.5, prerequisite course work.

Contact College of Nursing, Bon Secours Memorial College of Nursing, 8550 Magellan Parkway, Suite 1100, Richmond, VA 23227. *Telephone:* 804-627-5300.

Eastern Mennonite University

Department of Nursing
Harrisonburg, Virginia

Founded in 1917

DEGREES • BSN • MSN

Nursing Program Faculty 12 (25% with doctorates).

Baccalaureate Enrollment 146 Women 92.5% Men 7.5% Minority 8.2%

Graduate Enrollment 13 Women 84.6% Men 15.4% Minority 8% Part-time 8%

Distance Learning Courses Available.

Nursing Student Activities Sigma Theta Tau, Student Nurses' Association.

Nursing Student Resources Academic advising; academic or career counseling; assistance for students with disabilities; bookstore; campus computer network; career placement assistance; computer lab; computer-assisted instruction; e-mail services; employment services for current students; externships; housing assistance; interactive nursing skills videos; Internet; learning resource lab; library services; nursing audiovisuals; placement services for program completers; remedial services; resume preparation assistance; skills, simulation, or other laboratory; tutoring.

Library Facilities 168,802 volumes (1,256 in health, 926 in nursing); 843 periodical subscriptions (33 health-care related).

BACCALAUREATE PROGRAMS

Degree BSN

Available Programs ADN to Baccalaureate; Baccalaureate for Second Degree; Generic Baccalaureate; LPN to Baccalaureate; RN Baccalaureate.

Site Options Lancaster , PA.

Study Options Full-time and part-time.

Program Entrance Requirements Minimum overall college GPA of 2.8, transcript of college record, CPR certification, written essay, health exam, health insurance, high school chemistry, high school transcript, immunizations, 3 letters of recommendation, minimum high school GPA of 2.0, minimum GPA in nursing prerequisites of 2.8, professional liability insurance/malpractice insurance, prerequisite course work. Transfer students are accepted. *Application deadline:* 2/2 (fall), 6/1 (spring). Applications may be processed on a rolling basis for some programs.

Advanced Placement Credit by examination available. Credit given for nursing courses completed elsewhere dependent upon specific evaluations.

Contact *Telephone:* 800-368-2665. *Fax:* 540-432-4118.

GRADUATE PROGRAMS

Contact *Telephone:* 540-432-4000 Ext. 4192. *Fax:* 540-432-4000 Ext. 4444.

MASTER'S DEGREE PROGRAM

Degree MSN

Available Programs Master's; Master's for Nurses with Non-Nursing Degrees.

Concentrations Available Nursing administration.

Online Degree Options Yes (online only).

Program Entrance Requirements Clinical experience, computer literacy, minimum overall college GPA of 3.0, transcript of college record, written essay, 2 letters of recommendation, nursing research course. *Application deadline:* 4/1 (fall). Applications may be processed on a rolling basis for some programs. *Application fee:* $25.

Degree Requirements 37 total credit hours, thesis or project.

ECPI College of Technology

BSN Program
Virginia Beach, Virginia

http://www.medical.ecpi.edu/academics/programs.cfm?prgID=rnbsn

Founded in 1966

DEGREE • BSN

Distance Learning Courses Available.

Library Facilities 111,114 volumes; 293 periodical subscriptions.

BACCALAUREATE PROGRAMS

Degree BSN

Available Programs RN Baccalaureate.

Online Degree Options Yes.

Contact *Telephone:* 757-497-8400.

George Mason University

College of Health and Human Services
Fairfax, Virginia

http://chhs.gmu.edu/

Founded in 1957

DEGREES • BSN • MSN • PHD

Nursing Program Faculty 39 (69% with doctorates).

Baccalaureate Enrollment 359 Women 91% Men 9% Minority 51% International 3% Part-time 22%

Graduate Enrollment 187 Women 95% Men 5% Minority 33% International 2% Part-time 80%

Distance Learning Courses Available.

Nursing Student Activities Nursing Honor Society, Sigma Theta Tau, Student Nurses' Association.

Nursing Student Resources Academic advising; academic or career counseling; assistance for students with disabilities; bookstore; campus computer network; career placement assistance; computer lab; computer-assisted instruction; e-mail services; employment services for current students; housing assistance; interactive nursing skills videos; Internet; library services; nursing audiovisuals; remedial services; resume preparation assistance; skills, simulation, or other laboratory; tutoring.

Library Facilities 1.9 million volumes (16,172 in nursing); 77,565 periodical subscriptions (700 health-care related).

BACCALAUREATE PROGRAMS

Degree BSN

Available Programs Accelerated Baccalaureate for Second Degree; Generic Baccalaureate; RN Baccalaureate.

Study Options Full-time.

Online Degree Options Yes.

Program Entrance Requirements Minimum overall college GPA of 2.0, CPR certification, written essay, health exam, health insurance, immunizations, minimum high school GPA of 2.0, minimum GPA in nursing prerequisites of 3.0, professional liability insurance/malpractice insurance, prerequisite course work. Transfer students are accepted. *Application deadline:* 1/15 (fall). *Application fee:* $50.

Expenses (2012–13) *Tuition, state resident:* part-time $393 per credit hour. *Tuition, nonresident:* part-time $1149 per credit hour. *Room and board:* $10,034; room only: $6643 per academic year. *Required fees:* part-time $239 per credit.

Financial Aid 65% of baccalaureate students in nursing programs received some form of financial aid in 2011–12.

Contact Dr. Carol Urban, Assistant Dean, Division of Undergraduate Studies, School of Nursing, College of Health and Human Services, George Mason University, Mailstop 3C4, 4400 University Drive, Fairfax, VA 22030-4444. *Telephone:* 703-993-2991. *Fax:* 703-993-1949. *E-mail:* curban@gmu.edu.

GRADUATE PROGRAMS

Expenses (2012–13) *Tuition, state resident:* part-time $544 per credit hour. *Tuition, nonresident:* part-time $1208 per credit hour. *Room and board:* $10,033; room only: $6642 per academic year. *Required fees:* part-time $100 per term.

Financial Aid 1 fellowship (averaging $18,000 per year), 23 research assistantships (averaging $18,761 per year), 6 teaching assistantships

(averaging $13,554 per year) were awarded; career-related internships or fieldwork, Federal Work-Study, scholarships, unspecified assistantships, and health care benefits (full-time research or teaching assistantship recipients) also available.
Contact Dr. Margaret Rodan, Assistant Dean for Graduate Programs, College of Health and Human Services, George Mason University, Mailstop 3C4, 4400 University Drive, Fairfax, VA 22030-4444. *Telephone:* 703-993-1727. *Fax:* 703-993-1949. *E-mail:* mrodan@gmu.edu.

MASTER'S DEGREE PROGRAM
Degree MSN
Available Programs Master's; RN to Master's.
Concentrations Available Nursing administration; nursing education. *Clinical nurse specialist programs in:* acute care, adult health, cardiovascular, critical care, medical-surgical, oncology. *Nurse practitioner programs in:* adult health, family health, primary care.
Site Options Prince William County, VA.
Study Options Full-time and part-time.
Online Degree Options Yes (online only).
Program Entrance Requirements Clinical experience, minimum overall college GPA of 3.0, CPR certification, written essay, immunizations, 2 letters of recommendation, physical assessment course, statistics course. *Application deadline:* 4/1 (fall), 11/1 (spring). *Application fee:* $50.
Degree Requirements 44 total credit hours, thesis or project.

POST-MASTER'S PROGRAM
Areas of Study Nursing administration; nursing education.

DOCTORAL DEGREE PROGRAM
Degree PhD
Available Programs Doctorate.
Areas of Study Individualized study.
Online Degree Options Yes (online only).
Program Entrance Requirements Clinical experience, minimum overall college GPA of 3.5, interview, 3 letters of recommendation, MSN or equivalent, statistics course, writing sample, MAT. *Application deadline:* 3/1 (spring). *Application fee:* $60.
Degree Requirements 48 total credit hours, dissertation, written exam.

POSTDOCTORAL PROGRAM
Postdoctoral Program Contact Jean Sorrell, Coordinator, College of Health and Human Services, George Mason University, Mailstop 3C4, 4400 University Drive, Fairfax, VA 22030-4444. *Telephone:* 703-993-1944. *Fax:* 703-993-1942. *E-mail:* jsorrell@gmu.edu.

CONTINUING EDUCATION PROGRAM
Contact Dr. Janet Boyd, Assistant Dean, College of Health and Human Services, George Mason University, Mailstop 1B8, 4400 University Drive, Fairfax, VA 22030-4444. *Telephone:* 703-993-1910. *Fax:* 703-993-1622. *E-mail:* jboyd1@gmu.edu.

Hampton University
School of Nursing
Hampton, Virginia

http://nursing.hamptonu.edu/
Founded in 1868
DEGREES • BS • MS • PHD
Nursing Program Faculty 26 (51% with doctorates).
Baccalaureate Enrollment 470 **Women** 93% **Men** 7% **Minority** 90% **International** 4% **Part-time** 4%
Graduate Enrollment 66 **Women** 100% **Minority** 80% **Part-time** 25%
Distance Learning Courses Available.
Nursing Student Activities Sigma Theta Tau, Student Nurses' Association.
Nursing Student Resources Academic advising; bookstore; computer lab; e-mail services; interactive nursing skills videos; Internet; library services; skills, simulation, or other laboratory; tutoring.
Library Facilities 526,154 volumes (4,000 in health, 2,000 in nursing); 32,187 periodical subscriptions (500 health-care related).

BACCALAUREATE PROGRAMS
Degree BS

Available Programs Accelerated Baccalaureate; Generic Baccalaureate; LPN to Baccalaureate; LPN to RN Baccalaureate; RN Baccalaureate.
Site Options Virginia Beach, VA.
Study Options Full-time and part-time.
Program Entrance Requirements Minimum overall college GPA of 2.3, transcript of college record, CPR certification, written essay, health exam, health insurance, high school biology, high school chemistry, 3 years high school math, 2 years high school science, high school transcript, immunizations, 2 letters of recommendation, minimum high school GPA of 2.0, minimum high school rank 50%, minimum GPA in nursing prerequisites of 2.0, professional liability insurance/malpractice insurance. Transfer students are accepted. *Application deadline:* 3/1 (fall), 12/1 (spring).
Advanced Placement Credit by examination available. Credit given for nursing courses completed elsewhere dependent upon specific evaluations.
Contact *Telephone:* 757-727-5251.

GRADUATE PROGRAMS
Contact *Telephone:* 757-727-5251. *Fax:* 757-727-5423.

MASTER'S DEGREE PROGRAM
Degree MS
Available Programs Master's; RN to Master's.
Concentrations Available Health-care administration; nursing administration; nursing education. *Nurse practitioner programs in:* family health, gerontology, pediatric, primary care, women's health.
Study Options Full-time and part-time.
Online Degree Options Yes.
Program Entrance Requirements Clinical experience, computer literacy, minimum overall college GPA of 2.5, transcript of college record, written essay, interview, 2 letters of recommendation, nursing research course, physical assessment course, resume, statistics course, GRE General Test. *Application deadline:* 3/30 (fall), 11/1 (spring).
Advanced Placement Credit given for nursing courses completed elsewhere dependent upon specific evaluations.
Degree Requirements 46 total credit hours, thesis or project, comprehensive exam.

DOCTORAL DEGREE PROGRAM
Degree PhD
Available Programs Doctorate.
Areas of Study Family health.
Online Degree Options Yes (online only).
Program Entrance Requirements Minimum overall college GPA of 3.5, interview by faculty committee, interview, 3 letters of recommendation, MSN or equivalent, statistics course, vita, writing sample. *Application deadline:* 3/30 (fall).
Degree Requirements 44 total credit hours, dissertation, oral exam, written exam, residency.

James Madison University
Department of Nursing
Harrisonburg, Virginia

http://www.nursing.jmu.edu/
Founded in 1908
DEGREES • BSN • DNP • MSN
Nursing Program Faculty 37 (13% with doctorates).
Baccalaureate Enrollment 334 **Women** 93% **Men** 7% **Minority** 7%
Graduate Enrollment 63 **Women** 81% **Men** 19% **Minority** 3% **Part-time** 45%
Distance Learning Courses Available.
Nursing Student Activities Nursing Honor Society, Sigma Theta Tau, Student Nurses' Association.
Nursing Student Resources Academic advising; academic or career counseling; assistance for students with disabilities; bookstore; campus computer network; career placement assistance; computer lab; computer-assisted instruction; e-mail services; employment services for current students; externships; housing assistance; interactive nursing skills videos; Internet; learning resource lab; library services; nursing audiovisuals; paid internships; remedial services; resume preparation assistance; skills, simulation, or other laboratory; unpaid internships.
Library Facilities 714,959 volumes (67,716 in health, 12,054 in nursing); 12,339 periodical subscriptions.

BACCALAUREATE PROGRAMS

Degree BSN
Available Programs Generic Baccalaureate; RN Baccalaureate.
Study Options Full-time.
Program Entrance Requirements Minimum overall college GPA of 3.0, transcript of college record, CPR certification, health exam, immunizations, minimum GPA in nursing prerequisites of 2.0, prerequisite course work. Transfer students are accepted. *Application deadline:* 12/1 (fall), 7/1 (spring).
Advanced Placement Credit given for nursing courses completed elsewhere dependent upon specific evaluations.
Expenses (2012–13) *Tuition, state resident:* full-time $8808. *Tuition, nonresident:* full-time $22,796. *Required fees:* full-time $665.
Financial Aid 50% of baccalaureate students in nursing programs received some form of financial aid in 2011–12. *Gift aid (need-based):* Federal Pell, FSEOG, state, private, college/university gift aid from institutional funds. *Loans:* Federal Nursing Student Loans, Federal Direct (Subsidized and Unsubsidized Stafford PLUS), Perkins. *Work-study:* Federal Work-Study, part-time campus jobs. *Financial aid application deadline (priority):* 3/1.
Contact Ms. Becky Meadows, Administrative Assistant, Department of Nursing, James Madison University, 820 Madison Drive, Burruss Hall, MSC 4305, Harrisonburg, VA 22807. *Telephone:* 540-568-6314. *Fax:* 540-568-5613. *E-mail:* meadowra@jmu.edu.

GRADUATE PROGRAMS

Contact Dr. Patty Hale, Program Director, Department of Nursing, James Madison University, 820 Madison Drive, Burruss Hall, MSC 4305, Harrisonburg, VA 22807. *Telephone:* 540-568-6314. *Fax:* 540-568-7896. *E-mail:* halepj@jmu.edu.

MASTER'S DEGREE PROGRAM

Degree MSN
Available Programs Master's.
Concentrations Available Clinical nurse leader; nurse-midwifery; nursing administration. *Nurse practitioner programs in:* adult health, family health, gerontology.
Study Options Full-time and part-time.
Program Entrance Requirements Clinical experience, computer literacy, minimum overall college GPA of 2.8, transcript of college record, CPR certification, written essay, immunizations, 2 letters of recommendation, physical assessment course, prerequisite course work, resume, statistics course. *Application deadline:* 4/1 (fall), 10/1 (spring). Applications may be processed on a rolling basis for some programs. *Application fee:* $55.
Advanced Placement Credit given for nursing courses completed elsewhere dependent upon specific evaluations.
Degree Requirements 43 total credit hours.

POST-MASTER'S PROGRAM

Areas of Study Clinical nurse leader; nurse-midwifery; nursing administration. *Nurse practitioner programs in:* adult health, family health, gerontology.

DOCTORAL DEGREE PROGRAM

Degree DNP
Available Programs Doctorate.

Jefferson College of Health Sciences

Nursing Education Program
Roanoke, Virginia

http://www.jchs.edu/
Founded in 1982
DEGREES • BSN • MSN
Nursing Program Faculty 24 (17% with doctorates).
Baccalaureate Enrollment 260 **Women** 93% **Men** 7% **Minority** 15% **Part-time** 47%
Graduate Enrollment 32 **Women** 91% **Men** 9% **Minority** 9% **Part-time** 3%
Distance Learning Courses Available.
Nursing Student Activities Nursing Honor Society, Sigma Theta Tau, Student Nurses' Association.

Nursing Student Resources Academic advising; academic or career counseling; assistance for students with disabilities; bookstore; campus computer network; computer lab; computer-assisted instruction; e-mail services; externships; housing assistance; interactive nursing skills videos; Internet; learning resource lab; library services; nursing audiovisuals; skills, simulation, or other laboratory; tutoring.
Library Facilities 6,042 volumes (4,403 in health, 1,422 in nursing); 233 periodical subscriptions (277 health-care related).

BACCALAUREATE PROGRAMS

Degree BSN
Available Programs ADN to Baccalaureate; Generic Baccalaureate; RN Baccalaureate.
Site Options Roanoke, VA.
Study Options Full-time and part-time.
Program Entrance Requirements Minimum overall college GPA of 2.0, transcript of college record, CPR certification, health exam, health insurance, high school biology, high school chemistry, 2 years high school math, 2 years high school science, high school transcript, immunizations, minimum high school GPA of 2.0, prerequisite course work. Transfer students are accepted.
Advanced Placement Credit by examination available. Credit given for nursing courses completed elsewhere dependent upon specific evaluations.
Contact *Telephone:* 540-985-9083. *Fax:* 540-224-6703.

GRADUATE PROGRAMS

Contact *Telephone:* 540-985-9083. *Fax:* 540-224-6703.

MASTER'S DEGREE PROGRAM

Degree MSN
Available Programs Master's; Master's for Nurses with Non-Nursing Degrees.
Concentrations Available Nursing administration; nursing education.
Site Options Roanoke, VA.
Study Options Full-time.
Program Entrance Requirements Clinical experience, computer literacy, transcript of college record, 2 letters of recommendation, nursing research course, resume, statistics course.
Degree Requirements 37 total credit hours, thesis or project.

CONTINUING EDUCATION PROGRAM

Contact *Telephone:* 540-767-6072.

Liberty University

Department of Nursing
Lynchburg, Virginia

http://www.liberty.edu/
Founded in 1971
DEGREES • BSN • MSN
Nursing Program Faculty 25 (25% with doctorates).
Baccalaureate Enrollment 358 **Women** 93% **Men** 7% **Minority** 7% **International** 8%
Graduate Enrollment 280 **Women** 89% **Men** 11% **Minority** 29% **International** 3% **Part-time** 99%
Distance Learning Courses Available.
Nursing Student Activities Student Nurses' Association.
Nursing Student Resources Academic advising; academic or career counseling; assistance for students with disabilities; bookstore; campus computer network; career placement assistance; computer lab; e-mail services; externships; interactive nursing skills videos; Internet; learning resource lab; library services; nursing audiovisuals; resume preparation assistance; skills, simulation, or other laboratory; tutoring.
Library Facilities 354,920 volumes (3,632 in health, 3,000 in nursing); 97,105 periodical subscriptions (46 health-care related).

BACCALAUREATE PROGRAMS

Degree BSN
Available Programs Generic Baccalaureate; RN Baccalaureate.
Site Options Lynchburg, VA.
Study Options Full-time and part-time.
Program Entrance Requirements Minimum overall college GPA of 3.0, transcript of college record, CPR certification, written essay, immunizations, 2 letters of recommendation, minimum GPA in nursing prereq-

uisites of 3.0, professional liability insurance/malpractice insurance, prerequisite course work. Transfer students are accepted. *Application deadline:* 2/11 (spring).
Advanced Placement Credit given for nursing courses completed elsewhere dependent upon specific evaluations.
Contact *Telephone:* 804-582-2519. *Fax:* 804-582-7035.

GRADUATE PROGRAMS

Contact *Telephone:* 804-582-2519.

MASTER'S DEGREE PROGRAM
Degree MSN
Available Programs Master's.
Concentrations Available Nursing education. *Clinical nurse specialist programs in:* acute care.
Site Options Lynchburg, VA.
Study Options Full-time and part-time.
Online Degree Options Yes (online only).
Program Entrance Requirements Clinical experience, computer literacy, minimum overall college GPA of 3.0, transcript of college record, CPR certification, written essay, immunizations, interview, 3 letters of recommendation, nursing research course, physical assessment course, prerequisite course work, resume, statistics course. *Application deadline:* Applications may be processed on a rolling basis for some programs. *Application fee:* $50.
Degree Requirements 36 total credit hours, thesis or project.

Lynchburg College
School of Health Sciences and Human Performance
Lynchburg, Virginia

Founded in 1903
DEGREES • BS • MSN • MSN/MBA
Nursing Program Faculty 14 (38% with doctorates).
Baccalaureate Enrollment 95 **Women** 95% **Men** 5% **Minority** 8%
Graduate Enrollment 16 **Women** 90% **Men** 10% **Minority** 10% **International** 10% **Part-time** 90%
Distance Learning Courses Available.
Nursing Student Activities Nursing Honor Society, Sigma Theta Tau, Student Nurses' Association.
Nursing Student Resources Academic advising; academic or career counseling; assistance for students with disabilities; bookstore; campus computer network; career placement assistance; computer lab; computer-assisted instruction; e-mail services; employment services for current students; externships; housing assistance; interactive nursing skills videos; Internet; learning resource lab; library services; nursing audiovisuals; remedial services; resume preparation assistance; skills, simulation, or other laboratory; tutoring; unpaid internships.
Library Facilities 326,000 volumes (6,300 in health, 2,000 in nursing); 271 periodical subscriptions (100 health-care related).

BACCALAUREATE PROGRAMS

Degree BS
Available Programs Accelerated Baccalaureate; Baccalaureate for Second Degree; Generic Baccalaureate.
Study Options Full-time and part-time.
Program Entrance Requirements Transcript of college record, high school biology, high school chemistry, 3 years high school math, high school science, high school transcript, minimum GPA in nursing prerequisites of 3.0, prerequisite course work. Transfer students are accepted. *Application deadline:* 4/1 (fall), 4/1 (summer). *Application fee:* $30.
Advanced Placement Credit given for nursing courses completed elsewhere dependent upon specific evaluations.
Expenses (2012–13) *Tuition:* full-time $31,060; part-time $860 per contact hour. *Room and board:* $7440; room only: $3920 per academic year.
Financial Aid 97% of baccalaureate students in nursing programs received some form of financial aid in 2011–12. *Gift aid (need-based):* Federal Pell, FSEOG, state, private, college/university gift aid from institutional funds. *Loans:* Federal Direct (Subsidized and Unsubsidized Stafford PLUS), Perkins. *Work-study:* Federal Work-Study, part-time campus jobs. *Financial aid application deadline (priority):* 3/5.
Contact Dr. Ellen K. DeLuca, Director of Nursing Program and Associate Professor, School of Health Sciences and Human Performance, Lynchburg College, 1501 Lakeside Drive, McMillan Nursing Building,

Lynchburg, VA 24501-3199. *Telephone:* 434-544-8322. *Fax:* 434-544-8323. *E-mail:* deluca@lynchburg.edu.

GRADUATE PROGRAMS

Expenses (2012–13) *Tuition:* part-time $430 per credit hour. *Room and board:* $7440; room only: $3920 per academic year.
Financial Aid 50% of graduate students in nursing programs received some form of financial aid in 2011–12.
Contact Dr. Jean St. Clair, Director of Nursing Graduate Programs, School of Health Sciences and Human Performance, Lynchburg College, 1501 Lakeside Drive, Lynchburg, VA 24501. *Telephone:* 434-544-8740. *Fax:* 434-544-8323. *E-mail:* taylor.a@lynchburg.edu.

MASTER'S DEGREE PROGRAM
Degrees MSN; MSN/MBA
Available Programs Master's; RN to Master's.
Concentrations Available Clinical nurse leader; nursing education.
Study Options Full-time and part-time.
Program Entrance Requirements Clinical experience, minimum overall college GPA of 2.5, transcript of college record, 3 letters of recommendation, physical assessment course, statistics course. *Application deadline:* 4/1 (fall), 10/1 (winter), 4/1 (summer). Applications may be processed on a rolling basis for some programs. *Application fee:* $30.
Advanced Placement Credit given for nursing courses completed elsewhere dependent upon specific evaluations.
Degree Requirements 37 total credit hours, thesis or project.

Marymount University
Malek School of Health Professions
Arlington, Virginia

http://www.marymount.edu/academics/schools/shp
Founded in 1950
DEGREES • BSN • DNP • MSN
Nursing Program Faculty 20 (65% with doctorates).
Baccalaureate Enrollment 389 **Women** 90% **Men** 10% **Minority** 32% **International** 4% **Part-time** 17%
Graduate Enrollment 70 **Women** 91% **Men** 9% **Minority** 48% **International** 5% **Part-time** 84%
Distance Learning Courses Available.
Nursing Student Activities Sigma Theta Tau, Student Nurses' Association.
Nursing Student Resources Academic advising; academic or career counseling; assistance for students with disabilities; bookstore; campus computer network; career placement assistance; computer lab; computer-assisted instruction; e-mail services; externships; housing assistance; interactive nursing skills videos; Internet; learning resource lab; library services; nursing audiovisuals; paid internships; remedial services; resume preparation assistance; skills, simulation, or other laboratory; tutoring; unpaid internships.
Library Facilities 237,385 volumes (12,204 in health, 1,623 in nursing); 57,961 periodical subscriptions (2,906 health-care related).

BACCALAUREATE PROGRAMS

Degree BSN
Available Programs ADN to Baccalaureate; Accelerated Baccalaureate for Second Degree; Generic Baccalaureate; RN Baccalaureate.
Site Options Arlington, VA.
Study Options Full-time and part-time.
Program Entrance Requirements Minimum overall college GPA of 2.5, health exam, health insurance, high school transcript, 2 letters of recommendation, minimum high school GPA of 2.5. Transfer students are accepted. *Application deadline:* Applications may be processed on a rolling basis for some programs. *Application fee:* $40.
Advanced Placement Credit by examination available. Credit given for nursing courses completed elsewhere dependent upon specific evaluations.
Financial Aid 84% of baccalaureate students in nursing programs received some form of financial aid in 2011–12. *Gift aid (need-based):* Federal Pell, FSEOG, state, private, college/university gift aid from institutional funds. *Loans:* Federal Direct (Subsidized and Unsubsidized Stafford PLUS), Perkins. *Work-study:* Federal Work-Study. *Financial aid application deadline (priority):* 3/1.
Contact Admissions Counselor, Undergraduate Admissions, Malek School of Health Professions, Marymount University, 2807 North Glebe

Road, Arlington, VA 22207-4299. *Telephone:* 800-548-7638. *Fax:* 703-522-0349. *E-mail:* admissions@marymount.edu.

GRADUATE PROGRAMS

Financial Aid 57% of graduate students in nursing programs received some form of financial aid in 2011–12. Research assistantships with full and partial tuition reimbursements available, career-related internships or fieldwork, Federal Work-Study, scholarships, and unspecified assistantships available. Aid available to part-time students.

Contact Ms. Francesca Reed, Coordinator, Graduate Admissions, Malek School of Health Professions, Marymount University, 2807 North Glebe Road, Arlington, VA 22207-4299. *Telephone:* 703-284-5906. *E-mail:* francesca.reed@marymount.edu.

MASTER'S DEGREE PROGRAM
Degree MSN
Available Programs Master's.
Concentrations Available *Nurse practitioner programs in:* family health.
Site Options Arlington, VA.
Study Options Full-time and part-time.
Program Entrance Requirements Minimum overall college GPA of 3.0, transcript of college record, CPR certification, immunizations, interview, 2 letters of recommendation, professional liability insurance/malpractice insurance, resume, statistics course, GRE, MAT. *Application deadline:* 9/15 (fall), 4/1 (spring). Applications may be processed on a rolling basis for some programs. *Application fee:* $40.
Advanced Placement Credit given for nursing courses completed elsewhere dependent upon specific evaluations.
Degree Requirements 42 total credit hours, comprehensive exam.

POST-MASTER'S PROGRAM
Areas of Study *Nurse practitioner programs in:* family health.

DOCTORAL DEGREE PROGRAM
Degree DNP
Available Programs Doctorate; Post-Baccalaureate Doctorate.
Areas of Study Advanced practice nursing.
Site Options Arlington, VA.
Program Entrance Requirements Clinical experience, minimum overall college GPA of 3.3, interview by faculty committee, interview, 2 letters of recommendation, MSN or equivalent, vita, writing sample, GRE. *Application deadline:* 4/1 (fall). *Application fee:* $40.
Degree Requirements 32–76 total credit hours, residency.

Norfolk State University
Department of Nursing
Norfolk, Virginia

http://cset.nsu.edu/nursing/index.php/
Founded in 1935
DEGREE • BSN
Nursing Program Faculty 26 (40% with doctorates).
Baccalaureate Enrollment 133 **Women** 90% **Men** 10% **Minority** 85% **International** 15% **Part-time** 45%
Distance Learning Courses Available.
Nursing Student Activities Nursing Honor Society, Student Nurses' Association, nursing club.
Nursing Student Resources Academic advising; academic or career counseling; assistance for students with disabilities; bookstore; campus computer network; career placement assistance; computer lab; computer-assisted instruction; daycare for children of students; e-mail services; employment services for current students; externships; housing assistance; interactive nursing skills videos; Internet; learning resource lab; library services; nursing audiovisuals; paid internships; remedial services; resume preparation assistance; skills, simulation, or other laboratory; tutoring; unpaid internships.
Library Facilities 600 volumes in health, 300 volumes in nursing; 125 periodical subscriptions health-care related.

BACCALAUREATE PROGRAMS
Degree BSN
Available Programs Accelerated Baccalaureate for Second Degree; Accelerated LPN to Baccalaureate; RN Baccalaureate.
Site Options Virginia Beach , VA.
Study Options Full-time and part-time.

Program Entrance Requirements Minimum overall college GPA of 2.5, transcript of college record, CPR certification, health exam, health insurance, high school biology, high school chemistry, 2 years high school math, high school transcript, immunizations, minimum high school GPA of 2.5, minimum GPA in nursing prerequisites of 2.5, professional liability insurance/malpractice insurance, prerequisite course work. Transfer students are accepted. *Application deadline:* 8/1 (fall), 12/1 (winter), 2/1 (spring), 8/1 (summer).
Advanced Placement Credit by examination available. Credit given for nursing courses completed elsewhere dependent upon specific evaluations.
Contact *Telephone:* 757-823-9015. *Fax:* 757-823-2131.

Old Dominion University
Department of Nursing
Norfolk, Virginia

http://www.odu.edu/nursson
Founded in 1930
DEGREES • BSN • DNP • MSN
Nursing Program Faculty 27 (33% with doctorates).
Baccalaureate Enrollment 399 **Women** 91% **Men** 9% **Minority** 40% **Part-time** 46%
Graduate Enrollment 219 **Women** 92% **Men** 8% **Minority** 23% **Part-time** 47%
Distance Learning Courses Available.
Nursing Student Activities Sigma Theta Tau, Student Nurses' Association.
Nursing Student Resources Academic advising; academic or career counseling; assistance for students with disabilities; bookstore; campus computer network; career placement assistance; computer lab; computer-assisted instruction; e-mail services; externships; interactive nursing skills videos; Internet; learning resource lab; library services; nursing audiovisuals; paid internships; remedial services; resume preparation assistance; skills, simulation, or other laboratory; tutoring; unpaid internships.
Library Facilities 2.3 million volumes (44,144 in health, 3,622 in nursing); 40,874 periodical subscriptions (3,035 health-care related).

BACCALAUREATE PROGRAMS
Degree BSN
Available Programs Accelerated Baccalaureate; Generic Baccalaureate; RN Baccalaureate.
Site Options Olympia, WA; Yavapai, AZ.
Study Options Full-time.
Program Entrance Requirements Transcript of college record, CPR certification, immunizations, minimum GPA in nursing prerequisites of 2.5, prerequisite course work. Transfer students are accepted. *Application deadline:* 2/1 (fall). *Application fee:* $40.
Contact *Telephone:* 757-683-5245. *Fax:* 757-683-5253.

GRADUATE PROGRAMS
Contact *Telephone:* 757-683-4298. *Fax:* 757-683-5253.

MASTER'S DEGREE PROGRAM
Degree MSN
Available Programs Master's; RN to Master's.
Concentrations Available Nurse anesthesia; nurse-midwifery; nursing administration; nursing education. *Nurse practitioner programs in:* family health, women's health.
Site Options Athens, GA; Olympia, WA; Yavapai, AZ.
Study Options Full-time and part-time.
Online Degree Options Yes (online only).
Program Entrance Requirements Clinical experience, computer literacy, minimum overall college GPA of 3.0, transcript of college record, CPR certification, written essay, immunizations, interview, 3 letters of recommendation, physical assessment course, statistics course. *Application deadline:* 6/1 (fall), 12/1 (winter). *Application fee:* $40.
Advanced Placement Credit given for nursing courses completed elsewhere dependent upon specific evaluations.
Degree Requirements 47 total credit hours, comprehensive exam.

POST-MASTER'S PROGRAM
Areas of Study Nurse anesthesia; nurse-midwifery; nursing administration; nursing education. *Nurse practitioner programs in:* family health, women's health.

DOCTORAL DEGREE PROGRAM
Degree DNP
Available Programs Doctorate.
Areas of Study Advanced practice nursing.
Online Degree Options Yes (online only).
Program Entrance Requirements Clinical experience, minimum overall college GPA of 3.0, 3 letters of recommendation, MSN or equivalent, statistics course, vita, writing sample. *Application deadline:* 11/15 (fall), 11/15 (winter), 11/15 (spring).
Degree Requirements 36 total credit hours.

CONTINUING EDUCATION PROGRAM

Contact *Telephone:* 757-683-5261. *Fax:* 757-683-5253.

Radford University
School of Nursing
Radford, Virginia

http://www.radford.edu/nurs-web
Founded in 1910
DEGREES • BSN • DNP • MSN
Nursing Program Faculty 42 (31% with doctorates).
Baccalaureate Enrollment 227
Graduate Enrollment 58
Distance Learning Courses Available.
Nursing Student Activities Nursing Honor Society, Sigma Theta Tau, Student Nurses' Association.
Nursing Student Resources Academic advising; academic or career counseling; assistance for students with disabilities; bookstore; campus computer network; career placement assistance; computer lab; computer-assisted instruction; e-mail services; employment services for current students; externships; housing assistance; interactive nursing skills videos; Internet; learning resource lab; library services; nursing audiovisuals; resume preparation assistance; skills, simulation, or other laboratory; tutoring; unpaid internships.
Library Facilities 499,475 volumes; 9,865 periodical subscriptions.

BACCALAUREATE PROGRAMS

Degree BSN
Available Programs Baccalaureate for Second Degree; Generic Baccalaureate; RN Baccalaureate.
Site Options Roanoke, VA.
Study Options Full-time.
Online Degree Options Yes.
Program Entrance Requirements Minimum overall college GPA of 2.8, transcript of college record, CPR certification, written essay, health exam, health insurance, immunizations, prerequisite course work. Transfer students are accepted. *Application deadline:* 11/15 (fall), 8/1 (spring).
Advanced Placement Credit given for nursing courses completed elsewhere dependent upon specific evaluations.
Contact Dr. Anthony Ray Ramsey, Director, School of Nursing, Radford University, PO Box 6964, Radford, VA 24142. *Telephone:* 540-831-7700. *Fax:* 540-831-7716. *E-mail:* nurs-web@radford.edu.

GRADUATE PROGRAMS

Financial Aid 3 teaching assistantships (averaging $8,420 per year) were awarded; career-related internships or fieldwork, Federal Work-Study, institutionally sponsored loans, scholarships, and unspecified assistantships also available.
Contact Dr. Virginia Burggraf, Graduate Program Coordinator, School of Nursing, Radford University, PO Box 6964, Radford, VA 24142. *Telephone:* 540-831-7714. *Fax:* 540-831-7716. *E-mail:* nurs-web@radford.edu.

MASTER'S DEGREE PROGRAM
Degree MSN
Available Programs Master's.
Concentrations Available Nurse-midwifery. *Nurse practitioner programs in:* family health.
Study Options Full-time and part-time.
Program Entrance Requirements Clinical experience, computer literacy, transcript of college record, CPR certification, written essay, immunizations, interview, letters of recommendation, nursing research course, physical assessment course, professional liability insurance/mal-practice insurance, resume, statistics course, GRE. *Application deadline:* Applications may be processed on a rolling basis for some programs.
Degree Requirements Thesis or project.

POST-MASTER'S PROGRAM
Areas of Study Nurse-midwifery. *Nurse practitioner programs in:* family health.

DOCTORAL DEGREE PROGRAM
Degree DNP
Available Programs Doctorate; Post-Baccalaureate Doctorate.
Areas of Study Advanced practice nursing, clinical practice, faculty preparation, family health, gerontology, maternity-newborn.
Online Degree Options Yes (online only).
Program Entrance Requirements Clinical experience, minimum overall college GPA of 3.0, interview by faculty committee, interview, 3 letters of recommendation, statistics course, vita, writing sample. *Application deadline:* Applications may be processed on a rolling basis for some programs.
Degree Requirements Residency.

Sentara College of Health Sciences
Bachelor of Science in Nursing Program
Chesapeake, Virginia

DEGREE • BSN

BACCALAUREATE PROGRAMS

Degree BSN
Available Programs Generic Baccalaureate; LPN to Baccalaureate; RN Baccalaureate.
Study Options Full-time and part-time.
Online Degree Options Yes.
Program Entrance Requirements Prerequisite course work.
Contact Admission Recruiter, Bachelor of Science in Nursing Program, Sentara College of Health Sciences, Suite 105, 1441 Crossways Boulevard, Chesapeake, VA 23320. *Telephone:* 757-388-2862. *E-mail:* salamb@sentara.com.

Shenandoah University
Eleanor Wade Custer School of Nursing
Winchester, Virginia

http://www.nursing.su.edu/
Founded in 1875
DEGREES • BSN • DNP • MSN • MSN/MBA
Nursing Program Faculty 44 (30% with doctorates).
Baccalaureate Enrollment 350 **Women** 97% **Men** 3% **Minority** 10% **International** 3% **Part-time** 15%
Graduate Enrollment 120 **Women** 97% **Men** 3% **Minority** 10% **Part-time** 25%
Nursing Student Activities Nursing Honor Society, Sigma Theta Tau, Student Nurses' Association.
Nursing Student Resources Academic advising; academic or career counseling; assistance for students with disabilities; bookstore; campus computer network; computer lab; daycare for children of students; e-mail services; interactive nursing skills videos; Internet; learning resource lab; library services; nursing audiovisuals; resume preparation assistance; skills, simulation, or other laboratory; tutoring.
Library Facilities 211,976 volumes (500 in health, 200 in nursing); 56,719 periodical subscriptions (250 health-care related).

BACCALAUREATE PROGRAMS

Degree BSN
Available Programs ADN to Baccalaureate; Accelerated Baccalaureate for Second Degree; Generic Baccalaureate; RN Baccalaureate.
Site Options Leesburg, VA.
Study Options Full-time and part-time.
Program Entrance Requirements Minimum overall college GPA of 3.0, transcript of college record, CPR certification, health exam, health insurance, high school biology, high school chemistry, 2 years high

school math, high school transcript, immunizations, minimum high school GPA of 3.0, minimum GPA in nursing prerequisites of 3.0, prerequisite course work. Transfer students are accepted. *Application deadline:* Applications may be processed on a rolling basis for some programs.

Advanced Placement Credit by examination available. Credit given for nursing courses completed elsewhere dependent upon specific evaluations.

Financial Aid 80% of baccalaureate students in nursing programs received some form of financial aid in 2010–11. *Gift aid (need-based):* Federal Pell, FSEOG, state, private, college/university gift aid from institutional funds, Federal Nursing. *Loans:* Federal Nursing Student Loans, Federal Direct (Subsidized and Unsubsidized Stafford PLUS), Perkins, college/university.*Work-study:* Federal Work-Study, part-time campus jobs.*Financial aid application deadline (priority):* 2/15.

Contact Dr. Kathryn Ganske, Director, Eleanor Wade Custer School of Nursing, Shenandoah University, 1460 University Drive, Winchester, VA 22601. *Telephone:* 540-678-4381. *Fax:* 540-665-5519. *E-mail:* sralph@su.edu.

GRADUATE PROGRAMS

Financial Aid 85% of graduate students in nursing programs received some form of financial aid in 2010–11. 3 teaching assistantships with partial tuition reimbursements available (averaging $4,224 per year) were awarded; career-related internships or fieldwork, institutionally sponsored loans, scholarships, unspecified assistantships, and federal loans, alternative loans also available. Aid available to part-time students. *Financial aid application deadline:* 3/15.

Contact Dr. Patricia Krauskopf, Coordinator, FNP Graduate Program, Eleanor Wade Custer School of Nursing, Shenandoah University, 1775 North Sector Court, Winchester, VA 22601. *Telephone:* 540-665-5512. *Fax:* 540-665-5519. *E-mail:* pkrausko@su.edu.

MASTER'S DEGREE PROGRAM

Degrees MSN; MSN/MBA

Available Programs Master's; RN to Master's.

Concentrations Available Nurse case management; nurse-midwifery. *Clinical nurse specialist programs in:* psychiatric/mental health. *Nurse practitioner programs in:* family health, psychiatric/mental health.

Study Options Full-time and part-time.

Program Entrance Requirements Clinical experience, computer literacy, minimum overall college GPA of 3.0, transcript of college record, CPR certification, immunizations, interview, 3 letters of recommendation, nursing research course, physical assessment course, professional liability insurance/malpractice insurance, prerequisite course work, resume, statistics course, GRE General Test. *Application deadline:* Applications may be processed on a rolling basis for some programs.

Advanced Placement Credit given for nursing courses completed elsewhere dependent upon specific evaluations.

Degree Requirements 48 total credit hours, thesis or project.

POST-MASTER'S PROGRAM

Areas of Study Nurse-midwifery. *Nurse practitioner programs in:* family health, psychiatric/mental health.

DOCTORAL DEGREE PROGRAM

Degree DNP

Available Programs Doctorate; Post-Baccalaureate Doctorate.

Program Entrance Requirements Clinical experience, minimum overall college GPA of 3.0, interview by faculty committee, letters of recommendation, MSN or equivalent, statistics course, vita. *Application deadline:* Applications may be processed on a rolling basis for some programs.

Degree Requirements 30 total credit hours.

CONTINUING EDUCATION PROGRAM

Contact Dr. Jennifer Matthews, Professor, Division of Nursing, Eleanor Wade Custer School of Nursing, Shenandoah University, 1460 University Drive, Winchester, VA 22601. *Telephone:* 540-678-4374. *E-mail:* jmatthew@su.edu.

University of Virginia
School of Nursing
Charlottesville, Virginia

http://www.nursing.virginia.edu/
Founded in 1819
DEGREES • BSN • MSN • MSN/MBA • MSN/PHD • PHD
Nursing Program Faculty 99 (65% with doctorates).
Baccalaureate Enrollment 360 **Women** 95% **Men** 5% **Minority** 30% **International** 2% **Part-time** 5%
Graduate Enrollment 350 **Women** 88% **Men** 12% **Minority** 25% **International** 2% **Part-time** 50%
Distance Learning Courses Available.
Nursing Student Activities Nursing Honor Society, Sigma Theta Tau, Student Nurses' Association, nursing club.
Nursing Student Resources Academic advising; academic or career counseling; assistance for students with disabilities; bookstore; campus computer network; career placement assistance; computer-assisted instruction; e-mail services; employment services for current students; housing assistance; interactive nursing skills videos; Internet; learning resource lab; library services; nursing audiovisuals; placement services for program completers; remedial services; resume preparation assistance; skills, simulation, or other laboratory; tutoring.
Library Facilities 5.6 million volumes (200,000 in health); 185,729 periodical subscriptions (1,000 health-care related).

BACCALAUREATE PROGRAMS

Degree BSN
Available Programs ADN to Baccalaureate; Generic Baccalaureate; RN Baccalaureate.
Study Options Full-time.
Program Entrance Requirements Transcript of college record, written essay, health insurance, high school biology, 2 years high school math, 2 years high school science, high school transcript, 1 letter of recommendation, minimum high school GPA. Transfer students are accepted. *Application deadline:* 1/1 (fall). *Application fee:* $60.
Advanced Placement Credit by examination available.
Expenses (2012–13) *Tuition, state resident:* full-time $9622; part-time $320 per credit hour. *Tuition, nonresident:* full-time $34,952; part-time $1165 per credit hour. *International tuition:* $34,952 full-time. *Room and board:* $9440; room only: $5170 per academic year. *Required fees:* full-time $2592; part-time $2592 per term.
Financial Aid 60% of baccalaureate students in nursing programs received some form of financial aid in 2011–12. *Gift aid (need-based):* Federal Pell, FSEOG, state, private, college/university gift aid from institutional funds, Federal Nursing. *Loans:* Federal Nursing Student Loans, Perkins, college/university, private loans.*Work-study:* Federal Work-Study.*Financial aid application deadline (priority):* 3/1.
Contact Mr. Clay Hysell, Assistant Dean for Admissions and Financial Aid, School of Nursing, University of Virginia, Claude Moore Nursing Education Building, PO Box 800826, Charlottesville, VA 22908. *Telephone:* 888-283-8703. *Fax:* 434-924-0528. *E-mail:* nursing-admissions@virginia.edu.

GRADUATE PROGRAMS

Expenses (2012–13) *Tuition, state resident:* full-time $12,906; part-time $717 per credit hour. *Tuition, nonresident:* full-time $22,230; part-time $1235 per credit hour. *International tuition:* $22,230 full-time. *Required fees:* full-time $2402.
Financial Aid 80% of graduate students in nursing programs received some form of financial aid in 2011–12. Fellowships, research assistantships, teaching assistantships, Federal Work-Study and scholarships available.
Contact Mr. Clay D. Hysell, Assistant Dean for Admissions and Financial Aid, School of Nursing, University of Virginia, Claude Moore Nursing Education Building, PO Box 800826, Charlottesville, VA 22908. *Telephone:* 888-283-8703. *Fax:* 434-924-0528. *E-mail:* nursing-admissions@virginia.edu.

MASTER'S DEGREE PROGRAM
Degrees MSN; MSN/MBA; MSN/PhD
Available Programs Master's; Master's for Non-Nursing College Graduates; Master's for Nurses with Non-Nursing Degrees.
Concentrations Available Clinical nurse leader; nursing administration. *Clinical nurse specialist programs in:* acute care, medical-surgical, psychiatric/mental health. *Nurse practitioner programs in:* acute care, com-

munity health, family health, pediatric, primary care, psychiatric/mental health.
Study Options Full-time and part-time.
Program Entrance Requirements Clinical experience, minimum overall college GPA of 3.0, transcript of college record, written essay, 3 letters of recommendation, resume, statistics course, GRE General Test, MAT. *Application deadline:* 3/1 (fall). Applications may be processed on a rolling basis for some programs. *Application fee:* $60.
Advanced Placement Credit given for nursing courses completed elsewhere dependent upon specific evaluations.
Degree Requirements 34 total credit hours.

POST-MASTER'S PROGRAM
Areas of Study Nursing administration. *Clinical nurse specialist programs in:* acute care, medical-surgical, psychiatric/mental health. *Nurse practitioner programs in:* acute care, community health, family health, pediatric, primary care, psychiatric/mental health.

DOCTORAL DEGREE PROGRAM
Degree PhD
Available Programs Doctorate; Post-Baccalaureate Doctorate.
Areas of Study Advanced practice nursing, aging, bio-behavioral research, clinical practice, community health, critical care, ethics, faculty preparation, family health, forensic nursing, health policy, health promotion/disease prevention, health-care systems, information systems, maternity-newborn, nursing administration, nursing education, nursing policy, nursing research, nursing science, oncology, urban health, women's health.
Program Entrance Requirements Minimum overall college GPA of 3.0, interview by faculty committee, interview, 3 letters of recommendation, statistics course, vita, writing sample, GRE General Test. *Application deadline:* 12/15 (fall). Applications may be processed on a rolling basis for some programs. *Application fee:* $60.
Degree Requirements 46 total credit hours, dissertation, written exam, residency.

POSTDOCTORAL PROGRAM
Areas of Study Nursing research, nursing science.
Postdoctoral Program Contact Mr. Clay D. Hysell, Assistant Dean for Admissions and Financial Aid, School of Nursing, University of Virginia, McLeod Hall, PO Box 800826, Charlottesville, VA 22908. *Telephone:* 434-924-0141. *Fax:* 434-924-0528. *E-mail:* cdh6n@virginia.edu.

The University of Virginia's College at Wise
Department of Nursing
Wise, Virginia

http://www.uvawise.edu/
Founded in 1954
DEGREE • BSN
Nursing Program Faculty 10 (30% with doctorates).
Baccalaureate Enrollment 47 **Women** 79% **Men** 21% **Minority** 15% **Part-time** 5%
Nursing Student Activities Sigma Theta Tau, Student Nurses' Association.
Nursing Student Resources Academic advising; academic or career counseling; assistance for students with disabilities; bookstore; campus computer network; career placement assistance; computer lab; computer-assisted instruction; e-mail services; employment services for current students; externships; housing assistance; interactive nursing skills videos; Internet; learning resource lab; library services; nursing audiovisuals; resume preparation assistance; skills, simulation, or other laboratory; tutoring.
Library Facilities 160,378 volumes (4,654 in health, 2,761 in nursing); 3,131 periodical subscriptions (40 health-care related).

BACCALAUREATE PROGRAMS
Degree BSN
Available Programs ADN to Baccalaureate; Generic Baccalaureate; RN Baccalaureate.
Study Options Full-time.
Program Entrance Requirements Minimum overall college GPA of 2.75, transcript of college record, CPR certification, written essay, health exam, health insurance, immunizations, minimum GPA in nursing pre-

requisites of 2.75, professional liability insurance/malpractice insurance, prerequisite course work. Transfer students are accepted. *Application deadline:* 11/1 (spring). *Application fee:* $25.
Advanced Placement Credit given for nursing courses completed elsewhere dependent upon specific evaluations.
Financial Aid 90% of baccalaureate students in nursing programs received some form of financial aid in 2010–11.
Contact Dr. Cathleen A. Collins, Chair, Department of Nursing, The University of Virginia's College at Wise, One College Avenue, Wise, VA 24293-4400. *Telephone:* 276-328-0275. *Fax:* 276-376-4589. *E-mail:* cac8ff@uvawise.edu.

Virginia Commonwealth University
School of Nursing
Richmond, Virginia

http://www.nursing.vcu.edu/
Founded in 1838
DEGREES • BS • MS • PHD
Nursing Program Faculty 137 (30% with doctorates).
Baccalaureate Enrollment 547 **Women** 92% **Men** 8% **Minority** 32% **International** 1% **Part-time** 40%
Graduate Enrollment 319 **Women** 94% **Men** 6% **Minority** 24% **International** 1% **Part-time** 62%
Distance Learning Courses Available.
Nursing Student Activities Sigma Theta Tau, Student Nurses' Association, nursing club.
Nursing Student Resources Academic advising; academic or career counseling; assistance for students with disabilities; bookstore; campus computer network; career placement assistance; computer lab; computer-assisted instruction; daycare for children of students; e-mail services; employment services for current students; externships; housing assistance; interactive nursing skills videos; Internet; learning resource lab; library services; nursing audiovisuals; paid internships; placement services for program completers; remedial services; resume preparation assistance; skills, simulation, or other laboratory; tutoring.
Library Facilities 2.2 million volumes (484,644 in health, 12,472 in nursing); 61,000 periodical subscriptions (11,096 health-care related).

BACCALAUREATE PROGRAMS
Degree BS
Available Programs ADN to Baccalaureate; Accelerated Baccalaureate for Second Degree; Generic Baccalaureate.
Site Options Newport News, VA.
Study Options Full-time.
Program Entrance Requirements Minimum overall college GPA of 2.5, transcript of college record, CPR certification, written essay, immunizations, 3 letters of recommendation, minimum GPA in nursing prerequisites of 2.5, prerequisite course work. Transfer students are accepted. *Application deadline:* 2/1 (fall). *Application fee:* $40.
Advanced Placement Credit by examination available. Credit given for nursing courses completed elsewhere dependent upon specific evaluations.
Expenses (2012–13) *Tuition, state resident:* full-time $7860; part-time $328 per credit hour. *Tuition, nonresident:* full-time $21,275; part-time $886 per credit hour. *International tuition:* $21,275 full-time. *Room and board:* $9966; room only: $6148 per academic year. *Required fees:* full-time $1971; part-time $74 per credit.
Contact Mrs. Susan L. Lipp, Assistant Dean of Enrollment and Student Services, School of Nursing, Virginia Commonwealth University, 1100 East Leigh Street, PO Box 980567, Richmond, VA 23298-0567. *Telephone:* 804-828-5171. *Fax:* 804-828-7743. *E-mail:* slipp@vcu.edu.

GRADUATE PROGRAMS
Expenses (2012–13) *Tuition, state resident:* full-time $9530; part-time $529 per credit hour. *Tuition, nonresident:* full-time $19,594; part-time $1089 per credit hour. *International tuition:* $19,594 full-time. *Room and board:* $8214; room only: $5850 per academic year. *Required fees:* full-time $1971; part-time $74 per credit.
Financial Aid Fellowships, research assistantships, teaching assistantships, career-related internships or fieldwork and institutionally sponsored loans available.
Contact Mrs. Susan L. Lipp, Assistant Dean of Enrollment and Student Services, School of Nursing, Virginia Commonwealth University, 1100

East Leigh Street, PO Box 980567, Richmond, VA 23298-0567. *Telephone:* 804-828-5171. *Fax:* 804-828-7743. *E-mail:* slipp@vcu.edu.

MASTER'S DEGREE PROGRAM
Degree MS
Available Programs Master's; RN to Master's.
Concentrations Available Nursing administration. *Clinical nurse specialist programs in:* acute care. *Nurse practitioner programs in:* acute care, adult health, family health, pediatric, primary care, psychiatric/mental health, women's health.
Study Options Full-time and part-time.
Program Entrance Requirements Computer literacy, minimum overall college GPA of 3.0, transcript of college record, CPR certification, written essay, immunizations, 3 letters of recommendation, prerequisite course work, resume, statistics course, GRE General Test. *Application deadline:* 3/15 (fall), 9/15 (spring). *Application fee:* $50.
Advanced Placement Credit given for nursing courses completed elsewhere dependent upon specific evaluations.
Degree Requirements 55 total credit hours.

POST-MASTER'S PROGRAM
Areas of Study Nursing administration. *Clinical nurse specialist programs in:* acute care. *Nurse practitioner programs in:* acute care, adult health, family health, pediatric, primary care, psychiatric/mental health, women's health.

DOCTORAL DEGREE PROGRAM
Degree PhD
Available Programs Doctorate.
Areas of Study Bio-behavioral research.
Online Degree Options Yes (online only).
Program Entrance Requirements Minimum overall college GPA of 3.0, interview by faculty committee, interview, 3 letters of recommendation, MSN or equivalent, statistics course, vita, writing sample, GRE General Test. *Application deadline:* 2/1 (fall). *Application fee:* $50.
Degree Requirements 61 total credit hours, dissertation, written exam.

POSTDOCTORAL PROGRAM
Postdoctoral Program Contact Ms. Susan L. Lipp, Assistant Dean of Enrollment and Student Services, School of Nursing, Virginia Commonwealth University, 1100 East Leigh Street, PO Box 980567, Richmond, VA 23298-0567. *Telephone:* 804-828-5171. *Fax:* 804-828-7743. *E-mail:* slipp@vcu.edu.

WASHINGTON

Eastern Washington University
Intercollegiate College of Nursing/Washington State University
Cheney, Washington

See description of programs under Washington State University College of Nursing (Spokane, Washington).

Gonzaga University
Department of Nursing
Spokane, Washington

http://www.gonzaga.edu/nursing
Founded in 1887
DEGREES • BSN • MSN
Nursing Program Faculty 15 (73% with doctorates).
Baccalaureate Enrollment 233 **Women** 93% **Men** 7%
Graduate Enrollment 337 **Women** 94% **Men** 6% **Part-time** 14%
Distance Learning Courses Available.
Nursing Student Activities Sigma Theta Tau, Student Nurses' Association.
Nursing Student Resources Academic advising; academic or career counseling; assistance for students with disabilities; bookstore; campus

computer network; computer lab; computer-assisted instruction; e-mail services; housing assistance; interactive nursing skills videos; Internet; learning resource lab; library services; nursing audiovisuals; resume preparation assistance; skills, simulation, or other laboratory; tutoring.
Library Facilities 350,342 volumes (35,000 in health, 950 in nursing); 48,985 periodical subscriptions (206 health-care related).

BACCALAUREATE PROGRAMS
Degree BSN
Available Programs Generic Baccalaureate.
Study Options Full-time and part-time.
Program Entrance Requirements Minimum overall college GPA of 2.9, transcript of college record, written essay, high school biology, high school chemistry, 4 years high school math, 4 years high school science, high school transcript, 2 letters of recommendation, minimum high school GPA of 2.9, minimum GPA in nursing prerequisites of 2.0, prerequisite course work. Transfer students are accepted. *Application deadline:* 1/15 (fall), 9/15 (spring). *Application fee:* $50.
Advanced Placement Credit given for nursing courses completed elsewhere dependent upon specific evaluations.
Contact *Telephone:* 509-313-3580. *Fax:* 509-313-5827.

GRADUATE PROGRAMS
Contact *Telephone:* 509-313-6640. *Fax:* 509-323-5827.

MASTER'S DEGREE PROGRAM
Degree MSN
Available Programs Accelerated RN to Master's; Master's; Master's for Nurses with Non-Nursing Degrees.
Concentrations Available Health-care administration; nursing administration; nursing education. *Clinical nurse specialist programs in:* psychiatric/mental health. *Nurse practitioner programs in:* family health, primary care, psychiatric/mental health.
Study Options Full-time and part-time.
Online Degree Options Yes (online only).
Program Entrance Requirements Computer literacy, minimum overall college GPA of 3.0, transcript of college record, written essay, 2 letters of recommendation, resume, statistics course, MAT. *Application deadline:* Applications may be processed on a rolling basis for some programs.
Advanced Placement Credit given for nursing courses completed elsewhere dependent upon specific evaluations.
Degree Requirements 36 total credit hours.

POST-MASTER'S PROGRAM
Areas of Study Health-care administration; nursing administration; nursing education. *Clinical nurse specialist programs in:* psychiatric/mental health. *Nurse practitioner programs in:* family health, primary care, psychiatric/mental health.

Northwest University
The Mark and Huldah Buntain School of Nursing
Kirkland, Washington

http://www.northwestu.edu/schools/nursing/
Founded in 1934
DEGREE • BS
Nursing Program Faculty 24 (16% with doctorates).
Baccalaureate Enrollment 50 **Women** 87% **Men** 13% **Minority** 11%
Nursing Student Resources Academic advising; academic or career counseling; assistance for students with disabilities; bookstore; campus computer network; computer lab; computer-assisted instruction; e-mail services; employment services for current students; housing assistance; interactive nursing skills videos; Internet; learning resource lab; library services; nursing audiovisuals; other; remedial services; resume preparation assistance; skills, simulation, or other laboratory; tutoring; unpaid internships.
Library Facilities 100,356 volumes (1,922 in health, 387 in nursing); 13,443 periodical subscriptions (815 health-care related).

BACCALAUREATE PROGRAMS
Degree BS
Available Programs Generic Baccalaureate.
Study Options Full-time.
Program Entrance Requirements Minimum overall college GPA of 3.0, transcript of college record, CPR certification, written essay, health

exam, health insurance, high school transcript, immunizations, 2 letters of recommendation, minimum GPA in nursing prerequisites of 3.0, prerequisite course work. Transfer students are accepted. *Application deadline:* 1/30 (fall). *Application fee:* $35.
Contact *Telephone:* 800-669-3781 Ext. 7822. *Fax:* 425-889-7822.

Olympic College
Nursing Programs
Bremerton, Washington

Founded in 1946
DEGREE • BSN
Library Facilities 70,000 volumes.

BACCALAUREATE PROGRAMS

Degree BSN
Available Programs RN Baccalaureate.
Study Options Full-time and part-time.
Program Entrance Requirements Minimum overall college GPA of 2.5, minimum GPA in nursing prerequisites of 2.0, RN licensure.
Contact *Telephone:* 360-475-7748. *Fax:* 360-475-7628.

Pacific Lutheran University
School of Nursing
Tacoma, Washington

http://www.plu.edu/nursing/
Founded in 1890
DEGREES • BSN • MSN • MSN/MBA
Nursing Program Faculty 30 (40% with doctorates).
Baccalaureate Enrollment 242 **Women** 89% **Men** 11% **Minority** 15% **International** 2%
Graduate Enrollment 51 **Women** 82% **Men** 18% **Minority** 6% **International** 2%
Nursing Student Activities Nursing Honor Society, Sigma Theta Tau, Student Nurses' Association, nursing club.
Nursing Student Resources Academic advising; academic or career counseling; assistance for students with disabilities; bookstore; campus computer network; career placement assistance; computer lab; computer-assisted instruction; daycare for children of students; e-mail services; employment services for current students; housing assistance; interactive nursing skills videos; Internet; learning resource lab; library services; nursing audiovisuals; other; resume preparation assistance; skills, simulation, or other laboratory; tutoring; unpaid internships.
Library Facilities 337,167 volumes (15,000 in health, 6,500 in nursing); 5,808 periodical subscriptions (150 health-care related).

BACCALAUREATE PROGRAMS

Degree BSN
Available Programs Generic Baccalaureate; LPN to Baccalaureate.
Study Options Full-time.
Program Entrance Requirements Minimum overall college GPA of 3.0, transcript of college record, CPR certification, written essay, health exam, health insurance, high school foreign language, 2 years high school math, high school transcript, immunizations, 2 letters of recommendation, minimum GPA in nursing prerequisites of 2.75, professional liability insurance/malpractice insurance, prerequisite course work. Transfer students are accepted. *Application deadline:* 2/1 (fall), 2/1 (spring). Applications may be processed on a rolling basis for some programs.
Advanced Placement Credit by examination available. Credit given for nursing courses completed elsewhere dependent upon specific evaluations.
Financial Aid 90% of baccalaureate students in nursing programs received some form of financial aid in 2011–12. *Gift aid (need-based):* Federal Pell, FSEOG, state, private, college/university gift aid from institutional funds, Federal Nursing. *Loans:* Federal Nursing Student Loans, Federal Direct (Subsidized and Unsubsidized Stafford PLUS), Perkins, state. *Work-study:* Federal Work-Study, part-time campus jobs. *Financial aid application deadline (priority):* 1/31.
Contact Ms. Lindsay R. Burke, Admissions Coordinator, School of Nursing, Pacific Lutheran University, 12180 Park Avenue South, Tacoma, WA 98447-0029. *Telephone:* 253-535-7672. *Fax:* 253-535-7590. *E-mail:* burkelr@plu.edu.

GRADUATE PROGRAMS

Financial Aid 90% of graduate students in nursing programs received some form of financial aid in 2011–12. Fellowships, Federal Work-Study, scholarships, and unspecified assistantships available. *Financial aid application deadline:* 3/1.
Contact Ms. Lindsay R. Burke, Admissions Coordinator, School of Nursing, Pacific Lutheran University, 12180 Park Avenue South, Tacoma, WA 98447-0029. *Telephone:* 253-535-7672. *Fax:* 253-535-7590. *E-mail:* gradnurs@plu.edu.

MASTER'S DEGREE PROGRAM

Degrees MSN; MSN/MBA
Available Programs Accelerated Master's for Non-Nursing College Graduates; Master's.
Concentrations Available Clinical nurse leader; health-care administration; nurse case management; nursing administration; nursing education. *Nurse practitioner programs in:* family health.
Study Options Full-time.
Program Entrance Requirements Clinical experience, computer literacy, minimum overall college GPA of 3.0, transcript of college record, CPR certification, written essay, immunizations, interview, 2 letters of recommendation, professional liability insurance/malpractice insurance, prerequisite course work, resume, statistics course, GRE General Test. *Application deadline:* 11/15 (summer). Applications may be processed on a rolling basis for some programs. *Application fee:* $40.
Advanced Placement Credit given for nursing courses completed elsewhere dependent upon specific evaluations.
Degree Requirements 33 total credit hours, thesis or project.

CONTINUING EDUCATION PROGRAM

Contact Ms. Jessica J. Immerman, Coordinator, Continuing Nursing Education and Clinical Placements, School of Nursing, Pacific Lutheran University, 12180 Park Avenue South, Tacoma, WA 98447-0029. *Telephone:* 253-535-7683. *Fax:* 253-535-7590. *E-mail:* immermjJ@plu.edu.

Seattle Pacific University
School of Health Sciences
Seattle, Washington

http://www.spu.edu/depts/hsc
Founded in 1891
DEGREES • BS • MSN
Nursing Program Faculty 23 (39% with doctorates).
Baccalaureate Enrollment 98 **Women** 91% **Men** 9% **Minority** 21% **International** 2%
Graduate Enrollment 61 **Women** 89% **Men** 11% **Minority** 39% **Part-time** 49%
Nursing Student Activities Nursing Honor Society, Sigma Theta Tau, Student Nurses' Association, nursing club.
Nursing Student Resources Academic advising; academic or career counseling; assistance for students with disabilities; bookstore; campus computer network; career placement assistance; computer lab; computer-assisted instruction; e-mail services; employment services for current students; housing assistance; Internet; learning resource lab; library services; nursing audiovisuals; placement services for program completers; remedial services; resume preparation assistance; skills, simulation, or other laboratory; tutoring; unpaid internships.
Library Facilities 211,210 volumes (11,539 in health, 1,791 in nursing); 2,125 periodical subscriptions (274 health-care related).

BACCALAUREATE PROGRAMS

Degree BS
Available Programs Generic Baccalaureate; RN Baccalaureate.
Study Options Full-time.
Program Entrance Requirements Minimum overall college GPA of 2.75, transcript of college record, CPR certification, written essay, health exam, health insurance, high school transcript, immunizations, 1 letter of recommendation, minimum GPA in nursing prerequisites of 2.75, prerequisite course work. Transfer students are accepted. *Application deadline:* 1/15 (fall).

Advanced Placement Credit given for nursing courses completed elsewhere dependent upon specific evaluations.
Contact *Telephone:* 206-281-2612. *Fax:* 206-281-2767.

GRADUATE PROGRAMS

Contact *Telephone:* 206-281-2888. *Fax:* 206-378-5480.

MASTER'S DEGREE PROGRAM

Degree MSN
Available Programs Master's; Master's for Nurses with Non-Nursing Degrees.
Concentrations Available Nursing administration; nursing education. *Clinical nurse specialist programs in:* acute care, adult health, community health, critical care, gerontology, medical-surgical, oncology, palliative care, parent-child, pediatric, women's health. *Nurse practitioner programs in:* adult health, family health.
Study Options Full-time and part-time.
Program Entrance Requirements Clinical experience, computer literacy, minimum overall college GPA of 3.0, transcript of college record, CPR certification, written essay, immunizations, interview, 3 letters of recommendation, nursing research course, professional liability insurance/malpractice insurance, prerequisite course work, resume, statistics course, GRE General Test. *Application deadline:* 5/1 (fall). *Application fee:* $50.
Advanced Placement Credit given for nursing courses completed elsewhere dependent upon specific evaluations.
Degree Requirements 59 total credit hours, thesis or project, comprehensive exam.

POST-MASTER'S PROGRAM

Areas of Study Nursing education. *Nurse practitioner programs in:* adult health, family health.

Seattle University
College of Nursing
Seattle, Washington

http://www.seattleu.edu/nursing
Founded in 1891
DEGREES • BSN • DNP • MSN
Nursing Program Faculty 81 (42% with doctorates).
Baccalaureate Enrollment 418 **Women** 90% **Men** 10% **Minority** 37% **International** 1%
Graduate Enrollment 110 **Women** 89% **Men** 11% **Minority** 18% **International** 1%
Distance Learning Courses Available.
Nursing Student Activities Sigma Theta Tau, Student Nurses' Association.
Nursing Student Resources Academic advising; academic or career counseling; assistance for students with disabilities; bookstore; campus computer network; career placement assistance; computer lab; computer-assisted instruction; e-mail services; employment services for current students; housing assistance; interactive nursing skills videos; Internet; learning resource lab; library services; nursing audiovisuals; paid internships; remedial services; resume preparation assistance; skills, simulation, or other laboratory; tutoring.
Library Facilities 293,806 volumes; 1,569 periodical subscriptions.

BACCALAUREATE PROGRAMS

Degree BSN
Available Programs Baccalaureate for Second Degree; Generic Baccalaureate.
Study Options Full-time.
Program Entrance Requirements Minimum overall college GPA of 2.75, transcript of college record, CPR certification, written essay, health insurance, high school biology, high school chemistry, high school foreign language, 3 years high school math, 2 years high school science, high school transcript, immunizations, minimum GPA in nursing prerequisites of 3.0, professional liability insurance/malpractice insurance, prerequisite course work. Transfer students are accepted. *Application deadline:* 1/5 (winter). *Application fee:* $50.
Financial Aid 80% of baccalaureate students in nursing programs received some form of financial aid in 2011–12. *Gift aid (need-based):* Federal Pell, FSEOG, state, private, college/university gift aid from institutional funds, Federal Nursing. *Loans:* Federal Nursing Student Loans, Federal Direct (Subsidized and Unsubsidized Stafford PLUS),

Perkins. *Work-study:* Federal Work-Study, part-time campus jobs. *Financial aid application deadline (priority):* 2/1.
Contact Rita Tower, Pre-Major Advisor, College of Nursing, Seattle University, 901 12th Avenue, PO Box 222000, Seattle, WA 98122-1090. *Telephone:* 206-296-2242. *Fax:* 206-296-5544. *E-mail:* rstower@seattleu.edu.

GRADUATE PROGRAMS

Financial Aid 81% of graduate students in nursing programs received some form of financial aid in 2011–12. Fellowships, research assistantships, career-related internships or fieldwork and Federal Work-Study available. Aid available to part-time students.
Contact Dr. Anne Hirsch, Associate Dean for Graduate Education, College of Nursing, Seattle University, 901 12th Avenue, PO Box 222000, Seattle, WA 98122-1090. *Telephone:* 206-296-5660. *Fax:* 206-296-5544. *E-mail:* nurse@seattleu.edu.

MASTER'S DEGREE PROGRAM

Degree MSN
Available Programs Accelerated Master's for Nurses with Non-Nursing Degrees; Master's.
Concentrations Available *Clinical nurse specialist programs in:* community health. *Nurse practitioner programs in:* family health, gerontology, psychiatric/mental health.
Study Options Full-time.
Program Entrance Requirements Clinical experience, computer literacy, minimum overall college GPA of 3.0, transcript of college record, CPR certification, written essay, immunizations, interview, 2 letters of recommendation, professional liability insurance/malpractice insurance, prerequisite course work, resume, statistics course, GRE General Test. *Application deadline:* 12/1 (fall). *Application fee:* $55.
Advanced Placement Credit given for nursing courses completed elsewhere dependent upon specific evaluations.
Degree Requirements 110 total credit hours, thesis or project.

POST-MASTER'S PROGRAM

Areas of Study *Clinical nurse specialist programs in:* community health. *Nurse practitioner programs in:* family health, gerontology, psychiatric/mental health.

DOCTORAL DEGREE PROGRAM

Degree DNP
Available Programs Doctorate.
Areas of Study Advanced practice nursing, clinical practice, community health, critical care, family health, health policy, individualized study, information systems, nursing education, nursing policy, nursing research.
Program Entrance Requirements Clinical experience, minimum overall college GPA of 3.25, interview by faculty committee, 2 letters of recommendation, MSN or equivalent, writing sample. *Application deadline:* 5/1 (fall). Applications may be processed on a rolling basis for some programs. *Application fee:* $55.
Degree Requirements 40 total credit hours.

University of Washington
School of Nursing
Seattle, Washington

http://nursing.uw.edu/
Founded in 1861
DEGREES • BSN • DNP • MN • MN/MPH • PHD
Nursing Program Faculty 246 (78% with doctorates).
Baccalaureate Enrollment 559 **Women** 84% **Men** 16% **Minority** 26% **International** 2% **Part-time** 13%
Graduate Enrollment 565 **Women** 87% **Men** 13% **Minority** 25% **International** 5% **Part-time** 59%
Distance Learning Courses Available.
Nursing Student Activities Sigma Theta Tau, Student Nurses' Association.
Nursing Student Resources Academic advising; academic or career counseling; assistance for students with disabilities; bookstore; campus computer network; computer lab; computer-assisted instruction; e-mail services; employment services for current students; interactive nursing skills videos; Internet; learning resource lab; library services; nursing audiovisuals; skills, simulation, or other laboratory.
Library Facilities 350,000 volumes in health; 2,400 periodical subscriptions health-care related.

BACCALAUREATE PROGRAMS

Degree BSN
Available Programs ADN to Baccalaureate; Accelerated Baccalaureate; Generic Baccalaureate.
Site Options Bothell, WA; Tacoma, WA.
Study Options Full-time.
Program Entrance Requirements Minimum overall college GPA of 2.0, transcript of college record, CPR certification, written essay, 1 letter of recommendation, minimum GPA in nursing prerequisites of 2.8, prerequisite course work. *Application deadline:* 1/15 (fall).
Expenses (2012–13) *Tuition, state resident:* full-time $11,307; part-time $375 per credit. *Tuition, nonresident:* full-time $28,860; part-time $960 per credit. *International tuition:* $28,860 full-time. *Room and board:* $9316; room only: $5316 per academic year. *Required fees:* full-time $1080; part-time $131 per credit.
Contact Academic Services, School of Nursing, University of Washington, Box 357260, Health Sciences Building, Room T310, Seattle, WA 98195. *Telephone:* 206-543-8736. *Fax:* 206-543-3624. *E-mail:* sonas@u.washington.edu.

GRADUATE PROGRAMS

Expenses (2012–13) *Tuition, state resident:* full-time $21,432; part-time $1021 per credit. *Tuition, nonresident:* full-time $38,553; part-time $1836 per credit. *International tuition:* $38,553 full-time. *Room and board:* $16,942; room only: $11,626 per academic year. *Required fees:* full-time $1078; part-time $80 per credit.
Financial Aid Fellowships, research assistantships, teaching assistantships, Federal Work-Study, institutionally sponsored loans, scholarships, and traineeships available.
Contact Academic Services, School of Nursing, University of Washington, Box 357260, Health Sciences Building, Room T310, Seattle, WA 98195. *Telephone:* 206-543-8736. *Fax:* 206-543-3624. *E-mail:* sonas@u.washington.edu.

MASTER'S DEGREE PROGRAM

Degrees MN; MN/MPH
Available Programs Master's; Master's for Nurses with Non-Nursing Degrees.
Concentrations Available Nurse-midwifery; nursing education. *Clinical nurse specialist programs in:* adult health, community health, gerontology, maternity-newborn, perinatal. *Nurse practitioner programs in:* adult health, family health, neonatal health, pediatric, primary care, psychiatric/mental health.
Site Options Bothell, WA; Tacoma, WA.
Study Options Full-time and part-time.
Program Entrance Requirements Minimum overall college GPA of 3.0, transcript of college record, written essay, 3 letters of recommendation, resume, statistics course, GRE. *Application deadline:* 1/15 (fall). *Application fee:* $75.
Advanced Placement Credit given for nursing courses completed elsewhere dependent upon specific evaluations.
Degree Requirements 38 total credit hours, thesis or project.

Degree MS
Available Programs Master's; Master's for Nurses with Non-Nursing Degrees.
Concentrations Available Nursing informatics.
Study Options Full-time and part-time.
Program Entrance Requirements Minimum overall college GPA of 3.0, transcript of college record, written essay, resume, 3 letters of recommendation, statistics course. Application deadline: 5/1 (fall). Application fee: $75.
Advanced Placement Credit given for nursing courses completed elsewhere dependent upon specific evaluations.
Degree Requirements 46 total credit hours, thesis or project.

POST-MASTER'S PROGRAM

Areas of Study Nurse-midwifery. *Clinical nurse specialist programs in:* gerontology, maternity-newborn, perinatal. *Nurse practitioner programs in:* adult health, neonatal health, pediatric, primary care, psychiatric/mental health.

DOCTORAL DEGREE PROGRAM

Degree DNP
Available Programs Doctorate; Doctorate for Nurses with Non-Nursing Degrees; Post-Baccalaureate Doctorate.
Areas of Study Advanced practice nursing, community health, family health, gerontology, maternity-newborn.

Program Entrance Requirements Minimum overall college GPA of 3.0, 3 letters of recommendation, statistics course, vita, writing sample, GRE. *Application deadline:* 1/15 (fall). *Application fee:* $75.
Degree Requirements 90 total credit hours.

DOCTORAL DEGREE PROGRAM

Degree PhD
Available Programs Doctorate, Doctorate for Nurses with Non-Nursing Degrees, Post-Baccalaureate Doctorate.
Areas of Study Faculty preparation, individualized study, nursing research.
Program Entrance Requirements Minimum overall college GPA of 3.0, 3 letters of recommendation, vita, writing sample. *Application deadline:* 1/15 (fall). *Application fee:* $75.
Degree Requirements 93 total credit hours, dissertation, oral exam, residency.

POSTDOCTORAL PROGRAM

Areas of Study Aging, cancer care, chronic illness, gerontology, health promotion/disease prevention, infection prevention/skin care, neurobehavior, nursing interventions, nursing research, self-care.
Postdoctoral Program Contact Academic Services, School of Nursing, University of Washington, Box 357260, Health Sciences Building, Room T310, Seattle, WA 98195. *Telephone:* 206-543-8736. *Fax:* 206-685-1613. *E-mail:* sonas@u.washington.edu.

CONTINUING EDUCATION PROGRAM

Contact Martha Duhamel, Assistant Dean for Continuing Nursing Education, School of Nursing, University of Washington, Box 359440, Seattle, WA 98195-9440. *Telephone:* 206-543-1047. *Fax:* 206-543-6953. *E-mail:* marthadu@u.washington.edu.

Walla Walla University
School of Nursing
College Place, Washington

http://www.wallawalla.edu/nursing
Founded in 1892

DEGREE • BS

Nursing Program Faculty 28 (11% with doctorates).
Baccalaureate Enrollment 191 **Women** 81% **Men** 19% **Minority** 23% **International** 2% **Part-time** 2%
Nursing Student Activities Nursing Honor Society, nursing club.
Nursing Student Resources Academic advising; academic or career counseling; assistance for students with disabilities; bookstore; campus computer network; computer lab; e-mail services; Internet; learning resource lab; library services; nursing audiovisuals; resume preparation assistance; skills, simulation, or other laboratory; tutoring.
Library Facilities 10,000 volumes in health, 7,000 volumes in nursing; 450 periodical subscriptions health-care related.

BACCALAUREATE PROGRAMS

Degree BS
Available Programs ADN to Baccalaureate; Generic Baccalaureate; LPN to Baccalaureate; RN Baccalaureate.
Site Options Portland, OR.
Study Options Full-time.
Program Entrance Requirements Minimum overall college GPA of 2.75, transcript of college record, CPR certification, written essay, health exam, health insurance, high school biology, 3 years high school math, 2 years high school science, high school transcript, immunizations, 3 letters of recommendation, minimum high school GPA of 2.75, minimum GPA in nursing prerequisites of 2.75, prerequisite course work. Transfer students are accepted. *Application deadline:* 4/15 (fall), 2/1 (summer). *Application fee:* $40.
Advanced Placement Credit given for nursing courses completed elsewhere dependent upon specific evaluations.
Expenses (2012–13) *Tuition:* full-time $24,360; part-time $638 per quarter hour. *International tuition:* $24,360 full-time. *Room and board:* $5853; room only: $3288 per academic year. *Required fees:* full-time $540; part-time $180 per term.
Financial Aid 95% of baccalaureate students in nursing programs received some form of financial aid in 2011–12.
Contact Jan Thurnhofer, Student Program Advisor, School of Nursing, Walla Walla University, 10345 SE Market Street, Portland, OR 97216.

Telephone: 503-251-6115 Ext. 7304. *Fax:* 503-251-6249. *E-mail:* jant@
wallawalla.edu.

Washington State University

Intercollegiate College of Nursing/Washington
State University
Pullman, Washington

*See description of programs under Washington State
University College of Nursing (Spokane, Washington).*

Washington State University College of Nursing

Washington State University College of Nursing
Spokane, Washington

http://www.nursing.wsu.edu/

DEGREES • BSN • MN • PHD

Nursing Program Faculty 114 (39% with doctorates).
Baccalaureate Enrollment 759 **Women** 84% **Men** 16% **Minority** 22%
Part-time 29%
Graduate Enrollment 274 **Women** 89% **Men** 11% **Minority** 12%
International 1% **Part-time** 83%
Distance Learning Courses Available.
Nursing Student Activities Nursing Honor Society, Sigma Theta Tau,
Student Nurses' Association, nursing club.
Nursing Student Resources Academic advising; academic or career
counseling; assistance for students with disabilities; bookstore; campus
computer network; computer lab; computer-assisted instruction; e-mail
services; interactive nursing skills videos; Internet; learning resource lab;
library services; nursing audiovisuals; other; remedial services; resume
preparation assistance; skills, simulation, or other laboratory; tutoring;
unpaid internships.
Library Facilities 15,000 volumes in health, 7,000 volumes in nursing;
2,000 periodical subscriptions health-care related.

BACCALAUREATE PROGRAMS

Degree BSN
Available Programs Generic Baccalaureate; RN Baccalaureate.
Site Options Richland, WA; Yakima, WA; Vancouver, WA.
Study Options Full-time.
Program Entrance Requirements Minimum overall college GPA of
2.8, transcript of college record, CPR certification, health insurance,
immunizations, interview, minimum GPA in nursing prerequisites of 2.8,
professional liability insurance/malpractice insurance, prerequisite course
work. Transfer students are accepted. *Application deadline:* 1/15 (fall),
8/5 (spring). *Application fee:* $45.
Advanced Placement Credit given for nursing courses completed elsewhere dependent upon specific evaluations.
Expenses (2011–12) *Tuition, state resident:* full-time $9886; part-time
$494 per credit hour. *Tuition, nonresident:* full-time $21,164; part-time
$1058 per credit hour. *International tuition:* $21,164 full-time. *Required
fees:* full-time $1124.
Financial Aid 68% of baccalaureate students in nursing programs
received some form of financial aid in 2010–11.
Contact Ms. Renae J. Richter, Academic Coordinator, Washington State
University College of Nursing, PO Box 1495, Spokane, WA 99210-1495.
Telephone: 509-324-7337. *Fax:* 509-324-7336. *E-mail:* richre@wsu.edu.

GRADUATE PROGRAMS

Expenses (2011–12) *Tuition, state resident:* full-time $16,470; part-time
$824 per credit hour. *Tuition, nonresident:* full-time $31,232; part-time
$1562 per credit hour. *Required fees:* full-time $420.
Financial Aid 53% of graduate students in nursing programs received
some form of financial aid in 2010–11.
Contact Ms. Tamara Kelley, Principal Assistant, Washington State
University College of Nursing, PO Box 1495, Spokane, WA 99210-1495.
Telephone: 509-324-7334. *Fax:* 509-324-7336. *E-mail:* kelleyt@
wsu.edu.

MASTER'S DEGREE PROGRAM

Degree MN
Available Programs Accelerated Master's for Nurses with Non-Nursing
Degrees; Accelerated RN to Master's; Master's.
Concentrations Available Nurse case management; nursing administration; nursing education. *Clinical nurse specialist programs in:* community health. *Nurse practitioner programs in:* family health,
psychiatric/mental health.
Site Options Richland, WA; Yakima, WA; Vancouver, WA.
Study Options Full-time and part-time.
Program Entrance Requirements Computer literacy, minimum overall
college GPA of 3.0, transcript of college record, CPR certification,
written essay, immunizations, interview, 3 letters of recommendation,
physical assessment course, professional liability insurance/malpractice
insurance, prerequisite course work, statistics course. *Application
deadline:* 2/1 (fall), 10/1 (spring).
Advanced Placement Credit given for nursing courses completed elsewhere dependent upon specific evaluations.
Degree Requirements 45 total credit hours, thesis or project.

POST-MASTER'S PROGRAM

Areas of Study *Nurse practitioner programs in:* family health, psychi-
atric/mental health.

DOCTORAL DEGREE PROGRAM

Degree PhD
Available Programs Doctorate.
Areas of Study Nursing education, nursing research.
Program Entrance Requirements Minimum overall college GPA of
3.5, interview by faculty committee, 3 letters of recommendation, MSN
or equivalent, scholarly papers, statistics course, vita. *Application
deadline:* 1/10 (summer).
Degree Requirements 72 total credit hours, dissertation.

CONTINUING EDUCATION PROGRAM

Contact Mr. Ryan Townsend, Director of Professional Development,
Washington State University College of Nursing, PO Box 1495, Spokane,
WA 99210-1495. *Telephone:* 509-324-7354. *Fax:* 509-324-7341. *E-mail:*
cjohns@wsu.edu.

Whitworth College

Intercollegiate College of Nursing/Washington
State University
Spokane, Washington

*See description of programs under Washington State
University College of Nursing (Spokane, Washington).*

WEST VIRGINIA

Alderson-Broaddus College

Department of Nursing
Philippi, West Virginia

http://www.ab.edu/
Founded in 1871
DEGREE • BSN
Nursing Program Faculty 13 (1% with doctorates).
Baccalaureate Enrollment 96 **Women** 94% **Men** 6% **Minority** 2%
International 1% **Part-time** 2%
Nursing Student Activities Student Nurses' Association.
Nursing Student Resources Academic advising; academic or career
counseling; assistance for students with disabilities; bookstore; campus
computer network; career placement assistance; computer lab; computer-
assisted instruction; e-mail services; employment services for current students; Internet; learning resource lab; library services; nursing audiovisuals; remedial services; resume preparation assistance; skills,
simulation, or other laboratory; tutoring.

Library Facilities 60,000 volumes (6,000 in health, 1,000 in nursing); 11,000 periodical subscriptions (172 health-care related).

BACCALAUREATE PROGRAMS

Degree BSN

Available Programs Generic Baccalaureate; LPN to RN Baccalaureate; RN Baccalaureate.

Study Options Full-time.

Program Entrance Requirements Minimum overall college GPA of 2.0, transcript of college record, CPR certification, health exam, high school chemistry, high school transcript, immunizations, minimum GPA in nursing prerequisites of 2.25, professional liability insurance/malpractice insurance, prerequisite course work. Transfer students are accepted. *Application deadline:* 7/30 (fall), 1/5 (winter). Applications may be processed on a rolling basis for some programs. *Application fee:* $25.

Advanced Placement Credit by examination available. Credit given for nursing courses completed elsewhere dependent upon specific evaluations.

Contact *Telephone:* 304-457-6384. *Fax:* 304-457-6293.

Bluefield State College

Program in Nursing
Bluefield, West Virginia

http://www.bluefieldstate.edu/
Founded in 1895

DEGREE • BSN

Nursing Program Faculty 15

Baccalaureate Enrollment 4 **Women** 93% **Men** 7% **Part-time** 20%

Distance Learning Courses Available.

Nursing Student Activities Nursing Honor Society, Sigma Theta Tau, Student Nurses' Association.

Nursing Student Resources Academic advising; academic or career counseling; assistance for students with disabilities; bookstore; campus computer network; career placement assistance; computer lab; computer-assisted instruction; e-mail services; housing assistance; interactive nursing skills videos; Internet; learning resource lab; library services; nursing audiovisuals; resume preparation assistance; skills, simulation, or other laboratory; tutoring.

Library Facilities 5,649 volumes in health, 1,250 volumes in nursing; 200 periodical subscriptions health-care related.

BACCALAUREATE PROGRAMS

Degree BSN

Available Programs ADN to Baccalaureate; RN Baccalaureate.

Site Options Beckley, WV; Bluefield, WV.

Study Options Full-time and part-time.

Online Degree Options Yes (online only).

Program Entrance Requirements Minimum overall college GPA of 2.5, transcript of college record, CPR certification, health exam, health insurance, high school chemistry, immunizations, letters of recommendation, minimum high school GPA of 2.8, minimum GPA in nursing prerequisites of 2.0, prerequisite course work, RN licensure. Transfer students are accepted. *Application deadline:* 3/1 (fall), 4/15 (spring).

Expenses (2012–13) *Tuition, area resident:* full-time $2528; part-time $210 per credit hour. *Tuition, state resident:* full-time $3600; part-time $300 per credit hour. *Tuition, nonresident:* full-time $5534; part-time $461 per credit hour.

Financial Aid 35% of baccalaureate students in nursing programs received some form of financial aid in 2011–12.

Contact Ms. Beth Pritchett, Director, Program in Nursing, Bluefield State College, 219 Rock Street, Bluefield, WV 24701. *Telephone:* 304-327-4139. *Fax:* 304-327-4219. *E-mail:* bpritchett@bluefieldstate.edu.

Fairmont State University

School of Nursing and Allied Health Administration
Fairmont, West Virginia

http://www.fairmontstate.edu/
Founded in 1865

DEGREE • BSN

Nursing Program Faculty 4 (75% with doctorates).
Baccalaureate Enrollment 150 **Women** 96% **Men** 4% **International** 1% **Part-time** 40%
Distance Learning Courses Available.
Nursing Student Activities Sigma Theta Tau, Student Nurses' Association.
Nursing Student Resources Academic advising; academic or career counseling; assistance for students with disabilities; bookstore; campus computer network; career placement assistance; computer lab; computer-assisted instruction; e-mail services; housing assistance; interactive nursing skills videos; Internet; learning resource lab; library services; nursing audiovisuals; placement services for program completers; remedial services; resume preparation assistance; skills, simulation, or other laboratory; tutoring.
Library Facilities 280,000 volumes (9,000 in health, 1,100 in nursing); 895 periodical subscriptions (50 health-care related).

BACCALAUREATE PROGRAMS

Degree BSN

Available Programs ADN to Baccalaureate; Accelerated RN Baccalaureate; RN Baccalaureate.
Study Options Full-time and part-time.
Program Entrance Requirements Minimum overall college GPA of 2.0, transcript of college record, CPR certification, health exam, high school transcript, immunizations, minimum high school GPA of 2.0, RN licensure. Transfer students are accepted. *Application deadline:* 8/15 (fall), 8/15 (winter), 1/2 (spring), 5/15 (summer). Applications may be processed on a rolling basis for some programs.
Advanced Placement Credit by examination available. Credit given for nursing courses completed elsewhere dependent upon specific evaluations.
Financial Aid 80% of baccalaureate students in nursing programs received some form of financial aid in 2010–11.
Contact Dr. Tanya Lynn Rogers, Associate Professor/BSN Program Director, School of Nursing and Allied Health Administration, Fairmont State University, 1201 Locust Avenue, Fairmont, WV 26554. *Telephone:* 304-367-4074. *Fax:* 304-367-4268. *E-mail:* tanya.rogers@fairmontstate.edu.

CONTINUING EDUCATION PROGRAM

Contact Dr. Tanya Lynn Rogers, Associate Professor/BSN Program Director, School of Nursing and Allied Health Administration, Fairmont State University, 1201 Locust Avenue, Fairmont, WV 26554. *Telephone:* 304-367-4074. *Fax:* 304-367-4268. *E-mail:* tanya.rogers@fairmontstate.edu.

Marshall University

College of Health Professions
Huntington, West Virginia

http://www.marshall.edu/cohp
Founded in 1837

DEGREES • BSN • MSN

Nursing Program Faculty 35 (23% with doctorates).
Baccalaureate Enrollment 345 **Women** 80% **Men** 20% **Minority** 5% **Part-time** 35%
Graduate Enrollment 100 **Women** 90% **Men** 10% **Part-time** 60%
Nursing Student Activities Sigma Theta Tau, Student Nurses' Association, nursing club.
Nursing Student Resources Academic advising; academic or career counseling; assistance for students with disabilities; bookstore; campus computer network; career placement assistance; computer lab; computer-assisted instruction; daycare for children of students; e-mail services; employment services for current students; externships; housing assistance; interactive nursing skills videos; Internet; learning resource lab; library services; nursing audiovisuals; placement services for program

completers; remedial services; resume preparation assistance; skills, simulation, or other laboratory; tutoring.
Library Facilities 1.7 million volumes (20,200 in health, 6,400 in nursing); 24,652 periodical subscriptions (500 health-care related).

BACCALAUREATE PROGRAMS

Degree BSN
Available Programs Accelerated RN Baccalaureate; Generic Baccalaureate.
Study Options Full-time and part-time.
Program Entrance Requirements Minimum overall college GPA of 2.5, transcript of college record, high school transcript, minimum high school GPA of 2.5. Transfer students are accepted.
Advanced Placement Credit given for nursing courses completed elsewhere dependent upon specific evaluations.
Contact *Telephone:* 304-696-2639. *Fax:* 304-696-6739.

GRADUATE PROGRAMS

Contact *Telephone:* 304-696-2639. *Fax:* 304-696-6739.

MASTER'S DEGREE PROGRAM

Degree MSN
Available Programs Master's.
Concentrations Available Nursing administration; nursing education. *Nurse practitioner programs in:* family health.
Study Options Full-time and part-time.
Program Entrance Requirements Minimum overall college GPA of 3.0, transcript of college record, nursing research course, resume, statistics course, GRE General Test.
Advanced Placement Credit given for nursing courses completed elsewhere dependent upon specific evaluations.
Degree Requirements 36 total credit hours, thesis or project.

POST-MASTER'S PROGRAM

Areas of Study Nursing administration; nursing education. *Nurse practitioner programs in:* family health.

Shepherd University

Department of Nursing Education
Shepherdstown, West Virginia

http://www.shepherd.edu/nurseweb/
Founded in 1871
DEGREE • BSN
Nursing Program Faculty 8 (50% with doctorates).
Baccalaureate Enrollment 144 **Women** 92% **Men** 8% **Minority** 18%
International 4%
Nursing Student Activities Nursing Honor Society, Student Nurses' Association.
Nursing Student Resources Academic advising; academic or career counseling; assistance for students with disabilities; bookstore; campus computer network; career placement assistance; computer lab; computer-assisted instruction; e-mail services; interactive nursing skills videos; Internet; learning resource lab; library services; nursing audiovisuals; remedial services; resume preparation assistance; skills, simulation, or other laboratory; tutoring.
Library Facilities 285,494 volumes (4,997 in health, 462 in nursing); 45,260 periodical subscriptions (1,956 health-care related).

BACCALAUREATE PROGRAMS

Degree BSN
Available Programs ADN to Baccalaureate; Generic Baccalaureate; RN Baccalaureate.
Study Options Full-time.
Program Entrance Requirements Minimum overall college GPA of 2.5, transcript of college record, CPR certification, written essay, health exam, health insurance, immunizations, interview, minimum GPA in nursing prerequisites of 2.0, professional liability insurance/malpractice insurance, prerequisite course work. Transfer students are accepted.
Application deadline: 3/1 (fall), 10/1 (spring).
Advanced Placement Credit by examination available. Credit given for nursing courses completed elsewhere dependent upon specific evaluations.
Contact *Telephone:* 304-876-5341. *Fax:* 304-876-5169.

CONTINUING EDUCATION PROGRAM

Contact *Telephone:* 304-876-5341. *Fax:* 304-876-5169.

University of Charleston

Department of Nursing
Charleston, West Virginia

http://www.ucwv.edu/majors/nursing/
Founded in 1888
DEGREE • BSN
Nursing Program Faculty 6 (33% with doctorates).
Baccalaureate Enrollment 65 **Women** 97% **Men** 3% **Minority** 3%
International 1% **Part-time** 1%
Nursing Student Activities Nursing Honor Society, Sigma Theta Tau, Student Nurses' Association, nursing club.
Nursing Student Resources Academic advising; academic or career counseling; assistance for students with disabilities; bookstore; campus computer network; career placement assistance; computer lab; computer-assisted instruction; e-mail services; employment services for current students; externships; housing assistance; interactive nursing skills videos; Internet; learning resource lab; library services; nursing audiovisuals; paid internships; placement services for program completers; remedial services; resume preparation assistance; skills, simulation, or other laboratory; tutoring; unpaid internships.
Library Facilities 164,457 volumes (3,900 in health, 1,550 in nursing); 14,192 periodical subscriptions (75 health-care related).

BACCALAUREATE PROGRAMS

Degree BSN
Available Programs Generic Baccalaureate.
Study Options Full-time and part-time.
Program Entrance Requirements Minimum overall college GPA of 2.75, transcript of college record, CPR certification, health exam, high school biology, 1 year of high school math, high school transcript, immunizations, minimum high school GPA of 2.25, minimum GPA in nursing prerequisites of 2.75, professional liability insurance/malpractice insurance, prerequisite course work. Transfer students are accepted. *Application deadline:* Applications may be processed on a rolling basis for some programs.
Advanced Placement Credit given for nursing courses completed elsewhere dependent upon specific evaluations.
Expenses (2011–12) *Tuition:* full-time $19,500; part-time $900 per credit. *Room and board:* $9000; room only: $4900 per academic year. *Required fees:* full-time $1200.
Financial Aid 100% of baccalaureate students in nursing programs received some form of financial aid in 2010–11. *Gift aid (need-based):* Federal Pell, FSEOG, state, private, college/university gift aid from institutional funds, Academic Competitiveness Grants, National SMART Grants, TEACH Grants. *Loans:* Federal Nursing Student Loans, Federal Direct (Subsidized and Unsubsidized Stafford PLUS), Perkins, private loans. *Work-study:* Federal Work-Study, part-time campus jobs. *Financial aid application deadline:* 8/15(priority: 3/1).
Contact Joan Clark, Office of Undergraduate Admissions, Department of Nursing, University of Charleston, 2300 MacCorkle Avenue SE, Charleston, WV 25304. *Telephone:* 304-357-4750. *Fax:* 304-357-4781. *E-mail:* admissions@ucwv.edu.

West Liberty University

Department of Health Sciences
West Liberty, West Virginia

http://www.westliberty.edu/nursing/index.htm
Founded in 1837
DEGREE • BSN
Nursing Program Faculty 12 (33% with doctorates).
Baccalaureate Enrollment 123 **Women** 88% **Men** 12% **Minority** 3%
International 1%
Distance Learning Courses Available.
Nursing Student Activities Student Nurses' Association.
Nursing Student Resources Academic advising; academic or career counseling; assistance for students with disabilities; bookstore; campus computer network; career placement assistance; computer lab; computer-assisted instruction; e-mail services; externships; housing assistance;

interactive nursing skills videos; Internet; learning resource lab; library services; nursing audiovisuals; placement services for program completers; remedial services; resume preparation assistance; skills, simulation, or other laboratory; tutoring; unpaid internships.
Library Facilities 2,500 volumes in health, 750 volumes in nursing; 350 periodical subscriptions health-care related.

BACCALAUREATE PROGRAMS

Degree BSN
Available Programs Accelerated RN Baccalaureate; Generic Baccalaureate.
Site Options Triadelphia, WV.
Study Options Full-time and part-time.
Program Entrance Requirements Minimum overall college GPA of 3.0, transcript of college record, health exam, immunizations, minimum high school GPA of 3.0, minimum GPA in nursing prerequisites of 2.0, prerequisite course work. Transfer students are accepted. *Application deadline:* 3/31 (spring).
Advanced Placement Credit by examination available. Credit given for nursing courses completed elsewhere dependent upon specific evaluations.
Expenses (2012–13) *Tuition, state resident:* full-time $6422. *Tuition, nonresident:* full-time $13,990. *Room and board:* $8200 per academic year. *Required fees:* full-time $275.
Financial Aid 90% of baccalaureate students in nursing programs received some form of financial aid in 2011–12.
Contact Dr. Rose Kutlenios, Interim Program Director, Nursing, Department of Health Sciences, West Liberty University, 208 University Drive, College Union Box 140, West Liberty, WV 26074. *Telephone:* 304-336-8911. *Fax:* 304-336-5104. *E-mail:* rose.kutlenios@westliberty.edu.

West Virginia University
School of Nursing
Morgantown, West Virginia

http://nursing.hsc.wvu.edu/
Founded in 1867
DEGREES • BSN • DNP • MSN • PHD
Nursing Program Faculty 88 (53% with doctorates).
Baccalaureate Enrollment 653 **Women** 81% **Men** 19% **Minority** 4.6% **International** .3% **Part-time** 22%
Graduate Enrollment 193 **Women** 92% **Men** 8% **Minority** 5.3% **Part-time** 56%
Distance Learning Courses Available.
Nursing Student Activities Nursing Honor Society, Sigma Theta Tau, Student Nurses' Association.
Nursing Student Resources Academic advising; academic or career counseling; assistance for students with disabilities; bookstore; campus computer network; career placement assistance; computer lab; computer-assisted instruction; daycare for children of students; e-mail services; employment services for current students; externships; housing assistance; interactive nursing skills videos; Internet; learning resource lab; library services; nursing audiovisuals; other; paid internships; remedial services; resume preparation assistance; skills, simulation, or other laboratory; tutoring.
Library Facilities 1.9 million volumes (76,400 in health, 3,309 in nursing); 64,310 periodical subscriptions (72,384 health-care related).

BACCALAUREATE PROGRAMS

Degree BSN
Available Programs ADN to Baccalaureate; Accelerated Baccalaureate; Accelerated Baccalaureate for Second Degree; Generic Baccalaureate; RN Baccalaureate.
Site Options Glenville, WV; Montgomery, WV.
Study Options Full-time.
Program Entrance Requirements Minimum overall college GPA of 3.0, transcript of college record, CPR certification, health insurance, high school biology, high school chemistry, 3 years high school math, 3 years high school science, high school transcript, immunizations, interview, minimum high school GPA of 3.0, minimum GPA in nursing prerequisites of 3.0, prerequisite course work. Transfer students are accepted. *Application deadline:* 1/15 (fall), 5/15 (spring). *Application fee:* $30.
Advanced Placement Credit by examination available. Credit given for nursing courses completed elsewhere dependent upon specific evaluations.

Expenses (2012–13) *Tuition, state resident:* full-time $8194; part-time $682 per credit hour. *Tuition, nonresident:* full-time $23,222; part-time $1935 per credit hour. *Room and board:* $9808 per academic year.
Financial Aid 94% of baccalaureate students in nursing programs received some form of financial aid in 2011–12.
Contact Mrs. Kim McCourt, Recruiting and Outreach Coordinator, School of Nursing, West Virginia University, PO Box 9640, 6400 Health Sciences Center South, Morgantown, WV 26506-9600. *Telephone:* 304-293-1386. *Fax:* 304-293-2546. *E-mail:* kmccourt@hsc.wvu.edu.

GRADUATE PROGRAMS

Expenses (2012–13) *Tuition, state resident:* part-time $450 per credit hour. *Tuition, nonresident:* part-time $1758 per credit hour.
Financial Aid 88% of graduate students in nursing programs received some form of financial aid in 2011–12. 1 teaching assistantship with tuition reimbursement available (averaging $10,000 per year) was awarded; institutionally sponsored loans, tuition waivers (partial), and graduate administrative assistantships also available. *Financial aid application deadline:* 2/1.
Contact Mrs. Kim McCourt, Recruiting and Outreach Coordinator, School of Nursing, West Virginia University, PO Box 9640, 6400 RCB Health Sciences Center South, Morgantown, WV 26506-9600. *Telephone:* 304-293-1386. *Fax:* 304-293-2546. *E-mail:* kmccourt@hsc.wvu.edu.

MASTER'S DEGREE PROGRAM

Degree MSN
Available Programs Accelerated AD/RN to Master's; Accelerated Master's; Accelerated RN to Master's; Master's; RN to Master's.
Concentrations Available Nursing administration. *Nurse practitioner programs in:* family health, neonatal health, pediatric, women's health.
Site Options Charleston, WV.
Study Options Full-time and part-time.
Online Degree Options Yes (online only).
Program Entrance Requirements Computer literacy, minimum overall college GPA of 3.0, transcript of college record, CPR certification, written essay, immunizations, 3 letters of recommendation, nursing research course, physical assessment course, resume, statistics course. *Application deadline:* 3/1 (fall). *Application fee:* $60.
Advanced Placement Credit by examination available. Credit given for nursing courses completed elsewhere dependent upon specific evaluations.
Degree Requirements 44 total credit hours.

POST-MASTER'S PROGRAM

Areas of Study Nursing administration. *Nurse practitioner programs in:* family health, neonatal health, pediatric, women's health.

DOCTORAL DEGREE PROGRAM

Degree DNP
Available Programs Doctorate.
Areas of Study Addiction/substance abuse, advanced practice nursing, aging, bio-behavioral research, clinical practice, community health, ethics, family health, gerontology, health promotion/disease prevention, human health and illness, individualized study, maternity-newborn, neuro-behavior, nursing administration, oncology, women's health.
Online Degree Options Yes (online only).
Program Entrance Requirements Minimum overall college GPA of 3.0, 3 letters of recommendation, MSN or equivalent, statistics course, vita, writing sample. *Application deadline:* 3/1 (summer). *Application fee:* $50.
Degree Requirements 44 total credit hours, Capstone project, oral exam.

DOCTORAL DEGREE PROGRAM

Degree PhD
Available Programs Doctorate.
Areas of Study Addiction/substance abuse, aging, bio-behavioral research, community health, ethics, gerontology, health promotion/disease prevention, individualized study, nursing research, oncology, women's health.
Site Options Charleston, WV.
Program Entrance Requirements Minimum overall college GPA of 3.0, interview by faculty committee, 3 letters of recommendation, MSN or equivalent, statistics course, vita, writing sample, GRE General Test (PhD). *Application deadline:* 3/1 (summer). *Application fee:* $60.
Degree Requirements 55 total credit hours, dissertation, oral exam, written exam, residency.

CONTINUING EDUCATION PROGRAM

Contact Office of Extended Learning, School of Nursing, West Virginia University, PO Box 6800, 150 Clay Street, Morgantown, WV 26506-6800. *Telephone:* 800-253-2762. *Fax:* 304-293-4899. *E-mail:* elearn@mail.wvu.edu.

West Virginia Wesleyan College
School of Nursing
Buckhannon, West Virginia

http://www.wvwc.edu/
Founded in 1890
DEGREES • BSN • MSN
Nursing Program Faculty 11 (36% with doctorates).
Baccalaureate Enrollment 140 **Women** 94% **Men** 6% **Minority** 2%
Graduate Enrollment 20 **Women** 97% **Men** 3%
Nursing Student Activities Nursing Honor Society, Sigma Theta Tau, Student Nurses' Association.
Nursing Student Resources Academic advising; academic or career counseling; assistance for students with disabilities; bookstore; campus computer network; career placement assistance; computer-assisted instruction; e-mail services; employment services for current students; externships; interactive nursing skills videos; Internet; learning resource lab; library services; nursing audiovisuals; placement services for program completers; remedial services; resume preparation assistance; skills, simulation, or other laboratory; tutoring.
Library Facilities 130,000 volumes (4,000 in health, 600 in nursing); 14,500 periodical subscriptions (90 health-care related).

BACCALAUREATE PROGRAMS

Degree BSN
Available Programs Generic Baccalaureate.
Study Options Full-time and part-time.
Program Entrance Requirements Minimum overall college GPA of 3.0, transcript of college record, CPR certification, health exam, health insurance, high school transcript, immunizations, interview, minimum high school GPA of 2.5, minimum GPA in nursing prerequisites of 2.0, prerequisite course work. Transfer students are accepted. *Application deadline:* 6/15 (fall), 12/15 (spring). Applications may be processed on a rolling basis for some programs.
Advanced Placement Credit by examination available. Credit given for nursing courses completed elsewhere dependent upon specific evaluations.
Expenses (2012–13) *Tuition:* full-time $12,390; part-time $1040 per credit hour. *International tuition:* $12,390 full-time. *Room and board:* $7510; room only: $3840 per academic year. *Required fees:* full-time $1024; part-time $512 per term.
Financial Aid 95% of baccalaureate students in nursing programs received some form of financial aid in 2011–12. *Gift aid (need-based):* Federal Pell, FSEOG, state, private, college/university gift aid from institutional funds, Federal Nursing. *Loans:* Federal Nursing Student Loans, Federal Direct (Subsidized and Unsubsidized Stafford PLUS), Perkins.*Work-study:* Federal Work-Study, part-time campus jobs.*Financial aid application deadline (priority):* 2/15.
Contact Dr. Judith McKinney, Professor and Director, School of Nursing, West Virginia Wesleyan College, 59 College Avenue, Buckhannon, WV 26201-2995. *Telephone:* 304-473-8224. *Fax:* 304-473-8435. *E-mail:* mckinney@wvwc.edu.

GRADUATE PROGRAMS

Expenses (2012–13) *Tuition:* full-time $10,200; part-time $425 per credit hour. *International tuition:* $10,200 full-time. *Required fees:* full-time $780; part-time $195 per term.
Financial Aid 50% of graduate students in nursing programs received some form of financial aid in 2011–12.
Contact Dr. Sue Leight, Associate Professor and Director of MSN Program, School of Nursing, West Virginia Wesleyan College, 59 College Avenue, Buckhannon, WV 26201. *Telephone:* 304-473-8228. *E-mail:* leight@wvwc.edu.

MASTER'S DEGREE PROGRAM
Degree MSN
Available Programs Master's.

Concentrations Available Nurse-midwifery; nursing administration; nursing education. *Nurse practitioner programs in:* psychiatric/mental health.
Study Options Full-time and part-time.
Program Entrance Requirements Minimum overall college GPA of 3.0, transcript of college record, CPR certification, immunizations, interview, letters of recommendation, physical assessment course, professional liability insurance/malpractice insurance, resume, statistics course. *Application deadline:* 8/1 (fall), 12/10 (spring), 5/1 (summer). Applications may be processed on a rolling basis for some programs. *Application fee:* $50.
Degree Requirements 36 total credit hours, thesis or project.

Wheeling Jesuit University
Department of Nursing
Wheeling, West Virginia

http://www.wju.edu/
Founded in 1954
DEGREES • BSN • MSN
Nursing Program Faculty 18 (28% with doctorates).
Baccalaureate Enrollment 133 **Women** 93% **Men** 7% **Minority** 1% **International** 1% **Part-time** 52%
Graduate Enrollment 177 **Women** 94% **Men** 6% **Minority** 3% **Part-time** 88%
Distance Learning Courses Available.
Nursing Student Activities Sigma Theta Tau, Student Nurses' Association.
Nursing Student Resources Academic advising; academic or career counseling; assistance for students with disabilities; bookstore; campus computer network; career placement assistance; computer lab; computer-assisted instruction; e-mail services; employment services for current students; externships; housing assistance; Internet; learning resource lab; library services; nursing audiovisuals; placement services for program completers; remedial services; resume preparation assistance; skills, simulation, or other laboratory; tutoring.
Library Facilities 298,582 volumes (5,065 in nursing); 245 periodical subscriptions (90 health-care related).

BACCALAUREATE PROGRAMS

Degree BSN
Available Programs Accelerated Baccalaureate for Second Degree; Generic Baccalaureate; RN Baccalaureate.
Study Options Full-time and part-time.
Online Degree Options Yes.
Program Entrance Requirements Minimum overall college GPA of 2.75, transcript of college record, CPR certification, health exam, health insurance, immunizations, minimum GPA in nursing prerequisites of 2.0, prerequisite course work. Transfer students are accepted. *Application deadline:* Applications may be processed on a rolling basis for some programs.
Advanced Placement Credit by examination available. Credit given for nursing courses completed elsewhere dependent upon specific evaluations.
Expenses (2012–13) *Tuition:* full-time $25,360; part-time $695 per semester. *International tuition:* $25,360 full-time. *Required fees:* full-time $2210; part-time $1105 per term.
Financial Aid 97% of baccalaureate students in nursing programs received some form of financial aid in 2011–12.
Contact Admissions Office, Department of Nursing, Wheeling Jesuit University, 316 Washington Avenue, Wheeling, WV 26003-6233. *Telephone:* 304-243-2359. *Fax:* 304-243-2397.

GRADUATE PROGRAMS

Expenses (2012–13) *Tuition:* full-time $9990; part-time $555 per credit hour. *International tuition:* $9990 full-time. *Room and board:* $7160; room only: $4540 per academic year. *Required fees:* full-time $375; part-time $210 per term.
Financial Aid 95% of graduate students in nursing programs received some form of financial aid in 2011–12. Scholarships and unspecified assistantships available. *Financial aid application deadline:* 8/1.
Contact Mrs. Carol Carroll, Program Contact, Department of Nursing, Wheeling Jesuit University, 316 Washington Avenue, Wheeling, WV 26003-6233. *Telephone:* 304-243-2344. *Fax:* 304-243-2608. *E-mail:* ccarroll@wju.edu.

MASTER'S DEGREE PROGRAM

Degree MSN

Available Programs Master's; RN to Master's.

Concentrations Available Nursing administration; nursing education. *Nurse practitioner programs in:* family health.

Study Options Full-time and part-time.

Online Degree Options Yes (online only).

Program Entrance Requirements Computer literacy, minimum overall college GPA of 3.0, 3 letters of recommendation, statistics course, GRE General Test or MAT. *Application deadline:* Applications may be processed on a rolling basis for some programs.

Advanced Placement Credit given for nursing courses completed elsewhere dependent upon specific evaluations.

Degree Requirements 42 total credit hours, thesis or project, comprehensive exam.

POST-MASTER'S PROGRAM

Areas of Study Nursing administration; nursing education. *Nurse practitioner programs in:* family health.

WISCONSIN

Alverno College

Division of Nursing
Milwaukee, Wisconsin

http://www.alverno.edu/
Founded in 1887

DEGREES • BSN • MSN

Nursing Program Faculty 39 (5% with doctorates).

Baccalaureate Enrollment 763 **Women** 100% **Minority** 24% **Part-time** 22%

Graduate Enrollment 43 **Women** 96% **Men** 4% **Minority** 9% **Part-time** 62%

Nursing Student Activities Student Nurses' Association.

Nursing Student Resources Academic advising; academic or career counseling; assistance for students with disabilities; bookstore; campus computer network; career placement assistance; computer lab; computer-assisted instruction; daycare for children of students; e-mail services; employment services for current students; externships; housing assistance; interactive nursing skills videos; Internet; learning resource lab; library services; nursing audiovisuals; remedial services; resume preparation assistance; skills, simulation, or other laboratory; tutoring; unpaid internships.

Library Facilities 104,411 volumes; 36,986 periodical subscriptions.

BACCALAUREATE PROGRAMS

Degree BSN

Available Programs ADN to Baccalaureate; Baccalaureate for Second Degree; Generic Baccalaureate; LPN to Baccalaureate; RN Baccalaureate.

Study Options Full-time and part-time.

Program Entrance Requirements Minimum overall college GPA of 2.5, transcript of college record, written essay, high school biology, high school chemistry, 3 years high school math, 2 years high school science, high school transcript, minimum high school GPA of 2.0, prerequisite course work. Transfer students are accepted.

Advanced Placement Credit by examination available. Credit given for nursing courses completed elsewhere dependent upon specific evaluations.

Contact *Telephone:* 414-382-6276. *Fax:* 414-382-6279.

GRADUATE PROGRAMS

Contact *Telephone:* 414-382-6278. *Fax:* 414-382-6279.

MASTER'S DEGREE PROGRAM

Degree MSN

Available Programs Master's.

Concentrations Available Nursing education. *Clinical nurse specialist programs in:* adult health, gerontology, medical-surgical.

Study Options Full-time and part-time.

Program Entrance Requirements Clinical experience, transcript of college record, CPR certification, written essay, immunizations, 3 letters of recommendation, physical assessment course, statistics course.

Advanced Placement Credit given for nursing courses completed elsewhere dependent upon specific evaluations.

Degree Requirements 39 total credit hours, thesis or project.

CONTINUING EDUCATION PROGRAM

Contact *Telephone:* 414-382-6177. *Fax:* 414-382-6354.

Bellin College

Nursing Program
Green Bay, Wisconsin

http://www.bellincollege.edu/
Founded in 1909

DEGREES • BSN • MSN

Nursing Program Faculty 20 (21% with doctorates).

Baccalaureate Enrollment 274 **Women** 92% **Men** 8% **Minority** 5% **International** 1% **Part-time** 9%

Graduate Enrollment 32 **Women** 93% **Men** 7% **Minority** 2% **Part-time** 81%

Distance Learning Courses Available.

Nursing Student Activities Sigma Theta Tau, Student Nurses' Association.

Nursing Student Resources Academic advising; academic or career counseling; assistance for students with disabilities; career placement assistance; computer lab; computer-assisted instruction; e-mail services; interactive nursing skills videos; Internet; learning resource lab; library services; nursing audiovisuals; resume preparation assistance; skills, simulation, or other laboratory; tutoring.

Library Facilities 7,000 volumes (7,000 in health, 4,000 in nursing); 225 periodical subscriptions (190 health-care related).

BACCALAUREATE PROGRAMS

Degree BSN

Available Programs Accelerated Baccalaureate; Accelerated Baccalaureate for Second Degree; Baccalaureate for Second Degree; Generic Baccalaureate.

Study Options Full-time and part-time.

Program Entrance Requirements Minimum overall college GPA of 2.7, transcript of college record, CPR certification, health exam, health insurance, high school biology, high school chemistry, 3 years high school math, 3 years high school science, high school transcript, immunizations, interview, 3 letters of recommendation, minimum high school GPA of 3.25, minimum GPA in nursing prerequisites of 2.7. Transfer students are accepted. *Application deadline:* Applications may be processed on a rolling basis for some programs. *Application fee:* $30.

Advanced Placement Credit by examination available. Credit given for nursing courses completed elsewhere dependent upon specific evaluations.

Contact *Telephone:* 920-433-6651. *Fax:* 920-433-1922.

GRADUATE PROGRAMS

Contact *Telephone:* 920-433-3624. *Fax:* 920-433-1922.

MASTER'S DEGREE PROGRAM

Degree MSN

Available Programs Master's.

Concentrations Available Nursing administration; nursing education.

Study Options Full-time and part-time.

Online Degree Options Yes.

Program Entrance Requirements Computer literacy, minimum overall college GPA of 3.0, transcript of college record, written essay, interview, 3 letters of recommendation, nursing research course, resume, statistics course. *Application deadline:* Applications may be processed on a rolling basis for some programs. *Application fee:* $50.

Advanced Placement Credit given for nursing courses completed elsewhere dependent upon specific evaluations.

Degree Requirements 38 total credit hours, thesis or project.

Cardinal Stritch University
Ruth S. Coleman College of Nursing
Milwaukee, Wisconsin

http://www.stritch.edu/nursing
Founded in 1937

DEGREES • BSN • MSN

Nursing Program Faculty 36 (11% with doctorates).
Baccalaureate Enrollment 98 **Women** 90% **Men** 10% **Minority** 17% **International** 6%
Graduate Enrollment 15 **Women** 100% **Minority** 13%
Nursing Student Activities Student Nurses' Association.
Nursing Student Resources Academic advising; academic or career counseling; assistance for students with disabilities; bookstore; campus computer network; career placement assistance; computer lab; e-mail services; employment services for current students; interactive nursing skills videos; Internet; learning resource lab; library services; nursing audiovisuals; remedial services; resume preparation assistance; skills, simulation, or other laboratory; tutoring.
Library Facilities 124,897 volumes (4,500 in health, 600 in nursing); 667 periodical subscriptions (1,500 health-care related).

BACCALAUREATE PROGRAMS

Degree BSN
Available Programs ADN to Baccalaureate.
Site Options Menomonee Falls, WI; Milwaukee, WI.
Study Options Full-time and part-time.
Program Entrance Requirements Minimum overall college GPA of 2.33, transcript of college record, RN licensure. Transfer students are accepted. *Application deadline:* Applications may be processed on a rolling basis for some programs.
Advanced Placement Credit by examination available. Credit given for nursing courses completed elsewhere dependent upon specific evaluations.
Contact *Telephone:* 414-410-4966. *Fax:* 414-410-4049.

GRADUATE PROGRAMS

Contact *Telephone:* 414-410-4966. *Fax:* 414-410-4049.

MASTER'S DEGREE PROGRAM
Degree MSN
Available Programs Accelerated Master's.
Concentrations Available Nursing education.
Study Options Full-time.
Program Entrance Requirements Computer literacy, minimum overall college GPA of 3.0, transcript of college record, CPR certification, written essay, immunizations, interview, 3 letters of recommendation, nursing research course, resume. *Application deadline:* Applications may be processed on a rolling basis for some programs.
Advanced Placement Credit given for nursing courses completed elsewhere dependent upon specific evaluations.
Degree Requirements 36 total credit hours, thesis or project.

Carroll University
Nursing Program
Waukesha, Wisconsin

http://www.carrollu.edu/programs/nursing/
Founded in 1846

DEGREE • BSN

Nursing Program Faculty 14
Baccalaureate Enrollment 299 **Women** 93.31% **Men** 6.69% **Minority** 6% **International** 1% **Part-time** 8%
Nursing Student Activities Sigma Theta Tau, Student Nurses' Association.
Nursing Student Resources Academic advising; academic or career counseling; assistance for students with disabilities; bookstore; campus computer network; computer lab; computer-assisted instruction; e-mail services; housing assistance; interactive nursing skills videos; Internet; learning resource lab; library services; nursing audiovisuals; resume preparation assistance; skills, simulation, or other laboratory; tutoring.
Library Facilities 150,000 volumes; 65,200 periodical subscriptions.

BACCALAUREATE PROGRAMS

Degree BSN
Available Programs ADN to Baccalaureate; Generic Baccalaureate.
Study Options Full-time.
Program Entrance Requirements Minimum overall college GPA of 2.75, transcript of college record, written essay, health exam, health insurance, high school biology, high school chemistry, 3 years high school math, high school transcript, minimum high school GPA of 2.75, minimum GPA in nursing prerequisites of 2.75, prerequisite course work. Transfer students are accepted. *Application deadline:* Applications may be processed on a rolling basis for some programs.
Expenses (2012–13) *Tuition:* full-time $25,899; part-time $421 per credit. *International tuition:* $25,899 full-time. *Room and board:* $8314; room only: $4369 per academic year. *Required fees:* full-time $500; part-time $250 per term.
Financial Aid 98% of baccalaureate students in nursing programs received some form of financial aid in 2011–12. *Gift aid (need-based):* Federal Pell, FSEOG, state, private, college/university gift aid from institutional funds. *Loans:* Federal Direct (Subsidized and Unsubsidized Stafford PLUS), Perkins, state, college/university. *Work-study:* Federal Work-Study, part-time campus jobs. *Financial aid application deadline:* Continuous.
Contact Ms. Angela Rose Brindowski, Chair, Department of Nursing, Nursing Program, Carroll University, 100 North East Avenue, Waukesha, WI 53186. *Telephone:* 262-524-4927. *E-mail:* abrindow@carrollu.edu.

Columbia College of Nursing
Columbia College of Nursing/Mount Mary College Nursing Program
Milwaukee, Wisconsin

See description of programs under Columbia College of Nursing/Mount Mary College Nursing Program (Milwaukee, Wisconsin).

Columbia College of Nursing/Mount Mary College Nursing Program
Columbia College of Nursing/Mount Mary College Nursing Program
Milwaukee, Wisconsin

http://www.mtmary.edu/dept_nursing.htm
Founded in 2002

DEGREE • BSN

Nursing Program Faculty 20 (7% with doctorates).
Baccalaureate Enrollment 250 **Women** 95% **Men** 5% **Minority** 15% **Part-time** 20%
Nursing Student Activities Sigma Theta Tau, Student Nurses' Association.
Nursing Student Resources Academic advising; academic or career counseling; bookstore; campus computer network; career placement assistance; computer lab; computer-assisted instruction; daycare for children of students; e-mail services; employment services for current students; housing assistance; interactive nursing skills videos; Internet; learning resource lab; library services; nursing audiovisuals; resume preparation assistance; skills, simulation, or other laboratory; tutoring.

BACCALAUREATE PROGRAMS

Degree BSN
Available Programs Baccalaureate for Second Degree; Generic Baccalaureate; RN Baccalaureate.
Site Options Milwaukee, WI.
Study Options Full-time and part-time.
Program Entrance Requirements Minimum overall college GPA of 2.8, transcript of college record, health exam, health insurance, high school biology, high school chemistry, 2 years high school math, 2 years high school science, high school transcript, minimum high school GPA of 2.5, minimum high school rank 40%, minimum GPA in nursing prerequisites of 2.8, prerequisite course work. Transfer students are accepted.

Advanced Placement Credit by examination available. Credit given for nursing courses completed elsewhere dependent upon specific evaluations.
Contact *Telephone:* 414-256-1219 Ext. 193. *Fax:* 414-256-0180.

Concordia University Wisconsin
Program in Nursing
Mequon, Wisconsin

http://www.cuw.edu/
Founded in 1881
DEGREES • BSN • DNP • MSN
Nursing Program Faculty 12 (3% with doctorates).
Baccalaureate Enrollment 420 Women 92% Men 8% Minority 10% International 1% Part-time 32%
Graduate Enrollment 611 Women 95% Men 5% Minority 8% International 1% Part-time 44%
Distance Learning Courses Available.
Nursing Student Activities Nursing Honor Society, Sigma Theta Tau, Student Nurses' Association.
Nursing Student Resources Academic advising; academic or career counseling; assistance for students with disabilities; bookstore; campus computer network; career placement assistance; computer lab; computer-assisted instruction; e-mail services; employment services for current students; externships; interactive nursing skills videos; Internet; learning resource lab; library services; nursing audiovisuals; paid internships; placement services for program completers; resume preparation assistance; skills, simulation, or other laboratory; tutoring.
Library Facilities 3,893 volumes in health, 1,011 volumes in nursing; 922 periodical subscriptions health-care related.

BACCALAUREATE PROGRAMS

Degree BSN
Available Programs ADN to Baccalaureate; Generic Baccalaureate; LPN to RN Baccalaureate; RN Baccalaureate.
Site Options Mequon, WI; Milwaukee, WI.
Study Options Full-time.
Program Entrance Requirements Transcript of college record, CPR certification, health exam, health insurance, high school transcript, immunizations, minimum high school GPA of 2.75, minimum GPA in nursing prerequisites of 2.75, RN licensure. Transfer students are accepted. *Application deadline:* 7/15 (fall), 7/15 (winter), 10/15 (spring), 3/15 (summer). *Application fee:* $50.
Advanced Placement Credit given for nursing courses completed elsewhere dependent upon specific evaluations.
Expenses (2011–12) *Tuition:* full-time $23,050; part-time $960 per credit hour. *International tuition:* $23,050 full-time. *Room and board:* $8700 per academic year. *Required fees:* full-time $210; part-time $105 per term.
Financial Aid 98% of baccalaureate students in nursing programs received some form of financial aid in 2010–11. *Gift aid (need-based):* Federal Pell, FSEOG, state, private, college/university gift aid from institutional funds. *Loans:* Federal Direct (Subsidized and Unsubsidized Stafford PLUS), state. *Work-study:* Federal Work-Study. *Financial aid application deadline (priority):* 3/15.
Contact Mrs. Sandra Hannemann, Administrative Assistant, Nursing Department, Program in Nursing, Concordia University Wisconsin, 12800 North Lake Shore Drive, Mequon, WI 53097. *Telephone:* 262-243-4374. *Fax:* 262-243-4466. *E-mail:* sandy.hannemann@cuw.edu.

GRADUATE PROGRAMS

Expenses (2011–12) *Tuition:* full-time $8550; part-time $570 per credit hour. *International tuition:* $8550 full-time. *Required fees:* full-time $485; part-time $160 per term.
Financial Aid 96% of graduate students in nursing programs received some form of financial aid in 2010–11. *Application deadline:* 8/1.
Contact Dr. Teri Kaul, Director, Masters Program in Nursing and DNP, Program in Nursing, Concordia University Wisconsin, 12800 North Lake Shore Drive, Mequon, WI 53097. *Telephone:* 262-243-4538. *Fax:* 262-243-4506. *E-mail:* teri.kaul@cuw.edu.

MASTER'S DEGREE PROGRAM
Degree MSN
Available Programs Master's.
Concentrations Available Nursing education. *Nurse practitioner programs in:* adult health, family health, gerontology.

Site Options multiple cities and states; Mequon, WI; Milwaukee, WI.
Study Options Full-time and part-time.
Program Entrance Requirements Clinical experience, computer literacy, minimum overall college GPA of 3.0, transcript of college record, CPR certification, written essay, immunizations, interview, 2 letters of recommendation, physical assessment course, professional liability insurance/malpractice insurance, resume, statistics course. *Application deadline:* 6/1 (fall), 10/15 (spring). *Application fee:* $50.
Advanced Placement Credit given for nursing courses completed elsewhere dependent upon specific evaluations.
Degree Requirements 44 total credit hours, thesis or project.

POST-MASTER'S PROGRAM
Areas of Study *Nurse practitioner programs in:* family health.

DOCTORAL DEGREE PROGRAM
Degree DNP
Available Programs Doctorate.
Areas of Study Family health, gerontology.
Site Options multiple cities and states; Mequon, WI; Milwaukee, WI.
Online Degree Options Yes (online only).
Program Entrance Requirements Clinical experience, minimum overall college GPA of 3.0, 2 letters of recommendation, MSN or equivalent, vita, writing sample. *Application deadline:* 4/1 (spring). *Application fee:* $50.
Degree Requirements 35 total credit hours, dissertation.

Edgewood College
Program in Nursing
Madison, Wisconsin

http://nursing.edgewood.edu/
Founded in 1927
DEGREES • BS • MS • MSN/MBA
Nursing Program Faculty 36 (25% with doctorates).
Baccalaureate Enrollment 220 Women 90% Men 10% Minority 2% International 1% Part-time 35%
Graduate Enrollment 45 Women 86% Men 14% Minority 2% Part-time 100%
Distance Learning Courses Available.
Nursing Student Activities Sigma Theta Tau, Student Nurses' Association.
Nursing Student Resources Academic advising; academic or career counseling; assistance for students with disabilities; bookstore; campus computer network; career placement assistance; computer lab; computer-assisted instruction; e-mail services; employment services for current students; externships; housing assistance; interactive nursing skills videos; Internet; learning resource lab; library services; nursing audiovisuals; paid internships; remedial services; resume preparation assistance; skills, simulation, or other laboratory; tutoring; unpaid internships.
Library Facilities 92,145 volumes (4,500 in health, 1,000 in nursing); 26,700 periodical subscriptions (45 health-care related).

BACCALAUREATE PROGRAMS

Degree BS
Available Programs Accelerated Baccalaureate for Second Degree; Baccalaureate for Second Degree; Generic Baccalaureate.
Site Options Madison, WI.
Study Options Full-time and part-time.
Program Entrance Requirements Minimum overall college GPA of 2.75, transcript of college record, CPR certification, written essay, health exam, high school biology, high school chemistry, high school foreign language, high school math, high school transcript, immunizations, interview, minimum high school GPA of 2.75, minimum GPA in nursing prerequisites of 2.75, prerequisite course work. Transfer students are accepted. *Application deadline:* 1/15 (fall), 9/15 (spring). *Application fee:* $40.
Advanced Placement Credit given for nursing courses completed elsewhere dependent upon specific evaluations.
Contact *Telephone:* 608-663-2280. *Fax:* 608-663-2863.

GRADUATE PROGRAMS

Contact *Telephone:* 608-663-2280. *Fax:* 608-663-2863.

MASTER'S DEGREE PROGRAM
Degrees MS; MSN/MBA

Available Programs Master's.
Concentrations Available Nursing administration; nursing education.
Site Options Madison, WI.
Study Options Full-time and part-time.
Program Entrance Requirements Clinical experience, computer literacy, minimum overall college GPA of 3.0, transcript of college record, CPR certification, written essay, immunizations, interview, 2 letters of recommendation, nursing research course, prerequisite course work, resume, statistics course. *Application deadline:* Applications may be processed on a rolling basis for some programs.
Advanced Placement Credit given for nursing courses completed elsewhere dependent upon specific evaluations.
Degree Requirements 36 total credit hours, thesis or project.

Herzing University Online
Program in Nursing
Milwaukee, Wisconsin

DEGREE • BSN

BACCALAUREATE PROGRAMS

Degree BSN
Available Programs Generic Baccalaureate.
Online Degree Options Yes (online only).
Contact Nursing Information, Program in Nursing, Herzing University Online, Administrative Offices, W140 N8917 Lilly Road, Menomonee Falls, WI 53051. *Telephone:* 866-508-0748. *Fax:* 414-727-7090. *E-mail:* admissions@onl.herzing.edu.

Maranatha Baptist Bible College
Nursing Department
Watertown, Wisconsin

http://www.mbbc.edu
Founded in 1968
DEGREE • BSN
Baccalaureate Enrollment 58
Nursing Student Activities Student Nurses' Association.
Nursing Student Resources Academic advising; academic or career counseling; assistance for students with disabilities; bookstore; campus computer network; career placement assistance; computer lab; computer-assisted instruction; e-mail services; employment services for current students; housing assistance; interactive nursing skills videos; Internet; learning resource lab; library services; nursing audiovisuals; skills, simulation, or other laboratory; tutoring.
Library Facilities 124,000 volumes; 500 periodical subscriptions.

BACCALAUREATE PROGRAMS

Degree BSN
Available Programs RN Baccalaureate.
Program Entrance Requirements Minimum overall college GPA of 2.5, CPR certification, written essay, health exam, immunizations, interview, minimum high school GPA, minimum GPA in nursing prerequisites of 2.5, prerequisite course work. Transfer students are accepted. *Application deadline:* Applications may be processed on a rolling basis for some programs.
Contact *Telephone:* 920-206-4050.

Marian University
School of Nursing
Fond du Lac, Wisconsin

http://www.mariancollege.edu/
Founded in 1936
DEGREES • BSN • MSN
Baccalaureate Enrollment 221 **Women** 95% **Men** 5% **Minority** 1% **Part-time** 7%
Graduate Enrollment 39 **Women** 97% **Men** 3% **Part-time** 15%
Nursing Student Activities Student Nurses' Association.

Nursing Student Resources Academic advising; academic or career counseling; assistance for students with disabilities; bookstore; career placement assistance; computer lab; daycare for children of students; e-mail services; externships; interactive nursing skills videos; Internet; learning resource lab; library services; nursing audiovisuals.
Library Facilities 141,495 volumes (3,000 in health, 2,500 in nursing); 1,391 periodical subscriptions (91 health-care related).

BACCALAUREATE PROGRAMS

Degree BSN
Available Programs ADN to Baccalaureate; Generic Baccalaureate.
Site Options Appleton, WI; Beaver Dam, WI.
Study Options Full-time and part-time.
Program Entrance Requirements Transcript of college record, high school biology, high school chemistry, 3 years high school math, high school science, high school transcript, minimum high school GPA of 2.5. Transfer students are accepted.
Advanced Placement Credit given for nursing courses completed elsewhere dependent upon specific evaluations.
Contact *Telephone:* 920-923-8732. *Fax:* 920-923-8770.

GRADUATE PROGRAMS

Contact *Telephone:* 920-923-8094. *Fax:* 920-923-8094.

MASTER'S DEGREE PROGRAM
Degree MSN
Available Programs Master's.
Concentrations Available Nursing education. *Nurse practitioner programs in:* adult health.
Study Options Full-time and part-time.
Program Entrance Requirements Clinical experience, minimum overall college GPA of 3.0, transcript of college record, CPR certification, written essay, immunizations, 3 letters of recommendation, nursing research course, professional liability insurance/malpractice insurance, resume, statistics course.
Advanced Placement Credit given for nursing courses completed elsewhere dependent upon specific evaluations.
Degree Requirements 39 total credit hours, thesis or project.

POST-MASTER'S PROGRAM
Areas of Study Nursing education.

Marquette University
College of Nursing
Milwaukee, Wisconsin

http://www.marquette.edu/nursing
Founded in 1881
DEGREES • BSN • DNP • MSN • MSN/MBA • PHD
Nursing Program Faculty 60 (57% with doctorates).
Baccalaureate Enrollment 449 **Women** 94% **Men** 6% **Minority** 15% **International** .4% **Part-time** 1%
Graduate Enrollment 350 **Women** 92% **Men** 8% **Minority** 10% **International** .5% **Part-time** 71%
Distance Learning Courses Available.
Nursing Student Activities Nursing Honor Society, Sigma Theta Tau, Student Nurses' Association.
Nursing Student Resources Academic advising; academic or career counseling; assistance for students with disabilities; bookstore; campus computer network; career placement assistance; computer lab; computer-assisted instruction; daycare for children of students; e-mail services; employment services for current students; housing assistance; interactive nursing skills videos; Internet; learning resource lab; library services; nursing audiovisuals; placement services for program completers; remedial services; resume preparation assistance; skills, simulation, or other laboratory; tutoring.
Library Facilities 1.7 million volumes (51,164 in health, 9,127 in nursing); 34,416 periodical subscriptions (6,065 health-care related).

BACCALAUREATE PROGRAMS

Degree BSN
Available Programs Generic Baccalaureate.
Study Options Full-time and part-time.
Program Entrance Requirements Minimum overall college GPA of 3.0, transcript of college record, written essay, high school biology, high

school chemistry, 3 years high school math, high school transcript, 1 letter of recommendation, minimum high school GPA of 2.5, minimum high school rank 25%. *Application deadline:* 12/1 (fall).

Advanced Placement Credit given for nursing courses completed elsewhere dependent upon specific evaluations.

Expenses (2012–13) *Tuition:* full-time $32,818; part-time $955 per credit. *International tuition:* $32,818 full-time. *Room and board:* $10,360; room only: $6640 per academic year. *Required fees:* full-time $800.

Financial Aid 97% of baccalaureate students in nursing programs received some form of financial aid in 2011–12. *Gift aid (need-based):* Federal Pell, FSEOG, state, private, college/university gift aid from institutional funds. *Loans:* Federal Nursing Student Loans, Federal Direct (Subsidized and Unsubsidized Stafford PLUS), Perkins, state, college/university. *Work-study:* Federal Work-Study, part-time campus jobs. *Financial aid application deadline:* Continuous.

Contact Dr. Kerry Kosmoski-Goepfert, Associate Dean for Undergraduate Programs, College of Nursing, Marquette University, Clark Hall, PO Box 1881, Milwaukee, WI 53201-1881. *Telephone:* 414-288-3809. *Fax:* 414-288-1597. *E-mail:* kerry.goepfert@marquette.edu.

GRADUATE PROGRAMS

Expenses (2012–13) *Tuition:* part-time $985 per credit.

Financial Aid 90% of graduate students in nursing programs received some form of financial aid in 2011–12. 1 fellowship with partial tuition reimbursement available (averaging $17,500 per year), 2 research assistantships with full tuition reimbursements available (averaging $13,285 per year), 8 teaching assistantships with full tuition reimbursements available (averaging $13,912 per year) were awarded; career-related internships or fieldwork, Federal Work-Study, scholarships, tuition waivers (partial), and unspecified assistantships also available. Aid available to part-time students. *Financial aid application deadline:* 2/15.

Contact Dr. Maureen O'Brien, Associate Dean for Graduate Programs, College of Nursing, Marquette University, Clark Hall, PO Box 1881, Milwaukee, WI 53201-1881. *Telephone:* 414-288-3869. *Fax:* 414-288-1597. *E-mail:* maureen.obrien@marquette.edu.

MASTER'S DEGREE PROGRAM

Degrees MSN; MSN/MBA

Available Programs Master's; Master's for Non-Nursing College Graduates; Master's for Nurses with Non-Nursing Degrees; RN to Master's.

Concentrations Available Clinical nurse leader; nurse-midwifery; nursing administration. *Clinical nurse specialist programs in:* adult health, pediatric. *Nurse practitioner programs in:* acute care, adult health, gerontology, pediatric, primary care.

Study Options Full-time and part-time.

Program Entrance Requirements Minimum overall college GPA of 3.0, transcript of college record, CPR certification, written essay, immunizations, 3 letters of recommendation, nursing research course, physical assessment course, prerequisite course work, resume, statistics course, GRE General Test. *Application deadline:* 2/15 (fall), 11/15 (spring). Applications may be processed on a rolling basis for some programs. *Application fee:* $50.

Advanced Placement Credit given for nursing courses completed elsewhere dependent upon specific evaluations.

Degree Requirements 42 total credit hours, comprehensive exam.

POST-MASTER'S PROGRAM

Areas of Study Nurse-midwifery; nursing administration. *Clinical nurse specialist programs in:* adult health. *Nurse practitioner programs in:* acute care, adult health, gerontology, pediatric, primary care.

DOCTORAL DEGREE PROGRAM

Degree DNP

Available Programs Doctorate, Post-Baccalaureate Doctorate.

Areas of Study Advanced practice nursing, health-care systems, nursing administration.

Program Entrance Requirements Minimum overall college GPA of 3.2, clinical experience, letters of recommendation, MSN or equivalent, statistics course, vita. *Application deadline:* 2/15 (fall).

Degree Requirements 63-67 credits Post-BSN/30 credits Post-Masters, residency, written exam.

DOCTORAL DEGREE PROGRAM

Degree PhD

Available Programs Doctorate; Post-Baccalaureate Doctorate.

Areas of Study Aging, faculty preparation, health promotion/disease prevention, health-care systems, human health and illness, illness and transition, nursing administration, nursing education, nursing research, nursing science.

Program Entrance Requirements Minimum overall college GPA of 3.2, interview, 3 letters of recommendation, MSN or equivalent, statistics course, vita, writing sample, GRE General Test. *Application deadline:* 2/15 (fall), 11/15 (spring). Applications may be processed on a rolling basis for some programs. *Application fee:* $50.

Degree Requirements 51 total credit hours, dissertation, oral exam, written exam, residency.

See display on next page and full description on page 492.

Milwaukee School of Engineering
School of Nursing
Milwaukee, Wisconsin

http://www.msoe.edu/nursing

Founded in 1903

DEGREE • BSN

Nursing Program Faculty 26 (23% with doctorates).

Baccalaureate Enrollment 185 **Women** 85% **Men** 15% **Minority** 20% **Part-time** 3%

Nursing Student Activities Nursing Honor Society, Student Nurses' Association.

Nursing Student Resources Academic advising; academic or career counseling; assistance for students with disabilities; bookstore; campus computer network; career placement assistance; computer lab; computer-assisted instruction; e-mail services; externships; housing assistance; interactive nursing skills videos; Internet; learning resource lab; library services; nursing audiovisuals; placement services for program completers; remedial services; resume preparation assistance; skills, simulation, or other laboratory; tutoring.

Library Facilities 94,891 volumes (1,956 in health, 1,126 in nursing); 313 periodical subscriptions (116 health-care related).

BACCALAUREATE PROGRAMS

Degree BSN

Available Programs Generic Baccalaureate; RN Baccalaureate.

Study Options Full-time and part-time.

Program Entrance Requirements Minimum overall college GPA of 2.75, transcript of college record, CPR certification, health exam, health insurance, high school biology, high school chemistry, 3 years high school math, 3 years high school science, high school transcript, immunizations, minimum high school GPA of 2.8, professional liability insurance/malpractice insurance. Transfer students are accepted. *Application deadline:* 9/1 (fall), 12/1 (winter), 3/1 (spring). Applications may be processed on a rolling basis for some programs. *Application fee:* $25.

Advanced Placement Credit by examination available. Credit given for nursing courses completed elsewhere dependent upon specific evaluations.

Contact *Telephone:* 414-277-4516. *Fax:* 414-277-4540.

Mount Mary College
Columbia College of Nursing/Mount Mary College Nursing Program
Milwaukee, Wisconsin

See description of programs under Columbia College of Nursing/Mount Mary College Nursing Program (Milwaukee, Wisconsin).

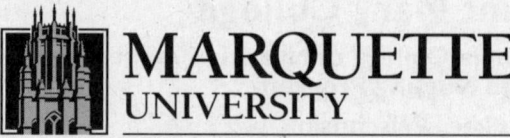
Silver Lake College of the Holy Family

Nursing Program
Manitowoc, Wisconsin

Founded in 1869
DEGREE • BSN
Nursing Program Faculty 8
Baccalaureate Enrollment 19 **Women** 80% **Men** 20% **Minority** 5% **Part-time** 100%
Distance Learning Courses Available.
Nursing Student Resources Academic advising; assistance for students with disabilities; bookstore; campus computer network; computer lab; computer-assisted instruction; e-mail services; interactive nursing skills videos; Internet; library services; nursing audiovisuals; tutoring.
Library Facilities 62,418 volumes; 259 periodical subscriptions.

BACCALAUREATE PROGRAMS

Degree BSN
Available Programs ADN to Baccalaureate.
Site Options Green Bay, WI.
Study Options Part-time.
Online Degree Options Yes.
Program Entrance Requirements Minimum overall college GPA of 2.0, transcript of college record, health insurance, immunizations, 1 letter of recommendation, prerequisite course work, RN licensure. Transfer students are accepted. *Application deadline:* Applications may be processed on a rolling basis for some programs.
Advanced Placement Credit given for nursing courses completed elsewhere dependent upon specific evaluations.
Expenses (2012–13) *Tuition:* part-time $420 per credit.
Financial Aid 25% of baccalaureate students in nursing programs received some form of financial aid in 2011–12. *Gift aid (need-based):* Federal Pell, FSEOG, state, private, college/university gift aid from institutional funds. *Loans:* Federal Direct (Subsidized and Unsubsidized Stafford PLUS), state. *Work-study:* Federal Work-Study, part-time campus jobs. *Financial aid application deadline (priority):* 3/15.
Contact Brianna Neuser, BSN Completion Program Director, Nursing Program, Silver Lake College of the Holy Family, 2406 South Alverno Road, Manitowoc, WI 54220. *Telephone:* 920-686-6213. *E-mail:* brianna.neuser@sl.edu.

University of Phoenix–Milwaukee Campus

College of Health and Human Services
Milwaukee, Wisconsin

http://www.phoenix.edu/campus-locations/wi/milwaukee-campus/milwaukee-campus.html
DEGREES • BSN • MSN • PHD

BACCALAUREATE PROGRAMS

Degree BSN
Available Programs RN Baccalaureate.
Contact *Telephone:* 262-785-0608.

GRADUATE PROGRAMS

Contact *Telephone:* 262-785-0608.

MASTER'S DEGREE PROGRAM
Degree MSN
Available Programs Master's.

DOCTORAL DEGREE PROGRAM
Degree PhD
Available Programs Doctorate.

University of Wisconsin–Eau Claire

College of Nursing and Health Sciences
Eau Claire, Wisconsin

http://www.uwec.edu/conhs/index.htm
Founded in 1916
DEGREES • BSN • DNP • MSN
Nursing Program Faculty 47 (28% with doctorates).
Baccalaureate Enrollment 401 **Women** 91% **Men** 9% **Minority** 4%
Part-time 20%
Graduate Enrollment 102 **Women** 96% **Men** 4% **Minority** 1% **Part-time** 61%
Distance Learning Courses Available.
Nursing Student Activities Sigma Theta Tau, Student Nurses' Association.
Nursing Student Resources Academic advising; academic or career counseling; assistance for students with disabilities; bookstore; campus computer network; career placement assistance; computer lab; computer-assisted instruction; daycare for children of students; e-mail services; employment services for current students; housing assistance; interactive nursing skills videos; Internet; learning resource lab; library services; nursing audiovisuals; other; placement services for program completers; remedial services; resume preparation assistance; skills, simulation, or other laboratory; tutoring.
Library Facilities 1.7 million volumes (17,256 in health, 1,984 in nursing); 36,768 periodical subscriptions (3,893 health-care related).

BACCALAUREATE PROGRAMS

Degree BSN
Available Programs ADN to Baccalaureate; Accelerated Baccalaureate for Second Degree; Generic Baccalaureate; RN Baccalaureate.
Site Options Marshfield, WI.
Study Options Full-time.
Program Entrance Requirements Minimum overall college GPA of 3.0, transcript of college record, CPR certification, written essay, health exam, high school biology, high school chemistry, high school foreign language, 3 years high school math, 3 years high school science, high school transcript, immunizations, minimum GPA in nursing prerequisites of 2.5, prerequisite course work. Transfer students are accepted. *Application deadline:* 5/1 (fall), 12/1 (spring). *Application fee:* $86.
Advanced Placement Credit given for nursing courses completed elsewhere dependent upon specific evaluations.
Contact *Telephone:* 715-836-5287. *Fax:* 715-836-5925.

GRADUATE PROGRAMS

Contact *Telephone:* 715-836-5287. *Fax:* 715-836-5925.

MASTER'S DEGREE PROGRAM
Degree MSN
Available Programs Master's; RN to Master's.
Concentrations Available Nursing administration; nursing education. *Clinical nurse specialist programs in:* adult health. *Nurse practitioner programs in:* adult health, family health, gerontology.
Site Options Marshfield, WI.
Study Options Full-time and part-time.
Program Entrance Requirements Clinical experience, minimum overall college GPA of 3.0, transcript of college record, CPR certification, written essay, immunizations, 3 letters of recommendation, physical assessment course, professional liability insurance/malpractice insurance, statistics course. *Application deadline:* 1/15 (summer). Applications may be processed on a rolling basis for some programs. *Application fee:* $86.
Advanced Placement Credit given for nursing courses completed elsewhere dependent upon specific evaluations.
Degree Requirements 42 total credit hours, thesis or project.

POST-MASTER'S PROGRAM
Areas of Study Nursing administration; nursing education. *Clinical nurse specialist programs in:* adult health. *Nurse practitioner programs in:* adult health, family health, gerontology.

DOCTORAL DEGREE PROGRAM
Degree DNP
Available Programs Doctorate; Post-Baccalaureate Doctorate.
Areas of Study Family health, gerontology, nursing administration.

Program Entrance Requirements Clinical experience, minimum overall college GPA of 3.00, 3 letters of recommendation, statistics course, vita, writing sample. *Application deadline:* 1/4 (summer). Applications may be processed on a rolling basis for some programs. *Application fee:* $86.
Degree Requirements 72 total credit hours.

CONTINUING EDUCATION PROGRAM

Contact *Telephone:* 715-836-5645. *Fax:* 715-836-5263.

University of Wisconsin–Green Bay

BSN–LINC Online RN–BSN Program
Green Bay, Wisconsin

http://www.uwgb.edu/nursing/
Founded in 1968
DEGREE • BSN
Nursing Program Faculty 10 (86% with doctorates).
Baccalaureate Enrollment 309 **Women** 91% **Men** 9% **Minority** 7% **International** 1% **Part-time** 97%
Distance Learning Courses Available.
Nursing Student Activities Sigma Theta Tau, Student Nurses' Association.
Nursing Student Resources Academic advising; academic or career counseling; assistance for students with disabilities; bookstore; campus computer network; career placement assistance; computer lab; computer-assisted instruction; e-mail services; employment services for current students; Internet; learning resource lab; library services; nursing audiovisuals; resume preparation assistance; skills, simulation, or other laboratory.
Library Facilities 360,795 volumes (1,000 in health, 675 in nursing); 4,452 periodical subscriptions (100 health-care related).

BACCALAUREATE PROGRAMS

Degree BSN
Available Programs RN Baccalaureate.
Site Options Marinette, WI; Rhinelander, WI.
Study Options Full-time and part-time.
Online Degree Options Yes.
Program Entrance Requirements Minimum overall college GPA of 2.5, transcript of college record, RN licensure. Transfer students are accepted. *Application fee:* $44.
Expenses (2012–13) *Tuition, area resident:* part-time $318 per credit hour. *Tuition, state resident:* part-time $452 per credit hour. *Tuition, non-resident:* part-time $415 per credit hour.
Financial Aid 45% of baccalaureate students in nursing programs received some form of financial aid in 2011–12.
Contact Ms. Sharon Gajeski, Advisor, BSN–LINC Online RN–BSN Program, University of Wisconsin–Green Bay, 2420 Nicolet Drive, Green Bay, WI 54311-7001. *Telephone:* 920-465-2570. *Fax:* 920-465-2854. *E-mail:* gajeskis@uwgb.edu.

University of Wisconsin–Madison

School of Nursing
Madison, Wisconsin

http://www.son.wisc.edu/
Founded in 1848
DEGREES • BS • PHD
Nursing Program Faculty 52 (35% with doctorates).
Baccalaureate Enrollment 384 **Women** 86% **Men** 14% **Minority** 11% **International** 2% **Part-time** 25%
Graduate Enrollment 164 **Women** 95% **Men** 5% **Minority** 7% **International** 4% **Part-time** 60%
Distance Learning Courses Available.
Nursing Student Activities Nursing Honor Society, Sigma Theta Tau, Student Nurses' Association, nursing club.
Nursing Student Resources Academic advising; academic or career counseling; assistance for students with disabilities; bookstore; campus computer network; career placement assistance; computer lab; computer-assisted instruction; e-mail services; externships; interactive nursing

skills videos; Internet; learning resource lab; library services; nursing audiovisuals; resume preparation assistance; skills, simulation, or other laboratory; tutoring.

Library Facilities 334,000 volumes in health, 8,300 volumes in nursing; 1,500 periodical subscriptions health-care related.

BACCALAUREATE PROGRAMS

Degree BS

Available Programs Generic Baccalaureate; RN Baccalaureate.

Site Options La Crosse, WI.

Study Options Full-time.

Program Entrance Requirements Minimum overall college GPA of 2.75, transcript of college record, CPR certification, written essay, high school chemistry, high school foreign language, 3 years high school math, 3 years high school science, high school transcript, immunizations, minimum GPA in nursing prerequisites of 2.75, prerequisite course work. Transfer students are accepted. *Application deadline:* 2/1 (fall). *Application fee:* $50.

Advanced Placement Credit by examination available. Credit given for nursing courses completed elsewhere dependent upon specific evaluations.

Expenses (2011–12) *Tuition, state resident:* full-time $9670; part-time $405 per credit. *Tuition, nonresident:* full-time $25,420; part-time $1062 per credit. *Room and board:* $7780 per academic year.

Financial Aid 65% of baccalaureate students in nursing programs received some form of financial aid in 2010–11.

Contact Nursing Admissions, School of Nursing, University of Wisconsin–Madison, 600 Highland Avenue, Room K6/146, Madison, WI 53792-2455. *Telephone:* 608-263-5202. *Fax:* 608-263-5296. *E-mail:* ugadmit@son.wisc.edu.

GRADUATE PROGRAMS

Expenses (2011–12) *Tuition, state resident:* full-time $11,374; part-time $713 per credit. *Tuition, nonresident:* full-time $25,132; part-time $1573 per credit. *Room and board:* $9370 per academic year.

Financial Aid 55% of graduate students in nursing programs received some form of financial aid in 2010–11. 8 fellowships with full tuition reimbursements available (averaging $26,900 per year), 8 research assistantships with full tuition reimbursements available (averaging $18,000 per year), 5 teaching assistantships with full tuition reimbursements available (averaging $11,000 per year) were awarded; career-related internships or fieldwork, Federal Work-Study, institutionally sponsored loans, scholarships, traineeships, and unspecified assistantships also available. Aid available to part-time students. *Financial aid application deadline:* 3/1.

Contact Ms. Marcia Voss, Graduate Program Coordinator, School of Nursing, University of Wisconsin–Madison, 600 Highland Avenue, Room K6/140, Clinical Science Center, Madison, WI 53792-2455. *Telephone:* 608-263-5258. *Fax:* 608-263-5296. *E-mail:* mlvoss@wisc.edu.

DOCTORAL DEGREE PROGRAM

Degree PhD

Available Programs Doctorate; Post-Baccalaureate Doctorate.

Areas of Study Aging, bio-behavioral research, biology of health and illness, community health, faculty preparation, family health, gerontology, health policy, health promotion/disease prevention, human health and illness, information systems, nursing education, nursing research, oncology, women's health.

Program Entrance Requirements Minimum overall college GPA of 3.0, interview, 3 letters of recommendation, scholarly papers, vita, writing sample, GRE General Test. *Application deadline:* 1/15 (fall), 9/15 (spring). *Application fee:* $56.

Degree Requirements 60 total credit hours, dissertation, written exam, residency.

POSTDOCTORAL PROGRAM

Areas of Study Adolescent health, aging, cancer care, chronic illness, community health, family health, gerontology, health promotion/disease prevention, individualized study, nursing informatics, nursing interventions, nursing research, vulnerable population, women's health.

Postdoctoral Program Contact Carol Aspinwall, Student Services Coordinator, School of Nursing, University of Wisconsin–Madison, 600 Highland Avenue, Room K6/133, Madison, WI 53792-2455. *Telephone:* 608-263-9109. *Fax:* 608-263-5296. *E-mail:* caaspinwall@wisc.edu.

CONTINUING EDUCATION PROGRAM

Contact Ms. Marilyn Haynes Brokopp, Clinical Associate Professor, School of Nursing, University of Wisconsin–Madison, 600 Highland Avenue, Room H6/158, Clinical Science Center, Madison, WI 53792-2455. *Telephone:* 608-262-1179. *Fax:* 608-263-5332. *E-mail:* haynesbrokop@wisc.edu.

University of Wisconsin–Milwaukee
College of Nursing
Milwaukee, Wisconsin

http://www.nursing.uwm.edu/
Founded in 1956

DEGREES • BSN • DNP • MN • PHD

Nursing Program Faculty 34 (100% with doctorates).

Baccalaureate Enrollment 1,197 **Women** 85% **Men** 15% **Minority** 25% **International** .75% **Part-time** 30%

Graduate Enrollment 229 **Women** 88% **Men** 12% **Minority** 12% **International** 3% **Part-time** 46%

Distance Learning Courses Available.

Nursing Student Activities Sigma Theta Tau, Student Nurses' Association.

Nursing Student Resources Academic advising; academic or career counseling; assistance for students with disabilities; bookstore; campus computer network; career placement assistance; computer lab; computer-assisted instruction; e-mail services; interactive nursing skills videos; Internet; learning resource lab; library services; nursing audiovisuals; remedial services; skills, simulation, or other laboratory; tutoring.

Library Facilities 2.2 million volumes (330,089 in health, 179,089 in nursing); 62,432 periodical subscriptions (926 health-care related).

BACCALAUREATE PROGRAMS

Degree BSN

Available Programs ADN to Baccalaureate; Generic Baccalaureate; RN Baccalaureate.

Site Options West Bend, WI; Kenosha, WI.

Study Options Full-time and part-time.

Program Entrance Requirements Minimum overall college GPA of 2.75, transcript of college record, written essay, high school biology, high school chemistry, high school foreign language, 3 years high school math, 3 years high school science, high school transcript, minimum high school GPA of 2.0, minimum GPA in nursing prerequisites of 2.75, prerequisite course work. Transfer students are accepted. *Application deadline:* 1/15 (fall), 8/15 (spring). *Application fee:* $44.

Advanced Placement Credit given for nursing courses completed elsewhere dependent upon specific evaluations.

Expenses (2012–13) *Tuition, state resident:* full-time $8092; part-time $337 per credit. *Tuition, nonresident:* full-time $17,820; part-time $742 per credit. *International tuition:* $17,820 full-time. *Room and board:* $8554; room only: $4983 per academic year. *Required fees:* full-time $1096; part-time $548 per term.

Financial Aid 95% of baccalaureate students in nursing programs received some form of financial aid in 2011–12. *Gift aid (need-based):* Federal Pell, FSEOG, state, private, college/university gift aid from institutional funds, Federal Nursing. *Loans:* Federal Nursing Student Loans, Federal Direct (Subsidized and Unsubsidized Stafford PLUS), Perkins, state, alternative loans. *Work-study:* Federal Work-Study. *Financial aid application deadline (priority):* 3/1.

Contact Ms. Donna Wier, Senior Advisor, College of Nursing, University of Wisconsin–Milwaukee, PO Box 413, Student Affairs, Milwaukee, WI 53201. *Telephone:* 414-229-5481. *Fax:* 414-229-5554. *E-mail:* ddw@uwm.edu.

GRADUATE PROGRAMS

Expenses (2012–13) *Tuition, state resident:* full-time $10,386; part-time $649 per credit. *Tuition, nonresident:* full-time $22,852; part-time $1428 per credit. *International tuition:* $22,852 full-time. *Room and board:* $10,131; room only: $6560 per academic year. *Required fees:* full-time $1096; part-time $548 per term.

Financial Aid 74% of graduate students in nursing programs received some form of financial aid in 2011–12. 3 fellowships, 1 research assistantship, 9 teaching assistantships were awarded; career-related internships or fieldwork, Federal Work-Study, unspecified assistantships, and project assistantships also available. Aid available to part-time students. *Financial aid application deadline:* 4/15.

Contact Ms. Robin Jens, Director, Student Services, College of Nursing, University of Wisconsin–Milwaukee, PO Box 413, Student Affairs, Milwaukee, WI 53201. *Telephone:* 414-229-2494. *Fax:* 414-229-5554. *E-mail:* rjens@uwm.edu.

MASTER'S DEGREE PROGRAM
Degree MN
Available Programs Master's; Master's for Non-Nursing College Graduates.
Concentrations Available Clinical nurse leader.
Site Options Kenosha, WI.
Study Options Full-time and part-time.
Program Entrance Requirements Minimum overall college GPA of 3.0, transcript of college record, written essay, 3 letters of recommendation, prerequisite course work, resume, statistics course, GRE General Test or MAT. *Application deadline:* 1/1 (fall), 9/1 (spring). *Application fee:* $56.
Advanced Placement Credit given for nursing courses completed elsewhere dependent upon specific evaluations.
Degree Requirements 33 total credit hours.

DOCTORAL DEGREE PROGRAM
Degree DNP
Available Programs Doctorate, Post-Baccalaureate Doctorate.
Areas of Study Advanced practice nursing, clinical practice, community health, family health, gerontology, health-care systems, human health and illness, individualized study, maternity-newborn, neuro-behavior, women's health.
Online Degree Options Yes.
Program Entrance Requirements Minimum overall college GPA of 3.2, interview, 3 letters of recommendation, scholarly papers, statistics course, vita, writing sample. *Application deadline:* 1/1 (fall), 9/1 (spring), 11/1 (summer). Applications may be processed on a rolling basis for some programs. *Application fee:* $56.
Degree Requirements 64 total credit hours, residency.

DOCTORAL DEGREE PROGRAM
Degree PhD
Available Programs Doctorate; Post-Baccalaureate Doctorate.

Areas of Study Health-care systems, individualized study, neuro-behavior, nursing research.
Online Degree Options Yes.
Program Entrance Requirements Minimum overall college GPA of 3.2, interview, 3 letters of recommendation, scholarly papers, statistics course, vita, writing sample, GRE. *Application deadline:* 1/1 (fall), 9/1 (spring), 11/1 (summer). Applications may be processed on a rolling basis for some programs. *Application fee:* $56.
Degree Requirements 64 total credit hours, dissertation, oral exam, written exam.

See display below and full description on page 510.

University of Wisconsin–Oshkosh
College of Nursing
Oshkosh, Wisconsin

http://www.uwosh.edu/con
Founded in 1871
DEGREES • BSN • DNP • MSN
Nursing Program Faculty 79 (19% with doctorates).
Baccalaureate Enrollment 1,369 **Women** 88% **Men** 12% **Minority** 10% **Part-time** 14%
Graduate Enrollment 100 **Women** 90% **Men** 10% **Minority** 4% **Part-time** 78%
Distance Learning Courses Available.
Nursing Student Activities Sigma Theta Tau, Student Nurses' Association, nursing club.
Nursing Student Resources Academic advising; academic or career counseling; assistance for students with disabilities; bookstore; campus computer network; career placement assistance; computer lab; computer-assisted instruction; daycare for children of students; e-mail services; employment services for current students; externships; housing assistance; interactive nursing skills videos; Internet; learning resource lab; library services; nursing audiovisuals; other; paid internships; placement services for program completers; remedial services; resume preparation assistance; skills, simulation, or other laboratory; tutoring; unpaid internships.
Library Facilities 446,774 volumes; 5,219 periodical subscriptions.

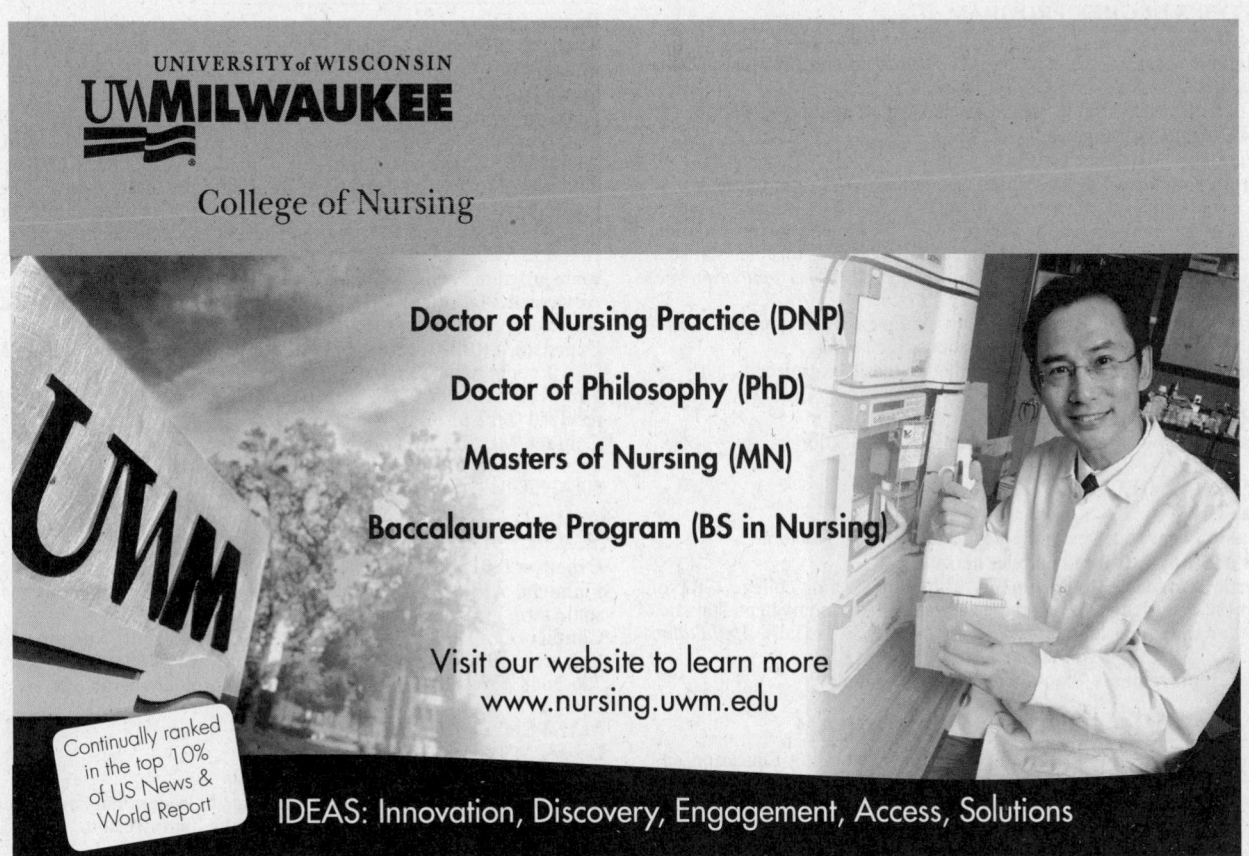

BACCALAUREATE PROGRAMS

Degree BSN

Available Programs ADN to Baccalaureate; Accelerated Baccalaureate; Accelerated Baccalaureate for Second Degree; Accelerated RN Baccalaureate; Baccalaureate for Second Degree; Generic Baccalaureate; RN Baccalaureate.

Site Options Sheboygan, WI; Wausau, WI; Manitowoc, WI.

Study Options Full-time and part-time.

Online Degree Options Yes.

Program Entrance Requirements Minimum overall college GPA of 2.75, transcript of college record, CPR certification, written essay, health exam, 3 years high school math, 3 years high school science, immunizations, interview, minimum high school rank 50%, minimum GPA in nursing prerequisites of 2.75, prerequisite course work. Transfer students are accepted. *Application deadline;* 1/30 (fall), 8/30 (spring).

Advanced Placement Credit by examination available. Credit given for nursing courses completed elsewhere dependent upon specific evaluations.

Financial Aid *Gift aid (need-based):* Federal Pell, FSEOG, state, private, college/university gift aid from institutional funds, United Negro College Fund, Federal Nursing. *Loans:* Federal Nursing Student Loans, Federal Direct (Subsidized and Unsubsidized Stafford PLUS), Perkins, state, college/university.*Work-study:* Federal Work-Study, part-time campus jobs.*Financial aid application deadline (priority):* 3/15.

Contact Dr. Suzanne Marnocha, Undergraduate Program Director, College of Nursing, University of Wisconsin–Oshkosh, 800 Algoma Boulevard, Oshkosh, WI 54901-8660. *Telephone:* 920-424-1028. *Fax:* 920-424-0123. *E-mail:* marnocha@uwosh.edu.

GRADUATE PROGRAMS

Financial Aid 40% of graduate students in nursing programs received some form of financial aid in 2011–12. Fellowships, research assistantships with partial tuition reimbursements available, institutionally sponsored loans, scholarships, traineeships, tuition waivers (partial), and unspecified assistantships available. *Financial aid application deadline:* 3/15.

Contact Ms. Susan Robl, Graduate Program Assistant, College of Nursing, University of Wisconsin–Oshkosh, College of Nursing, 800 Algoma Boulevard, Oshkosh, WI 54901-8660. *Telephone:* 920-424-2106. *Fax:* 920-424-0123. *E-mail:* congrad@uwosh.edu.

MASTER'S DEGREE PROGRAM

Degree MSN

Available Programs Accelerated AD/RN to Master's; Master's; RN to Master's.

Concentrations Available Clinical nurse leader; nursing education.

Study Options Full-time and part-time.

Online Degree Options Yes (online only).

Program Entrance Requirements Computer literacy, minimum overall college GPA of 3.0, transcript of college record, CPR certification, written essay, immunizations, interview, 3 letters of recommendation, professional liability insurance/malpractice insurance, resume, statistics course. *Application deadline:* 3/1 (fall), 11/1 (spring). *Application fee:* $56.

Advanced Placement Credit given for nursing courses completed elsewhere dependent upon specific evaluations.

Degree Requirements 37 total credit hours, thesis or project.

POST-MASTER'S PROGRAM

Areas of Study Clinical nurse leader; nursing education.

DOCTORAL DEGREE PROGRAM

Degree DNP

Available Programs Doctorate; Post-Baccalaureate Doctorate.

Areas of Study Advanced practice nursing.

Program Entrance Requirements Minimum overall college GPA of 3.0, interview, 3 letters of recommendation, MSN or equivalent, statistics course, vita, writing sample. *Application deadline:* 3/1 (fall). *Application fee:* $56.

Degree Requirements 74 total credit hours, residency.

CONTINUING EDUCATION PROGRAM

Contact Dr. Karen Heikel, Acting Director, Continuing Education and Extension, College of Nursing, University of Wisconsin–Oshkosh, 800 Algoma Boulevard, Oshkosh, WI 54901-8660. *Telephone:* 920-424-1463. *Fax:* 920-424-1803. *E-mail:* heikelk@uwosh.edu.

University of Wisconsin–Waukesha

Columbia College of Nursing/Mount Mary College Nursing Program

Waukesha, Wisconsin

See description of programs under Columbia College of Nursing/Mount Mary College Nursing Program (Milwaukee, Wisconsin).

Viterbo University

School of Nursing
La Crosse, Wisconsin

http://www.viterbo.edu/

Founded in 1890

DEGREES • BSN • MSN

Nursing Program Faculty 32 (8% with doctorates).

Baccalaureate Enrollment 688 **Women** 94% **Men** 6% **Minority** 3% **International** 1% **Part-time** 5%

Graduate Enrollment 60 **Women** 99% **Men** 1% **Minority** 1% **Part-time** 15%

Nursing Student Activities Sigma Theta Tau, Student Nurses' Association.

Nursing Student Resources Academic advising; academic or career counseling; assistance for students with disabilities; bookstore; campus computer network; career placement assistance; computer lab; computer-assisted instruction; e-mail services; interactive nursing skills videos; Internet; learning resource lab; library services; nursing audiovisuals; remedial services; resume preparation assistance; skills, simulation, or other laboratory; tutoring.

Library Facilities 5,200 volumes in health, 3,398 volumes in nursing; 312 periodical subscriptions health-care related.

BACCALAUREATE PROGRAMS

Degree BSN

Available Programs Generic Baccalaureate; RN Baccalaureate.

Site Options Rochester, MN; Madison, WI; Janesville, WI.

Study Options Full-time and part-time.

Program Entrance Requirements Minimum overall college GPA of 2.75, transcript of college record, CPR certification, health exam, high school chemistry, 2 years high school math, 2 years high school science, high school transcript, immunizations, minimum high school GPA of 3.0, minimum high school rank 55%, minimum GPA in nursing prerequisites of 2.75, prerequisite course work. Transfer students are accepted. *Application deadline:* Applications may be processed on a rolling basis for some programs. *Application fee:* $25.

Advanced Placement Credit given for nursing courses completed elsewhere dependent upon specific evaluations.

Expenses (2012–13) *Tuition:* full-time $22,080. *Room and board:* $6410; room only: $3310 per academic year.

Financial Aid 98% of baccalaureate students in nursing programs received some form of financial aid in 2011–12.

Contact Mr. Robert Forget, Dean of Admission, School of Nursing, Viterbo University, 900 Viterbo Drive, La Crosse, WI 54601. *Telephone:* 608-796-3012. *Fax:* 608-796-3050. *E-mail:* rlforget@viterbo.edu.

GRADUATE PROGRAMS

Expenses (2012–13) *Tuition:* part-time $680 per credit.

Financial Aid 33% of graduate students in nursing programs received some form of financial aid in 2011–12.

Contact Dr. Bonnie Nesbitt, Director, School of Nursing, Viterbo University, 900 Viterbo Drive, La Crosse, WI 54601. *Telephone:* 608-796-3688. *Fax:* 608-796-3668. *E-mail:* bjnesbitt@viterbo.edu.

MASTER'S DEGREE PROGRAM

Degree MSN

Available Programs Master's.

Concentrations Available Clinical nurse leader; nursing education. *Nurse practitioner programs in:* adult health, family health.

Study Options Full-time and part-time.

Program Entrance Requirements Clinical experience, computer literacy, minimum overall college GPA of 3.0, transcript of college record, CPR certification, written essay, immunizations, interview, 3 letters of recommendation, nursing research course, physical assessment course, resume, statistics course. *Application deadline:* 2/15 (fall). *Application fee:* $50.

Advanced Placement Credit given for nursing courses completed elsewhere dependent upon specific evaluations.

Degree Requirements 40 total credit hours, thesis or project.

POST-MASTER'S PROGRAM

Areas of Study Nursing education. *Nurse practitioner programs in:* adult health, family health.

CONTINUING EDUCATION PROGRAM

Contact Ms. Delayne Vogel, Continuing Education Coordinator, School of Nursing, Viterbo University, 900 Viterbo Drive, La Crosse, WI 54601. *Telephone:* 608-796-3692. *Fax:* 608-796-3668. *E-mail:* dgvogel@viterbo.edu.

Wisconsin Lutheran College

Nursing Program
Milwaukee, Wisconsin

Founded in 1973
DEGREE • BSN
Nursing Program Faculty 2
Baccalaureate Enrollment 14
Nursing Student Activities Student Nurses' Association.
Nursing Student Resources Academic advising; academic or career counseling; assistance for students with disabilities; bookstore; campus computer network; career placement assistance; computer lab; computer-assisted instruction; e-mail services; externships; housing assistance; interactive nursing skills videos; Internet; learning resource lab; library services; nursing audiovisuals; skills, simulation, or other laboratory; tutoring.
Library Facilities 78,107 volumes; 310 periodical subscriptions.

BACCALAUREATE PROGRAMS

Degree BSN
Available Programs Generic Baccalaureate.
Study Options Full-time.
Program Entrance Requirements Minimum overall college GPA of 2.75, transcript of college record, written essay, high school foreign language, interview, 3 letters of recommendation, minimum GPA in nursing prerequisites of 2.0, prerequisite course work. Transfer students are accepted. *Application deadline:* 3/15 (spring).
Contact *Telephone:* 414-443-8800.

CONTINUING EDUCATION PROGRAM

Contact *Telephone:* 414-443-8800.

WYOMING

University of Wyoming

Fay W. Whitney School of Nursing
Laramie, Wyoming

http://www.uwyo.edu/nursing
Founded in 1886
DEGREES • BSN • DNP • MS
Nursing Program Faculty 48 (25% with doctorates).
Baccalaureate Enrollment 516 **Women** 89% **Men** 11% **Minority** 10%
International 1% **Part-time** 73%
Graduate Enrollment 46 **Women** 93% **Men** 7% **Part-time** 61%

Distance Learning Courses Available.
Nursing Student Activities Sigma Theta Tau, Student Nurses' Association.
Nursing Student Resources Academic advising; academic or career counseling; assistance for students with disabilities; bookstore; campus computer network; career placement assistance; computer lab; computer-assisted instruction; e-mail services; employment services for current students; externships; housing assistance; interactive nursing skills videos; Internet; learning resource lab; library services; nursing audiovisuals; paid internships; remedial services; resume preparation assistance; skills, simulation, or other laboratory; tutoring; unpaid internships.
Library Facilities 3.9 million volumes (56,231 in health); 89,028 periodical subscriptions (1,689 health-care related).

BACCALAUREATE PROGRAMS

Degree BSN
Available Programs ADN to Baccalaureate; Accelerated Baccalaureate for Second Degree; Generic Baccalaureate.
Study Options Full-time.
Online Degree Options Yes.
Program Entrance Requirements Transcript of college record, CPR certification, written essay, immunizations, 2 letters of recommendation, minimum GPA in nursing prerequisites of 2.75, professional liability insurance/malpractice insurance, prerequisite course work. Transfer students are accepted. *Application deadline:* 2/1 (fall). *Application fee:* $30.
Advanced Placement Credit given for nursing courses completed elsewhere dependent upon specific evaluations.
Expenses (2012–13) *Tuition, state resident:* part-time $106 per credit hour. *Tuition, nonresident:* part-time $413 per credit hour.
Contact Ms. Debbie A. Shoefelt, Credentials Analyst/Academic Advisor, Fay W. Whitney School of Nursing, University of Wyoming, Department 3065, 1000 East University Avenue, Laramie, WY 82071. *Telephone:* 307-766-4292. *Fax:* 307-766-4294. *E-mail:* basicbsn@uwyo.edu.

GRADUATE PROGRAMS

Expenses (2012–13) *Tuition, state resident:* part-time $206 per credit hour. *Tuition, nonresident:* part-time $602 per credit hour. *Required fees:* part-time $40 per credit.
Financial Aid Research assistantships (averaging $10,062 per year), teaching assistantships (averaging $10,062 per year) were awarded; career-related internships or fieldwork, institutionally sponsored loans, scholarships, traineeships, and unspecified assistantships also available.
Contact Ms. Crystal McFadden, Office Associate, Fay W. Whitney School of Nursing, University of Wyoming, Department 3065, 1000 East University Avenue, Laramie, WY 82071. *Telephone:* 307-766-6568. *Fax:* 307-766-4294. *E-mail:* gradnurse@uwyo.edu.

MASTER'S DEGREE PROGRAM

Degree MS
Available Programs Master's; Master's for Nurses with Non-Nursing Degrees.
Concentrations Available Nursing education.
Study Options Part-time.
Online Degree Options Yes (online only).
Program Entrance Requirements Clinical experience, minimum overall college GPA of 3.0, transcript of college record, CPR certification, written essay, immunizations, 3 letters of recommendation, professional liability insurance/malpractice insurance, resume, statistics course, GRE General Test. *Application deadline:* 2/1 (fall). *Application fee:* $50.
Degree Requirements 36 total credit hours.

POST-MASTER'S PROGRAM

Areas of Study Nursing education.

DOCTORAL DEGREE PROGRAM

Degree DNP
Available Programs Doctorate.
Areas of Study Advanced practice nursing, clinical practice, ethics, family health, health policy, health promotion/disease prevention, human health and illness, individualized study, information systems, nursing policy, women's health.

Program Entrance Requirements Minimum overall college GPA of 3.5, interview by faculty committee, 3 letters of recommendation, vita, writing sample. *Application deadline:* 2/1 (fall). *Application fee:* $50.
Degree Requirements 84 total credit hours.

CANADA

ALBERTA

Athabasca University
Centre for Nursing and Health Studies
Athabasca, Alberta

http://www.athabascau.ca/cnhs/
Founded in 1970
DEGREES • BN • MN • MN/MBA • MN/MHSA
Nursing Program Faculty 115 (49% with doctorates).
Baccalaureate Enrollment 3,349
Graduate Enrollment 1,325
Distance Learning Courses Available.
Nursing Student Activities Student Nurses' Association.
Nursing Student Resources Academic advising; academic or career counseling; assistance for students with disabilities; bookstore; campus computer network; computer lab; computer-assisted instruction; e-mail services; interactive nursing skills videos; Internet; library services; nursing audiovisuals; remedial services; skills, simulation, or other laboratory; tutoring.
Library Facilities 178,808 volumes; 32,619 periodical subscriptions.

BACCALAUREATE PROGRAMS

Degree BN
Available Programs Generic Baccalaureate; LPN to RN Baccalaureate; RN Baccalaureate.
Site Options Calgary, AB.
Study Options Full-time and part-time.
Program Entrance Requirements Minimum overall college GPA of 2.5, transcript of college record, CPR certification, high school biology, 3 years high school math, 3 years high school science, high school transcript, immunizations, minimum high school GPA of 2.0, minimum GPA in nursing prerequisites of 2.0, RN licensure. Transfer students are accepted. *Application deadline:* Applications may be processed on a rolling basis for some programs.
Advanced Placement Credit by examination available. Credit given for nursing courses completed elsewhere dependent upon specific evaluations.
Expenses (2012–13) *Tuition, state resident:* part-time CAN$663 per course. *Tuition, nonresident:* part-time CAN$768 per course. *International tuition:* CAN$1240 full-time.
Contact Gayle Deren-Purdy, Undergraduate Student Advisor, Centre for Nursing and Health Studies, Athabasca University, 1 University Drive, Athabasca, AB T9S 3A3. *Telephone:* 800-788-9041 Ext. 6446. *Fax:* 780-675-6468. *E-mail:* gayled@athabascau.ca.

GRADUATE PROGRAMS

Expenses (2012–13) *Tuition, state resident:* part-time CAN$1370 per course. *Tuition, nonresident:* part-time CAN$1370 per course. *International tuition:* CAN$1570 full-time.
Contact Ms. Donna Dunn Hart, Graduate Student Advisor, Centre for Nursing and Health Studies, Athabasca University, 1 University Drive, Athabasca, AB T9S 3A3. *Telephone:* 800-788-9041 Ext. 6300. *Fax:* 780-675-6468. *E-mail:* donnad@athabascau.ca.

MASTER'S DEGREE PROGRAM
Degrees MN; MN/MBA; MN/MHSA

Available Programs Master's; Master's for Nurses with Non-Nursing Degrees.
Concentrations Available Nursing administration; nursing education. *Nurse practitioner programs in:* community health, family health, primary care.
Study Options Full-time and part-time.
Online Degree Options Yes.
Program Entrance Requirements Clinical experience, computer literacy, minimum overall college GPA of 3.0, transcript of college record, written essay, 3 letters of recommendation, resume. *Application deadline:* 3/1 (fall), 12/1 (spring). *Application fee:* CAN$150.
Advanced Placement Credit given for nursing courses completed elsewhere dependent upon specific evaluations.
Degree Requirements 33 total credit hours, thesis or project, comprehensive exam.

POST-MASTER'S PROGRAM
Areas of Study *Nurse practitioner programs in:* community health, family health.

University of Alberta
Faculty of Nursing
Edmonton, Alberta

http://www.nursing.ualberta.ca/
Founded in 1906
DEGREES • BSCN • MN • PHD
Nursing Program Faculty 109 (50% with doctorates).
Baccalaureate Enrollment 1,600 **Women** 93% **Men** 7% **International** 1% **Part-time** 7%
Graduate Enrollment 200 **Women** 90% **Men** 10% **International** 7% **Part-time** 60%
Distance Learning Courses Available.
Nursing Student Activities Nursing Honor Society, Sigma Theta Tau, Student Nurses' Association.
Nursing Student Resources Academic advising; academic or career counseling; assistance for students with disabilities; bookstore; campus computer network; career placement assistance; computer lab; computer-assisted instruction; daycare for children of students; e-mail services; employment services for current students; housing assistance; interactive nursing skills videos; Internet; learning resource lab; library services; nursing audiovisuals; other; paid internships; remedial services; resume preparation assistance; skills, simulation, or other laboratory; tutoring; unpaid internships.
Library Facilities 9.7 million volumes (115,000 in health, 19,000 in nursing); 2,400 periodical subscriptions health-care related.

BACCALAUREATE PROGRAMS

Degree BScN
Available Programs Accelerated Baccalaureate for Second Degree; Baccalaureate for Second Degree; Generic Baccalaureate; RN Baccalaureate; RPN to Baccalaureate.
Site Options Fort McMurray, AB; Grande Prairie, AB; Red Deer, AB.
Study Options Full-time.
Program Entrance Requirements Minimum overall college GPA of 3.0, transcript of college record, CPR certification, health exam, high school biology, high school chemistry, 3 years high school math, 3 years high school science, high school transcript, immunizations, minimum high school rank 80%. Transfer students are accepted. *Application*

deadline: 5/1 (fall). Applications may be processed on a rolling basis for some programs. *Application fee:* CAN$115.

Advanced Placement Credit given for nursing courses completed elsewhere dependent upon specific evaluations.

Contact Ms. Kristan Morin, Student Recruiter, Faculty of Nursing, University of Alberta, 3 Edmonton Clinic Health Authority, Edmonton, AB T6G 1C9. *Telephone:* 780-492-1242. *Fax:* 780-492-2551. *E-mail:* undergraduate@nurs.ualberta.ca.

GRADUATE PROGRAMS

Financial Aid 47% of graduate students in nursing programs received some form of financial aid in 2011–12. 12 fellowships with partial tuition reimbursements available (averaging $23,868 per year), 27 research assistantships with partial tuition reimbursements available (averaging $6,186 per year), 12 teaching assistantships with partial tuition reimbursements available (averaging $2,365 per year) were awarded; institutionally sponsored loans and scholarships also available.

Contact Yvette Labiuk, Graduate Services Administrator, Faculty of Nursing, University of Alberta, 4-171 Edmonton Clinic Health Academy, 11405 87 Avenue, Edmonton, AB T6G 1C9. *Telephone:* 780-492-9546. *Fax:* 780-492-2551. *E-mail:* nursing.graduate@ualberta.ca.

MASTER'S DEGREE PROGRAM
Degree MN
Available Programs Master's.
Concentrations Available *Nurse practitioner programs in:* adult health, gerontology.
Study Options Full-time and part-time.
Program Entrance Requirements Clinical experience, computer literacy, minimum overall college GPA of 3.0, transcript of college record, CPR certification, 3 letters of recommendation, nursing research course, physical assessment course, resume, statistics course. *Application deadline:* 2/1 (fall). *Application fee:* CAN$100.
Advanced Placement Credit given for nursing courses completed elsewhere dependent upon specific evaluations.
Degree Requirements 39 total credit hours, thesis or project.

POST-MASTER'S PROGRAM
Areas of Study *Nurse practitioner programs in:* adult health, gerontology.

DOCTORAL DEGREE PROGRAM
Degree PhD
Available Programs Doctorate.
Areas of Study Aging, community health, ethics, family health, gerontology, health policy, health promotion/disease prevention, health-care systems, nursing education, nursing policy, nursing research.
Program Entrance Requirements Clinical experience, minimum overall college GPA of 3.0, 3 letters of recommendation, MSN or equivalent, scholarly papers, statistics course, vita, writing sample. *Application deadline:* 2/1 (fall). *Application fee:* CAN$100.
Degree Requirements 36 total credit hours, dissertation, oral exam, written exam, residency.

POSTDOCTORAL PROGRAM
Postdoctoral Program Contact Dr. Phyllis Giovannetti, Associate Dean, Graduate Education, Faculty of Nursing, University of Alberta, Clinical Sciences Building, 3rd Floor, Edmonton, AB T6G 2G3. *Telephone:* 780-492-6764. *Fax:* 780-492-2551. *E-mail:* phyllis.giovannetti@ualberta.ca.

University of Calgary
Faculty of Nursing
Calgary, Alberta

http://www.ucalgary.ca/nu
Founded in 1945
DEGREES • BN • MN • PHD
Nursing Program Faculty 50 (85% with doctorates).
Baccalaureate Enrollment 930 **Women** 90% **Men** 10% **Minority** 5% **International** 1%
Graduate Enrollment 110 **Women** 95% **Men** 5% **Minority** 1% **International** 1% **Part-time** 21%
Nursing Student Activities Student Nurses' Association.
Nursing Student Resources Academic advising; academic or career counseling; assistance for students with disabilities; bookstore; campus computer network; career placement assistance; computer lab; computer-assisted instruction; daycare for children of students; e-mail services; externships; housing assistance; interactive nursing skills videos; Internet; learning resource lab; library services; nursing audiovisuals; remedial services; resume preparation assistance; skills, simulation, or other laboratory; tutoring.
Library Facilities 3.3 million volumes; 37,285 periodical subscriptions.

BACCALAUREATE PROGRAMS
Degree BN
Available Programs Accelerated Baccalaureate; Accelerated Baccalaureate for Second Degree; Baccalaureate for Second Degree; Generic Baccalaureate; RN Baccalaureate.
Site Options Medicine Hat, AB.
Study Options Full-time.
Program Entrance Requirements Minimum overall college GPA of 3.3, transcript of college record, CPR certification, health exam, high school biology, high school chemistry, 3 years high school math, high school transcript, immunizations, minimum high school rank 78%. Transfer students are accepted.
Advanced Placement Credit by examination available. Credit given for nursing courses completed elsewhere dependent upon specific evaluations.
Contact *Telephone:* 403-220-4636. *Fax:* 403-284-4803.

GRADUATE PROGRAMS

Contact *Telephone:* 403-220-6241. *Fax:* 403-284-4803.

MASTER'S DEGREE PROGRAM
Degree MN
Available Programs Master's; RN to Master's.
Concentrations Available *Clinical nurse specialist programs in:* acute care, adult health, cardiovascular, community health, critical care, family health, gerontology, maternity-newborn, medical-surgical, parent-child, pediatric, perinatal, psychiatric/mental health, public health, rehabilitation, women's health. *Nurse practitioner programs in:* acute care, adult health, neonatal health.
Study Options Full-time and part-time.
Program Entrance Requirements Clinical experience, computer literacy, minimum overall college GPA of 3.0, transcript of college record, CPR certification, written essay, 3 letters of recommendation, nursing research course, statistics course.
Advanced Placement Credit given for nursing courses completed elsewhere dependent upon specific evaluations.
Degree Requirements 30 total credit hours, thesis or project, comprehensive exam.

POST-MASTER'S PROGRAM
Areas of Study *Nurse practitioner programs in:* acute care, adult health, neonatal health.

DOCTORAL DEGREE PROGRAM
Degree PhD
Available Programs Doctorate; Doctorate for Nurses with Non-Nursing Degrees.
Areas of Study Advanced practice nursing, aging, clinical practice, community health, critical care, ethics, family health, gerontology, health promotion/disease prevention, health-care systems, human health and illness, illness and transition, individualized study, maternity-newborn, neuro-behavior, nursing research, women's health.
Program Entrance Requirements Clinical experience, minimum overall college GPA of 3.0, 3 letters of recommendation, MSN or equivalent, scholarly papers, statistics course, vita, writing sample.
Degree Requirements Dissertation, oral exam, written exam.

University of Lethbridge
Faculty of Health Sciences
Lethbridge, Alberta

http://www.uleth.ca/healthsciences/
Founded in 1967
DEGREES • BN • M SC
Nursing Program Faculty 41 (17% with doctorates).
Baccalaureate Enrollment 709 **Women** 97.6% **Men** 2.4%
Graduate Enrollment 11 **Women** 82% **Men** 18%
Nursing Student Activities Nursing club.

Nursing Student Resources Academic advising; academic or career counseling; assistance for students with disabilities; bookstore; campus computer network; career placement assistance; computer lab; computer-assisted instruction; daycare for children of students; e-mail services; employment services for current students; housing assistance; interactive nursing skills videos; Internet; learning resource lab; library services; nursing audiovisuals; other; remedial services; resume preparation assistance; skills, simulation, or other laboratory; tutoring; unpaid internships.
Library Facilities 602,148 volumes (14,743 in health, 2,554 in nursing); 6,533 periodical subscriptions (11,168 health-care related).

BACCALAUREATE PROGRAMS

Degree BN
Available Programs Accelerated Baccalaureate; Baccalaureate for Second Degree; Generic Baccalaureate.
Site Options Lethbridge, AB.
Study Options Full-time.
Program Entrance Requirements CPR certification, high school biology, high school chemistry, 3 years high school math, 3 years high school science, high school transcript, immunizations, minimum high school rank 70%. Transfer students are accepted. *Application deadline:* 3/1 (fall). *Application fee:* CAN$100.
Advanced Placement Credit given for nursing courses completed elsewhere dependent upon specific evaluations.
Financial Aid *Gift aid (need-based):* private, college/university gift aid from institutional funds. *Financial aid application deadline:* Continuous.
Contact Sherry Hogeweide, Academic Advisor, Faculty of Health Sciences, University of Lethbridge, 4401 University Drive, Lethbridge, AB T1K 3M4. *Telephone:* 403-329-2220. *Fax:* 403-329-2668. *E-mail:* health.sciences@uleth.ca.

GRADUATE PROGRAMS

Contact Dr. Brad Hagen, Graduate Studies Coordinator, Faculty of Health Sciences, University of Lethbridge, 4401 University Drive, Lethbridge, AB T1K 3M4. *Telephone:* 403-329-2299. *Fax:* 403-329-2668. *E-mail:* brad.hagen@uleth.ca.

MASTER'S DEGREE PROGRAM

Degree M Sc
Available Programs Master's.
Study Options Full-time and part-time.
Program Entrance Requirements Clinical experience, computer literacy, minimum overall college GPA of 3.0, transcript of college record, CPR certification, immunizations, interview. *Application deadline:* 3/1 (fall).
Degree Requirements Thesis or project, comprehensive exam.

BRITISH COLUMBIA

British Columbia Institute of Technology
School of Health Sciences
Burnaby, British Columbia

http://www.health.bcit.ca/nursing/
Founded in 1964
DEGREE • BSN
Nursing Program Faculty 94
Baccalaureate Enrollment 510 **Women** 90% **Men** 10%
Distance Learning Courses Available.
Nursing Student Activities Student Nurses' Association.
Nursing Student Resources Academic advising; academic or career counseling; assistance for students with disabilities; bookstore; campus computer network; computer lab; computer-assisted instruction; e-mail services; housing assistance; interactive nursing skills videos; Internet; learning resource lab; library services; nursing audiovisuals; paid internships; resume preparation assistance; skills, simulation, or other laboratory; tutoring; unpaid internships.
Library Facilities 169,404 volumes (10,000 in health, 2,600 in nursing); 1,080 periodical subscriptions (110 health-care related).

BACCALAUREATE PROGRAMS

Degree BSN
Available Programs RN Baccalaureate; RPN to Baccalaureate.
Study Options Full-time.
Program Entrance Requirements Transcript of college record, CPR certification, high school biology, high school chemistry, 11 years high school math, 12 years high school science, high school transcript, immunizations, 2 letters of recommendation, prerequisite course work. Transfer students are accepted. *Application deadline:* 12/15 (fall), 7/15 (winter). *Application fee:* CAN$60.
Advanced Placement Credit given for nursing courses completed elsewhere dependent upon specific evaluations.
Expenses (2012–13) *Tuition, area resident:* full-time CAN$5700. *Room and board:* room only: CAN$5400 per academic year. *Required fees:* full-time CAN$900.
Financial Aid 70% of baccalaureate students in nursing programs received some form of financial aid in 2011–12. *Financial aid application deadline:* Continuous.
Contact Ms. Loreen Martin, Administrative Coordinator, School of Health Sciences, British Columbia Institute of Technology, 3700 Willingdon Avenue, SE12, Room 418, Burnaby, BC V5G 3H2. *Telephone:* 604-432-8884. *Fax:* 604-436-9590. *E-mail:* loreen_martin@bcit.ca.

CONTINUING EDUCATION PROGRAM

Contact Ms. Pauline O'Reilly, Program Head, School of Health Sciences, British Columbia Institute of Technology, 3700 Willingdon Avenue, SE12, Room 328, Burnaby, BC V5G 3H2. *Telephone:* 604-451-7115. *E-mail:* pauline_o'reilly@bcit.ca.

Kwantlen Polytechnic University
Faculty of Community and Health Sciences
Surrey, British Columbia

http://www.kwantlen.ca/
Founded in 1981
DEGREE • BSN
Nursing Program Faculty 60 (13% with doctorates).
Baccalaureate Enrollment 360 **Women** 90% **Men** 10% **Part-time** 13%
Nursing Student Activities Student Nurses' Association.
Nursing Student Resources Academic advising; academic or career counseling; assistance for students with disabilities; bookstore; campus computer network; career placement assistance; computer lab; computer-assisted instruction; e-mail services; employment services for current students; interactive nursing skills videos; Internet; learning resource lab; library services; nursing audiovisuals; remedial services; resume preparation assistance; skills, simulation, or other laboratory.

BACCALAUREATE PROGRAMS

Degree BSN
Available Programs Accelerated Baccalaureate for Second Degree; Generic Baccalaureate; RN Baccalaureate.
Study Options Full-time.
Program Entrance Requirements CPR certification, health insurance, high school biology, high school chemistry, high school math, 2 years high school science, high school transcript, immunizations. Transfer students are accepted.
Advanced Placement Credit given for nursing courses completed elsewhere dependent upon specific evaluations.
Expenses (2012–13) *Tuition, area resident:* full-time CAN$4000. *Required fees:* full-time CAN$200.
Financial Aid 40% of baccalaureate students in nursing programs received some form of financial aid in 2011–12. *Gift aid (need-based):* college/university gift aid from institutional funds. *Loans:* Federal Direct (Subsidized and Unsubsidized Stafford PLUS), provincial loans. *Financial aid application deadline:* Continuous.
Contact Ms. Pam Kubossek, Admissions Assistant, Faculty of Community and Health Sciences, Kwantlen Polytechnic University, 12666 72nd Avenue, Surrey, BC V3W 2M8. *Telephone:* 604-599-2141. *E-mail:* Pam.Kubossek@kwantlen.ca.

Thompson Rivers University
School of Nursing
Kamloops, British Columbia

http://www.tru.ca/nursing.html
Founded in 1970
DEGREE • BSN
Nursing Program Faculty 56
Library Facilities 285,426 volumes (7,326 in health, 2,275 in nursing); 9,585 periodical subscriptions (89 health-care related).

BACCALAUREATE PROGRAMS

Degree BSN
Study Options Full-time and part-time.
Program Entrance Requirements Minimum overall college GPA of 2.7, transcript of college record, CPR certification, health exam, high school biology, high school chemistry, high school foreign language, high school math, high school science, high school transcript, immunizations, interview, 2 letters of recommendation, minimum high school GPA of 2.3, minimum GPA in nursing prerequisites of 2.3. Transfer students are accepted.
Advanced Placement Credit given for nursing courses completed elsewhere dependent upon specific evaluations.
Contact *Telephone:* 250-828-5435. *Fax:* 250-828-5450.

CONTINUING EDUCATION PROGRAM

Contact *Telephone:* 250-828-5210. *Fax:* 250-371-5510.

Trinity Western University
Department of Nursing
Langley, British Columbia

http://www.twu.ca/
Founded in 1962
DEGREES • BSCN • MSN
Nursing Program Faculty 12 (60% with doctorates).
Baccalaureate Enrollment 182 **Women** 91% **Men** 9% **Minority** 18% **International** 10% **Part-time** 1%
Graduate Enrollment 63 **Women** 100% **Minority** 32% **International** .5% **Part-time** 6%
Distance Learning Courses Available.
Nursing Student Activities Student Nurses' Association.
Nursing Student Resources Academic advising; academic or career counseling; assistance for students with disabilities; bookstore; campus computer network; career placement assistance; computer lab; computer-assisted instruction; e-mail services; employment services for current students; housing assistance; interactive nursing skills videos; Internet; learning resource lab; library services; nursing audiovisuals; remedial services; resume preparation assistance; skills, simulation, or other laboratory; tutoring.
Library Facilities 190,565 volumes (2,500 in health, 800 in nursing); 11,000 periodical subscriptions (369 health-care related).

BACCALAUREATE PROGRAMS

Degree BScN
Available Programs Generic Baccalaureate.
Study Options Full-time.
Program Entrance Requirements Minimum overall college GPA of 2.0, CPR certification, health insurance, high school biology, high school chemistry, 1 year of high school math, 2 years high school science, high school transcript, immunizations, 2 letters of recommendation, minimum high school GPA of 2.7, minimum GPA in nursing prerequisites of 2.3. Transfer students are accepted. *Application deadline:* 2/28 (fall).
Advanced Placement Credit given for nursing courses completed elsewhere dependent upon specific evaluations.
Expenses (2012–13) *Tuition:* full-time CAN$21,450; part-time CAN$715 per credit hour. *Room and board:* CAN$7550 per academic year. *Required fees:* full-time CAN$1600.
Financial Aid 70% of baccalaureate students in nursing programs received some form of financial aid in 2011–12. *Gift aid (need-based):* private, college/university gift aid from institutional funds. *Loans:* federal and provincial loans. *Financial aid application deadline (priority):* 2/28.

Contact Dr. Landa Terblanche, Dean, Department of Nursing, Trinity Western University, 7600 Glover Road, Langley, BC V2Y 1Y1. *Telephone:* 604-888-7511 Ext. 3268. *Fax:* 604-513-2012. *E-mail:* landa.terblanche@twu.ca.

GRADUATE PROGRAMS

Financial Aid 20% of graduate students in nursing programs received some form of financial aid in 2011–12.
Contact Ms. Guelda Redman, MSN Administrative Assistant, Department of Nursing, Trinity Western University, 7600 Glover Road, Langley, BC V2Y 1Y1. *Telephone:* 604-888-7511 Ext. 3270. *Fax:* 604-513-2012. *E-mail:* guelda.redman@twu.ca.

MASTER'S DEGREE PROGRAM

Degree MSN
Available Programs Master's.
Concentrations Available Clinical nurse leader; health-care administration; nursing administration; nursing education. *Clinical nurse specialist programs in:* gerontology. *Nurse practitioner programs in:* gerontology.
Study Options Full-time and part-time.
Program Entrance Requirements Minimum overall college GPA of 3.0, transcript of college record, written essay, 3 letters of recommendation, resume, statistics course. *Application deadline:* 5/1 (summer).
Advanced Placement Credit given for nursing courses completed elsewhere dependent upon specific evaluations.
Degree Requirements 30 total credit hours, thesis or project.

The University of British Columbia
Program in Nursing
Vancouver, British Columbia

http://www.nursing.ubc.ca/
Founded in 1915
DEGREES • BSN • MSN • PHD
Nursing Program Faculty 55 (51% with doctorates).
Baccalaureate Enrollment 242 **Women** 84.7% **Men** 15.3% **International** 1%
Graduate Enrollment 206 **Women** 92.3% **Men** 7.7% **International** 10% **Part-time** 27%
Nursing Student Activities Nursing Honor Society, Sigma Theta Tau, Student Nurses' Association, nursing club.
Nursing Student Resources Academic advising; academic or career counseling; assistance for students with disabilities; bookstore; campus computer network; career placement assistance; computer lab; computer-assisted instruction; e-mail services; employment services for current students; housing assistance; interactive nursing skills videos; Internet; learning resource lab; library services; nursing audiovisuals; skills, simulation, or other laboratory.
Library Facilities 6.4 million volumes (160,000 in health, 11,000 in nursing); 778,063 periodical subscriptions (17,000 health-care related).

BACCALAUREATE PROGRAMS

Degree BSN
Available Programs Accelerated Baccalaureate; Accelerated Baccalaureate for Second Degree.
Study Options Full-time.
Program Entrance Requirements Minimum overall college GPA of 2.8, transcript of college record, CPR certification, written essay, health exam, health insurance, high school transcript, immunizations, interview, professional liability insurance/malpractice insurance, prerequisite course work. *Application deadline:* 12/1 (winter). *Application fee:* CAN$215.
Expenses (2012–13) *Tuition, state resident:* full-time CAN$7521. *Tuition, nonresident:* full-time CAN$7521. *International tuition:* CAN$36,194 full-time. *Room and board:* CAN$8345; room only: CAN$6645 per academic year. *Required fees:* full-time CAN$953.
Financial Aid *Gift aid (need-based):* state, private, college/university gift aid from institutional funds, provincial scholarships/grants, Federal Canada Study Grants. *Loans:* college/university, Canadian government student loans (for Canadian citizens), provincial student loans. *Work-study:* part-time campus jobs. *Financial aid application deadline:* 9/15(priority: 4/15).
Contact Ruxandra Vasiljevic, Undergraduate Admissions Assistant, Program in Nursing, The University of British Columbia, T201-2211

Wesbrook Mall, Vancouver, BC V6T 2B5. *Telephone:* 604-822-9754. *Fax:* 604-822-7466. *E-mail:* information@nursing.ubc.ca.

GRADUATE PROGRAMS

Expenses (2012–13) *Tuition, state resident:* full-time CAN$4350. *Tuition, nonresident:* full-time CAN$4350. *International tuition:* CAN$7641 full-time. *Room and board:* CAN$11,000; room only: CAN$8580 per academic year. *Required fees:* full-time CAN$953.
Financial Aid 10% of graduate students in nursing programs received some form of financial aid in 2011–12. 4 fellowships (averaging $8,000 per year), 14 research assistantships (averaging $800 per year), 3 teaching assistantships were awarded.
Contact Mr. Drew St. Laurent, Graduate Records Officer, Program in Nursing, The University of British Columbia, T201-2211 Wesbrook Mall, Vancouver, BC V6T 2B5. *Telephone:* 604-822-7446. *E-mail:* student.services@nursing.ubc.ca.

MASTER'S DEGREE PROGRAM

Degree MSN
Available Programs Master's.
Concentrations Available Nursing administration; nursing education. *Clinical nurse specialist programs in:* adult health, cardiovascular, community health, family health, gerontology, maternity-newborn, oncology, parent-child, pediatric, perinatal, psychiatric/mental health, public health, women's health. *Nurse practitioner programs in:* community health, family health, primary care.
Study Options Full-time and part-time.
Program Entrance Requirements Computer literacy, minimum overall college GPA of 3.3, transcript of college record, 3 letters of recommendation, resume, GRE. *Application deadline:* 1/31 (winter). Applications may be processed on a rolling basis for some programs. *Application fee:* CAN$93.
Advanced Placement Credit given for nursing courses completed elsewhere dependent upon specific evaluations.
Degree Requirements 33 total credit hours, thesis or project.

DOCTORAL DEGREE PROGRAM

Degree PhD
Available Programs Doctorate.
Areas of Study Addiction/substance abuse, advanced practice nursing, aging, clinical practice, community health, ethics, faculty preparation, family health, gerontology, health policy, health promotion/disease prevention, health-care systems, human health and illness, illness and transition, individualized study, information systems, maternity-newborn, nursing administration, nursing education, nursing policy, nursing research, nursing science, oncology, urban health, women's health.
Program Entrance Requirements interview, 3 letters of recommendation, MSN or equivalent, vita, writing sample, GRE. *Application deadline:* 1/31 (fall). Applications may be processed on a rolling basis for some programs. *Application fee:* CAN$153.
Degree Requirements 18 total credit hours, dissertation, oral exam.

POSTDOCTORAL PROGRAM

Areas of Study Addiction/substance abuse, adolescent health, aging, cancer care, chronic illness, community health, family health, gerontology, health promotion/disease prevention, individualized study, infection prevention/skin care, information systems, neuro-behavior, nursing informatics, nursing interventions, nursing research, nursing science, outcomes, self-care, vulnerable population, women's health.
Postdoctoral Program Contact Dr. Elizabeth Saewyc, Associate Director, Research, Program in Nursing, The University of British Columbia, T201-2211 Wesbrook Mall, Vancouver, BC V6T 2B5. *Telephone:* 604-822-7505. *Fax:* 604-822-7466. *E-mail:* elizabeth.saewyc@nursing.ubc.ca.

University of Northern British Columbia

Nursing Programme
Prince George, British Columbia

http://www.unbc.ca/nursing/
Founded in 1994

DEGREES • BSCN • M SC N
Nursing Program Faculty 40 (18% with doctorates).
Baccalaureate Enrollment 600

Graduate Enrollment 60
Distance Learning Courses Available.
Nursing Student Activities Student Nurses' Association.
Nursing Student Resources Academic advising; academic or career counseling; assistance for students with disabilities; bookstore; campus computer network; computer lab; computer-assisted instruction; e-mail services; employment services for current students; externships; Internet; learning resource lab; library services; nursing audiovisuals; skills, simulation, or other laboratory.
Library Facilities 310,433 volumes (4,000 in health, 2,000 in nursing); 19,570 periodical subscriptions (300 health-care related).

BACCALAUREATE PROGRAMS

Degree BScN
Available Programs Generic Baccalaureate; RN Baccalaureate.
Site Options Prince George, BC; Quesnel, BC; Terrace, BC.
Study Options Full-time.
Program Entrance Requirements Minimum overall college GPA of 2.33, transcript of college record, CPR certification, health exam, high school biology, high school chemistry, 1 year of high school math, 4 years high school science, high school transcript, immunizations, minimum high school GPA of 2.3, minimum high school rank 65%, minimum GPA in nursing prerequisites of 2.0, professional liability insurance/malpractice insurance. Transfer students are accepted. *Application deadline:* 3/31 (fall). *Application fee:* CAN$35.
Advanced Placement Credit given for nursing courses completed elsewhere dependent upon specific evaluations.
Contact *Telephone:* 250-960-5645.

GRADUATE PROGRAMS

Contact *Telephone:* 250-960-5848. *Fax:* 250-960-6410.

MASTER'S DEGREE PROGRAM

Degree M Sc N
Available Programs Master's.
Concentrations Available *Nurse practitioner programs in:* family health.
Study Options Full-time and part-time.
Program Entrance Requirements Clinical experience, minimum overall college GPA of 3.0, transcript of college record, CPR certification, written essay, 3 letters of recommendation, nursing research course, professional liability insurance/malpractice insurance, prerequisite course work. *Application deadline:* 2/15 (fall). *Application fee:* CAN$75.
Advanced Placement Credit given for nursing courses completed elsewhere dependent upon specific evaluations.
Degree Requirements 51 total credit hours, thesis or project.

POSTDOCTORAL PROGRAM

Areas of Study Chronic illness, community health, family health, health promotion/disease prevention, individualized study, nursing interventions, nursing research, nursing science, outcomes, vulnerable population.
Postdoctoral Program Contact *Telephone:* 250-960-6507. *Fax:* 250-960-6410.

University of Victoria

School of Nursing
Victoria, British Columbia

http://web.uvic.ca/nurs/
Founded in 1963

DEGREES • BSN • MN • PHD
Nursing Program Faculty 21 (95% with doctorates).
Baccalaureate Enrollment 1,100 **Women** 95% **Men** 5% **Part-time** 50%
Nursing Student Activities Student Nurses' Association.
Nursing Student Resources Academic advising; assistance for students with disabilities; bookstore; campus computer network; computer lab; e-mail services; employment services for current students; interactive nursing skills videos; Internet; library services; nursing audiovisuals; remedial services; resume preparation assistance; unpaid internships.
Library Facilities 1.8 million volumes; 14,000 periodical subscriptions.

BACCALAUREATE PROGRAMS

Degree BSN

Site Options Vancouver, BC.
Program Entrance Requirements Minimum overall college GPA of 3.5, transcript of college record, CPR certification, high school transcript, immunizations, prerequisite course work. Transfer students are accepted.
Contact *Telephone:* 250-721-7961. *Fax:* 250-721-6231.

GRADUATE PROGRAMS

Contact *Telephone:* 250-721-7961. *Fax:* 250-721-6231.

MASTER'S DEGREE PROGRAM
Degree MN
Available Programs Master's.
Site Options Victoria.
Study Options Full-time and part-time.
Program Entrance Requirements Clinical experience, transcript of college record, letters of recommendation.
Advanced Placement Credit given for nursing courses completed elsewhere dependent upon specific evaluations.
Degree Requirements 18 total credit hours, thesis or project.

DOCTORAL DEGREE PROGRAM
Degree PhD
Program Entrance Requirements Clinical experience, MSN or equivalent.
Degree Requirements Dissertation.

Vancouver Island University
Department of Nursing
Nanaimo, British Columbia

http://www.viu.ca/calendar/Health/bscnursing.asp
Founded in 1969
DEGREE • BSCN
Nursing Program Faculty 34 (14% with doctorates).
Baccalaureate Enrollment 275 Women 92% Men 8% Minority 6%
Nursing Student Activities Student Nurses' Association.
Nursing Student Resources Academic advising; academic or career counseling; assistance for students with disabilities; bookstore; campus computer network; computer lab; computer-assisted instruction; e-mail services; employment services for current students; housing assistance; interactive nursing skills videos; Internet; learning resource lab; library services; nursing audiovisuals; remedial services; resume preparation assistance; skills, simulation, or other laboratory; tutoring; unpaid internships.
Library Facilities 9,475 volumes in health, 1,299 volumes in nursing; 800 periodical subscriptions health-care related.

BACCALAUREATE PROGRAMS

Degree BScN
Available Programs Generic Baccalaureate.
Study Options Full-time.
Program Entrance Requirements CPR certification, health insurance, high school biology, high school chemistry, 11 years high school math, high school transcript, immunizations, minimum GPA in nursing prerequisites of 3.0, prerequisite course work, RN licensure. Transfer students are accepted. *Application deadline:* 2/28 (fall). *Application fee:* CAN$35.
Advanced Placement Credit given for nursing courses completed elsewhere dependent upon specific evaluations.
Expenses (2011–12) *Tuition, area resident:* full-time CAN$2600. *International tuition:* CAN$12,500 full-time. *Room and board:* room only: CAN$4000 per academic year.
Financial Aid 53% of baccalaureate students in nursing programs received some form of financial aid in 2010–11. *Gift aid (need-based):* private, college/university gift aid from institutional funds. *Loans:* government student loans.
Contact Dr. France Bouthillette, Chair of Bachelor of Science in Nursing Programs, Department of Nursing, Vancouver Island University, 900 Fifth Street, Nanaimo, BC V9R 5S5. *Telephone:* 250-740-6260. *Fax:* 250-740-6468. *E-mail:* france.bouthillette@viu.ca.

CONTINUING EDUCATION PROGRAM

Contact Ms. Cheryl Dill, Program Coordinator, Department of Nursing, Vancouver Island University, 900 Fifth Street, Nanaimo, BC V9R 5S5. *Telephone:* 250-740-6327. *E-mail:* Cheryl.Dill@viu.ca.

MANITOBA

Brandon University
School of Health Studies
Brandon, Manitoba

http://www.brandonu.ca/health-studies/
Founded in 1899
DEGREE • BN
Nursing Program Faculty 20 (40% with doctorates).
Baccalaureate Enrollment 480 Women 95% Men 5% Minority 10% Part-time 25%
Distance Learning Courses Available.
Nursing Student Activities Nursing Honor Society, Sigma Theta Tau, Student Nurses' Association.
Nursing Student Resources Academic advising; academic or career counseling; assistance for students with disabilities; bookstore; campus computer network; career placement assistance; computer lab; computer-assisted instruction; e-mail services; employment services for current students; housing assistance; interactive nursing skills videos; Internet; library services; resume preparation assistance; skills, simulation, or other laboratory; tutoring.
Library Facilities 238,816 volumes; 1,699 periodical subscriptions.

BACCALAUREATE PROGRAMS

Degree BN
Available Programs Baccalaureate for Second Degree; Generic Baccalaureate; LPN to Baccalaureate; RN Baccalaureate.
Site Options Winnipeg, MB.
Study Options Full-time and part-time.
Program Entrance Requirements Minimum overall college GPA of 2.0, CPR certification, immunizations, minimum GPA in nursing prerequisites of 2.0, prerequisite course work. Transfer students are accepted. *Application deadline:* 5/1 (fall).
Advanced Placement Credit given for nursing courses completed elsewhere dependent upon specific evaluations.
Contact *Telephone:* 204-571-8567. *Fax:* 204-571-8568.

University of Manitoba
Faculty of Nursing
Winnipeg, Manitoba

http://www.umanitoba.ca/faculties/nursing/
Founded in 1877
DEGREES • BN • MN • PHD
Nursing Program Faculty 54 (53% with doctorates).
Baccalaureate Enrollment 962 Women 87% Men 13% Part-time 25%
Graduate Enrollment 84 Women 92% Men 8% Part-time 38%
Distance Learning Courses Available.
Nursing Student Activities Nursing Honor Society, Sigma Theta Tau, Student Nurses' Association.
Nursing Student Resources Academic advising; academic or career counseling; assistance for students with disabilities; bookstore; campus computer network; computer lab; computer-assisted instruction; daycare for children of students; e-mail services; employment services for current students; housing assistance; interactive nursing skills videos; Internet; learning resource lab; library services; skills, simulation, or other laboratory; unpaid internships.
Library Facilities 2 million volumes (137,100 in health, 5,000 in nursing); 47,299 periodical subscriptions (2,208 health-care related).

BACCALAUREATE PROGRAMS

Degree BN
Available Programs Baccalaureate for Second Degree; Generic Baccalaureate; RN Baccalaureate.
Site Options Thompson, MB; The Pas, MB.
Study Options Full-time and part-time.
Program Entrance Requirements Minimum overall college GPA of 2.5, transcript of college record, CPR certification, high school chemistry, high school math, high school science, high school transcript, immunizations, minimum high school GPA of 2.5, prerequisite course work. Transfer students are accepted. *Application deadline:* 4/1 (fall).

Advanced Placement Credit given for nursing courses completed elsewhere dependent upon specific evaluations.

Expenses (2012–13) *Tuition, area resident:* full-time CAN$12,000.

Contact Dr. Marion McKay, Associate Dean, Undergraduate Program, Faculty of Nursing, University of Manitoba, 277 Helen Glass Centre for Nursing, Winnipeg, MB R3T 2N2. *Telephone:* 204-474-6220. *Fax:* 204-474-7682. *E-mail:* marion_mckay@umanitoba.ca.

GRADUATE PROGRAMS

Expenses (2012–13) *Tuition, area resident:* full-time CAN$4283. *International tuition:* CAN$8566 full-time.

Contact Dr. Jo-Ann Sawatzky, Associate Dean, Graduate Programs, Faculty of Nursing, University of Manitoba, 281-89 Curry Place, Winnipeg, MB R3T 2N2. *Telephone:* 204-474-9317. *Fax:* 204-474-7682. *E-mail:* joann.sawatzky@ad.umanitoba.ca.

MASTER'S DEGREE PROGRAM

Degree MN

Available Programs Master's.

Concentrations Available Nursing administration. *Clinical nurse specialist programs in:* acute care, family health, gerontology, perinatal, women's health. *Nurse practitioner programs in:* primary care.

Study Options Full-time and part-time.

Program Entrance Requirements Clinical experience, minimum overall college GPA of 3.0, transcript of college record, written essay, 3 letters of recommendation, nursing research course, resume, statistics course. *Application deadline:* 4/1 (fall).

Advanced Placement Credit given for nursing courses completed elsewhere dependent upon specific evaluations.

Degree Requirements 27 total credit hours, thesis or project, comprehensive exam.

DOCTORAL DEGREE PROGRAM

Degree PhD

Available Programs Doctorate.

Areas of Study Nursing science.

Program Entrance Requirements Clinical experience, letters of recommendation, MSN or equivalent. *Application deadline:* 4/1 (fall).

Degree Requirements 21 total credit hours, dissertation.

CONTINUING EDUCATION PROGRAM

Contact Dr. Beverly O'Connell, Professor, Faculty of Nursing, University of Manitoba, 293 Helen Glass Centre for Nursing, Winnipeg, MB R3T 2N2. *Telephone:* 204-474-9201. *Fax:* 204-474-7500. *E-mail:* beverly.oconnell@ad.umanitoba.ca.

NEW BRUNSWICK

Université de Moncton
School of Nursing
Moncton, New Brunswick

http://www.umoncton.ca/umcm-fsssc-scienceinfirmiere
Founded in 1963

DEGREES • BSCN • M SC N

Nursing Program Faculty 64 (17% with doctorates).

Baccalaureate Enrollment 548 **Women** 86% **Men** 14% **Minority** 4% **International** 6% **Part-time** 1%

Graduate Enrollment 56 **Women** 89% **Men** 11% **Minority** 2% **International** 2% **Part-time** 100%

Distance Learning Courses Available.

Nursing Student Activities Student Nurses' Association.

Nursing Student Resources Academic or career counseling; assistance for students with disabilities; bookstore; campus computer network; career placement assistance; computer lab; computer-assisted instruction; daycare for children of students; e-mail services; employment services for current students; externships; housing assistance; Internet; library services; nursing audiovisuals; placement services for program completers; resume preparation assistance; skills, simulation, or other laboratory; tutoring; unpaid internships.

Library Facilities 789,046 volumes (10,757 in health, 3,807 in nursing); 2,059 periodical subscriptions (210 health-care related).

BACCALAUREATE PROGRAMS

Degree BScN

Available Programs RN Baccalaureate.

Site Options Edmundston, NB; Bathurst, NB; Moncton, NB.

Study Options Full-time.

Program Entrance Requirements Transcript of college record, CPR certification, high school biology, high school chemistry, 30411 years high school math, high school science, high school transcript, immunizations, minimum high school rank 65%. Transfer students are accepted. *Application deadline:* 4/1 (winter). *Application fee:* CAN$50.

Advanced Placement Credit given for nursing courses completed elsewhere dependent upon specific evaluations.

Expenses (2012–13) *Tuition, state resident:* full-time CAN$5292; part-time CAN$178 per credit. *Tuition, nonresident:* full-time CAN$5292; part-time CAN$178 per credit. *International tuition:* CAN$8972 full-time. *Room and board:* CAN$5162; room only: CAN$3937 per academic year. *Required fees:* full-time CAN$338.

Financial Aid 50% of baccalaureate students in nursing programs received some form of financial aid in 2011–12. *Gift aid (need-based):* state, private, college/university gift aid from institutional funds. *Loans:* Federal Direct (Subsidized and Unsubsidized Stafford PLUS), college/university, federal and provincial student loans. *Work-study:* part-time campus jobs. *Financial aid application deadline:* 3/9.

Contact Yoland Bordeleau, Bureau de recrutement, School of Nursing, Université de Moncton, Pavillon Leopold Taillon, Moncton, NB E1A 3E9. *Telephone:* 506-858-4443. *Fax:* 506-858-4538. *E-mail:* yoland.bordeleau@umoncton.ca.

GRADUATE PROGRAMS

Expenses (2012–13) *Tuition:* part-time CAN$206 per credit. *Room and board:* CAN$5162; room only: CAN$3937 per academic year.

Financial Aid 4% of graduate students in nursing programs received some form of financial aid in 2011–12.

Contact Yoland Bordeleau, Bureau de recrutement, School of Nursing, Université de Moncton, Pavillon Leopold Taillon, Moncton, NB E1A 3E9. *Telephone:* 506-858-4443. *Fax:* 506-858-4538. *E-mail:* yoland.bordeleau@umoncton.ca.

MASTER'S DEGREE PROGRAM

Degree M Sc N

Available Programs Master's; RN to Master's.

Concentrations Available Health-care administration; nurse case management; nursing administration; nursing education. *Clinical nurse specialist programs in:* community health, family health, home health care, occupational health, pediatric, psychiatric/mental health, public health, school health. *Nurse practitioner programs in:* adult health, community health, family health, oncology, primary care.

Site Options Moncton, NB.

Study Options Full-time and part-time.

Program Entrance Requirements Minimum overall college GPA of 3.0, transcript of college record, CPR certification, written essay, immunizations, 2 letters of recommendation, resume, statistics course. *Application deadline:* 6/1 (summer). *Application fee:* CAN$50.

Advanced Placement Credit given for nursing courses completed elsewhere dependent upon specific evaluations.

Degree Requirements 45 total credit hours, thesis or project.

CONTINUING EDUCATION PROGRAM

Contact Mrs. Denise Savoie, Directrice du service la clientle, School of Nursing, Université de Moncton, ducation permanente, 18 avenue Antonine-Maillet, Moncton, NB E1A 3E9. *Telephone:* 506-858-4621. *Fax:* 506-858-4480. *E-mail:* denise.savoie@umoncton.ca.

University of New Brunswick Fredericton
Faculty of Nursing
Fredericton, New Brunswick

http://www.unbf.ca/nursing/
Founded in 1785

DEGREES • BN • MN

Nursing Program Faculty 75 (17% with doctorates).

Baccalaureate Enrollment 740 **Women** 94% **Men** 6% **International** 1%

Graduate Enrollment 53 **Women** 96% **Men** 4% **Part-time** 30%

Distance Learning Courses Available.

Nursing Student Activities Student Nurses' Association, nursing club.

Nursing Student Resources Academic advising; academic or career counseling; assistance for students with disabilities; bookstore; campus computer network; computer lab; computer-assisted instruction; daycare for children of students; e-mail services; employment services for current students; interactive nursing skills videos; Internet; learning resource lab; library services; nursing audiovisuals; resume preparation assistance; skills, simulation, or other laboratory; tutoring.

Library Facilities 1.7 million volumes (12,547 in health, 1,910 in nursing); 37,550 periodical subscriptions (250 health-care related).

BACCALAUREATE PROGRAMS

Degree BN

Available Programs Accelerated Baccalaureate; Generic Baccalaureate.

Site Options Bathurst, NB; Moncton, NB; Fredericton, NB.

Study Options Full-time.

Program Entrance Requirements Minimum overall college GPA of 3.0, transcript of college record, CPR certification, written essay, health exam, high school biology, high school chemistry, 60 years high school math, high school transcript, immunizations, interview, minimum high school rank 70%, prerequisite course work. Transfer students are accepted. *Application deadline:* 3/31 (fall). *Application fee:* CAN$55.

Advanced Placement Credit given for nursing courses completed elsewhere dependent upon specific evaluations.

Contact Ms. Pam Wiebe, Administrative Assistant, Faculty of Nursing, University of New Brunswick Fredericton, PO Box 4400, Fredericton, NB E3B 5A3. *Telephone:* 506-458-7670. *Fax:* 506-453-3512. *E-mail:* pwiebe@unb.ca.

GRADUATE PROGRAMS

Contact Mr. Francis Perry, Graduate Assistant, Faculty of Nursing, University of New Brunswick Fredericton, PO Box 4400, Fredericton, NB E3B 5A3. *Telephone:* 506-451-6844. *Fax:* 506-447-3374. *E-mail:* fperry@unb.ca.

MASTER'S DEGREE PROGRAM

Degree MN

Available Programs Master's.

Concentrations Available Nurse case management; nursing administration; nursing education; nursing informatics. *Clinical nurse specialist programs in:* acute care, adult health, cardiovascular, community health, critical care, family health, gerontology, maternity-newborn, medical-surgical, oncology, parent-child, pediatric, psychiatric/mental health, public health, school health, women's health. *Nurse practitioner programs in:* acute care, adult health, community health, family health, gerontology, neonatal health, pediatric, primary care, psychiatric/mental health, women's health.

Site Options Fredericton, NB.

Study Options Full-time and part-time.

Program Entrance Requirements Clinical experience, computer literacy, minimum overall college GPA of 3.3, transcript of college record, written essay, 3 letters of recommendation, nursing research course, physical assessment course, prerequisite course work, statistics course. *Application deadline:* 1/2 (winter). *Application fee:* CAN$50.

Advanced Placement Credit given for nursing courses completed elsewhere dependent upon specific evaluations.

Degree Requirements 27 total credit hours, thesis or project.

CONTINUING EDUCATION PROGRAM

Contact Mr. Lee Heenan, Administrative Assistant, Faculty of Nursing, University of New Brunswick Fredericton, PO Box 4400, Fredericton, NB E3B 5A3. *Telephone:* 506-458-7625. *Fax:* 506-447-3057. *E-mail:* nursing@unb.ca.

NEWFOUNDLAND AND LABRADOR

Memorial University of Newfoundland
School of Nursing
St. John's, Newfoundland and Labrador

http://www.nurs.mun.ca/
Founded in 1925

DEGREES • BN • MN

Nursing Program Faculty 42 (30% with doctorates).

Baccalaureate Enrollment 642 **Women** 92% **Men** 8% **International** 2% **Part-time** 50%

Graduate Enrollment 100 **Women** 91% **Men** 9% **International** 1% **Part-time** 82%

Distance Learning Courses Available.

Nursing Student Activities Student Nurses' Association.

Nursing Student Resources Academic advising; academic or career counseling; assistance for students with disabilities; bookstore; campus computer network; computer lab; computer-assisted instruction; daycare for children of students; e-mail services; externships; interactive nursing skills videos; Internet; learning resource lab; library services; nursing audiovisuals; remedial services; skills, simulation, or other laboratory; tutoring.

Library Facilities 1.9 million volumes (40,000 in health, 5,000 in nursing); 17,170 periodical subscriptions (3,800 health-care related).

BACCALAUREATE PROGRAMS

Degree BN

Available Programs Accelerated Baccalaureate; Generic Baccalaureate; LPN to Baccalaureate; RN Baccalaureate.

Study Options Full-time.

Program Entrance Requirements Minimum overall college GPA of 3.0, transcript of college record, written essay, high school biology, high school chemistry, high school foreign language, high school math, high school science, high school transcript, 2 letters of recommendation, minimum high school rank 80%. Transfer students are accepted. *Application deadline:* 3/1 (fall).

Contact *Telephone:* 709-737-6871. *Fax:* 709-737-3890.

GRADUATE PROGRAMS

Contact *Telephone:* 709-777-6679. *Fax:* 709-777-7037.

MASTER'S DEGREE PROGRAM

Degree MN

Available Programs Master's.

Concentrations Available Nursing education. *Nurse practitioner programs in:* acute care.

Study Options Full-time and part-time.

Online Degree Options Yes (online only).

Program Entrance Requirements Clinical experience, minimum overall college GPA of 3.0, transcript of college record, written essay, 2 letters of recommendation, nursing research course, professional liability insurance/malpractice insurance, prerequisite course work, resume, statistics course. *Application deadline:* 2/15 (fall). *Application fee:* CAN$40.

Advanced Placement Credit given for nursing courses completed elsewhere dependent upon specific evaluations.

Degree Requirements 28 total credit hours, thesis or project.

POST-MASTER'S PROGRAM

Areas of Study *Nurse practitioner programs in:* acute care.

NOVA SCOTIA

St. Francis Xavier University
Department of Nursing
Antigonish, Nova Scotia

http://www.stfx.ca/
Founded in 1853
DEGREE • BSCN
Nursing Program Faculty 67 (10% with doctorates).
Baccalaureate Enrollment 1,067 **Women** 90% **Men** 10% **Minority** 5%
International 1% **Part-time** 40%
Nursing Student Activities Student Nurses' Association, nursing club.
Nursing Student Resources Academic advising; academic or career counseling; assistance for students with disabilities; bookstore; campus computer network; career placement assistance; computer lab; computer-assisted instruction; daycare for children of students; e-mail services; employment services for current students; externships; housing assistance; interactive nursing skills videos; Internet; learning resource lab; library services; nursing audiovisuals; other; paid internships; placement services for program completers; remedial services; resume preparation assistance; skills, simulation, or other laboratory; tutoring; unpaid internships.
Library Facilities 320,317 volumes (4,000 in health, 4,000 in nursing); 24,293 periodical subscriptions (1,015 health-care related).

BACCALAUREATE PROGRAMS
Degree BScN
Available Programs Accelerated Baccalaureate; Accelerated Baccalaureate for Second Degree; Accelerated LPN to Baccalaureate; Generic Baccalaureate; RN Baccalaureate.
Site Options Sydney, NS.
Study Options Full-time.
Program Entrance Requirements Transcript of college record, CPR certification, health exam, high school biology, high school chemistry, 2 years high school math, 2 years high school science, high school transcript, immunizations, minimum high school GPA, prerequisite course work. Transfer students are accepted.
Advanced Placement Credit given for nursing courses completed elsewhere dependent upon specific evaluations.
Contact *Telephone:* 902-867-5386. *Fax:* 902-867-2329.

CONTINUING EDUCATION PROGRAM
Contact *Telephone:* 902-867-5186. *Fax:* 902-867-5154.

ONTARIO

Brock University
Department of Nursing
St. Catharines, Ontario

http://www.brocku.ca/nursing/
Founded in 1964
DEGREE • BSCN
Nursing Program Faculty 27
Nursing Student Activities Student Nurses' Association, nursing club.
Nursing Student Resources Academic advising; academic or career counseling; assistance for students with disabilities; bookstore; campus computer network; computer lab; computer-assisted instruction; daycare for children of students; e-mail services; employment services for current students; housing assistance; interactive nursing skills videos; Internet; learning resource lab; library services; nursing audiovisuals; other; resume preparation assistance; skills, simulation, or other laboratory; tutoring.
Library Facilities 769,873 volumes.

BACCALAUREATE PROGRAMS
Degree BScN
Available Programs Generic Baccalaureate; RN Baccalaureate.

Study Options Full-time.
Program Entrance Requirements High school biology, high school chemistry.
Contact *Telephone:* 905-688-5550 Ext. 4660.

Lakehead University
School of Nursing
Thunder Bay, Ontario

http://www.lakeheadu.ca/
Founded in 1965
DEGREE • BSCN
Nursing Program Faculty 15 (20% with doctorates).
Baccalaureate Enrollment 575 **Women** 82% **Men** 18%
Distance Learning Courses Available.
Nursing Student Activities Student Nurses' Association.
Nursing Student Resources Academic advising; academic or career counseling; assistance for students with disabilities; bookstore; campus computer network; career placement assistance; computer lab; daycare for children of students; e-mail services; employment services for current students; externships; housing assistance; interactive nursing skills videos; Internet; library services; nursing audiovisuals; resume preparation assistance; skills, simulation, or other laboratory; tutoring; unpaid internships.
Library Facilities 715,276 volumes; 44,533 periodical subscriptions.

BACCALAUREATE PROGRAMS
Degree BScN
Available Programs Accelerated Baccalaureate; Generic Baccalaureate; RN Baccalaureate.
Study Options Full-time and part-time.
Online Degree Options Yes.
Program Entrance Requirements Transcript of college record, CPR certification, health insurance, high school biology, high school chemistry, 4 years high school math, high school transcript, immunizations, minimum high school GPA. Transfer students are accepted. *Application deadline:* 1/12 (winter). Applications may be processed on a rolling basis for some programs.
Advanced Placement Credit given for nursing courses completed elsewhere dependent upon specific evaluations.
Contact *Telephone:* 807-343-8439. *Fax:* 807-343-8246.

Laurentian University
School of Nursing
Sudbury, Ontario

http://www.laurentian.ca/content/program/nursing/overview
Founded in 1960
DEGREES • BSCN • M SC N
Nursing Program Faculty 25 (20% with doctorates).
Baccalaureate Enrollment 1,000 **Women** 90% **Men** 10% **Minority** 5%
International 5%
Graduate Enrollment 70
Distance Learning Courses Available.
Nursing Student Activities Student Nurses' Association.
Nursing Student Resources Academic advising; academic or career counseling; assistance for students with disabilities; bookstore; campus computer network; career placement assistance; computer lab; computer-assisted instruction; daycare for children of students; e-mail services; employment services for current students; externships; interactive nursing skills videos; Internet; learning resource lab; library services; nursing audiovisuals; resume preparation assistance; skills, simulation, or other laboratory; tutoring; unpaid internships.

BACCALAUREATE PROGRAMS
Degree BScN
Available Programs Accelerated Baccalaureate; Baccalaureate for Second Degree; Generic Baccalaureate; RN Baccalaureate.
Site Options Timmins, ON; Sault Ste. Marie, ON; Cornwall/Kingston/Brockville, ON.
Study Options Full-time and part-time.
Online Degree Options Yes (online only).

Program Entrance Requirements CPR certification, health exam, high school biology, high school chemistry, high school transcript, immunizations. Transfer students are accepted.
Advanced Placement Credit by examination available. Credit given for nursing courses completed elsewhere dependent upon specific evaluations.
Financial Aid *Gift aid (need-based):* state, private, college/university gift aid from institutional funds. *Loans:* college/university.*Work-study:* part-time campus jobs.*Financial aid application deadline:* Continuous.
Contact Ms. Fran Guilbeault, Administrative Assistant, School of Nursing, Laurentian University, 935 Ramsey Lake Road, Sudbury, ON P3E 2C6. *Telephone:* 705-675-1151 Ext. 3800. *Fax:* 705-675-4861. *E-mail:* fguilbeault@laurentian.ca.

GRADUATE PROGRAMS

Contact Fran Guilbeault, Administrative Assistant, School of Nursing, Laurentian University, 935 Ramsey Lake Road, Sudbury, ON P3E 2C6. *Telephone:* 705-675-1151 Ext. 3800. *Fax:* 705-675-4861. *E-mail:* fguilbeault@laurentian.ca.

MASTER'S DEGREE PROGRAM
Degree M Sc N
Available Programs Master's.
Study Options Full-time and part-time.
Program Entrance Requirements Clinical experience, computer literacy, transcript of college record, CPR certification, written essay, immunizations, interview, letters of recommendation, resume.
Degree Requirements Thesis or project.

CONTINUING EDUCATION PROGRAM

Contact Mrs. Fran Guilbeault, Administrative Assistant, School of Nursing, Laurentian University, 935 Ramsey Lake Road, Sudbury, ON P3E 2C6. *Telephone:* 705-675-1151 Ext. 3800. *Fax:* 705-675-4861. *E-mail:* fguilbeault@laurentian.ca.

McMaster University
School of Nursing
Hamilton, Ontario

http://www.fhs.mcmaster.ca/nursing
Founded in 1887
DEGREES • BSCN • M SC • MSN/PHD • PHD
Nursing Program Faculty 53 (47% with doctorates).
Baccalaureate Enrollment 548 **Women** 90% **Men** 10% **Part-time** 20%
Nursing Student Activities Student Nurses' Association.
Nursing Student Resources Academic advising; academic or career counseling; assistance for students with disabilities; bookstore; campus computer network; career placement assistance; computer lab; daycare for children of students; e-mail services; employment services for current students; housing assistance; Internet; learning resource lab; library services; nursing audiovisuals; placement services for program completers; remedial services; resume preparation assistance; skills, simulation, or other laboratory; tutoring.
Library Facilities 1.7 million volumes (150,446 in health); 57,487 periodical subscriptions (89,267 health-care related).

BACCALAUREATE PROGRAMS

Degree BScN
Available Programs Baccalaureate for Second Degree; Generic Baccalaureate; RN Baccalaureate.
Site Options Kitchener, ON.
Study Options Full-time and part-time.
Program Entrance Requirements CPR certification, health exam, high school biology, high school chemistry, 4 years high school math, 4 years high school science, high school transcript, immunizations, minimum high school GPA of 3.0, minimum high school rank 75%. Transfer students are accepted.
Advanced Placement Credit by examination available. Credit given for nursing courses completed elsewhere dependent upon specific evaluations.
Contact *Telephone:* 905-525-9140 Ext. 22232. *Fax:* 905-528-4727.

GRADUATE PROGRAMS

Contact *Telephone:* 905-525-9140 Ext. 22982. *Fax:* 905-546-1129.

MASTER'S DEGREE PROGRAM
Degrees M Sc; MSN/PhD
Available Programs Master's.
Concentrations Available *Clinical nurse specialist programs in:* perinatal. *Nurse practitioner programs in:* neonatal health.
Study Options Full-time and part-time.
Program Entrance Requirements Transcript of college record, written essay, 2 letters of recommendation.
Advanced Placement Credit given for nursing courses completed elsewhere dependent upon specific evaluations.
Degree Requirements Thesis or project.

DOCTORAL DEGREE PROGRAM
Degree PhD
Available Programs Doctorate.
Program Entrance Requirements 2 letters of recommendation, MSN or equivalent, vita.
Degree Requirements Dissertation, oral exam.

Nipissing University
Nursing Department
North Bay, Ontario

http://www.nipissingu.ca/nursing/
Founded in 1992
DEGREE • BSCN
Nursing Program Faculty 12 (3% with doctorates).
Baccalaureate Enrollment 378 **Women** 91% **Men** 9%
Distance Learning Courses Available.
Nursing Student Activities Student Nurses' Association.
Nursing Student Resources Academic advising; academic or career counseling; assistance for students with disabilities; bookstore; campus computer network; career placement assistance; computer lab; computer-assisted instruction; e-mail services; employment services for current students; housing assistance; interactive nursing skills videos; Internet; learning resource lab; library services; nursing audiovisuals; placement services for program completers; remedial services; resume preparation assistance; skills, simulation, or other laboratory; tutoring; unpaid internships.
Library Facilities 715,494 volumes (2,800 in health, 1,820 in nursing); 19,115 periodical subscriptions (2,430 health-care related).

BACCALAUREATE PROGRAMS

Degree BScN
Available Programs RN Baccalaureate; RPN to Baccalaureate.
Study Options Full-time.
Online Degree Options Yes.
Program Entrance Requirements Minimum overall college GPA of 3.0, transcript of college record, CPR certification, high school biology, high school chemistry, high school transcript, immunizations, minimum high school rank 70%. Transfer students are accepted. *Application deadline:* 4/1 (fall). Applications may be processed on a rolling basis for some programs. *Application fee:* CAN$130.
Advanced Placement Credit given for nursing courses completed elsewhere dependent upon specific evaluations.
Expenses (2012–13) *Tuition, area resident:* full-time CAN$5380. *International tuition:* CAN$14,500 full-time. *Room and board:* room only: CAN$5875 per academic year. *Required fees:* full-time CAN$1257.
Financial Aid 44% of baccalaureate students in nursing programs received some form of financial aid in 2011–12.
Contact Registrar's Office, Nursing Department, Nipissing University, 100 College Drive, PO Box 5002, North Bay, ON P1B 8L7. *Telephone:* 705-474-3450 Ext. 4521. *E-mail:* registrar@nipssingu.ca.

Queen's University at Kingston
School of Nursing
Kingston, Ontario

http://nursing.queensu.ca/
Founded in 1841
DEGREES • BNSC • M SC • PHD
Nursing Program Faculty 20 (80% with doctorates).

Baccalaureate Enrollment 400 **Women** 95% **Men** 5% **Minority** 4% **International** 2%

Graduate Enrollment 51 **Women** 99% **Men** 1% **Minority** 5% **International** 5%

Distance Learning Courses Available.

Nursing Student Activities Student Nurses' Association.

Nursing Student Resources Academic advising; academic or career counseling; assistance for students with disabilities; bookstore; campus computer network; career placement assistance; computer lab; computer-assisted instruction; e-mail services; employment services for current students; housing assistance; interactive nursing skills videos; Internet; learning resource lab; library services; nursing audiovisuals; resume preparation assistance; skills, simulation, or other laboratory; tutoring; unpaid internships.

Library Facilities 3.5 million volumes (5,209 in health, 3,652 in nursing); 16,109 periodical subscriptions (1,054 health-care related).

BACCALAUREATE PROGRAMS

Degree BNSc

Available Programs Accelerated Baccalaureate; Generic Baccalaureate.

Study Options Full-time.

Program Entrance Requirements CPR certification, high school biology, high school chemistry, high school math, high school science, high school transcript, immunizations, minimum high school GPA, minimum high school rank. Transfer students are accepted. *Application deadline:* 2/1 (fall). *Application fee:* CAN$120.

Advanced Placement Credit given for nursing courses completed elsewhere dependent upon specific evaluations.

Financial Aid 41% of baccalaureate students in nursing programs received some form of financial aid in 2010–11.

Contact Prof. Cheryl Pulling, Chair, Admissions Committee, School of Nursing, Queen's University at Kingston, Cataraqui Building, 92 Barrie Street, Kingston, ON K7L 3N6. *Telephone:* 613-533-2668. *Fax:* 613-533-6770. *E-mail:* cap1@queensu.ca.

GRADUATE PROGRAMS

Financial Aid 100% of graduate students in nursing programs received some form of financial aid in 2010–11. 25 fellowships (averaging $6,636 per year), 4 research assistantships, 9 teaching assistantships (averaging $2,592 per year) were awarded; institutionally sponsored loans and scholarships also available. *Financial aid application deadline:* 2/1.

Contact Dr. Dana Edge, Graduate Coordinator, School of Nursing, Queen's University at Kingston, Cataraqui Building, 92 Barrie Street, Kingston, ON K7L 3N6. *Telephone:* 613-533-6000 Ext. 74765. *Fax:* 613-533-6770. *E-mail:* dana.edge@queensu.ca.

MASTER'S DEGREE PROGRAM

Degree M Sc

Available Programs Master's.

Concentrations Available *Nurse practitioner programs in:* primary care.

Study Options Full-time.

Program Entrance Requirements Minimum overall college GPA of 3.0, transcript of college record, 2 letters of recommendation, nursing research course, prerequisite course work, resume, statistics course. *Application deadline:* 2/1 (fall). *Application fee:* CAN$105.

Degree Requirements 15 total credit hours, thesis or project.

DOCTORAL DEGREE PROGRAM

Degree PhD

Available Programs Doctorate.

Areas of Study Illness and transition, nursing science.

Program Entrance Requirements Minimum overall college GPA of 3.2, 2 letters of recommendation, MSN or equivalent, statistics course, vita. *Application deadline:* 2/1 (fall). *Application fee:* CAN$105.

Degree Requirements 15 total credit hours, dissertation, oral exam, written exam, residency.

Ryerson University
Program in Nursing
Toronto, Ontario

http://www.ryerson.ca/nursing
Founded in 1948
DEGREES • BSCN • MN
Nursing Program Faculty 80 (94% with doctorates).
Baccalaureate Enrollment 1,953 **Women** 89% **Men** 11% **International** 1% **Part-time** 25.75%
Graduate Enrollment 168 **Women** 89% **Men** 11% **Part-time** 28%
Distance Learning Courses Available.
Nursing Student Activities Sigma Theta Tau, Student Nurses' Association, nursing club.
Nursing Student Resources Academic advising; academic or career counseling; assistance for students with disabilities; bookstore; campus computer network; career placement assistance; computer lab; computer-assisted instruction; daycare for children of students; e-mail services; employment services for current students; housing assistance; interactive nursing skills videos; Internet; learning resource lab; library services; nursing audiovisuals; remedial services; resume preparation assistance; skills, simulation, or other laboratory; tutoring.
Library Facilities 487,361 volumes (29,163 in health, 4,963 in nursing); 28,075 periodical subscriptions (5,567 health-care related).

BACCALAUREATE PROGRAMS

Degree BScN
Available Programs Generic Baccalaureate; International Nurse to Baccalaureate; RN Baccalaureate; RPN to Baccalaureate.
Study Options Full-time.
Program Entrance Requirements Transcript of college record, CPR certification, health exam, health insurance, high school biology, high school chemistry, high school foreign language, 3 years high school math, 4 years high school science, high school transcript, immunizations, minimum high school rank, minimum GPA in nursing prerequisites of 3.0. *Application deadline:* 3/1 (fall). *Application fee:* CAN$215.
Advanced Placement Credit given for nursing courses completed elsewhere dependent upon specific evaluations.
Financial Aid *Gift aid (need-based):* college/university gift aid from institutional funds. *Loans:* Federal Direct (Subsidized and Unsubsidized Stafford).*Financial aid application deadline:* 1/15.
Contact Heather Palmer, Senior Admission Officer, Program in Nursing, Ryerson University, 350 Victoria Street, Toronto, ON M5B 2K3. *Telephone:* 416-979-5000 Ext. 4122. *Fax:* 416-979-5221. *E-mail:* hpalmer@ryerson.ca.

GRADUATE PROGRAMS

Financial Aid 11% of graduate students in nursing programs received some form of financial aid in 2011–12.
Contact Mr. Gerry Warner, Program Administrator, Program in Nursing, Ryerson University, 350 Victoria Street, Toronto, ON M5B 2K3. *Telephone:* 416-979-5000 Ext. 7852. *Fax:* 416-979-5332. *E-mail:* gerry.warner@ryerson.ca.

MASTER'S DEGREE PROGRAM
Degree MN
Available Programs Master's.
Concentrations Available *Clinical nurse specialist programs in:* adult health, community health, family health, public health. *Nurse practitioner programs in:* primary care.
Study Options Full-time and part-time.
Program Entrance Requirements Minimum overall college GPA of 3.33, transcript of college record, written essay, immunizations, 2 letters of recommendation, nursing research course, physical assessment course, resume. *Application deadline:* 1/31 (fall). Applications may be processed on a rolling basis for some programs. *Application fee:* CAN$110.
Advanced Placement Credit given for nursing courses completed elsewhere dependent upon specific evaluations.
Degree Requirements 10 total credit hours, thesis or project.

CONTINUING EDUCATION PROGRAM
Contact Paula Mastrilli, Program Manager, Program in Nursing, Ryerson University, 297 Victoria Street, POD 481-D, Toronto, ON M5B 2K3. *Telephone:* 416-979-0000 Ext. 5178. *Fax:* 416-542-5878. *E-mail:* pmastril@gwemail.ryerson.ca.

Trent University
Nursing Program
Peterborough, Ontario

http://www.trentu.ca/nursing/
Founded in 1963
DEGREE • BSCN
Nursing Program Faculty 45 (10% with doctorates).
Baccalaureate Enrollment 523
Distance Learning Courses Available.
Nursing Student Activities Student Nurses' Association.
Nursing Student Resources Academic advising; academic or career counseling; assistance for students with disabilities; bookstore; campus computer network; computer lab; computer-assisted instruction; e-mail services; employment services for current students; housing assistance; interactive nursing skills videos; Internet; learning resource lab; library services; nursing audiovisuals; remedial services; resume preparation assistance; skills, simulation, or other laboratory; tutoring.
Library Facilities 6,393 volumes in health, 1,281 volumes in nursing; 360 periodical subscriptions health-care related.

BACCALAUREATE PROGRAMS

Degree BScN
Available Programs Accelerated Baccalaureate; Generic Baccalaureate.
Site Options Peterborough, ON.
Study Options Full-time.
Program Entrance Requirements CPR certification, health exam, high school biology, high school chemistry, 4 years high school math, 4 years high school science, high school transcript, immunizations, minimum high school rank 70%. Transfer students are accepted.
Advanced Placement Credit given for nursing courses completed elsewhere dependent upon specific evaluations.
Contact *Telephone:* 705-748-1011 Ext. 7809. *Fax:* 705-748-1088.

University of Ottawa
School of Nursing
Ottawa, Ontario

http://www.health.uottawa.ca/sn/
Founded in 1848
DEGREES • BSCN • M SC N • PHD
Nursing Program Faculty 125 (33% with doctorates).
Baccalaureate Enrollment 1,655 **Women** 94% **Men** 6% **Part-time** 21%
Graduate Enrollment 214 **Women** 90% **Men** 10% **Part-time** 55%
Distance Learning Courses Available.
Nursing Student Activities Sigma Theta Tau, Student Nurses' Association.
Nursing Student Resources Academic advising; academic or career counseling; assistance for students with disabilities; bookstore; campus computer network; career placement assistance; computer lab; computer-assisted instruction; e-mail services; employment services for current students; housing assistance; interactive nursing skills videos; Internet; learning resource lab; library services; nursing audiovisuals; remedial services; resume preparation assistance; skills, simulation, or other laboratory; tutoring.
Library Facilities 3.6 million volumes (54,000 in health, 7,000 in nursing); 79,499 periodical subscriptions (1,050 health-care related).

BACCALAUREATE PROGRAMS

Degree BScN
Available Programs Baccalaureate for Second Degree; Generic Baccalaureate; International Nurse to Baccalaureate; LPN to Baccalaureate; RN Baccalaureate; RPN to Baccalaureate.
Site Options Montreal , QC; Pembroke, ON; Montreal, QC.
Study Options Full-time.
Program Entrance Requirements Transcript of college record, CPR certification, high school biology, high school chemistry, high school math, high school transcript, immunizations, minimum high school rank 72%. Transfer students are accepted. *Application deadline:* 2/15 (winter).
Advanced Placement Credit given for nursing courses completed elsewhere dependent upon specific evaluations.
Expenses (2012–13) *Tuition, area resident:* full-time CAN$2833; part-time CAN$225 per credit. *International tuition:* CAN$9646 full-time. *Room and board:* room only: CAN$5500 per academic year.

Financial Aid *Gift aid (need-based):* state, private, college/university gift aid from institutional funds. *Loans:* Federal Direct (Subsidized and Unsubsidized Stafford PLUS).*Work-study:* part-time campus jobs.*Financial aid application deadline:* 1/31.
Contact Ms. Julie Monette, Academic Advisor, School of Nursing, University of Ottawa, 125 Universit, Ottawa, ON K1N 6N5. *Telephone:* 613-562-5800 Ext. 4238. *Fax:* 613-562-5149. *E-mail:* jmonette@uottawa.ca.

GRADUATE PROGRAMS

Expenses (2012–13) *Tuition, area resident:* full-time CAN$2472; part-time CAN$268 per credit. *International tuition:* CAN$5444 full-time. *Room and board:* room only: CAN$5500 per academic year. *Required fees:* full-time CAN$659; part-time CAN$109 per credit.
Financial Aid Fellowships, research assistantships, teaching assistantships, career-related internships or fieldwork, Federal Work-Study, scholarships, traineeships, tuition waivers (full and partial), and unspecified assistantships available.
Contact Dr. Jocelyne Tourigny, Assistant Director of Graduate Program, School of Nursing, University of Ottawa, 451 Smyth Road, Ottawa, ON K1H 8M5. *Telephone:* 613-562-5800 Ext. 8422. *Fax:* 613-562-5473. *E-mail:* jtourign@uottawa.ca.

MASTER'S DEGREE PROGRAM

Degree M Sc N
Available Programs Master's.
Concentrations Available *Clinical nurse specialist programs in:* acute care, adult health, cardiovascular, community health, critical care, family health, forensic nursing, gerontology, home health care, maternity-newborn, medical-surgical, occupational health, oncology, palliative care, parent-child, pediatric, perinatal, psychiatric/mental health, public health, rehabilitation, school health, women's health. *Nurse practitioner programs in:* primary care.
Study Options Full-time and part-time.
Program Entrance Requirements Clinical experience, minimum overall college GPA of 3.0, transcript of college record, written essay, immunizations, 3 letters of recommendation, nursing research course, physical assessment course, prerequisite course work, resume, statistics course. *Application deadline:* 2/15 (winter).
Advanced Placement Credit given for nursing courses completed elsewhere dependent upon specific evaluations.
Degree Requirements 24 total credit hours, thesis or project.

DOCTORAL DEGREE PROGRAM

Degree PhD
Available Programs Doctorate; Doctorate for Nurses with Non-Nursing Degrees.
Areas of Study Aging, community health, critical care, ethics, forensic nursing, gerontology, health policy, health promotion/disease prevention, health-care systems, human health and illness, illness and transition, maternity-newborn, nursing education, nursing policy, nursing research, nursing science, oncology, women's health.
Program Entrance Requirements Minimum overall college GPA of 3.5, 3 letters of recommendation, MSN or equivalent, statistics course, vita, writing sample.
Degree Requirements 18 total credit hours, dissertation, oral exam, written exam, residency.

POSTDOCTORAL PROGRAM

Areas of Study Addiction/substance abuse, aging, cancer care, chronic illness, community health, health promotion/disease prevention, information systems, nursing interventions, nursing research, nursing science, outcomes, vulnerable population, women's health.
Postdoctoral Program Contact Dr. Jocelyn Tourigny, Assistant Director of Graduate Program, School of Nursing, University of Ottawa, 451 Smyth Road, Ottawa, ON K1H 8M5. *Telephone:* 613-562-5800. *E-mail:* jtourign@uottawa.ca.

University of Toronto
Faculty of Nursing
Toronto, Ontario

http://bloomberg.nursing.utoronto.ca/
Founded in 1827
DEGREES • BSCN • MN • PHD
Nursing Program Faculty 250 (50% with doctorates).

Baccalaureate Enrollment 340 **Women** 87% **Men** 13% **International** 5%
Graduate Enrollment 360
Distance Learning Courses Available.
Nursing Student Activities Sigma Theta Tau, Student Nurses' Association, nursing club.
Nursing Student Resources Academic advising; academic or career counseling; assistance for students with disabilities; bookstore; campus computer network; career placement assistance; computer lab; computer-assisted instruction; daycare for children of students; e-mail services; employment services for current students; externships; housing assistance; interactive nursing skills videos; Internet; learning resource lab; library services; nursing audiovisuals; paid internships; remedial services; resume preparation assistance; skills, simulation, or other laboratory; tutoring.
Library Facilities 14.5 million volumes; 97,753 periodical subscriptions.

BACCALAUREATE PROGRAMS

Degree BScN
Available Programs Accelerated Baccalaureate; Accelerated Baccalaureate for Second Degree; Accelerated RN Baccalaureate; Baccalaureate for Second Degree.
Study Options Full-time.
Program Entrance Requirements Minimum overall college GPA of 3.0, CPR certification, written essay, immunizations, 2 letters of recommendation, minimum GPA in nursing prerequisites of 3.0, prerequisite course work. *Application deadline:* 2/1 (fall).
Expenses (2011–12) *International tuition:* CAN$27,572 full-time. *Room and board:* CAN$11,000; room only: CAN$6500 per academic year. *Required fees:* full-time CAN$1302.
Financial Aid *Work-study:* Federal Work-Study.
Contact Student Services, Faculty of Nursing, University of Toronto, 155 College Street, Toronto, ON M5T 1P8. *Telephone:* 416-978-2392. *Fax:* 416-978-8222. *E-mail:* inquiry.nursing@utoronto.ca.

GRADUATE PROGRAMS

Expenses (2011–12) *International tuition:* CAN$25,808 full-time. *Room and board:* CAN$11,000; room only: CAN$6370 per academic year. *Required fees:* full-time CAN$1636.
Contact Student Services, Faculty of Nursing, University of Toronto, 155 College Street, Toronto, ON M5T 1P8. *Telephone:* 416-978-2392. *Fax:* 416-978-8222. *E-mail:* connect.nursing@utoronto.ca.

MASTER'S DEGREE PROGRAM

Degree MN
Available Programs Master's.
Concentrations Available Clinical nurse leader; health-care administration; nurse anesthesia; nursing administration; nursing education; nursing informatics. *Clinical nurse specialist programs in:* acute care, adult health, cardiovascular, community health, critical care, family health, gerontology, maternity-newborn, medical-surgical, occupational health, oncology, palliative care, parent-child, pediatric, perinatal, psychiatric/mental health, public health, rehabilitation, school health, women's health. *Nurse practitioner programs in:* acute care, adult health, family health, gerontology, neonatal health, oncology, pediatric, primary care.
Study Options Full-time.
Online Degree Options Yes.
Program Entrance Requirements Clinical experience, minimum overall college GPA of 3.0, transcript of college record, CPR certification, written essay, 2 letters of recommendation, prerequisite course work, resume, statistics course. *Application deadline:* 3/15 (fall).
Degree Requirements 9 total credit hours.

POST-MASTER'S PROGRAM

Areas of Study Nurse anesthesia. *Clinical nurse specialist programs in:* acute care, adult health, gerontology, maternity-newborn, pediatric. *Nurse practitioner programs in:* acute care, adult health, pediatric, primary care.

DOCTORAL DEGREE PROGRAM

Degree PhD
Available Programs Doctorate; Doctorate for Nurses with Non-Nursing Degrees; Post-Baccalaureate Doctorate.
Areas of Study Addiction/substance abuse, advanced practice nursing, aging, bio-behavioral research, biology of health and illness, community health, critical care, ethics, faculty preparation, family health, gerontology, health policy, health promotion/disease prevention, health-care

systems, human health and illness, individualized study, information systems, maternity-newborn, neuro-behavior, nurse case management, nursing administration, nursing education, nursing policy, nursing research, nursing science, oncology, urban health, women's health.
Program Entrance Requirements Minimum overall college GPA of 3.3, interview by faculty committee, 2 letters of recommendation, MSN or equivalent, scholarly papers, statistics course, vita, writing sample. *Application deadline:* 2/1 (fall).
Degree Requirements 6 total credit hours, dissertation, oral exam.

POSTDOCTORAL PROGRAM

Postdoctoral Program Contact Graduate Department, Faculty of Nursing, University of Toronto, 50 St. George Street, Toronto, ON M5S 3H4. *Telephone:* 416-978-8069.

CONTINUING EDUCATION PROGRAM

Contact The Bloomberg Centre for Advanced Studies in Professional Practice, Faculty of Nursing, University of Toronto, 155 College Street, Suite 130, Toronto, ON M5T 1P8. *E-mail:* caspp.nursing@utoronto.ca.

The University of Western Ontario
School of Nursing
London, Ontario

http://www.uwo.ca/fhs/nursing
Founded in 1878
DEGREES • BSCN • M SC N • PHD
Nursing Program Faculty 101 (18% with doctorates).
Baccalaureate Enrollment 1,153 **Women** 93.24% **Men** 6.76% **Part-time** 13.53%
Graduate Enrollment 54 **Women** 89% **Men** 11% **Part-time** 28%
Nursing Student Activities Nursing Honor Society, Sigma Theta Tau, Student Nurses' Association.
Nursing Student Resources Academic advising; academic or career counseling; assistance for students with disabilities; bookstore; campus computer network; computer lab; computer-assisted instruction; daycare for children of students; e-mail services; employment services for current students; housing assistance; interactive nursing skills videos; Internet; learning resource lab; library services; nursing audiovisuals; resume preparation assistance; unpaid internships.
Library Facilities 4.5 million volumes (357,263 in health, 40 in nursing); 105,556 periodical subscriptions (250 health-care related).

BACCALAUREATE PROGRAMS

Degree BScN
Available Programs Accelerated Baccalaureate; Generic Baccalaureate; RN Baccalaureate.
Study Options Full-time.
Program Entrance Requirements CPR certification, high school biology, high school chemistry, 4 years high school math, high school science, high school transcript, immunizations, minimum high school rank 80%. Transfer students are accepted.
Advanced Placement Credit given for nursing courses completed elsewhere dependent upon specific evaluations.
Contact *Telephone:* 519-661-2111 Ext. 86564. *Fax:* 519-661-3928.

GRADUATE PROGRAMS

Contact *Telephone:* 519-661-3409. *Fax:* 519-661-3928.

MASTER'S DEGREE PROGRAM

Degree M Sc N
Available Programs Master's.
Concentrations Available Health-care administration; nursing administration; nursing education. *Clinical nurse specialist programs in:* acute care, adult health, community health, psychiatric/mental health, public health, women's health. *Nurse practitioner programs in:* community health.
Study Options Full-time and part-time.
Program Entrance Requirements Minimum overall college GPA of 3.5, transcript of college record, written essay, interview, 2 letters of recommendation, nursing research course, prerequisite course work, resume, statistics course.

Advanced Placement Credit given for nursing courses completed elsewhere dependent upon specific evaluations.
Degree Requirements 7 total credit hours, thesis or project.

DOCTORAL DEGREE PROGRAM
Degree PhD
Available Programs Doctorate.
Areas of Study Addiction/substance abuse, advanced practice nursing, aging, clinical practice, community health, faculty preparation, health policy, health promotion/disease prevention, health-care systems, human health and illness, individualized study, nurse case management, nursing administration, nursing education, nursing research, nursing science, women's health.
Program Entrance Requirements Clinical experience, minimum overall college GPA of 3.5, interview by faculty committee, interview, 2 letters of recommendation, MSN or equivalent, scholarly papers, statistics course, vita, writing sample.
Degree Requirements 4 total credit hours, dissertation, written exam.

POSTDOCTORAL PROGRAM
Areas of Study Addiction/substance abuse, community health, health promotion/disease prevention, vulnerable population, women's health.
Postdoctoral Program Contact *Telephone:* 519-661-2111 Ext. 86573.

University of Windsor
Faculty of Nursing
Windsor, Ontario

http://www.uwindsor.ca/nursing
Founded in 1857
DEGREES • BSCN • M SC
Nursing Program Faculty 188 (8% with doctorates).
Baccalaureate Enrollment 868 **Women** 81% **Men** 19% **International** .5% **Part-time** 6%
Graduate Enrollment 62 **Women** 89% **Men** 11% **International** 3% **Part-time** 34%
Distance Learning Courses Available.
Nursing Student Activities Nursing Honor Society, Sigma Theta Tau, Student Nurses' Association, nursing club.
Nursing Student Resources Academic advising; academic or career counseling; assistance for students with disabilities; bookstore; campus computer network; career placement assistance; computer lab; computer-assisted instruction; e-mail services; employment services for current students; interactive nursing skills videos; Internet; learning resource lab; library services; nursing audiovisuals; placement services for program completers; remedial services; resume preparation assistance; skills, simulation, or other laboratory; tutoring.
Library Facilities 2.8 million volumes (65,328 in nursing); 25,458 periodical subscriptions.

BACCALAUREATE PROGRAMS
Degree BScN
Available Programs Generic Baccalaureate.
Study Options Full-time.
Program Entrance Requirements CPR certification, health exam, health insurance, high school biology, high school chemistry, high school math, 4 years high school science, high school transcript, immunizations, minimum high school rank 80%. Transfer students are accepted. *Application deadline:* 1/16 (fall). *Application fee:* CAN$130.
Advanced Placement Credit given for nursing courses completed elsewhere dependent upon specific evaluations.
Expenses (2012–13) *Tuition, area resident:* full-time CAN$5557; part-time CAN$556 per course. *International tuition:* CAN$19,210 full-time. *Room and board:* CAN$9502; room only: CAN$7332 per academic year. *Required fees:* full-time CAN$995; part-time CAN$32 per credit; part-time CAN$372 per term.
Financial Aid 31% of baccalaureate students in nursing programs received some form of financial aid in 2011–12.
Contact Nursing Contact, Faculty of Nursing, University of Windsor, 401 Sunset Avenue, Windsor, ON N9B 3P4. *Telephone:* 519-253-3000 Ext. 2258. *Fax:* 519-973-7084. *E-mail:* nurse@uwindsor.ca.

GRADUATE PROGRAMS
Expenses (2012–13) *Tuition, area resident:* full-time CAN$5111; part-time CAN$1278 per term. *International tuition:* CAN$11,550 full-time. *Room and board:* CAN$9502; room only: CAN$7332 per academic year. *Required fees:* full-time CAN$1061; part-time CAN$13 per credit; part-time CAN$86 per term.
Financial Aid 24% of graduate students in nursing programs received some form of financial aid in 2011–12.
Contact Dr. Debbie Kane, Graduate Coordinator, Faculty of Nursing, University of Windsor, 401 Sunset Avenue, Windsor, ON N9B 3P4. *Telephone:* 519-253-3000 Ext. 2268. *Fax:* 519-973-7084. *E-mail:* dkane@uwindsor.ca.

MASTER'S DEGREE PROGRAM
Degree M Sc, MN
Available Programs Master's.
Concentrations Available *Nurse practitioner programs in:* primary care.
Study Options Full-time and part-time.
Program Entrance Requirements Minimum overall college GPA of 3.0, transcript of college record, written essay, 3 letters of recommendation, nursing research course, physical assessment course, statistics course. *Application deadline:* 2/15 (fall). *Application fee:* CAN$135.
Advanced Placement Credit given for nursing courses completed elsewhere dependent upon specific evaluations.
Degree Requirements 10 total credit hours, thesis or project.

POST-MASTER'S PROGRAM
Areas of Study *Clinical nurse specialist programs in:* oncology, palliative care.

CONTINUING EDUCATION PROGRAM
Contact Nursing Main Office, Faculty of Nursing, University of Windsor, 401 Sunset Avenue, Windsor, ON N9B 3P4. *Telephone:* 519-253-3000 Ext. 2258. *Fax:* 519-973-7084. *E-mail:* nurse@uwindsor.ca.

York University
School of Nursing
Toronto, Ontario

Founded in 1959
DEGREE • BSCN
Nursing Program Faculty 19 (79% with doctorates).
Baccalaureate Enrollment 850 **Women** 96% **Men** 4% **Minority** 30% **International** 1% **Part-time** 15%
Nursing Student Resources Academic advising; academic or career counseling; assistance for students with disabilities; bookstore; campus computer network; career placement assistance; computer lab; computer-assisted instruction; daycare for children of students; e-mail services; employment services for current students; housing assistance; interactive nursing skills videos; Internet; learning resource lab; library services; nursing audiovisuals; skills, simulation, or other laboratory; unpaid internships.
Library Facilities 6.5 million volumes; 540,000 periodical subscriptions.

BACCALAUREATE PROGRAMS
Degree BScN
Available Programs Generic Baccalaureate; RN Baccalaureate.
Site Options King City, ON; Barrie, ON; Oshawa, ON.
Study Options Full-time and part-time.
Program Entrance Requirements CPR certification, written essay, health exam, high school biology, high school chemistry, high school math, high school science, high school transcript, immunizations, 1 letter of recommendation, minimum high school GPA, minimum GPA in nursing prerequisites. Transfer students are accepted.
Advanced Placement Credit by examination available. Credit given for nursing courses completed elsewhere dependent upon specific evaluations.
Contact *Telephone:* 416-736-5271 Ext. 66351. *Fax:* 416-736-5714.

CONTINUING EDUCATION PROGRAM
Contact *Telephone:* 416-736-5271. *Fax:* 416-736-5714.

PRINCE EDWARD ISLAND

University of Prince Edward Island

School of Nursing
Charlottetown, Prince Edward Island

Founded in 1834
DEGREE • BSCN
Nursing Program Faculty 10 (2% with doctorates).
Baccalaureate Enrollment 211 **Women** 97% **Men** 3% **International** 1%
Nursing Student Activities Nursing Honor Society, Student Nurses' Association, nursing club.
Nursing Student Resources Academic advising; academic or career counseling; assistance for students with disabilities; bookstore; campus computer network; career placement assistance; computer lab; computer-assisted instruction; daycare for children of students; e-mail services; employment services for current students; housing assistance; interactive nursing skills videos; Internet; learning resource lab; library services; nursing audiovisuals; placement services for program completers; remedial services; resume preparation assistance; skills, simulation, or other laboratory; tutoring.
Library Facilities 402,808 volumes; 26,196 periodical subscriptions.

BACCALAUREATE PROGRAMS

Degree BScN
Available Programs Generic Baccalaureate.
Study Options Full-time and part-time.
Program Entrance Requirements Transcript of college record, CPR certification, high school chemistry, high school math, high school science, high school transcript, immunizations, minimum high school GPA of 3.0, minimum high school rank 75%, minimum GPA in nursing prerequisites of 3.0, prerequisite course work. Transfer students are accepted.
Advanced Placement Credit given for nursing courses completed elsewhere dependent upon specific evaluations.
Contact *Telephone:* 902-566-0733. *Fax:* 902-566-0777.

QUEBEC

McGill University

School of Nursing
Montréal, Quebec

http://www.mcgill.ca/
Founded in 1821
DEGREES • BSCN • M SC • PHD
Nursing Program Faculty 163 (13% with doctorates).
Baccalaureate Enrollment 438 **Women** 90% **Men** 10% **International** 2% **Part-time** 25%
Graduate Enrollment 93 **Women** 90% **Men** 10% **International** 5% **Part-time** 26%
Nursing Student Activities Student Nurses' Association.
Nursing Student Resources Academic advising; academic or career counseling; assistance for students with disabilities; bookstore; campus computer network; career placement assistance; computer lab; e-mail services; Internet; learning resource lab; library services; nursing audiovisuals; skills, simulation, or other laboratory; tutoring; unpaid internships.
Library Facilities 4.2 million volumes; 49,433 periodical subscriptions.

BACCALAUREATE PROGRAMS

Degree BScN
Available Programs Accelerated RN Baccalaureate; Generic Baccalaureate; RN Baccalaureate.
Study Options Full-time.
Program Entrance Requirements Minimum overall college GPA of 3.0, transcript of college record, high school chemistry, 4 years high school math, 4 years high school science, high school transcript, minimum high school GPA of 3.3, minimum high school rank 25%. Transfer students are accepted. *Application deadline:* 1/15 (fall), 11/1 (winter). *Application fee:* CAN$85.
Advanced Placement Credit given for nursing courses completed elsewhere dependent upon specific evaluations.
Contact *Telephone:* 514-398-3784. *Fax:* 514-398-8455.

GRADUATE PROGRAMS

Contact *Telephone:* 514-398-4151. *Fax:* 514-398-8455.

MASTER'S DEGREE PROGRAM
Degree M Sc
Available Programs Master's; Master's for Non-Nursing College Graduates.
Concentrations Available Nursing administration. *Clinical nurse specialist programs in:* acute care, adult health, cardiovascular, community health, critical care, family health, gerontology, home health care, maternity-newborn, medical-surgical, oncology, parent-child, pediatric, perinatal, psychiatric/mental health, public health, rehabilitation, women's health. *Nurse practitioner programs in:* neonatal health, primary care.
Study Options Full-time.
Program Entrance Requirements Clinical experience, minimum overall college GPA of 3.0, transcript of college record, CPR certification, written essay, immunizations, interview, 3 letters of recommendation, resume, statistics course. *Application deadline:* 1/15 (fall). *Application fee:* CAN$85.
Degree Requirements 53 total credit hours, thesis or project.

DOCTORAL DEGREE PROGRAM
Degree PhD
Available Programs Doctorate; Post-Baccalaureate Doctorate.
Areas of Study Family health, health-care systems, human health and illness, nursing administration, nursing research, oncology.
Program Entrance Requirements Minimum overall college GPA of 3.3, interview, 2 letters of recommendation, MSN or equivalent, statistics course, vita, writing sample. *Application deadline:* 1/15 (fall). *Application fee:* CAN$85.
Degree Requirements 90 total credit hours, dissertation, oral exam, written exam, residency.

POSTDOCTORAL PROGRAM
Areas of Study Cancer care, chronic illness.
Postdoctoral Program Contact *Telephone:* 514-398-4157. *Fax:* 514-398-8455.

Université de Montréal

Faculty of Nursing
Montréal, Quebec

http://www.scinf.umontreal.ca/
Founded in 1920
DEGREES • BSCN • M SC • PHD
Nursing Program Faculty 40 (95% with doctorates).
Baccalaureate Enrollment 850 **Women** 70% **Men** 30% **Minority** 30% **International** 3% **Part-time** 20%
Graduate Enrollment 360 **Women** 75% **Men** 25% **Minority** 20% **International** 3%
Distance Learning Courses Available.
Nursing Student Activities Student Nurses' Association.
Nursing Student Resources Academic advising; academic or career counseling; assistance for students with disabilities; bookstore; campus computer network; career placement assistance; computer lab; computer-assisted instruction; daycare for children of students; e-mail services; employment services for current students; externships; housing assistance; interactive nursing skills videos; Internet; learning resource lab; library services; nursing audiovisuals; other; placement services for program completers; remedial services; resume preparation assistance; skills, simulation, or other laboratory; tutoring.
Library Facilities 4 million volumes (32,536 in health, 32,536 in nursing); 18,330 periodical subscriptions (1,319 health-care related).

BACCALAUREATE PROGRAMS

Degree BScN
Available Programs RN Baccalaureate.

Site Options Laval, QC.

Study Options Full-time.

Program Entrance Requirements Transcript of college record, CPR certification, high school biology, high school chemistry, immunizations, minimum high school GPA. Transfer students are accepted. *Application deadline:* 3/1 (fall), 10/3 (winter). *Application fee:* CAN$85.

Advanced Placement Credit given for nursing courses completed elsewhere dependent upon specific evaluations.

Contact Catherine Sarrazin, Assistant to Vice Dean, Faculty of Nursing, Université de Montréal, Pav. Marg. d'Youville, CP 6128 Succursale Centre-Ville, Montreal, QC H3C 3J7. *Telephone:* 514-343-6439. *Fax:* 514-343-2306. *E-mail:* catherine.sarrazin@umontreal.ca.

GRADUATE PROGRAMS

Expenses (2011–12) *Tuition:* full-time CAN$3252. *International tuition:* CAN$21,842 full-time. *Required fees:* full-time CAN$550.

Financial Aid 30% of graduate students in nursing programs received some form of financial aid in 2010–11. Fellowships, research assistantships, teaching assistantships, career-related internships or fieldwork, Federal Work-Study, and institutionally sponsored loans available.

Contact Suzanne Pinel, Assistant to the Vice Dean of Studies, Faculty of Nursing, Université de Montréal, Pav. Marg. d'Youville, CP 6128 Succursale Centre-Ville, Montreal, QC H3C 3J7. *Telephone:* 514-343-6111 Ext. 7098. *Fax:* 514-343-6111 Ext. 2705. *E-mail:* suzanne.pinel@umontreal.ca.

MASTER'S DEGREE PROGRAM

Degree M Sc

Available Programs Master's; RN to Master's.

Concentrations Available Clinical nurse leader; nursing administration; nursing education. *Clinical nurse specialist programs in:* acute care, adult health, cardiovascular, community health, family health, gerontology, maternity-newborn, medical-surgical, occupational health, oncology, palliative care, parent-child, psychiatric/mental health, public health, rehabilitation, women's health. *Nurse practitioner programs in:* acute care, family health, primary care.

Study Options Full-time and part-time.

Program Entrance Requirements Transcript of college record, CPR certification, nursing research course, statistics course. *Application deadline:* 3/1 (fall). *Application fee:* CAN$85.

Degree Requirements 45 total credit hours, thesis or project.

POST-MASTER'S PROGRAM

Areas of Study *Nurse practitioner programs in:* acute care, family health, primary care.

DOCTORAL DEGREE PROGRAM

Degree PhD

Available Programs Doctorate.

Areas of Study Addiction/substance abuse, aging, bio-behavioral research, clinical practice, community health, critical care, family health, gerontology, health policy, health promotion/disease prevention, healthcare systems, human health and illness, illness and transition, maternity-newborn, neuro-behavior, nursing administration, nursing education, nursing policy, nursing research, nursing science, oncology, urban health, women's health.

Program Entrance Requirements Minimum overall college GPA of 3.4, letters of recommendation, MSN or equivalent, statistics course. *Application deadline:* 3/1 (fall). *Application fee:* CAN$85.

Degree Requirements 90 total credit hours, dissertation, oral exam.

POSTDOCTORAL PROGRAM

Areas of Study Adolescent health, aging, cancer care, chronic illness, community health, family health, gerontology, health promotion/disease prevention, individualized study, neuro-behavior, nursing informatics, nursing interventions, nursing research, nursing science, outcomes, self-care, vulnerable population, women's health.

Postdoctoral Program Contact Ms. Chantal Cara, Vice Dean, Research, Faculty of Nursing, Université de Montréal, Pav. Marg. d'Youville, CP 6128 Succursale Centre-Ville, Montreal, QC H3C 3J7. *Telephone:* 514-343-5835. *Fax:* 514-343-2306. *E-mail:* chantal.cara@umontreal.ca.

CONTINUING EDUCATION PROGRAM

Contact Ms. Jocelyne Labarre, Program Coordinator, Faculty of Nursing, Université de Montréal, Pav. Marg. d'Youville, CP 6128 Succursale Centre-Ville, Montreal, QC H3C 3J7. *Telephone:* 514-343-7723. *Fax:* 514-343-2306. *E-mail:* jocyelyne.labarre@umontreal.ca.

Université de Sherbrooke
Department of Nursing
Sherbrooke, Quebec

http://www.usherbrooke.ca/scinf/
Founded in 1954

DEGREES • BSCN • M SC • PHD

Nursing Program Faculty 17 (76% with doctorates).

Baccalaureate Enrollment 482 **Women** 90% **Men** 10% **Minority** .5% **Part-time** 30%

Graduate Enrollment 61 **Women** 95% **Men** 5% **Part-time** 50%

Nursing Student Activities Student Nurses' Association.

Nursing Student Resources Academic advising; academic or career counseling; assistance for students with disabilities; bookstore; computer lab; computer-assisted instruction; e-mail services; externships; housing assistance; Internet; learning resource lab; library services; nursing audiovisuals; tutoring.

Library Facilities 1.2 million volumes (40,000 in health, 4,000 in nursing); 43,478 periodical subscriptions (3,000 health-care related).

BACCALAUREATE PROGRAMS

Degree BScN

Available Programs RN Baccalaureate.

Site Options Longueuil, QC.

Study Options Full-time and part-time.

Program Entrance Requirements Transcript of college record, high school chemistry, 4 years high school math, immunizations, professional liability insurance/malpractice insurance, RN licensure. Transfer students are accepted.

Advanced Placement Credit given for nursing courses completed elsewhere dependent upon specific evaluations.

Contact *Telephone:* 819-563-5355. *Fax:* 819-820-6816.

GRADUATE PROGRAMS

Contact *Telephone:* 819-564-5354. *Fax:* 819-820-6816.

MASTER'S DEGREE PROGRAM

Degree M Sc

Available Programs Master's.

Concentrations Available *Clinical nurse specialist programs in:* acute care, community health, family health, gerontology.

Site Options Longueuil, QC.

Study Options Full-time and part-time.

Program Entrance Requirements Transcript of college record, interview, 3 letters of recommendation, nursing research course, professional liability insurance/malpractice insurance, resume.

Degree Requirements 45 total credit hours, thesis or project.

DOCTORAL DEGREE PROGRAM

Degree PhD

Available Programs Doctorate.

Areas of Study Advanced practice nursing, aging, biology of health and illness, clinical practice, community health, critical care, family health, gerontology, health promotion/disease prevention, human health and illness, illness and transition, information systems, maternity-newborn, neuro-behavior, nurse case management, nursing administration, nursing education, nursing policy, nursing research, nursing science, oncology, women's health.

Site Options Longueuil, QC.

Program Entrance Requirements Clinical experience, interview, 3 letters of recommendation, MSN or equivalent, statistics course, vita, writing sample.

Degree Requirements 90 total credit hours, dissertation, oral exam, written exam.

POSTDOCTORAL PROGRAM

Postdoctoral Program Contact *Telephone:* 819-564-5355. *Fax:* 819-820-6816.

Université du Québec à Chicoutimi

Program in Nursing
Chicoutimi, Quebec

Founded in 1969

DEGREES • BNSC • MS/MPH • MSN

Nursing Program Faculty 12 (30% with doctorates).
Baccalaureate Enrollment 600 **Women** 90% **Men** 10% **Minority** 5% **Part-time** 75%
Graduate Enrollment 30 **Women** 90% **Men** 10% **Minority** 2% **Part-time** 80%
Distance Learning Courses Available.
Nursing Student Activities Nursing Honor Society, Student Nurses' Association.
Nursing Student Resources Academic advising; academic or career counseling; assistance for students with disabilities; bookstore; campus computer network; computer lab; computer-assisted instruction; e-mail services; employment services for current students; externships; housing assistance; interactive nursing skills videos; Internet; learning resource lab; library services; nursing audiovisuals; resume preparation assistance; skills, simulation, or other laboratory; tutoring; unpaid internships.
Library Facilities 689,214 volumes (8,000 in health, 6,300 in nursing); 5,092 periodical subscriptions (5,250 health-care related).

BACCALAUREATE PROGRAMS

Degree BNSc
Available Programs Accelerated RN Baccalaureate; RN Baccalaureate.
Site Options Sept-Iles, QC; Alma, QC; St. Felicien, QC.
Study Options Full-time and part-time.
Program Entrance Requirements Transcript of college record, health exam, high school biology, high school chemistry, high school math, immunizations, interview. Transfer students are accepted. *Application deadline:* 3/1 (fall), 3/1 (winter). *Application fee:* CAN$50.
Advanced Placement Credit given for nursing courses completed elsewhere dependent upon specific evaluations.
Expenses (2012–13) *Tuition, area resident:* full-time CAN$2662; part-time CAN$1331 per term. *Required fees:* part-time CAN$163 per credit.
Financial Aid 5% of baccalaureate students in nursing programs received some form of financial aid in 2011–12. *Gift aid (need-based):* private, college/university gift aid from institutional funds. *Loans:* college/university.*Work-study:* part-time campus jobs.
Contact Mme. Anna Gauthier, Secretary, Program in Nursing, Université du Québec à Chicoutimi, 555 Boulevard de l'Universite, Chicoutimi, QC G7H 2B1. *Telephone:* 418-545-5011 Ext. 5315. *Fax:* 418-615-1205. *E-mail:* anna_gauthier@uqac.ca.

GRADUATE PROGRAMS

Expenses (2012–13) *Tuition, area resident:* part-time CAN$324 per course.
Financial Aid 2% of graduate students in nursing programs received some form of financial aid in 2011–12.
Contact Mrs. Francoise Courville, Director of Masters Degree Program, Program in Nursing, Université du Québec à Chicoutimi, UQAC, 555 Boulevard de l'Universit, Saguenay, QC G7H 2B1. *Telephone:* 418-545-5011 Ext. 2374. *Fax:* 418-545-5012. *E-mail:* francoise_courville@uqac.ca.

MASTER'S DEGREE PROGRAM

Degrees MS/MPH; MSN
Available Programs Accelerated RN to Master's; Master's; RN to Master's.
Concentrations Available *Clinical nurse specialist programs in:* acute care, adult health, cardiovascular, community health, critical care, family health, gerontology, home health care, maternity-newborn, medical-surgical, occupational health, oncology, parent-child, pediatric, perinatal, psychiatric/mental health, public health, rehabilitation, school health, women's health. *Nurse practitioner programs in:* primary care.
Site Options Sept-Iles, QC; Alma, QC; St. Felicien, QC.
Study Options Full-time and part-time.
Program Entrance Requirements Clinical experience, minimum overall college GPA of 3.2, transcript of college record, written essay, interview, 3 letters of recommendation, nursing research course, professional liability insurance/malpractice insurance, resume, statistics course. *Application deadline:* 2/1 (fall), 11/1 (winter). *Application fee:* CAN$50.

Advanced Placement Credit given for nursing courses completed elsewhere dependent upon specific evaluations.
Degree Requirements 45 total credit hours, thesis or project, comprehensive exam.

Université du Québec à Rimouski

Program in Nursing
Rimouski, Quebec

http://www.uquebec.ca/mscinf/
Founded in 1973

DEGREES • BSCN • M SC N

Nursing Program Faculty 17 (53% with doctorates).
Baccalaureate Enrollment 750 **Women** 90% **Men** 10% **Part-time** 74%
Graduate Enrollment 24 **Women** 96% **Men** 4% **Part-time** 92%
Distance Learning Courses Available.
Nursing Student Activities Student Nurses' Association.
Nursing Student Resources Academic advising; academic or career counseling; assistance for students with disabilities; bookstore; campus computer network; career placement assistance; computer lab; daycare for children of students; e-mail services; employment services for current students; housing assistance; Internet; learning resource lab; library services; nursing audiovisuals; other; placement services for program completers; resume preparation assistance; skills, simulation, or other laboratory; tutoring.
Library Facilities 263,142 volumes (5,200 in health, 1,100 in nursing); 3,951 periodical subscriptions (1,300 health-care related).

BACCALAUREATE PROGRAMS

Degree BScN
Available Programs RN Baccalaureate.
Site Options Rimouski, QC; Lvis, QC.
Study Options Full-time and part-time.
Program Entrance Requirements Transcript of college record, professional liability insurance/malpractice insurance, prerequisite course work. Transfer students are accepted.
Advanced Placement Credit by examination available.
Contact *Telephone:* 418-723-1986 Ext. 1568. *Fax:* 418-724-1450.

GRADUATE PROGRAMS

Contact *Telephone:* 418-723-1986 Ext. 1345. *Fax:* 418-724-1450.

MASTER'S DEGREE PROGRAM

Degree M Sc N
Available Programs Master's.
Concentrations Available *Clinical nurse specialist programs in:* community health, critical care, gerontology, psychiatric/mental health.
Site Options Rimouski, QC; Lvis, QC.
Study Options Full-time and part-time.
Program Entrance Requirements Clinical experience, transcript of college record, interview, 3 letters of recommendation, nursing research course, prerequisite course work, statistics course.
Advanced Placement Credit given for nursing courses completed elsewhere dependent upon specific evaluations.
Degree Requirements 45 total credit hours, thesis or project.

CONTINUING EDUCATION PROGRAM

Contact *Telephone:* 418-723-1986 Ext. 1818. *Fax:* 418-724-1525.

Université du Québec à Trois-Rivières

Program in Nursing
Trois-Rivières, Quebec

http://www.uqtr.ca/
Founded in 1969

DEGREES • BSN • MSN

Nursing Program Faculty 28 (30% with doctorates).
Baccalaureate Enrollment 180 **Women** 95% **Men** 5% **Minority** 5% **International** 1% **Part-time** 75%

Graduate Enrollment 50 **Women** 97% **Men** 3% **Minority** 1% **Part-time** 90%
Distance Learning Courses Available.
Nursing Student Activities Student Nurses' Association.
Nursing Student Resources Academic advising; academic or career counseling; assistance for students with disabilities; bookstore; campus computer network; career placement assistance; computer lab; computer-assisted instruction; daycare for children of students; e-mail services; employment services for current students; externships; interactive nursing skills videos; Internet; learning resource lab; library services; nursing audiovisuals; placement services for program completers; resume preparation assistance; skills, simulation, or other laboratory; tutoring; unpaid internships.
Library Facilities 464,338 volumes (2,000 in health, 500 in nursing); 2,000 periodical subscriptions health-care related.

BACCALAUREATE PROGRAMS

Degree BSN
Available Programs Generic Baccalaureate; RN Baccalaureate.
Study Options Full-time and part-time.
Program Entrance Requirements Transcript of college record, CPR certification, high school biology, high school chemistry, prerequisite course work, RN licensure. Transfer students are accepted. *Application deadline:* 3/1 (fall). Applications may be processed on a rolling basis for some programs. *Application fee:* CAN$30.
Advanced Placement Credit given for nursing courses completed elsewhere dependent upon specific evaluations.
Contact *Telephone:* 819-376-5011 Ext. 3471. *Fax:* 819-376-5048.

GRADUATE PROGRAMS

Contact *Telephone:* 819-376-5011 Ext. 3460.

MASTER'S DEGREE PROGRAM

Degree MSN
Available Programs Master's.
Concentrations Available *Clinical nurse specialist programs in:* acute care, adult health, community health, critical care, family health, home health care, maternity-newborn, medical-surgical, pediatric, perinatal, psychiatric/mental health, public health. *Nurse practitioner programs in:* primary care.
Study Options Full-time and part-time.
Program Entrance Requirements Minimum overall college GPA of 3, transcript of college record, CPR certification, immunizations, 3 letters of recommendation, nursing research course, physical assessment course, prerequisite course work, statistics course. *Application deadline:* 8/29 (fall), 11/29 (winter), 4/29 (spring). Applications may be processed on a rolling basis for some programs. *Application fee:* CAN$30.
Advanced Placement Credit by examination available.
Degree Requirements 45 total credit hours, thesis or project.

Université du Québec en Abitibi-Témiscamingue
Département des sciences sociales et de la santé
Rouyn-Noranda, Quebec

http://www.uqat.ca/en/
Founded in 1983
DEGREE • BN
Nursing Program Faculty 12
Baccalaureate Enrollment 78 **Women** 95% **Men** 5% **Part-time** 64%
Nursing Student Resources Academic advising; assistance for students with disabilities; bookstore; campus computer network; computer lab; computer-assisted instruction; housing assistance; Internet; library services; resume preparation assistance; skills, simulation, or other laboratory.
Library Facilities 135,882 volumes (3,239 in health, 715 in nursing); 302 periodical subscriptions (17 health-care related).

BACCALAUREATE PROGRAMS

Degree BN
Program Entrance Requirements Transfer students are accepted.
Contact *Telephone:* 819-762-0971 Ext. 2370. *Fax:* 819-797-4727.

Université du Québec en Outaouais
Département des Sciences Infirmières
Gatineau, Quebec

http://uqo.ca/
Founded in 1981
DEGREES • BSCN • M SC N
Nursing Program Faculty 13 (38% with doctorates).
Baccalaureate Enrollment 700 **Women** 90% **Men** 10% **Minority** 20% **Part-time** 40%
Graduate Enrollment 40 **Women** 99% **Men** 1% **Minority** 6% **Part-time** 100%
Nursing Student Activities Student Nurses' Association.
Nursing Student Resources Academic advising; academic or career counseling; bookstore; campus computer network; computer lab; daycare for children of students; e-mail services; employment services for current students; externships; housing assistance; Internet; learning resource lab; library services; nursing audiovisuals; placement services for program completers; skills, simulation, or other laboratory.
Library Facilities 230,910 volumes; 12,351 periodical subscriptions.

BACCALAUREATE PROGRAMS

Degree BScN
Available Programs Generic Baccalaureate; RN Baccalaureate.
Site Options St. Jerome, QC.
Study Options Full-time and part-time.
Program Entrance Requirements CPR certification, high school chemistry, immunizations, interview, RN licensure. Transfer students are accepted. *Application deadline:* 3/1 (fall). *Application fee:* CAN$30.
Advanced Placement Credit by examination available. Credit given for nursing courses completed elsewhere dependent upon specific evaluations.
Contact *Telephone:* 819-595-3900 Ext. 2345. *Fax:* 819-595-3801.

GRADUATE PROGRAMS

Contact *Telephone:* 819-595-3900 Ext. 2347. *Fax:* 819-595-2202.

MASTER'S DEGREE PROGRAM

Degree M Sc N
Available Programs Master's.
Concentrations Available Health-care administration. *Clinical nurse specialist programs in:* community health, critical care, psychiatric/mental health, rehabilitation. *Nurse practitioner programs in:* primary care.
Site Options St. Jerome, QC.
Study Options Full-time and part-time.
Program Entrance Requirements Computer literacy, 3 letters of recommendation, nursing research course, resume, statistics course. *Application deadline:* 5/1 (fall), 11/1 (winter), 3/1 (spring). *Application fee:* CAN$30.
Advanced Placement Credit given for nursing courses completed elsewhere dependent upon specific evaluations.
Degree Requirements 45 total credit hours, thesis or project.

Université Laval
Faculty of Nursing
Québec, Quebec

http://www.fsi.ulaval.ca/
Founded in 1852
DEGREES • BSCN • MSN • PHD
Nursing Program Faculty 25 (64% with doctorates).
Baccalaureate Enrollment 798 **Women** 94% **Men** 6% **Minority** 18% **International** 12% **Part-time** 32%
Graduate Enrollment 116 **Women** 72% **Men** 28% **Minority** 32% **International** 24% **Part-time** 22%
Distance Learning Courses Available.
Nursing Student Activities Student Nurses' Association, nursing club.
Nursing Student Resources Academic advising; academic or career counseling; assistance for students with disabilities; bookstore; campus computer network; career placement assistance; computer lab; computer-assisted instruction; daycare for children of students; e-mail services;

employment services for current students; externships; housing assistance; interactive nursing skills videos; Internet; learning resource lab; library services; nursing audiovisuals; placement services for program completers; resume preparation assistance; skills, simulation, or other laboratory; tutoring.

Library Facilities 3 million volumes (118,994 in health, 3,781 in nursing); 13,928 periodical subscriptions (624 health-care related).

BACCALAUREATE PROGRAMS

Degree BScN

Available Programs Accelerated Baccalaureate; Accelerated RN Baccalaureate; Generic Baccalaureate; RN Baccalaureate.

Study Options Full-time and part-time.

Program Entrance Requirements Transcript of college record, high school biology, high school chemistry, 5 years high school math, high school transcript, immunizations, minimum high school GPA. Transfer students are accepted.

Advanced Placement Credit given for nursing courses completed elsewhere dependent upon specific evaluations.

Contact *Telephone:* 418-656-2131 Ext. 7930. *Fax:* 418-656-7747.

GRADUATE PROGRAMS

Contact *Telephone:* 418-656-3356. *Fax:* 418-656-7304.

MASTER'S DEGREE PROGRAM

Degree MSN

Available Programs Accelerated Master's; Master's.

Concentrations Available Clinical nurse leader; health-care administration; nursing administration. *Clinical nurse specialist programs in:* acute care, adult health, cardiovascular, community health, critical care, family health, gerontology, oncology, palliative care, parent-child, pediatric, perinatal, psychiatric/mental health, public health, rehabilitation. *Nurse practitioner programs in:* adult health, primary care.

Study Options Full-time and part-time.

Program Entrance Requirements Clinical experience, transcript of college record, 2 letters of recommendation, nursing research course, resume, statistics course, French exam.

Advanced Placement Credit given for nursing courses completed elsewhere dependent upon specific evaluations.

Degree Requirements 45 total credit hours, thesis or project.

POST-MASTER'S PROGRAM

Areas of Study *Clinical nurse specialist programs in:* acute care, adult health, cardiovascular, community health, critical care, family health, gerontology, oncology, palliative care, parent-child, pediatric, perinatal, psychiatric/mental health, public health, rehabilitation. *Nurse practitioner programs in:* adult health, primary care.

DOCTORAL DEGREE PROGRAM

Degree PhD

Available Programs Doctorate.

Areas of Study Community health, nursing science.

Program Entrance Requirements Clinical experience, interview, 2 letters of recommendation, MSN or equivalent, scholarly papers, statistics course, vita, writing sample.

Degree Requirements 96 total credit hours, dissertation, oral exam, written exam.

POSTDOCTORAL PROGRAM

Areas of Study Aging, cancer care, community health, gerontology, health promotion/disease prevention, nursing interventions, nursing research, nursing science, outcomes.

Postdoctoral Program Contact *Telephone:* 418-656-3356. *Fax:* 418-656-7747.

CONTINUING EDUCATION PROGRAM

Contact *Telephone:* 418-656-2131 Ext. 6712. *Fax:* 418-656-7747.

SASKATCHEWAN

University of Saskatchewan
College of Nursing
Saskatoon, Saskatchewan

http://www.usask.ca/nursing/
Founded in 1907

DEGREES • BSN • MN • PHD
Nursing Program Faculty 134 (20% with doctorates).
Baccalaureate Enrollment 1,678 **Women** 93% **Men** 7% **Minority** 5% **Part-time** 17%
Graduate Enrollment 50 **Women** 94% **Men** 6% **Minority** 2% **Part-time** 62%
Distance Learning Courses Available.
Nursing Student Activities Student Nurses' Association.
Nursing Student Resources Academic advising; academic or career counseling; assistance for students with disabilities; bookstore; campus computer network; computer lab; computer-assisted instruction; daycare for children of students; e-mail services; employment services for current students; interactive nursing skills videos; Internet; learning resource lab; library services; nursing audiovisuals; other; remedial services; resume preparation assistance; skills, simulation, or other laboratory; tutoring.
Library Facilities 2.5 million volumes (92,505 in health, 3,932 in nursing); 47,055 periodical subscriptions (3,069 health-care related).

BACCALAUREATE PROGRAMS

Degree BSN

Available Programs Accelerated Baccalaureate; Accelerated RN Baccalaureate; Baccalaureate for Second Degree; Generic Baccalaureate; RN Baccalaureate.
Site Options Regina , SK; Prince Albert, SK; Saskatoon , SK.
Study Options Full-time and part-time.
Program Entrance Requirements Transcript of college record, CPR certification, high school biology, high school chemistry, 4 years high school math, 4 years high school science, high school transcript, immunizations, minimum high school GPA of 2.0. Transfer students are accepted. *Application deadline:* 1/15 (fall). *Application fee:* CAN$90.
Advanced Placement Credit given for nursing courses completed elsewhere dependent upon specific evaluations.
Contact *Telephone:* 306-966-6231. *Fax:* 306-966-6621.

GRADUATE PROGRAMS

Contact *Telephone:* 306-966-1477. *Fax:* 306-966-6703.

MASTER'S DEGREE PROGRAM
Degree MN
Available Programs Master's.
Concentrations Available Nursing education. *Nurse practitioner programs in:* primary care.
Site Options Saskatoon , SK.
Study Options Full-time and part-time.
Program Entrance Requirements Minimum overall college GPA of 2.5, transcript of college record, 3 letters of recommendation, nursing research course, statistics course. *Application deadline:* 11/15 (fall). *Application fee:* CAN$75.
Advanced Placement Credit given for nursing courses completed elsewhere dependent upon specific evaluations.
Degree Requirements 24 total credit hours, thesis or project.

POST-MASTER'S PROGRAM
Areas of Study *Nurse practitioner programs in:* primary care.

DOCTORAL DEGREE PROGRAM
Degree PhD
Available Programs Doctorate.
Areas of Study Individualized study.
Site Options Saskatoon , SK.
Program Entrance Requirements Minimum overall college GPA of 4, 3 letters of recommendation, MSN or equivalent, statistics course, vita. *Application deadline:* 11/15 (fall). *Application fee:* CAN$75.

Degree Requirements 18 total credit hours, dissertation, oral exam, written exam.

CONTINUING EDUCATION PROGRAM

Contact *Telephone:* 306-966-6261. *Fax:* 306-966-7673.

TWO-PAGE DESCRIPTIONS

ADELPHI UNIVERSITY

SCHOOL OF NURSING

Leading to New Horizons in Nursing

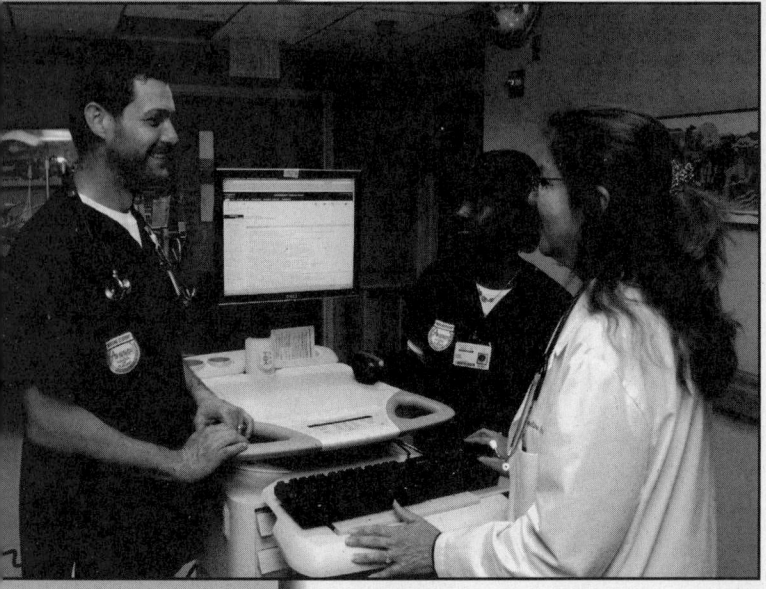

Adelphi School of Nursing students benefit from a progressive curriculum, unique partnerships, and hands-on clinical training.

Established 70 years ago, Adelphi's School of Nursing has educated competent clinicians and leaders in the healthcare field. Preparing students to lead the transformation of healthcare in the 21st century, the School provides them with a progressive curriculum, unique partnerships, and focused clinical training.

The nationally accredited School—dedicated to providing students with the skills, knowledge, and specialized education to succeed as qualified caregivers and leaders in the nursing profession—offers three basic undergraduate programs leading to a Bachelor of Science in Nursing. The basic curriculum is for those seeking a B.S. in Nursing and to meet the New York State licensing requirements as a registered professional nurse (R.N.). A second curriculum (ASCEND) is for current registered nurses continuing their education to receive a B.S. in Nursing. This one-day-a-week R.N. to B.S. program includes not only classroom, but some online courses as well.

The third program, the Professional Acceleration to Healthcare (PATH) program, is

a 14-month intensive program for those who have a bachelor's degree in another discipline and are now seeking a degree in nursing. Candidates for the accelerated PATH program must have all of their prerequisites completed with a grade of C+ or better at the time of application submission.

Adelphi's nursing programs combine theory, clinical practice, and community service. The School's students partner with community healthcare providers and receive innovative clinical education with esteemed faculty members who have a passion for teaching and the profession of nursing. Adelphi maintains an extensive network of partnerships in more than 100 healthcare settings, from acute care to community environments.

Adelphi has clinical affiliations with all the major health systems, hospitals, and community agencies in the metropolitan New York area.

On Adelphi's Garden City campus and at the Manhattan Center, students have access to the Nursing Resource Center, which features learning labs designed to simulate hospital settings and simulation labs for real-time problem scenario learning.

Candidates seeking admission as freshmen must meet the general admission requirements of Adelphi University. Those who have college credits or an associate degree may apply as transfer students. A minimum cumulative GPA of 3.0 is required for admission to the ASCEND program. A maximum of 64 credits may be transferred from a regionally accredited community college, and a maximum of 90 credits may be transferred from a regionally accredited university.

Successful completion of the Test of Essential Academic Skills (TEAS), Version V, is an admission prerequisite for transfer students to the School of Nursing B.S. program.

At the graduate level, the emphasis is on the development of scholarly critical thinkers with a focus on a specialty practice area and the ability to translate knowledge into practice. In Adelphi's nurse practitioner program, through the process of critical thinking, students learn to understand the nature of complex human and environmental systems and to develop strategies for effective intervention. In addition, the core of the master's curriculum provides the knowledge base and experience needed to develop specific specialty skills, evaluate research designs and methodologies, and to utilize findings providing evidence-based practice.

Graduate programs include the following: M.S. Adult/Geriatric Nurse Practitioner; M.S. in Nursing Administration; M.S. in Nursing Education; M.S. in Nutrition (fully online); Master of Public Health; Ph.D. in Nursing; and M.S. in Healthcare Informatics. Post-master's certificates are available in most of the above.

Graduate applicants must submit a completed application, an essay, letters of reference, and a $50 nonrefundable application fee. In addition, they must have official copies of standardized test scores forwarded to Adelphi, as well as official transcripts from all colleges and universities previously attended.

- *2012–13 UNDERGRADUATE TUITION & FEES FOR FULL-TIME (12–17 CREDITS PER SEMESTER) NURSING UPPER DIVISION STUDENTS:*

  Resident (living on campus): $41,470

  Nonresident: $29,550

- *2012–13 GRADUATE TUITION & FEES FOR PART-TIME (6 CREDITS PER SEMESTER) STUDENTS:*

  Nonresident: $1,060 per credit hour (Graduate nursing students do not live on campus)

- *APPLICATION DEADLINES:*

  Ph.D. program (fall admission only): January 15

  All other programs (fall semester only): Rolling admission

  Exception: PATH program has a May start; application deadline is January 15.

- *FACULTY INFORMATION:*

  http://nursing.adelphi.edu/faculty

- *MULTIMEDIA:*

  http://nursing.adelphi.edu/about

CONTACT INFORMATION

Adelphi University School of Nursing
One South Avenue
Garden City, NY 11530
Phone: 516-877-4533
800-ADELPHI (toll-free)
E-mail: nursing@adelphi.edu
Website: http://nursing.adelphi.edu

UNDERGRADUATE NURSING PROGRAM:
Phone: 516-877-3050
E-mail: admissions@adelphi.edu

GRADUATE NURSING PROGRAM:
Phone: 516-877-3050
E-mail: graduateadmissions@adelphi.edu

Find us on Facebook®: facebook.com/AdelphiU
Follow us on Twitter™: twitter.com/adelphiu

Alumnae Hall is home to Adelphi's School of Nursing, which has prepared students for dedicated careers since its founding in 1942.

Louise Herrington School of Nursing

Learn. Lead. Serve.

Baylor University is the world's largest Baptist university and is the oldest continuously operating university in Texas. Established in 1909, the Louise Herrington School of Nursing has an outstanding reputation based on excellent faculty, curriculum, and students.

Baylor School of Nursing has always been committed to providing students with premier education and clinical experience in a faith-based environment. Baylor's curriculum challenges students to think and act like nurses long before they graduate.

The undergraduate program consists of 131 semester hours and awards the Bachelor Science in Nursing (B.S.N.) degree. This includes 66 semester hours of prerequisites, which may be taken on the Baylor-Waco campus or at any other accredited college or university. The upper-level (junior and senior years) of the program consists of 65 semester hours completed on the School of Nursing campus in Dallas. Baylor's FastBacc is a twelve-month accelerated track that is designed for individuals who have already completed a bachelor's degree in a non-nursing discipline. It is an intensive full-time program that begins each summer with a combination of teaching methodologies, including traditional classroom, online course component, clinical and lab experiences, and hybrid interactive learning courses.

The Louise Herrington School of Nursing.

Baylor's graduate studies program is ranked nationally by *US News & World Report* for its academic reputation and offers part- or full-time study in one of three advanced practice majors: Family Nurse Practitioner (FNP), Neonatal Nursing (NNP) and Midwifery (CNM). Students completing the Nurse-Midwife track are awarded a Doctor of Nursing Practice (DNP) degree. Caring for the medically underserved is a special focus for the Baylor graduate program.

The School and all its programs have received full, national accreditation by the Commission on Collegiate Nursing Education (CCNE) and are approved by the Texas Board of Nurses. The Accreditation Commission for Midwifery Education (ACME) accredits the Midwifery program.

At the heart of the Louise Herrington School of Nursing is an exceptional faculty, each member committed to the success of Baylor's students. The faculty is a unique group— researchers, authors, winners of countless national awards, presidents of national organizations, former missionaries and administrators, and experts in their specialties. Faculty members are always accessible and are always focused on the needs of their students.

Located on the Baylor University Medical Center campus near downtown Dallas, the four-story complex includes a student computer lab (open 24 hours a day, 7 days a week), spacious classrooms wired for multimedia and video presentations, quiet study lounges, and the high-fidelity Don A. and Ruth Buchholz Patient Simulation Lab.

The Learning Resource Center, staffed by professional medical librarians, provides support services exclusively to Baylor's students and faculty members. The Barnabas Student Success Center, Student Ministry, and other student organizations are here to provide students with all the tools and resources they need to succeed in their education.

Classes are small and clinical experiences individualized to student needs. Financial support often is available. The School offers a comprehensive program that includes merit-based and need-based scholarships as well as grants, loans and part-time employment to ease the financial burdens of undergraduate nursing students.

The need is great. A career in nursing is one in which you choose to make a difference. You choose to serve. You choose to care. You have the potential to do extraordinary good, to make the world a better place. Our goal is to prepare the next generation of nurses. There's never been a more exciting time in medicine or health care. There's never been a greater need for the best and the brightest. Join us, and through a life of leadership and service, become an unstoppable force for good. When you are ready, Baylor is the next step in your calling to Learn, Lead, and Serve.

- *2012–13 UNDERGRADUATE TUITION & FEES:*

    Tuition: $30,586 per academic year

    Courses Fees (approximate): $700

    General Student Fee: $3130

    For more information: http://www.Baylor.edu/sfs

- *2012–13 GRADUATE TUITION & FEES:*

    Tuition: $1274 per semester hour

    General Student Fee (12 hours or more per semester): $1565

    General Student Fee (less than 12 hours): $131 per semester hour

    Course Fees: (varies) minimum $50

    For more information: http://www.Baylor.edu/sfs

- *APPLICATION DEADLINES:*

    Traditional Baccalaureate: January 15 (fall semester); May 31 (spring semester)

    FastBacc Track: January 5

    Graduate Program: February 1 (fall admission only); April 15 (early admission)

CONTACT INFORMATION
Louise Herrington School of Nursing
Baylor University
3700 Worth Street
Dallas, Texas 75246
Phone: 214-820-3361
Fax: 214-820-3835
E-mail: BU_Nursing@baylor.edu
Web site: http://www.baylor.edu/Nursing

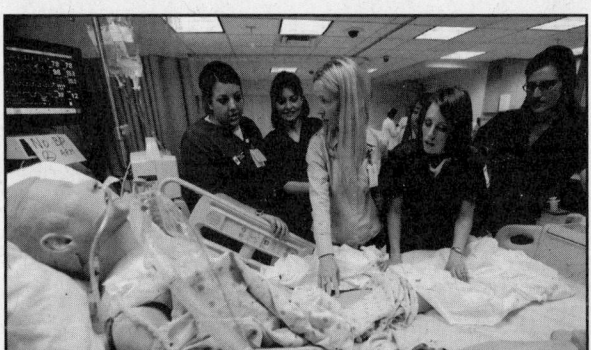

Students and instructor in the Simulation Lab.

DUQUESNE UNIVERSITY
SCHOOL OF NURSING
NLN Center *of* **Excellence**
2011-2015

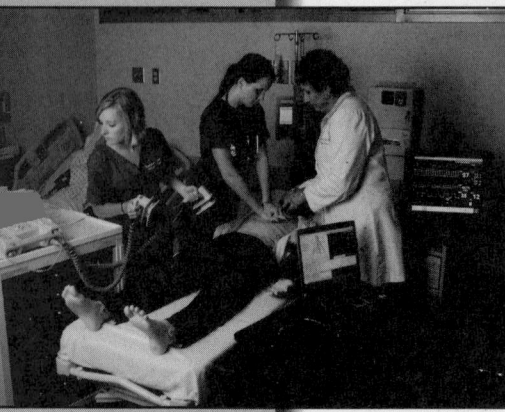

In the instructive environment of Duquesne's high-tech nursing labs, students acquire clinical knowledge and decision-making skills.

The Duquesne University School of Nursing was the first nursing school in Pennsylvania to offer a Bachelor of Science in Nursing degree and the first in the nation with an entirely online doctorate in nursing program.

Twice recognized as a National League for Nursing Center of Excellence, the School of Nursing is accredited by the Commission on Collegiate Nursing Education and the Pennsylvania State Board of Nursing.

Since its founding in 1878, Duquesne University has earned a reputation for academic excellence and having a faculty that is committed to teaching and to helping students succeed. Today, Duquesne is experiencing an exciting period of growth and increased recognition:

U.S. News & World Report:

- Duquesne University School of Nursing online Graduate Programs ranked 7th of 72 ranked/96 total schools in 2013.

- A top-tier university among the 1,600 American institutions considered for 2013.

- The only private university in Pennsylvania listed among the 20 most financially efficient top-ranked schools.

- Among the nation's top 100 popular schools. For the third time, Duquesne is described as having a "top reputation and students are highly motivated to go there."

- Offering high academic quality at a good price, Duquesne appears as number 44 on the 2013 Great Schools at Great Prices list.

Princeton Review

- Among The Best 377 Colleges for 2013, which profiles only 15 percent of American four-year colleges.

- One of the Best in the Northeast, Duquesne was one of only 220 institutions chosen for 2012.

- Named for the second year in the *Guide to 311 Green Colleges* as one of America's most environmentally responsible schools.

In addition, Duquesne University is 16th in the nation among small research universities, according to a Chronicle of Higher Education index that measured faculty productivity among more than 7,300 doctoral programs

From the beginning, Duquesne has worked diligently to improve the quality of life for the people of Pittsburgh. To that end, the School of Nursing operates a Nurse-Managed Wellness Center for underserved communities, where nurses and other health-care providers promote health and wellness and monitor chronic medical conditions. These clinics offer students an invaluable learning experience as well as an opportunity for community service. The School of Nursing is also home to the Center for Nursing Research, which supports qualitative and quantitative inquiry in areas related to health disparities, cultural competence, and chronic deviations from health.

Duquesne's green, self-contained, 49-acre campus—centrally located in a city with an international reputation for leadership in medicine and technology—has superb recreational facilities and student services and is only minutes away from Pittsburgh's rich cultural, sports, and entertainment offerings.

Bachelor of Science in Nursing (B.S.N.) Program

Clinical experiences, which begin in the sophomore year, create a strong foundation for nursing practice, and Duquesne's students complete over 1,170 clinical hours in hospitals and community health facilities. The clinical faculty-to-student ratio is 1:8.

Duquesne's nursing labs have the latest nursing simulators for helping students gain patient-care skills in a controlled environment designed to improve decision making and develop teamwork, communications, and leadership skills.

Nursing students can add international perspectives by participating in faculty-led, summertime study-abroad programs or for-credit learning experiences in Nicaragua during spring break. The University offers semester-long programs at a satellite campus in Italy and at an International Study Center in Ireland.

Second Degree B.S.N. Program

The Second Degree Bachelor of Science in Nursing (B.S.N.) program enables the non-nurse with a baccalaureate degree to obtain a B.S.N. in twelve months. The program includes three semesters of course work and over 850 hours of clinical experience.

Graduate Programs

All graduate nursing programs are offered exclusively online in a user-friendly, asynchronous format. Online learning provides flexibility for professional nurses with busy schedules and permits students to earn degrees in a reasonable length of time. Course work is highly interactive, so students communicate often with instructors and class-mates. Online flexibility plus academic rigor make the Duquesne University School of Nursing the ideal choice for graduate nursing education.

Master of Science in Nursing (M.S.N.)
Family Nurse Practitioner (FNP)
Forensic Nursing
Nursing Education
Post-Master's Certificates
Family Nurse Practitioner (FNP)
Forensic Nursing
Ph.D. in Nursing
Doctor of Nursing Practice (D.N.P.)

Visit www.duq.edu/nursing for complete admission requirements and application instructions, or call 412-396-4945 or e-mail nursing@duq.edu.

- *2012–13 FULL-TIME UNDERGRADUATE TUITION & FEES: $30,034 ($994 per credit)*
- *2012–13 FULL-TIME GRADUATE TUITION & FEES: $1083 per credit*
- *APPLICATION DEADLINES:*

  B.S.N.: May 1

  B.S.N. (transfer students): April 1 (fall admission); November 1 (spring admission)

  Second Degree B.S.N.: December 1

  M.S.N.: March 1

  Ph.D.: January 15

  D.N.P.: February 1

  Visit www.duq.edu/nursing for complete admission requirements and application instructions.

- *FACULTY INFORMATION: www.duq.edu/nursing*

CONTACT INFORMATION

Susan Hardner, Nurse Recruiter
545-A Fisher Hall
Duquesne University
600 Forbes Avenue
Pittsburgh, Pennsylvania 15282
Phone: 412-396-4945
Fax: 412-396-6346
E-mail: nursing@duq.edu
Web site: http://www.duq.edu/nursing
**   www.facebook.com/DUNursing**

A Duquesne nursing student with Nicaraguan children during her international nursing experience.

D'Youville COLLEGE
Educating for life

School of Nursing

Educating competent, compassionate, knowledgeable, professional nurses.

D'Youville College is a private, co-educational liberal arts and professional college offering students a high-quality education in more than thirty undergraduate and graduate degree programs. Founded in 1908 by the Grey Nuns as the first college for women in western New York to offer baccalaureate degrees to women, it was named for their founder, Saint Marguerite D'Youville. The current enrollment is 3,100 men and women; the student-faculty ratio is 14:1, allowing for individual attention and student support by faculty. The College is committed to helping its students grow academically, socially, and personally throughout their college experience. The Learning Center and other college-wide support services are available to enhance students' opportunity for success. Many student organizations, including pre-professional student associations, expand the learning environment.

D'Youville College has been growing and attracting students from all over the world since 1908, particularly in the areas of professional health-related programs. D'Youville College has been educating and preparing professional nurses for careers since 1942; the first Bachelor of Science in Nursing (B.S.N.) class graduated in 1946. Since then, nursing education programs at D'Youville have continued to grow, and the school of nursing is now the largest single education entity on campus. D'Youville offers a four-year Bachelor of Science in Nursing. The B.S.N. program combines a liberal arts foundation with professional nursing classroom and clinical instruction. An active Student Nurses Association orients students to the role that professional organizations play in life-long professional practice and promotion of health for populations.

Classroom instruction concentrates on preparing students for critical thinking and clinical decision making required for clinical practice. Students begin their clinical experiences at area hospitals, long-term care facilities, community agencies, and other health-related facilities and services. On-campus nursing laboratory instruction and practice with low-, mid-, and high-fidelity simulators; standardized patients; and inter-professional learning opportunities help to prepare students for actual clinical practice. Clinical practice begins in the sophomore year. Areas of clinical experience include geriatrics, pediatrics, obstetrics/gynecology, behavioral health, community health, and medical/surgical nursing. Some area hospital systems provide paid competitive internship opportunities for students between their junior and senior years. D'Youville enjoys partnerships and active affiliations with area health-care facilities and agencies where students develop their clinical competencies. Within a narrow geographic area surrounding the college campus and its nearby suburbs are several institutions of the Catholic Health System; Erie County Medical Center (including WNY's Level 1 Trauma and Burn Center); Buffalo Psychiatric Center, Kaleida Health Care System (including Women and Children's Hospital of Buffalo and the Gates Vascular Institute); the Visiting Nurses Association of Western New York; the world-renowned Roswell Park Cancer Institute; and numerous community health agencies and services that provide for primary care and population health. Opportunity is available for service-learning locally and in third-world locations.

In 1957, the RN to B.S.N. program was initiated, offering a specialized curriculum for licensed professional nurses with nursing diplomas and associate degrees. Professional nurses can complete a two-year RN to B.S.N. program or opt for the RN to B.S.N./M.S in nursing. The RN to BSN/MS requires an additional year of study and completion of a master's project or thesis after which students graduate with both degrees conferred at the same time. Convenient class scheduling provides professional nurses opportunity to study full-time by attending only two days a week,

The Koessler Administration Building dates back to 1872 when it was the home of Holy Angels Academy, a private boarding school for young ladies in elementary and secondary grades. In 1908, a charter established D'Youville College and the Academy of the Holy Angels. As the College grew, the Academy moved to another location in Buffalo in 1930. Today, the landmark building houses the President's suite and other administrative offices.

while still being able to maintain their professional employment.

Graduate programs offer several options for baccalaureate–prepared nurses to continue their professional development: the Master of Science (M.S.) in community health nursing, with concentrations in advanced clinical nursing, nursing management, or nursing education; the M.S. in nursing, with choice of clinical focus; the M.S. in family nurse practitioner studies; and a post-master's certificate in family nurse practitioner studies. Begun in fall 2012, D'Youville now offers a Doctor of Nursing Practice (DNP). The DNP can be taken as a post-baccalaureate degree or as a post-master's degree. Admission and progression in the program is individualized to the student's prior preparation.

All baccalaureate and masters programs offered by the School of Nursing are fully accredited by the Commission on Collegiate Nursing Education (CCNE) and approved by the New York State Education Department. The DNP program is approved by the New York State Education Department; the application for accreditation by CCNE will be made one year prior to the graduation of the first class, which is the standard procedure for new programs.

The nursing faculty members are committed, dedicated educators who pride themselves on providing individual attention to students. Faculty members represent diverse educational and clinical preparation and expertise. Their active practice in a variety of specialty practice areas, their research and other scholarly work, and their participation in professional organizations enrich the teaching/learning opportunities provided at D'Youville.

D'Youville College admits students on a rolling admissions basis but recommends students submit applications well before the start of the semester. Applications are reviewed as they are received by the Admissions Office. Undergraduate applicants must submit a completed application; official high school transcripts, and SAT or ACT scores. Transfer students must also submit official transcripts from all colleges previously attended. Graduate and doctorate applicants present evidence of their undergraduate education from an accredited college or university and their current unrestricted license to practice

as a professional registered nurse and/or nurse practitioner.

- *2012–13 UNDERGRADUATE TUITION & FEES: FULL-TIME: $21,930 ROOM AND BOARD: $10,000 PER YEAR*
- *2012–13 GRADUATE TUITION & FEES: $810 per credit*
- *APPLICATION DEADLINES: Rolling admissions*
- *FACULTY: http://www.dyc.edu/academics/ nursing/faculty.asp*

CONTACT INFORMATION

Dr. Judith Lewis
School of Nursing
D'Youville College
320 Porter Avenue
Buffalo, New York 14201
Phone: 716-829-7600
        800-777-3921 (toll-free)
Fax: 716-829-7900
E-mail: admissions@dyc.edu
Web site: http://www.dyc.edu/academics/ nursing/
UNDERGRADUATE NURSING PROGRAM
Dr. Steve Smith, Director of Admissions
Phone: 716-829-7600
E-mail: admissions@dyc.edu

GRADUATE NURSING PROGRAM
Linda Fisher, Director of Graduate Admissions
Phone: 716-829-8400
E-mail: graduateadmissions@dyc.edu

Find us on Facebook®: http://www.dyc.edu/facebook
Follow us on Twitter™: http://twitter.com/uanursing

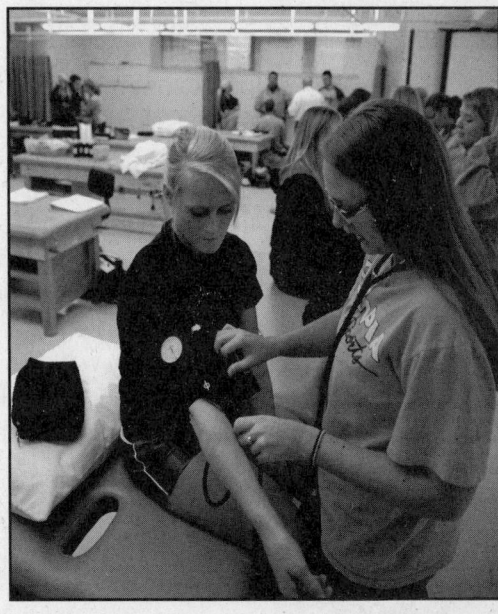

D'Youville College is internationally known for its wide array of health-care academic offerings. Majors include nursing, physician assistant, occupational and physical therapy, pharmacy, chiropractic, and dietetics. All majors include a strong liberal arts component.

EMMANUEL COLLEGE

Students benefit from small, interactive classes.

UNDERGRADUATE AND GRADUATE PROGRAMS IN NURSING

Emmanuel College's undergraduate and graduate programs for registered nurses (RN) open new doors in the field of nursing. Emmanuel College offers a Bachelor of Science in Nursing (BSN) and a Master of Science in Nursing (MSN). Both programs offer curricula specifically developed to meet students' learning needs, as well as individualized plans of nursing study to prepare RNs for the next step in their professional careers.

The Bachelor of Science in Nursing program prepares students to think critically, appreciate diverse human experience, and use personal and professional values in everyday life. Emmanuel College's program is health promotion–based, enabling students to meet career goals in a constantly changing health-care environment. Teaching and learning strategies throughout Emmanuel College's BSN and MSN courses prepare graduates with the knowledge, skills, and attitudes necessary to continuously improve the quality and safety of the health-care systems in which they work. The RN-to-BSN program is fully accredited by the Commission on Collegiate Nursing Education (CCNE).

The Master of Science in Nursing program prepares students for an advanced role as a nurse educator or nurse manager/administrator. These distinctive tracks offer students the knowledge and expertise to thrive in a wide variety of clinical settings and to work with diverse populations. Students who choose the education concentration are qualified to pursue roles in clinical education, staff development, and as nursing faculty members; graduates of the management track are prepared for management/administration positions such as nurse administrator, manager, director, coordinator, and case manager.

Emmanuel College's Boston campus is located in the heart of the Longwood Medical and Academic Area (LMA), adjacent to some of the most respected health-care institutions in the nation. Its proximity to these health-care institutions allows Emmanuel College to form strategic partnerships, including on-site classes with employers such as Brigham and Women's Hospital and the Caritas Christi Health Care System. Emmanuel College is the recipient of the University Professional and Continuing Education Association's (UPCEA) 2010 Community of Practice Award for Outreach and Engagement for Employer and Association Partnerships.

As respected professionals with years of experience in nursing, Emmanuel College faculty members maintain a strong and up-to-date command in their areas of expertise in research and teaching. As understanding nurse educators, they cultivate lively dialogue so that students share first-hand perspectives on patient care, health-care issues, and other key subjects. Emmanuel College professors are clinicians, researchers and teachers who serve as true advocates. Each student works directly with a full-time member of the nursing faculty as a dedicated advisor. This provides students with the individual attention necessary to get the most from their plan of study.

With an average class size of 15 students, students have the ability to engage in lively classroom discussions, to share their unique experiences as RNs, and to exchange views and clinical knowledge. Classes meet evenings or Saturday mornings every other week, enabling students to fit academics into their professional and personal schedules. All modified accelerated courses include independent study, and students can set their own pace with flexible program scheduling. Graduate nursing classes meet seven times during the semester and are offered at Emmanuel College's Boston campus. Undergraduate nursing classes meet six times during a semester and are offered at Emmanuel College's easy-to-reach Boston and Woburn campuses.

The BSN program has enrollment and application opportunities multiple times per year and is also available by request at employer sites. The MSN has a new cohort beginning each fall semester, and the application deadline for the MSN is April 30.

- *2012–13 TUITION & FEES*:

   Bachelor of Science in Nursing (BSN):

   $1772 per 4-credit course

   Master of Science in Nursing (MSN):

   $2518 per 3-credit course

   There are no additional fees associated with either program.

- *APPLICATION DEADLINES*

   Bachelor of Science in Nursing (BSN):

   There are enrollment opportunities multiple times per year. An application form must be submitted prior to enrollment.

   Master of Science in Nursing (MSN):

   The preferred application deadline is April 30th for enrollment in the fall semester.
   The Graduate Nursing Admissions Committee will review only completed applications.

   There is no application fee.

- *FACULTY INFORMATION*

   http://gpp.emmanuel.edu

CONTACT INFORMATION

Helen Muterperl, Assistant Director
Graduate Admissions /Nursing Programs
Emmanuel College
Graduate and Professional Programs
400 The Fenway
Boston, Massachusetts 02115
Phone: 617-735-9700
E-mail: gpp@emmanuel.edu
Web site: http://gpp.emmanuel.edu/nursing

Find us on Facebook®: http://www.facebook.com/emmanuelgpp

Emmanuel's Boston campus is located in the world-renowned Longwood Medical and Academic Area.

GANNON

UNIVERSITY

Believe in the possibilities.

Villa Maria School of Nursing

Graduates of the Villa Maria School of Nursing at Gannon University enjoyed a 100% job placement rate last year.

The Villa Maria School of Nursing offers baccalaureate, master's, and Doctor of Nursing Practice (DNP) degree programs to prepare students for life as well as for the practice of professional nursing. The community-based baccalaureate program provides competencies, knowledge, values, and roles that prepare professional nurses to provide high-quality care to diverse populations in and across various environments.

Gannon's nursing faculty members have graduate preparation in their clinical areas of specializations and are skilled clinical practitioners. Gannon's nursing curriculum maintains a balanced study of natural and social sciences and the humanities within the context of professional education, fostering creative thinking and effective communication, and promoting caring, respect, and concern for individuals, communities, and society. All programs are accredited by the Commission on Collegiate Nursing Education (CCNE).

Nursing students can participate in clinical experiences at more than forty local hospitals, clinics, and community agencies. First-attempt NCLEX-RN (licensure examination) pass rates have averaged 96 percent over the last four years.

The Villa Maria School of Nursing accepts an entering freshman baccalaureate class of 70 each year. Transfer students are evaluated on an individual basis. Freshman students begin the investigation into the profession of nursing with seminar courses. Clinical course work begins in the sophomore year, increasing in number of hours over the junior and senior years of study.

Gannon also offers a graduate program in nursing. The Master of Science in Nursing (MSN) program integrates nursing education, research, and practice and is designed so that graduates are able to respond to the challenges facing nursing and the healthcare system through advanced clinical practice and scientific inquiry.

The MSN degree is awarded to graduates who complete requirements for a specific advanced practice option in an identified area of nursing practice. Currently, students may select from family nurse practitioner, nurse anesthetist, and nursing administration.

Each graduate student is expected to conduct research and prepare a research thesis or project. The program may be completed by enrolling on a full-time or part-time basis, with the exception of the nurse anesthesia option, which can be completed only by enrolling full-time.

Options for registered nurses are available, including RN to BSN (also available as an online program) and RN to MSN. Students follow a course of study that includes challenge exams, transfer credits, and validation of prior learning via student-created portfolios. The portfolio options focus on non-duplication of previously learned nursing knowledge and are offered at a greatly reduced cost.

The Villa Maria School of Nursing offers a Post-Bachelor's (BSN) certification program for school nurses in cooperation with the School of Education. The certification, which is available to currently registered nurses licensed in the Commonwealth of Pennsylvania who hold an earned BSN with a minimum cumulative grade point average of 3.0.

Gannon University is a Catholic, Diocesan, student-centered university with more than 4,000 students, providing a caring environment that fosters inclusiveness and cultural diversity. With a low, faculty-to-staff ratio of 14:1, Gannon's outstanding, values-based education combines liberal arts with professional specializations to prepare students for leadership roles in their careers, society, and church. A range of campus organizations and activities encourages academic interests, community service, and moral and spiritual growth. Gannon also offers students a broad program of intramural and intercollegiate athletics.

Gannon University offers degrees in more than seventy academic majors in the sciences, health sciences, engineering, humanities, business, and education.

- *2013–14 UNDERGRADUATE TUITION & FEES:*

  For current information, visit http://gannon.edu/ Financial-Aid/Tuition-and-Fees.

- *2013–14 GRADUATE TUITION & FEES:*

  For current information, visit http://gannon.edu/ Financial-Aid/Tuition-and-Fees.

- *APPLICATION DEADLINES:*

  Gannon University offers rolling admissions. For current information, visit http://gannon.edu/ Admissions.

- *FACULTY INFORMATION:*

  www.gannon.edu/Academic-Offerings/ Health-Professions-and-Sciences/ Villa-Maria-School-of-Nursing

- *MULTIMEDIA:*

  www.gannon.edu/simcenter

CONTACT INFORMATION

Kathleen T. Patterson, Ph.D., R.N.
Director, Villa Maria School of Nursing
Gannon University
109 University Square
Erie, Pennsylvania 16541-0001
Phone: 814-871-5520
            800-GANNON-U
            [800-426-6668 (toll-free)]
E-mail: patterso018@gannon.edu
Web site: www.gannon.edu/nursing

UNDERGRADUATE NURSING PROGRAM:
Patricia Marshall
Director, Undergraduate Program
Morosky College of Health Professions and
     Sciences
Phone: 814-871-5470
E-mail: marshall001@gannon.edu

GRADUATE NURSING PROGRAM:
Kathleen T. Patterson, Ph.D., R.N.
Director, Villa Maria School of Nursing
Morosky College of Health Professions and
     Sciences
Phone: 814-871-5520
E-mail: patterso018@gannon.edu

Find us on Facebook®: http://www.facebook.com/gannonu
Follow us on Twitter™: @GannonU

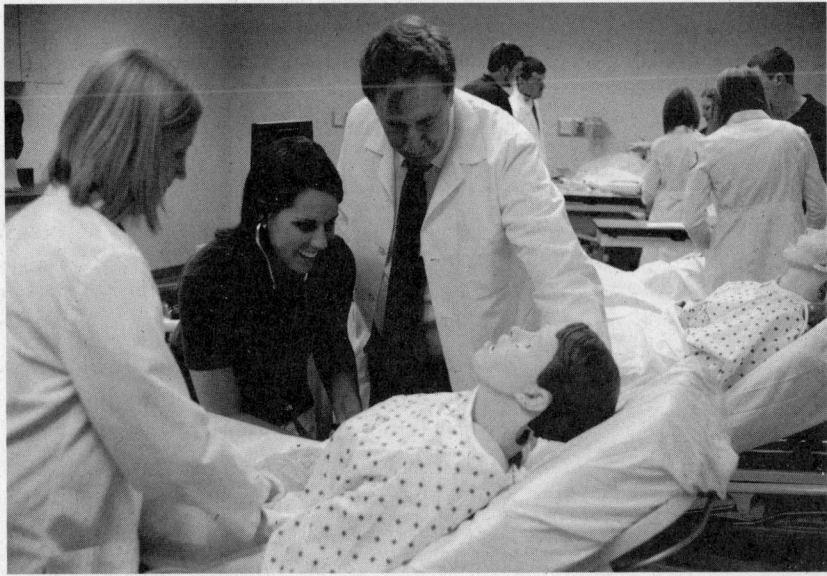

The Villa Maria School of Nursing's Patient Simulation center has 14 mid- and hi-fidelity manikins in a multidisciplinary setting.

JOHNS HOPKINS
UNIVERSITY

SCHOOL OF NURSING

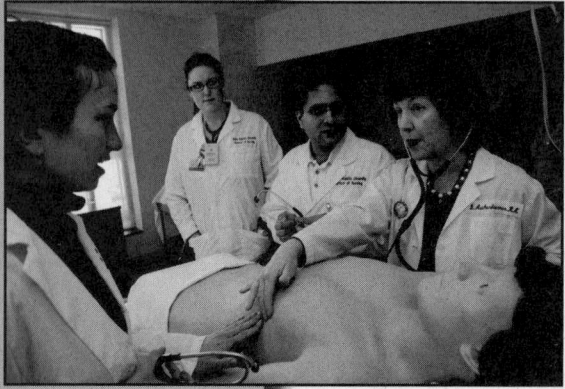

Students engage the "SimMan," a universal patient simulator.

The Johns Hopkins University School of Nursing is a place where exceptional people discover possibilities that forever change their lives and the world. With more than a century of established excellence in connection with The Johns Hopkins Hospital and the University, the School of Nursing is both connected to the past and focused on the future. It attracts students and faculty from around the world to collaborate, research, and learn the best practices to advance the science and art of nursing. Hopkins students enjoy the advantages of an education at an institution with a worldwide reputation and an outstanding network of alumni who are willing to serve as guides and mentors. A rigorous academic curriculum, which includes a strong scientific orientation, gives students the background to understand the healthcare decisions they will make as professionals.

Recognized as a leader by its peers, the School of Nursing ranked first in the nation for Community Health Nursing Programs and first overall for Graduate Programs in the 2012 edition of *U.S. News & World Report*. The School is ranked first among nursing schools in the United States in the National Institutes of Health (NIH) research funding. Named a Center of Excellence in Nursing Education in 2010 by the National League for Nursing, the School is located adjacent to the top-ranked Johns Hopkins University schools of Medicine and Public Health and The Johns Hopkins Hospital.

Johns Hopkins University is accredited by Middle States Commission on Higher Education. The bachelor's and master's programs of the School of Nursing are fully accredited by the National League for Nursing Accrediting Commission (NLNAC) and the Commission on Collegiate Nursing Education (CCNE). In addition, the bachelor's and master's programs are approved by the Maryland State Board of Examiners of Nurses. The bachelor's, master's, and doctoral programs are endorsed by the Maryland State Board for Higher Education. The School's Doctor of Nursing Practice (DNP) program went through the accreditation process with the Commission on Collegiate Nursing Education (CCNE) in fall 2009 and received full accreditation until 2015. The School is also proud to be the only Paul D. Coverdell Fellows Program in nursing.

A complete bachelor's and master's application consists of an application form and a nonrefundable $75 application fee. Doctoral applicants pay an application fee of $100. Applicants to the bachelor's program are required to submit three letters of recommendation and official college- or university-level transcripts. A grade point average (GPA) above 3.0 (on a 4.0 scale) is recommended. Personal interviews may be requested.

Applicants to the master's program are required to have graduated from a bachelor's or master's degree program in nursing with a GPA above 3.0 (on a 4.0 scale), a current Maryland state nursing license, academic and professional references, written expression of goals, and official transcripts from all previous colleges/universities attended. Personal interviews may be requested.

• *2013–14 UNDERGRADUATE TUITION & FEES:*
Summer-Entry Accelerated Bachelor's Program:
Tuition: $65,700 (for entire 13-month program)
Housing, food, books, fees, and other costs: $29,632

Fall-Entry Accelerated Bachelor's Program:
Tuition: $66,193 (for entire 17-month program)
Housing, food, books, fees, and other costs: $33,412

Accelerated BS-MSN with Paid Clinical Residency Program: *Bachelor's tuition: $66,193 (full-time—12 credit hours/semester). Housing, food, books, fees, and other costs: $33,412. Master's tuition dependent on track.*

- *2013–14 GRADUATE TUITION & FEES:*

MSN Program:
Tuition: $33,168 (full-time—12 credit hours/semester); $1,382 per credit (part-time). Housing, food, books, fees, and other costs: $18,866

MSN/MPH Program:
Tuition: $52,614 (full-time—16 credit hours/semester); $1,385 per credit (part-time). Housing, food, books, fees, and other costs: $23,110

PhD Program:
Tuition: $40,626 (full-time—9 credit hours/semester); $2,257 per credit (part-time). Housing, food, books, fees, and other costs: $18,866

DNP Program:
Tuition: $55,000 (for entire 40 credit program); $1,375 per credit (part-time). Housing, food, books, fees, and other costs: $18,866

- *APPLICATION DEADLINES:*

Bachelor's Program: *November 1 (early decision); November 15 (summer entry); January 15 (fall entry)*

Accelerated BS-MSN with Paid Clinical Residency Program: *May 1 (fall entry)*

Master's Program: *March 15 (fall entry); September 1 (spring entry); January 15 (summer entry)*

Special Deadlines:

> *MSN/MPH and MSN/MPH Nurse Practitioner: December 1 (summer entry)*

> *MSN in Public Health Nursing/Nurse-Midwifery Track: December 1 (fall entry)*

> *MSN Primary Care Nurse Practitioner (Adult-Geriatric, Family, Pediatric): December 1 (fall entry)*

Note: BS to MSN students who are enrolled in the Bachelor's degree portion of the program must confirm their planned fall enrollment in the MSN program by February 1.

- **Post-Degree Options**

Family Primary Care Nurse Practitioner: December 1 (fall entry)

Applied Health Informatics: June 1 (fall entry)

Forensic Nursing: November 1 (spring entry); June 1 (fall entry)

Nurse Educator: July 15 (fall entry); December 1 (spring entry); May 1 (summer entry)

Adult-Gerontology Acute Care, Pediatric Primary Care, and Adult-Geriatric Nurse Practitioner: January 15 (fall entry)

Accelerated Acute Care Nurse Practitioner: September 1 (spring entry)

PhD Program:
March 1 (fall entry); September 1 (spring entry); January 15 (for full eligibility for scholarship opportunities).

DNP Program:
January 1 (summer entry)

- *FACULTY INFORMATION:*
  http://nursing.jhu.edu/faculty

- *MULTIMEDIA:*
  http://youtube.com/hopkinsnursing

CONTACT INFORMATION

Office of Admissions and Student Services
Johns Hopkins University School of Nursing
525 North Wolfe Street
Baltimore, Maryland 21205
Phone: 410-955-7548
Fax: 410-614-7086
E-mail: jhuson@jhu.edu
Web site: www.nursing.jhu.edu

Find us on Facebook®: www.facebook.com/jhunursing
Follow us on Twitter™: twitter.com/JHUNursing

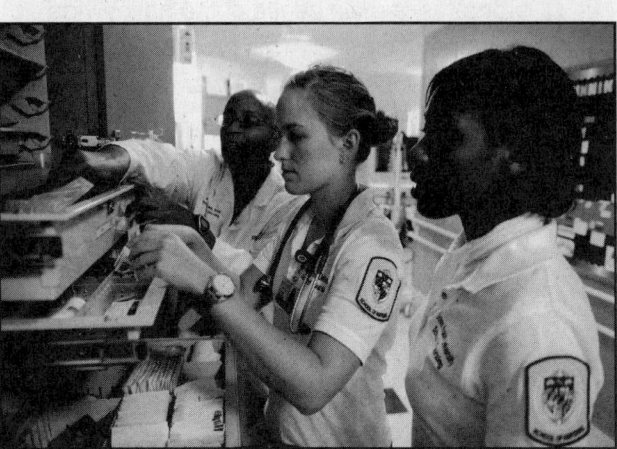

Students work closely with clinical instructors at The Johns Hopkins Hospital.

SCHOOL OF HEALTH PROFESSIONS AND NURSING

Find Out How Good You Really Are: Nursing Education Program at LIU Post

Convenient "Blended Learning" M.S. Program for Nurse Educators

Danielle Coppola, an LIU Post alumna, loves her job as a nurse at Saint Francis Hospital in Roslyn, New York. When the opportunity to train some of her colleagues emerged, she quickly discovered the part of nursing she likes best: teaching. "I definitely want to teach," she said. "That's where my heart is."

The LIU Post School of Health Professions and Nursing launched the Nursing Education master's degree program in 2006 to help address the scarcity of nursing education programs, a main cause of the nationwide shortage of nurses. "This program was perfect," Coppola said. "It was very hands-on, and the professors were all nursing educators who taught from experience. Because the classes were small, it was very intimate, and that helped me learn the material. We could ask many questions and really discuss the subjects." Coppola's degree qualifies her for a variety of nursing education roles in hospitals, schools, and colleges.

The Master of Science (M.S.) program is offered in a Blended Learning Format, which combines the convenience of online learning with the benefits of live classroom discussion

Nursing Education Class: Students in LIU Post's Nursing Education program benefit from online courses and hands-on instruction.

and interaction. Nearly half of each course in the M.S. in Nursing Education program is taught online, with the balance occurring in a traditional classroom setting. The core curriculum includes course work in nursing theory, issues in professional nursing for advanced practice nurses and nurse educators, and nursing research. As part of their degree requirements, students are required to complete a research proposal, 12 credits of core courses, and 21 credits of specialty courses.

The 33-credit program can be completed in five semesters of part-time study and one summer session. Nurse Educator candidates complete two semesters of preceptored teaching practice.

Additional Nursing Programs for RNs

The M.S. in Nursing Education programs qualifies graduates to teach in nursing programs at the LPN, associate, bachelor's, and master's levels and to serve as staff educators in health-care facilities. It is open to nurses who need specific education courses to qualify for New York State certification as secondary school health education teachers.

The School of Health Professions and Nursing also offers a B.S. program exclusively for RNs, and M.S. degrees in Family Nurse Practitioner and Advanced Practice Nursing: Clinical Nurse Specialist. Post-master's advanced certificates include Family Nurse Practitioner and Nursing Education. The B.S. and M.S. programs are fully accredited by the Commission on Collegiate Nursing Education.

Hands-On Learning with Leading Faculty

LIU Post nursing students actively participate in clinical practice at well-respected medical centers and hospitals, including North Shore-Long Island Jewish Health System and Memorial Sloan-Kettering Cancer Center, as well as some of the nation's top pharmaceutical companies. Graduates have secured rewarding positions with the region's leading health-care providers, including hospitals and private practices. Students in the LIU Post nursing program benefit from the faculty's professional experience and career counseling support. Faculty members are dedicated to preparing students for lifelong learning in order to meet the increasing demands of the expanding environment of nursing practice. Graduates of the Department of Nursing will have developed the values and competencies that are in high demand in the industry: critical thinking, culturally competent care, autonomy, communication, and decision making within a framework of professional and ethical principles essential to delivering nursing care in a global environment. LIU Post programs offer individualized attention and small classes to accommodate the needs of busy RNs.

About LIU Post

LIU Post (formerly the C.W. Post Campus of Long Island University) is one of the most beautiful, historic, and scholarly settings in the country. Located on the north shore of Long Island, in the Village of Brookville, LIU Post has grown to include 260 degree programs, five schools of study, 8,700 students, and more than 300 faculty members. Conveniently located just 50 minutes from New York City, LIU Post's academic programs carry elite accreditations, signifying they meet the highest standards of quality. For directions, visit www.liu.edu/post/directions.

- *2012–13 UNDERGRADUATE TUITION & FEES:*

  Bachelor's Degree & Undergraduate Studies, 12–18 credits: $15,601

  University Fee (12 or more credits): $720

  University Fee (11.9 credits or less): $360

  Student Activity Fee (12 or more credits): $110

  Student Activity Fee (4.1 to 11.9 credits): $85

- *2012–13 GRADUATE TUITION & FEES:*

  Master's Degree and Graduate Studies: $1068 per credit

  University Fee (12 or more credits): $720

  University Fee (11.9 credits or less): $360

  Student Activity Fee (12 or more credits): $110

  Student Activity Fee (4.1 to 11.9 credits): $85

- *APPLICATION DEADLINES:*

  LIU Post offers rolling admissions for its nursing programs. Students are encouraged to apply as early as possible for the Fall and Spring semesters by using the online application at www.liu.edu/post/apply.

- *FACULTY INFORMATION:*
  www.liu.edu/post/nursing

CONTACT INFORMATION
Mary T. Infantino, Ph.D., Chair
Department of Nursing
LIU Post
Northern Boulevard
Brookville, New York 11548
Phone: 516-299-2320
Fax: 516-299-2527
E-mail: healprof@liu.edu
Web site: www.liu.edu/post/nursing

Find us on Facebook® @LIUPostAdmissions

Danielle Coppola is a Nursing Education student who is using her new skills at St. Francis Hospital in Roslyn, New York.

LUTHER COLLEGE

Department of Nursing

The nursing major at Luther College offers an integrated program of liberal arts and 14 professional nursing courses, giving students a broad approach to nursing and providing a base for graduate study or immediate entry into the profession. Students gain clinical experience at healthcare sites such as St. Marys Hospital, an affiliate of Mayo Clinic in Rochester, Minnesota.

The goal of Luther's nursing faculty is to prepare nurses to function autonomously and interdependently with individuals, families, groups, and communities to promote, maintain, and restore optimal health in a variety of health-care settings. The nursing major, therefore, offers an integrated program of liberal arts and 14 professional nursing courses. The program gives students a broad approach to nursing, providing a base for graduate study or immediate entry into the nursing profession.

Following graduation, Luther nursing students may take the National Council Licensure Examination for Registered Nurses (NCLEX-RN). More information is available upon request.

The first year at Luther provides a foundation in the liberal arts and sciences. All nursing majors are assigned a faculty adviser to help each student decide whether to pursue a nursing curriculum plan. All students interested in nursing are invited to participate in the Luther Student Nurses Association (LSNA).

Clinical nursing courses begin in the fall of the sophomore year. Nursing courses at this level emphasize health assessment, health promotion, clinical reasoning, and fundamental skills throughout the life span in a variety of settings. These learning experiences develop new communication and interpersonal skills.

Third-year students experience a concentrated study of nursing concepts by caring for children and adults with physical and emotional problems. The sites for this clinical experience are Rochester Methodist Hospital and St. Marys Hospital, affiliates of Mayo Clinic; the Federal Medical Center; and a variety of community-based health-care agencies in Rochester, Minnesota.

The senior year provides final preparation for entry into the practice of professional nursing. Courses focus on promoting health and preventing illness in childbearing families and in community groups. Students further develop leadership management and research skills through selected areas of nursing.

Minimum academic requirements must be met to be considered for enrollment in nursing courses. However, meeting the minimum requirements does not guarantee placement in the courses. Decisions affecting progression in the major are made at the end of each semester.

The study of nursing at Luther incorporates academic classroom learning, based in the newly renovated Valders Hall of Science, and clinical experience in several community facilities. These include Winneshiek Medical Center; the Decorah Free Clinic; Mayo Clinic: Methodist Hospital and Mayo Clinic: Saint Marys Hospital; the Federal Medical Center; and a variety of community-based health-care agencies in Decorah, Iowa and Rochester, Minnesota.

Nursing scholarships are available to incoming students on a competitive basis upon admission. Selection of recipients is based on academic information submitted on the application and the high school transcript. Scholarship renewal is based on satisfactory academic and clinical performance in the major.

All nursing students benefit from the Bernice Fischer Cross and Bert S. Cross Perpetual Endowment for the Luther College Mayo Nursing Program and Health Sciences Program. This is used for equal-share assistance for the Luther College nursing students enrolled in the curriculum provided at Mayo Clinic in Rochester, Minnesota. The endowment is not a need-based scholarship.

Located in the northeast Iowa town of Decorah (resident population: 8,100), Luther College is an undergraduate liberal arts institution of about 2,500 students that is affiliated with the Lutheran church (ELCA). The Upper Iowa River—the only waterway in the state designated as wild and scenic—flows through the lower portion of Luther's 200-acre central campus and borders Decorah's business district. Decorah is known nationwide for its recreational opportunities, numerous cultural heritage events and festivals, pedestrian-friendly village center, and its conscious efforts to thrive as a small town. Public transportation includes commercial airports in Rochester (Minnesota), Waterloo (Iowa), and La Crosse (Wisconsin); a municipal airport in Decorah; and train and bus depots in La Crosse, Wisconsin.

- *2013–14 UNDERGRADUATE TUITION & FEES:*

  The comprehensive fee is $43,940 ($37,330 tuition, $3,000 room, $3,610 board).

- *APPLICATION DEADLINES:*

  Luther College operates on rolling admission. There is no application deadline.

- *FACULTY INFORMATION:*

  http://www.luther.edu/nursing/faculty/

- *MULTIMEDIA:*

  http://www.luther.edu/video/

CONTACT INFORMATION

**M. Patricia Donahue, Interim Head
Department of Nursing
Luther College
700 College Drive
Decorah, Iowa 52101
Phone: 563-387-1057
           800-458-8437 (toll-free)
E-mail: donama01@luther.edu
Web site: http://www.luther.edu/nursing/**

Find us on Facebook®: www.facebook.com/luthercollege1861
Follow us on Twitter™: www.twitter.com/luthercollege

Luther College students learn in a community that emphasizes rigorous academics, a world-class music program, champion athletics, and opportunities to put their classroom learning to the test through internships, independent research, and study abroad. Typically, 96 percent of Luther graduates are employed, attending graduate school, or engaged in an internship or volunteer work within eight months of graduation.

College of Nursing

*Simulated
Cardiac Arrest
Resuscitation*

The four-year Bachelor of Science in Nursing (B.S.N.) degree program at Marquette University provides a strong academic foundation in nursing, natural and social science, and humanities. Preparation for a professional nursing role is emphasized through the development of clinical, cognitive, and leadership skills and personal and professional values. Students are **admitted directly as freshmen** into the College of Nursing, which **assures placement in clinical nursing courses.** Nursing courses begin on the first day of enrollment. Clinical reasoning, introduced in the first year through course assignments and simulation experiences, is further developed through five clinical rotations in health-care agencies across the sophomore, junior, and senior years. A low student-teacher ratio (8:1) affords personal attention in all clinical rotations, including maternity, community health, nursing care for children and adults with chronic and acute conditions, and transition into professional practice.
The 128-credit B.S.N. program includes courses in the humanities, physical-biological sciences, and social-behavioral sciences as well as electives and courses in the nursing major. A University Core of Common Studies is foundational for all majors at Marquette University. Lower-division nursing courses are Dimensions of Professional Nursing in the Jesuit Tradition, Nursing and Health in the Jesuit Tradition, Health Assessment and Fundamentals I and II, Pathophysiology I and II, and Concepts and Interventions for the Promotion of Mental Health. Upper-division

courses include Pharmacology, Evidence-Based Practice and Nursing Research, Maternity Nursing and Women's Health, Family and Community-Centered Nursing*, Community and Population Health Nursing, Nursing Concepts and Interventions for the Care of Adults—Older Adults I and II, Nursing Care for Persons with Chronic and Acute Conditions*, Family Centered Nursing of Children, Quality and Safety in Nursing, Leadership in Professional Nursing Practice, Transition into Professional Nursing*, and Palliative Care. [The asterisk (*) denotes clinical practice courses.]

Marquette University College of Nursing offers the Master of Science in Nursing (M.S.N.) degree and post-master's certificates that prepare graduates for advanced practice roles or leadership roles within health-care systems. Individuals may enter through three pathways: post-B.S.N.; Direct Entry (DE), a combined RN and M.S.N. for those with non-nursing bachelor's degrees; and ADN-prepared nurses with bachelor's degrees in other disciplines. Graduates are academically eligible to seek formal professional certification as nurse practitioners, clinical nurse specialists, nurse midwives, nurse administrators, or clinical nurse leaders. Seven specialty options are available: systems leadership and health care quality, clinical nurse leader, and advanced practice programs in nurse midwifery, adult-older adult primary or acute care, adult-older adult clinical nurse specialist, and pediatric primary or acute care. Full-time students complete the 39–49 credit programs in four to six semesters.

At the Ph.D. program level, a 69-credit B.S.N. to Ph.D. program and a 51-credit post-M.S.N./Ph.D. program to prepare nurse scientists as teachers/scholars who focus on knowledge generation related to vulnerable populations.

At the Doctor of Nursing Practice (D.N.P.) level, a 63–69 credit B.S.N. to D.N.P. program or a 33-credit post-M.S.N. program, is another route to leadership in advanced practice nursing. The program emphasizes translational research, epidemiology, informatics, health policy, statistics, and professional issues. All students complete a two-semester capstone clinical project. A residency course is also required.

The College is affiliated with more than ninety health-care agencies in Wisconsin and the surrounding states. These agencies include hospitals, clinics, home care facilities, public health departments, schools, parishes, long-term-care facilities, and hospice. Many of these agencies offer excellent student employment opportunities as well as financial aid and loan forgiveness programs once students graduate from the program.

Marquette is located on an 80-acre campus with excellent facilities. The College of Nursing has many technology-enhanced classrooms and a well-equipped Center for Clinical Simulation, including SIM-MAN G, a birthing simulator, and many other advanced simulation technology models for student learning. The Simulation Center provides media resources and practice labs supplied with state-of-the-art models and equipment necessary to develop a solid foundation for clinical practice. Students participate in simulation exercises that are videotaped for maximal learning before entering into complex health-care systems. A new Simulation Center is being planned for the fall of 2012.

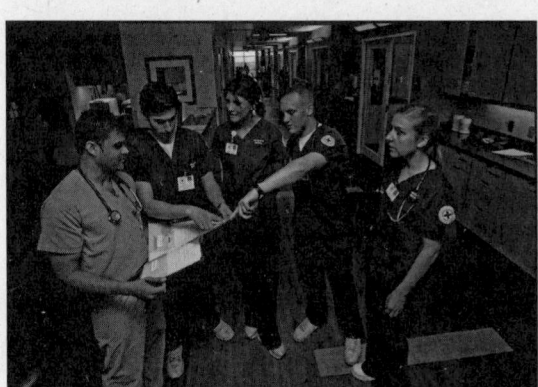

Intensive Care Unit Patient Consultation.

- *2012–13 UNDERGRADUATE TUITION & FEES:*

  Full-time tuition: $34,200

  Typical room and board: $10,670; Fees: $805

- *2012–13 GRADUATE TUITION & FEES:*

  $1,025 per credit hour

  15-Month Direct Entry Pre-MSN Program: $52,480 paid in four payments (summer, fall, spring, and summer)

- *APPLICATION DEADLINES:*

  Undergraduate: December 1

  Graduate and Post-Grad: August 1 for fall; November 1 for spring

  D.N.P.: February 15

  Direct Entry (DE) Master's: December 31 for May start

- *FACULTY INFORMATION:*

  http://www.mu.edu/facstaff

- *MULTIMEDIA: http://www.mu.edu/nursing*

CONTACT INFORMATION

Undergraduate Nursing Program:

Mary Grant
Undergraduate Program Assistant
Phone: 414-288-3809
E-mail: mary.grant@mu.edu

Graduate Nursing Program:

Karen Nest
Graduate Program Coordinator
Phone: 414-288-3810
E-mail: Karen.nest@mu.edu

Bridget O'Meara
Graduate Program & Communication Coordinator
College of Nursing
Marquette University
P.O. Box 1881
Milwaukee, Wisconsin 53233
Phone: 414-288-3869
Fax: 414-288-1939
E-mail: bridget.omeara@mu.edu
Web site: http://www.mu.edu/nursing

Find us on Facebook®: http://www.facebook.com/MarquetteU
Follow us on Twitter™: http://www.twitter.com/marquetteu

Division of Nursing

Molloy's undergraduate nursing program is the fifth largest in the United States, and the College also offers multiple graduate programs, including a Ph.D. in Nursing.

An Emphasis on Human Compassion, Dignity, and Respect

At Molloy, nursing is both art and science. One of the country's largest and most respected programs, Molloy's Nursing Division curriculum immerses students in clinical practice with an emphasis on human compassion, dignity, and respect for the patient. Molloy's programs proactively respond to the changing needs of today's health-care environment, providing students with individualized attention from an expert faculty that is easily accessible and always committed to students' success.

From Molloy's fully equipped, state-of-the-art learning laboratory to its innovative clinical practice opportunities, at Molloy students can find all the resources and support they need to become an effective, humanistic health-care provider—whether students are just beginning their nursing education or are professionals who are ready to take their career to the next level. At Molloy, students benefit from a comprehensive array of:

- Undergraduate programs. Offering a wealth of hands-on clinical experiences beginning in a student's sophomore year,

Molloy's bachelor's degree program prepares students for a vital role in health care. Already working in health care or in another career? Consider one of Molloy's dual-degree programs, the degree completion program for registered nurses, the LPN to B.S./RN career mobility program, or the accelerated dual-degree program for second degree students holding a non-nursing baccalaureate or higher degree.

- Graduate programs. Focused on advanced theory and its application in a selected area of nursing, Molloy offers seven distinct tracks leading to master's degrees and nine master's certificates concentrating on advanced clinical practice, administrative and informatics expertise, and specialty training in education. Nurse Practitioner tracks are available in Pediatrics, Adult, Family or Psychiatry, Clinical Nurse Specialist (CNS): Adult Health, Nursing Education, or Nursing Administration with Informatics.

- Doctoral program. Molloy's first doctoral program is designed to prepare doctoral students to become leaders, advancing the profession of nursing through research, education, administration, and health policy.

Molloy College launched its first doctoral program, a Ph.D. in Nursing, in fall 2010. According to Veronica Feeg, Ph.D., RN, FAAN, Associate Dean and Director of the Doctoral Program, "Doctoral education is important for our profession and the Ph.D. at Molloy will produce the researchers and scholars who will lead the discipline."

"2010 was the International Year of the Nurse, so the timing was ideal for launching our Nursing Ph.D. program," said Jeannine D. Muldoon, Ph.D., RN, Dean of the Division of Nursing. "We expect that our Ph.D. graduates will leave Molloy prepared to serve our communities, develop the next generation of nursing leaders and have a strong voice in health policy decisions that affect us all."

"This milestone event further demonstrates the College's commitment to academic excellence," said Valerie H. Collins, Ph.D., Vice President of Academic Affairs and Dean of Faculty. "Molloy's Nursing programs have always been among the finest in the country—the undergraduate program is the fifth largest in the United States—so we are pleased that the College's first doctoral program comes from this Division."

A Ph.D. from Molloy prepares nurses for leadership roles in academia, health policy formulation, health-care administration, and clinical practice. The curriculum focuses on theory, research, the humanities, and methodology. Essential elements of the curriculum feature leadership through caring, both in educational and organizational/policy settings, as well as theory and research in the nursing profession. Students are required to complete 45 credits of course work and a dissertation.

- *2012–13 UNDERGRADUATE TUITION & FEES:*

  Tuition: $23,410

  Fees: $1,010

- *2012–13 GRADUATE TUITION & FEES:*

  Master's program:
  Tuition: $895 per credit

  Fees: $720 (if taking 1–4 credits); $880 (if taking 5 or more credits)

  Ph.D. program: $1,000/credit; fees same as for Master's program

- *APPLICATION DEADLINES:*

  Undergraduate: Rolling admissions

  Master's program: Rolling admissions

  Ph.D. program: February 1

CONTACT INFORMATION

Molloy College
1000 Hempstead Avenue
Rockville Centre, New York 11571
Phone: 888-4-MOLLOY (toll-free)
Web site: http://www.molloy.edu

Undergraduate Admissions
Phone: 516-678-5000, Ext. 6230
E-mail: admissions@molloy.edu

Graduate and Ph.D. Admissions
Alina Haitz
Phone: 516-678-5000, Ext. 6399
E-mail: ahaitz@molloy.edu

Find us on Facebook®: http://www.facebook.com/GoMolloy
Follow us on Twitter™: http://www.twitter.com/MolloyCollege

Molloy College recently celebrated the launch of its new Ph.D. program with a series of lectures and a "nursing fashion show" that featured students wearing uniforms from various decades.

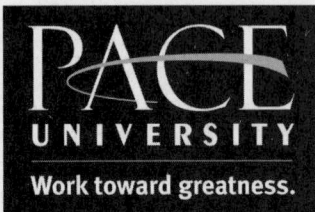

College of Health Professions

LIENHARD SCHOOL OF NURSING

PACE UNIVERSITY

Work toward greatness.

Discover unlimited opportunities in the health professions at Pace!

Professor Elizabeth Berro, MA, RN, with with Lienhard School of Nursing students.

The College of Health Professions

The Lienhard School of Nursing is part of Pace University's College of Health Professions, which was established in 2010 in an effort to showcase the breadth of health profession majors at Pace University. The College is made up of the Lienhard School of Nursing and the Pace University–Lenox Hill Hospital Physician Assistant Studies Program. The College's vision is innovative leadership in education, practice, and scholarship for the health professions. Its mission is to educate and challenge students for the health professions to be innovators and leaders who will positively impact global health care.

The Lienhard School of Nursing

Set within urban and suburban settings, the Lienhard School of Nursing (LSN) partners with many well-known primary, acute, and tertiary care facilities and community agencies to foster human growth and dignity and provide primary health care. The School is committed to helping individuals, families, and communities at local, national, and international levels that strive to meet health-care demands now and in the future. Lienhard's vision is to be a leader in innovation and excellence in education, research, and practice in primary health care.

The Lienhard School of Nursing considers teaching and learning its highest priorities and is committed to the integration of scholarship and practice. Graduates have the competitive edge through the School's focus on highly developed clinical skills and critical thinking, evidence-based practice, cultural competence, and leadership. LSN's primary health-care focus is intended to promote improved health outcomes for clients.

For more than 47 years, The Lienhard School of Nursing has been educating practitioners to deliver health care to indi-viduals and families. Its master's program is nationally ranked by *U.S. News & World Report.* In addition, its DNP program prepares nurses for the most advanced level of clinical practice.

Lienhard School of Nursing graduates are prepared to be leaders in both academic and health-care settings.

The Lienhard School of Nursing has many distinguished programs, faculty members, and services that give students a great start to nursing practice. The following programs are available:

- 4-year B.S. (Pleasantville campus only)
- Bridge Program to Advanced Degree (for RNs with a bachelor's degree in a field other than nursing)
- Combined Degree Program (CDP)—Accelerated BSN for non-nurse college graduates

- iPace RN/BS Completion Program for RNs with an associate degree or diploma in nursing

- MS/Family Nurse Practitioner (FNP)—Certificates of Advanced Graduate Studies (CAGS) also offered

- MA in Nursing Education (offered in a blended online and in-class format) —Certificates of Advanced Graduate Studies (CAGS) also offered

- Doctor of Nursing Practice (DNP) (New York City campus only)

What makes Lienhard School of Nursing programs unique?

- NCLEX pass rates are excellent and consistently exceed state and national averages.

- Students in the RN-4 program start nursing classes in their freshman year and clinicals in their sophomore year—earlier than many other programs, giving them an edge.

- The faculty is composed of excellent teachers/clinicians who partner with New York's premier hospitals and health-care organizations to share their expertise while creating unparalleled clinical experiences for Lienhard students. Graduates are prepared to be leaders in both academic and health-care settings.

Pace University's motto is *Opportunitas,* and it is the foundation of the LSN philosophy—offering students the *opportunity* to discover and fulfill their potential and offering a distinguished faculty and an outstanding staff the *opportunity* to achieve excellence.

Based on Lienhard School of Nursing's long and rich history of educating nurses, students can be confident that they will be prepared for positions of responsibility in all areas of health care and nursing education.

- *2012–13 UNDERGRADUATE TUITION & FEES:*

  For up-to-date, detailed information, visit:

  www.pace.edu/prospectivestudents/ undergraduate/tuition-fees

- *2012–13 GRADUATE TUITION & FEES:*

  For up-to-date, detailed information, visit:

  http://www.pace.edu/prospectivestudents/ graduate/tuition-fees

- *APPLICATION DEADLINES (domestic students):*

  RN-4 Program—February 15
  CDP 1-Year FT Program (Fall)—March 1
  CDP 1-Year FT Program (Spring)—September 1
  CDP 2-Year Program (Fall)—March 1
  CDP 2-Year Program (Spring)—September 1
  FNP Program (Fall)—March 1
  Nursing Education (Fall)—March 1
  DNP Program (Fall 2013 Cohort)—March 1

- *FACULTY INFORMATION:*

  www.pace.edu/lienhard/faculty

- *MULTIMEDIA:*

  www.pace.edu/lienhard

CONTACT INFORMATION

Sally Hay, Staff Assistant
Lienhard School of Nursing, College of Health Professions
Pace University
861 Bedford Road
Pleasantville, New York 10570
Phone: 914-773-3552
866-722-3338 (general info; toll-free)
E-mail: nursing@pace.edu
Web site: www.pace.edu/lienhard

Find Lienhard on Facebook®: https://www.facebook.com/lienhardnursing
Follow Pace University on Twitter™: http://twitter.com/paceuniversity

Professor Andrea Sonenberg, DNSc, RN, with Lienhard School of Nursing students.

QUINNIPIAC
UNIVERSITY

School of Nursing

Education with a Personal Touch.

Professional nursing courses take place in the Graduate and Health Sciences building on Quinnipiac's 104-acre North Haven campus.

Quinnipiac University (QU), located in Hamden, Connecticut, just 8 miles from New Haven and midway between New York City and Boston, has 6,200 undergraduate and 2,000 graduate students. QU offers the B.S. in Nursing, an Accelerated B.S.N. for those who hold a non-nursing college degree, the M.S.N. in Nursing (Nurse Practitioner) and the graduate D.N.P. Doctorate of Nursing Practice plus two post-master's tracks.

Our view of nursing as a profession is that it is research-based and goal-directed as well as creative and concerned with the health and dignity of the whole person. The art of delivering high-quality nursing care depends on the successful mastery and application of intellectually rigorous nursing knowledge. Quinnipiac takes this a step further in developing an approach to health care that broadens awareness and encompasses other health-care majors in the School of Health Sciences and the Frank H. Netter MD School of Medicine by fostering a teamwork approach in providing health care to patients of all ages, abilities, and backgrounds.

Accredited by the National League for Nursing Accrediting Commission (NLNAC), Quinnipiac's bachelor's degree program in nursing offers the theoretical and clinical education students need to enter professional nursing practice. Graduates of the program are eligible to take the NCLEX-RN exam and are well prepared for graduate study in nursing. The nursing curriculum fosters professional socialization for future roles and responsibilities within the profession. Graduates of the program are prepared as generalists to begin the practice of holistic professional nursing, with sound theoretical foundations and nearly 800 hours of diverse clinical practice and laboratory experiences. In addition to the traditional four-year program, an innovative accelerated second degree option is available to non-nurse college graduates.

The graduate nursing program prepares professional nurses at an advanced theoretical and clinical practice level in order to address present and potential societal health needs. The Master of Science in Nursing broadens the scope of practice and provides for the acquisition of expertise in an area of specialization (Adult-Gerontology Nurse Practitioner or Family Nurse Practitioner). The D.N.P. program prepares students for leadership roles in advanced specialty practice, nursing leadership, and organizational management. The program commences a clinical doctorate resulting in the Doctorate of Nursing Practice (D.N.P.) degree. Two available tracks are Adult-Gerontology Nurse Practitioner and Family Nurse Practitioner. The following Post-master's tracks are also available: the Care of Individuals (for licensed APRNs) and the Care of Populations (for master's prepared nurses who are not APRNs). The graduate nursing program includes core courses that cover advanced concepts and theoretical foundations of nursing, epidemiology, and health-care policy and economics.

Quinnipiac's strong affiliates with health-care providers in the area allow students to complete clinical work at such institutions as Yale-New Haven Hospital, Connecticut Children's Medical Center, the Hospital of St. Raphael, and MidState Medical Center as well as in private practices, clinics, and other health-care centers.

Quinnipiac's Mount Carmel Campus is the main location for housing, recreation, and course work for undergraduates in their first two years. Starting in the junior year, the professional courses in nursing take place on the nearby 104-acre North Haven campus in the Graduate and Health Sciences building, which houses a remarkable facility with state-of-the-art technologies to prepare health-care professionals in a variety of fields. The

Clinical Simulation Labs house "patients" that are lifelike simulation mannequins. Cameras capture the simulation for student assessment. The Pediatric/Neonatal Lab is filled with infant mannequins and introduces students to this special area of health care in the acute setting. The Clinical Skills labs and the Intensive Care Unit create real-world conditions to prepare students for clinical training assignments. The Physical Diagnosis Lab, Physical Exam Suite, and Health Assessment Lab duplicate care in an outpatient primary care setting, such as an emergency room or doctor's office.

For more on the North Haven campus, see www.quinnipiac.edu/resources-facilities/.

Students applying as freshmen into the nursing program should file their application for admission by November 15. Information regarding admission requirements can be found at http://www.quinnipiac.edu/apply. Transfer students must have a minimum 3.0 GPA and are considered on a space-available basis.

The accelerated (second degree) nursing program begins in August. The complete application and all supporting documents must be filed by January 1. See www.quinnipiac.edu/accelerated for details.

Graduate admission information for the D.N.P. and the post-master's tracks can be found at www.quinnipiac.edu/gradnursing.

- *2013–14 UNDERGRADUATE TUITION & FEES:*

  Full-time: $39,330 (tuition and fees); $14,250 (room and board)

  Part-time: $900 per credit

- *2013–14 GRADUATE TUITION: $895 per credit plus $35 per credit student fee.*

- *APPLICATION DEADLINES:*

  Undergraduate applicants should apply by Nov. 1 for fall admission

  Graduate students should contact the Office of Graduate Admissions for deadline information

- *FACULTY INFORMATION:*

  http://www.quinnipiac.edu/nursing

- *MULTIMEDIA:*

  http://www.quinnipiac.edu/prebuilt/vtour/vtour. html

In the pediatrics maternity lab, students learn about fetal development and birthing. Students are taught to bathe and swaddle infants as well as how to educate new mothers about infant care.

CONTACT INFORMATION

Joan Isaac Mohr
VP for Admissions & Financial Aid
Admissions Office
Quinnipiac University
275 Mt. Carmel Avenue
Hamden, Connecticut 06518
Phone: 203-582-8600
              800-462-1944 (toll-free)
Fax: 203-582-8906
E-mail: admissions@quinnipiac.edu
Web site: http://www.quinnipiac.edu

Undergraduate Nursing Program:
Office of Undergraduate Admissions
Phone: 203-582-8600
E-mail: admissions@quinnipiac.edu

Graduate Nursing Program:
Office of Graduate Admissions
Phone: 203-582-8672
E-mail: graduate@quinnipiac.edu

ROBERTS
WESLEYAN COLLEGE
Education for Character Since 1866

DEPARTMENT OF NURSING

Nurses know . . . one degree can make a difference!

The Roberts Wesleyan College Department of Nursing enjoys an excellent reputation for preparing graduates who are respected and sought-after in the healthcare community. Students also find that the experience of attending Roberts Wesleyan College impacts their view of the world and helps them to think more about what it means to be a Christian professional in the contemporary healthcare environment.

In addition to the traditional undergraduate program, Roberts meets the needs of working RNs who are looking to advance their knowledge of nursing science, leadership, and education. Working RNs who hold an associate degree and want to earn a bachelor's degree in nursing, as well as nurses who hold bachelor's degrees and want to earn their master's degree in nursing, find the nursing programs of Roberts Wesleyan College beneficial to their careers and professional lives in general.

RN-BS PROGRAM

The Modular R.N. to B.S. Program is a unique alternative to the traditional method of pursuing a college degree. Recognizing the needs of adult learners, the Department of Nursing at Roberts Wesleyan has designed a curriculum that is stimulating, relevant, challenging, and rewarding. It is designed specifically for registered nurses who want to earn their bachelor's degree while continuing to work. The program is completed while attending class just one night per week or online for 15 months.

- Offered at Clifton Springs Hospital in Clifton Springs, New York; Noyes Memorial Hospital in Dansville, New York; St. Ann's Community and Unity at Ridgeway, in Rochester, New York; as well as in Weedsport and Williamsville, New York

- Available to take completely online three times a year in March, July, and October

- College credit granted for life and work experience

- Curriculum and teaching style are great preparation for master's degree

- No tests

- Your practice experience is met in the workplace and through other course work

MASTER OF SCIENCE IN NURSING PROGRAMS

The Roberts Wesleyan Department of Nursing graduate programs are designed specifically for bachelor's-prepared, working RNs. Based on nursing science, the programs can be completed in 20 months completely online or by attending class just one night per week.

Students in the Master of Science in Nursing Education (MSNE) Program:

- Develop expertise through practice teaching in an area of choice

- Implement evidence-based teaching

- Prepare to work in multiple teaching settings

- Design a curriculum

- Master the latest technological advances in education

Students in the Master of Science in Nursing Leadership & Administration (MSNLA) Program:

- Sharpen their knowledge of administration and management in nursing

- Develop their visionary leadership skills and their impact on healthcare system improvement

- Prepare to lead in multiple settings

- Gain new expertise through internships in areas of choice

- Benefit from a significant focus on the business aspect of health care

POST-MASTERS CERTIFICATES

These programs are offered to nurses who have a master's degree in nursing. Nurses who desire expertise in education and the teaching/learning of nursing students or nursing staff can enroll in the Nursing Education Certificate Program. The Post-Masters certificate in Nursing Leadership & Administration is for those who desire specialized knowledge in the business aspects of healthcare. The 18-credit hours of study in each program may fulfill the education criteria for certification exams.

• *2012–13 TUITION & FEES*

Undergraduate Nursing Program:

Tuition: $25,350*; Fees: $974**; Room: $5932; Board: $3332; Total: $35.588

*The cost of books and fees for certain courses are in addition to tuition charges.
**A one-time student fee of $375 is also charged to all incoming students.

Non-Traditional Modular RN to BS Program:
$22,554 including books and fees

Graduate Nursing Program:
$29,238 including books and fees

• *APPLICATION DEADLINES*

Traditional Undergraduate Priority Deadline:
February 1 (applications are reviewed after this date if space is available)

Non-Traditional Modular RN to BS Program:
Applications are accepted continuously

Graduate Nursing Program:
Applications are accepted continuously

• *FACULTY INFORMATION:*
http://www.roberts.edu/academics/divisions/ nursing/Division_Info/faculty_staff.asp

CONTACT INFORMATION

Department of Nursing
Roberts Wesleyan College
2301 Westside Drive
Rochester, New York 14624
Phone: 585-594-6000
800-777-4792 (4RWC; toll-free)
Web site: www.roberts.edu/nursing

Undergraduate Nursing Program:
Phone: 585-594-6330
Fax: 585-594-6593

Non-Traditional Modular RN to BS Program:
Stephanie Sheets
Phone: 585-594-6634
Fax: 585-594-6599
E-mail: SheetsS@Roberts.edu

Graduate Nursing Program:
Brenda Mutton
Phone: 585-594-6686
Fax: 585-594-6593
E-mail: Mutton_Brenda@Roberts.edu

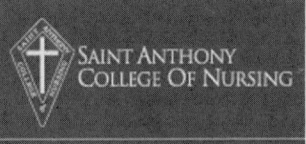

SAINT ANTHONY COLLEGE OF NURSING

Personal, individualized attention in a caring environment.

SACN students attain a broad spectrum of scientific, critical thinking, humanistic, communication, and leadership concepts and experiences expected of today's medical professionals.

Saint Anthony College of Nursing (SACN) is a specialized college granting the Bachelor of Science in Nursing (B.S.N.) and Master of Science in Nursing (M.S.N.) degrees. The College is located in Rockford, Illinois, in the north-central part of the state. The surrounding area provides much to see and do. Students receive excellent academic instruction along with abundant clinical experience.

Striving for excellence in nursing education, SACN's upper-division baccalaureate nursing program integrates Christian ideals, values, and practices, while building on a broad foundation of general education courses in the humanities and sciences.

SACN students are admitted as juniors, entering with the prerequisite credits from another regionally accredited college or university. They complete the last two years of a four-year Bachelor of Science in Nursing (B.S.N.) degree, which provides a broad spectrum of scientific, critical thinking, humanistic, communication, and leadership concepts and experiences expected of today's medical professionals. These last two years build on the broad base of two academic years (64 semester hours) transferred

from another regionally accredited college or university. To this end, cooperative agreements have been reached with several of the community colleges in the area. Prospective students are encouraged to work with the SACN admissions office at the beginning of their college career to ensure transfer of credits.

Clinical sites for B.S.N. students include Carrie Lynn Children's Center, Walter Lawson's Children's Home, Rosecrance Treatment Centers, Northern Illinois Hospice, Rockford Memorial Hospital, Rockford Public Schools, OSF Saint Anthony Medical Center, Visiting Nurses Association, Winnebago County Health Department, Winnebago County Housing Authority, and many other institutions.

Registered Nurses with an associate degree or diploma in nursing may apply for admission to the RN-to-BSN program. This program is designed with the working nurse in mind. Courses are held one night per week with a hybrid format (partially online and partially face-to-face), allowing the student flexibility and convenience. The RN-to-BSN program is offered on the main campus as well as in Freeport, Illinois, on Highland Community College's campus.

Graduate students enroll in a program designed for the part-time student to complete within three or four years, leading to a Master of Science in Nursing degree for nurse educators, clinical nurse leaders, clinical nurse specialists in adult health concepts, and family nurse practitioners. The faculty and staff members are well known for their ability to provide personal, individualized attention in a caring environment. Classes are generally held one night per week, with additional work done online.

Students entering the master's program must enter with a bachelor's degree. Students may present with a baccalaureate degree in nursing (B.S.N.) or a baccalaureate in a field other than nursing. Licensure as a registered nurse is required for the state in which they will partake of their clinical practicum. If the student's baccalaureate degree is not in nursing, he or she must successfully complete an undergraduate nursing concepts course and nursing research course from a regionally accredited college or university prior to enrolling in the master's-level nursing concepts course or nursing research course.

A post-master's certificate is available for those who already have earned an M.S.N. degree but would like to take courses toward eligibility for the Nurse Educator Certificate. Student-at-Large status is available for graduate students. Interested students should contact the Graduate Affairs Office for details.

The student-to-faculty ratio at SACN is less than 8:1, and the NCLEX-RN pass rate for 2012 was 100 percent. In addition, 85 percent of all undergraduate students applied for and received financial aid. Because SACN is a nonresidential facility, students commute from their homes or find a residence in the Rockford area.

Saint Anthony College of Nursing is accredited by the Higher Learning Commission, member of the North Central Association of Colleges and Schools (NCA). The B.S.N. and M.S.N. programs are accredited by the Commission on Collegiate Nursing Education.

- *2012–13 UNDERGRADUATE TUITION & FEES*

  Full-time: $10,067 per semester

  Part-time: $630 per credit

  Testing fees vary from $93–$120

  Supplies fee: $60 (first semester)

  Graduation fee: $160

- *2012–13 GRADUATE TUITION & FEES:*
  $767 per credit

- *APPLICATION DEADLINES:*

  Undergraduate students: September 15 (spring admission); February 15 (fall admission)

  Graduate students: February 1

- *FACULTY INFORMATION:*
  http://www.sacn.edu/contact/

- *MULTIMEDIA:*
  http://www.sacn.edu

CONTACT INFORMATION

Nancy Sanders, Associate Dean
Saint Anthony College of Nursing
5658 E. State Street
Rockford, Illinois 61108-2468
Phone: 815-395-5100
Fax: 815-395-2275
E-mail: admissions@sacn.edu
Web site: http://www.sacn.edu

UNDERGRADUATE NURSING PROGRAM:
Cheryl Delgado
Supervisor of Enrollment Management
Phone: 815-227-2141
E-mail: cheryldelgado@sacn.edu

GRADUATE NURSING PROGRAM:
Melissa Aukes
Student Affairs Specialist–Graduate Affairs
Phone: 815-395-5476
E-mail: melissawrolstad@sacn.edu

Saint Anthony College of Nursing students have a high graduation rate—92 percent of all students who attend the first day of class (full-time and part-time) will graduate.

ST.FRANCIS COLLEGE
THE SMALL COLLEGE OF BIG DREAMS

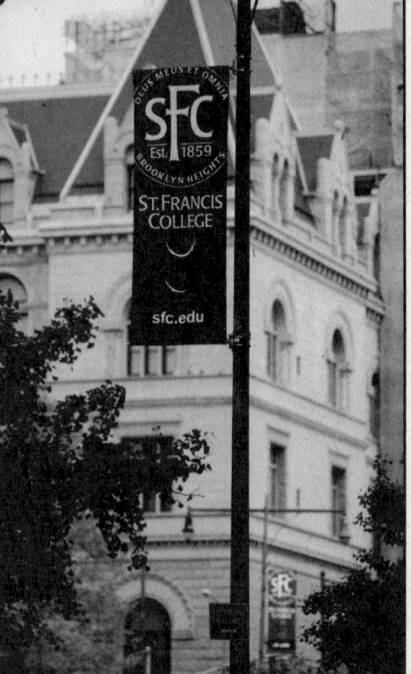

St. Francis College has been recognized by "U.S. News & World Report" among the best regional colleges in the north and was named by Forbes.com to its America's Best Colleges List.

NURSING PROGRAM

Building a foundation of knowledge that will contribute to the development of the nursing profession and society as a whole.

Quality Private Education

Graduates of the St. Francis College Nursing Program go on to a wide variety of nursing careers at many of the best hospitals and health-care institutions in New York and nationally. St. Francis students are accepted into top graduate programs in nursing that include Columbia University Teacher's College, Long Island University, New York University, Pace University, and SUNY Downstate, among others. The College's well-rounded nursing program prepares its graduates for graduate school admission into careers as nurse practitioners, clinical specialists, administrators, and nurse educators.

Academic Excellence

St. Francis College consistently makes the grade when it comes to college rankings. *U.S. News & World Report* classifies St. Francis as one of the "best regional colleges in the North," while Forbes.com just placed St. Francis on its America's Top Colleges list for the fourth year in a row.

Prepare Yourself for the Future of Nursing

The Nursing program at St. Francis College offers a Bachelor of Science degree to qualified transfer students with a valid New York State RN license. St. Francis is registered with the New York State Education Department

and accredited by the Commission on Collegiate Nursing Education (CCNE), the accrediting arm of the American Association of Colleges of Nursing (AACN). In addition to nursing courses that include physical assessment, leadership, research and community health, and informatics, nursing students gain valuable knowledge and skill in liberal arts and sciences through courses focused on mathematics, natural sciences, social sciences, advanced writing, and oral communication.

Flexible scheduling allows for full- or part-time study. In fact, the program is designed for nurses who wish to keep working while continuing their education. Courses are scheduled to best fit the time commitments of working nurses. All students are required to complete the program within a maximum five-year period.

Department Mission

The mission of the Department of Nursing is consistent with the overall mission of the College—to promote the development of the whole person by integrating a liberal arts education with preprofessional programs designed to prepare nurses for the rigors of an increasingly technological and globalized marketplace and society. The department's mission encompasses the Franciscan and Catholic traditions that underpin its commitment to academic excellence, spiritual and moral values, physical fitness, social responsibility, and lifelong learning. These traditions include The Franciscan tradition of service, equality, aesthetics, freedom, honor, dignity, justice, and truth that are demonstrated within the context of professional nursing standards at the baccalaureate level (AACN Baccalaureate Essentials; ANA Standards of Clinical Nursing Practice). This nursing program builds a foundation of knowledge that will contribute to the development of the nursing profession as well as society as a whole.

Students who successfully complete the St. Francis Nursing program are able to:

- Integrate knowledge from bio/psycho/social/spiritual dimensions in caring for individuals, families, groups, and communities.

- Apply the nursing process in the delivery of culturally competent nursing care.

- Apply principles of leadership and management in caring for individuals, families, groups, and communities.

- Demonstrate accountability and responsibility for individual nursing actions.

- Collaborate as a member of a multidisciplinary healthcare team.

- Analyze research findings and technological advances for their applicability to clinical practice.

- Analyze national and international health policy initiatives for their impact on service, equality, aesthetics, freedom, human dignity, justice, and health of populations.

- Critically analyze the rationale for the nursing care provided.

- Incorporate the Franciscan tradition of service, equality, aesthetics, freedom, honor, dignity, justice, and truth into daily nursing practice.

- Recognize the legal and ethical health policy ramifications central to the delivery of health care.

- Demonstrate proficiency in the use of technology in the delivery of nursing care.

For details on tuition and fees, application deadlines, and more information, please visit the College's Web site at www.sfc.edu.

- *FACULTY:*

www.sfc.edu/nursing

- *APPLICATION INFORMATION:*

Students are encouraged to apply through Nursing CA, the national centralized application service for students applying to registered nursing programs in the United States. Apply online at www.nursingcas.org.

Online applications are also available at www.sfc.edu.

CONTACT INFORMATION

Office of Admissions
St. Francis College
180 Remsen Street
Brooklyn Heights, NY 11201
Phone: 718-489-5200
Web sites: www.sfc.edu
           www.sfc.edu/nursing

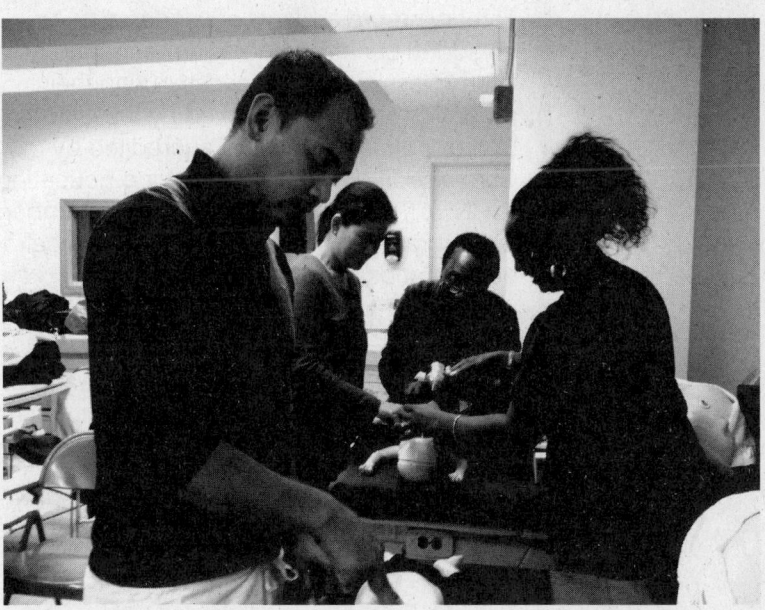

Hands-on work with Sim Baby exposes St. Francis Nursing students to real-world medical scenarios.

The University of Akron

Transforming Lives through Caring, Competence, and Commitment.

University of Akron Nursing students engaged in a simulation of basic nursing skills and assessment.

Founded in 1967, originally as the College of Nursing, in 2012 it became the School of Nursing within the College of Health Professions. The School of Nursing at The University of Akron (UA) offers multiple programs for students aspiring to become professional nurses and practicing nurses seeking career and professional advancement. As an added benefit, students are engaged in interprofessional experiences during their programs of study. Approved by the Ohio Board of Nursing and fully accredited by the Commission on Collegiate Nursing Education (CCNE), the School employs faculty members with a broad range of research and clinical backgrounds.

The basic Baccalaureate program is a four-year program. Clinical experiences are required in each semester of the program after the first year. The senior year features a senior practicum designed to give the student greater depth in an area of the student's choosing. A fifteen-month Accelerated B.S.N. program is open to students who hold a bachelor's degree.

The LPN/B.S.N. for the licensed LPN features testing for advanced placement. The LPN can finish the B.S.N. in five semesters.

The RN/B.S.N. sequence for the registered nurse (RN) features a full-time or part-time option and flexible hours for clinical requirements. Students can select from one of two options of delivery: the totally online option or via distance learning at one of UA's sites offered at the Lorain County Community College campus, Wayne College, Lakeland Community College, UA Lakewood, and Medina County University Center (MCUC). For the distance learning option, classes are scheduled to meet one day per week.

The Master of Science in Nursing (M.S.N.) program prepares graduates for advanced practice or administration. Students may choose adult/gerontological health nursing, family behavioral health nursing, child and adolescent health nursing acute or primary care, or nurse anesthesia tracks. Advanced practice options include nurse practitioner (NP) or clinical nurse specialist (CNS). A post-masters certificate is also available for the Family Nurse Practitioner.

The RN/M.S.N. sequence is designed for RNs who meet graduate admission criteria. Students take three years to complete both the B.S.N. and master's course work.

A Doctor of Nursing Practice (D.N.P.) program is approved and enrolling students for the fall 2013 semester. This post-master's degree program for advanced practice nurses is clinically focused, preparing students to generate clinical evidence, translate research, and develop evidence-based guidelines for practice in varied healthcare environments. The D.N.P. is offered in a hybrid format with a blend of intensive face-to-face (2 weekends per semester) and distance and/or asynchronous learning modalities. The student can complete the program in two years of full-time study (two courses per semester). Part-time options are also available.

The University of Akron and Kent State University offer a Joint Ph.D. in Nursing (JPDN) program.

The School has a state-of-the-art Learning Resources Center (LRC) that includes simulated patient-care areas and a computer laboratory. The simulation area includes a birthing suite, an advanced clinical unit, and a control room providing video capture for students to review their work with faculty members.

The Nursing Center for Community Health links the School to the community and is used by the underinsured and medically vulnerable populations in the area for health-care services and by the faculty and students as a practice and research site.

Students applying for all baccalaureate programs must have completed prerequisite college/university courses. Basic B.S.N. candidates must have earned at least a 2.75 grade point average (GPA) in prerequisite and science courses. Course work begins in the fall.

Students entering the LPN/B.S.N. sequence must hold a current Ohio LPN license with a minimum prerequisite and science GPA of 2.75. Course work begins in January.

Requirements for the RN/B.S.N. sequence include a prerequisite GPA of 2.75 (or 3.0 for RN/M.S.N.) and current Ohio RN licensure. Course work begins in May.

Students applying to the M.S.N. program must hold a baccalaureate degree in nursing from an accredited nursing program; complete prerequisite courses; submit scores from the CCRN (CRNA program only), an essay, and three letters of reference; and hold a current Ohio RN license.

- *2012–13 UNDERGRADUATE TUITION & FEES (full year):* $10,300 (Ohio Resident/full-time); $5260 (Ohio Resident/part-time); $18,200 (Nonresident/full-time); $9100 (Nonresident/part-time)

- *2012–13 GRADUATE TUITION & FEES (full year):* $8065 (Ohio Resident/full-time); $4140 (Ohio Resident/part-time); $12,900 (Nonresident/full-time); $5920 (Nonresident/part-time)

- *APPLICATION DEADLINES: The University of Akron has rolling admissions year round. Contact the appropriate Admissions Office for specific deadlines for each semester: http://www.uakron.edu/admissions/.*

- *FACULTY INFORMATION: http://www.uakron.edu/nursing/about-us/*

- *MULTIMEDIA: http://www.uakron.edu/nursing/*

CONTACT INFORMATION

Dr. Elaine Fisher
Interim Director, School of Nursing
College of Health Professions
The University of Akron
302 Buchtel Common
Akron, Ohio 44325-3701
Phone: 330-972-6674
        888-477-7887 (toll-free)
Fax: 330-972-5493
E-mail: nursinginfo@uakron.edu
Web site: www.uakron.edu/nursing

Graduate Nursing Program:
Marlene Huff, Assistant Director of Graduate Programs
Phone: 330-972-5930
        888-477-7887 (toll-free)
Fax: 330-972-5493
E-mail: mhuff@uakron.edu
Web site: www.uakron.edu/nursing

Find us on Facebook®: http://www.facebook.com/uanursing
Follow us on Twitter™: http://twitter.com/uanursing

Using various models, UA Nursing students practice their skills.

University of San Diego®

HAHN SCHOOL OF NURSING AND HEALTH SCIENCE

A Private School with a Public Conscience.

Excellence in Nursing.

Since 1974, the University of San Diego's Hahn School of Nursing and Health Science has provided high-quality education to more than 2,100 alumni and 260 doctorally prepared nurse scientists. With an impressive global network of clinical partners, preceptors, and granting agencies, the School consistently ranks in the top tier of graduate nursing programs nationwide.

Faculty members prepare nurse scientists and leaders in education and practice in a research-intensive community of progressive scholars. The School seeks to deepen its commitment to social justice and health care as a human right by influencing health policy and promoting an ethical approach to nursing characterized by compassion and respect for the dignity of the individual.

International clinical, research, and cultural immersion experiences are available in Mexico, the Dominican Republic, India, and Pacific Rim countries. Participating students are accompanied by faculty members who are experts in international health.

The Hahn School of Nursing offers the Doctor of Philosophy (Ph.D.) and Doctor of Nursing Practice (D.N.P.) degrees as well as the Master of Science in Nursing (M.S.N.) degree for RNs. MSN specialties include Clinical Nurse Leader, Executive Nurse Leader, Health Care Informatics, Adult-Gerontology Clinical Nurse Specialist and Primary Care Nurse Practitioner. For those with a non-nursing degree (baccalaureate or higher), the School offers a Master's Entry Program in Nursing (MEPN). In addition, the School offers a Post-BSN-DNP program for RNs who desire preparation in primary care as a Family, Dual Pediatric/Family, or Dual Adult-Gerontology/ Family Nurse Practitioner, in Family/Lifespan Psychiatric-Mental Health as a Nurse Practitioner or dual preparation as a Nurse Practitioner/Clinical Nurse Specialist, and preparation in Adult-Gerontology as a Clinical Nurse Specialist.

Classes are offered in traditional fifteen-week semesters in spring and fall and also in concentrated intersession and summer semesters.

The School provides mentoring in a research-intensive environment and specializes in personalized attention and small classes, labs, and clinical practicums taught by doctorally prepared and/or clinically certified faculty members. The students—women and men who represent many faiths, ethnic groups, and geographical regions—share in common intellectual curiosity, critical thinking skills, and compassion for their patients.

The Hahn School of Nursing and Health Science occupies a recently renovated 18,000-square-foot, two-story building and the newly renovated and equipped 5,000-square-foot Simulation and Standardized Patient Nursing Laboratory, a unique educational resource in Southern California. With a trauma center, birthing area, and nursing station, this state-of-the art facility uses trained "patient" actors and programmed robotic equipment to simulate primary-care, acute-care, and emergency situations to ensure that students develop the full range of clinical skills. Student performances are digitally recorded and evaluated by peers and the clinical instructors. The School is one of the few nursing schools in the country with the Standardized Patient Program.

The School is affiliated with a wide variety of clinical resources, including UCSD Medical Center, Sharp Health Care (Hospitals and Clinics), Palomar Health Care System, Scripps Health (Hospitals and Clinics), Children's Hospital, Veterans Administration Hospital, Kaiser Permanente, and Balboa Naval Hospital. Many community agencies are also utilized, including schools, home health agencies, the San Diego Department of Health Services, HMOs, and community clinics.

The University of San Diego, a Catholic institution of higher learning chartered in 1949, enrolls some 8,200 undergraduate and graduate students and is known for its commitment to teaching, the liberal arts, the formation of values and community service.

Nursing programs are fully accredited by the Commission on Collegiate Nursing Education (CCNE) and the California Board of Registered Nursing.

- *2012–13 GRADUATE TUITION & FEES*
  Master's Programs: $1285 per unit
  Doctoral Programs: $1315 per unit
  Living Expenses: Approximately $15,000 per year
  Other Educational Expenses: Approximately $5000 per year

- *FOR MORE INFORMATION:*
  http://www.sandiego.edu/nursing

- *APPLICATION DEADLINES:*
  Ph.D.: February 1
  D.N.P.: March 1
  Master's Entry Program in Nursing: November 1
  M.S.N. Programs: March 1 (fall entry); November 1 (spring entry)
  [Note: Spring entry is not available for the Nurse Practitioner programs]

- *FACULTY INFORMATION:*
  http://www.sandiego.edu/nursing/faculty/

- *MULTIMEDIA: http://www.sandiego.edu/ nursing/programs/video_overview.php*

CONTACT INFORMATION

Hahn School of Nursing and Health Science
University of San Diego
5998 Alcala Park
San Diego, California 92110-2492
Phone: 619-260-4548
Fax: 619-260-6814
Web site:
    http://www.sandiego.edu/nursing

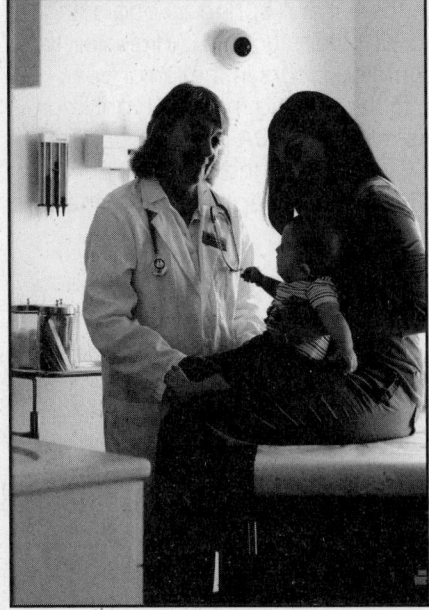

The University of San Diego provides excellent and diverse clinical/research experiences.

UNIVERSITY of WISCONSIN

UW MILWAUKEE

College of Nursing

Graduate students are key research partners and clinical partners in the College of Nursing at UW-Milwaukee.

IDEAS: Innovation, Discovery, Engagement, Access, Solutions.

As Wisconsin's largest nursing program, the University of Wisconsin–Milwaukee College of Nursing has made its home in the commercial, cultural, and economic capital of Wisconsin since 1965. Across Southeastern Wisconsin, our competitive, collaborative nursing program is valued for its ability to prepare science-based, compassionate nurse leaders through innovative, high-quality educational programs. The College is a vibrant, innovative environment for teaching, research, practice, and service to the community and the profession. The largest nursing school in Wisconsin, the College is one of three institutions in the state to offer students the full range of nursing degrees: Bachelor of Science in Nursing (B.S.), Master of Nursing (M.N.), Doctor of Philosophy in Nursing (Ph.D.) and Doctor of Nursing Practice (D.N.P.). The College of Nursing has an enrollment of 1,197 undergraduate students as well as 219 graduate students.

The College of Nursing's faculty members create innovative classroom environments and provide the latest technological teaching tools. The College is consistently ranked in the top 10 percent for its academic excellence by the *U.S. News and World Report* of colleges with Graduate Nursing Programs. Faculty members also embrace practice by engaging regional and global communities to develop solutions in improving health care.

The College enjoys clinical practice and research partnerships with over 130 clinical facilities throughout Southeastern Wisconsin and beyond. The College's Community Nursing Centers address the health needs of at-risk urban populations, engaging with community members to establish health-care solutions to fit their needs. Nationally recognized initiatives include the Collaborative for Intelligent Health Information Systems Initiative (CIHISI), a research center dedicated to creating health information technology solutions that improve the access, quality, and costs of health care. The Pediatric Nursing Research Consortium, a partnership with Children's Hospital of Wisconsin, the Medical College of Wisconsin, and Marquette University, combines the resources of clinical and academic researchers to create translational research in the care of children and families. The Self Management Science Center, a continuation of NIH Funded P20, expands research aimed at enhancing the science of the self-management in individuals and families. Faculty members have also extended the scope of international research to health care in rural Malawi and Kenya. The College also maintains a close relationship with two sister nursing schools in South Korea.

The baccalaureate, master, and doctorate programs are accredited by the Commission on Collegiate Nursing Education. The College of Nursing is also affiliated with Sigma Theta Tau International, Eta Nu Chapter, and the Nursing Centers Research Network.

The undergraduate nursing program is built upon a rigorous science-based curriculum and requires a dedication to scholarship and a passion for health care. Individuals may be considered for admission as pre-nursing students in the fall and spring as beginning freshmen or transfer students. Admission to the clinical major occurs in the junior year. Admission to the nursing major is highly competitive; the minimum GPA required can be significantly higher than the stated minimum GPA of 2.75 needed for application to the nursing major.

The College of Nursing continues to expand and enhance its graduate program opportunities. The College offers the Master in Nursing (M.N.) with two entry options. Entry to the Master of Nursing degree is for nurses and non-nurses who hold a bachelor's degree. The program provides the groundwork for practice as a clinical nurse leader, public health nurse, clinical research manager, informatician, or nurse manager. In addition to the Master of Nursing, the College offers a Doctor of Nursing Practice (D.N.P.) and Doctor of Philosophy in Nursing (Ph.D.) in face-to-face and online formats.

Graduate program application deadlines depend on the program of interest. Generally, applications are due to UWM by February 1 for fall enrollment and October 1 for spring semester enrollment. Prospective students are encouraged to visit the College Web site for more detailed information about admission requirements.

- *2012–13 UNDERGRADUATE TUITION & FEES:*
  Annual Full-time: $9187 (residents)
  $18,915 (nonresidents)

  Additional tuition differential fee of $32 per credit is due upon admission to the clinical major.

- *2012–13 GRADUATE TUITION & FEES:*
  Annual Full-time: $11,482 (residents)
  $23,948 (nonresidents)

- *APPLICATION DEADLINES:*
  Undergraduate: August 15 for spring admission to clinical major; January 15 for fall admission to clinical major.

  Graduate: February 1 for fall admission; October 1 for spring admission

- *FACULTY INFORMATION:*
  http://www4.uwm.edu/nursing/

CONTACT INFORMATION

Robin Jens, Director of Student Affairs
University of Wisconsin–Milwaukee
College of Nursing
1921 East Hartford Avenue
P.O. Box 413
Milwaukee, Wisconsin 53201
Phone: 414-229-5047
Fax: 414-229-5554
E-mail: asknursing@uwm.edu
Web site: www.nursing.uwm.edu

UNDERGRADUATE NURSING PROGRAM:
Deatra Holloway, Advisor
Undergraduate Pre-Nursing
Student Affairs Office
Room 129 – Cunningham hall
Phone: 414-229-5484
E-mail: hdd@uwm.edu

Donna Wier, Senior Advisor
Undergraduate Admissions
Student Affairs Office
Room 129-Cunningham Hall
Phone: 414-229-5481
E-mail: ddw@uwm.edu

GRADUATE NURSING PROGRAM:
Jennifer Daood, Advisor
Graduate Admissions
Student Affairs Office
Room 129–Cunningham Hall
Phone: 414-229-5474
E-mail: daood@uwm.edu

Find us on Facebook®: http://on.fb.me/UWM_Nursing

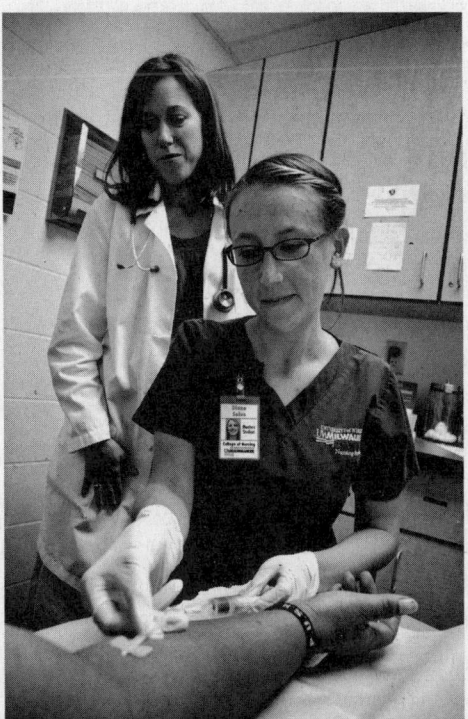

Undergraduate nursing education at UW–Milwaukee maximizes hands-on learning, technological innovation and training, and a comprehensive survey of nursing theory and practice.

Ursuline

VALUES·VOICE·VISION

Breen School of Nursing

Transforming health through reflection and healing.

Located on a beautiful, 100-acre wooded campus in Pepper Pike, Ohio, just 15 miles east of Cleveland, Ursuline's campus is safe, intimate, and easily accessible.

Nursing has been a vital program at Ursuline College since 1975. Today, the Breen School of Nursing has the largest academic program on campus. An individualized approach enables students to enjoy personalized instruction while learning the material in greater depth by gaining experience in a wide variety of health-care environments. Breen School graduates are highly sought by employers who find them to be well prepared and flexible in adapting to new settings.

The Breen School of Nursing offers the Bachelor of Science in Nursing (B.S.N.), Master of Science in Nursing (M.S.N.), and Doctor of Nursing Practice (D.N.P.) degree programs, as well as post-master's certificates. The total nursing enrollment is approximately 600 students per year. The School's NCLEX-RN exam first-time pass rate is 98% for traditional B.S.N. graduates and 100% for the Second Degree Accelerated B.S.N. Program graduates. The M.S.N. program offers the following Advanced Practice Registered Nurse (APRN) role and population-focused education tracks: Adult Health Clinical Nurse Specialist, Adult Nurse Practitioner, and Family Nurse Practitioner. Nursing education and palliative care are also offered as additional subspecialty

components to the M.S.N. or D.N.P. tracks. The focus of the post-M.S.N. and D.N.P. degree is leadership in evidence-based practice and policy development.

The B.S.N. and M.S.N. programs are accredited by the Commission on Collegiate Nursing Education (CCNE). The D.N.P. program, which was initiated in fall 2010, is approved by the Ohio Board of Regents and accredited by the Higher Learning Commission of North Central Association of Colleges and Schools. A CCNE-accreditation visit to review the D.N.P. program was made in November 2011 and full approval was conferred.

The Breen School of Nursing is affiliated with numerous internationally renowned health-care agencies that include the Cleveland Clinic Health Care System and the University Case Medical Center and Health System. M.S.N. and D.N.P. students may elect to complete their practicum and capstone experiences in another state or country.

The School's Nursing Resource Center (NRC) lab has four mid-fidelity manikins and four low-fidelity manikins for practicing skills, vital signs, health assessment, and simulation. The lab has a virtual IV computer that enables students to train on intravenous catheter insertion with a variety of scenarios as well as to complete an IV competency. Individual workstations allow nursing students to practice skills such as intramuscular, intravenous, and subcutaneous injections.

Undergraduate applications are accepted on a rolling basis. In addition to meeting the criteria for clear admission to the College, applicants seeking admission to the B.S.N. program directly from high school need to have a GPA of 2.75 or higher and minimum ACT scores of 20 or SAT composite scores of 1000. Students must also demonstrate proficiency by achieving a grade of at least C+ in algebra, biology with lab, and chemistry with lab. Transfer students need a strong recommendation from a counselor or teacher and at least a 2.5 cumulative GPA average in all completed college work. Applicants who have attended or are currently attending other nursing programs are also required to submit a letter of good standing from the program's dean or director.

Students applying to the RN to B.S.N. program must meet the criteria for clear admission to the College, have graduated from an accredited associate or diploma program, and hold an active RN license in the state of Ohio. Second Degree Accelerated B.S.N. applicants must clearly meet all Ursuline College admission criteria, supply proof of a bachelor's degree from an accredited college or university, have earned at least a minimum GPA of 2.5 in their first degree program, and provide a letter of rec-ommendation regarding their suitability for this program.

- *2012–13 UNDERGRADUATE TUITION & FEES:*
  Generic B.S.N.: Resident/nonresident full-time tuition: $851 per credit hour

  Accelerated Second Degree B.S.N.: Resident/ nonresident full-time tuition: $668 per credit hour

Ursuline College graduates are aggressively recruited by top Cleveland hospitals because of their caring and values-based approach to nursing.

- *2012–13 GRADUATE (M.S.N. and D.N.P.) NURSING TUITION & FEES:*
  Resident/nonresident full-time tuition: $906 per credit hour

- *APPLICATION DEADLINES*
  B.S.N. programs: Rolling admissions

  M.S.N. and D.N.P. programs: Mid-July (fall semester); mid-November (spring semester)

- *FACULTY INFORMATION: http://www.ursuline. edu/Academics/Nursing/Faculty/index.html*

CONTACT INFORMATION
Breen School of Nursing
Ursuline College
2550 Lander Road
Pepper Pike, Ohio 44124-4398
Phone: 440-646-8166
**   888-URSULINE (toll-free)**
Fax: 440-449-4267
Web site: http://www.ursuline.edu/Academics/ Nursing/index.html

Undergraduate Nursing Program:
Betsy Beach, Coordinator
BSN Enrollment & Clinical Placement
Undergraduate Nursing Program
Phone: 440-646-8171
E-mail: ebeach@ursuline.edu

Graduate Nursing Program:
Barbara Dussing, Administrative Assistant
Graduate Nursing Program
Phone: 440-684-6051
E-mail: bdussing@ursuline.edu

Find us on Facebook®:
Undergraduate: http://on.fb.me/ursuline_college
Graduate: http://on.fb.me/Ursuline_Coll_gradadmit

Follow us on Twitter™:
Undergraduate: http://twitter.com/UrsulineAdmit
Graduate: http://twitter.com/UrsulineGradStu

INDEXES

BACCALAUREATE PROGRAMS

ACCELERATED BACCALAUREATE

U.S. AND U.S. TERRITORIES

Alabama

University of South Alabama, College of Nursing, *Mobile (BSN)*

Arizona

Chamberlain College of Nursing, *Phoenix (BSN)*

University of Phoenix–Online Campus, Online Campus, *Phoenix (BSN)*

University of Phoenix–Phoenix Main Campus, College of Nursing, *Tempe (BSN)*

University of Phoenix–Southern Arizona Campus, College of Social Sciences, *Tucson (BSN)*

California

American University of Health Sciences, School of Nursing, *Signal Hill (BSN)*

Azusa Pacific University, School of Nursing, *Azusa (BSN)*

California State University, Long Beach, School of Nursing, *Long Beach (BSN)*

California State University, Northridge, Nursing Program, *Northridge (BSN)*

California State University, San Marcos, School of Nursing, *San Marcos (BSN)*

Mount St. Mary's College, Department of Nursing, *Los Angeles (BSN, BSc PN)*

Samuel Merritt University, School of Nursing, *Oakland (BSN)*

University of Phoenix–Bay Area Campus, College of Nursing, *San Jose (BSN)*

University of Phoenix–Sacramento Valley Campus, College of Nursing, *Sacramento (BSN)*

University of Phoenix–San Diego Campus, College of Nursing, *San Diego (BSN)*

University of Phoenix–Southern California Campus, College of Nursing, *Costa Mesa (BSN)*

Colorado

Denver College of Nursing, *Denver (BSN)*

Platt College, School of Nursing, *Aurora (BSN)*

Regis University, School of Nursing, *Denver (BSN)*

University of Colorado Denver, College of Nursing, *Aurora (BS)*

University of Northern Colorado, School of Nursing, *Greeley (BS)*

University of Phoenix–Denver Campus, College of Nursing, *Lone Tree (BSN)*

Connecticut

Southern Connecticut State University, Department of Nursing, *New Haven (BS)*

District of Columbia

The Catholic University of America, School of Nursing, *Washington (BSN)*

Florida

Barry University, Division of Nursing, *Miami Shores (BSN)*

Florida Southern College, School of Nursing & Health Sciences, *Lakeland (BSN)*

Florida State University, College of Nursing, *Tallahassee (BSN)*

Jacksonville University, School of Nursing, *Jacksonville (BSN)*

University of Phoenix–Central Florida Campus, College of Nursing, *Maitland (BSN)*

University of Phoenix–North Florida Campus, College of Nursing, *Jacksonville (BSN)*

University of Phoenix–West Florida Campus, College of Nursing, *Temple Terrace (BSN)*

Georgia

College of Coastal Georgia, Department of Nursing and Health Sciences, *Brunswick (BS)*

Emory University, Nell Hodgson Woodruff School of Nursing, *Atlanta (BSN)*

Kennesaw State University, School of Nursing, *Kennesaw (BSN)*

Hawaii

University of Phoenix–Hawaii Campus, College of Nursing, *Honolulu (BSN)*

Illinois

Olivet Nazarene University, Division of Nursing, *Bourbonnais (BSN)*

Resurrection University, *Oak Park (BSN)*

Southern Illinois University Edwardsville, School of Nursing, *Edwardsville (BS)*

Trinity College of Nursing and Health Sciences, *Rock Island (BSN)*

Indiana

Marian University, School of Nursing, *Indianapolis (BSN)*

Purdue University North Central, Department of Nursing, *Westville (BS)*

Saint Mary's College, Department of Nursing, *Notre Dame (BS)*

Valparaiso University, College of Nursing, *Valparaiso (BSN)*

Iowa

Allen College, Program in Nursing, *Waterloo (BSN)*

Kansas

MidAmerica Nazarene University, Division of Nursing, *Olathe (BSN)*

Wichita State University, School of Nursing, *Wichita (BSN)*

Louisiana

University of Phoenix–Louisiana Campus, College of Nursing, *Metairie (BSN)*

Maine

University of Maine at Fort Kent, Department of Nursing, *Fort Kent (BSN)*

Maryland

Bowie State University, Department of Nursing, *Bowie (BSN)*

The Johns Hopkins University, School of Nursing, *Baltimore (BS)*

Massachusetts

Massachusetts College of Pharmacy and Health Sciences, School of Nursing, *Boston (BSN)*

MGH Institute of Health Professions, School of Nursing, *Boston (BSN)*

Regis College, School of Nursing, Science and Health Professions, *Weston (BSN)*

Simmons College, School of Nursing and Health Sciences, *Boston (BS)*

Michigan

Northern Michigan University, College of Nursing and Allied Health Science, *Marquette (BSN)*

University of Phoenix–Metro Detroit Campus, College of Nursing, *Southfield (BSN)*

Missouri

Cox College, Department of Nursing, *Springfield (BSN)*

Goldfarb School of Nursing at Barnes-Jewish College, *St. Louis (BSN)*

Graceland University, School of Nursing, *Independence (BSN)*

Maryville University of Saint Louis, Nursing Program, School of Health Professions, *St. Louis (BSN)*

Research College of Nursing, College of Nursing, *Kansas City (BSN)*

Saint Louis University, School of Nursing, *St. Louis (BSN)*

University of Missouri, Sinclair School of Nursing, *Columbia (BSN)*

University of Missouri–Kansas City, School of Nursing, *Kansas City (BSN)*

University of Missouri–St. Louis, College of Nursing, *St. Louis (BSN)*

William Jewell College, Department of Nursing, *Liberty (BS)*

Nebraska

University of Nebraska Medical Center, College of Nursing, *Omaha (BSN)*

Nevada

Roseman University of Health Sciences, College of Nursing, *Henderson (BSN)*

University of Nevada, Las Vegas, School of Nursing, *Las Vegas (BSN)*

University of Nevada, Reno, Orvis School of Nursing, *Reno (BSN)*

New Mexico

University of Phoenix–New Mexico Campus, College of Nursing, *Albuquerque (BSN)*

New York

Columbia University, School of Nursing, *New York (BS)*

Hartwick College, Department of Nursing, *Oneonta (BS)*

Hunter College of the City University of New York, Hunter-Bellevue School of Nursing, *New York (BSN)*

Mount Saint Mary College, Division of Nursing, *Newburgh (BSN)*

The Sage Colleges, Department of Nursing, *Troy (BS)*

State University of New York Institute of Technology, School of Nursing and Health Systems, *Utica (BS)*

Stony Brook University, State University of New York, School of Nursing, *Stony Brook (BS)*

North Carolina

Queens University of Charlotte, Presbyterian School of Nursing, *Charlotte (BSN)*

The University of North Carolina at Chapel Hill, School of Nursing, *Chapel Hill (BSN)*

Western Carolina University, School of Nursing, *Cullowhee (BSN)*

Ohio

Ashland University, Dwight Schar College of Nursing and Health Sciences, *Ashland (BSN)*

Chamberlain College of Nursing, *Columbus (BSN)*

Kent State University, College of Nursing, *Kent (BSN)*

University of Phoenix–Cleveland Campus, College of Nursing, *Independence (BSN)*

Walsh University, Department of Nursing, *North Canton (BSN)*

Oklahoma

Northwestern Oklahoma State University, Division of Nursing, *Alva (BSN)*

Oklahoma City University, Kramer School of Nursing, *Oklahoma City (BSN)*

Oregon

Oregon Health & Science University, School of Nursing, *Portland (BS)*

Pennsylvania

DeSales University, Department of Nursing and Health, *Center Valley (BSN)*

Drexel University, College of Nursing and Health Professions, *Philadelphia (BSN)*

Edinboro University of Pennsylvania, Department of Nursing, *Edinboro (BS)*

Thomas Jefferson University, Department of Nursing, *Philadelphia (BSN)*

University of Pennsylvania, School of Nursing, *Philadelphia (BSN)*

Waynesburg University, Department of Nursing, *Waynesburg (BSN)*

Puerto Rico

Inter American University of Puerto Rico, Metropolitan Campus, Carmen Torres de Tiburcio School of Nursing, *San Juan (BSN)*

South Carolina

Clemson University, School of Nursing, *Clemson (BS)*

516

Lander University, School of Nursing, *Greenwood* (BSN)

Medical University of South Carolina, College of Nursing, *Charleston* (BSN)

South Dakota

South Dakota State University, College of Nursing, *Brookings* (BS)

University of Sioux Falls, School of Nursing, *Sioux Falls* (BSN)

Tennessee

Belmont University, School of Nursing, *Nashville* (BSN)

Carson-Newman University, Department of Nursing, *Jefferson City* (BSN)

Cumberland University, Rudy School of Nursing and Health Professions, *Lebanon* (BSN)

Lincoln Memorial University, Caylor School of Nursing, *Harrogate* (BSN)

University of Memphis, Loewenberg School of Nursing, *Memphis* (BSN)

The University of Tennessee, College of Nursing, *Knoxville* (BSN)

Texas

The University of Texas at Arlington, College of Nursing, *Arlington* (BSN)

The University of Texas at El Paso, School of Nursing, *El Paso* (BSN)

Utah

University of Utah, College of Nursing, *Salt Lake City* (BS)

Western Governors University, Online College of Health Professions, *Salt Lake City* (BS)

Virginia

Hampton University, School of Nursing, *Hampton* (BS)

Lynchburg College, School of Health Sciences and Human Performance, *Lynchburg* (BS)

Old Dominion University, Department of Nursing, *Norfolk* (BSN)

Washington

University of Washington, School of Nursing, *Seattle* (BSN)

West Virginia

West Virginia University, School of Nursing, *Morgantown* (BSN)

Wisconsin

Bellin College, Nursing Program, *Green Bay* (BSN)

University of Wisconsin–Oshkosh, College of Nursing, *Oshkosh* (BSN)

CANADA

Alberta

University of Calgary, Faculty of Nursing, *Calgary* (BN)

University of Lethbridge, Faculty of Health Sciences, *Lethbridge* (BN)

British Columbia

The University of British Columbia, Program in Nursing, *Vancouver* (BSN)

New Brunswick

University of New Brunswick Fredericton, Faculty of Nursing, *Fredericton* (BN)

Newfoundland and Labrador

Memorial University of Newfoundland, School of Nursing, *St. John's* (BN)

Nova Scotia

St. Francis Xavier University, Department of Nursing, *Antigonish* (BScN)

Ontario

Lakehead University, School of Nursing, *Thunder Bay* (BScN)

Laurentian University, School of Nursing, *Sudbury* (BScN)

Queen's University at Kingston, School of Nursing, *Kingston* (BNSc)

Trent University, Nursing Program, *Peterborough* (BScN)

University of Toronto, Faculty of Nursing, *Toronto* (BScN)

The University of Western Ontario, School of Nursing, *London* (BScN)

Quebec

Université Laval, Faculty of Nursing, *Québec* (BScN)

Saskatchewan

University of Saskatchewan, College of Nursing, *Saskatoon* (BSN)

ACCELERATED BACCALAUREATE FOR SECOND DEGREE

U.S. AND U.S. TERRITORIES

Alabama

Samford University, Ida V. Moffett School of Nursing, *Birmingham* (BSN)

Arizona

Arizona State University at the Downtown Phoenix Campus, College of Nursing, *Phoenix* (BSN)

Chamberlain College of Nursing, *Phoenix* (BSN)

Northern Arizona University, School of Nursing, *Flagstaff* (BSN)

Arkansas

Arkansas State University, Department of Nursing, *State University* (BSN)

California

Concordia University, Bachelor of Science in Nursing Program, *Irvine* (BSN)

Loma Linda University, School of Nursing, *Loma Linda* (BS)

Colorado

Colorado State University–Pueblo, Department of Nursing, *Pueblo* (BSN)

Denver College of Nursing, *Denver* (BSN)

Metropolitan State University of Denver, Department of Health Professions, *Denver* (BSN)

University of Colorado at Colorado Springs, Beth-El College of Nursing and Health Sciences, *Colorado Springs* (BSN)

Connecticut

Fairfield University, School of Nursing, *Fairfield* (BS)

Quinnipiac University, School of Nursing, *Hamden* (BSN)

University of Connecticut, School of Nursing, *Storrs* (BS)

Delaware

University of Delaware, School of Nursing, *Newark* (BSN)

District of Columbia

The Catholic University of America, School of Nursing, *Washington* (BSN)

Georgetown University, School of Nursing and Health Studies, *Washington* (BSN)

The George Washington University, School of Nursing, *Washington* (BSN)

Florida

Barry University, Division of Nursing, *Miami Shores* (BSN)

Florida Atlantic University, Christine E. Lynn College of Nursing, *Boca Raton* (BSN)

Florida International University, Graduate Nursing Programs, *Miami* (BSN)

Florida Southern College, School of Nursing & Health Sciences, *Lakeland* (BSN)

Jacksonville University, School of Nursing, *Jacksonville* (BSN)

Remington College of Nursing, *Lake Mary* (BSN)

University of Central Florida, College of Nursing, *Orlando* (BSN)

University of Florida, College of Nursing, *Gainesville* (BSN)

University of Miami, School of Nursing and Health Studies, *Coral Gables* (BSN)

University of North Florida, School of Nursing, *Jacksonville* (BSN)

University of South Florida, College of Nursing, *Tampa* (BS)

Georgia

Albany State University, College of Sciences and Health Professions, *Albany* (BSN)

Emory University, Nell Hodgson Woodruff School of Nursing, *Atlanta* (BSN)

Kennesaw State University, School of Nursing, *Kennesaw* (BSN)

Idaho

Idaho State University, Department of Nursing, *Pocatello* (BSN)

Illinois

Blessing–Rieman College of Nursing, *Quincy* (BSN)

Bradley University, Department of Nursing, *Peoria* (BSN, BSc PN)

Illinois State University, Mennonite College of Nursing, *Normal* (BSN)

Lewis University, Program in Nursing, *Romeoville* (BSN)

Loyola University Chicago, Marcella Niehoff School of Nursing, *Maywood* (BSN)

Methodist College, *Peoria* (BSN)

Resurrection University, *Oak Park* (BSN)

Trinity College of Nursing and Health Sciences, *Rock Island* (BSN)

Indiana

Ball State University, School of Nursing, *Muncie* (BS)

Indiana State University, Department of Nursing, *Terre Haute* (BS)

Indiana University–Purdue University Indianapolis, School of Nursing, *Indianapolis* (BSN)

Indiana University South Bend, College of Health Sciences, *South Bend* (BSN)

Indiana Wesleyan University, School of Nursing, *Marion* (BSN)

Marian University, School of Nursing, *Indianapolis* (BSN)

Purdue University, School of Nursing, *West Lafayette* (BS)

Purdue University Calumet, School of Nursing, *Hammond* (BS)

Purdue University North Central, Department of Nursing, *Westville* (BS)

Saint Joseph's College, St. Elizabeth School of Nursing, *Rensselaer* (BSN)

University of Indianapolis, School of Nursing, *Indianapolis* (BSN)

Iowa

Allen College, Program in Nursing, *Waterloo* (BSN)

Kansas

MidAmerica Nazarene University, Division of Nursing, *Olathe* (BSN)

Wichita State University, School of Nursing, *Wichita* (BSN)

Kentucky

Bellarmine University, Donna and Allan Lansing School of Nursing and Health Sciences, *Louisville* (BSN, MSCE)

Northern Kentucky University, Department of Nursing, *Highland Heights* (BSN)

Spalding University, School of Nursing, *Louisville* (BSN)

University of Louisville, School of Nursing, *Louisville* (BSN)

Louisiana

Louisiana State University Health Sciences Center, School of Nursing, *New Orleans* (BSN)

Our Lady of the Lake College, Division of Nursing, *Baton Rouge* (BSN)

Southeastern Louisiana University, School of Nursing, *Hammond* (BS)

University of Louisiana at Lafayette, College of Nursing, *Lafayette (BSN)*

Maine
University of Southern Maine, School of Nursing, *Portland (BS)*

Maryland
The Johns Hopkins University, School of Nursing, *Baltimore (BS)*

Salisbury University, Program in Nursing, *Salisbury (BS)*

Massachusetts
Curry College, Division of Nursing, *Milton (BS)*

Massachusetts College of Pharmacy and Health Sciences, School of Nursing, *Boston (BSN)*

Regis College, School of Nursing, Science and Health Professions, *Weston (BSN)*

Salem State University, Program in Nursing, *Salem (BSN)*

Simmons College, School of Nursing and Health Sciences, *Boston (BS)*

University of Massachusetts Amherst, School of Nursing, *Amherst (BS)*

University of Massachusetts Boston, College of Nursing and Health Sciences, *Boston (BS)*

Michigan
Ferris State University, School of Nursing, *Big Rapids (BSN)*

Michigan State University, College of Nursing, *East Lansing (BSN)*

Saginaw Valley State University, Crystal M. Lange College of Health and Human Services, *University Center (BSN)*

University of Detroit Mercy, McAuley School of Nursing, *Detroit (BSN)*

University of Michigan, School of Nursing, *Ann Arbor (BSN)*

University of Michigan–Flint, Department of Nursing, *Flint (BSN)*

Wayne State University, College of Nursing, *Detroit (BSN)*

Minnesota
The College of St. Scholastica, Department of Nursing, *Duluth (BS)*

Concordia College, Department of Nursing, *Moorhead (BA)*

Minnesota State University Mankato, School of Nursing, *Mankato (BS)*

Mississippi
University of Mississippi Medical Center, Program in Nursing, *Jackson (BSN)*

Missouri
Cox College, Department of Nursing, *Springfield (BSN)*

Goldfarb School of Nursing at Barnes-Jewish College, *St. Louis (BSN)*

Research College of Nursing, College of Nursing, *Kansas City (BSN)*

Saint Louis University, School of Nursing, *St. Louis (BSN)*

Southeast Missouri State University, Department of Nursing, *Cape Girardeau (BSN)*

University of Missouri, Sinclair School of Nursing, *Columbia (BSN)*

Montana
Montana State University, College of Nursing, *Bozeman (BSN)*

Nebraska
Creighton University, School of Nursing, *Omaha (BSN)*

Nebraska Methodist College, Department of Nursing, *Omaha (BSN)*

University of Nebraska Medical Center, College of Nursing, *Omaha (BSN)*

Nevada
Nevada State College at Henderson, Nursing Program, *Henderson (BSN)*

Roseman University of Health Sciences, College of Nursing, *Henderson (BSN)*

New Jersey
Fairleigh Dickinson University, Metropolitan Campus, Henry P. Becton School of Nursing and Allied Health, *Teaneck (BSN)*

Felician College, Division of Nursing and Health Management, *Lodi (BSN)*

New Jersey City University, Department of Nursing, *Jersey City (BSN)*

Rutgers, The State University of New Jersey, College of Nursing, *Newark (BS)*

Seton Hall University, College of Nursing, *South Orange (BSN)*

University of Medicine and Dentistry of New Jersey, School of Nursing, *Newark (BSN)*

William Paterson University of New Jersey, Department of Nursing, *Wayne (BSN)*

New Mexico
University of New Mexico, College of Nursing, *Albuquerque (BSN)*

New York
Adelphi University, School of Nursing, *Garden City (BS)*

The College of New Rochelle, School of Nursing, *New Rochelle (BSN)*

Columbia University, School of Nursing, *New York (BS)*

Concordia College–New York, Nursing Program, *Bronxville (BS)*

Dominican College, Department of Nursing, *Orangeburg (BSN)*

Hartwick College, Department of Nursing, *Oneonta (BS)*

Lehman College of the City University of New York, Department of Nursing, *Bronx (BS)*

Long Island University–Brooklyn Campus, School of Nursing, *Brooklyn (BS)*

Molloy College, Division of Nursing, *Rockville Centre (BS)*

New York University, College of Nursing, *New York (BS)*

Pace University, Lienhard School of Nursing, *New York (BS)*

The Sage Colleges, Department of Nursing, *Troy (BS)*

State University of New York Downstate Medical Center, College of Nursing, *Brooklyn (BS)*

University at Buffalo, the State University of New York, School of Nursing, *Buffalo (BS)*

University of Rochester, School of Nursing, *Rochester (BS)*

Utica College, Department of Nursing, *Utica (BS)*

North Carolina
Duke University, School of Nursing, *Durham (BSN)*

North Carolina Agricultural and Technical State University, School of Nursing, *Greensboro (BSN)*

Queens University of Charlotte, Presbyterian School of Nursing, *Charlotte (BSN)*

The University of North Carolina at Chapel Hill, School of Nursing, *Chapel Hill (BSN)*

North Dakota
University of North Dakota, College of Nursing, *Grand Forks (BSN)*

Ohio
Ashland University, Dwight Schar College of Nursing and Health Sciences, *Ashland (BSN)*

Capital University, School of Nursing, *Columbus (BSN)*

Chamberlain College of Nursing, *Columbus (BSN)*

Cleveland State University, School of Nursing, *Cleveland (BSN)*

Kent State University, College of Nursing, *Kent (BSN)*

Mount Carmel College of Nursing, Nursing Programs, *Columbus (BSN)*

The University of Akron, College of Nursing, *Akron (BSN)*

University of Cincinnati, College of Nursing, *Cincinnati (BSN)*

Ursuline College, The Breen School of Nursing, *Pepper Pike (BSN)*

Walsh University, Department of Nursing, *North Canton (BSN)*

Wright State University, College of Nursing and Health, *Dayton (BSN)*

Oklahoma
Oklahoma City University, Kramer School of Nursing, *Oklahoma City (BSN)*

University of Oklahoma Health Sciences Center, College of Nursing, *Oklahoma City (BSN)*

Oregon
Linfield College, School of Nursing, *McMinnville (BSN)*

Pennsylvania
Drexel University, College of Nursing and Health Professions, *Philadelphia (BSN)*

Duquesne University, School of Nursing, *Pittsburgh (BSN)*

Edinboro University of Pennsylvania, Department of Nursing, *Edinboro (BS)*

Thomas Jefferson University, Department of Nursing, *Philadelphia (BSN)*

University of Pennsylvania, School of Nursing, *Philadelphia (BSN)*

University of Pittsburgh, School of Nursing, *Pittsburgh (BSN)*

Villanova University, College of Nursing, *Villanova (BSN)*

Waynesburg University, Department of Nursing, *Waynesburg (BSN)*

West Chester University of Pennsylvania, Department of Nursing, *West Chester (BSN)*

Wilkes University, Department of Nursing, *Wilkes-Barre (BS)*

South Carolina
Lander University, School of Nursing, *Greenwood (BSN)*

Medical University of South Carolina, College of Nursing, *Charleston (BSN)*

Tennessee
Belmont University, School of Nursing, *Nashville (BSN)*

Carson-Newman University, Department of Nursing, *Jefferson City (BSN)*

Cumberland University, Rudy School of Nursing and Health Professions, *Lebanon (BSN)*

East Tennessee State University, College of Nursing, *Johnson City (BSN)*

Union University, School of Nursing, *Jackson (BSN)*

University of Memphis, Loewenberg School of Nursing, *Memphis (BSN)*

Texas
Baylor University, Louise Herrington School of Nursing, *Waco (BSN)*

Texas A&M Health Science Center, College of Nursing, *College Station (BSN)*

Texas A&M University–Corpus Christi, College of Nursing and Health Sciences, *Corpus Christi (BSN)*

Texas Christian University, Harris College of Nursing, *Fort Worth (BSN)*

Texas Tech University Health Sciences Center, School of Nursing, *Lubbock (BSN)*

University of Houston–Victoria, School of Nursing, *Victoria (BSN)*

The University of Texas at Arlington, College of Nursing, *Arlington (BSN)*

The University of Texas Health Science Center at Houston, School of Nursing, *Houston (BSN)*

The University of Texas Health Science Center at San Antonio, School of Nursing, *San Antonio (BSN)*

The University of Texas Medical Branch, School of Nursing, *Galveston (BSN)*

Virginia
George Mason University, College of Health and Human Services, *Fairfax (BSN)*

Marymount University, Malek School of Health Professions, *Arlington (BSN)*

Norfolk State University, Department of Nursing, *Norfolk (BSN)*

Shenandoah University, Eleanor Wade Custer School of Nursing, *Winchester (BSN)*
Virginia Commonwealth University, School of Nursing, *Richmond (BS)*

West Virginia

West Virginia University, School of Nursing, *Morgantown (BSN)*
Wheeling Jesuit University, Department of Nursing, *Wheeling (BSN)*

Wisconsin

Bellin College, Nursing Program, *Green Bay (BSN)*
Edgewood College, Program in Nursing, *Madison (BS)*
University of Wisconsin–Eau Claire, College of Nursing and Health Sciences, *Eau Claire (BSN)*
University of Wisconsin–Oshkosh, College of Nursing, *Oshkosh (BSN)*

Wyoming

University of Wyoming, Fay W. Whitney School of Nursing, *Laramie (BSN)*

CANADA

Alberta

University of Alberta, Faculty of Nursing, *Edmonton (BScN)*
University of Calgary, Faculty of Nursing, *Calgary (BN)*

British Columbia

Kwantlen Polytechnic University, Faculty of Community and Health Sciences, *Surrey (BSN)*
The University of British Columbia, Program in Nursing, *Vancouver (BSN)*

Nova Scotia

St. Francis Xavier University, Department of Nursing, *Antigonish (BScN)*

Ontario

University of Toronto, Faculty of Nursing, *Toronto (BScN)*

ACCELERATED LPN TO BACCALAUREATE

U.S. AND U.S. TERRITORIES

California

San Francisco State University, School of Nursing, *San Francisco (BSN)*

Kansas

MidAmerica Nazarene University, Division of Nursing, *Olathe (BSN)*

Massachusetts

Fitchburg State University, Department of Nursing, *Fitchburg (BS)*

New York

Dominican College, Department of Nursing, *Orangeburg (BSN)*

Oklahoma

Northwestern Oklahoma State University, Division of Nursing, *Alva (BSN)*

Pennsylvania

Wilkes University, Department of Nursing, *Wilkes-Barre (BS)*

South Dakota

Mount Marty College, Nursing Program, *Yankton (BSN)*

Virginia

Norfolk State University, Department of Nursing, *Norfolk (BSN)*

CANADA

Nova Scotia

St. Francis Xavier University, Department of Nursing, *Antigonish (BScN)*

ACCELERATED RN BACCALAUREATE

U.S. AND U.S. TERRITORIES

Arizona

Arizona State University at the Downtown Phoenix Campus, College of Nursing, *Phoenix (BSN)*

Arkansas

University of Arkansas for Medical Sciences, College of Nursing, *Little Rock (BSN)*

California

Azusa Pacific University, School of Nursing, *Azusa (BSN)*
Loma Linda University, School of Nursing, *Loma Linda (BS)*
West Coast University, Nursing Programs, *North Hollywood (BSN)*

Colorado

Colorado State University–Pueblo, Department of Nursing, *Pueblo (BSN)*

Delaware

Wilmington University, College of Health Professions, *New Castle (BSN)*

Florida

Northwest Florida State College, RN to BSN Degree Program, *Niceville (BSN)*

Georgia

Georgia State University, Byrdine F. Lewis School of Nursing and Health Professions, *Atlanta (BS)*
Thomas University, Division of Nursing, *Thomasville (BSN)*
University of West Georgia, School of Nursing, *Carrollton (BSN)*

Idaho

Boise State University, Department of Nursing, *Boise (BS)*

Illinois

Benedictine University, Department of Nursing, *Lisle (BSN)*
Lakeview College of Nursing, *Danville (BSN)*
Lewis University, Program in Nursing, *Romeoville (BSN)*
Resurrection University, *Oak Park (BSN)*
University of St. Francis, Leach College of Nursing, *Joliet (BSN)*

Indiana

Indiana University Kokomo, Indiana University School of Nursing, *Kokomo (BSN)*
Marian University, School of Nursing, *Indianapolis (BSN)*
Purdue University Calumet, School of Nursing, *Hammond (BS)*

Iowa

Allen College, Program in Nursing, *Waterloo (BSN)*
Mount Mercy University, Department of Nursing, *Cedar Rapids (BSN)*

Kansas

MidAmerica Nazarene University, Division of Nursing, *Olathe (BSN)*
Southwestern College, Nursing Program, *Winfield (BSN)*
Tabor College, Department of Nursing, *Hillsboro (BSN)*

Kentucky

Eastern Kentucky University, Department of Baccalaureate and Graduate Nursing, *Richmond (BSN)*
Midway College, Program in Nursing (Baccalaureate), *Midway (BSN)*
Spalding University, School of Nursing, *Louisville (BSN)*

Maine

University of New England, Department of Nursing, *Biddeford (BSN)*

Maryland

Coppin State University, Helene Fuld School of Nursing, *Baltimore (BSN)*
Notre Dame of Maryland University, Department of Nursing, *Baltimore (BS)*
Stevenson University, Nursing Division, *Stevenson (BS)*
Washington Adventist University, Nursing Department, *Takoma Park (BS)*

Massachusetts

Regis College, School of Nursing, Science and Health Professions, *Weston (BSN)*
University of Massachusetts Amherst, School of Nursing, *Amherst (BS)*

Michigan

Ferris State University, School of Nursing, *Big Rapids (BSN)*

Missouri

Chamberlain College of Nursing, *St. Louis (BSN)*
Maryville University of Saint Louis, Nursing Program, School of Health Professions, *St. Louis (BSN)*
Missouri State University, Department of Nursing, *Springfield (BSN)*

Nebraska

Clarkson College, Master of Science in Nursing Program, *Omaha (BSN)*
Nebraska Methodist College, Department of Nursing, *Omaha (BSN)*
Nebraska Wesleyan University, Department of Nursing, *Lincoln (BSN)*
University of Nebraska Medical Center, College of Nursing, *Omaha (BSN)*

New Jersey

College of Saint Elizabeth, Department of Nursing, *Morristown (BSN)*
Rutgers School of Nursing–Camden, *Camden (BS)*

New York

Binghamton University, State University of New York, Decker School of Nursing, *Binghamton (BS)*
The College of New Rochelle, School of Nursing, *New Rochelle (BSN)*
Daemen College, Department of Nursing, *Amherst (BS)*
Dominican College, Department of Nursing, *Orangeburg (BSN)*
Keuka College, Division of Nursing, *Keuka Park (BS)*
Lehman College of the City University of New York, Department of Nursing, *Bronx (BS)*
Medgar Evers College of the City University of New York, Department of Nursing, *Brooklyn (BSN)*
Mercy College, Programs in Nursing, *Dobbs Ferry (BS)*
Molloy College, Division of Nursing, *Rockville Centre (BS)*
Mount Saint Mary College, Division of Nursing, *Newburgh (BSN)*
St. John Fisher College, Wegmans School of Nursing, *Rochester (BS)*
State University of New York Institute of Technology, School of Nursing and Health Systems, *Utica (BS)*
University of Rochester, School of Nursing, *Rochester (BS)*

North Carolina

Winston-Salem State University, Department of Nursing, *Winston-Salem (BSN)*

Ohio

College of Mount St. Joseph, Department of Nursing, *Cincinnati (BSN)*
Kent State University, College of Nursing, *Kent (BSN)*
Otterbein University, Department of Nursing, *Westerville (BSN)*
The University of Akron, College of Nursing, *Akron (BSN)*

Ursuline College, The Breen School of Nursing, *Pepper Pike (BSN)*

Oklahoma

Bacone College, Department of Nursing, *Muskogee (BSN)*

Northeastern State University, Department of Nursing, *Tahlequah (BSN)*

Northwestern Oklahoma State University, Division of Nursing, *Alva (BSN)*

Oklahoma Wesleyan University, School of Nursing, *Bartlesville (BSN)*

Pennsylvania

Carlow University, School of Nursing, *Pittsburgh (BSN)*

DeSales University, Department of Nursing and Health, *Center Valley (BSN)*

Eastern University, Program in Nursing, *St. Davids (BSN)*

Gwynedd-Mercy College, School of Nursing, *Gwynedd Valley (BSN)*

Holy Family University, School of Nursing and Allied Health Professions, *Philadelphia (BSN)*

Immaculata University, Department of Nursing, *Immaculata (BSN)*

La Roche College, Department of Nursing and Nursing Management, *Pittsburgh (BSN)*

Misericordia University, Department of Nursing, *Dallas (BSN)*

Mount Aloysius College, Division of Nursing, *Cresson (BSN)*

Neumann University, Program in Nursing and Health Sciences, *Aston (BS)*

Thomas Jefferson University, Department of Nursing, *Philadelphia (BSN)*

University of Pennsylvania, School of Nursing, *Philadelphia (BSN)*

Wilkes University, Department of Nursing, *Wilkes-Barre (BS)*

South Carolina

Lander University, School of Nursing, *Greenwood (BSN)*

Tennessee

Aquinas College, School of Nursing, *Nashville (BSN)*

Cumberland University, Rudy School of Nursing and Health Professions, *Lebanon (BSN)*

East Tennessee State University, College of Nursing, *Johnson City (BSN)*

King College, School of Nursing, *Bristol (BSN)*

University of Memphis, Loewenberg School of Nursing, *Memphis (BSN)*

The University of Tennessee, College of Nursing, *Knoxville (BSN)*

Texas

The University of Texas at Arlington, College of Nursing, *Arlington (BSN)*

The University of Texas at Tyler, Program in Nursing, *Tyler (BSN)*

Utah

Western Governors University, Online College of Health Professions, *Salt Lake City (BS)*

West Virginia

Fairmont State University, School of Nursing and Allied Health Administration, *Fairmont (BSN)*

Marshall University, College of Health Professions, *Huntington (BSN)*

West Liberty University, Department of Health Sciences, *West Liberty (BSN)*

Wisconsin

University of Wisconsin–Oshkosh, College of Nursing, *Oshkosh (BSN)*

CANADA

Ontario

University of Toronto, Faculty of Nursing, *Toronto (BScN)*

Quebec

McGill University, School of Nursing, *Montréal (BScN)*

Université du Québec à Chicoutimi, Program in Nursing, *Chicoutimi (BNSc)*

Université Laval, Faculty of Nursing, *Québec (BScN)*

Saskatchewan

University of Saskatchewan, College of Nursing, *Saskatoon (BSN)*

ADN TO BACCALAUREATE

U.S. AND U.S. TERRITORIES

Alabama

Tuskegee University, Program in Nursing, *Tuskegee (BSN)*

University of Mobile, School of Nursing, *Mobile (BSN)*

University of South Alabama, College of Nursing, *Mobile (BSN)*

Arizona

Grand Canyon University, College of Nursing and Health Sciences, *Phoenix (BSN)*

Northern Arizona University, School of Nursing, *Flagstaff (BSN)*

Arkansas

Arkansas Tech University, Program in Nursing, *Russellville (BSN)*

Harding University, College of Nursing, *Searcy (BSN)*

Henderson State University, Department of Nursing, *Arkadelphia (BSN)*

Southern Arkansas University–Magnolia, Department of Nursing, *Magnolia (BSN)*

University of Arkansas at Monticello, School of Nursing, *Monticello (BSN)*

University of Arkansas for Medical Sciences, College of Nursing, *Little Rock (BSN)*

University of Arkansas–Fort Smith, Carol McKelvey Moore School of Nursing, *Fort Smith (BSN)*

University of Central Arkansas, Department of Nursing, *Conway (BSN)*

California

Azusa Pacific University, School of Nursing, *Azusa (BSN)*

Biola University, Department of Nursing, *La Mirada (BSN)*

California Baptist University, School of Nursing, *Riverside (BSN)*

California State University, Bakersfield, Program in Nursing, *Bakersfield (BSN)*

California State University, Chico, School of Nursing, *Chico (BSN)*

California State University, East Bay, Department of Nursing and Health Sciences, *Hayward (BS)*

California State University, Fresno, Department of Nursing, *Fresno (BSN)*

California State University, Fullerton, Department of Nursing, *Fullerton (BSN)*

California State University, Long Beach, School of Nursing, *Long Beach (BSN)*

California State University, Northridge, Nursing Program, *Northridge (BSN)*

California State University, Sacramento, School of Nursing, *Sacramento (BSN)*

California State University, Stanislaus, Department of Nursing, *Turlock (BSN)*

Loma Linda University, School of Nursing, *Loma Linda (BS)*

Mount St. Mary's College, Department of Nursing, *Los Angeles (BSN, BSc PN)*

National University, Department of Nursing, *La Jolla (BSN)*

Pacific Union College, Department of Nursing, *Angwin (BSN)*

Point Loma Nazarene University, School of Nursing, *San Diego (BSN)*

San Diego State University, School of Nursing, *San Diego (BSN)*

San Francisco State University, School of Nursing, *San Francisco (BSN)*

Colorado

Colorado Mesa University, Department of Nursing and Radiologic Sciences, *Grand Junction (BSN)*

Colorado State University–Pueblo, Department of Nursing, *Pueblo (BSN)*

Denver College of Nursing, *Denver (BSN)*

Metropolitan State University of Denver, Department of Health Professions, *Denver (BSN)*

Connecticut

Southern Connecticut State University, Department of Nursing, *New Haven (BS)*

University of Hartford, College of Education, Nursing, and Health Professions, *West Hartford (BSN)*

Florida

Barry University, Division of Nursing, *Miami Shores (BSN)*

Jacksonville University, School of Nursing, *Jacksonville (BSN)*

Northwest Florida State College, RN to BSN Degree Program, *Niceville (BSN)*

St. Petersburg College, Department of Nursing, *St. Petersburg (BSN)*

University of South Florida, College of Nursing, *Tampa (BS)*

The University of Tampa, Department of Nursing, *Tampa (BSN)*

University of West Florida, Department of Nursing, *Pensacola (BSN)*

Georgia

Albany State University, College of Sciences and Health Professions, *Albany (BSN)*

Armstrong Atlantic State University, Program in Nursing, *Savannah (BSN)*

Brenau University, College of Health and Science, *Gainesville (BSN)*

Georgia Southern University, School of Nursing, *Statesboro (BSN)*

Kennesaw State University, School of Nursing, *Kennesaw (BSN)*

Macon State College, School of Nursing and Health Sciences, *Macon (BSN)*

Thomas University, Division of Nursing, *Thomasville (BSN)*

University of North Georgia, Department of Nursing, *Dahlonega (BSN)*

Guam

University of Guam, School of Nursing and Health Sciences, *Mangilao (BSN)*

Hawaii

University of Hawaii at Hilo, Department in Nursing, *Hilo (BSN)*

University of Hawaii at Manoa, School of Nursing and Dental Hygiene, *Honolulu (BSN)*

Idaho

Idaho State University, Department of Nursing, *Pocatello (BSN)*

Lewis-Clark State College, Division of Nursing and Health Sciences, *Lewiston (BSN)*

Illinois

Blessing–Rieman College of Nursing, *Quincy (BSN)*

Bradley University, Department of Nursing, *Peoria (BSN, BSc PN)*

Eastern Illinois University, Nursing Program, *Charleston (BSN)*

MacMurray College, Department of Nursing, *Jacksonville (BSN)*

McKendree University, Department of Nursing, *Lebanon (BSN)*

Northern Illinois University, School of Nursing and Health Studies, *De Kalb (BS)*

Resurrection University, *Oak Park (BSN)*

Rockford College, Department of Nursing, *Rockford (BSN)*

Southern Illinois University Edwardsville, School of Nursing, *Edwardsville (BS)*

Trinity College of Nursing and Health Sciences, *Rock Island (BSN)*

University of Illinois at Chicago, College of Nursing, *Chicago (BSN)*

Indiana

Anderson University, School of Nursing, *Anderson (BSN)*

Bethel College, School of Nursing, *Mishawaka (BSN)*

Huntington University, Department of Nursing, *Huntington (BSN)*

Indiana University East, School of Nursing, *Richmond (BSN)*

Indiana University–Purdue University Indianapolis, School of Nursing, *Indianapolis (BSN)*

Purdue University, School of Nursing, *West Lafayette (BS)*

Purdue University North Central, Department of Nursing, *Westville (BS)*

University of Indianapolis, School of Nursing, *Indianapolis (BSN)*

University of Saint Francis, Department of Nursing, *Fort Wayne (BSN)*

Iowa

Allen College, Program in Nursing, *Waterloo (BSN)*

Briar Cliff University, Department of Nursing, *Sioux City (BSN)*

Iowa Wesleyan College, Division of Nursing, *Mount Pleasant (BSN)*

Mercy College of Health Sciences, Division of Nursing, *Des Moines (BSN)*

Mount Mercy University, Department of Nursing, *Cedar Rapids (BSN)*

Kansas

Emporia State University, Newman Division of Nursing, *Emporia (BSN)*

Kansas Wesleyan University, Department of Nursing Education, *Salina (BSN)*

MidAmerica Nazarene University, Division of Nursing, *Olathe (BSN)*

Tabor College, Department of Nursing, *Hillsboro (BSN)*

The University of Kansas, School of Nursing, *Kansas City (BSN)*

Washburn University, School of Nursing, *Topeka (BSN)*

Wichita State University, School of Nursing, *Wichita (BSN)*

Kentucky

Kentucky State University, School of Nursing, *Frankfort (BSN)*

Midway College, Program in Nursing (Baccalaureate), *Midway (BSN)*

Morehead State University, Department of Nursing, *Morehead (BSN)*

Western Kentucky University, School of Nursing, *Bowling Green (BSN)*

Louisiana

McNeese State University, College of Nursing, *Lake Charles (BSN)*

Northwestern State University of Louisiana, College of Nursing and Allied Health, *Shreveport (BSN)*

Our Lady of the Lake College, Division of Nursing, *Baton Rouge (BSN)*

University of Louisiana at Lafayette, College of Nursing, *Lafayette (BSN)*

University of Louisiana at Monroe, Nursing, *Monroe (BS)*

Maine

University of Southern Maine, School of Nursing, *Portland (BS)*

Maryland

Salisbury University, Program in Nursing, *Salisbury (BS)*

Stevenson University, Nursing Division, *Stevenson (BS)*

University of Maryland, Baltimore, Master's Program in Nursing, *Baltimore (BSN)*

Massachusetts

American International College, Division of Nursing, *Springfield (BSN)*

Anna Maria College, Department of Nursing, *Paxton (BSN)*

Framingham State University, Department of Nursing, *Framingham (BS)*

Regis College, School of Nursing, Science and Health Professions, *Weston (BSN)*

Salem State University, Program in Nursing, *Salem (BSN)*

Simmons College, School of Nursing and Health Sciences, *Boston (BS)*

Michigan

Andrews University, Department of Nursing, *Berrien Springs (BS)*

Davenport University, Division of Nursing, *Grand Rapids (BSN)*

Grand Valley State University, Kirkhof College of Nursing, *Allendale (BSN)*

Lake Superior State University, Department of Nursing, *Sault Sainte Marie (BSN)*

Madonna University, College of Nursing and Health, *Livonia (BSN)*

Saginaw Valley State University, Crystal M. Lange College of Health and Human Services, *University Center (BSN)*

Spring Arbor University, Program in Nursing, *Spring Arbor (BSN)*

Western Michigan University, College of Health and Human Services, *Kalamazoo (BSN)*

Minnesota

Augsburg College, Program in Nursing, *Minneapolis (BS)*

The College of St. Scholastica, Department of Nursing, *Duluth (BS)*

Minnesota State University Moorhead, School of Nursing and Healthcare Leadership, *Moorhead (BSN)*

Mississippi

Delta State University, School of Nursing, *Cleveland (BSN)*

Mississippi University for Women, College of Nursing and Speech Language Pathology, *Columbus (BSN)*

University of Mississippi Medical Center, Program in Nursing, *Jackson (BSN)*

University of Southern Mississippi, School of Nursing, *Hattiesburg (BSN)*

William Carey University, School of Nursing, *Hattiesburg (BSN)*

Missouri

Chamberlain College of Nursing, *St. Louis (BSN)*

Cox College, Department of Nursing, *Springfield (BSN)*

Goldfarb School of Nursing at Barnes-Jewish College, *St. Louis (BSN)*

Graceland University, School of Nursing, *Independence (BSN)*

Missouri Southern State University, Department of Nursing, *Joplin (BSN)*

Missouri State University, Department of Nursing, *Springfield (BSN)*

Missouri Western State University, Department of Nursing, *St. Joseph (BSN)*

University of Central Missouri, Department of Nursing, *Warrensburg (BS)*

University of Missouri, Sinclair School of Nursing, *Columbia (BSN)*

Webster University, Department of Nursing, *St. Louis (BSN)*

Montana

Montana State University–Northern, College of Nursing, *Havre (BSN)*

Nebraska

Clarkson College, Master of Science in Nursing Program, *Omaha (BSN)*

College of Saint Mary, Division of Health Care Professions, *Omaha (BSN)*

Midland University, Department of Nursing, *Fremont (BSN)*

Nebraska Wesleyan University, Department of Nursing, *Lincoln (BSN)*

Union College, Division of Health Sciences, *Lincoln (BSN)*

University of Nebraska Medical Center, College of Nursing, *Omaha (BSN)*

Nevada

Great Basin College, BSN Program, *Elko (BSN)*

Touro University, School of Nursing, *Henderson (BSN)*

University of Nevada, Reno, Orvis School of Nursing, *Reno (BSN)*

New Hampshire

Franklin Pierce University, Master of Science in Nursing, *Rindge (BS)*

Rivier University, Division of Nursing, *Nashua (BS)*

New Jersey

College of Saint Elizabeth, Department of Nursing, *Morristown (BSN)*

Kean University, Department of Nursing, *Union (BSN)*

Monmouth University, Marjorie K. Unterberg School of Nursing, *West Long Branch (BSN)*

Saint Peter's University, Nursing Program, *Jersey City (BSN)*

William Paterson University of New Jersey, Department of Nursing, *Wayne (BSN)*

New York

The College at Brockport, State University of New York, Department of Nursing, *Brockport (BSN)*

Daemen College, Department of Nursing, *Amherst (BS)*

Elmira College, Program in Nursing Education, *Elmira (BS)*

Lehman College of the City University of New York, Department of Nursing, *Bronx (BS)*

Le Moyne College, Nursing Programs, *Syracuse (BS)*

Long Island University–Brooklyn Campus, School of Nursing, *Brooklyn (BS)*

Medgar Evers College of the City University of New York, Department of Nursing, *Brooklyn (BSN)*

Molloy College, Division of Nursing, *Rockville Centre (BS)*

The Sage Colleges, Department of Nursing, *Troy (BS)*

St. Francis College, Department of Nursing, *Brooklyn Heights (BS)*

St. John Fisher College, Wegmans School of Nursing, *Rochester (BS)*

State University of New York at Plattsburgh, Department of Nursing, *Plattsburgh (BS)*

State University of New York Institute of Technology, School of Nursing and Health Systems, *Utica (BS)*

State University of New York Upstate Medical University, College of Nursing, *Syracuse (BS)*

University of Rochester, School of Nursing, *Rochester (BS)*

York College of the City University of New York, Program in Nursing, *Jamaica (BS)*

North Carolina

Barton College, School of Nursing, *Wilson (BSN)*

East Carolina University, College of Nursing, *Greenville (BSN)*

Gardner-Webb University, School of Nursing, *Boiling Springs (BSN)*

Lees-McRae College, Nursing Program, *Banner Elk (BSN)*

Lenoir-Rhyne University, Program in Nursing, *Hickory (BS)*

Queens University of Charlotte, Presbyterian School of Nursing, *Charlotte (BSN)*

The University of North Carolina at Charlotte, School of Nursing, *Charlotte (BSN)*

The University of North Carolina at Greensboro, School of Nursing, *Greensboro (BSN)*

Winston-Salem State University, Department of Nursing, *Winston-Salem (BSN)*

North Dakota

Dickinson State University, Department of Nursing, *Dickinson (BSN)*

North Dakota State University, Department of Nursing, *Fargo (BSN)*

University of North Dakota, College of Nursing, *Grand Forks (BSN)*

Ohio

Ashland University, Dwight Schar College of Nursing and Health Sciences, *Ashland (BSN)*

Capital University, School of Nursing, *Columbus (BSN)*

Kent State University, College of Nursing, *Kent (BSN)*

Malone University, School of Nursing, *Canton (BSN)*

Miami University, Department of Nursing, *Hamilton (BSN)*

Shawnee State University, Department of Nursing, *Portsmouth (BSN)*

The University of Akron, College of Nursing, *Akron (BSN)*

University of Cincinnati, College of Nursing, *Cincinnati (BSN)*

The University of Toledo, College of Nursing, *Toledo (BSN)*

Urbana University, College of Nursing and Allied Health, *Urbana (BSN)*

Ursuline College, The Breen School of Nursing, *Pepper Pike (BSN)*

Oklahoma

East Central University, Department of Nursing, *Ada (BS)*

Northwestern Oklahoma State University, Division of Nursing, *Alva (BSN)*

Oklahoma Baptist University, School of Nursing, *Shawnee (BSN)*

Oklahoma City University, Kramer School of Nursing, *Oklahoma City (BSN)*

Oklahoma Panhandle State University, Bachelor of Science in Nursing Program, *Goodwell (BSN)*

Oklahoma Wesleyan University, School of Nursing, *Bartlesville (BSN)*

Oral Roberts University, Anna Vaughn School of Nursing, *Tulsa (BSN)*

Rogers State University, Nursing Program, *Claremore (BSN)*

Southern Nazarene University, School of Nursing, *Bethany (BS)*

Southwestern Oklahoma State University, School of Nursing, *Weatherford (BSN)*

University of Oklahoma Health Sciences Center, College of Nursing, *Oklahoma City (BSN)*

Oregon

Linfield College, School of Nursing, *McMinnville (BSN)*

Pennsylvania

Bloomsburg University of Pennsylvania, Department of Nursing, *Bloomsburg (BSN)*

Clarion University of Pennsylvania, School of Nursing, *Oil City (BSN)*

DeSales University, Department of Nursing and Health, *Center Valley (BSN)*

Edinboro University of Pennsylvania, Department of Nursing, *Edinboro (BS)*

Gannon University, Villa Maria School of Nursing, *Erie (BSN)*

Gwynedd-Mercy College, School of Nursing, *Gwynedd Valley (BSN)*

Holy Family University, School of Nursing and Allied Health Professions, *Philadelphia (BSN)*

Marywood University, Department of Nursing, *Scranton (BSN)*

Mount Aloysius College, Division of Nursing, *Cresson (BSN)*

Neumann University, Program in Nursing and Health Sciences, *Aston (BS)*

Penn State University Park, School of Nursing, *University Park (BS)*

Slippery Rock University of Pennsylvania, Department of Nursing, *Slippery Rock (BSN)*

Thomas Jefferson University, Department of Nursing, *Philadelphia (BSN)*

University of Pennsylvania, School of Nursing, *Philadelphia (BSN)*

Villanova University, College of Nursing, *Villanova (BSN)*

Widener University, School of Nursing, *Chester (BSN)*

Wilkes University, Department of Nursing, *Wilkes-Barre (BSN)*

York College of Pennsylvania, Department of Nursing, *York (BS)*

Puerto Rico

Inter American University of Puerto Rico, Metropolitan Campus, Carmen Torres de Tiburcio School of Nursing, *San Juan (BSN)*

University of Puerto Rico, Medical Sciences Campus, School of Nursing, *San Juan (BSN)*

Rhode Island

University of Rhode Island, College of Nursing, *Kingston (BS)*

South Carolina

Charleston Southern University, Wingo School of Nursing, *Charleston (BSN)*

Francis Marion University, Department of Nursing, *Florence (BSN)*

University of South Carolina Aiken, School of Nursing, *Aiken (BSN)*

South Dakota

Mount Marty College, Nursing Program, *Yankton (BSN)*

Presentation College, Department of Nursing, *Aberdeen (BSN)*

Tennessee

Austin Peay State University, School of Nursing, *Clarksville (BSN)*

Belmont University, School of Nursing, *Nashville (BSN)*

Bethel University, Nursing Program, *McKenzie (BSN)*

Cumberland University, Rudy School of Nursing and Health Professions, *Lebanon (BSN)*

East Tennessee State University, College of Nursing, *Johnson City (BSN)*

Lincoln Memorial University, Caylor School of Nursing, *Harrogate (BSN)*

Milligan College, Department of Nursing, *Milligan College (BSN)*

Southern Adventist University, School of Nursing, *Collegedale (BS)*

Tennessee Technological University, Whitson-Hester School of Nursing, *Cookeville (BSN)*

Tennessee Wesleyan College, Fort Sanders Nursing Department, *Knoxville (BSN)*

University of Memphis, Loewenberg School of Nursing, *Memphis (BSN)*

The University of Tennessee at Chattanooga, School of Nursing, *Chattanooga (BSN)*

The University of Tennessee at Martin, Department of Nursing, *Martin (BSN)*

Texas

Lamar University, Department of Nursing, *Beaumont (BSN)*

Midwestern State University, Nursing Program, *Wichita Falls (BSN)*

Tarleton State University, Department of Nursing, *Stephenville (BSN)*

Texas A&M Health Science Center, College of Nursing, *College Station (BSN)*

Texas A&M University–Corpus Christi, College of Nursing and Health Sciences, *Corpus Christi (BSN)*

Texas A&M University–Texarkana, Nursing Department, *Texarkana (BSN)*

University of Mary Hardin-Baylor, College of Nursing, *Belton (BSN)*

The University of Texas at Brownsville, Department of Nursing, *Brownsville (BSN)*

The University of Texas at Tyler, Program in Nursing, *Tyler (BSN)*

The University of Texas Health Science Center at Houston, School of Nursing, *Houston (BS)*

The University of Texas–Pan American, Department of Nursing, *Edinburg (BSN)*

University of the Incarnate Word, Program in Nursing, *San Antonio (BSN)*

West Texas A&M University, Department of Nursing, *Canyon (BSN)*

Utah

Utah Valley University, Department of Nursing, *Orem (BSN)*

Weber State University, Program in Nursing, *Ogden (BSN)*

Vermont

Norwich University, Department of Nursing, *Northfield (BSN)*

Southern Vermont College, Department of Nursing, *Bennington (BSN)*

University of Vermont, Department of Nursing, *Burlington (BS)*

Virgin Islands

University of the Virgin Islands, Division of Nursing, *Saint Thomas (BSN)*

Virginia

Eastern Mennonite University, Department of Nursing, *Harrisonburg (BSN)*

Jefferson College of Health Sciences, Nursing Education Program, *Roanoke (BSN)*

Marymount University, Malek School of Health Professions, *Arlington (BSN)*

Shenandoah University, Eleanor Wade Custer School of Nursing, *Winchester (BSN)*

University of Virginia, School of Nursing, *Charlottesville (BSN)*

The University of Virginia's College at Wise, Department of Nursing, *Wise (BSN)*

Virginia Commonwealth University, School of Nursing, *Richmond (BS)*

Washington

University of Washington, School of Nursing, *Seattle (BSN)*

Walla Walla University, School of Nursing, *College Place (BS)*

West Virginia

Bluefield State College, Program in Nursing, *Bluefield (BSN)*

Fairmont State University, School of Nursing and Allied Health Administration, *Fairmont (BSN)*

Shepherd University, Department of Nursing Education, *Shepherdstown (BSN)*

West Virginia University, School of Nursing, *Morgantown (BSN)*

Wisconsin

Alverno College, Division of Nursing, *Milwaukee (BSN)*

Cardinal Stritch University, Ruth S. Coleman College of Nursing, *Milwaukee (BSN)*

Carroll University, Nursing Program, *Waukesha (BSN)*

Concordia University Wisconsin, Program in Nursing, *Mequon (BSN)*

Marian University, School of Nursing, *Fond du Lac (BSN)*

Silver Lake College of the Holy Family, Nursing Program, *Manitowoc (BSN)*

University of Wisconsin–Eau Claire, College of Nursing and Health Sciences, *Eau Claire (BSN)*

University of Wisconsin–Milwaukee, College of Nursing, *Milwaukee (BSN)*

University of Wisconsin–Oshkosh, College of Nursing, *Oshkosh (BSN)*

Wyoming

University of Wyoming, Fay W. Whitney School of Nursing, *Laramie (BSN)*

BACCALAUREATE FOR SECOND DEGREE

U.S. AND U.S. TERRITORIES

Alabama

Samford University, Ida V. Moffett School of Nursing, *Birmingham (BSN)*

Spring Hill College, Division of Nursing, *Mobile*
(BSN)
The University of Alabama, Capstone College of
Nursing, *Tuscaloosa (BSN)*
The University of Alabama at Birmingham,
School of Nursing, *Birmingham (BSN)*
The University of Alabama in Huntsville, College
of Nursing, *Huntsville (BSN)*

Arizona
Arizona State University at the Downtown
Phoenix Campus, College of Nursing, *Phoenix*
(BSN)

Arkansas
Arkansas Tech University, Program in Nursing,
Russellville (BSN)
University of Arkansas for Medical Sciences,
College of Nursing, *Little Rock (BSN)*

California
California State University, Chico, School of
Nursing, *Chico (BSN)*
California State University, Dominguez Hills,
Program in Nursing, *Carson (BSN)*
California State University, Fullerton, Department
of Nursing, *Fullerton (BSN)*
California State University, Long Beach, School
of.Nursing, *Long Beach (BSN)*
California State University, Sacramento, School of
Nursing, *Sacramento (BSN)*
Dominican University of California, Program in
Nursing, *San Rafael (BSN)*
Loma Linda University, School of Nursing,
Loma Linda (BS)
National University, Department of Nursing,
La Jolla (BSN)

Colorado
Colorado State University–Pueblo, Department of
Nursing, *Pueblo (BSN)*

Connecticut
University of Saint Joseph, Department of
Nursing, *West Hartford (BS)*

Florida
Barry University, Division of Nursing,
Miami Shores (BSN)
Florida Southern College, School of Nursing &
Health Sciences, *Lakeland (BSN)*
Jacksonville University, School of Nursing,
Jacksonville (BSN)
University of Miami, School of Nursing and
Health Studies, *Coral Gables (BSN)*

Georgia
Armstrong Atlantic State University, Program in
Nursing, *Savannah (BSN)*
Emory University, Nell Hodgson Woodruff School
of Nursing, *Atlanta (BSN)*
Georgia Southwestern State University, School of
Nursing, *Americus (BSN)*
Kennesaw State University, School of Nursing,
Kennesaw (BSN)

Illinois
Methodist College, *Peoria (BSN)*
Millikin University, School of Nursing, *Decatur*
(BSN)
Resurrection University, *Oak Park (BSN)*
Saint Anthony College of Nursing, *Rockford*
(BSN)
University of Illinois at Chicago, College of
Nursing, *Chicago (BSN)*

Indiana
Ball State University, School of Nursing, *Muncie*
(BS)
Indiana University Bloomington, Department of
Nursing–Bloomington Division, *Bloomington*
(BSN)
Indiana University Northwest, School of Nursing
and Health Professions, *Gary (BSN)*
Marian University, School of Nursing,
Indianapolis (BSN)
Purdue University, School of Nursing,
West Lafayette (BS)

Purdue University North Central, Department of
Nursing, *Westville (BS)*

Iowa
Allen College, Program in Nursing, *Waterloo*
(BSN)
Clarke University, Department of Nursing and
Health, *Dubuque (BS)*
Iowa Wesleyan College, Division of Nursing,
Mount Pleasant (BSN)
Morningside College, Department of Nursing
Education, *Sioux City (BSN)*

Kansas
MidAmerica Nazarene University, Division of
Nursing, *Olathe (BSN)*
Washburn University, School of Nursing, *Topeka*
(BSN)

Kentucky
Eastern Kentucky University, Department of
Baccalaureate and Graduate Nursing, *Richmond*
(BSN)
University of Kentucky, Graduate School
Programs in the College of Nursing, *Lexington*
(BSN)
Western Kentucky University, School of Nursing,
Bowling Green (BSN)

Maryland
Coppin State University, Helene Fuld School of
Nursing, *Baltimore (BSN)*
Stevenson University, Nursing Division,
Stevenson (BS)

Massachusetts
Regis College, School of Nursing, Science and
Health Professions, *Weston (BSN)*
Simmons College, School of Nursing and Health
Sciences, *Boston (BS)*

Michigan
Eastern Michigan University, School of Nursing,
Ypsilanti (BSN)
Ferris State University, School of Nursing,
Big Rapids (BSN)
Grand Valley State University, Kirkhof College of
Nursing, *Allendale (BSN)*
Saginaw Valley State University, Crystal M. Lange
College of Health and Human Services,
University Center (BSN)

Minnesota
St. Catherine University, Department of Nursing,
St. Paul (BS)

Missouri
Cox College, Department of Nursing, *Springfield*
(BSN)
Missouri Southern State University, Department of
Nursing, *Joplin (BSN)*
Research College of Nursing, College of Nursing,
Kansas City (BSN)
University of Missouri–St. Louis, College of
Nursing, *St. Louis (BSN)*

Montana
Montana State University, College of Nursing,
Bozeman (BSN)

Nebraska
Clarkson College, Master of Science in Nursing
Program, *Omaha (BSN)*
University of Nebraska Medical Center, College
of Nursing, *Omaha (BSN)*

New Jersey
Caldwell College, Nursing Programs, *Caldwell*
(BSN)
Rutgers, The State University of New Jersey,
College of Nursing, *Newark (BS)*
Seton Hall University, College of Nursing,
South Orange (BSN)

New York
College of Mount Saint Vincent, Department of
Nursing, *Riverdale (BS)*
The College of New Rochelle, School of Nursing,
New Rochelle (BSN)

Lehman College of the City University of New
York, Department of Nursing, *Bronx (BS)*
Molloy College, Division of Nursing,
Rockville Centre (BS)
The Sage Colleges, Department of Nursing, *Troy*
(BS)
St. John Fisher College, Wegmans School of
Nursing, *Rochester (BS)*
Wagner College, Department of Nursing,
Staten Island (BS)

North Carolina
Queens University of Charlotte, Presbyterian
School of Nursing, *Charlotte (BSN)*
The University of North Carolina at Chapel Hill,
School of Nursing, *Chapel Hill (BSN)*
The University of North Carolina at Greensboro,
School of Nursing, *Greensboro (BSN)*
Winston-Salem State University, Department of
Nursing, *Winston-Salem (BSN)*

North Dakota
University of North Dakota, College of Nursing,
Grand Forks (BSN)

Ohio
Ashland University, Dwight Schar College of
Nursing and Health Sciences, *Ashland (BSN)*
Kent State University, College of Nursing, *Kent*
(BSN)
Wright State University, College of Nursing and
Health, *Dayton (BSN)*

Oklahoma
Northwestern Oklahoma State University,
Division of Nursing, *Alva (BSN)*
Oklahoma Baptist University, School of Nursing,
Shawnee (BSN)
Oklahoma City University, Kramer School of
Nursing, *Oklahoma City (BSN)*
Oklahoma Wesleyan University, School of
Nursing, *Bartlesville (BSN)*
Southern Nazarene University, School of Nursing,
Bethany (BS)

Oregon
Linfield College, School of Nursing, *McMinnville*
(BSN)

Pennsylvania
Bloomsburg University of Pennsylvania,
Department of Nursing, *Bloomsburg (BSN)*
Carlow University, School of Nursing, *Pittsburgh*
(BSN)
Cedar Crest College, Department of Nursing,
Allentown (BS)
DeSales University, Department of Nursing and
Health, *Center Valley (BSN)*
Eastern University, Program in Nursing,
St. Davids (BSN)
Edinboro University of Pennsylvania, Department
of Nursing, *Edinboro (BS)*
Gannon University, Villa Maria School of
Nursing, *Erie (BSN)*
Indiana University of Pennsylvania, Department
of Nursing and Allied Health, *Indiana (BSN)*
La Salle University, School of Nursing and Health
Sciences, *Philadelphia (BSN)*
Misericordia University, Department of Nursing,
Dallas (BSN)
Neumann University, Program in Nursing and
Health Sciences, *Aston (BS)*
Robert Morris University, School of Nursing and
Health Sciences, *Moon Township (BSN)*
Thomas Jefferson University, Department of
Nursing, *Philadelphia (BSN)*
University of Pennsylvania, School of Nursing,
Philadelphia (BSN)
The University of Scranton, Department of
Nursing, *Scranton (BS)*
Villanova University, College of Nursing,
Villanova (BSN)

Rhode Island
Rhode Island College, Department of Nursing,
Providence (BSN)

South Carolina

Lander University, School of Nursing, *Greenwood* (BSN)

South Dakota

Presentation College, Department of Nursing, *Aberdeen (BSN)*

Tennessee

Austin Peay State University, School of Nursing, *Clarksville (BSN)*

Belmont University, School of Nursing, *Nashville* (BSN)

Cumberland University, Rudy School of Nursing and Health Professions, *Lebanon (BSN)*

Milligan College, Department of Nursing, *Milligan College (BSN)*

Tennessee Technological University, Whitson-Hester School of Nursing, *Cookeville (BSN)*

University of Memphis, Loewenberg School of Nursing, *Memphis (BSN)*

The University of Tennessee at Chattanooga, School of Nursing, *Chattanooga (BSN)*

Texas

Texas A&M University–Corpus Christi, College of Nursing and Health Sciences, *Corpus Christi* (BSN)

Texas State University–San Marcos, St. David's School of Nursing, *San Marcos (BSN)*

Texas Woman's University, College of Nursing, *Denton (BS)*

The University of Texas at Arlington, College of Nursing, *Arlington (BSN)*

University of the Incarnate Word, Program in Nursing, *San Antonio (BSN)*

Utah

Westminster College, School of Nursing and Health Sciences, *Salt Lake City (BSN)*

Virginia

Eastern Mennonite University, Department of Nursing, *Harrisonburg (BSN)*

Lynchburg College, School of Health Sciences and Human Performance, *Lynchburg (BS)*

Radford University, School of Nursing, *Radford* (BSN)

Washington

Seattle University, College of Nursing, *Seattle* (BSN)

Wisconsin

Alverno College, Division of Nursing, *Milwaukee* (BSN)

Bellin College, Nursing Program, *Green Bay* (BSN)

Columbia College of Nursing/Mount Mary College Nursing Program, *Milwaukee (BSN)*

Edgewood College, Program in Nursing, *Madison* (BS)

University of Wisconsin–Oshkosh, College of Nursing, *Oshkosh (BSN)*

CANADA

Alberta

University of Alberta, Faculty of Nursing, *Edmonton (BScN)*

University of Calgary, Faculty of Nursing, *Calgary (BN)*

University of Lethbridge, Faculty of Health Sciences, *Lethbridge (BN)*

Manitoba

Brandon University, School of Health Studies, *Brandon (BN)*

University of Manitoba, Faculty of Nursing, *Winnipeg (BN)*

Ontario

Laurentian University, School of Nursing, *Sudbury (BScN)*

McMaster University, School of Nursing, *Hamilton (BScN)*

University of Ottawa, School of Nursing, *Ottawa* (BScN)

University of Toronto, Faculty of Nursing, *Toronto* (BScN)

Saskatchewan

University of Saskatchewan, College of Nursing, *Saskatoon (BSN)*

GENERIC BACCALAUREATE

U.S. AND U.S. TERRITORIES

Alabama

Auburn University, School of Nursing, *Auburn University (BSN)*

Auburn University Montgomery, School of Nursing, *Montgomery (BSN)*

Jacksonville State University, College of Nursing and Health Sciences, *Jacksonville (BSN)*

Oakwood University, Department of Nursing, *Huntsville (BS)*

Samford University, Ida V. Moffett School of Nursing, *Birmingham (BSN)*

Spring Hill College, Division of Nursing, *Mobile* (BSN)

Troy University, School of Nursing, *Troy (BSN)*

Tuskegee University, Program in Nursing, *Tuskegee (BSN)*

The University of Alabama, Capstone College of Nursing, *Tuscaloosa (BSN)*

The University of Alabama at Birmingham, School of Nursing, *Birmingham (BSN)*

The University of Alabama in Huntsville, College of Nursing, *Huntsville (BSN)*

University of Mobile, School of Nursing, *Mobile (BSN)*

University of North Alabama, College of Nursing and Allied Health, *Florence (BSN)*

University of South Alabama, College of Nursing, *Mobile (BSN)*

Alaska

University of Alaska Anchorage, School of Nursing, *Anchorage (BS)*

Arizona

Arizona State University at the Downtown Phoenix Campus, College of Nursing, *Phoenix* (BSN)

Northern Arizona University, School of Nursing, *Flagstaff (BSN)*

The University of Arizona, College of Nursing, *Tucson (BSN)*

Arkansas

Arkansas State University, Department of Nursing, *State University (BSN)*

Arkansas Tech University, Program in Nursing, *Russellville (BSN)*

Harding University, College of Nursing, *Searcy* (BSN)

Henderson State University, Department of Nursing, *Arkadelphia (BSN)*

Southern Arkansas University–Magnolia, Department of Nursing, *Magnolia (BSN)*

University of Arkansas, Eleanor Mann School of Nursing, *Fayetteville (BSN)*

University of Arkansas at Monticello, School of Nursing, *Monticello (BSN)*

University of Arkansas at Pine Bluff, Department of Nursing, *Pine Bluff (BSN)*

University of Arkansas for Medical Sciences, College of Nursing, *Little Rock (BSN)*

University of Arkansas–Fort Smith, Carol McKelvey Moore School of Nursing, *Fort Smith* (BSN)

University of Central Arkansas, Department of Nursing, *Conway (BSN)*

California

American University of Health Sciences, School of Nursing, *Signal Hill (BSN)*

Azusa Pacific University, School of Nursing, *Azusa (BSN)*

Biola University, Department of Nursing, *La Mirada (BSN)*

California Baptist University, School of Nursing, *Riverside (BSN)*

California State University, Bakersfield, Program in Nursing, *Bakersfield (BSN)*

California State University Channel Islands, Nursing Program, *Camarillo (BSN)*

California State University, Chico, School of Nursing, *Chico (BSN)*

California State University, East Bay, Department of Nursing and Health Sciences, *Hayward (BS)*

California State University, Fresno, Department of Nursing, *Fresno (BSN)*

California State University, Fullerton, Department of Nursing, *Fullerton (BSN)*

California State University, Long Beach, School of Nursing, *Long Beach (BSN)*

California State University, Los Angeles, School of Nursing, *Los Angeles (BSN)*

California State University, Sacramento, School of Nursing, *Sacramento (BSN)*

California State University, San Bernardino, Department of Nursing, *San Bernardino (BSN)*

California State University, San Marcos, School of Nursing, *San Marcos (BSN)*

California State University, Stanislaus, Department of Nursing, *Turlock (BSN)*

Dominican University of California, Program in Nursing, *San Rafael (BSN)*

Loma Linda University, School of Nursing, *Loma Linda (BS)*

Mount St. Mary's College, Department of Nursing, *Los Angeles (BSN, BSc PN)*

National University, Department of Nursing, *La Jolla (BSN)*

Point Loma Nazarene University, School of Nursing, *San Diego (BSN)*

Samuel Merritt University, School of Nursing, *Oakland (BSN)*

San Diego State University, School of Nursing, *San Diego (BSN)*

San Francisco State University, School of Nursing, *San Francisco (BSN)*

San Jose State University, The Valley Foundation School of Nursing, *San Jose (BS)*

Sonoma State University, Department of Nursing, *Rohnert Park (BSN)*

University of California, Irvine, Program in Nursing Science, *Irvine (BS)*

University of California, Los Angeles, School of Nursing, *Los Angeles (BS)*

University of San Francisco, School of Nursing and Health Professions, *San Francisco (BSN)*

Colorado

Adams State University, Nursing Program, *Alamosa (BSN)*

Colorado Christian University, Nursing Programs, *Lakewood (BSN)*

Colorado Mesa University, Department of Nursing and Radiologic Sciences, *Grand Junction (BSN)*

Colorado State University–Pueblo, Department of Nursing, *Pueblo (BSN)*

Denver College of Nursing, *Denver (BSN)*

Regis University, School of Nursing, *Denver* (BSN)

University of Colorado at Colorado Springs, Beth-El College of Nursing and Health Sciences, *Colorado Springs (BSN)*

University of Colorado Denver, College of Nursing, *Aurora (BS)*

University of Northern Colorado, School of Nursing, *Greeley (BS)*

Connecticut

Central Connecticut State University, Department of Nursing, *New Britain (BSN)*

Fairfield University, School of Nursing, *Fairfield* (BS)

Quinnipiac University, School of Nursing, *Hamden (BSN)*

Sacred Heart University, Program in Nursing, *Fairfield (BSN)*

Southern Connecticut State University, Department of Nursing, *New Haven (BS)*

University of Connecticut, School of Nursing, *Storrs (BS)*

University of Saint Joseph, Department of Nursing, *West Hartford (BS)*

Western Connecticut State University, Department of Nursing, *Danbury (BS)*

Delaware

Delaware State University, Department of Nursing, *Dover (BSN)*

University of Delaware, School of Nursing, *Newark (BSN)*

Wesley College, Nursing Program, *Dover (BSN)*

District of Columbia

The Catholic University of America, School of Nursing, *Washington (BSN)*

Georgetown University, School of Nursing and Health Studies, *Washington (BSN)*

Howard University, Division of Nursing, *Washington (BSN)*

Trinity Washington University, Nursing Program, *Washington (BSN)*

Florida

Adventist University of Health Sciences, Department of Nursing, *Orlando (BSN)*

Barry University, Division of Nursing, *Miami Shores (BSN)*

Bethune-Cookman University, School of Nursing, *Daytona Beach (BSN)*

Florida Agricultural and Mechanical University, School of Nursing, *Tallahassee (BSN)*

Florida Atlantic University, Christine E. Lynn College of Nursing, *Boca Raton (BSN)*

Florida Gulf Coast University, School of Nursing, *Fort Myers (BSN)*

Florida International University, Graduate Nursing Programs, *Miami (BSN)*

Florida Southern College, School of Nursing & Health Sciences, *Lakeland (BSN)*

Florida State University, College of Nursing, *Tallahassee (BSN)*

Jacksonville University, School of Nursing, *Jacksonville (BSN)*

Kaplan University Online, The School of Nursing Online, *Fort Lauderdale (BSN)*

Nova Southeastern University, College of Health Care Sciences, *Fort Lauderdale (BSN)*

South University, Nursing Program, *Royal Palm Beach (BSN)*

University of Central Florida, College of Nursing, *Orlando (BSN)*

University of Florida, College of Nursing, *Gainesville (BSN)*

University of Miami, School of Nursing and Health Studies, *Coral Gables (BSN)*

University of North Florida, School of Nursing, *Jacksonville (BSN)*

University of South Florida, College of Nursing, *Tampa (BS)*

The University of Tampa, Department of Nursing, *Tampa (BSN)*

University of West Florida, Department of Nursing, *Pensacola (BSN)*

Georgia

Albany State University, College of Sciences and Health Professions, *Albany (BSN)*

Armstrong Atlantic State University, Program in Nursing, *Savannah (BSN)*

Augusta State University, Department of Nursing, *Augusta (BSN)*

Brenau University, College of Health and Science, *Gainesville (BSN)*

Clayton State University, Department of Nursing, *Morrow (BSN)*

College of Coastal Georgia, Department of Nursing and Health Sciences, *Brunswick (BS)*

Columbus State University, Nursing Program, *Columbus (BSN)*

Emory University, Nell Hodgson Woodruff School of Nursing, *Atlanta (BSN)*

Georgia College & State University, College of Health Sciences, *Milledgeville (BSN)*

Georgia Regents University, School of Nursing, *Augusta (BSN)*

Georgia Southern University, School of Nursing, *Statesboro (BSN)*

Georgia Southwestern State University, School of Nursing, *Americus (BSN)*

Georgia State University, Byrdine F. Lewis School of Nursing and Health Professions, *Atlanta (BS)*

Kennesaw State University, School of Nursing, *Kennesaw (BSN)*

LaGrange College, Department of Nursing, *LaGrange (BSN)*

Macon State College, School of Nursing and Health Sciences, *Macon (BSN)*

Mercer University Georgia Baptist College of Nursing, *Atlanta (BSN)*

Piedmont College, School of Nursing, *Demorest (BSN)*

Shorter University, School of Nursing, *Rome (BSN)*

University of West Georgia, School of Nursing, *Carrollton (BSN)*

Valdosta State University, College of Nursing, *Valdosta (BSN)*

Guam

University of Guam, School of Nursing and Health Sciences, *Mangilao (BSN)*

Hawaii

Chaminade University of Honolulu, Nursing Program, *Honolulu (BSN)*

Hawai'i Pacific University, College of Nursing and Health Sciences, *Honolulu (BSN)*

University of Hawaii at Hilo, Department in Nursing, *Hilo (BSN)*

University of Hawaii at Manoa, School of Nursing and Dental Hygiene, *Honolulu (BSN)*

Idaho

Boise State University, Department of Nursing, *Boise (BS)*

Idaho State University, Department of Nursing, *Pocatello (BSN)*

Lewis-Clark State College, Division of Nursing and Health Sciences, *Lewiston (BSN)*

Northwest Nazarene University, School of Health and Science, *Nampa (BSN)*

Illinois

Aurora University, School of Nursing, *Aurora (BSN)*

Blessing–Rieman College of Nursing, *Quincy (BSN)*

Bradley University, Department of Nursing, *Peoria (BSN, BSc PN)*

Chicago State University, Department of Nursing, *Chicago (BSN)*

Elmhurst College, Deicke Center for Nursing Education, *Elmhurst (BS)*

Illinois State University, Mennonite College of Nursing, *Normal (BSN)*

Illinois Wesleyan University, School of Nursing, *Bloomington (BSN)*

Lakeview College of Nursing, *Danville (BSN)*

Lewis University, Program in Nursing, *Romeoville (BSN)*

Loyola University Chicago, Marcella Niehoff School of Nursing, *Maywood (BSN)*

MacMurray College, Department of Nursing, *Jacksonville (BSN)*

Methodist College, *Peoria (BSN)*

Millikin University, School of Nursing, *Decatur (BSN)*

Northern Illinois University, School of Nursing and Health Studies, *De Kalb (BS)*

North Park University, School of Nursing, *Chicago (BS)*

Olivet Nazarene University, Division of Nursing, *Bourbonnais (BSN)*

Rockford College, Department of Nursing, *Rockford (BSN)*

Saint Anthony College of Nursing, *Rockford (BSN)*

Saint Francis Medical Center College of Nursing, Baccalaureate Nursing Program, *Peoria (BSN)*

St. John's College, Department of Nursing, *Springfield (BSN)*

Saint Xavier University, School of Nursing, *Chicago (BSN)*

Southern Illinois University Edwardsville, School of Nursing, *Edwardsville (BS)*

Trinity Christian College, Department of Nursing, *Palos Heights (BSN)*

Trinity College of Nursing and Health Sciences, *Rock Island (BSN)*

University of Illinois at Chicago, College of Nursing, *Chicago (BSN)*

University of St. Francis, Leach College of Nursing, *Joliet (BSN)*

Western Illinois University, School of Nursing, *Macomb (BSN)*

Indiana

Anderson University, School of Nursing, *Anderson (BSN)*

Ball State University, School of Nursing, *Muncie (BS)*

Bethel College, School of Nursing, *Mishawaka (BSN)*

Goshen College, Department of Nursing, *Goshen (BSN)*

Huntington University, Department of Nursing, *Huntington (BSN)*

Indiana State University, Department of Nursing, *Terre Haute (BS)*

Indiana University Bloomington, Department of Nursing–Bloomington Division, *Bloomington (BSN)*

Indiana University East, School of Nursing, *Richmond (BSN)*

Indiana University Kokomo, Indiana University School of Nursing, *Kokomo (BSN)*

Indiana University Northwest, School of Nursing and Health Professions, *Gary (BSN)*

Indiana University–Purdue University Fort Wayne, Department of Nursing, *Fort Wayne (BS)*

Indiana University–Purdue University Indianapolis, School of Nursing, *Indianapolis (BSN)*

Indiana University South Bend, College of Health Sciences, *South Bend (BSN)*

Indiana University Southeast, Division of Nursing, *New Albany (BSN)*

Indiana Wesleyan University, School of Nursing, *Marion (BSN)*

Marian University, School of Nursing, *Indianapolis (BSN)*

Purdue University, School of Nursing, *West Lafayette (BS)*

Purdue University Calumet, School of Nursing, *Hammond (BS)*

Saint Mary's College, Department of Nursing, *Notre Dame (BS)*

University of Evansville, Department of Nursing, *Evansville (BSN)*

University of Indianapolis, School of Nursing, *Indianapolis (BSN)*

University of Saint Francis, Department of Nursing, *Fort Wayne (BSN)*

University of Southern Indiana, College of Nursing and Health Professions, *Evansville (BSN)*

Valparaiso University, College of Nursing, *Valparaiso (BSN)*

Iowa

Allen College, Program in Nursing, *Waterloo (BSN)*

Briar Cliff University, Department of Nursing, *Sioux City (BSN)*

Clarke University, Department of Nursing and Health, *Dubuque (BS)*

Coe College, Department of Nursing, *Cedar Rapids (BSN)*

Dordt College, Nursing Program, *Sioux Center (BSN)*

Grand View University, Division of Nursing, *Des Moines (BSN)*

Iowa Wesleyan College, Division of Nursing, *Mount Pleasant (BSN)*

Luther College, Department of Nursing, *Decorah (BA)*

Morningside College, Department of Nursing Education, *Sioux City (BSN)*

Mount Mercy University, Department of Nursing, *Cedar Rapids (BSN)*

Northwestern College, Nursing Program, *Orange City (BSN)*

St. Ambrose University, Program in Nursing (BSN), *Davenport (BSN)*

The University of Iowa, College of Nursing, *Iowa City (BSN)*

Kansas

Baker University, School of Nursing, *Topeka (BSN)*

Benedictine College, Department of Nursing, *Atchison (BSN)*

Bethel College, Department of Nursing, *North Newton (BSN)*

Emporia State University, Newman Division of Nursing, *Emporia (BSN)*

Fort Hays State University, Department of Nursing, *Hays (BSN)*

Kansas Wesleyan University, Department of Nursing Education, *Salina (BSN)*

MidAmerica Nazarene University, Division of Nursing, *Olathe (BSN)*

Newman University, Division of Nursing, *Wichita (BSN)*

Pittsburg State University, Department of Nursing, *Pittsburg (BSN)*

Southwestern College, Nursing Program, *Winfield (BSN)*

The University of Kansas, School of Nursing, *Kansas City (BSN)*

University of Saint Mary, Bachelor of Science in Nursing Program, *Leavenworth (BSN)*

Washburn University, School of Nursing, *Topeka (BSN)*

Wichita State University, School of Nursing, *Wichita (BSN)*

Kentucky

Bellarmine University, Donna and Allan Lansing School of Nursing and Health Sciences, *Louisville (BSN, MSCE)*

Berea College, Department of Nursing, *Berea (BSN)*

Eastern Kentucky University, Department of Baccalaureate and Graduate Nursing, *Richmond (BSN)*

Kentucky Christian University, School of Nursing, *Grayson (BSN)*

Morehead State University, Department of Nursing, *Morehead (BSN)*

Murray State University, Program in Nursing, *Murray (BSN)*

Northern Kentucky University, Department of Nursing, *Highland Heights (BSN)*

Spalding University, School of Nursing, *Louisville (BSN)*

Thomas More College, Program in Nursing, *Crestview Hills (BSN)*

University of Kentucky, Graduate School Programs in the College of Nursing, *Lexington (BSN)*

University of Louisville, School of Nursing, *Louisville (BSN)*

Western Kentucky University, School of Nursing, *Bowling Green (BSN)*

Louisiana

Dillard University, Division of Nursing, *New Orleans (BSN)*

Grambling State University, School of Nursing, *Grambling (BSN)*

Louisiana College, Department of Nursing, *Pineville (BSN)*

Louisiana State University Health Sciences Center, School of Nursing, *New Orleans (BSN)*

McNeese State University, College of Nursing, *Lake Charles (BSN)*

Nicholls State University, Department of Nursing, *Thibodaux (BSN)*

Northwestern State University of Louisiana, College of Nursing and Allied Health, *Shreveport (BSN)*

Our Lady of Holy Cross College, Division of Nursing, *New Orleans (BSN)*

Our Lady of the Lake College, Division of Nursing, *Baton Rouge (BSN)*

Southeastern Louisiana University, School of Nursing, *Hammond (BS)*

Southern University and Agricultural and Mechanical College, School of Nursing, *Baton Rouge (BSN)*

University of Louisiana at Lafayette, College of Nursing, *Lafayette (BSN)*

University of Louisiana at Monroe, Nursing, *Monroe (BS)*

Maine

Husson University, School of Nursing, *Bangor (BSN)*

Saint Joseph's College of Maine, Master of Science in Nursing Program, *Standish (BSN)*

University of Maine, School of Nursing, *Orono (BSN)*

University of Maine at Fort Kent, Department of Nursing, *Fort Kent (BSN)*

University of New England, Department of Nursing, *Biddeford (BSN)*

University of Southern Maine, School of Nursing, *Portland (BS)*

Maryland

Bowie State University, Department of Nursing, *Bowie (BSN)*

Coppin State University, Helene Fuld School of Nursing, *Baltimore (BSN)*

Salisbury University, Program in Nursing, *Salisbury (BS)*

Stevenson University, Nursing Division, *Stevenson (BS)*

Towson University, Department of Nursing, *Towson (BS)*

University of Maryland, Baltimore, Master's Program in Nursing, *Baltimore (BSN)*

Washington Adventist University, Nursing Department, *Takoma Park (BS)*

Massachusetts

American International College, Division of Nursing, *Springfield (BSN)*

Boston College, William F. Connell School of Nursing, *Chestnut Hill (BS)*

Curry College, Division of Nursing, *Milton (BS)*

Elms College, Division of Nursing, *Chicopee (BS)*

Endicott College, Major in Nursing, *Beverly (BS)*

Fitchburg State University, Department of Nursing, *Fitchburg (BS)*

Northeastern University, School of Nursing, *Boston (BSN)*

Regis College, School of Nursing, Science and Health Professions, *Weston (BSN)*

Salem State University, Program in Nursing, *Salem (BSN)*

Simmons College, School of Nursing and Health Sciences, *Boston (BS)*

University of Massachusetts Amherst, School of Nursing, *Amherst (BS)*

University of Massachusetts Boston, College of Nursing and Health Sciences, *Boston (BS)*

University of Massachusetts Dartmouth, College of Nursing, *North Dartmouth (BSN)*

University of Massachusetts Lowell, Department of Nursing, *Lowell (BS)*

Worcester State University, Department of Nursing, *Worcester (BS)*

Michigan

Andrews University, Department of Nursing, *Berrien Springs (BS)*

Calvin College, Department of Nursing, *Grand Rapids (BSN)*

Davenport University, Division of Nursing, *Grand Rapids (BSN)*

Davenport University, Bachelor of Science in Nursing Program, *Kalamazoo (BSN)*

Eastern Michigan University, School of Nursing, *Ypsilanti (BSN)*

Finlandia University, College of Professional Studies, *Hancock (BSN)*

Grand Valley State University, Kirkhof College of Nursing, *Allendale (BSN)*

Hope College, Department of Nursing, *Holland (BSN)*

Lake Superior State University, Department of Nursing, *Sault Sainte Marie (BSN)*

Madonna University, College of Nursing and Health, *Livonia (BSN)*

Michigan State University, College of Nursing, *East Lansing (BSN)*

Northern Michigan University, College of Nursing and Allied Health Science, *Marquette (BSN)*

Oakland University, School of Nursing, *Rochester (BSN)*

Rochester College, School of Nursing, *Rochester Hills (BSN)*

Saginaw Valley State University, Crystal M. Lange College of Health and Human Services, *University Center (BSN)*

Siena Heights University, Nursing Program, *Adrian (BSN)*

University of Detroit Mercy, McAuley School of Nursing, *Detroit (BSN)*

University of Michigan, School of Nursing, *Ann Arbor (BSN)*

University of Michigan–Flint, Department of Nursing, *Flint (BSN)*

Wayne State University, College of Nursing, *Detroit (BSN)*

Western Michigan University, College of Health and Human Services, *Kalamazoo (BSN)*

Minnesota

Bemidji State University, Department of Nursing, *Bemidji (BS)*

Bethel University, Department of Nursing, *St. Paul (BSN)*

College of Saint Benedict, Department of Nursing, *Saint Joseph (BS)*

The College of St. Scholastica, Department of Nursing, *Duluth (BS)*

Concordia College, Department of Nursing, *Moorhead (BA)*

Crown College, Nursing Department, *St. Bonifacius (BSN)*

Globe University–Woodbury, Bachelor of Science in Nursing, *Woodbury (BS)*

Gustavus Adolphus College, Department of Nursing, *St. Peter (BA)*

Herzing University, Nursing Program, *Minneapolis (BSN)*

Minnesota Intercollegiate Nursing Consortium, *Northfield (BA)*

Minnesota State University Mankato, School of Nursing, *Mankato (BS)*

St. Catherine University, Department of Nursing, *St. Paul (BS)*

St. Cloud State University, Department of Nursing Science, *St. Cloud (BS)*

St. Olaf College, Department of Nursing, *Northfield (BA)*

University of Minnesota, Twin Cities Campus, School of Nursing, *Minneapolis (BSN)*

Winona State University, College of Nursing and Health Sciences, *Winona (BS)*

Mississippi

Alcorn State University, School of Nursing, *Natchez (BSN)*

Delta State University, School of Nursing, *Cleveland (BSN)*

Mississippi College, School of Nursing, *Clinton (BSN)*

Mississippi University for Women, College of Nursing and Speech Language Pathology, *Columbus (BSN)*

University of Mississippi Medical Center, Program in Nursing, *Jackson (BSN)*

University of Southern Mississippi, School of Nursing, *Hattiesburg (BSN)*

William Carey University, School of Nursing, *Hattiesburg (BSN)*

Missouri

Avila University, School of Nursing, *Kansas City (BSN)*

Central Methodist University, College of Liberal Arts and Sciences, *Fayette (BN)*

Chamberlain College of Nursing, *St. Louis (BSN)*

College of the Ozarks, Armstrong McDonald School of Nursing, *Point Lookout (BSN)*

Cox College, Department of Nursing, *Springfield (BSN)*

Goldfarb School of Nursing at Barnes-Jewish College, *St. Louis (BSN)*

Graceland University, School of Nursing, *Independence (BSN)*

Maryville University of Saint Louis, Nursing Program, School of Health Professions, *St. Louis (BSN)*

Missouri Southern State University, Department of Nursing, *Joplin (BSN)*

Missouri State University, Department of Nursing, *Springfield (BSN)*

Missouri Western State University, Department of Nursing, *St. Joseph (BSN)*

Research College of Nursing, College of Nursing, *Kansas City (BSN)*

Saint Louis University, School of Nursing, *St. Louis (BSN)*

Saint Luke's College of Health Sciences, Nursing College, *Kansas City (BSN)*

Southeast Missouri State University, Department of Nursing, *Cape Girardeau (BSN)*

Truman State University, Program in Nursing, *Kirksville (BSN)*

University of Central Missouri, Department of Nursing, *Warrensburg (BS)*

University of Missouri, Sinclair School of Nursing, *Columbia (BSN)*

University of Missouri–Kansas City, School of Nursing, *Kansas City (BSN)*

University of Missouri–St. Louis, College of Nursing, *St. Louis (BSN)*

William Jewell College, Department of Nursing, *Liberty (BS)*

Montana

Carroll College, Department of Nursing, *Helena (BS)*

Montana State University, College of Nursing, *Bozeman (BSN)*

Nebraska

BryanLGH College of Health Sciences, School of Nursing, *Lincoln (BSN)*

Clarkson College, Master of Science in Nursing Program, *Omaha (BSN)*

College of Saint Mary, Division of Health Care Professions, *Omaha (BSN)*

Creighton University, School of Nursing, *Omaha (BSN)*

Midland University, Department of Nursing, *Fremont (BSN)*

Nebraska Methodist College, Department of Nursing, *Omaha (BSN)*

Union College, Division of Health Sciences, *Lincoln (BSN)*

University of Nebraska Medical Center, College of Nursing, *Omaha (BSN)*

Nevada

Nevada State College at Henderson, Nursing Program, *Henderson (BSN)*

Roseman University of Health Sciences, College of Nursing, *Henderson (BSN)*

Touro University, School of Nursing, *Henderson (BSN)*

University of Nevada, Las Vegas, School of Nursing, *Las Vegas (BSN)*

University of Nevada, Reno, Orvis School of Nursing, *Reno (BSN)*

New Hampshire

Colby-Sawyer College, Department of Nursing, *New London (BSN)*

Rivier University, Division of Nursing, *Nashua (BS)*

University of New Hampshire, Department of Nursing, *Durham (BS)*

New Jersey

Bloomfield College, Division of Nursing, *Bloomfield (BS)*

Caldwell College, Nursing Programs, *Caldwell (BSN)*

The College of New Jersey, School of Nursing, Health and Exercise Science, *Ewing (BSN)*

Fairleigh Dickinson University, Metropolitan Campus, Henry P. Becton School of Nursing and Allied Health, *Teaneck (BSN)*

Felician College, Division of Nursing and Health Management, *Lodi (BSN)*

Ramapo College of New Jersey, Master of Science in Nursing Program, *Mahwah (BSN)*

Rutgers School of Nursing–Camden, *Camden (BS)*

Rutgers, The State University of New Jersey, College of Nursing, *Newark (BS)*

Saint Peter's University, Nursing Program, *Jersey City (BSN)*

Seton Hall University, College of Nursing, *South Orange (BSN)*

Thomas Edison State College, School of Nursing, *Trenton (BSN)*

William Paterson University of New Jersey, Department of Nursing, *Wayne (BSN)*

New Mexico

New Mexico State University, School of Nursing, *Las Cruces (BSN)*

University of New Mexico, College of Nursing, *Albuquerque (BSN)*

New York

Adelphi University, School of Nursing, *Garden City (BS)*

Binghamton University, State University of New York, Decker School of Nursing, *Binghamton (BS)*

The College at Brockport, State University of New York, Department of Nursing, *Brockport (BSN)*

College of Mount Saint Vincent, Department of Nursing, *Riverdale (BS)*

The College of New Rochelle, School of Nursing, *New Rochelle (BSN)*

Concordia College–New York, Nursing Program, *Bronxville (BS)*

Dominican College, Department of Nursing, *Orangeburg (BSN)*

D'Youville College, School of Nursing, *Buffalo (BSN)*

Elmira College, Program in Nursing Education, *Elmira (BS)*

Farmingdale State College, Nursing Department, *Farmingdale (BS)*

Hartwick College, Department of Nursing, *Oneonta (BS)*

Hunter College of the City University of New York, Hunter-Bellevue School of Nursing, *New York (BSN)*

Lehman College of the City University of New York, Department of Nursing, *Bronx (BS)*

Long Island University–Brooklyn Campus, School of Nursing, *Brooklyn (BS)*

Molloy College, Division of Nursing, *Rockville Centre (BS)*

Mount Saint Mary College, Division of Nursing, *Newburgh (BSN)*

Nazareth College of Rochester, Department of Nursing, *Rochester (BS)*

New York Institute of Technology, Department of Nursing, *Old Westbury (BSN)*

New York University, College of Nursing, *New York (BS)*

Pace University, Lienhard School of Nursing, *New York (BS)*

Roberts Wesleyan College, Division of Nursing, *Rochester (BScN)*

The Sage Colleges, Department of Nursing, *Troy (BS)*

St. John Fisher College, Wegmans School of Nursing, *Rochester (BS)*

State University of New York at Plattsburgh, Department of Nursing, *Plattsburgh (BS)*

Stony Brook University, State University of New York, School of Nursing, *Stony Brook (BS)*

University at Buffalo, the State University of New York, School of Nursing, *Buffalo (BS)*

Utica College, Department of Nursing, *Utica (BS)*

Wagner College, Department of Nursing, *Staten Island (BS)*

North Carolina

Appalachian State University, Department of Nursing, *Boone (BSN)*

Barton College, School of Nursing, *Wilson (BSN)*

East Carolina University, College of Nursing, *Greenville (BSN)*

Fayetteville State University, Program in Nursing, *Fayetteville (BSN)*

Gardner-Webb University, School of Nursing, *Boiling Springs (BSN)*

Lenoir-Rhyne University, Program in Nursing, *Hickory (BS)*

North Carolina Agricultural and Technical State University, School of Nursing, *Greensboro (BSN)*

North Carolina Central University, Department of Nursing, *Durham (BSN)*

Queens University of Charlotte, Presbyterian School of Nursing, *Charlotte (BSN)*

The University of North Carolina at Chapel Hill, School of Nursing, *Chapel Hill (BSN)*

The University of North Carolina at Charlotte, School of Nursing, *Charlotte (BSN)*

The University of North Carolina at Greensboro, School of Nursing, *Greensboro (BSN)*

The University of North Carolina at Pembroke, Nursing Program, *Pembroke (BSN)*

The University of North Carolina Wilmington, School of Nursing, *Wilmington (BSN)*

Western Carolina University, School of Nursing, *Cullowhee (BSN)*

Winston-Salem State University, Department of Nursing, *Winston-Salem (BSN)*

North Dakota

Minot State University, Department of Nursing, *Minot (BSN)*

North Dakota State University, Department of Nursing, *Fargo (BSN)*

University of Mary, Division of Nursing, *Bismarck (BSN)*

University of North Dakota, College of Nursing, *Grand Forks (BSN)*

Ohio

Capital University, School of Nursing, *Columbus (BSN)*

Case Western Reserve University, Frances Payne Bolton School of Nursing, *Cleveland (BSN)*

Cleveland State University, School of Nursing, *Cleveland (BSN)*

College of Mount St. Joseph, Department of Nursing, *Cincinnati (BSN)*

Defiance College, Bachelor's Degree in Nursing, *Defiance (BSN)*

Franciscan University of Steubenville, Department of Nursing, *Steubenville (BSN)*

Hiram College, Nursing Department, *Hiram (BSN)*

Kent State University, College of Nursing, *Kent (BSN)*

Kettering College, Division of Nursing, *Kettering (BSN)*

Lourdes University, School of Nursing, *Sylvania (BSN)*

Malone University, School of Nursing, *Canton (BSN)*

Mercy College of Ohio, Division of Nursing, *Toledo (BSN)*

Miami University, Department of Nursing, *Hamilton (BSN)*

Miami University Hamilton, Bachelor of Science in Nursing Program, *Hamilton (BSN)*

Mount Carmel College of Nursing, Nursing Programs, *Columbus (BSN)*

Mount Vernon Nazarene University, School of Nursing and Health Sciences, *Mount Vernon (BS)*

Muskingum University, Department of Nursing, *New Concord (BSN)*

Notre Dame College, Nursing Department, *South Euclid (BSN)*

The Ohio State University, College of Nursing, *Columbus (BSN)*

Ohio University, School of Nursing, *Athens (BSN)*

Otterbein University, Department of Nursing, *Westerville (BSN)*

The University of Akron, College of Nursing, *Akron (BSN)*

University of Cincinnati, College of Nursing, *Cincinnati (BSN)*

The University of Toledo, College of Nursing, *Toledo (BSN)*

Ursuline College, The Breen School of Nursing, *Pepper Pike (BSN)*

Walsh University, Department of Nursing, *North Canton (BSN)*

Wright State University, College of Nursing and Health, *Dayton (BSN)*

Xavier University, School of Nursing, *Cincinnati (BSN)*

Oklahoma

East Central University, Department of Nursing, *Ada (BSN)*

Langston University, School of Nursing and Health Professions, *Langston (BSN)*

Northwestern Oklahoma State University, Division of Nursing, *Alva (BSN)*

Oklahoma Baptist University, School of Nursing, *Shawnee (BSN)*

Oklahoma Christian University, Nursing Program, *Oklahoma City (BSN)*

Oklahoma City University, Kramer School of Nursing, *Oklahoma City (BSN)*

Oklahoma Wesleyan University, School of Nursing, *Bartlesville (BSN)*

Oral Roberts University, Anna Vaughn School of Nursing, *Tulsa (BSN)*

Southern Nazarene University, School of Nursing, *Bethany (BS)*

Southwestern Oklahoma State University, School of Nursing, *Weatherford (BSN)*

University of Central Oklahoma, Department of Nursing, *Edmond (BSN)*

University of Oklahoma Health Sciences Center, College of Nursing, *Oklahoma City (BSN)*

University of Tulsa, School of Nursing, *Tulsa (BSN)*

Oregon

George Fox University, Nursing Department, *Newberg (BSN)*

Linfield College, School of Nursing, *McMinnville (BSN)*

Oregon Health & Science University, School of Nursing, *Portland (BS)*

University of Portland, School of Nursing, *Portland (BSN)*

Pennsylvania

Alvernia University, Nursing, *Reading (BSN)*

Bloomsburg University of Pennsylvania, Department of Nursing, *Bloomsburg (BSN)*

Carlow University, School of Nursing, *Pittsburgh (BSN)*

Cedar Crest College, Department of Nursing, *Allentown (BS)*

DeSales University, Department of Nursing and Health, *Center Valley (BSN)*

Drexel University, College of Nursing and Health Professions, *Philadelphia (BSN)*

Duquesne University, School of Nursing, *Pittsburgh (BSN)*

Eastern University, Program in Nursing, *St. Davids (BSN)*

East Stroudsburg University of Pennsylvania, Department of Nursing, *East Stroudsburg (BS)*

Edinboro University of Pennsylvania, Department of Nursing, *Edinboro (BS)*

Gannon University, Villa Maria School of Nursing, *Erie (BSN)*

Holy Family University, School of Nursing and Allied Health Professions, *Philadelphia (BSN)*

Immaculata University, Department of Nursing, *Immaculata (BSN)*

Indiana University of Pennsylvania, Department of Nursing and Allied Health, *Indiana (BSN)*

La Salle University, School of Nursing and Health Sciences, *Philadelphia (BSN)*

Mansfield University of Pennsylvania, Department of Health Sciences–Nursing, *Mansfield (BSN)*

Marywood University, Department of Nursing, *Scranton (BSN)*

Messiah College, Department of Nursing, *Mechanicsburg (BSN)*

Misericordia University, Department of Nursing, *Dallas (BSN)*

Moravian College, St. Luke's School of Nursing, *Bethlehem (BS)*

Neumann University, Program in Nursing and Health Sciences, *Aston (BS)*

Penn State University Park, School of Nursing, *University Park (BS)*

Robert Morris University, School of Nursing and Health Sciences, *Moon Township (BSN)*

Saint Francis University, Department of Nursing, *Loretto (BSN)*

Temple University, Department of Nursing, *Philadelphia (BSN)*

Thomas Jefferson University, Department of Nursing, *Philadelphia (BSN)*

University of Pennsylvania, School of Nursing, *Philadelphia (BSN)*

University of Pittsburgh, School of Nursing, *Pittsburgh (BSN)*

University of Pittsburgh at Bradford, Department of Nursing, *Bradford (BSN)*

The University of Scranton, Department of Nursing, *Scranton (BS)*

Villanova University, College of Nursing, *Villanova (BSN)*

Waynesburg University, Department of Nursing, *Waynesburg (BSN)*

West Chester University of Pennsylvania, Department of Nursing, *West Chester (BSN)*

Widener University, School of Nursing, *Chester (BSN)*

Wilkes University, Department of Nursing, *Wilkes-Barre (BS)*

York College of Pennsylvania, Department of Nursing, *York (BS)*

Puerto Rico

Inter American University of Puerto Rico, Arecibo Campus, Nursing Program, *Arecibo (BS)*

Inter American University of Puerto Rico, Metropolitan Campus, Carmen Torres de Tiburcio School of Nursing, *San Juan (BSN)*

Pontifical Catholic University of Puerto Rico, Department of Nursing, *Ponce (BSN)*

Universidad Adventista de las Antillas, Department of Nursing, *Mayagüez (BSN)*

Universidad del Turabo, Nursing Program, *Gurabo (BS)*

University of Puerto Rico at Arecibo, Department of Nursing, *Arecibo (BSN)*

University of Puerto Rico at Humacao, Department of Nursing, *Humacao (BS)*

University of Puerto Rico, Mayagüez Campus, Department of Nursing, *Mayagüez (BSN)*

University of Puerto Rico, Medical Sciences Campus, School of Nursing, *San Juan (BSN)*

University of the Sacred Heart, Program in Nursing, *San Juan (BSN)*

Rhode Island

Rhode Island College, Department of Nursing, *Providence (BSN)*

Salve Regina University, Department of Nursing, *Newport (BS)*

University of Rhode Island, College of Nursing, *Kingston (BS)*

South Carolina

Charleston Southern University, Wingo School of Nursing, *Charleston (BSN)*

Clemson University, School of Nursing, *Clemson (BS)*

Francis Marion University, Department of Nursing, *Florence (BSN)*

Lander University, School of Nursing, *Greenwood (BSN)*

South Carolina State University, Department of Nursing, *Orangeburg (BSN)*

University of South Carolina, College of Nursing, *Columbia (BSN)*

University of South Carolina Aiken, School of Nursing, *Aiken (BSN)*

University of South Carolina Beaufort, Nursing Program, *Bluffton (BSN)*

University of South Carolina Upstate, Mary Black School of Nursing, *Spartanburg (BSN)*

South Dakota

Augustana College, Department of Nursing, *Sioux Falls (BA)*

Mount Marty College, Nursing Program, *Yankton (BSN)*

National American University, School of Nursing, *Rapid City (BSN)*

Presentation College, Department of Nursing, *Aberdeen (BSN)*

South Dakota State University, College of Nursing, *Brookings (BS)*

University of Sioux Falls, School of Nursing, *Sioux Falls (BSN)*

Tennessee

Austin Peay State University, School of Nursing, *Clarksville (BSN)*

Baptist College of Health Sciences, Nursing Division, *Memphis (BSN)*

Belmont University, School of Nursing, *Nashville (BSN)*

Bethel University, Nursing Program, *McKenzie (BSN)*

Carson-Newman University, Department of Nursing, *Jefferson City (BSN)*

Cumberland University, Rudy School of Nursing and Health Professions, *Lebanon (BSN)*

East Tennessee State University, College of Nursing, *Johnson City (BSN)*

King College, School of Nursing, *Bristol (BSN)*

Lincoln Memorial University, Caylor School of Nursing, *Harrogate (BSN)*

Lipscomb University, Department of Nursing, *Nashville (BSN)*

Martin Methodist College, Division of Nursing, *Pulaski (BSN)*

Middle Tennessee State University, School of Nursing, *Murfreesboro (BSN)*

Milligan College, Department of Nursing, *Milligan College (BSN)*

South College, Department of Nursing, *Knoxville (BSN)*

Tennessee State University, School of Nursing, *Nashville (BSN)*

Tennessee Technological University, Whitson-Hester School of Nursing, *Cookeville (BSN)*

Tennessee Wesleyan College, Fort Sanders Nursing Department, *Knoxville (BSN)*

Union University, School of Nursing, *Jackson (BSN)*

University of Memphis, Loewenberg School of Nursing, *Memphis (BSN)*

The University of Tennessee, College of Nursing, *Knoxville (BSN)*

The University of Tennessee at Chattanooga, School of Nursing, *Chattanooga (BSN)*

The University of Tennessee at Martin, Department of Nursing, *Martin (BSN)*

Texas

Angelo State University, Department of Nursing and Rehabilitation Sciences, *San Angelo (BSN)*

Baylor University, Louise Herrington School of Nursing, *Waco (BSN)*

East Texas Baptist University, Department of Nursing, *Marshall (BSN)*

Lamar University, Department of Nursing, *Beaumont (BSN)*

Midwestern State University, Nursing Program, *Wichita Falls (BSN)*

Patty Hanks Shelton School of Nursing, *Abilene (BSN)*

Prairie View A&M University, College of Nursing, *Houston (BSN)*

Southwestern Adventist University, Department of Nursing, *Keene (BS)*

Tarleton State University, Department of Nursing, *Stephenville (BSN)*

Texas A&M Health Science Center, College of Nursing, *College Station (BSN)*

Texas A&M International University, Canseco School of Nursing, *Laredo (BSN)*

Texas A&M University–Corpus Christi, College of Nursing and Health Sciences, *Corpus Christi (BSN)*

Texas Christian University, Harris College of Nursing, *Fort Worth (BSN)*

Texas State University–San Marcos, St. David's School of Nursing, *San Marcos (BSN)*

Texas Tech University Health Sciences Center, School of Nursing, *Lubbock (BSN)*

Texas Woman's University, College of Nursing, *Denton (BS)*

University of Mary Hardin-Baylor, College of Nursing, *Belton (BSN)*

The University of Texas at Arlington, College of Nursing, *Arlington (BSN)*

The University of Texas at Austin, School of Nursing, *Austin (BSN)*

The University of Texas at El Paso, School of Nursing, *El Paso (BSN)*

The University of Texas at Tyler, Program in Nursing, *Tyler (BSN)*

The University of Texas Health Science Center at Houston, School of Nursing, *Houston (BSN)*

The University of Texas Health Science Center at San Antonio, School of Nursing, *San Antonio (BSN)*

The University of Texas Medical Branch, School of Nursing, *Galveston (BSN)*

The University of Texas–Pan American, Department of Nursing, *Edinburg (BSN)*

University of the Incarnate Word, Program in Nursing, *San Antonio (BSN)*

West Texas A&M University, Department of Nursing, *Canyon (BSN)*

Utah

Southern Utah University, Department of Nursing, *Cedar City (BSN)*

University of Utah, College of Nursing, *Salt Lake City (BS)*

Western Governors University, Online College of Health Professions, *Salt Lake City (BS)*

Westminster College, School of Nursing and Health Sciences, *Salt Lake City (BSN)*

Vermont

Norwich University, Department of Nursing, *Northfield (BSN)*

University of Vermont, Department of Nursing, *Burlington (BS)*

Virgin Islands

University of the Virgin Islands, Division of Nursing, *Saint Thomas (BSN)*

Virginia

Bon Secours Memorial College of Nursing, *Richmond (BSN)*

Eastern Mennonite University, Department of Nursing, *Harrisonburg (BSN)*

George Mason University, College of Health and Human Services, *Fairfax (BSN)*

Hampton University, School of Nursing, *Hampton (BS)*

James Madison University, Department of Nursing, *Harrisonburg (BSN)*

Jefferson College of Health Sciences, Nursing Education Program, *Roanoke (BSN)*

Liberty University, Department of Nursing, *Lynchburg (BSN)*

Lynchburg College, School of Health Sciences and Human Performance, *Lynchburg (BS)*

Marymount University, Malek School of Health Professions, *Arlington (BSN)*

Old Dominion University, Department of Nursing, *Norfolk (BSN)*

Radford University, School of Nursing, *Radford (BSN)*

Sentara College of Health Sciences, Bachelor of Science in Nursing Program, *Chesapeake (BSN)*

Shenandoah University, Eleanor Wade Custer School of Nursing, *Winchester (BSN)*

University of Virginia, School of Nursing, *Charlottesville (BSN)*

The University of Virginia's College at Wise, Department of Nursing, *Wise (BSN)*

Virginia Commonwealth University, School of Nursing, *Richmond (BS)*

Washington

Gonzaga University, Department of Nursing, *Spokane (BSN)*

Northwest University, The Mark and Huldah Buntain School of Nursing, *Kirkland (BS)*

Pacific Lutheran University, School of Nursing, *Tacoma (BSN)*

Seattle Pacific University, School of Health Sciences, *Seattle (BS)*

Seattle University, College of Nursing, *Seattle (BSN)*

University of Washington, School of Nursing, *Seattle (BSN)*

Walla Walla University, School of Nursing, *College Place (BS)*

Washington State University College of Nursing, *Spokane (BSN)*

West Virginia

Alderson-Broaddus College, Department of Nursing, *Philippi (BSN)*

Marshall University, College of Health Professions, *Huntington (BSN)*

Shepherd University, Department of Nursing Education, *Shepherdstown (BSN)*

University of Charleston, Department of Nursing, *Charleston (BSN)*

West Liberty University, Department of Health Sciences, *West Liberty (BSN)*

West Virginia University, School of Nursing, *Morgantown (BSN)*

West Virginia Wesleyan College, School of Nursing, *Buckhannon (BSN)*

Wheeling Jesuit University, Department of Nursing, *Wheeling (BSN)*

Wisconsin

Alverno College, Division of Nursing, *Milwaukee (BSN)*

Bellin College, Nursing Program, *Green Bay (BSN)*

Carroll University, Nursing Program, *Waukesha (BSN)*

Columbia College of Nursing/Mount Mary College Nursing Program, *Milwaukee (BSN)*

Concordia University Wisconsin, Program in Nursing, *Mequon (BSN)*

Edgewood College, Program in Nursing, *Madison (BS)*

Herzing University Online, Program in Nursing, *Milwaukee (BSN)*

Marian University, School of Nursing, *Fond du Lac (BSN)*

Marquette University, College of Nursing, *Milwaukee (BSN)*

Milwaukee School of Engineering, School of Nursing, *Milwaukee (BSN)*

University of Wisconsin–Eau Claire, College of Nursing and Health Sciences, *Eau Claire (BSN)*

University of Wisconsin–Madison, School of Nursing, *Madison (BS)*

University of Wisconsin–Milwaukee, College of Nursing, *Milwaukee (BSN)*

University of Wisconsin–Oshkosh, College of Nursing, *Oshkosh (BSN)*

Viterbo University, School of Nursing, *La Crosse (BSN)*

Wisconsin Lutheran College, Nursing Program, *Milwaukee (BSN)*

Wyoming

University of Wyoming, Fay W. Whitney School of Nursing, *Laramie (BSN)*

CANADA

Alberta

Athabasca University, Centre for Nursing and Health Studies, *Athabasca (BN)*

University of Alberta, Faculty of Nursing, *Edmonton (BScN)*

University of Calgary, Faculty of Nursing, *Calgary (BN)*

University of Lethbridge, Faculty of Health Sciences, *Lethbridge (BN)*

British Columbia

Kwantlen Polytechnic University, Faculty of Community and Health Sciences, *Surrey (BSN)*

Trinity Western University, Department of Nursing, *Langley (BScN)*

University of Northern British Columbia, Nursing Programme, *Prince George (BScN)*

Vancouver Island University, Department of Nursing, *Nanaimo (BScN)*

Manitoba

Brandon University, School of Health Studies, *Brandon (BN)*

University of Manitoba, Faculty of Nursing, *Winnipeg (BN)*

New Brunswick

University of New Brunswick Fredericton, Faculty of Nursing, *Fredericton (BN)*

Newfoundland and Labrador

Memorial University of Newfoundland, School of Nursing, *St. John's (BN)*

Nova Scotia

St. Francis Xavier University, Department of Nursing, *Antigonish (BScN)*

Ontario

Brock University, Department of Nursing, *St. Catharines (BScN)*

Lakehead University, School of Nursing, *Thunder Bay (BScN)*

Laurentian University, School of Nursing, *Sudbury (BScN)*

McMaster University, School of Nursing, *Hamilton (BScN)*

Queen's University at Kingston, School of Nursing, *Kingston (BNSc)*

Ryerson University, Program in Nursing, *Toronto (BScN)*

Trent University, Nursing Program, *Peterborough (BScN)*

University of Ottawa, School of Nursing, *Ottawa (BScN)*

The University of Western Ontario, School of Nursing, *London (BScN)*

University of Windsor, Faculty of Nursing, *Windsor (BScN)*

York University, School of Nursing, *Toronto (BScN)*

Prince Edward Island

University of Prince Edward Island, School of Nursing, *Charlottetown (BScN)*

Quebec

McGill University, School of Nursing, *Montréal (BScN)*

Université du Québec à Trois-Rivières, Program in Nursing, *Trois-Rivières (BSN)*

Université du Québec en Outaouais, Département des Sciences Infirmières, *Gatineau (BScN)*

Université Laval, Faculty of Nursing, *Québec (BScN)*

Saskatchewan

University of Saskatchewan, College of Nursing, *Saskatoon (BSN)*

INTERNATIONAL NURSE TO BACCALAUREATE

U.S. AND U.S. TERRITORIES

Delaware

Wesley College, Nursing Program, *Dover (BSN)*

Wilmington University, College of Health Professions, *New Castle (BSN)*

Georgia

Thomas University, Division of Nursing, *Thomasville (BSN)*

Hawaii

Hawai`i Pacific University, College of Nursing and Health Sciences, *Honolulu (BSN)*

Iowa

Morningside College, Department of Nursing Education, *Sioux City (BSN)*

Massachusetts

Salem State University, Program in Nursing, *Salem (BSN)*

Nebraska

Nebraska Wesleyan University, Department of Nursing, *Lincoln (BSN)*

University of Nebraska Medical Center, College of Nursing, *Omaha (BSN)*

New Jersey

College of Saint Elizabeth, Department of Nursing, *Morristown (BSN)*

New York

College of Mount Saint Vincent, Department of Nursing, *Riverdale (BS)*

Daemen College, Department of Nursing, *Amherst (BS)*

Lehman College of the City University of New York, Department of Nursing, *Bronx (BS)*

The Sage Colleges, Department of Nursing, *Troy (BS)*

St. Francis College, Department of Nursing, *Brooklyn Heights (BS)*

Oklahoma

Oklahoma City University, Kramer School of Nursing, *Oklahoma City (BSN)*

Oklahoma Wesleyan University, School of Nursing, *Bartlesville (BSN)*

Pennsylvania

Eastern University, Program in Nursing, *St. Davids (BSN)*

Edinboro University of Pennsylvania, Department of Nursing, *Edinboro (BS)*

Gannon University, Villa Maria School of Nursing, *Erie (BSN)*

Holy Family University, School of Nursing and Allied Health Professions, *Philadelphia (BSN)*

Marywood University, Department of Nursing, *Scranton (BSN)*

Neumann University, Program in Nursing and Health Sciences, *Aston (BS)*

Villanova University, College of Nursing, *Villanova (BSN)*

South Carolina

University of South Carolina Aiken, School of Nursing, *Aiken (BSN)*

South Dakota

Mount Marty College, Nursing Program, *Yankton (BSN)*

Texas

The University of Texas at Tyler, Program in Nursing, *Tyler (BSN)*

CANADA

Ontario

Ryerson University, Program in Nursing, *Toronto (BScN)*

University of Ottawa, School of Nursing, *Ottawa (BScN)*

LPN TO BACCALAUREATE

U.S. AND U.S. TERRITORIES

Arizona

University of Phoenix–Phoenix Main Campus, College of Nursing, *Tempe (BSN)*

University of Phoenix–Southern Arizona Campus, College of Social Sciences, *Tucson (BSN)*

Arkansas

Arkansas State University, Department of Nursing, *State University (BSN)*

Arkansas Tech University, Program in Nursing, *Russellville (BSN)*

Harding University, College of Nursing, *Searcy (BSN)*

Henderson State University, Department of Nursing, *Arkadelphia (BSN)*

University of Arkansas, Eleanor Mann School of Nursing, *Fayetteville (BSN)*

University of Arkansas at Monticello, School of Nursing, *Monticello (BSN)*

University of Arkansas for Medical Sciences, College of Nursing, *Little Rock (BSN)*

University of Central Arkansas, Department of Nursing, *Conway (BSN)*

California

Biola University, Department of Nursing, *La Mirada (BSN)*

California State University, Fullerton, Department of Nursing, *Fullerton (BSN)*

California State University, Long Beach, School of Nursing, *Long Beach (BSN)*

California State University, San Bernardino, Department of Nursing, *San Bernardino (BSN)*

California State University, Stanislaus, Department of Nursing, *Turlock (BSN)*

Loma Linda University, School of Nursing, *Loma Linda (BS)*

National University, Department of Nursing, *La Jolla (BSN)*

University of Phoenix–Sacramento Valley Campus, College of Nursing, *Sacramento (BSN)*

Colorado

Colorado Mesa University, Department of Nursing and Radiologic Sciences, *Grand Junction (BSN)*

Colorado State University–Pueblo, Department of Nursing, *Pueblo (BSN)*

University of Phoenix–Denver Campus, College of Nursing, *Lone Tree (BSN)*

Delaware

Delaware State University, Department of Nursing, *Dover (BSN)*

Wesley College, Nursing Program, *Dover (BSN)*

District of Columbia

Howard University, Division of Nursing, *Washington (BSN)*

Florida

Barry University, Division of Nursing, *Miami Shores (BSN)*

Georgia

Armstrong Atlantic State University, Program in Nursing, *Savannah (BSN)*

Augusta State University, Department of Nursing, *Augusta (BSN)*

Piedmont College, School of Nursing, *Demorest (BSN)*

Hawaii

Hawai`i Pacific University, College of Nursing and Health Sciences, *Honolulu (BSN)*

University of Phoenix–Hawaii Campus, College of Nursing, *Honolulu (BSN)*

Idaho

Boise State University, Department of Nursing, *Boise (BS)*

Idaho State University, Department of Nursing, *Pocatello (BSN)*

Lewis-Clark State College, Division of Nursing and Health Sciences, *Lewiston (BSN)*

Illinois

Bradley University, Department of Nursing, *Peoria (BSN, BSc PN)*

Chicago State University, Department of Nursing, *Chicago (BSN)*

Indiana

Ball State University, School of Nursing, *Muncie (BS)*

Indiana State University, Department of Nursing, *Terre Haute (BS)*

Purdue University Calumet, School of Nursing, *Hammond (BS)*

Purdue University North Central, Department of Nursing, *Westville (BS)*

Iowa

Allen College, Program in Nursing, *Waterloo (BSN)*

Briar Cliff University, Department of Nursing, *Sioux City (BSN)*

Iowa Wesleyan College, Division of Nursing, *Mount Pleasant (BSN)*

Morningside College, Department of Nursing Education, *Sioux City (BSN)*

Kansas

Bethel College, Department of Nursing, *North Newton (BSN)*

Emporia State University, Newman Division of Nursing, *Emporia (BSN)*

Newman University, Division of Nursing, *Wichita (BSN)*

Southwestern College, Nursing Program, *Winfield (BSN)*

Washburn University, School of Nursing, *Topeka (BSN)*

Louisiana

Dillard University, Division of Nursing, *New Orleans (BSN)*

McNeese State University, College of Nursing, *Lake Charles (BSN)*

Nicholls State University, Department of Nursing, *Thibodaux (BSN)*

Northwestern State University of Louisiana, College of Nursing and Allied Health, *Shreveport (BSN)*

Our Lady of the Lake College, Division of Nursing, *Baton Rouge (BSN)*

University of Louisiana at Lafayette, College of Nursing, *Lafayette (BSN)*

University of Louisiana at Monroe, Nursing, *Monroe (BS)*

University of Phoenix–Louisiana Campus, College of Nursing, *Metairie (BSN)*

Massachusetts

Salem State University, Program in Nursing, *Salem (BSN)*

Simmons College, School of Nursing and Health Sciences, *Boston (BS)*

Michigan

Lake Superior State University, Department of Nursing, *Sault Sainte Marie (BSN)*

Madonna University, College of Nursing and Health, *Livonia (BSN)*

Northern Michigan University, College of Nursing and Allied Health Science, *Marquette (BSN)*

Missouri

Cox College, Department of Nursing, *Springfield (BSN)*

Maryville University of Saint Louis, Nursing Program, School of Health Professions, *St. Louis (BSN)*

Missouri Southern State University, Department of Nursing, *Joplin (BSN)*

Missouri State University, Department of Nursing, *Springfield (BSN)*

Montana

Montana State University, College of Nursing, *Bozeman (BSN)*

Nebraska

Clarkson College, Master of Science in Nursing Program, *Omaha (BSN)*

Nebraska Methodist College, Department of Nursing, *Omaha (BSN)*

Union College, Division of Health Sciences, *Lincoln (BSN)*

University of Nebraska Medical Center, College of Nursing, *Omaha (BSN)*

New Hampshire

Rivier University, Division of Nursing, *Nashua (BS)*

New Jersey
William Paterson University of New Jersey, Department of Nursing, *Wayne (BSN)*

New York
College of Mount Saint Vincent, Department of Nursing, *Riverdale (BS)*
Dominican College, Department of Nursing, *Orangeburg (BSN)*
Molloy College, Division of Nursing, *Rockville Centre (BS)*
Nazareth College of Rochester, Department of Nursing, *Rochester (BS)*
The Sage Colleges, Department of Nursing, *Troy (BS)*

North Carolina
The University of North Carolina at Greensboro, School of Nursing, *Greensboro (BSN)*
Winston-Salem State University, Department of Nursing, *Winston-Salem (BSN)*

North Dakota
Dickinson State University, Department of Nursing, *Dickinson (BSN)*
North Dakota State University, Department of Nursing, *Fargo (BSN)*
University of Mary, Division of Nursing, *Bismarck (BSN)*
University of North Dakota, College of Nursing, *Grand Forks (BSN)*

Ohio
Lourdes University, School of Nursing, *Sylvania (BSN)*
Otterbein University, Department of Nursing, *Westerville (BSN)*
The University of Akron, College of Nursing, *Akron (BSN)*

Oklahoma
Langston University, School of Nursing and Health Professions, *Langston (BSN)*
Northwestern Oklahoma State University, Division of Nursing, *Alva (BSN)*
Oklahoma Wesleyan University, School of Nursing, *Bartlesville (BSN)*
Southern Nazarene University, School of Nursing, *Bethany (BS)*
University of Central Oklahoma, Department of Nursing, *Edmond (BSN)*

Pennsylvania
Alvernia University, Nursing, *Reading (BSN)*
Cedar Crest College, Department of Nursing, *Allentown (BS)*
Indiana University of Pennsylvania, Department of Nursing and Allied Health, *Indiana (BSN)*
La Salle University, School of Nursing and Health Sciences, *Philadelphia (BSN)*
Marywood University, Department of Nursing, *Scranton (BSN)*
Neumann University, Program in Nursing and Health Sciences, *Aston (BS)*
Waynesburg University, Department of Nursing, *Waynesburg (BSN)*
York College of Pennsylvania, Department of Nursing, *York (BS)*

South Carolina
University of South Carolina Aiken, School of Nursing, *Aiken (BSN)*

South Dakota
Mount Marty College, Nursing Program, *Yankton (BSN)*

Tennessee
Baptist College of Health Sciences, Nursing Division, *Memphis (BSN)*
Carson-Newman University, Department of Nursing, *Jefferson City (BSN)*
East Tennessee State University, College of Nursing, *Johnson City (BSN)*
Milligan College, Department of Nursing, *Milligan College (BSN)*
Union University, School of Nursing, *Jackson (BSN)*

Texas
Prairie View A&M University, College of Nursing, *Houston (BSN)*
Tarleton State University, Department of Nursing, *Stephenville (BSN)*
The University of Texas at Tyler, Program in Nursing, *Tyler (BSN)*
West Texas A&M University, Department of Nursing, *Canyon (BSN)*

Virgin Islands
University of the Virgin Islands, Division of Nursing, *Saint Thomas (BSN)*

Virginia
Eastern Mennonite University, Department of Nursing, *Harrisonburg (BSN)*
Hampton University, School of Nursing, *Hampton (BS)*
Sentara College of Health Sciences, Bachelor of Science in Nursing Program, *Chesapeake (BSN)*

Washington
Pacific Lutheran University, School of Nursing, *Tacoma (BSN)*
Walla Walla University, School of Nursing, *College Place (BS)*

Wisconsin
Alverno College, Division of Nursing, *Milwaukee (BSN)*

CANADA

Manitoba
Brandon University, School of Health Studies, *Brandon (BN)*

Newfoundland and Labrador
Memorial University of Newfoundland, School of Nursing, *St. John's (BN)*

Ontario
University of Ottawa, School of Nursing, *Ottawa (BScN)*

LPN TO RN BACCALAUREATE

U.S. AND U.S. TERRITORIES

Arkansas
Harding University, College of Nursing, *Searcy (BSN)*
University of Arkansas, Eleanor Mann School of Nursing, *Fayetteville (BSN)*
University of Central Arkansas, Department of Nursing, *Conway (BSN)*

California
California State University, Chico, School of Nursing, *Chico (BSN)*
California State University, Los Angeles, School of Nursing, *Los Angeles (BSN)*
California State University, Sacramento, School of Nursing, *Sacramento (BSN)*
Holy Names University, Department of Nursing, *Oakland (BSN)*
Point Loma Nazarene University, School of Nursing, *San Diego (BSN)*

Colorado
Colorado Mesa University, Department of Nursing and Radiologic Sciences, *Grand Junction (BSN)*
Colorado State University–Pueblo, Department of Nursing, *Pueblo (BSN)*
Denver College of Nursing, *Denver (BSN)*

Florida
Barry University, Division of Nursing, *Miami Shores (BSN)*

Georgia
Georgia Southern University, School of Nursing, *Statesboro (BSN)*
Georgia Southwestern State University, School of Nursing, *Americus (BSN)*

Idaho
Lewis-Clark State College, Division of Nursing and Health Sciences, *Lewiston (BSN)*

Illinois
MacMurray College, Department of Nursing, *Jacksonville (BSN)*
Saint Xavier University, School of Nursing, *Chicago (BSN)*

Iowa
Iowa Wesleyan College, Division of Nursing, *Mount Pleasant (BSN)*

Kansas
Wichita State University, School of Nursing, *Wichita (BSN)*

Louisiana
Dillard University, Division of Nursing, *New Orleans (BSN)*
Grambling State University, School of Nursing, *Grambling (BSN)*
McNeese State University, College of Nursing, *Lake Charles (BSN)*
Southeastern Louisiana University, School of Nursing, *Hammond (BS)*

Massachusetts
Salem State University, Program in Nursing, *Salem (BSN)*

Michigan
Lake Superior State University, Department of Nursing, *Sault Sainte Marie (BSN)*

Mississippi
Alcorn State University, School of Nursing, *Natchez (BSN)*

Missouri
Chamberlain College of Nursing, *St. Louis (BSN)*
Cox College, Department of Nursing, *Springfield (BSN)*

Nebraska
Clarkson College, Master of Science in Nursing Program, *Omaha (BSN)*
Midland University, Department of Nursing, *Fremont (BSN)*
Nebraska Methodist College, Department of Nursing, *Omaha (BSN)*
University of Nebraska Medical Center, College of Nursing, *Omaha (BSN)*

New Hampshire
Rivier University, Division of Nursing, *Nashua (BS)*

New York
College of Mount Saint Vincent, Department of Nursing, *Riverdale (BS)*
Molloy College, Division of Nursing, *Rockville Centre (BS)*

North Carolina
The University of North Carolina at Greensboro, School of Nursing, *Greensboro (BSN)*

North Dakota
Dickinson State University, Department of Nursing, *Dickinson (BSN)*

Ohio
The University of Akron, College of Nursing, *Akron (BSN)*

Oklahoma
Northwestern Oklahoma State University, Division of Nursing, *Alva (BSN)*
Oklahoma Baptist University, School of Nursing, *Shawnee (BSN)*
University of Oklahoma Health Sciences Center, College of Nursing, *Oklahoma City (BSN)*
University of Tulsa, School of Nursing, *Tulsa (BSN)*

Pennsylvania
Alvernia University, Nursing, *Reading (BSN)*
Bloomsburg University of Pennsylvania, Department of Nursing, *Bloomsburg (BSN)*
La Roche College, Department of Nursing and Nursing Management, *Pittsburgh (BSN)*
Neumann University, Program in Nursing and Health Sciences, *Aston (BS)*

The University of Scranton, Department of Nursing, *Scranton (BS)*

Wilkes University, Department of Nursing, *Wilkes-Barre (BS)*

South Dakota

Mount Marty College, Nursing Program, *Yankton (BSN)*

Presentation College, Department of Nursing, *Aberdeen (BSN)*

Tennessee

Belmont University, School of Nursing, *Nashville (BSN)*

Carson-Newman University, Department of Nursing, *Jefferson City (BSN)*

Middle Tennessee State University, School of Nursing, *Murfreesboro (BSN)*

Milligan College, Department of Nursing, *Milligan College (BSN)*

The University of Tennessee at Martin, Department of Nursing, *Martin (BSN)*

Texas

Southwestern Adventist University, Department of Nursing, *Keene (BS)*

The University of Texas at Tyler, Program in Nursing, *Tyler (BSN)*

Utah

Western Governors University, Online College of Health Professions, *Salt Lake City (BS)*

Virginia

Hampton University, School of Nursing, *Hampton (BS)*

West Virginia

Alderson-Broaddus College, Department of Nursing, *Philippi (BSN)*

Wisconsin

Concordia University Wisconsin, Program in Nursing, *Mequon (BSN)*

CANADA

Alberta

Athabasca University, Centre for Nursing and Health Studies, *Athabasca (BN)*

RN BACCALAUREATE

U.S. AND U.S. TERRITORIES

Alabama

Auburn University Montgomery, School of Nursing, *Montgomery (BSN)*

Jacksonville State University, College of Nursing and Health Sciences, *Jacksonville (BSN)*

Oakwood University, Department of Nursing, *Huntsville (BS)*

Stillman College, Nursing Major, *Tuscaloosa (BSN)*

Troy University, School of Nursing, *Troy (BSN)*

Tuskegee University, Program in Nursing, *Tuskegee (BSN)*

The University of Alabama, Capstone College of Nursing, *Tuscaloosa (BSN)*

The University of Alabama at Birmingham, School of Nursing, *Birmingham (BSN)*

The University of Alabama in Huntsville, College of Nursing, *Huntsville (BSN)*

University of Mobile, School of Nursing, *Mobile (BSN)*

University of North Alabama, College of Nursing and Allied Health, *Florence (BSN)*

University of South Alabama, College of Nursing, *Mobile (BSN)*

Alaska

University of Alaska Anchorage, School of Nursing, *Anchorage (BS)*

Arizona

Arizona State University at the Downtown Phoenix Campus, College of Nursing, *Phoenix (BSN)*

Chamberlain College of Nursing, *Phoenix (BSN)*

Grand Canyon University, College of Nursing and Health Sciences, *Phoenix (BSN)*

Northern Arizona University, School of Nursing, *Flagstaff (BSN)*

Arkansas

Arkansas State University, Department of Nursing, *State University (BSN)*

Arkansas Tech University, Program in Nursing, *Russellville (BSN)*

Harding University, College of Nursing, *Searcy (BSN)*

Southern Arkansas University–Magnolia, Department of Nursing, *Magnolia (BSN)*

University of Arkansas, Eleanor Mann School of Nursing, *Fayetteville (BSN)*

University of Arkansas at Little Rock, BSN Programs, *Little Rock (BSN)*

University of Arkansas at Monticello, School of Nursing, *Monticello (BSN)*

University of Arkansas for Medical Sciences, College of Nursing, *Little Rock (BSN)*

University of Central Arkansas, Department of Nursing, *Conway (BSN)*

California

Biola University, Department of Nursing, *La Mirada (BSN)*

Brandman University, School of Nursing and Health Professions, *Irvine (BSN)*

California Baptist University, School of Nursing, *Riverside (BSN)*

California State University Channel Islands, Nursing Program, *Camarillo (BSN)*

California State University, Chico, School of Nursing, *Chico (BSN)*

California State University, Dominguez Hills, Program in Nursing, *Carson (BSN)*

California State University, Fullerton, Department of Nursing, *Fullerton (BSN)*

California State University, Los Angeles, School of Nursing, *Los Angeles (BSN)*

California State University, San Bernardino, Department of Nursing, *San Bernardino (BSN)*

Concordia University, Bachelor of Science in Nursing Program, *Irvine (BSN)*

Dominican University of California, Program in Nursing, *San Rafael (BSN)*

Fresno Pacific University, RN to BSN Program, *Fresno (BSN)*

Holy Names University, Department of Nursing, *Oakland (BSN)*

Loma Linda University, School of Nursing, *Loma Linda (BS)*

National University, Department of Nursing, *La Jolla (BSN)*

Point Loma Nazarene University, School of Nursing, *San Diego (BSN)*

San Diego State University, School of Nursing, *San Diego (BSN)*

San Francisco State University, School of Nursing, *San Francisco (BSN)*

University of Phoenix–Central Valley Campus, College of Health and Human Services, *Fresno (BSN)*

Vanguard University of Southern California, Nursing Program, *Costa Mesa (BSN)*

West Coast University, Nursing Programs, *North Hollywood (BSN)*

Colorado

Adams State University, Nursing Program, *Alamosa (BSN)*

American Sentinel University, RN to Bachelor of Science Nursing, *Aurora (BSN)*

Colorado Christian University, Nursing Programs, *Lakewood (BSN)*

Colorado Mesa University, Department of Nursing and Radiologic Sciences, *Grand Junction (BSN)*

Colorado State University–Pueblo, Department of Nursing, *Pueblo (BSN)*

Colorado Technical University Online, Nursing Program, *Colorado Springs (BSN)*

Denver College of Nursing, *Denver (BSN)*

Regis University, School of Nursing, *Denver (BSN)*

University of Colorado at Colorado Springs, Beth-El College of Nursing and Health Sciences, *Colorado Springs (BSN)*

University of Colorado Denver, College of Nursing, *Aurora (BS)*

University of Northern Colorado, School of Nursing, *Greeley (BS)*

Connecticut

Central Connecticut State University, Department of Nursing, *New Britain (BSN)*

Fairfield University, School of Nursing, *Fairfield (BS)*

Sacred Heart University, Program in Nursing, *Fairfield (BSN)*

Southern Connecticut State University, Department of Nursing, *New Haven (BS)*

University of Hartford, College of Education, Nursing, and Health Professions, *West Hartford (BSN)*

University of Saint Joseph, Department of Nursing, *West Hartford (BS)*

Western Connecticut State University, Department of Nursing, *Danbury (BS)*

Delaware

Delaware State University, Department of Nursing, *Dover (BSN)*

University of Delaware, School of Nursing, *Newark (BSN)*

Wilmington University, College of Health Professions, *New Castle (BSN)*

District of Columbia

Howard University, Division of Nursing, *Washington (BSN)*

Trinity Washington University, Nursing Program, *Washington (BSN)*

University of the District of Columbia, Nursing Education Program, *Washington (BSN)*

Florida

Adventist University of Health Sciences, Department of Nursing, *Orlando (BSN)*

Barry University, Division of Nursing, *Miami Shores (BSN)*

Bethune-Cookman University, School of Nursing, *Daytona Beach (BSN)*

Broward College, Nursing Program, *Fort Lauderdale (BSN)*

Edison State College, Bachelor of Science in Nursing Program, *Fort Myers (BSN)*

Florida Atlantic University, Christine E. Lynn College of Nursing, *Boca Raton (BSN)*

Florida International University, Graduate Nursing Programs, *Miami (BSN)*

Florida Southern College, School of Nursing & Health Sciences, *Lakeland (BSN)*

Florida State College at Jacksonville, Nursing Department, *Jacksonville (BSN)*

Indian River State College, Bachelor of Science in Nursing Program, *Fort Pierce (BSN)*

Keiser University, Nursing Programs, *Fort Lauderdale (BSN)*

Keiser University, Nursing Programs, *Fort Myers (BSN)*

Keiser University, Nursing Programs, *Jacksonville (BSN)*

Keiser University, Nursing Programs, *Lakeland (BSN)*

Keiser University, Nursing Programs, *Melbourne (BSN)*

Keiser University, Nursing Programs, *Miami (BSN)*

Keiser University, Nursing Programs, *Orlando (BSN)*

Keiser University, Nursing Program, *Pembroke Pines (BSN)*

Keiser University, Nursing Programs, *Port St. Lucie (BSN)*

Keiser University, Nursing Programs, *Sarasota (BSN)*

Keiser University, Nursing Programs, *Tallahassee (BSN)*

Keiser University, Nursing Programs, *Tampa (BSN)*

Keiser University, Nursing Programs, *West Palm Beach (BSN)*

Miami Dade College, School of Nursing, *Miami (BSN)*

Northwest Florida State College, RN to BSN Degree Program, *Niceville (BSN)*

Nova Southeastern University, College of Health Care Sciences, *Fort Lauderdale (BSN)*

Palm Beach Atlantic University, School of Nursing, *West Palm Beach (BSN)*

St. Petersburg College, Department of Nursing, *St. Petersburg (BSN)*

South University, Nursing Program, *Royal Palm Beach (BSN)*

South University, College of Nursing, *Tampa (BSN)*

State College of Florida Manatee-Sarasota, Nursing Degree Program, *Bradenton (BSN)*

University of Central Florida, College of Nursing, *Orlando (BSN)*

University of Miami, School of Nursing and Health Studies, *Coral Gables (BSN)*

University of North Florida, School of Nursing, *Jacksonville (BSN)*

University of Phoenix–South Florida Campus, College of Nursing, *Fort Lauderdale (BSN)*

The University of Tampa, Department of Nursing, *Tampa (BSN)*

University of West Florida, Department of Nursing, *Pensacola (BSN)*

Georgia

Armstrong Atlantic State University, Program in Nursing, *Savannah (BSN)*

Augusta State University, Department of Nursing, *Augusta (BSN)*

Brenau University, College of Health and Science, *Gainesville (BSN)*

Clayton State University, Department of Nursing, *Morrow (BSN)*

College of Coastal Georgia, Department of Nursing and Health Sciences, *Brunswick (BS)*

Columbus State University, Nursing Program, *Columbus (BSN)*

Georgia College & State University, College of Health Sciences, *Milledgeville (BSN)*

Georgia Southwestern State University, School of Nursing, *Americus (BSN)*

Gordon State College, Division of Nursing and Health Sciences, *Barnesville (BSN)*

Kennesaw State University, School of Nursing, *Kennesaw (BSN)*

LaGrange College, Department of Nursing, *LaGrange (BSN)*

Mercer University Georgia Baptist College of Nursing, *Atlanta (BSN)*

Piedmont College, School of Nursing, *Demorest (BSN)*

Thomas University, Division of Nursing, *Thomasville (BSN)*

Valdosta State University, College of Nursing, *Valdosta (BSN)*

Guam

University of Guam, School of Nursing and Health Sciences, *Mangilao (BSN)*

Hawaii

Hawai`i Pacific University, College of Nursing and Health Sciences, *Honolulu (BSN)*

University of Hawaii at Hilo, Department in Nursing, *Hilo (BSN)*

University of Hawaii at Manoa, School of Nursing and Dental Hygiene, *Honolulu (BSN)*

Idaho

Boise State University, Department of Nursing, *Boise (BS)*

Brigham Young University–Idaho, Department of Nursing, *Rexburg (BSN)*

Illinois

Aurora University, School of Nursing, *Aurora (BSN)*

Blessing–Rieman College of Nursing, *Quincy (BSN)*

Bradley University, Department of Nursing, *Peoria (BSN, BSc PN)*

Chicago State University, Department of Nursing, *Chicago (BSN)*

Elmhurst College, Deicke Center for Nursing Education, *Elmhurst (BS)*

Governors State University, College of Health and Human Services, *University Park (BS)*

Illinois State University, Mennonite College of Nursing, *Normal (BSN)*

Lakeview College of Nursing, *Danville (BSN)*

Loyola University Chicago, Marcella Niehoff School of Nursing, *Maywood (BSN)*

Methodist College, *Peoria (BSN)*

Millikin University, School of Nursing, *Decatur (BSN)*

Northern Illinois University, School of Nursing and Health Studies, *De Kalb (BS)*

North Park University, School of Nursing, *Chicago (BS)*

Olivet Nazarene University, Division of Nursing, *Bourbonnais (BSN)*

Resurrection University, *Oak Park (BSN)*

Rockford College, Department of Nursing, *Rockford (BSN)*

Saint Anthony College of Nursing, *Rockford (BSN)*

Saint Francis Medical Center College of Nursing, Baccalaureate Nursing Program, *Peoria (BSN)*

Trinity Christian College, Department of Nursing, *Palos Heights (BSN)*

Trinity College of Nursing and Health Sciences, *Rock Island (BSN)*

University of Illinois at Chicago, College of Nursing, *Chicago (BSN)*

Western Illinois University, School of Nursing, *Macomb (BSN)*

Indiana

Ball State University, School of Nursing, *Muncie (BS)*

Bethel College, School of Nursing, *Mishawaka (BSN)*

Goshen College, Department of Nursing, *Goshen (BSN)*

Huntington University, Department of Nursing, *Huntington (BSN)*

Indiana State University, Department of Nursing, *Terre Haute (BS)*

Indiana University Bloomington, Department of Nursing–Bloomington Division, *Bloomington (BSN)*

Indiana University East, School of Nursing, *Richmond (BSN)*

Indiana University Northwest, School of Nursing and Health Professions, *Gary (BSN)*

Indiana University–Purdue University Fort Wayne, Department of Nursing, *Fort Wayne (BS)*

Indiana University–Purdue University Indianapolis, School of Nursing, *Indianapolis (BSN)*

Indiana University South Bend, College of Health Sciences, *South Bend (BSN)*

Indiana University Southeast, Division of Nursing, *New Albany (BSN)*

Indiana Wesleyan University, School of Nursing, *Marion (BSN)*

Marian University, School of Nursing, *Indianapolis (BSN)*

Purdue University, School of Nursing, *West Lafayette (BS)*

Purdue University North Central, Department of Nursing, *Westville (BS)*

Saint Joseph's College, St. Elizabeth School of Nursing, *Rensselaer (BSN)*

University of Evansville, Department of Nursing, *Evansville (BSN)*

University of Indianapolis, School of Nursing, *Indianapolis (BSN)*

University of Saint Francis, Department of Nursing, *Fort Wayne (BSN)*

University of Southern Indiana, College of Nursing and Health Professions, *Evansville (BSN)*

Valparaiso University, College of Nursing, *Valparaiso (BSN)*

Vincennes University, Department of Nursing, *Vincennes (BSN)*

Iowa

Allen College, Program in Nursing, *Waterloo (BSN)*

Briar Cliff University, Department of Nursing, *Sioux City (BSN)*

Clarke University, Department of Nursing and Health, *Dubuque (BS)*

Grand View University, Division of Nursing, *Des Moines (BSN)*

Iowa Wesleyan College, Division of Nursing, *Mount Pleasant (BSN)*

Morningside College, Department of Nursing Education, *Sioux City (BSN)*

St. Ambrose University, Program in Nursing (BSN), *Davenport (BSN)*

University of Dubuque, School of Professional Programs, *Dubuque (BSN)*

The University of Iowa, College of Nursing, *Iowa City (BSN)*

Upper Iowa University, RN-BSN Nursing Program, *Fayette (BSN)*

Kansas

Baker University, School of Nursing, *Topeka (BSN)*

Bethel College, Department of Nursing, *North Newton (BSN)*

Emporia State University, Newman Division of Nursing, *Emporia (BSN)*

Fort Hays State University, Department of Nursing, *Hays (BSN)*

Kansas Wesleyan University, Department of Nursing Education, *Salina (BSN)*

MidAmerica Nazarene University, Division of Nursing, *Olathe (BSN)*

Newman University, Division of Nursing, *Wichita (BSN)*

Pittsburg State University, Department of Nursing, *Pittsburg (BSN)*

Southwestern College, Nursing Program, *Winfield (BSN)*

The University of Kansas, School of Nursing, *Kansas City (BSN)*

University of Saint Mary, Bachelor of Science in Nursing Program, *Leavenworth (BSN)*

Washburn University, School of Nursing, *Topeka (BSN)*

Wichita State University, School of Nursing, *Wichita (BSN)*

Kentucky

Bellarmine University, Donna and Allan Lansing School of Nursing and Health Sciences, *Louisville (BSN, MSCE)*

Eastern Kentucky University, Department of Baccalaureate and Graduate Nursing, *Richmond (BSN)*

Midway College, Program in Nursing (Baccalaureate), *Midway (BSN)*

Morehead State University, Department of Nursing, *Morehead (BSN)*

Murray State University, Program in Nursing, *Murray (BSN)*

Northern Kentucky University, Department of Nursing, *Highland Heights (BSN)*

University of Kentucky, Graduate School Programs in the College of Nursing, *Lexington (BSN)*

University of Louisville, School of Nursing, *Louisville (BSN)*

Western Kentucky University, School of Nursing, *Bowling Green (BSN)*

Louisiana

Dillard University, Division of Nursing, *New Orleans (BSN)*

Grambling State University, School of Nursing, *Grambling (BSN)*

Louisiana State University at Alexandria, Nursing Program, *Alexandria (BSN)*

Louisiana State University Health Sciences Center, School of Nursing, *New Orleans (BSN)*

Loyola University New Orleans, School of Nursing, *New Orleans (BSN)*

Nicholls State University, Department of Nursing, *Thibodaux (BSN)*

Northwestern State University of Louisiana, College of Nursing and Allied Health, *Shreveport (BSN)*

Our Lady of the Lake College, Division of Nursing, *Baton Rouge (BSN)*

Southeastern Louisiana University, School of Nursing, *Hammond (BS)*

University of Louisiana at Monroe, Nursing, *Monroe (BS)*

Maine

Saint Joseph's College of Maine, Master of Science in Nursing Program, *Standish (BSN)*

University of Maine, School of Nursing, *Orono (BSN)*

University of Maine at Fort Kent, Department of Nursing, *Fort Kent (BSN)*

University of New England, Department of Nursing, *Biddeford (BSN)*

University of Southern Maine, School of Nursing, *Portland (BS)*

Maryland

Bowie State University, Department of Nursing, *Bowie (BSN)*

Coppin State University, Helene Fuld School of Nursing, *Baltimore (BSN)*

Frostburg State University, Nursing Department, *Frostburg (BSN)*

Notre Dame of Maryland University, Department of Nursing, *Baltimore (BS)*

Salisbury University, Program in Nursing, *Salisbury (BS)*

Stevenson University, Nursing Division, *Stevenson (BS)*

Towson University, Department of Nursing, *Towson (BS)*

University of Maryland, Baltimore, Master's Program in Nursing, *Baltimore (BSN)*

Massachusetts

American International College, Division of Nursing, *Springfield (BSN)*

Anna Maria College, Department of Nursing, *Paxton (BSN)*

Curry College, Division of Nursing, *Milton (BS)*

Elms College, Division of Nursing, *Chicopee (BS)*

Emmanuel College, Department of Nursing, *Boston (BS)*

Endicott College, Major in Nursing, *Beverly (BS)*

Fitchburg State University, Department of Nursing, *Fitchburg (BS)*

Regis College, School of Nursing, Science and Health Professions, *Weston (BSN)*

Simmons College, School of Nursing and Health Sciences, *Boston (BS)*

University of Massachusetts Boston, College of Nursing and Health Sciences, *Boston (BS)*

University of Massachusetts Dartmouth, College of Nursing, *North Dartmouth (BSN)*

University of Massachusetts Lowell, Department of Nursing, *Lowell (BS)*

Worcester State University, Department of Nursing, *Worcester (BS)*

Michigan

Davenport University, Division of Nursing, *Grand Rapids (BSN)*

Davenport University, Bachelor of Science in Nursing Program, *Kalamazoo (BSN)*

Eastern Michigan University, School of Nursing, *Ypsilanti (BSN)*

Ferris State University, School of Nursing, *Big Rapids (BSN)*

Finlandia University, College of Professional Studies, *Hancock (BS)*

Grand Valley State University, Kirkhof College of Nursing, *Allendale (BSN)*

Lake Superior State University, Department of Nursing, *Sault Sainte Marie (BSN)*

Madonna University, College of Nursing and Health, *Livonia (BSN)*

Michigan State University, College of Nursing, *East Lansing (BSN)*

Northern Michigan University, College of Nursing and Allied Health Science, *Marquette (BSN)*

Oakland University, School of Nursing, *Rochester (BSN)*

The Robert B. Miller College, School of Nursing, *Battle Creek (BSN)*

Rochester College, School of Nursing, *Rochester Hills (BSN)*

Saginaw Valley State University, Crystal M. Lange College of Health and Human Services, *University Center (BSN)*

Siena Heights University, Nursing Program, *Adrian (BSN)*

University of Detroit Mercy, McAuley School of Nursing, *Detroit (BSN)*

University of Michigan, School of Nursing, *Ann Arbor (BSN)*

University of Michigan–Flint, Department of Nursing, *Flint (BSN)*

Minnesota

Bemidji State University, Department of Nursing, *Bemidji (BS)*

Bethel University, Department of Nursing, *St. Paul (BSN)*

Capella University, Nursing Programs, *Minneapolis (BSN)*

Minnesota State University Mankato, School of Nursing, *Mankato (BS)*

Minnesota State University Moorhead, School of Nursing and Healthcare Leadership, *Moorhead (BSN)*

St. Catherine University, Department of Nursing, *St. Paul (BS)*

Saint Mary's University of Minnesota, B.S. in Nursing, *Winona (BS)*

Walden University, Nursing Programs, *Minneapolis (BSN)*

Winona State University, College of Nursing and Health Sciences, *Winona (BS)*

Mississippi

Alcorn State University, School of Nursing, *Natchez (BSN)*

Mississippi College, School of Nursing, *Clinton (BSN)*

Missouri

Chamberlain College of Nursing, *St. Louis (BSN)*

Cox College, Department of Nursing, *Springfield (BSN)*

Goldfarb School of Nursing at Barnes-Jewish College, *St. Louis (BSN)*

Graceland University, School of Nursing, *Independence (BSN)*

Lincoln University, Department of Nursing, *Jefferson City (BSN)*

Maryville University of Saint Louis, Nursing Program, School of Health Professions, *St. Louis (BSN)*

Missouri Southern State University, Department of Nursing, *Joplin (BSN)*

Missouri State University, Department of Nursing, *Springfield (BSN)*

Saint Louis University, School of Nursing, *St. Louis (BSN)*

Southeast Missouri State University, Department of Nursing, *Cape Girardeau (BSN)*

Southwest Baptist University, College of Nursing, *Bolivar (BSN)*

University of Central Missouri, Department of Nursing, *Warrensburg (BS)*

University of Missouri, Sinclair School of Nursing, *Columbia (BSN)*

University of Missouri–Kansas City, School of Nursing, *Kansas City (BSN)*

University of Missouri–St. Louis, College of Nursing, *St. Louis (BSN)*

Webster University, Department of Nursing, *St. Louis (BSN)*

Montana

Montana State University–Northern, College of Nursing, *Havre (BSN)*

Salish Kootenai College, Nursing Department, *Pablo (BS)*

University of Great Falls, B.S. in Nursing Degree Completion Program, *Great Falls (BSN)*

Nebraska

BryanLGH College of Health Sciences, School of Nursing, *Lincoln (BSN)*

Clarkson College, Master of Science in Nursing Program, *Omaha (BSN)*

Creighton University, School of Nursing, *Omaha (BSN)*

Midland University, Department of Nursing, *Fremont (BSN)*

Nebraska Methodist College, Department of Nursing, *Omaha (BSN)*

Nebraska Wesleyan University, Department of Nursing, *Lincoln (BSN)*

University of Nebraska Medical Center, College of Nursing, *Omaha (BSN)*

Nevada

Great Basin College, BSN Program, *Elko (BSN)*

Nevada State College at Henderson, Nursing Program, *Henderson (BSN)*

Touro University, School of Nursing, *Henderson (BSN)*

University of Nevada, Reno, Orvis School of Nursing, *Reno (BSN)*

New Hampshire

Franklin Pierce University, Master of Science in Nursing, *Rindge (BS)*

Rivier University, Division of Nursing, *Nashua (BS)*

Saint Anselm College, Department of Nursing, *Manchester (BSN)*

University of New Hampshire, Department of Nursing, *Durham (BS)*

New Jersey

Bloomfield College, Division of Nursing, *Bloomfield (BS)*

Caldwell College, Nursing Programs, *Caldwell (BSN)*

The College of New Jersey, School of Nursing, Health and Exercise Science, *Ewing (BSN)*

College of Saint Elizabeth, Department of Nursing, *Morristown (BSN)*

Fairleigh Dickinson University, Metropolitan Campus, Henry P. Becton School of Nursing and Allied Health, *Teaneck (BSN)*

Kean University, Department of Nursing, *Union (BSN)*

Monmouth University, Marjorie K. Unterberg School of Nursing, *West Long Branch (BSN)*

New Jersey City University, Department of Nursing, *Jersey City (BSN)*

Ramapo College of New Jersey, Master of Science in Nursing Program, *Mahwah (BSN)*

The Richard Stockton College of New Jersey, Program in Nursing, *Pomona (BSN)*

Rowan University, RN to BSN Program, *Glassboro (BSN)*

Rutgers School of Nursing–Camden, *Camden (BS)*

Rutgers, The State University of New Jersey, College of Nursing, *Newark (BS)*

Saint Peter's University, Nursing Program, *Jersey City (BSN)*

Seton Hall University, College of Nursing, *South Orange (BSN)*

University of Medicine and Dentistry of New Jersey, School of Nursing, *Newark (BSN)*

William Paterson University of New Jersey, Department of Nursing, *Wayne (BSN)*

New Mexico

New Mexico Highlands University, Department of Nursing, *Las Vegas (BSN)*

New Mexico State University, School of Nursing, *Las Cruces (BSN)*

Northern New Mexico College, College of Nursing and Health Sciences, *Espa&nnola (BSN)*

University of New Mexico, College of Nursing, *Albuquerque (BSN)*

Western New Mexico University, Nursing Department, *Silver City (BSN)*

New York

Adelphi University, School of Nursing, *Garden City (BS)*

The College of New Rochelle, School of Nursing, *New Rochelle (BSN)*

College of Staten Island of the City University of New York, Department of Nursing, *Staten Island (BS)*

Daemen College, Department of Nursing, *Amherst (BS)*

Dominican College, Department of Nursing, *Orangeburg (BSN)*

D'Youville College, School of Nursing, *Buffalo (BSN)*

Elmira College, Program in Nursing Education, *Elmira (BS)*

Excelsior College, School of Nursing, *Albany (BS)*

Farmingdale State College, Nursing Department, *Farmingdale (BS)*

Hartwick College, Department of Nursing, *Oneonta (BS)*

Hunter College of the City University of New York, Hunter-Bellevue School of Nursing, *New York (BSN)*

Lehman College of the City University of New York, Department of Nursing, *Bronx (BS)*

Le Moyne College, Nursing Programs, *Syracuse (BS)*

Long Island University–C. W. Post Campus, Department of Nursing, *Brookville (BS)*

Mercy College, Programs in Nursing, *Dobbs Ferry (BS)*

Molloy College, Division of Nursing, *Rockville Centre (BS)*

Mount Saint Mary College, Division of Nursing, *Newburgh (BSN)*

Nazareth College of Rochester, Department of Nursing, *Rochester (BS)*

New York City College of Technology of the City University of New York, Department of Nursing, *Brooklyn (BS)*

New York University, College of Nursing, *New York (BS)*

Niagara University, Department of Nursing, *Niagara University (BS)*

Roberts Wesleyan College, Division of Nursing, *Rochester (BScN)*

The Sage Colleges, Department of Nursing, *Troy (BS)*

St. John Fisher College, Wegmans School of Nursing, *Rochester (BS)*

St. Joseph's College, New York, Department of Nursing, *Brooklyn (BSN)*

State University of New York at Plattsburgh, Department of Nursing, *Plattsburgh (BS)*

State University of New York College of Technology at Delhi, Bachelor of Science in Nursing Program, *Delhi (BSN)*

State University of New York Downstate Medical Center, College of Nursing, *Brooklyn (BS)*

State University of New York Empire State College, Bachelor of Science in Nursing Program, *Saratoga Springs (BS)*

State University of New York Institute of Technology, School of Nursing and Health Systems, *Utica (BS)*

Stony Brook University, State University of New York, School of Nursing, *Stony Brook (BS)*

University at Buffalo, the State University of New York, School of Nursing, *Buffalo (BS)*

University of Rochester, School of Nursing, *Rochester (BS)*

Utica College, Department of Nursing, *Utica (BS)*

York College of the City University of New York, Program in Nursing, *Jamaica (BS)*

North Carolina

Appalachian State University, Department of Nursing, *Boone (BSN)*

Barton College, School of Nursing, *Wilson (BSN)*

Cabarrus College of Health Sciences, Louise Harkey School of Nursing, *Concord (BSN)*

Fayetteville State University, Program in Nursing, *Fayetteville (BSN)*

North Carolina Agricultural and Technical State University, School of Nursing, *Greensboro (BSN)*

Queens University of Charlotte, Presbyterian School of Nursing, *Charlotte (BSN)*

The University of North Carolina at Charlotte, School of Nursing, *Charlotte (BSN)*

The University of North Carolina at Greensboro, School of Nursing, *Greensboro (BSN)*

The University of North Carolina at Pembroke, Nursing Program, *Pembroke (BSN)*

The University of North Carolina Wilmington, School of Nursing, *Wilmington (BS)*

Western Carolina University, School of Nursing, *Cullowhee (BSN)*

Winston-Salem State University, Department of Nursing, *Winston-Salem (BSN)*

North Dakota

Dickinson State University, Department of Nursing, *Dickinson (BSN)*

Minot State University, Department of Nursing, *Minot (BSN)*

Sanford College of Nursing, *Bismarck (BSN)*

University of Mary, Division of Nursing, *Bismarck (BSN)*

Ohio

Ashland University, Dwight Schar College of Nursing and Health Sciences, *Ashland (BSN)*

Capital University, School of Nursing, *Columbus (BSN)*

Cedarville University, Department of Nursing, *Cedarville (BSN)*

Chamberlain College of Nursing, *Columbus (BSN)*

Cleveland State University, School of Nursing, *Cleveland (BSN)*

Defiance College, Bachelor's Degree in Nursing, *Defiance (BSN)*

Franciscan University of Steubenville, Department of Nursing, *Steubenville (BSN)*

Kent State University, College of Nursing, *Kent (BSN)*

Kettering College, Division of Nursing, *Kettering (BSN)*

Lourdes University, School of Nursing, *Sylvania (BSN)*

Malone University, School of Nursing, *Canton (BSN)*

Mercy College of Ohio, Division of Nursing, *Toledo (BSN)*

Miami University, Department of Nursing, *Hamilton (BSN)*

Miami University Hamilton, Bachelor of Science in Nursing Program, *Hamilton (BSN)*

Mount Carmel College of Nursing, Nursing Programs, *Columbus (BSN)*

Notre Dame College, Nursing Department, *South Euclid (BSN)*

Ohio Northern University, Nursing Program, *Ada (BSN)*

The Ohio State University, College of Nursing, *Columbus (BSN)*

Ohio University, School of Nursing, *Athens (BSN)*

Otterbein University, Department of Nursing, *Westerville (BSN)*

Shawnee State University, Department of Nursing, *Portsmouth (BSN)*

University of Cincinnati, College of Nursing, *Cincinnati (BSN)*

University of Rio Grande, Holzer School of Nursing, *Rio Grande (BSN)*

The University of Toledo, College of Nursing, *Toledo (BSN)*

Walsh University, Department of Nursing, *North Canton (BSN)*

Wright State University, College of Nursing and Health, *Dayton (BSN)*

Oklahoma

Langston University, School of Nursing and Health Professions, *Langston (BSN)*

Northeastern State University, Department of Nursing, *Tahlequah (BSN)*

Northwestern Oklahoma State University, Division of Nursing, *Alva (BSN)*

Oklahoma Baptist University, School of Nursing, *Shawnee (BSN)*

Oklahoma City University, Kramer School of Nursing, *Oklahoma City (BSN)*

Oklahoma Wesleyan University, School of Nursing, *Bartlesville (BSN)*

Oral Roberts University, Anna Vaughn School of Nursing, *Tulsa (BSN)*

Southwestern Oklahoma State University, School of Nursing, *Weatherford (BSN)*

University of Central Oklahoma, Department of Nursing, *Edmond (BSN)*

University of Tulsa, School of Nursing, *Tulsa (BSN)*

Oregon

Oregon Health & Science University, School of Nursing, *Portland (BS)*

Pennsylvania

Alvernia University, Nursing, *Reading (BSN)*

Bloomsburg University of Pennsylvania, Department of Nursing, *Bloomsburg (BSN)*

California University of Pennsylvania, Department of Nursing, *California (BSN)*

Cedar Crest College, Department of Nursing, *Allentown (BS)*

Chatham University, Nursing Programs, *Pittsburgh (BSN)*

Clarion University of Pennsylvania, School of Nursing, *Oil City (BSN)*

DeSales University, Department of Nursing and Health, *Center Valley (BSN)*

Drexel University, College of Nursing and Health Professions, *Philadelphia (BSN)*

East Stroudsburg University of Pennsylvania, Department of Nursing, *East Stroudsburg (BS)*

Gannon University, Villa Maria School of Nursing, *Erie (BSN)*

Gwynedd-Mercy College, School of Nursing, *Gwynedd Valley (BSN)*

Immaculata University, Department of Nursing, *Immaculata (BSN)*

Lancaster General College of Nursing & Health Sciences, Bachelor of Science in Nursing Program, *Lancaster (BSN)*

La Roche College, Department of Nursing and Nursing Management, *Pittsburgh (BSN)*

La Salle University, School of Nursing and Health Sciences, *Philadelphia (BSN)*

Mansfield University of Pennsylvania, Department of Health Sciences–Nursing, *Mansfield (BSN)*

Marywood University, Department of Nursing, *Scranton (BSN)*

Millersville University of Pennsylvania, Department of Nursing, *Millersville (BSN)*

Misericordia University, Department of Nursing, *Dallas (BSN)*

Moravian College, St. Luke's School of Nursing, *Bethlehem (BSN)*

Penn State University Park, School of Nursing, *University Park (BS)*

Pennsylvania College of Technology, School of Health Sciences, *Williamsport (BSN)*

Slippery Rock University of Pennsylvania, Department of Nursing, *Slippery Rock (BSN)*

Temple University, Department of Nursing, *Philadelphia (BSN)*

Thomas Jefferson University, Department of Nursing, *Philadelphia (BSN)*

University of Pennsylvania, School of Nursing, *Philadelphia (BSN)*

University of Pittsburgh, School of Nursing, *Pittsburgh (BSN)*

University of Pittsburgh at Bradford, Department of Nursing, *Bradford (BSN)*

The University of Scranton, Department of Nursing, *Scranton (BS)*

Villanova University, College of Nursing, *Villanova (BSN)*

West Chester University of Pennsylvania, Department of Nursing, *West Chester (BSN)*

Widener University, School of Nursing, *Chester (BSN)*

Wilkes University, Department of Nursing, *Wilkes-Barre (BS)*

York College of Pennsylvania, Department of Nursing, *York (BS)*

Puerto Rico

Inter American University of Puerto Rico, Aguadilla Campus, Nursing Program, *Aguadilla (BSN)*

Universidad Adventista de las Antillas, Department of Nursing, *Mayagüez (BSN)*

Rhode Island

Rhode Island College, Department of Nursing, *Providence (BSN)*

Salve Regina University, Department of Nursing, *Newport (BS)*

University of Rhode Island, College of Nursing, *Kingston (BS)*

South Carolina

Charleston Southern University, Wingo School of Nursing, *Charleston (BSN)*

Clemson University, School of Nursing, *Clemson (BS)*

Coastal Carolina University, Nursing Completion Program, *Conway (BSN)*

Lander University, School of Nursing, *Greenwood (BSN)*

Newberry College, Department of Nursing, *Newberry (BSN)*

South Carolina State University, Department of Nursing, *Orangeburg (BSN)*

University of South Carolina Aiken, School of Nursing, *Aiken (BSN)*

University of South Carolina Beaufort, Nursing Program, *Bluffton (BSN)*

University of South Carolina Upstate, Mary Black School of Nursing, *Spartanburg (BSN)*

South Dakota

Mount Marty College, Nursing Program, *Yankton (BSN)*

Presentation College, Department of Nursing, *Aberdeen (BSN)*

South Dakota State University, College of Nursing, *Brookings (BS)*

University of Sioux Falls, School of Nursing, *Sioux Falls (BSN)*

Tennessee

Austin Peay State University, School of Nursing, *Clarksville (BSN)*

Baptist College of Health Sciences, Nursing Division, *Memphis (BSN)*

Belmont University, School of Nursing, *Nashville (BSN)*

Carson-Newman University, Department of Nursing, *Jefferson City (BSN)*

Cumberland University, Rudy School of Nursing and Health Professions, *Lebanon (BSN)*

East Tennessee State University, College of Nursing, *Johnson City (BSN)*

Lincoln Memorial University, Caylor School of Nursing, *Harrogate (BSN)*

Middle Tennessee State University, School of Nursing, *Murfreesboro (BSN)*

Milligan College, Department of Nursing, *Milligan College (BSN)*

Tennessee State University, School of Nursing, *Nashville (BSN)*

Tennessee Technological University, Whitson-Hester School of Nursing, *Cookeville (BSN)*

Tennessee Wesleyan College, Fort Sanders Nursing Department, *Knoxville (BSN)*

Union University, School of Nursing, *Jackson (BSN)*

University of Memphis, Loewenberg School of Nursing, *Memphis (BSN)*

Texas

Angelo State University, Department of Nursing and Rehabilitation Sciences, *San Angelo (BSN)*

Houston Baptist University, School of Nursing and Allied Health, *Houston (BSN)*

Lamar University, Department of Nursing, *Beaumont (BSN)*

Lubbock Christian University, Department of Nursing, *Lubbock (BSN)*

Patty Hanks Shelton School of Nursing, *Abilene (BSN)*

Prairie View A&M University, College of Nursing, *Houston (BSN)*

Southwestern Adventist University, Department of Nursing, *Keene (BS)*

Stephen F. Austin State University, Richard and Lucille Dewitt School of Nursing, *Nacogdoches (BSN)*

Texas A&M Health Science Center, College of Nursing, *College Station (BSN)*

Texas A&M International University, Canseco School of Nursing, *Laredo (BSN)*

Texas A&M University–Corpus Christi, College of Nursing and Health Sciences, *Corpus Christi (BSN)*

Texas Tech University Health Sciences Center, School of Nursing, *Lubbock (BSN)*

Texas Woman's University, College of Nursing, *Denton (BS)*

University of Houston–Victoria, School of Nursing, *Victoria (BSN)*

The University of Texas at Arlington, College of Nursing, *Arlington (BSN)*

The University of Texas at Austin, School of Nursing, *Austin (BSN)*

The University of Texas at El Paso, School of Nursing, *El Paso (BSN)*

The University of Texas at Tyler, Program in Nursing, *Tyler (BSN)*

The University of Texas Medical Branch, School of Nursing, *Galveston (BSN)*

The University of Texas–Pan American, Department of Nursing, *Edinburg (BSN)*

Wayland Baptist University, Bachelor of Science in Nursing Program, *Plainview (BSN)*

Utah

Brigham Young University, College of Nursing, *Provo (BS)*

Dixie State College of Utah, Nursing Department, *St. George (BSN)*

Southern Utah University, Department of Nursing, *Cedar City (BSN)*

University of Utah, College of Nursing, *Salt Lake City (BS)*

Western Governors University, Online College of Health Professions, *Salt Lake City (BS)*

Westminster College, School of Nursing and Health Sciences, *Salt Lake City (BSN)*

Vermont

Norwich University, Department of Nursing, *Northfield (BSN)*

Southern Vermont College, Department of Nursing, *Bennington (BSN)*

Virgin Islands

University of the Virgin Islands, Division of Nursing, *Saint Thomas (BSN)*

Virginia

Bon Secours Memorial College of Nursing, *Richmond (BSN)*

Eastern Mennonite University, Department of Nursing, *Harrisonburg (BSN)*

ECPI College of Technology, BSN Program, *Virginia Beach (BSN)*

George Mason University, College of Health and Human Services, *Fairfax (BSN)*

Hampton University, School of Nursing, *Hampton (BS)*

James Madison University, Department of Nursing, *Harrisonburg (BSN)*

Jefferson College of Health Sciences, Nursing Education Program, *Roanoke (BSN)*

Liberty University, Department of Nursing, *Lynchburg (BSN)*

Marymount University, Malek School of Health Professions, *Arlington (BSN)*

Norfolk State University, Department of Nursing, *Norfolk (BSN)*

Old Dominion University, Department of Nursing, *Norfolk (BSN)*

Radford University, School of Nursing, *Radford (BSN)*

Sentara College of Health Sciences, Bachelor of Science in Nursing Program, *Chesapeake (BSN)*

Shenandoah University, Eleanor Wade Custer School of Nursing, *Winchester (BSN)*

University of Virginia, School of Nursing, *Charlottesville (BSN)*

The University of Virginia's College at Wise, Department of Nursing, *Wise (BSN)*

Washington

Olympic College, Nursing Programs, *Bremerton (BSN)*

Seattle Pacific University, School of Health Sciences, *Seattle (BS)*

Walla Walla University, School of Nursing, *College Place (BS)*

Washington State University College of Nursing, *Spokane (BSN)*

West Virginia

Alderson-Broaddus College, Department of Nursing, *Philippi (BSN)*

Bluefield State College, Program in Nursing, *Bluefield (BSN)*

Fairmont State University, School of Nursing and Allied Health Administration, *Fairmont (BSN)*

Shepherd University, Department of Nursing Education, *Shepherdstown (BSN)*

West Virginia University, School of Nursing, *Morgantown (BSN)*

Wheeling Jesuit University, Department of Nursing, *Wheeling (BSN)*

Wisconsin

Alverno College, Division of Nursing, *Milwaukee (BSN)*

Columbia College of Nursing/Mount Mary College Nursing Program, *Milwaukee (BSN)*

Concordia University Wisconsin, Program in Nursing, *Mequon (BSN)*

Maranatha Baptist Bible College, Nursing Department, *Watertown (BSN)*

Milwaukee School of Engineering, School of Nursing, *Milwaukee (BSN)*

University of Phoenix–Milwaukee Campus, College of Health and Human Services, *Milwaukee (BSN)*

University of Wisconsin–Eau Claire, College of Nursing and Health Sciences, *Eau Claire (BSN)*

University of Wisconsin–Green Bay, BSN–LINC Online RN–BSN Program, *Green Bay (BSN)*

University of Wisconsin–Madison, School of Nursing, *Madison (BS)*

University of Wisconsin–Milwaukee, College of Nursing, *Milwaukee (BSN)*

University of Wisconsin–Oshkosh, College of Nursing, *Oshkosh (BSN)*

Viterbo University, School of Nursing, *La Crosse (BSN)*

CANADA

Alberta

Athabasca University, Centre for Nursing and Health Studies, *Athabasca (BN)*

University of Alberta, Faculty of Nursing, *Edmonton (BScN)*

University of Calgary, Faculty of Nursing, *Calgary (BN)*

British Columbia

British Columbia Institute of Technology, School of Health Sciences, *Burnaby (BSN)*

Kwantlen Polytechnic University, Faculty of Community and Health Sciences, *Surrey (BSN)*

University of Northern British Columbia, Nursing Programme, *Prince George (BScN)*

Manitoba

Brandon University, School of Health Studies, *Brandon (BN)*

University of Manitoba, Faculty of Nursing, *Winnipeg (BN)*

New Brunswick

Université de Moncton, School of Nursing, *Moncton (BScN)*

Newfoundland and Labrador

Memorial University of Newfoundland, School of Nursing, *St. John's (BN)*

Nova Scotia

St. Francis Xavier University, Department of Nursing, *Antigonish (BScN)*

Ontario

Brock University, Department of Nursing, *St. Catharines (BScN)*

Lakehead University, School of Nursing, *Thunder Bay (BScN)*

Laurentian University, School of Nursing, *Sudbury (BScN)*

McMaster University, School of Nursing, *Hamilton (BScN)*

Nipissing University, Nursing Department, *North Bay (BScN)*

Ryerson University, Program in Nursing, *Toronto (BScN)*

University of Ottawa, School of Nursing, *Ottawa (BScN)*

The University of Western Ontario, School of Nursing, *London (BScN)*

York University, School of Nursing, *Toronto (BScN)*

Quebec

McGill University, School of Nursing, *Montréal (BScN)*

Université de Montréal, Faculty of Nursing, *Montréal (BScN)*

Université de Sherbrooke, Department of Nursing, *Sherbrooke (BScN)*

Université du Québec à Chicoutimi, Program in Nursing, *Chicoutimi (BNSc)*

Université du Québec à Rimouski, Program in Nursing, *Rimouski (BScN)*

Université du Québec à Trois-Rivières, Program in Nursing, *Trois-Rivières (BSN)*

Université du Québec en Outaouais, Département des Sciences Infirmières, *Gatineau (BScN)*

Université Laval, Faculty of Nursing, *Québec (BScN)*

Saskatchewan

University of Saskatchewan, College of Nursing, *Saskatoon (BSN)*

RPN TO BACCALAUREATE

U.S. AND U.S. TERRITORIES

California

San Jose State University, The Valley Foundation School of Nursing, *San Jose (BS)*

Massachusetts

Curry College, Division of Nursing, *Milton (BS)*

Michigan

Lake Superior State University, Department of Nursing, *Sault Sainte Marie (BSN)*

Nebraska

University of Nebraska Medical Center, College of Nursing, *Omaha (BSN)*

New Mexico

Eastern New Mexico University, Department of Allied Health–Nursing, *Portales (BSN)*

Ohio

Franciscan University of Steubenville, Department of Nursing, *Steubenville (BSN)*

Pennsylvania

Chatham University, Nursing Programs, *Pittsburgh (BSN)*

CANADA

Alberta

University of Alberta, Faculty of Nursing, *Edmonton (BScN)*

British Columbia

British Columbia Institute of Technology, School of Health Sciences, *Burnaby (BSN)*

Ontario

Nipissing University, Nursing Department, *North Bay (BScN)*

Ryerson University, Program in Nursing, *Toronto (BScN)*

University of Ottawa, School of Nursing, *Ottawa (BScN)*

MASTER'S DEGREE PROGRAMS

ACCELERATED AD/RN TO MASTER'S

U.S. AND U.S. TERRITORIES

Alabama

Spring Hill College, Division of Nursing, *Mobile (MSN)*

The University of Alabama at Birmingham, School of Nursing, *Birmingham (MSN, MSN/ MPH)*

California

University of San Francisco, School of Nursing and Health Professions, *San Francisco (MSN)*

Western University of Health Sciences, College of Graduate Nursing, *Pomona (MSN)*

Delaware

Wesley College, Nursing Program, *Dover (MSN)*

Wilmington University, College of Health Professions, *New Castle (MSN, MSN/MBA, MSN/MS)*

Florida

Florida International University, Graduate Nursing Programs, *Miami (MSN)*

Georgia

Albany State University, College of Sciences and Health Professions, *Albany (MSN)*

Brenau University, College of Health and Science, *Gainesville (MSN)*

Idaho

Idaho State University, Department of Nursing, *Pocatello (MS)*

Kentucky

Frontier Nursing University, Nursing Degree Programs, *Hyden (MSN)*

Massachusetts

Regis College, School of Nursing, Science and Health Professions, *Weston (MSN)*

Michigan

Ferris State University, School of Nursing, *Big Rapids (MSN, MSN/MBA)*

Saginaw Valley State University, Crystal M. Lange College of Health and Human Services, *University Center (MSN)*

University of Detroit Mercy, McAuley School of Nursing, *Detroit (MSN)*

Mississippi

University of Mississippi Medical Center, Program in Nursing, *Jackson (MSN)*

Missouri

Missouri State University, Department of Nursing, *Springfield (MSN)*

Nebraska

Nebraska Wesleyan University, Department of Nursing, *Lincoln (MSN)*

New York

Daemen College, Department of Nursing, *Amherst (MS)*

State University of New York Institute of Technology, School of Nursing and Health Systems, *Utica (MS)*

University of Rochester, School of Nursing, *Rochester (MS, MSN/PhD)*

Ohio

Case Western Reserve University, Frances Payne Bolton School of Nursing, *Cleveland (MSN, MSN/MA, MSN/MBA, MSN/MPH)*

Walsh University, Department of Nursing, *North Canton (MSN)*

Oklahoma

Oklahoma City University, Kramer School of Nursing, *Oklahoma City (MSN, MSN/MBA)*

Pennsylvania

DeSales University, Department of Nursing and Health, *Center Valley (MSN, MSN/MBA)*

Gannon University, Villa Maria School of Nursing, *Erie (MSN)*

The University of Scranton, Department of Nursing, *Scranton (MSN)*

Wilkes University, Department of Nursing, *Wilkes-Barre (MS)*

Tennessee

Carson-Newman University, Department of Nursing, *Jefferson City (MSN)*

Middle Tennessee State University, School of Nursing, *Murfreesboro (MSN)*

Texas

The University of Texas at Tyler, Program in Nursing, *Tyler (MSN, MSN/MBA)*

University of the Incarnate Word, Program in Nursing, *San Antonio (MSN)*

West Virginia

West Virginia University, School of Nursing, *Morgantown (MSN)*

Wisconsin

University of Wisconsin–Oshkosh, College of Nursing, *Oshkosh (MSN)*

ACCELERATED MASTER'S

U.S. AND U.S. TERRITORIES

Alabama

University of South Alabama, College of Nursing, *Mobile (MSN)*

Arizona

The University of Arizona, College of Nursing, *Tucson (MSN)*

California

California State University, Fresno, Department of Nursing, *Fresno (MSN)*

California State University, Long Beach, School of Nursing, *Long Beach (MSN, MSN/MHA)*

University of Phoenix–Sacramento Valley Campus, College of Nursing, *Sacramento (MSN, MSN/MHA)*

Western University of Health Sciences, College of Graduate Nursing, *Pomona (MSN)*

Georgia

Albany State University, College of Sciences and Health Professions, *Albany (MSN)*

Thomas University, Division of Nursing, *Thomasville (MSN, MSN/MBA)*

Hawaii

University of Hawaii at Manoa, School of Nursing and Dental Hygiene, *Honolulu (MS, MSN/MBA)*

Illinois

Benedictine University, Department of Nursing, *Lisle (MSN)*

Lewis University, Program in Nursing, *Romeoville (MSN, MSN/MBA)*

Kansas

MidAmerica Nazarene University, Division of Nursing, *Olathe (MSN)*

Maryland

Stevenson University, Nursing Division, *Stevenson (MS)*

Massachusetts

Boston College, William F. Connell School of Nursing, *Chestnut Hill (MS, MSN/MA, MSN/ MBA, MSN/PhD)*

Regis College, School of Nursing, Science and Health Professions, *Weston (MSN)*

Simmons College, School of Nursing and Health Sciences, *Boston (MS)*

University of Massachusetts Lowell, Department of Nursing, *Lowell (MS)*

Nebraska

Nebraska Wesleyan University, Department of Nursing, *Lincoln (MSN)*

New York

The Sage Colleges, Department of Nursing, *Troy (MS, MS/MBA)*

Ohio

Ursuline College, The Breen School of Nursing, *Pepper Pike (MSN)*

Oklahoma

Oklahoma City University, Kramer School of Nursing, *Oklahoma City (MSN, MSN/MBA)*

Southern Nazarene University, School of Nursing, *Bethany (MS)*

Pennsylvania

Carlow University, School of Nursing, *Pittsburgh (MSN)*

Thomas Jefferson University, Department of Nursing, *Philadelphia (MSN)*

Waynesburg University, Department of Nursing, *Waynesburg (MSN, MSN/MBA)*

Utah

Western Governors University, Online College of Health Professions, *Salt Lake City (MS)*

West Virginia

West Virginia University, School of Nursing, *Morgantown (MSN)*

Wisconsin

Cardinal Stritch University, Ruth S. Coleman College of Nursing, *Milwaukee (MSN)*

CANADA

Quebec

Université Laval, Faculty of Nursing, *Québec (MSN)*

ACCELERATED MASTER'S FOR NON-NURSING COLLEGE GRADUATES

U.S. AND U.S. TERRITORIES

Alabama

The University of Alabama at Birmingham, School of Nursing, *Birmingham (MSN, MSN/ MPH)*

Arizona

The University of Arizona, College of Nursing, *Tucson (MSN)*

California

Azusa Pacific University, School of Nursing, *Azusa (MSN)*

California Baptist University, School of Nursing, *Riverside (MSN)*

San Francisco State University, School of Nursing, *San Francisco (MSN)*

University of San Diego, Hahn School of Nursing and Health Science, *San Diego (MSN)*

University of San Francisco, School of Nursing and Health Professions, *San Francisco (MSN)*

Western University of Health Sciences, College of Graduate Nursing, *Pomona (MSN)*

Georgia

Georgia Regents University, School of Nursing, *Augusta (MSN)*

Illinois

Millikin University, School of Nursing, *Decatur (MSN)*

Indiana

University of Indianapolis, School of Nursing, *Indianapolis (MSN, MSN/MALAS, MSN/MS, MSN/MSBA)*

Maryland

University of Maryland, Baltimore, Master's Program in Nursing, *Baltimore (MS, MSN/MBA, MSN/MPH)*

Massachusetts

Boston College, William F. Connell School of Nursing, *Chestnut Hill (MS, MSN/MA, MSN/MBA, MSN/PhD)*

Regis College, School of Nursing, Science and Health Professions, *Weston (MSN)*

Salem State University, Program in Nursing, *Salem (MSN, MSN/MBA)*

Simmons College, School of Nursing and Health Sciences, *Boston (MS)*

University of Massachusetts Worcester, Graduate School of Nursing, *Worcester (MS)*

Missouri

Saint Louis University, School of Nursing, *St. Louis (MSN, MN/MPH)*

New York

Columbia University, School of Nursing, *New York (MS, MSN/MBA, MSN/MPH)*

Mercy College, Programs in Nursing, *Dobbs Ferry (MS)*

University of Rochester, School of Nursing, *Rochester (MS, MSN/PhD)*

North Carolina

East Carolina University, College of Nursing, *Greenville (MSN)*

Ohio

College of Mount St. Joseph, Department of Nursing, *Cincinnati (MN)*

The Ohio State University, College of Nursing, *Columbus (MS, MS/MPH)*

University of Cincinnati, College of Nursing, *Cincinnati (MSN, MSN/MBA, MSN/PhD)*

Xavier University, School of Nursing, *Cincinnati (MSN, MSN/MBA, MSN/Ed D)*

Oregon

Oregon Health & Science University, School of Nursing, *Portland (MS, MN/MPH)*

Pennsylvania

University of Pennsylvania, School of Nursing, *Philadelphia (MSN, MSN/MBA, MSN/MPH, MSN/PhD)*

Tennessee

The University of Tennessee Health Science Center, College of Nursing, *Memphis (MSN)*

Washington

Pacific Lutheran University, School of Nursing, *Tacoma (MSN, MSN/MBA)*

ACCELERATED MASTER'S FOR NURSES WITH NON-NURSING DEGREES

U.S. AND U.S. TERRITORIES

California

Azusa Pacific University, School of Nursing, *Azusa (MSN)*

California State University, Los Angeles, School of Nursing, *Los Angeles (MSN)*

Charles Drew University of Medicine and Science, School of Nursing, *Los Angeles (MSN)*

San Francisco State University, School of Nursing, *San Francisco (MSN)*

Delaware

Wilmington University, College of Health Professions, *New Castle (MSN, MSN/MBA, MSN/MS)*

Illinois

Lewis University, Program in Nursing, *Romeoville (MSN, MSN/MBA)*

Resurrection University, *Oak Park (MSN)*

Kentucky

Western Kentucky University, School of Nursing, *Bowling Green (MSN)*

Massachusetts

Boston College, William F. Connell School of Nursing, *Chestnut Hill (MS, MSN/MA, MSN/MBA, MSN/PhD)*

Regis College, School of Nursing, Science and Health Professions, *Weston (MSN)*

Simmons College, School of Nursing and Health Sciences, *Boston (MS)*

New Jersey

Kean University, Department of Nursing, *Union (MSN, MSN/MPA)*

Seton Hall University, College of Nursing, *South Orange (MSN, MSN/MA, MSN/MBA)*

New York

Mercy College, Programs in Nursing, *Dobbs Ferry (MS)*

North Carolina

East Carolina University, College of Nursing, *Greenville (MSN)*

Ohio

The Ohio State University, College of Nursing, *Columbus (MS, MS/MPH)*

Oklahoma

Oklahoma City University, Kramer School of Nursing, *Oklahoma City (MSN, MSN/MBA)*

Southern Nazarene University, School of Nursing, *Bethany (MS)*

Pennsylvania

Waynesburg University, Department of Nursing, *Waynesburg (MSN, MSN/MBA)*

Tennessee

University of Memphis, Loewenberg School of Nursing, *Memphis (MSN)*

The University of Tennessee, College of Nursing, *Knoxville (MSN)*

Washington

Seattle University, College of Nursing, *Seattle (MSN)*

Washington State University College of Nursing, *Spokane (MN)*

ACCELERATED RN TO MASTER'S

U.S. AND U.S. TERRITORIES

California

California State University, Los Angeles, School of Nursing, *Los Angeles (MSN)*

Delaware

Wesley College, Nursing Program, *Dover (MSN)*

Georgia

Brenau University, College of Health and Science, *Gainesville (MSN)*

University of West Georgia, School of Nursing, *Carrollton (MSN)*

Illinois

Lewis University, Program in Nursing, *Romeoville (MSN, MSN/MBA)*

Saint Francis Medical Center College of Nursing, Baccalaureate Nursing Program, *Peoria (MSN)*

Iowa

The University of Iowa, College of Nursing, *Iowa City (MSN, MSN/MBA, MSN/MPH)*

Kentucky

Spalding University, School of Nursing, *Louisville (MSN)*

Maryland

Stevenson University, Nursing Division, *Stevenson (MS)*

Massachusetts

Regis College, School of Nursing, Science and Health Professions, *Weston (MSN)*

University of Massachusetts Lowell, Department of Nursing, *Lowell (MS)*

Michigan

Ferris State University, School of Nursing, *Big Rapids (MSN, MSN/MBA)*

University of Michigan, School of Nursing, *Ann Arbor (MS, MSN/MBA, MSN/MPH)*

University of Michigan–Flint, Department of Nursing, *Flint (MSN)*

Minnesota

Capella University, Nursing Programs, *Minneapolis (MSN)*

Minnesota State University Mankato, School of Nursing, *Mankato (MSN, MSN/MS)*

Missouri

Maryville University of Saint Louis, Nursing Program, School of Health Professions, *St. Louis (MSN)*

Nebraska

Nebraska Wesleyan University, Department of Nursing, *Lincoln (MSN)*

New Jersey

Fairleigh Dickinson University, Metropolitan Campus, Henry P. Becton School of Nursing and Allied Health, *Teaneck (MSN)*

Felician College, Division of Nursing and Health Management, *Lodi (MSN, MA/MSM)*

New York

Daemen College, Department of Nursing, *Amherst (MS)*

Mercy College, Programs in Nursing, *Dobbs Ferry (MS)*

The Sage Colleges, Department of Nursing, *Troy (MS, MS/MBA)*

State University of New York Institute of Technology, School of Nursing and Health Systems, *Utica (MS)*

State University of New York Upstate Medical University, College of Nursing, *Syracuse (MS)*

University of Rochester, School of Nursing, *Rochester (MS, MSN/PhD)*

Ohio

Kent State University, College of Nursing, *Kent (MSN, MSN/MBA, MSN/MPA)*

The Ohio State University, College of Nursing, *Columbus (MS, MS/MPH)*

Oklahoma

Oklahoma City University, Kramer School of Nursing, *Oklahoma City (MSN, MSN/MBA)*

Pennsylvania

Gannon University, Villa Maria School of Nursing, *Erie (MSN)*

Thomas Jefferson University, Department of Nursing, *Philadelphia (MSN)*

University of Pennsylvania, School of Nursing, *Philadelphia (MSN, MSN/MBA, MSN/MPH, MSN/PhD)*

The University of Scranton, Department of Nursing, *Scranton (MSN)*

Waynesburg University, Department of Nursing, *Waynesburg (MSN, MSN/MBA)*

Wilkes University, Department of Nursing, *Wilkes-Barre (MS)*

Tennessee

King College, School of Nursing, *Bristol (MSN, MSN/MBA)*

Southern Adventist University, School of Nursing, *Collegedale (MSN, MSN/MBA)*

The University of Tennessee, College of Nursing, *Knoxville (MSN)*

Texas

The University of Texas at Tyler, Program in Nursing, *Tyler (MSN, MSN/MBA)*

Utah

Western Governors University, Online College of Health Professions, *Salt Lake City (MS)*

Washington

Gonzaga University, Department of Nursing, *Spokane (MSN)*

Washington State University College of Nursing, *Spokane (MN)*

West Virginia

West Virginia University, School of Nursing, *Morgantown (MSN)*

CANADA

Quebec

Université du Québec à Chicoutimi, Program in Nursing, *Chicoutimi (MSN, MS/MPH)*

JOINT DEGREES

U.S. AND U.S. TERRITORIES

Alabama

Samford University, Ida V. Moffett School of Nursing, *Birmingham (MSN, MSN/MBA)*

The University of Alabama, Capstone College of Nursing, *Tuscaloosa (MSN, MSN/MA, MSN/Ed D)*

The University of Alabama at Birmingham, School of Nursing, *Birmingham (MSN, MSN/MPH)*

Arizona

Arizona State University at the Downtown Phoenix Campus, College of Nursing, *Phoenix (MS, MS/MPH)*

Grand Canyon University, College of Nursing and Health Sciences, *Phoenix (MS, MSN/MBA)*

University of Phoenix–Online Campus, Online Campus, *Phoenix (MSN, MSN/MBA, MSN/MHA)*

University of Phoenix–Phoenix Main Campus, College of Nursing, *Tempe (MSN, MSN/MBA, MSN/MHA)*

California

California State University, Long Beach, School of Nursing, *Long Beach (MSN, MSN/MHA)*

Holy Names University, Department of Nursing, *Oakland (MSN, MSN/MBA)*

University of California, Los Angeles, School of Nursing, *Los Angeles (MSN, MSN/MBA)*

University of Phoenix–Bay Area Campus, College of Nursing, *San Jose (MSN, MSN/MBA, MSN/MHA)*

University of Phoenix–Sacramento Valley Campus, College of Nursing, *Sacramento (MSN, MSN/MHA)*

University of Phoenix–Southern California Campus, College of Nursing, *Costa Mesa (MSN, MSN/MBA, MSN/MHA)*

Colorado

University of Phoenix–Denver Campus, College of Nursing, *Lone Tree (MSN, MSN/MHA, MSN/Ed D)*

Connecticut

University of Connecticut, School of Nursing, *Storrs (MS, MS/MBA)*

University of Hartford, College of Education, Nursing, and Health Professions, *West Hartford (MSN, MSN/MSOB)*

Yale University, School of Nursing, *New Haven (MSN, MSN/MPH, MSN/MDIV)*

Delaware

Wilmington University, College of Health Professions, *New Castle (MSN, MSN/MBA, MSN/MS)*

District of Columbia

The Catholic University of America, School of Nursing, *Washington (MSN, MA/MSM)*

Florida

Barry University, Division of Nursing, *Miami Shores (MSN, MSN/MBA)*

Florida Southern College, School of Nursing & Health Sciences, *Lakeland (MSN, MSN/MBA)*

Jacksonville University, School of Nursing, *Jacksonville (MSN, MSN/MBA)*

University of Florida, College of Nursing, *Gainesville (MSN, MSN/PhD)*

University of Phoenix–North Florida Campus, College of Nursing, *Jacksonville (MSN, MSN/MHA, MSN/Ed D)*

University of Phoenix–South Florida Campus, College of Nursing, *Fort Lauderdale (MSN, MSN/MBA, MSN/MHA)*

University of South Florida, College of Nursing, *Tampa (MS, MS/MPH)*

Georgia

Armstrong Atlantic State University, Program in Nursing, *Savannah (MSN, MS/MHSA)*

Emory University, Nell Hodgson Woodruff School of Nursing, *Atlanta (MSN, MSN/MPH)*

Thomas University, Division of Nursing, *Thomasville (MSN, MSN/MBA)*

Hawaii

Hawai`i Pacific University, College of Nursing and Health Sciences, *Honolulu (MSN, MSN/MBA)*

University of Hawaii at Manoa, School of Nursing and Dental Hygiene, *Honolulu (MS, MSN/MBA)*

Idaho

Boise State University, Department of Nursing, *Boise (MSN, MSN/MS)*

Illinois

Elmhurst College, Deicke Center for Nursing Education, *Elmhurst (MS, MSN/MBA)*

Lewis University, Program in Nursing, *Romeoville (MSN, MSN/MBA)*

Loyola University Chicago, Marcella Niehoff School of Nursing, *Maywood (MSN, MSN/MBA)*

Northern Illinois University, School of Nursing and Health Studies, *De Kalb (MS, MSN/MPH)*

North Park University, School of Nursing, *Chicago (MS, MSN/MA, MSN/MBA, MSN/MM)*

Saint Xavier University, School of Nursing, *Chicago (MSN, MSN/MBA)*

University of Illinois at Chicago, College of Nursing, *Chicago (MS, MS/MBA, MS/MPH)*

Indiana

Anderson University, School of Nursing, *Anderson (MSN, MSN/MBA)*

Indiana University–Purdue University Indianapolis, School of Nursing, *Indianapolis (MSN, MSN/MPH)*

University of Indianapolis, School of Nursing, *Indianapolis (MSN, MSN/MALAS, MSN/MS, MSN/MSBA)*

Valparaiso University, College of Nursing, *Valparaiso (MSN, MSN/MBA)*

Iowa

The University of Iowa, College of Nursing, *Iowa City (MSN, MSN/MBA, MSN/MPH)*

Kansas

The University of Kansas, School of Nursing, *Kansas City (MS, MS/MHSA, MS/MPH)*

Kentucky

Bellarmine University, Donna and Allan Lansing School of Nursing and Health Sciences, *Louisville (Certificate of Completion, MSN, MSN/MBA)*

Maine

Saint Joseph's College of Maine, Master of Science in Nursing Program, *Standish (MSN, MSN/MHA)*

University of Southern Maine, School of Nursing, *Portland (MS, MS/MBA)*

Maryland

The Johns Hopkins University, School of Nursing, *Baltimore (MSN, MSN/MBA, MSN/MPH, MSN/PhD)*

University of Maryland, Baltimore, Master's Program in Nursing, *Baltimore (MS, MSN/MBA, MSN/MPH)*

Massachusetts

Boston College, William F. Connell School of Nursing, *Chestnut Hill (MS, MSN/MA, MSN/MBA, MSN/PhD)*

Salem State University, Program in Nursing, *Salem (MSN, MSN/MBA)*

Michigan

Ferris State University, School of Nursing, *Big Rapids (MSN, MSN/MBA)*

Madonna University, College of Nursing and Health, *Livonia (MSN, MSN/MBA)*

Spring Arbor University, Program in Nursing, *Spring Arbor (MSN, MSN/MBA)*

University of Michigan, School of Nursing, *Ann Arbor (MS, MSN/MBA, MSN/MPH)*

Minnesota

Minnesota State University Mankato, School of Nursing, *Mankato (MSN, MSN/MS)*

Missouri

Saint Louis University, School of Nursing, *St. Louis (MSN, MN/MPH)*

University of Missouri, Sinclair School of Nursing, *Columbia (MSN, MSN/PhD)*

Nevada

University of Nevada, Reno, Orvis School of Nursing, *Reno (MSN, MSN/MPH)*

New Jersey

Felician College, Division of Nursing and Health Management, *Lodi (MSN, MA/MSM)*

Kean University, Department of Nursing, *Union (MSN, MSN/MPA)*

Rutgers, The State University of New Jersey, College of Nursing, *Newark (MS, MS/MPH)*

Seton Hall University, College of Nursing, *South Orange (MSN, MSN/MA, MSN/MBA)*

University of Medicine and Dentistry of New Jersey, School of Nursing, *Newark (MSN, MSN/MPH)*

New Mexico

University of New Mexico, College of Nursing, *Albuquerque (MSN, MSN/MPH)*

New York

Adelphi University, School of Nursing, *Garden City (MS, MS/MBA)*

Columbia University, School of Nursing, *New York (MS, MSN/MBA, MSN/MPH)*

Hunter College of the City University of New York, Hunter-Bellevue School of Nursing, *New York (MS, MSN/MPA, MSN/MPH)*

New York University, College of Nursing, *New York (MS, MS/MA, MS/MPH)*

The Sage Colleges, Department of Nursing, *Troy (MS, MS/MBA)*

State University of New York Downstate Medical Center, College of Nursing, *Brooklyn (MS, MS/MPH)*

University of Rochester, School of Nursing, *Rochester (MS, MSN/PhD)*

North Carolina

Duke University, School of Nursing, *Durham (MSN, MSN/MBA)*

Gardner-Webb University, School of Nursing, *Boiling Springs (MSN, MSN/MBA)*

Queens University of Charlotte, Presbyterian School of Nursing, *Charlotte (MSN, MSN/MBA)*

The University of North Carolina at Greensboro, School of Nursing, *Greensboro (MSN, MSN/MBA)*

Ohio

Capital University, School of Nursing, *Columbus (MSN, MN/MBA, MSN/JD, MSN/MDIV)*

Case Western Reserve University, Frances Payne Bolton School of Nursing, *Cleveland (MSN, MSN/MA, MSN/MBA, MSN/MPH)*

Cleveland State University, School of Nursing, *Cleveland (MSN, MSN/MBA)*

Kent State University, College of Nursing, *Kent (MSN, MSN/MBA, MSN/MPA)*

The Ohio State University, College of Nursing, *Columbus (MS, MS/MPH)*

University of Cincinnati, College of Nursing, *Cincinnati (MSN, MSN/MBA, MSN/PhD)*

Wright State University, College of Nursing and Health, *Dayton (MS, MS/MBA)*

Xavier University, School of Nursing, *Cincinnati (MSN, MSN/MBA, MSN/Ed D)*

Oklahoma

Oklahoma City University, Kramer School of Nursing, *Oklahoma City (MSN, MSN/MBA)*

Oregon

Oregon Health & Science University, School of Nursing, *Portland (MS, MN/MPH)*

Pennsylvania

Bloomsburg University of Pennsylvania, Department of Nursing, *Bloomsburg (MSN, MSN/MBA)*

DeSales University, Department of Nursing and Health, *Center Valley (MSN, MSN/MBA)*

La Salle University, School of Nursing and Health Sciences, *Philadelphia (MSN, MSN/MBA)*

Marywood University, Department of Nursing, *Scranton (MSN, MSN/MBA)*

Penn State University Park, School of Nursing, *University Park (MS, MSN/PhD)*

University of Pennsylvania, School of Nursing, *Philadelphia (MSN, MSN/MBA, MSN/MPH, MSN/PhD)*

Waynesburg University, Department of Nursing, *Waynesburg (MSN, MSN/MBA)*

Widener University, School of Nursing, *Chester (MSN, MSN/PhD)*

Tennessee

King College, School of Nursing, *Bristol (MSN, MSN/MBA)*

Southern Adventist University, School of Nursing, *Collegedale (MSN, MSN/MBA)*

Vanderbilt University, Vanderbilt University School of Nursing, *Nashville (MSN, MSN/MDIV, MSN/MTS)*

Texas

Lamar University, Department of Nursing, *Beaumont (MSN, MSN/MBA)*

Texas Woman's University, College of Nursing, *Denton (MS, MSN/MHA)*

The University of Texas at Arlington, College of Nursing, *Arlington (MSN, MSN/MBA, MSN/MHA, MSN/MPH)*

The University of Texas at Austin, School of Nursing, *Austin (MSN, MSN/MBA)*

The University of Texas at Tyler, Program in Nursing, *Tyler (MSN, MSN/MBA)*

The University of Texas Health Science Center at Houston, School of Nursing, *Houston (MSN, MSN/MPH)*

Virginia

Lynchburg College, School of Health Sciences and Human Performance, *Lynchburg (MSN, MSN/MBA)*

Shenandoah University, Eleanor Wade Custer School of Nursing, *Winchester (MSN, MSN/MBA)*

University of Virginia, School of Nursing, *Charlottesville (MSN, MSN/MBA, MSN/PhD)*

Washington

Pacific Lutheran University, School of Nursing, *Tacoma (MSN, MSN/MBA)*

University of Washington, School of Nursing, *Seattle (MN, MN/MPH, MS)*

Wisconsin

Edgewood College, Program in Nursing, *Madison (MS, MSN/MBA)*

Marquette University, College of Nursing, *Milwaukee (MSN, MSN/MBA)*

CANADA

Alberta

Athabasca University, Centre for Nursing and Health Studies, *Athabasca (MN, MN/MHSA, MN/MBA)*

Ontario

McMaster University, School of Nursing, *Hamilton (M Sc, MSN/PhD)*

Quebec

Université du Québec à Chicoutimi, Program in Nursing, *Chicoutimi (MSN, MS/MPH)*

MASTER'S

U.S. AND U.S. TERRITORIES

Alabama

Auburn University, School of Nursing, *Auburn University (MSN)*

Auburn University Montgomery, School of Nursing, *Montgomery (MSN)*

Jacksonville State University, College of Nursing and Health Sciences, *Jacksonville (MSN)*

Samford University, Ida V. Moffett School of Nursing, *Birmingham (MSN, MSN/MBA)*

Spring Hill College, Division of Nursing, *Mobile (MSN)*

Troy University, School of Nursing, *Troy (MSN)*

The University of Alabama, Capstone College of Nursing, *Tuscaloosa (MSN, MSN/MA, MSN/Ed D)*

The University of Alabama at Birmingham, School of Nursing, *Birmingham (MSN, MSN/MPH)*

The University of Alabama in Huntsville, College of Nursing, *Huntsville (MSN)*

University of Mobile, School of Nursing, *Mobile (MSN)*

University of North Alabama, College of Nursing and Allied Health, *Florence (MSN)*

University of South Alabama, College of Nursing, *Mobile (MSN)*

Alaska

University of Alaska Anchorage, School of Nursing, *Anchorage (MS)*

Arizona

Arizona State University at the Downtown Phoenix Campus, College of Nursing, *Phoenix (MS, MS/MPH)*

Chamberlain College of Nursing, *Phoenix (MSN)*

Grand Canyon University, College of Nursing and Health Sciences, *Phoenix (MS, MSN/MBA)*

Northern Arizona University, School of Nursing, *Flagstaff (MS)*

University of Phoenix–Online Campus, Online Campus, *Phoenix (MSN, MSN/MBA, MSN/MHA)*

University of Phoenix–Phoenix Main Campus, College of Nursing, *Tempe (MSN, MSN/MBA, MSN/MHA)*

University of Phoenix–Southern Arizona Campus, College of Social Sciences, *Tucson (MSN)*

Arkansas

Arkansas State University, Department of Nursing, *State University (MSN)*

Arkansas Tech University, Program in Nursing, *Russellville (MSN)*

University of Arkansas, Eleanor Mann School of Nursing, *Fayetteville (MSN)*

University of Arkansas for Medical Sciences, College of Nursing, *Little Rock (MN Sc)*

University of Central Arkansas, Department of Nursing, *Conway (MSN)*

California

Azusa Pacific University, School of Nursing, *Azusa (MSN)*

Brandman University, School of Nursing and Health Professions, *Irvine (MS)*

California Baptist University, School of Nursing, *Riverside (MSN)*

California State University, Chico, School of Nursing, *Chico (MSN)*

California State University, Dominguez Hills, Program in Nursing, *Carson (MSN)*

California State University, Fresno, Department of Nursing, *Fresno (MSN)*

California State University, Fullerton, Department of Nursing, *Fullerton (MSN)*

California State University, Long Beach, School of Nursing, *Long Beach (MSN, MSN/MHA)*

California State University, Los Angeles, School of Nursing, *Los Angeles (MSN)*

California State University, Sacramento, School of Nursing, *Sacramento (MS)*

California State University, San Bernardino, Department of Nursing, *San Bernardino (MSN)*

Charles Drew University of Medicine and Science, School of Nursing, *Los Angeles (MSN)*

Dominican University of California, Program in Nursing, *San Rafael (MSN)*

Holy Names University, Department of Nursing, *Oakland (MSN, MSN/MBA)*

Loma Linda University, School of Nursing, *Loma Linda (MS)*

Mount St. Mary's College, Department of Nursing, *Los Angeles (MSN)*

National University, Department of Nursing, *La Jolla (MSN)*

Point Loma Nazarene University, School of Nursing, *San Diego (MSN)*

Samuel Merritt University, School of Nursing, *Oakland (MSN)*

San Diego State University, School of Nursing, *San Diego (MSN)*

San Francisco State University, School of Nursing, *San Francisco (MSN)*

San Jose State University, The Valley Foundation School of Nursing, *San Jose (MS)*

University of California, Davis, The Betty Irene Moore School of Nursing, *Davis (MS)*

University of California, Irvine, Program in Nursing Science, *Irvine (MS)*

University of California, Los Angeles, School of Nursing, *Los Angeles (MSN, MSN/MBA)*

University of California, San Francisco, School of Nursing, *San Francisco (MS)*

University of Phoenix–Bay Area Campus, College of Nursing, *San Jose (MSN, MSN/MBA, MSN/MHA)*

University of Phoenix–San Diego Campus, College of Nursing, *San Diego (MSN, MSN/Ed D)*

University of Phoenix–Southern California Campus, College of Nursing, *Costa Mesa (MSN, MSN/MBA, MSN/MHA)*

University of San Diego, Hahn School of Nursing and Health Science, *San Diego (MSN)*

Western University of Health Sciences, College of Graduate Nursing, *Pomona (MSN)*

Colorado

American Sentinel University, RN to Bachelor of Science Nursing, *Aurora (MSN)*

Aspen University, Graduate School of Health Professions and Studies, *Denver (MSN)*

Colorado State University–Pueblo, Department of Nursing, *Pueblo (MS)*

Regis University, School of Nursing, *Denver (MS)*

University of Colorado at Colorado Springs, Beth-El College of Nursing and Health Sciences, *Colorado Springs (MSN)*

University of Colorado Denver, College of Nursing, *Aurora (MS)*

University of Northern Colorado, School of Nursing, *Greeley (MS)*

University of Phoenix–Denver Campus, College of Nursing, *Lone Tree (MSN, MSN/MHA, MSN/Ed D)*

Connecticut

Fairfield University, School of Nursing, *Fairfield (MSN)*

Quinnipiac University, School of Nursing, *Hamden (MSN)*

Sacred Heart University, Program in Nursing, *Fairfield (MSN)*

Southern Connecticut State University, Department of Nursing, *New Haven (MSN)*

University of Connecticut, School of Nursing, *Storrs (MS, MS/MBA)*

University of Hartford, College of Education, Nursing, and Health Professions, *West Hartford (MSN, MSN/MSOB)*

University of Saint Joseph, Department of Nursing, *West Hartford (MS)*

Western Connecticut State University, Department of Nursing, *Danbury (MS)*

Yale University, School of Nursing, *New Haven (MSN, MSN/MPH, MSN/MDIV)*

Delaware

Delaware State University, Department of Nursing, *Dover (MS)*

University of Delaware, School of Nursing, *Newark (MSN)*

Wesley College, Nursing Program, *Dover (MSN)*

Wilmington University, College of Health Professions, *New Castle (MSN, MSN/MBA, MSN/MS)*

District of Columbia

The Catholic University of America, School of Nursing, *Washington (MSN, MA/MSM)*

Georgetown University, School of Nursing and Health Studies, *Washington (MS)*

The George Washington University, School of Nursing, *Washington (MSN)*

Howard University, Division of Nursing, *Washington (MSN)*

Florida

Barry University, Division of Nursing, *Miami Shores (MSN, MSN/MBA)*

Florida Agricultural and Mechanical University, School of Nursing, *Tallahassee (MSN)*

Florida Atlantic University, Christine E. Lynn College of Nursing, *Boca Raton (MS)*

Florida Gulf Coast University, School of Nursing, *Fort Myers (MSN)*

Florida International University, Graduate Nursing Programs, *Miami (MSN)*

Florida Southern College, School of Nursing & Health Sciences, *Lakeland (MSN, MSN/MBA)*

Florida State University, College of Nursing, *Tallahassee (MSN)*

Jacksonville University, School of Nursing, *Jacksonville (MSN, MSN/MBA)*

Kaplan University Online, The School of Nursing Online, *Fort Lauderdale (MSN)*

Keiser University, Nursing Programs, *Fort Lauderdale (MSN)*

Keiser University, Nursing Programs, *Fort Myers (MSN)*

Keiser University, Nursing Programs, *Jacksonville (MSN)*

Keiser University, Nursing Programs, *Lakeland (MSN)*

Keiser University, Nursing Programs, *Melbourne (MSN)*

Keiser University, Nursing Programs, *Miami (MSN)*

Keiser University, Nursing Programs, *Orlando (MSN)*

Keiser University, Nursing Program, *Pembroke Pines (MSN)*

Keiser University, Nursing Programs, *Port St. Lucie (MSN)*

Keiser University, Nursing Programs, *Sarasota (MSN)*

Keiser University, Nursing Programs, *Tallahassee (MSN)*

Keiser University, Nursing Programs, *Tampa (MSN)*

Keiser University, Nursing Programs, *West Palm Beach (MSN)*

Nova Southeastern University, College of Health Care Sciences, *Fort Lauderdale (MSN)*

South University, Nursing Program, *Royal Palm Beach (MSN)*

South University, College of Nursing, *Tampa (MS)*

University of Central Florida, College of Nursing, *Orlando (MSN)*

University of Florida, College of Nursing, *Gainesville (MSN, MSN/PhD)*

University of Miami, School of Nursing and Health Studies, *Coral Gables (MSN)*

University of North Florida, School of Nursing, *Jacksonville (MSN)*

University of Phoenix–Central Florida Campus, College of Nursing, *Maitland (MSN, MSN/Ed D)*

University of Phoenix–North Florida Campus, College of Nursing, *Jacksonville (MSN, MSN/MHA, MSN/Ed D)*

University of Phoenix–South Florida Campus, College of Nursing, *Fort Lauderdale (MSN, MSN/MBA, MSN/MHA)*

University of South Florida, College of Nursing, *Tampa (MS, MS/MPH)*

The University of Tampa, Department of Nursing, *Tampa (MSN)*

University of West Florida, Department of Nursing, *Pensacola (MSN)*

Georgia

Albany State University, College of Sciences and Health Professions, *Albany (MSN)*

Armstrong Atlantic State University, Program in Nursing, *Savannah (MSN, MS/MHSA)*

Brenau University, College of Health and Science, *Gainesville (MSN)*

Clayton State University, Department of Nursing, *Morrow (MSN)*

Emory University, Nell Hodgson Woodruff School of Nursing, *Atlanta (MSN, MSN/MPH)*

Georgia College & State University, College of Health Sciences, *Milledgeville (MSN)*

Georgia Regents University, School of Nursing, *Augusta (MSN)*

Georgia Southern University, School of Nursing, *Statesboro (MSN)*

Georgia Southwestern State University, School of Nursing, *Americus (MSN)*

Georgia State University, Byrdine F. Lewis School of Nursing and Health Professions, *Atlanta (MSN)*

Kennesaw State University, School of Nursing, *Kennesaw (MSN)*

Mercer University Georgia Baptist College of Nursing, *Atlanta (MSN)*

Thomas University, Division of Nursing, *Thomasville (MSN, MSN/MBA)*

University of North Georgia, Department of Nursing, *Dahlonega (MS)*

University of West Georgia, School of Nursing, *Carrollton (MSN)*

Valdosta State University, College of Nursing, *Valdosta (MSN)*

Hawaii

Hawai`i Pacific University, College of Nursing and Health Sciences, *Honolulu (MSN, MSN/MBA)*

University of Hawaii at Manoa, School of Nursing and Dental Hygiene, *Honolulu (MS, MSN/MBA)*

University of Phoenix–Hawaii Campus, College of Nursing, *Honolulu (MSN, MSN/Ed D)*

Idaho

Boise State University, Department of Nursing, *Boise (MSN, MSN/MS)*

Idaho State University, Department of Nursing, *Pocatello (MS)*

Northwest Nazarene University, School of Health and Science, *Nampa (MSN)*

Illinois

Aurora University, School of Nursing, *Aurora (MSN)*

Benedictine University, Department of Nursing, *Lisle (MSN)*

Blessing–Rieman College of Nursing, *Quincy (MSN)*

Bradley University, Department of Nursing, *Peoria (MSN)*

DePaul University, Department of Nursing, *Chicago (MS)*

Elmhurst College, Deicke Center for Nursing Education, *Elmhurst (MS, MSN/MBA)*

Governors State University, College of Health and Human Services, *University Park (MS)*

Illinois State University, Mennonite College of Nursing, *Normal (MSN)*

Loyola University Chicago, Marcella Niehoff School of Nursing, *Maywood (MSN, MSN/MBA)*

McKendree University, Department of Nursing, *Lebanon (MSN)*

Millikin University, School of Nursing, *Decatur (MSN)*

Northern Illinois University, School of Nursing and Health Studies, *De Kalb (MS, MSN/MPH)*

North Park University, School of Nursing, *Chicago (MS, MSN/MA, MSN/MBA, MSN/MM)*

Olivet Nazarene University, Division of Nursing, *Bourbonnais (MSN)*

Resurrection University, *Oak Park (MSN)*

Rush University, College of Nursing, *Chicago (MSN)*

Saint Anthony College of Nursing, *Rockford (MSN)*

Saint Francis Medical Center College of Nursing, Baccalaureate Nursing Program, *Peoria (MSN)*

Saint Xavier University, School of Nursing, *Chicago (MSN, MSN/MBA)*

Southern Illinois University Edwardsville, School of Nursing, *Edwardsville (MS)*

University of Illinois at Chicago, College of Nursing, *Chicago (MS, MS/MBA, MS/MPH)*

University of St. Francis, Leach College of Nursing, *Joliet (MSN)*

Indiana

Anderson University, School of Nursing, *Anderson (MSN, MSN/MBA)*

Ball State University, School of Nursing, *Muncie (MS)*

Bethel College, School of Nursing, *Mishawaka (MSN)*

Goshen College, Department of Nursing, *Goshen (MSN)*

Indiana State University, Department of Nursing, *Terre Haute (MS)*

Indiana University–Purdue University Fort Wayne, Department of Nursing, *Fort Wayne (MS)*

Indiana University–Purdue University Indianapolis, School of Nursing, *Indianapolis (MSN, MSN/MPH)*

Indiana University South Bend, College of Health Sciences, *South Bend (MSN)*

Indiana Wesleyan University, School of Nursing, *Marion (MSN)*

Purdue University, School of Nursing, *West Lafayette (MS)*

Purdue University Calumet, School of Nursing, *Hammond (MS)*

University of Indianapolis, School of Nursing, *Indianapolis (MSN, MSN/MALAS, MSN/MS, MSN/MSBA)*

University of Saint Francis, Department of Nursing, *Fort Wayne (MSN)*

University of Southern Indiana, College of Nursing and Health Professions, *Evansville (MSN)*

Valparaiso University, College of Nursing, *Valparaiso (MSN, MSN/MBA)*

Iowa

Allen College, Program in Nursing, *Waterloo (MSN)*

Briar Cliff University, Department of Nursing, *Sioux City (MSN)*

Clarke University, Department of Nursing and Health, *Dubuque (MSN)*

Grand View University, Division of Nursing, *Des Moines (MS)*

Mount Mercy University, Department of Nursing, *Cedar Rapids (MSN)*

St. Ambrose University, Program in Nursing (BSN), *Davenport (MSN)*

The University of Iowa, College of Nursing, *Iowa City (MSN, MSN/MBA, MSN/MPH)*

Kansas

Fort Hays State University, Department of Nursing, *Hays (MSN, MSN/Ed D)*

MidAmerica Nazarene University, Division of Nursing, *Olathe (MSN)*

Pittsburg State University, Department of Nursing, *Pittsburg (MSN)*

The University of Kansas, School of Nursing, *Kansas City (MS, MS/MHSA, MS/MPH)*

Washburn University, School of Nursing, *Topeka (MSN)*

Kentucky

Bellarmine University, Donna and Allan Lansing School of Nursing and Health Sciences, *Louisville (Certificate of Completion, MSN, MSN/MBA)*

Eastern Kentucky University, Department of Baccalaureate and Graduate Nursing, *Richmond (MSN)*

Murray State University, Program in Nursing, *Murray (MSN)*

Northern Kentucky University, Department of Nursing, *Highland Heights (MSN)*

Spalding University, School of Nursing, *Louisville (MSN)*

University of Kentucky, Graduate School Programs in the College of Nursing, *Lexington (MSN)*

University of Louisville, School of Nursing, *Louisville (MSN)*

Western Kentucky University, School of Nursing, *Bowling Green (MSN)*

Louisiana

Grambling State University, School of Nursing, *Grambling (MSN)*

Louisiana State University Health Sciences Center, School of Nursing, *New Orleans (MN)*

Loyola University New Orleans, School of Nursing, *New Orleans (MSN)*

McNeese State University, College of Nursing, *Lake Charles (MSN)*

Northwestern State University of Louisiana, College of Nursing and Allied Health, *Shreveport (MSN)*

Our Lady of the Lake College, Division of Nursing, *Baton Rouge (MSN)*

Southeastern Louisiana University, School of Nursing, *Hammond (MSN)*

Southern University and Agricultural and Mechanical College, School of Nursing, *Baton Rouge (MSN)*

University of Louisiana at Lafayette, College of Nursing, *Lafayette (MSN)*

Maine

Husson University, School of Nursing, *Bangor (MSN)*

Saint Joseph's College of Maine, Master of Science in Nursing Program, *Standish (MSN, MSN/MHA)*

University of Maine, School of Nursing, *Orono (MSN)*

University of Southern Maine, School of Nursing, *Portland (MS, MS/MBA)*

Maryland

Bowie State University, Department of Nursing, *Bowie (MSN)*

Coppin State University, Helene Fuld School of Nursing, *Baltimore (MSN)*

The Johns Hopkins University, School of Nursing, *Baltimore (MSN, MSN/MBA, MSN/MPH, MSN/PhD)*

Salisbury University, Program in Nursing, *Salisbury (MS)*

Towson University, Department of Nursing, *Towson (MS)*

University of Maryland, Baltimore, Master's Program in Nursing, *Baltimore (MS, MSN/MBA, MSN/MPH)*

Massachusetts

American International College, Division of Nursing, *Springfield (MSN)*

Boston College, William F. Connell School of Nursing, *Chestnut Hill (MS, MSN/MA, MSN/MBA, MSN/PhD)*

Curry College, Division of Nursing, *Milton (MSN)*

Elms College, Division of Nursing, *Chicopee (MSN)*

Emmanuel College, Department of Nursing, *Boston (MS)*

Endicott College, Major in Nursing, *Beverly (MSN)*

Fitchburg State University, Department of Nursing, *Fitchburg (MS)*

Framingham State University, Department of Nursing, *Framingham (MSN)*

MGH Institute of Health Professions, School of Nursing, *Boston (MS)*

Northeastern University, School of Nursing, *Boston (MS)*

Regis College, School of Nursing, Science and Health Professions, *Weston (MSN)*

Salem State University, Program in Nursing, *Salem (MSN, MSN/MBA)*

Simmons College, School of Nursing and Health Sciences, *Boston (MS)*

University of Massachusetts Amherst, School of Nursing, *Amherst (MS)*

University of Massachusetts Boston, College of Nursing and Health Sciences, *Boston (MS)*

University of Massachusetts Dartmouth, College of Nursing, *North Dartmouth (MS)*

University of Massachusetts Lowell, Department of Nursing, *Lowell (MS)*

University of Massachusetts Worcester, Graduate School of Nursing, *Worcester (MS)*

Worcester State University, Department of Nursing, *Worcester (MS)*

Michigan

Andrews University, Department of Nursing, *Berrien Springs (MS)*

Eastern Michigan University, School of Nursing, *Ypsilanti (MSN)*

Ferris State University, School of Nursing, *Big Rapids (MSN, MSN/MBA)*

Grand Valley State University, Kirkhof College of Nursing, *Allendale (MSN)*

Madonna University, College of Nursing and Health, *Livonia (MSN, MSN/MBA)*

Michigan State University, College of Nursing, *East Lansing (MSN)*

Northern Michigan University, College of Nursing and Allied Health Science, *Marquette (MSN)*

Oakland University, School of Nursing, *Rochester (MSN)*

Saginaw Valley State University, Crystal M. Lange College of Health and Human Services, *University Center (MSN)*

Spring Arbor University, Program in Nursing, *Spring Arbor (MSN, MSN/MBA)*

University of Detroit Mercy, McAuley School of Nursing, *Detroit (MSN)*

University of Michigan, School of Nursing, *Ann Arbor (MS, MSN/MBA, MSN/MPH)*

University of Phoenix–Metro Detroit Campus, College of Nursing, *Southfield (MSN)*

Wayne State University, College of Nursing, *Detroit (MSN)*

Western Michigan University, College of Health and Human Services, *Kalamazoo (MSN)*

Minnesota

Augsburg College, Program in Nursing, *Minneapolis (MA)*

Bethel University, Department of Nursing, *St. Paul (MA)*

Capella University, Nursing Programs, *Minneapolis (MSN)*

The College of St. Scholastica, Department of Nursing, *Duluth (MA)*

Concordia College, Department of Nursing, *Moorhead (MS)*

Minnesota State University Mankato, School of Nursing, *Mankato (MSN, MSN/MS)*

Minnesota State University Moorhead, School of Nursing and Healthcare Leadership, *Moorhead (MS)*

St. Catherine University, Department of Nursing, *St. Paul (MA)*

Walden University, Nursing Programs, *Minneapolis (MSN)*

Winona State University, College of Nursing and Health Sciences, *Winona (MS)*

Mississippi

Alcorn State University, School of Nursing, *Natchez (MSN)*

Delta State University, School of Nursing, *Cleveland (MSN)*

Mississippi University for Women, College of Nursing and Speech Language Pathology, *Columbus (MSN)*

University of Mississippi Medical Center, Program in Nursing, *Jackson (MSN)*

University of Southern Mississippi, School of Nursing, *Hattiesburg (MSN)*

William Carey University, School of Nursing, *Hattiesburg (MSN)*

Missouri

Central Methodist University, College of Liberal Arts and Sciences, *Fayette (MSN)*

Cox College, Department of Nursing, *Springfield (MSN)*

Goldfarb School of Nursing at Barnes-Jewish College, *St. Louis (MSN)*

Graceland University, School of Nursing, *Independence (MSN)*

Maryville University of Saint Louis, Nursing Program, School of Health Professions, *St. Louis (MSN)*

Missouri Southern State University, Department of Nursing, *Joplin (MSN)*

Missouri State University, Department of Nursing, *Springfield (MSN)*

Missouri Western State University, Department of Nursing, *St. Joseph (MSN)*

Research College of Nursing, College of Nursing, *Kansas City (MSN)*

Saint Louis University, School of Nursing, *St. Louis (MSN, MN/MPH)*

Southeast Missouri State University, Department of Nursing, *Cape Girardeau (MSN)*

Southwest Baptist University, College of Nursing, *Bolivar (MSN)*

University of Central Missouri, Department of Nursing, *Warrensburg (MS)*

University of Missouri, Sinclair School of Nursing, *Columbia (MSN, MSN/PhD)*

University of Missouri–Kansas City, School of Nursing, *Kansas City (MSN)*

University of Missouri–St. Louis, College of Nursing, *St. Louis (MSN)*

Webster University, Department of Nursing, *St. Louis (MSN)*

Montana

Montana State University, College of Nursing, *Bozeman (MN)*

Nebraska

BryanLGH College of Health Sciences, School of Nursing, *Lincoln (MS)*

Clarkson College, Master of Science in Nursing Program, *Omaha (MSN)*

Creighton University, School of Nursing, *Omaha (MSN)*

Nebraska Methodist College, Department of Nursing, *Omaha (MSN)*

Nebraska Wesleyan University, Department of Nursing, *Lincoln (MSN)*

University of Nebraska Medical Center, College of Nursing, *Omaha (MSN)*

Nevada

Touro University, School of Nursing, *Henderson (MSN)*

University of Nevada, Las Vegas, School of Nursing, *Las Vegas (MSN)*

University of Nevada, Reno, Orvis School of Nursing, *Reno (MSN, MSN/MPH)*

New Hampshire

Franklin Pierce University, Master of Science in Nursing, *Rindge (MSN)*

Rivier University, Division of Nursing, *Nashua (MS)*

University of New Hampshire, Department of Nursing, *Durham (MS)*

New Jersey

The College of New Jersey, School of Nursing, Health and Exercise Science, *Ewing (MSN)*

Fairleigh Dickinson University, Metropolitan Campus, Henry P. Becton School of Nursing and Allied Health, *Teaneck (MSN)*

Felician College, Division of Nursing and Health Management, *Lodi (MSN, MA/MSM)*

Kean University, Department of Nursing, *Union (MSN, MSN/MPA)*

Monmouth University, Marjorie K. Unterberg School of Nursing, *West Long Branch (MSN)*

Ramapo College of New Jersey, Master of Science in Nursing Program, *Mahwah (MSN)*

Rutgers, The State University of New Jersey, College of Nursing, *Newark (MS, MS/MPH)*

Saint Peter's University, Nursing Program, *Jersey City (MSN)*

Seton Hall University, College of Nursing, *South Orange (MSN, MSN/MA, MSN/MBA)*

Thomas Edison State College, School of Nursing, *Trenton (MSN)*

University of Medicine and Dentistry of New Jersey, School of Nursing, *Newark (MSN, MSN/MPH)*

William Paterson University of New Jersey, Department of Nursing, *Wayne (MSN)*

New Mexico

New Mexico State University, School of Nursing, *Las Cruces (MSN)*

University of New Mexico, College of Nursing, *Albuquerque (MSN, MSN/MPH)*

University of Phoenix–New Mexico Campus, College of Nursing, *Albuquerque (MSN, MSN/Ed D)*

New York

Adelphi University, School of Nursing, *Garden City (MS, MS/MBA)*

Binghamton University, State University of New York, Decker School of Nursing, *Binghamton (MS)*

College of Mount Saint Vincent, Department of Nursing, *Riverdale (MSN)*

The College of New Rochelle, School of Nursing, *New Rochelle (MS)*

College of Staten Island of the City University of New York, Department of Nursing, *Staten Island (MS)*

Columbia University, School of Nursing, *New York (MS, MSN/MBA, MSN/MPH)*

Daemen College, Department of Nursing, *Amherst (MS)*

Dominican College, Department of Nursing, *Orangeburg (M Sc N)*

D'Youville College, School of Nursing, *Buffalo (MS)*

Excelsior College, School of Nursing, *Albany (MS)*

Hunter College of the City University of New York, Hunter-Bellevue School of Nursing, *New York (MS, MSN/MPA, MSN/MPH)*

Lehman College of the City University of New York, Department of Nursing, *Bronx (MS)*

Le Moyne College, Nursing Programs, *Syracuse (MS)*

Long Island University–Brooklyn Campus, School of Nursing, *Brooklyn (MS)*

Long Island University–C. W. Post Campus, Department of Nursing, *Brookville (MS)*

Mercy College, Programs in Nursing, *Dobbs Ferry (MS)*

Molloy College, Division of Nursing, *Rockville Centre (MS)*

Mount Saint Mary College, Division of Nursing, *Newburgh (MS)*

New York University, College of Nursing, *New York (MS, MS/MA, MS/MPH)*

Pace University, Lienhard School of Nursing, *New York (MS)*

Roberts Wesleyan College, Division of Nursing, *Rochester (M Sc N)*

The Sage Colleges, Department of Nursing, *Troy (MS, MS/MBA)*

St. John Fisher College, Wegmans School of Nursing, *Rochester (MS)*

St. Joseph's College, New York, Department of Nursing, *Brooklyn (MS)*

State University of New York Downstate Medical Center, College of Nursing, *Brooklyn (MS, MS/MPH)*

State University of New York Institute of Technology, School of Nursing and Health Systems, *Utica (MS)*

State University of New York Upstate Medical University, College of Nursing, *Syracuse (MS)*

Stony Brook University, State University of New York, School of Nursing, *Stony Brook (MS)*

University of Rochester, School of Nursing, *Rochester (MS, MSN/PhD)*

North Carolina

Duke University, School of Nursing, *Durham (MSN, MSN/MBA)*

East Carolina University, College of Nursing, *Greenville (MSN)*

Gardner-Webb University, School of Nursing, *Boiling Springs (MSN, MSN/MBA)*

Lenoir-Rhyne University, Program in Nursing, *Hickory (MSN)*

Queens University of Charlotte, Presbyterian School of Nursing, *Charlotte (MSN, MSN/MBA)*

The University of North Carolina at Chapel Hill, School of Nursing, *Chapel Hill (MSN)*

The University of North Carolina at Charlotte, School of Nursing, *Charlotte (MSN)*

The University of North Carolina at Greensboro, School of Nursing, *Greensboro (MSN, MSN/MBA)*

The University of North Carolina Wilmington, School of Nursing, *Wilmington (MSN)*

Western Carolina University, School of Nursing, *Cullowhee (MS)*

Winston-Salem State University, Department of Nursing, *Winston-Salem (MSN)*

North Dakota

North Dakota State University, Department of Nursing, *Fargo (MS)*

University of Mary, Division of Nursing, *Bismarck (MSN)*

University of North Dakota, College of Nursing, *Grand Forks (MS)*

Ohio

Capital University, School of Nursing, *Columbus (MSN, MN/MBA, MSN/JD, MSN/MDIV)*

Case Western Reserve University, Frances Payne Bolton School of Nursing, *Cleveland (MSN, MSN/MA, MSN/MBA, MSN/MPH)*

Cedarville University, Department of Nursing, *Cedarville (MSN)*

Chamberlain College of Nursing, *Columbus (MSN)*

Cleveland State University, School of Nursing, *Cleveland (MSN, MSN/MBA)*

Franciscan University of Steubenville, Department of Nursing, *Steubenville (MSN)*

Kent State University, College of Nursing, *Kent (MSN, MSN/MBA, MSN/MPA)*

Lourdes University, School of Nursing, *Sylvania (MSN)*

Malone University, School of Nursing, *Canton (MSN)*

Mount Carmel College of Nursing, Nursing Programs, *Columbus (MS)*

The Ohio State University, College of Nursing, *Columbus (MS, MS/MPH)*

Ohio University, School of Nursing, *Athens (MSN)*

Otterbein University, Department of Nursing, *Westerville (MSN)*

The University of Akron, College of Nursing, *Akron (MSN)*

University of Cincinnati, College of Nursing, *Cincinnati (MSN, MSN/MBA, MSN/PhD)*

University of Phoenix–Cleveland Campus, College of Nursing, *Independence (MSN)*

The University of Toledo, College of Nursing, *Toledo (MSN)*

Urbana University, College of Nursing and Allied Health, *Urbana (MSN)*

Ursuline College, The Breen School of Nursing, *Pepper Pike (MSN)*

Walsh University, Department of Nursing, *North Canton (MSN)*

Wright State University, College of Nursing and Health, *Dayton (MS, MS/MBA)*

Xavier University, School of Nursing, *Cincinnati (MSN, MSN/MBA, MSN/Ed D)*

Oklahoma

Northeastern State University, Department of Nursing, *Tahlequah (MSN)*

Oklahoma Baptist University, School of Nursing, *Shawnee (MSN)*

Oklahoma City University, Kramer School of Nursing, *Oklahoma City (MSN, MSN/MBA)*

University of Oklahoma Health Sciences Center, College of Nursing, *Oklahoma City (MS)*

Oregon

Oregon Health & Science University, School of Nursing, *Portland (MS, MN/MPH)*

University of Portland, School of Nursing, *Portland (MS)*

Pennsylvania

Bloomsburg University of Pennsylvania, Department of Nursing, *Bloomsburg (MSN, MSN/MBA)*

Carlow University, School of Nursing, *Pittsburgh (MSN)*

Cedar Crest College, Department of Nursing, *Allentown (MSN)*

Chatham University, Nursing Programs, *Pittsburgh (MSN)*

Clarion University of Pennsylvania, School of Nursing, *Oil City (MSN)*

DeSales University, Department of Nursing and Health, *Center Valley (MSN, MSN/MBA)*

Drexel University, College of Nursing and Health Professions, *Philadelphia (MSN)*

Duquesne University, School of Nursing, *Pittsburgh (MSN)*

Gannon University, Villa Maria School of Nursing, *Erie (MSN)*

Gwynedd-Mercy College, School of Nursing, *Gwynedd Valley (MSN)*

Holy Family University, School of Nursing and Allied Health Professions, *Philadelphia (MSN)*

Immaculata University, Department of Nursing, *Immaculata (MSN)*

Indiana University of Pennsylvania, Department of Nursing and Allied Health, *Indiana (MS)*

La Roche College, Department of Nursing and Nursing Management, *Pittsburgh (MSN)*

La Salle University, School of Nursing and Health Sciences, *Philadelphia (MSN, MSN/MBA)*

Mansfield University of Pennsylvania, Department of Health Sciences–Nursing, *Mansfield (MSN)*

Marywood University, Department of Nursing, *Scranton (MSN, MSN/MPH)*

Millersville University of Pennsylvania, Department of Nursing, *Millersville (MSN)*

Misericordia University, Department of Nursing, *Dallas (MSN)*

Moravian College, St. Luke's School of Nursing, *Bethlehem (MS)*

Neumann University, Program in Nursing and Health Sciences, *Aston (MS)*

Penn State University Park, School of Nursing, *University Park (MS, MSN/PhD)*

Robert Morris University, School of Nursing and Health Sciences, *Moon Township (MSN)*

Temple University, Department of Nursing, *Philadelphia (MSN)*

Thomas Jefferson University, Department of Nursing, *Philadelphia (MSN)*

University of Pennsylvania, School of Nursing, *Philadelphia (MSN, MSN/MBA, MSN/MPH, MSN/PhD)*

University of Pittsburgh, School of Nursing, *Pittsburgh (MSN)*

The University of Scranton, Department of Nursing, *Scranton (MSN)*

Villanova University, College of Nursing, *Villanova (MSN)*

West Chester University of Pennsylvania, Department of Nursing, *West Chester (MSN)*

Widener University, School of Nursing, *Chester (MSN, MSN/PhD)*

Wilkes University, Department of Nursing, *Wilkes-Barre (MS)*

York College of Pennsylvania, Department of Nursing, *York (MS)*

Puerto Rico

University of Puerto Rico, Medical Sciences Campus, School of Nursing, *San Juan (MSN)*

University of the Sacred Heart, Program in Nursing, *San Juan (MSN)*

Rhode Island

Rhode Island College, Department of Nursing, *Providence (MSN)*

University of Rhode Island, College of Nursing, *Kingston (MS)*

South Carolina

Charleston Southern University, Wingo School of Nursing, *Charleston (MSN)*

Clemson University, School of Nursing, *Clemson (MS)*

Medical University of South Carolina, College of Nursing, *Charleston (MSN)*

University of South Carolina, College of Nursing, *Columbia (MSN)*

South Dakota

South Dakota State University, College of Nursing, *Brookings (MS)*

Tennessee

Aquinas College, School of Nursing, *Nashville (MSN)*

Austin Peay State University, School of Nursing, *Clarksville (MSN)*

Belmont University, School of Nursing, *Nashville (MSN)*

Carson-Newman University, Department of Nursing, *Jefferson City (MSN)*

East Tennessee State University, College of Nursing, *Johnson City (MSN)*

King College, School of Nursing, *Bristol (MSN, MSN/MBA)*

Lincoln Memorial University, Caylor School of Nursing, *Harrogate (MSN)*

Middle Tennessee State University, School of Nursing, *Murfreesboro (MSN)*

Southern Adventist University, School of Nursing, *Collegedale (MSN, MSN/MBA)*

Tennessee Technological University, Whitson-Hester School of Nursing, *Cookeville (MSN, M Sc N)*

Union University, School of Nursing, *Jackson (MSN)*

University of Memphis, Loewenberg School of Nursing, *Memphis (MSN)*

The University of Tennessee, College of Nursing, *Knoxville (MSN)*

The University of Tennessee at Chattanooga, School of Nursing, *Chattanooga (MSN)*

Vanderbilt University, Vanderbilt University School of Nursing, *Nashville (MSN, MSN/MDIV, MSN/MTS)*

Texas

Angelo State University, Department of Nursing and Rehabilitation Sciences, *San Angelo (MSN)*

Baylor University, Louise Herrington School of Nursing, *Waco (MSN)*

Lamar University, Department of Nursing, *Beaumont (MSN, MSN/MBA)*

Midwestern State University, Nursing Program, *Wichita Falls (MSN)*

Patty Hanks Shelton School of Nursing, *Abilene (MSN)*

Prairie View A&M University, College of Nursing, *Houston (MSN)*

Texas A&M International University, Canseco School of Nursing, *Laredo (MSN)*

Texas A&M University–Corpus Christi, College of Nursing and Health Sciences, *Corpus Christi (MSN)*

Texas A&M University–Texarkana, Nursing Department, *Texarkana (MSN)*

Texas Christian University, Harris College of Nursing, *Fort Worth (MSN)*

Texas State University–San Marcos, St. David's School of Nursing, *San Marcos (MSN)*

Texas Tech University Health Sciences Center, School of Nursing, *Lubbock (MSN)*

Texas Woman's University, College of Nursing, *Denton (MS, MSN/MHA)*

University of Houston–Victoria, School of Nursing, *Victoria (MSN)*

University of Mary Hardin-Baylor, College of Nursing, *Belton (MSN)*

The University of Texas at Arlington, College of Nursing, *Arlington (MSN, MSN/MBA, MSN/MHA, MSN/MPH)*

The University of Texas at Austin, School of Nursing, *Austin (MSN, MSN/MBA)*

The University of Texas at Brownsville, Department of Nursing, *Brownsville (MSN)*

The University of Texas at El Paso, School of Nursing, *El Paso (MSN)*

The University of Texas at Tyler, Program in Nursing, *Tyler (MSN, MSN/MBA)*

The University of Texas Health Science Center at Houston, School of Nursing, *Houston (MSN, MSN/MPH)*

The University of Texas Health Science Center at San Antonio, School of Nursing, *San Antonio (MSN)*

The University of Texas Medical Branch, School of Nursing, *Galveston (MSN)*

The University of Texas–Pan American, Department of Nursing, *Edinburg (MSN)*

University of the Incarnate Word, Program in Nursing, *San Antonio (MSN)*

West Texas A&M University, Department of Nursing, *Canyon (MSN)*

Utah

Brigham Young University, College of Nursing, *Provo (MS)*

University of Utah, College of Nursing, *Salt Lake City (MS)*

Weber State University, Program in Nursing, *Ogden (MSN)*

Western Governors University, Online College of Health Professions, *Salt Lake City (MS)*

Westminster College, School of Nursing and Health Sciences, *Salt Lake City (MSN)*

Vermont

University of Vermont, Department of Nursing, *Burlington (MS)*

Virginia

Eastern Mennonite University, Department of Nursing, *Harrisonburg (MSN)*

George Mason University, College of Health and Human Services, *Fairfax (MSN)*

Hampton University, School of Nursing, *Hampton (MS)*

James Madison University, Department of Nursing, *Harrisonburg (MSN)*

Jefferson College of Health Sciences, Nursing Education Program, *Roanoke (MSN)*

Liberty University, Department of Nursing, *Lynchburg (MSN)*

Lynchburg College, School of Health Sciences and Human Performance, *Lynchburg (MSN, MSN/MBA)*

Marymount University, Malek School of Health Professions, *Arlington (MSN)*

Old Dominion University, Department of Nursing, *Norfolk (MSN)*

Radford University, School of Nursing, *Radford (MSN)*

Shenandoah University, Eleanor Wade Custer School of Nursing, *Winchester (MSN, MSN/MBA)*

University of Virginia, School of Nursing, *Charlottesville (MSN, MSN/MBA, MSN/PhD)*

Virginia Commonwealth University, School of Nursing, *Richmond (MS)*

Washington

Gonzaga University, Department of Nursing, *Spokane (MSN)*

Pacific Lutheran University, School of Nursing, *Tacoma (MSN, MSN/MBA)*

Seattle Pacific University, School of Health Sciences, *Seattle (MSN)*

Seattle University, College of Nursing, *Seattle (MSN)*

University of Washington, School of Nursing, *Seattle (MN, MN/MPH)*

Washington State University College of Nursing, *Spokane (MN)*

West Virginia

Marshall University, College of Health Professions, *Huntington (MSN)*

West Virginia University, School of Nursing, *Morgantown (MSN)*

West Virginia Wesleyan College, School of Nursing, *Buckhannon (MSN)*

Wheeling Jesuit University, Department of Nursing, *Wheeling (MSN)*

Wisconsin

Alverno College, Division of Nursing, *Milwaukee (MSN)*

Bellin College, Nursing Program, *Green Bay (MSN)*

Concordia University Wisconsin, Program in Nursing, *Mequon (MSN)*

Edgewood College, Program in Nursing, *Madison (MS, MSN/MBA)*

Marian University, School of Nursing, *Fond du Lac (MSN)*

Marquette University, College of Nursing, *Milwaukee (MSN, MSN/MBA)*

University of Phoenix–Milwaukee Campus, College of Health and Human Services, *Milwaukee (MSN)*

University of Wisconsin–Eau Claire, College of Nursing and Health Sciences, *Eau Claire (MSN)*

University of Wisconsin–Milwaukee, College of Nursing, *Milwaukee (MN)*

University of Wisconsin–Oshkosh, College of Nursing, *Oshkosh (MSN)*

Viterbo University, School of Nursing, *La Crosse (MSN)*

Wyoming

University of Wyoming, Fay W. Whitney School of Nursing, *Laramie (MS)*

CANADA

Alberta

Athabasca University, Centre for Nursing and Health Studies, *Athabasca (MN, MN/MHSA, MN/MBA)*

University of Alberta, Faculty of Nursing, *Edmonton (MN)*

University of Calgary, Faculty of Nursing, *Calgary (MN)*

University of Lethbridge, Faculty of Health Sciences, *Lethbridge (M Sc)*

British Columbia

Trinity Western University, Department of Nursing, *Langley (MSN)*

The University of British Columbia, Program in Nursing, *Vancouver (MSN)*

University of Northern British Columbia, Nursing Programme, *Prince George (M Sc N)*

University of Victoria, School of Nursing, *Victoria (MN)*

Manitoba

University of Manitoba, Faculty of Nursing, *Winnipeg (MN)*

New Brunswick

Université de Moncton, School of Nursing, *Moncton (M Sc N)*

University of New Brunswick Fredericton, Faculty of Nursing, *Fredericton (MN)*

Newfoundland and Labrador

Memorial University of Newfoundland, School of Nursing, *St. John's (MN)*

Ontario

Laurentian University, School of Nursing, *Sudbury (M Sc N)*

McMaster University, School of Nursing, *Hamilton (M Sc, MSN/PhD)*

Queen's University at Kingston, School of Nursing, *Kingston (M Sc)*

Ryerson University, Program in Nursing, *Toronto (MN)*

University of Ottawa, School of Nursing, *Ottawa (M Sc N)*

University of Toronto, Faculty of Nursing, *Toronto (MN)*

The University of Western Ontario, School of Nursing, *London (M Sc N)*

University of Windsor, Faculty of Nursing, *Windsor (MN, M Sc)*

Quebec

McGill University, School of Nursing, *Montréal (M Sc)*

Université de Montréal, Faculty of Nursing, *Montréal (M Sc)*

Université de Sherbrooke, Department of Nursing, *Sherbrooke (M Sc)*

Université du Québec à Chicoutimi, Program in Nursing, *Chicoutimi (MSN, MS/MPH)*

Université du Québec à Rimouski, Program in Nursing, *Rimouski (M Sc N)*

Université du Québec à Trois-Rivières, Program in Nursing, *Trois-Rivières (MSN)*

Université du Québec en Outaouais, Département des Sciences Infirmières, *Gatineau (M Sc N)*

Université Laval, Faculty of Nursing, *Québec (MSN)*

Saskatchewan

University of Saskatchewan, College of Nursing, *Saskatoon (MN)*

MASTER'S FOR NON-NURSING COLLEGE GRADUATES

U.S. AND U.S. TERRITORIES

California

California State University, Dominguez Hills, Program in Nursing, *Carson (MSN)*

California State University, Fullerton, Department of Nursing, *Fullerton (MSN)*

California State University, Long Beach, School of Nursing, *Long Beach (MSN, MSN/MHA)*

California State University, Los Angeles, School of Nursing, *Los Angeles (MSN)*

Samuel Merritt University, School of Nursing, *Oakland (MSN)*

San Francisco State University, School of Nursing, *San Francisco (MSN)*

University of California, Los Angeles, School of Nursing, *Los Angeles (MSN, MSN/MBA)*

University of California, San Francisco, School of Nursing, *San Francisco (MS)*

Connecticut

Yale University, School of Nursing, *New Haven (MSN, MSN/MPH, MSN/MDIV)*

District of Columbia

Georgetown University, School of Nursing and Health Studies, *Washington (MS)*

Hawaii

University of Hawaii at Manoa, School of Nursing and Dental Hygiene, *Honolulu (MS, MSN/MBA)*

Illinois

DePaul University, Department of Nursing, *Chicago (MS)*

University of Illinois at Chicago, College of Nursing, *Chicago (MS, MS/MBA, MS/MPH)*

Maine

University of Southern Maine, School of Nursing, *Portland (MS, MS/MBA)*

Massachusetts

MGH Institute of Health Professions, School of Nursing, *Boston (MS)*

Regis College, School of Nursing, Science and Health Professions, *Weston (MSN)*

Nebraska

University of Nebraska Medical Center, College of Nursing, *Omaha (MSN)*

New York

Columbia University, School of Nursing, *New York (MS, MSN/MBA, MSN/MPH)*

Mercy College, Programs in Nursing, *Dobbs Ferry (MS)*

North Carolina

Gardner-Webb University, School of Nursing, *Boiling Springs (MSN, MSN/MBA)*

Ohio

Case Western Reserve University, Frances Payne Bolton School of Nursing, *Cleveland (MSN, MSN/MA, MSN/MBA, MSN/MPH)*

The Ohio State University, College of Nursing, *Columbus (MS, MS/MPH)*

The University of Toledo, College of Nursing, *Toledo (MSN)*

Oklahoma

University of Oklahoma Health Sciences Center, College of Nursing, *Oklahoma City (MS)*

Pennsylvania

Immaculata University, Department of Nursing, *Immaculata (MSN)*

Thomas Jefferson University, Department of Nursing, *Philadelphia (MSN)*

Wilkes University, Department of Nursing, *Wilkes-Barre (MS)*

Tennessee

University of Memphis, Loewenberg School of Nursing, *Memphis (MSN)*

The University of Tennessee, College of Nursing, *Knoxville (MSN)*

Vanderbilt University, Vanderbilt University School of Nursing, *Nashville (MSN, MSN/MDIV, MSN/MTS)*

Texas

Angelo State University, Department of Nursing and Rehabilitation Sciences, *San Angelo (MSN)*

The University of Texas at Austin, School of Nursing, *Austin (MSN, MSN/MBA)*

Vermont

University of Vermont, Department of Nursing, *Burlington (MS)*

Virginia

University of Virginia, School of Nursing, *Charlottesville (MSN, MSN/MBA, MSN/PhD)*

Wisconsin

Marquette University, College of Nursing, *Milwaukee (MSN, MSN/MBA)*

University of Wisconsin–Milwaukee, College of Nursing, *Milwaukee (MN)*

CANADA

Quebec

McGill University, School of Nursing, *Montréal (M Sc)*

MASTER'S FOR NURSES WITH NON-NURSING DEGREES

U.S. AND U.S. TERRITORIES

Alabama

University of South Alabama, College of Nursing, *Mobile (MSN)*

Arizona

University of Phoenix–Online Campus, Online Campus, *Phoenix (MSN, MSN/MBA, MSN/MHA)*

Arkansas

Arkansas Tech University, Program in Nursing, *Russellville (MSN)*

University of Arkansas for Medical Sciences, College of Nursing, *Little Rock (MN Sc)*

California

California State University, Dominguez Hills, Program in Nursing, *Carson (MSN)*

California State University, Fresno, Department of Nursing, *Fresno (MSN)*

Dominican University of California, Program in Nursing, *San Rafael (MSN)*

Holy Names University, Department of Nursing, *Oakland (MSN, MSN/MBA)*

Samuel Merritt University, School of Nursing, *Oakland (MSN)*

San Francisco State University, School of Nursing, *San Francisco (MSN)*

University of California, San Francisco, School of Nursing, *San Francisco (MS)*

University of San Diego, Hahn School of Nursing and Health Science, *San Diego (MSN)*

University of San Francisco, School of Nursing and Health Professions, *San Francisco (MSN)*

Connecticut

Fairfield University, School of Nursing, *Fairfield (MSN)*

University of Hartford, College of Education, Nursing, and Health Professions, *West Hartford (MSN, MSN/MSOB)*

University of Saint Joseph, Department of Nursing, *West Hartford (MS)*

Yale University, School of Nursing, *New Haven (MSN, MSN/MPH, MSN/MDIV)*

Florida

Florida Atlantic University, Christine E. Lynn College of Nursing, *Boca Raton (MS)*

Florida International University, Graduate Nursing Programs, *Miami (MSN)*

Florida Southern College, School of Nursing & Health Sciences, *Lakeland (MSN, MSN/MBA)*

University of South Florida, College of Nursing, *Tampa (MS, MS/MPH)*

Illinois

Resurrection University, *Oak Park (MSN)*

Rush University, College of Nursing, *Chicago (MSN)*

University of Illinois at Chicago, College of Nursing, *Chicago (MS, MS/MBA, MS/MPH)*

University of St. Francis, Leach College of Nursing, *Joliet (MSN)*

Indiana

University of Saint Francis, Department of Nursing, *Fort Wayne (MSN)*

Iowa

Allen College, Program in Nursing, *Waterloo (MSN)*

The University of Iowa, College of Nursing, *Iowa City (MSN, MSN/MBA, MSN/MPH)*

Kentucky

Bellarmine University, Donna and Allan Lansing School of Nursing and Health Sciences, *Louisville (Certificate of Completion, MSN, MSN/MBA)*

Louisiana

Loyola University New Orleans, School of Nursing, *New Orleans (MSN)*

Maine

Husson University, School of Nursing, *Bangor (MSN)*

Saint Joseph's College of Maine, Master of Science in Nursing Program, *Standish (MSN, MSN/MHA)*

University of Southern Maine, School of Nursing, *Portland (MS, MS/MBA)*

Massachusetts

Fitchburg State University, Department of Nursing, *Fitchburg (MS)*

MGH Institute of Health Professions, School of Nursing, *Boston (MS)*

Regis College, School of Nursing, Science and Health Professions, *Weston (MSN)*

Salem State University, Program in Nursing, *Salem (MSN, MSN/MBA)*

Worcester State University, Department of Nursing, *Worcester (MS)*

Michigan

University of Detroit Mercy, McAuley School of Nursing, *Detroit (MSN)*

Minnesota

Metropolitan State University, College of Health, Community and Professional Studies, *St. Paul (MSN)*

Minnesota State University Mankato, School of Nursing, *Mankato (MSN, MSN/MS)*

Winona State University, College of Nursing and Health Sciences, *Winona (MS)*

Mississippi

Delta State University, School of Nursing, *Cleveland (MSN)*

Missouri

Saint Louis University, School of Nursing, *St. Louis (MSN, MN/MPH)*

Nebraska

Nebraska Methodist College, Department of Nursing, *Omaha (MSN)*

New Hampshire

Franklin Pierce University, Master of Science in Nursing, *Rindge (MSN)*

Rivier University, Division of Nursing, *Nashua (MS)*

University of New Hampshire, Department of Nursing, *Durham (MS)*

New Jersey

The College of New Jersey, School of Nursing, Health and Exercise Science, *Ewing (MSN)*

Kean University, Department of Nursing, *Union (MSN, MSN/MPA)*

Monmouth University, Marjorie K. Unterberg School of Nursing, *West Long Branch (MSN)*

Saint Peter's University, Nursing Program, *Jersey City (MSN)*

Seton Hall University, College of Nursing, *South Orange (MSN, MSN/MA, MSN/MBA)*

University of Medicine and Dentistry of New Jersey, School of Nursing, *Newark (MSN, MSN/MPH)*

William Paterson University of New Jersey, Department of Nursing, *Wayne (MSN)*

New Mexico

New Mexico State University, School of Nursing, *Las Cruces (MSN)*

New York

Daemen College, Department of Nursing, *Amherst (MS)*

Lehman College of the City University of New York, Department of Nursing, *Bronx (MS)*

Le Moyne College, Nursing Programs, *Syracuse (MS)*

Long Island University–C. W. Post Campus, Department of Nursing, *Brookville (MS)*

Mercy College, Programs in Nursing, *Dobbs Ferry (MS)*

Pace University, Lienhard School of Nursing, *New York (MS)*

State University of New York Upstate Medical University, College of Nursing, *Syracuse (MS)*

Ohio

The Ohio State University, College of Nursing, *Columbus (MS, MS/MPH)*

The University of Toledo, College of Nursing, *Toledo (MSN)*

Urbana University, College of Nursing and Allied Health, *Urbana (MSN)*

Wright State University, College of Nursing and Health, *Dayton (MS, MS/MBA)*

Xavier University, School of Nursing, *Cincinnati (MSN, MSN/MBA, MSN/Ed D)*

Oklahoma

Oklahoma City University, Kramer School of Nursing, *Oklahoma City (MSN, MSN/MBA)*

Pennsylvania

Bloomsburg University of Pennsylvania, Department of Nursing, *Bloomsburg (MSN, MSN/MBA)*

Holy Family University, School of Nursing and Allied Health Professions, *Philadelphia (MSN)*

Indiana University of Pennsylvania, Department of Nursing and Allied Health, *Indiana (MS)*

Moravian College, St. Luke's School of Nursing, *Bethlehem (MS)*

Thomas Jefferson University, Department of Nursing, *Philadelphia (MSN)*

Widener University, School of Nursing, *Chester (MSN, MSN/PhD)*

Tennessee

East Tennessee State University, College of Nursing, *Johnson City (MSN)*

Tennessee Technological University, Whitson-Hester School of Nursing, *Cookeville (MSN, M Sc N)*

University of Memphis, Loewenberg School of Nursing, *Memphis (MSN)*

The University of Tennessee, College of Nursing, *Knoxville (MSN)*

Texas

The University of Texas at Austin, School of Nursing, *Austin (MSN, MSN/MBA)*

The University of Texas at Brownsville, Department of Nursing, *Brownsville (MSN)*

Vermont

University of Vermont, Department of Nursing, *Burlington (MS)*

Virginia

Eastern Mennonite University, Department of Nursing, *Harrisonburg (MSN)*

Jefferson College of Health Sciences, Nursing Education Program, *Roanoke (MSN)*

University of Virginia, School of Nursing, *Charlottesville (MSN, MSN/MBA, MSN/PhD)*

Washington

Gonzaga University, Department of Nursing, *Spokane (MSN)*

Seattle Pacific University, School of Health Sciences, *Seattle (MSN)*

University of Washington, School of Nursing, *Seattle (MN, MN/MPH)*

Wisconsin

Marquette University, College of Nursing, *Milwaukee (MSN, MSN/MBA)*

Wyoming

University of Wyoming, Fay W. Whitney School of Nursing, *Laramie (MS)*

CANADA

Alberta

Athabasca University, Centre for Nursing and Health Studies, *Athabasca (MN, MN/MHSA, MN/MBA)*

RN TO MASTER'S

U.S. AND U.S. TERRITORIES

Alabama

Samford University, Ida V. Moffett School of Nursing, *Birmingham (MSN, MSN/MBA)*

Spring Hill College, Division of Nursing, *Mobile (MSN)*

The University of Alabama, Capstone College of Nursing, *Tuscaloosa (MSN, MSN/MA, MSN/Ed D)*

The University of Alabama in Huntsville, College of Nursing, *Huntsville (MSN)*

Arizona

The University of Arizona, College of Nursing, *Tucson (MSN)*

Arkansas

Arkansas Tech University, Program in Nursing, *Russellville (MSN)*

University of Arkansas for Medical Sciences, College of Nursing, *Little Rock (MN Sc)*

University of Central Arkansas, Department of Nursing, *Conway (MSN)*

California

Dominican University of California, Program in Nursing, *San Rafael (MSN)*

Loma Linda University, School of Nursing, *Loma Linda (MS)*

Mount St. Mary's College, Department of Nursing, *Los Angeles (MSN)*

Point Loma Nazarene University, School of Nursing, *San Diego (MSN)*

University of San Francisco, School of Nursing and Health Professions, *San Francisco (MSN)*

Colorado

Aspen University, Graduate School of Health Professions and Studies, *Denver (MSN)*

Regis University, School of Nursing, *Denver (MS)*

Connecticut

Sacred Heart University, Program in Nursing, *Fairfield (MSN)*

Southern Connecticut State University, Department of Nursing, *New Haven (MSN)*

University of Connecticut, School of Nursing, *Storrs (MS, MS/MBA)*

Delaware

University of Delaware, School of Nursing, *Newark (MSN)*

Wesley College, Nursing Program, *Dover (MSN)*

Florida

Florida Atlantic University, Christine E. Lynn College of Nursing, *Boca Raton (MS)*

Kaplan University Online, The School of Nursing Online, *Fort Lauderdale (MSN)*

Nova Southeastern University, College of Health Care Sciences, *Fort Lauderdale (MSN)*

South University, Nursing Program, *Royal Palm Beach (MSN)*

University of Central Florida, College of Nursing, *Orlando (MSN)*

University of North Florida, School of Nursing, *Jacksonville (MSN)*

University of South Florida, College of Nursing, *Tampa (MS, MS/MPH)*

The University of Tampa, Department of Nursing, *Tampa (MSN)*

Georgia

Albany State University, College of Sciences and Health Professions, *Albany (MSN)*

Armstrong Atlantic State University, Program in Nursing, *Savannah (MSN, MS/MHSA)*

Brenau University, College of Health and Science, *Gainesville (MSN)*

Clayton State University, Department of Nursing, *Morrow (MSN)*

Emory University, Nell Hodgson Woodruff School of Nursing, *Atlanta (MSN, MSN/MPH)*

Georgia Southern University, School of Nursing, *Statesboro (MSN)*

Georgia Southwestern State University, School of Nursing, *Americus (MSN)*

Georgia State University, Byrdine F. Lewis School of Nursing and Health Professions, *Atlanta (MSN)*

Thomas University, Division of Nursing, *Thomasville (MSN, MSN/MBA)*

Valdosta State University, College of Nursing, *Valdosta (MSN)*

Hawaii

Hawai`i Pacific University, College of Nursing and Health Sciences, *Honolulu (MSN, MSN/MBA)*

University of Hawaii at Manoa, School of Nursing and Dental Hygiene, *Honolulu (MS, MSN/MBA)*

Idaho
Northwest Nazarene University, School of Health and Science, *Nampa (MSN)*

Illinois
Blessing–Rieman College of Nursing, *Quincy (MSN)*

Bradley University, Department of Nursing, *Peoria (MSN)*

Lewis University, Program in Nursing, *Romeoville (MSN, MSN/MBA)*

Loyola University Chicago, Marcella Niehoff School of Nursing, *Maywood (MSN, MSN/MBA)*

McKendree University, Department of Nursing, *Lebanon (MSN)*

North Park University, School of Nursing, *Chicago (MS, MSN/MA, MSN/MBA, MSN/MM)*

Resurrection University, *Oak Park (MSN)*

Indiana
Anderson University, School of Nursing, *Anderson (MSN, MSN/MBA)*

Ball State University, School of Nursing, *Muncie (MS)*

Indiana University–Purdue University Indianapolis, School of Nursing, *Indianapolis (MSN, MSN/MPH)*

University of Southern Indiana, College of Nursing and Health Professions, *Evansville (MSN)*

Valparaiso University, College of Nursing, *Valparaiso (MSN, MSN/MBA)*

Iowa
Allen College, Program in Nursing, *Waterloo (MSN)*

Kansas
The University of Kansas, School of Nursing, *Kansas City (MS, MS/MHSA, MS/MPH)*

Kentucky
Bellarmine University, Donna and Allan Lansing School of Nursing and Health Sciences, *Louisville (Certificate of Completion, MSN, MSN/MBA)*

University of Kentucky, Graduate School Programs in the College of Nursing, *Lexington (MSN)*

Louisiana
Loyola University New Orleans, School of Nursing, *New Orleans (MSN)*

University of Louisiana at Lafayette, College of Nursing, *Lafayette (MSN)*

Maine
Saint Joseph's College of Maine, Master of Science in Nursing Program, *Standish (MSN, MSN/MHA)*

University of Maine, School of Nursing, *Orono (MSN)*

University of Southern Maine, School of Nursing, *Portland (MS, MS/MBA)*

Maryland
Salisbury University, Program in Nursing, *Salisbury (MS)*

Stevenson University, Nursing Division, *Stevenson (MS)*

University of Maryland, Baltimore, Master's Program in Nursing, *Baltimore (MS, MSN/MBA, MSN/MPH)*

Massachusetts
Boston College, William F. Connell School of Nursing, *Chestnut Hill (MS, MSN/MA, MSN/MBA, MSN/PhD)*

Curry College, Division of Nursing, *Milton (MSN)*

Elms College, Division of Nursing, *Chicopee (MSN)*

MGH Institute of Health Professions, School of Nursing, *Boston (MS)*

Regis College, School of Nursing, Science and Health Professions, *Weston (MSN)*

Simmons College, School of Nursing and Health Sciences, *Boston (MS)*

Worcester State University, Department of Nursing, *Worcester (MS)*

Michigan
Ferris State University, School of Nursing, *Big Rapids (MSN, MSN/MBA)*

Saginaw Valley State University, Crystal M. Lange College of Health and Human Services, *University Center (MSN)*

University of Michigan, School of Nursing, *Ann Arbor (MS, MSN/MBA, MSN/MPH)*

University of Michigan–Flint, Department of Nursing, *Flint (MSN)*

Minnesota
Metropolitan State University, College of Health, Community and Professional Studies, *St. Paul (MSN)*

Minnesota State University Mankato, School of Nursing, *Mankato (MSN, MSN/MS)*

Walden University, Nursing Programs, *Minneapolis (MSN)*

Winona State University, College of Nursing and Health Sciences, *Winona (MS)*

Mississippi
University of Mississippi Medical Center, Program in Nursing, *Jackson (MSN)*

University of Southern Mississippi, School of Nursing, *Hattiesburg (MSN)*

Missouri
Cox College, Department of Nursing, *Springfield (MSN)*

Graceland University, School of Nursing, *Independence (MSN)*

Maryville University of Saint Louis, Nursing Program, School of Health Professions, *St. Louis (MSN)*

Missouri State University, Department of Nursing, *Springfield (MSN)*

Research College of Nursing, College of Nursing, *Kansas City (MSN)*

Webster University, Department of Nursing, *St. Louis (MSN)*

Nebraska
Clarkson College, Master of Science in Nursing Program, *Omaha (MSN)*

Nebraska Methodist College, Department of Nursing, *Omaha (MSN)*

Nebraska Wesleyan University, Department of Nursing, *Lincoln (MSN)*

University of Nebraska Medical Center, College of Nursing, *Omaha (MSN)*

New Hampshire
Franklin Pierce University, Master of Science in Nursing, *Rindge (MSN)*

Rivier University, Division of Nursing, *Nashua (MS)*

New Jersey
The College of New Jersey, School of Nursing, Health and Exercise Science, *Ewing (MSN)*

Fairleigh Dickinson University, Metropolitan Campus, Henry P. Becton School of Nursing and Allied Health, *Teaneck (MSN)*

Monmouth University, Marjorie K. Unterberg School of Nursing, *West Long Branch (MSN)*

Seton Hall University, College of Nursing, *South Orange (MSN, MSN/MA, MSN/MBA)*

Thomas Edison State College, School of Nursing, *Trenton (MSN)*

University of Medicine and Dentistry of New Jersey, School of Nursing, *Newark (MSN, MSN/MPH)*

New York
The College of New Rochelle, School of Nursing, *New Rochelle (MS)*

Daemen College, Department of Nursing, *Amherst (MS)*

D'Youville College, School of Nursing, *Buffalo (MS)*

Excelsior College, School of Nursing, *Albany (MS)*

Hunter College of the City University of New York, Hunter-Bellevue School of Nursing, *New York (MS, MSN/MPA, MSN/MPH)*

Long Island University–Brooklyn Campus, School of Nursing, *Brooklyn (MS)*

New York University, College of Nursing, *New York (MS, MS/MA, MS/MPH)*

St. John Fisher College, Wegmans School of Nursing, *Rochester (MS)*

State University of New York Institute of Technology, School of Nursing and Health Systems, *Utica (MS)*

State University of New York Upstate Medical University, College of Nursing, *Syracuse (MS)*

Stony Brook University, State University of New York, School of Nursing, *Stony Brook (MS)*

North Carolina
Duke University, School of Nursing, *Durham (MSN, MSN/MBA)*

East Carolina University, College of Nursing, *Greenville (MSN)*

Gardner-Webb University, School of Nursing, *Boiling Springs (MSN, MSN/MBA)*

Lenoir-Rhyne University, Program in Nursing, *Hickory (MSN)*

Queens University of Charlotte, Presbyterian School of Nursing, *Charlotte (MSN, MSN/MBA)*

The University of North Carolina at Chapel Hill, School of Nursing, *Chapel Hill (MSN)*

The University of North Carolina at Charlotte, School of Nursing, *Charlotte (MSN)*

North Dakota
University of Mary, Division of Nursing, *Bismarck (MSN)*

Ohio
Capital University, School of Nursing, *Columbus (MSN, MN/MBA, MSN/JD, MSN/MDIV)*

Case Western Reserve University, Frances Payne Bolton School of Nursing, *Cleveland (MSN, MSN/MA, MSN/MBA, MSN/MPH)*

Franciscan University of Steubenville, Department of Nursing, *Steubenville (MSN)*

Lourdes University, School of Nursing, *Sylvania (MSN)*

The University of Akron, College of Nursing, *Akron (MSN)*

Urbana University, College of Nursing and Allied Health, *Urbana (MSN)*

Xavier University, School of Nursing, *Cincinnati (MSN, MSN/MBA, MSN/Ed D)*

Oklahoma
Oklahoma City University, Kramer School of Nursing, *Oklahoma City (MSN, MSN/MBA)*

Pennsylvania
Bloomsburg University of Pennsylvania, Department of Nursing, *Bloomsburg (MSN, MSN/MBA)*

Carlow University, School of Nursing, *Pittsburgh (MSN)*

Clarion University of Pennsylvania, School of Nursing, *Oil City (MSN)*

DeSales University, Department of Nursing and Health, *Center Valley (MSN, MSN/MBA)*

Drexel University, College of Nursing and Health Professions, *Philadelphia (MSN)*

Gannon University, Villa Maria School of Nursing, *Erie (MSN)*

Gwynedd-Mercy College, School of Nursing, *Gwynedd Valley (MSN)*

La Roche College, Department of Nursing and Nursing Management, *Pittsburgh (MSN)*

La Salle University, School of Nursing and Health Sciences, *Philadelphia (MSN, MSN/MBA)*

Misericordia University, Department of Nursing, *Dallas (MSN)*

Thomas Jefferson University, Department of Nursing, *Philadelphia (MSN)*

University of Pittsburgh, School of Nursing, *Pittsburgh (MSN)*

The University of Scranton, Department of Nursing, *Scranton (MSN)*

Wilkes University, Department of Nursing, *Wilkes-Barre (MS)*

York College of Pennsylvania, Department of Nursing, *York (MS)*

Rhode Island

University of Rhode Island, College of Nursing, *Kingston (MS)*

South Carolina

Charleston Southern University, Wingo School of Nursing, *Charleston (MSN)*

South Dakota

South Dakota State University, College of Nursing, *Brookings (MS)*

Tennessee

Tennessee State University, School of Nursing, *Nashville (MSN)*

The University of Tennessee, College of Nursing, *Knoxville (MSN)*

Vanderbilt University, Vanderbilt University School of Nursing, *Nashville (MSN, MSN/MDIV, MSN/MTS)*

Texas

Angelo State University, Department of Nursing and Rehabilitation Sciences, *San Angelo (MSN)*

Midwestern State University, Nursing Program, *Wichita Falls (MSN)*

Texas A&M University–Corpus Christi, College of Nursing and Health Sciences, *Corpus Christi (MSN)*

Texas Woman's University, College of Nursing, *Denton (MS, MSN/MHA)*

University of Houston–Victoria, School of Nursing, *Victoria (MSN)*

The University of Texas at El Paso, School of Nursing, *El Paso (MSN)*

The University of Texas at Tyler, Program in Nursing, *Tyler (MSN, MSN/MBA)*

The University of Texas Health Science Center at San Antonio, School of Nursing, *San Antonio (MSN)*

West Texas A&M University, Department of Nursing, *Canyon (MSN)*

Utah

University of Utah, College of Nursing, *Salt Lake City (MS)*

Western Governors University, Online College of Health Professions, *Salt Lake City (MS)*

Vermont

University of Vermont, Department of Nursing, *Burlington (MS)*

Virginia

George Mason University, College of Health and Human Services, *Fairfax (MSN)*

Hampton University, School of Nursing, *Hampton (MS)*

Lynchburg College, School of Health Sciences and Human Performance, *Lynchburg (MSN, MSN/MBA)*

Old Dominion University, Department of Nursing, *Norfolk (MSN)*

Shenandoah University, Eleanor Wade Custer School of Nursing, *Winchester (MSN, MSN/MBA)*

Virginia Commonwealth University, School of Nursing, *Richmond (MS)*

West Virginia

West Virginia University, School of Nursing, *Morgantown (MSN)*

Wheeling Jesuit University, Department of Nursing, *Wheeling (MSN)*

Wisconsin

Marquette University, College of Nursing, *Milwaukee (MSN, MSN/MBA)*

University of Wisconsin–Eau Claire, College of Nursing and Health Sciences, *Eau Claire (MSN)*

University of Wisconsin–Oshkosh, College of Nursing, *Oshkosh (MSN)*

CANADA

Alberta

University of Calgary, Faculty of Nursing, *Calgary (MN)*

New Brunswick

Université de Moncton, School of Nursing, *Moncton (M Sc N)*

Quebec

Université de Montréal, Faculty of Nursing, *Montréal (M Sc)*

Université du Québec à Chicoutimi, Program in Nursing, *Chicoutimi (MSN, MS/MPH)*

CASE MANAGEMENT

American Sentinel University, CO
Boise State University, ID
Carlow University, PA
Duke University, NC
The Johns Hopkins University, MD
Lewis University, IL
Loyola University New Orleans, LA
Pacific Lutheran University, WA
Regis College, MA
Saint Peter's University, NJ
Samuel Merritt University, CA
San Francisco State University, CA
Seton Hall University, NJ
Shenandoah University, VA
Université de Moncton, NB
The University of Alabama, AL
University of Central Florida, FL
University of Kentucky, KY
University of Nebraska Medical Center, NE
University of New Brunswick Fredericton, NB
Ursuline College, OH
Valdosta State University, GA
Washington State University College of
   Nursing, WA

CLINICAL NURSE LEADER

Boise State University, ID
Brenau University, GA
California Baptist University, CA
California State University, Dominguez Hills, CA
Cleveland State University, OH
The College of New Jersey, NJ
Cox College, MO
Creighton University, NE
Curry College, MA
Dominican University of California, CA
Drexel University, PA
East Tennessee State University, TN
Elmhurst College, IL
Fairfield University, CT
Florida Atlantic University, FL
The George Washington University, DC
Georgia Regents University, GA
Grand Valley State University, MI
Grand View University, IA
Hunter College of the City University of New
   York, NY
Idaho State University, ID
Illinois State University, IL
James Madison University, VA
Lynchburg College, VA
Marquette University, WI
Millikin University, IL
Montana State University, MT
Moravian College, PA
The Ohio State University, OH
Pacific Lutheran University, WA
Pittsburg State University, KS
Queens University of Charlotte, NC
Regis College, MA
Research College of Nursing, MO
Resurrection University, IL
Rush University, IL
Sacred Heart University, CT
Saginaw Valley State University, MI
Saint Anthony College of Nursing, IL
Saint Francis Medical Center College of
   Nursing, IL
Saint Xavier University, IL
Salem State University, MA
Seton Hall University, NJ
South Dakota State University, SD
Southern Connecticut State University, CT
Spring Hill College, AL
Texas Christian University, TX
Texas Woman's University, TX
Trinity Western University, BC
Université de Montréal, QC
Université Laval, QC
The University of Alabama, AL
The University of Alabama at Birmingham, AL

The University of Alabama in Huntsville, AL
University of California, Los Angeles, CA
University of Connecticut, CT
University of Florida, FL
University of Mary Hardin-Baylor, TX
University of Maryland, Baltimore, MD
University of Massachusetts Amherst, MA
University of Medicine and Dentistry of New
   Jersey, NJ
University of Nevada, Reno, NV
The University of North Carolina at
   Chapel Hill, NC
University of Oklahoma Health Sciences
   Center, OK
University of Pittsburgh, PA
University of Portland, OR
University of Rhode Island, RI
University of Rochester, NY
University of San Diego, CA
University of San Francisco, CA
University of Southern Maine, ME
University of South Florida, FL
The University of Tennessee Health Science
   Center, TN
The University of Texas Health Science Center at
   San Antonio, TX
The University of Texas Medical Branch, TX
University of the Incarnate Word, TX
The University of Toledo, OH
University of Toronto, ON
University of Virginia, VA
University of West Georgia, GA
University of Wisconsin–Milwaukee, WI
University of Wisconsin–Oshkosh, WI
Viterbo University, WI
Walsh University, OH
Western Governors University, UT
Western University of Health Sciences, CA
Wright State University, OH
Xavier University, OH

CLINICAL NURSE SPECIALIST PROGRAMS

Acute Care

Arizona State University at the Downtown
   Phoenix Campus, AZ
Armstrong Atlantic State University, GA
Colorado State University–Pueblo, CO
George Mason University, VA
Georgetown University, DC
Indiana University–Purdue University
   Indianapolis, IN
The Johns Hopkins University, MD
King College, TN
Liberty University, VA
Loyola University Chicago, IL
McGill University, QC
Mercer University Georgia Baptist College of
   Nursing, GA
MGH Institute of Health Professions, MA
Regis College, MA
Rhode Island College, RI
The Sage Colleges, NY
Seattle Pacific University, WA
Thomas Jefferson University, PA
Université de Montréal, QC
Université de Sherbrooke, QC
Université du Québec à Chicoutimi, QC
Université du Québec à Trois-Rivières, QC
Université Laval, QC
University of Arkansas, AR
University of Arkansas for Medical Sciences, AR
University of Calgary, AB
University of California, Los Angeles, CA
University of Central Florida, FL
University of Connecticut, CT
University of Illinois at Chicago, IL
University of Kentucky, KY
University of Manitoba, MB
University of Maryland, Baltimore, MD
University of Massachusetts Boston, MA
University of Missouri, MO

University of Nebraska Medical Center, NE
University of New Brunswick Fredericton, NB
University of Oklahoma Health Sciences
   Center, OK
University of Ottawa, ON
University of Pennsylvania, PA
University of San Diego, CA
University of South Alabama, AL
The University of Texas Health Science Center at
   Houston, TX
University of Toronto, ON
University of Virginia, VA
The University of Western Ontario, ON
Virginia Commonwealth University, VA
Wayne State University, MI
Widener University, PA

Adult Health

Alverno College, WI
Angelo State University, TX
Arizona State University at the Downtown
   Phoenix Campus, AZ
Arkansas State University, AR
Armstrong Atlantic State University, GA
Auburn University, AL
Auburn University Montgomery, AL
Azusa Pacific University, CA
Ball State University, IN
Boston College, MA
California Baptist University, CA
California State University, Fresno, CA
California State University, Long Beach, CA
Capital University, OH
The Catholic University of America, DC
The College of New Jersey, NJ
The College of St. Scholastica, MN
College of Staten Island of the City University of
   New York, NY
Creighton University, NE
DeSales University, PA
East Carolina University, NC
Eastern Michigan University, MI
Florida Southern College, FL
George Mason University, VA
Georgia State University, GA
Governors State University, IL
Grambling State University, LA
Grand Canyon University, AZ
Hunter College of the City University of New
   York, NY
Idaho State University, ID
Indiana University–Purdue University
   Indianapolis, IN
The Johns Hopkins University, MD
Kennesaw State University, GA
Kent State University, OH
King College, TN
La Salle University, PA
Lehman College of the City University of New
   York, NY
Loma Linda University, CA
Long Island University–C. W. Post Campus, NY
Louisiana State University Health Sciences
   Center, LA
Loyola University Chicago, IL
Malone University, OH
Marquette University, WI
McGill University, QC
Mercer University Georgia Baptist College of
   Nursing, GA
MGH Institute of Health Professions, MA
Michigan State University, MI
Minnesota State University Mankato, MN
Minnesota State University Moorhead, MN
Molloy College, NY
Mount Carmel College of Nursing, OH
Mount Saint Mary College, NY
Mount St. Mary's College, CA
Murray State University, KY
North Dakota State University, ND
Northern Illinois University, IL
Northwestern State University of Louisiana, LA
The Ohio State University, OH

Otterbein University, OH
Penn State University Park, PA
Purdue University Calumet, IN
Rhode Island College, RI
Rush University, IL
Rutgers, The State University of New Jersey, College of Nursing, NJ
Ryerson University, ON
The Sage Colleges, NY
Saint Anthony College of Nursing, IL
St. John Fisher College, NY
St. Joseph's College, New York, NY
San Diego State University, CA
San Francisco State University, CA
Seattle Pacific University, WA
Southeast Missouri State University, MO
State University of New York Downstate Medical Center, NY
Stony Brook University, State University of New York, NY
Thomas Jefferson University, PA
Troy University, AL
Union University, TN
Université de Montréal, QC
Université du Québec à Chicoutimi, QC
Université du Québec à Trois-Rivières, QC
Université Laval, QC
The University of Akron, OH
The University of Alabama in Huntsville, AL
University of Arkansas for Medical Sciences, AR
The University of British Columbia, BC
University of Calgary, AB
University of Cincinnati, OH
University of Colorado at Colorado Springs, CO
University of Colorado Denver, CO
University of Delaware, DE
University of Illinois at Chicago, IL
The University of Iowa, IA
The University of Kansas, KS
University of Kentucky, KY
University of Louisiana at Lafayette, LA
University of Massachusetts Boston, MA
University of Massachusetts Dartmouth, MA
University of Missouri, MO
University of Nebraska Medical Center, NE
University of New Brunswick Fredericton, NB
University of New Hampshire, NH
University of North Florida, FL
University of Ottawa, ON
University of Pennsylvania, PA
University of Puerto Rico, Medical Sciences Campus, PR
University of San Diego, CA
The University of Scranton, PA
University of Southern Indiana, IN
The University of Tennessee, TN
The University of Texas at Austin, TX
The University of Texas Health Science Center at Houston, TX
The University of Texas–Pan American, TX
University of the Incarnate Word, TX
University of Toronto, ON
University of Washington, WA
The University of Western Ontario, ON
University of Wisconsin–Eau Claire, WI
Ursuline College, OH
Valdosta State University, GA
Valparaiso University, IN
Western Connecticut State University, CT
Widener University, PA
Winona State University, MN
Wright State University, OH
York College of Pennsylvania, PA

Cardiovascular

Creighton University, NE
George Mason University, VA
McGill University, QC
The Ohio State University, OH
The Sage Colleges, NY
Université de Montréal, QC
Université du Québec à Chicoutimi, QC
Université Laval, QC
The University of British Columbia, BC
University of Calgary, AB
University of California, San Francisco, CA

University of Illinois at Chicago, IL
University of Missouri, MO
University of Nebraska Medical Center, NE
University of New Brunswick Fredericton, NB
University of North Florida, FL
University of Ottawa, ON
University of Toronto, ON

Community Health

Arizona State University at the Downtown Phoenix Campus, AZ
Augsburg College, MN
Binghamton University, State University of New York, NY
Boston College, MA
California State University, San Bernardino, CA
The Catholic University of America, DC
Cleveland State University, OH
D'Youville College, NY
Georgia Southern University, GA
Hawai'i Pacific University, HI
Hunter College of the City University of New York, NY
Indiana University–Purdue University Indianapolis, IN
Jacksonville State University, AL
Kean University, NJ
Louisiana State University Health Sciences Center, LA
McGill University, QC
Mount Mercy University, IA
Mount St. Mary's College, CA
Northern Illinois University, IL
North Park University, IL
The Ohio State University, OH
Penn State University Park, PA
Rhode Island College, RI
Rush University, IL
Rutgers, The State University of New Jersey, College of Nursing, NJ
Ryerson University, ON
The Sage Colleges, NY
Salem State University, MA
San Diego State University, CA
Seattle Pacific University, WA
Seattle University, WA
Stony Brook University, State University of New York, NY
Thomas Jefferson University, PA
Université de Moncton, NB
Université de Montréal, QC
Université de Sherbrooke, QC
Université du Québec à Chicoutimi, QC
Université du Québec à Rimouski, QC
Université du Québec à Trois-Rivières, QC
Université du Québec en Outaouais, QC
Université Laval, QC
University of Alaska Anchorage, AK
The University of British Columbia, BC
University of Calgary, AB
University of California, San Francisco, CA
University of Illinois at Chicago, IL
The University of Iowa, IA
University of Kentucky, KY
University of Maryland, Baltimore, MD
University of Massachusetts Dartmouth, MA
University of Michigan, MI
University of Missouri, MO
University of Nebraska Medical Center, NE
University of New Brunswick Fredericton, NB
The University of North Carolina at Charlotte, NC
University of North Florida, FL
University of Ottawa, ON
University of Puerto Rico, Medical Sciences Campus, PR
University of South Alabama, AL
University of Toronto, ON
University of Washington, WA
The University of Western Ontario, ON
Washington State University College of Nursing, WA
Wayne State University, MI
Wesley College, DE
William Paterson University of New Jersey, NJ
Worcester State University, MA
Wright State University, OH

Critical Care

George Mason University, VA
Georgetown University, DC
Indiana University–Purdue University Indianapolis, IN
Loyola University Chicago, IL
McGill University, QC
Mercer University Georgia Baptist College of Nursing, GA
Murray State University, KY
Northwestern State University of Louisiana, LA
Purdue University Calumet, IN
Rush University, IL
The Sage Colleges, NY
San Diego State University, CA
Seattle Pacific University, WA
Stony Brook University, State University of New York, NY
Thomas Jefferson University, PA
Université du Québec à Chicoutimi, QC
Université du Québec à Rimouski, QC
Université du Québec à Trois-Rivières, QC
Université du Québec en Outaouais, QC
Université Laval, QC
University of Calgary, AB
University of California, San Francisco, CA
University of Central Florida, FL
University of Cincinnati, OH
University of Kentucky, KY
University of Maryland, Baltimore, MD
University of Massachusetts Boston, MA
University of Missouri, MO
University of Nebraska Medical Center, NE
University of New Brunswick Fredericton, NB
University of North Florida, FL
University of Ottawa, ON
University of Puerto Rico, Medical Sciences Campus, PR
University of San Diego, CA
The University of Texas Health Science Center at Houston, TX
University of Toronto, ON
Wayne State University, MI
Widener University, PA

Family Health

Binghamton University, State University of New York, NY
Cedarville University, OH
Cox College, MO
Creighton University, NE
Loma Linda University, CA
McGill University, QC
MGH Institute of Health Professions, MA
Minnesota State University Mankato, MN
Misericordia University, PA
Missouri Southern State University, MO
Pittsburg State University, KS
Point Loma Nazarene University, CA
Rivier University, NH
Ryerson University, ON
The Sage Colleges, NY
Saginaw Valley State University, MI
Saint Francis Medical Center College of Nursing, IL
Southern University and Agricultural and Mechanical College, LA
Université de Moncton, NB
Université de Montréal, QC
Université de Sherbrooke, QC
Université du Québec à Chicoutimi, QC
Université du Québec à Trois-Rivières, QC
Université Laval, QC
The University of British Columbia, BC
University of Calgary, AB
University of Illinois at Chicago, IL
University of Manitoba, MB
University of Massachusetts Lowell, MA
University of Nebraska Medical Center, NE
University of New Brunswick Fredericton, NB
University of Northern Colorado, CO
University of Ottawa, ON
University of South Alabama, AL
University of Toronto, ON
Valdosta State University, GA
Webster University, MO

Forensic Nursing

Boston College, MA
Cleveland State University, OH
Duquesne University, PA
Fitchburg State University, MA
Monmouth University, NJ
National University, CA
University of Ottawa, ON
Xavier University, OH

Gerontology

Alverno College, WI
Auburn University, AL
Auburn University Montgomery, AL
Binghamton University, State University of New
    York, NY
Boston College, MA
California State University, Dominguez Hills, CA
California State University, Fresno, CA
Capella University, MN
The College of St. Scholastica, MN
College of Staten Island of the City University of
    New York, NY
Creighton University, NE
Florida Southern College, FL
Gwynedd-Mercy College, PA
Hunter College of the City University of New
    York, NY
The Johns Hopkins University, MD
Kent State University, OH
Lehman College of the City University of New
    York, NY
McGill University, QC
Mercer University Georgia Baptist College of
    Nursing, GA
MGH Institute of Health Professions, MA
Minnesota State University Moorhead, MN
Penn State University Park, PA
Point Loma Nazarene University, CA
Rush University, IL
The Sage Colleges, NY
St. John Fisher College, NY
San Diego State University, CA
San Jose State University, CA
Seattle Pacific University, WA
Texas Christian University, TX
Trinity Western University, BC
Université de Montréal, QC
Université de Sherbrooke, QC
Université du Québec à Chicoutimi, QC
Université du Québec à Rimouski, QC
Université Laval, QC
The University of Akron, OH
The University of British Columbia, BC
University of Calgary, AB
University of California, San Francisco, CA
University of Cincinnati, OH
University of Illinois at Chicago, IL
The University of Iowa, IA
The University of Kansas, KS
University of Kentucky, KY
University of Manitoba, MB
University of Massachusetts Boston, MA
University of Michigan, MI
University of Nebraska Medical Center, NE
University of New Brunswick Fredericton, NB
University of North Dakota, ND
University of North Florida, FL
University of Ottawa, ON
University of Puerto Rico, Medical Sciences
    Campus, PR
University of Rhode Island, RI
University of South Alabama, AL
The University of Texas Health Science Center at
    Houston, TX
University of Toronto, ON
University of Washington, WA
Valparaiso University, IN
Widener University, PA
Wilkes University, PA

Home Health Care

Carlow University, PA
McGill University, QC
Thomas Jefferson University, PA
Université de Moncton, NB

Université du Québec à Chicoutimi, QC
Université du Québec à Trois-Rivières, QC
University of Michigan, MI
University of Missouri, MO
University of Ottawa, ON

Maternity-newborn

Creighton University, NE
Grambling State University, LA
Loma Linda University, CA
McGill University, QC
San Diego State University, CA
State University of New York Downstate Medical
    Center, NY
Troy University, AL
Université de Montréal, QC
Université du Québec à Chicoutimi, QC
Université du Québec à Trois-Rivières, QC
The University of British Columbia, BC
University of Calgary, AB
University of Connecticut, CT
University of Illinois at Chicago, IL
University of Missouri, MO
University of Nebraska Medical Center, NE
University of New Brunswick Fredericton, NB
University of North Florida, FL
University of Ottawa, ON
University of Pennsylvania, PA
University of Puerto Rico, Medical Sciences
    Campus, PR
University of South Alabama, AL
University of Toronto, ON
University of Washington, WA

Medical-surgical

Alverno College, WI
Angelo State University, TX
Azusa Pacific University, CA
George Mason University, VA
Loma Linda University, CA
Malone University, OH
McGill University, QC
Murray State University, KY
Point Loma Nazarene University, CA
Saint Francis Medical Center College of Nursing,
    IL
Seattle Pacific University, WA
State University of New York Upstate Medical
    University, NY
Thomas Jefferson University, PA
Université de Montréal, QC
Université du Québec à Chicoutimi, QC
Université du Québec à Trois-Rivières, QC
University of Arkansas, AR
University of Calgary, AB
University of Central Arkansas, AR
University of Cincinnati, OH
University of Illinois at Chicago, IL
University of Kentucky, KY
University of Michigan, MI
University of Nebraska Medical Center, NE
University of New Brunswick Fredericton, NB
University of North Florida, FL
University of Ottawa, ON
University of San Diego, CA
University of Toronto, ON
University of Virginia, VA

Occupational Health

Université de Moncton, NB
Université de Montréal, QC
Université du Québec à Chicoutimi, QC
University of California, San Francisco, CA
University of Cincinnati, OH
University of Illinois at Chicago, IL
The University of Iowa, IA
University of Michigan, MI
University of Ottawa, ON
University of Toronto, ON

Oncology

Case Western Reserve University, OH
Creighton University, NE
George Mason University, VA
Gwynedd-Mercy College, PA
Indiana University–Purdue University
    Indianapolis, IN

King College, TN
Loyola University Chicago, IL
McGill University, QC
The Ohio State University, OH
Rutgers, The State University of New Jersey,
    College of Nursing, NJ
The Sage Colleges, NY
Seattle Pacific University, WA
Thomas Jefferson University, PA
Université de Montréal, QC
Université du Québec à Chicoutimi, QC
Université Laval, QC
The University of British Columbia, BC
University of California, Los Angeles, CA
University of California, San Francisco, CA
University of Kentucky, KY
University of Missouri, MO
University of Nebraska Medical Center, NE
University of New Brunswick Fredericton, NB
University of Ottawa, ON
University of Toronto, ON

Palliative Care

Boston College, MA
D'Youville College, NY
The Sage Colleges, NY
Seattle Pacific University, WA
Université de Montréal, QC
Université Laval, QC
University of Missouri, MO
University of Ottawa, ON
University of San Diego, CA
University of Toronto, ON
Ursuline College, OH

Parent-child

Azusa Pacific University, CA
California State University, Dominguez Hills, CA
Lehman College of the City University of New
    York, NY
Loma Linda University, CA
Louisiana State University Health Sciences
    Center, LA
McGill University, QC
Rutgers, The State University of New Jersey,
    College of Nursing, NJ
Seattle Pacific University, WA
Stony Brook University, State University of New
    York, NY
Université de Montréal, QC
Université du Québec à Chicoutimi, QC
Université Laval, QC
The University of British Columbia, BC
University of Calgary, AB
University of Kentucky, KY
University of Nebraska Medical Center, NE
University of New Brunswick Fredericton, NB
University of Ottawa, ON
University of Toronto, ON

Pediatric

Arizona State University at the Downtown
    Phoenix Campus, AZ
Auburn University, AL
Auburn University Montgomery, AL
Azusa Pacific University, CA
Boston College, MA
California State University, Fresno, CA
Creighton University, NE
Georgia State University, GA
Grambling State University, LA
Gwynedd-Mercy College, PA
Indiana University–Purdue University
    Indianapolis, IN
The Johns Hopkins University, MD
Kent State University, OH
Loma Linda University, CA
Marquette University, WI
McGill University, QC
Mercer University Georgia Baptist College of
    Nursing, GA
MGH Institute of Health Professions, MA
Minnesota State University Mankato, MN
Rush University, IL
St. John Fisher College, NY
Seattle Pacific University, WA

Stony Brook University, State University of New York, NY
Texas Christian University, TX
Thomas Jefferson University, PA
Union University, TN
Université de Moncton, NB
Université du Québec à Chicoutimi, QC
Université du Québec à Trois-Rivières, QC
Université Laval, QC
The University of Akron, OH
University of Arkansas for Medical Sciences, AR
The University of British Columbia, BC
University of Calgary, AB
University of California, Los Angeles, CA
University of California, San Francisco, CA
University of Delaware, DE
University of Illinois at Chicago, IL
University of Kentucky, KY
University of Missouri, MO
University of Nebraska Medical Center, NE
University of New Brunswick Fredericton, NB
University of North Florida, FL
University of Ottawa, ON
University of Pennsylvania, PA
University of Puerto Rico, Medical Sciences Campus, PR
University of South Alabama, AL
The University of Tennessee, TN
University of Toronto, ON
Wright State University, OH

Perinatal
Georgia State University, GA
Loma Linda University, CA
McGill University, QC
McMaster University, ON
San Francisco State University, CA
Stony Brook University, State University of New York, NY
Université du Québec à Chicoutimi, QC
Université du Québec à Trois-Rivières, QC
Université Laval, QC
The University of British Columbia, BC
University of Calgary, AB
University of California, San Francisco, CA
University of Illinois at Chicago, IL
University of Kentucky, KY
University of Manitoba, MB
University of Nebraska Medical Center, NE
University of Ottawa, ON
University of Toronto, ON
University of Washington, WA

Psychiatric/mental Health
Arizona State University at the Downtown Phoenix Campus, AZ
Binghamton University, State University of New York, NY
Boston College, MA
California State University, Los Angeles, CA
Colorado State University–Pueblo, CO
Georgia State University, GA
Gonzaga University, WA
Hunter College of the City University of New York, NY
Husson University, ME
Indiana University–Purdue University Indianapolis, IN
Kent State University, OH
Louisiana State University Health Sciences Center, LA
McGill University, QC
MGH Institute of Health Professions, MA
The Ohio State University, OH
Point Loma Nazarene University, CA
Rivier University, NH
Rutgers, The State University of New Jersey, College of Nursing, NJ
The Sage Colleges, NY
Shenandoah University, VA
Stony Brook University, State University of New York, NY
Temple University, PA
Université de Moncton, NB
Université de Montréal, QC
Université du Québec à Chicoutimi, QC

Université du Québec à Rimouski, QC
Université du Québec à Trois-Rivières, QC
Université du Québec en Outaouais, QC
Université Laval, QC
The University of Akron, OH
University of Alaska Anchorage, AK
The University of British Columbia, BC
University of Calgary, AB
University of California, San Francisco, CA
University of Florida, FL
University of Hawaii at Manoa, HI
University of Illinois at Chicago, IL
The University of Iowa, IA
University of Kentucky, KY
University of Louisiana at Lafayette, LA
University of Massachusetts Lowell, MA
University of Michigan, MI
University of Nebraska Medical Center, NE
University of New Brunswick Fredericton, NB
University of North Dakota, ND
University of North Florida, FL
University of Ottawa, ON
University of Puerto Rico, Medical Sciences Campus, PR
University of Rhode Island, RI
University of South Alabama, AL
The University of Tennessee, TN
University of Toronto, ON
University of Virginia, VA
The University of Western Ontario, ON
Valdosta State University, GA
Wayne State University, MI
Wilkes University, PA

Public Health
Delaware State University, DE
Eastern Kentucky University, KY
Emory University, GA
Hunter College of the City University of New York, NY
La Salle University, PA
McGill University, QC
Mount Mercy University, IA
The Ohio State University, OH
Rush University, IL
Ryerson University, ON
Salem State University, MA
San Francisco State University, CA
Thomas Jefferson University, PA
Université de Moncton, NB
Université de Montréal, QC
Université du Québec à Chicoutimi, QC
Université du Québec à Trois-Rivières, QC
Université Laval, QC
The University of British Columbia, BC
University of Calgary, AB
University of Cincinnati, OH
University of Florida, FL
University of Hartford, CT
University of Illinois at Chicago, IL
University of Kentucky, KY
University of Missouri, MO
University of Nebraska Medical Center, NE
University of New Brunswick Fredericton, NB
University of North Dakota, ND
University of Ottawa, ON
The University of Texas at Brownsville, TX
University of Toronto, ON
The University of Western Ontario, ON
West Chester University of Pennsylvania, PA
Worcester State University, MA
Wright State University, OH

Rehabilitation
McGill University, QC
Salem State University, MA
Université de Montréal, QC
Université du Québec à Chicoutimi, QC
Université du Québec en Outaouais, QC
Université Laval, QC
University of Calgary, AB
University of Missouri, MO
University of Ottawa, ON
University of Toronto, ON

School Health
Azusa Pacific University, CA

California State University, Fullerton, CA
Kean University, NJ
Monmouth University, NJ
San Diego State University, CA
San Jose State University, CA
Seton Hall University, NJ
Université de Moncton, NB
Université du Québec à Chicoutimi, QC
University of Illinois at Chicago, IL
University of Missouri, MO
University of New Brunswick Fredericton, NB
University of Ottawa, ON
University of Toronto, ON
Wright State University, OH
Xavier University, OH

Women's Health
Drexel University, PA
Georgia State University, GA
Kent State University, OH
McGill University, QC
St. John Fisher College, NY
San Diego State University, CA
Seattle Pacific University, WA
Stony Brook University, State University of New York, NY
Université de Montréal, QC
Université du Québec à Chicoutimi, QC
The University of British Columbia, BC
University of Calgary, AB
University of Illinois at Chicago, IL
University of Kentucky, KY
University of Manitoba, MB
University of Missouri, MO
University of Nebraska Medical Center, NE
University of New Brunswick Fredericton, NB
University of North Florida, FL
University of Ottawa, ON
University of South Alabama, AL
University of Toronto, ON
The University of Western Ontario, ON
Valparaiso University, IN
Wesley College, DE

HEALTH-CARE ADMINISTRATION
Adelphi University, NY
Boise State University, ID
California State University, Long Beach, CA
Clarkson College, NE
The College of New Rochelle, NY
Daemen College, NY
Duke University, NC
Fairfield University, CT
Georgetown University, DC
The George Washington University, DC
Goldfarb School of Nursing at Barnes-Jewish College, MO
Gonzaga University, WA
Hampton University, VA
The Johns Hopkins University, MD
Kaplan University Online, FL
Kean University, NJ
Kent State University, OH
Lenoir-Rhyne University, NC
Loma Linda University, CA
Long Island University–Brooklyn Campus, NY
Louisiana State University Health Sciences Center, LA
Loyola University New Orleans, LA
Mercy College, NY
MidAmerica Nazarene University, KS
Missouri Western State University, MO
Mount Mercy University, IA
The Ohio State University, OH
Pacific Lutheran University, WA
Regis College, MA
Regis University, CO
Resurrection University, IL
The Sage Colleges, NY
St. Ambrose University, IA
Salisbury University, MD
Seton Hall University, NJ
Southern Illinois University Edwardsville, IL
Southern University and Agricultural and Mechanical College, LA
Stevenson University, MD

Texas Woman's University, TX
Thomas University, GA
Towson University, MD
Trinity Western University, BC
Université de Moncton, NB
Université du Québec en Outaouais, QC
Université Laval, QC
The University of Alabama at Birmingham, AL
The University of Alabama in Huntsville, AL
University of Alaska Anchorage, AK
University of Delaware, DE
University of Illinois at Chicago, IL
The University of Kansas, KS
University of Louisiana at Lafayette, LA
University of Maine, ME
University of Michigan, MI
University of Nebraska Medical Center, NE
The University of North Carolina at
   Chapel Hill, NC
University of Oklahoma Health Sciences
   Center, OK
University of Pennsylvania, PA
University of Phoenix–Bay Area Campus, CA
University of Phoenix–Hawaii Campus, HI
University of Phoenix–Metro Detroit Campus, MI
University of Phoenix–North Florida Campus, FL
University of Phoenix–Online Campus, AZ
University of Phoenix–Phoenix Main Campus, AZ
University of Phoenix–Sacramento Valley
   Campus, CA
University of Phoenix–San Diego Campus, CA
University of Phoenix–Southern Arizona
   Campus, AZ
University of Phoenix–Southern California
   Campus, CA
University of Phoenix–South Florida Campus, FL
University of Rochester, NY
The University of Texas at Arlington, TX
University of Toronto, ON
The University of Western Ontario, ON
Vanderbilt University, TN
Villanova University, PA
Western Governors University, UT
Wright State University, OH

LEGAL NURSE CONSULTANT

Capital University, OH
Wilmington University, DE

NURSE ANESTHESIA

Arkansas State University, AR
Bloomsburg University of Pennsylvania, PA
Boston College, MA
Bradley University, IL
BryanLGH College of Health Sciences, NE
California State University, Fullerton, CA
Case Western Reserve University, OH
Clarkson College, NE
Columbia University, NY
DePaul University, IL
Drexel University, PA
Duke University, NC
East Carolina University, NC
Fairfield University, CT
Florida Gulf Coast University, FL
Florida International University, FL
Gannon University, PA
Georgetown University, DC
Georgia Regents University, GA
Goldfarb School of Nursing at Barnes-Jewish
   College, MO
La Salle University, PA
Lincoln Memorial University, TN
Loma Linda University, CA
Louisiana State University Health Sciences
   Center, LA
Lourdes University, OH
Michigan State University, MI
Millikin University, IL
Murray State University, KY
National University, CA
Oakland University, MI
Old Dominion University, VA
Oregon Health & Science University, OR
Our Lady of the Lake College, LA

Rush University, IL
Samford University, AL
Samuel Merritt University, CA
Southern Illinois University Edwardsville, IL
State University of New York Downstate Medical
   Center, NY
Thomas Jefferson University, PA
Union University, TN
The University of Akron, OH
The University of Alabama at Birmingham, AL
University of Cincinnati, OH
The University of Iowa, IA
University of Maryland, Baltimore, MD
University of Medicine and Dentistry of New
   Jersey, NJ
University of Miami, FL
University of Michigan–Flint, MI
The University of North Carolina at Charlotte, NC
The University of North Carolina at
   Greensboro, NC
University of North Dakota, ND
University of Pennsylvania, PA
University of Pittsburgh, PA
University of Puerto Rico, Medical Sciences
   Campus, PR
The University of Scranton, PA
University of South Florida, FL
The University of Tennessee, TN
The University of Tennessee at Chattanooga, TN
The University of Texas Health Science Center at
   Houston, TX
University of Toronto, ON
Villanova University, PA
Western Carolina University, NC
York College of Pennsylvania, PA
Youngstown State University, OH

NURSE-MIDWIFERY

California State University, Fullerton, CA
Case Western Reserve University, OH
Columbia University, NY
East Carolina University, NC
Emory University, GA
Georgetown University, DC
James Madison University, VA
The Johns Hopkins University, MD
Marquette University, WI
New York University, NY
The Ohio State University, OH
Old Dominion University, VA
Oregon Health & Science University, OR
Radford University, VA
San Diego State University, CA
Shenandoah University, VA
State University of New York Downstate Medical
   Center, NY
Stony Brook University, State University of New
   York, NY
Texas Tech University Health Sciences Center, TX
University of California, San Francisco, CA
University of Cincinnati, OH
University of Colorado Denver, CO
University of Florida, FL
University of Illinois at Chicago, IL
University of Indianapolis, IN
The University of Kansas, KS
University of Medicine and Dentistry of New
   Jersey, NJ
University of Miami, FL
University of Michigan, MI
University of New Mexico, NM
University of Pennsylvania, PA
University of Washington, WA
Vanderbilt University, TN
Wayne State University, MI
West Virginia Wesleyan College, WV
Yale University, CT

NURSE PRACTITIONER PROGRAMS

Acute Care

Allen College, IA
Arizona State University at the Downtown
   Phoenix Campus, AZ
Armstrong Atlantic State University, GA

Barry University, FL
California State University, Los Angeles, CA
Case Western Reserve University, OH
The Catholic University of America, DC
Colorado State University–Pueblo, CO
Columbia University, NY
Creighton University, NE
Drexel University, PA
Duke University, NC
Emory University, GA
Florida Gulf Coast University, FL
Georgetown University, DC
Goldfarb School of Nursing at Barnes-Jewish
   College, MO
Grand Canyon University, AZ
Indiana University–Purdue University
   Indianapolis, IN
The Johns Hopkins University, MD
Kent State University, OH
Loyola University Chicago, IL
Madonna University, MI
Marquette University, WI
Memorial University of Newfoundland, NL
MGH Institute of Health Professions, MA
New York University, NY
Northern Kentucky University, KY
Northwestern State University of Louisiana, LA
The Ohio State University, OH
Rhode Island College, RI
Rush University, IL
Rutgers, The State University of New Jersey,
   College of Nursing, NJ
The Sage Colleges, NY
Saint Louis University, MO
San Diego State University, CA
Southern Adventist University, TN
Texas Tech University Health Sciences Center, TX
Texas Woman's University, TX
Thomas Jefferson University, PA
Université de Montréal, QC
The University of Akron, OH
The University of Alabama at Birmingham, AL
The University of Alabama in Huntsville, AL
University of Arkansas for Medical Sciences, AR
University of Calgary, AB
University of California, Los Angeles, CA
University of California, San Francisco, CA
University of Connecticut, CT
University of Florida, FL
University of Illinois at Chicago, IL
University of Kentucky, KY
University of Louisville, KY
University of Maryland, Baltimore, MD
University of Massachusetts Worcester, MA
University of Medicine and Dentistry of New
   Jersey, NJ
University of Miami, FL
University of Michigan, MI
University of Mississippi Medical Center, MS
University of Nebraska Medical Center, NE
University of New Brunswick Fredericton, NB
University of New Mexico, NM
University of Pennsylvania, PA
University of Rochester, NY
University of South Alabama, AL
University of South Carolina, SC
University of Southern Indiana, IN
University of South Florida, FL
The University of Texas at Arlington, TX
The University of Texas Health Science Center at
   Houston, TX
University of Toronto, ON
University of Virginia, VA
Vanderbilt University, TN
Virginia Commonwealth University, VA
Wayne State University, MI
Wright State University, OH
Yale University, CT

Adult Health

Adelphi University, NY
Allen College, IA
Arizona State University at the Downtown
   Phoenix Campus, AZ
Armstrong Atlantic State University, GA
Azusa Pacific University, CA

Ball State University, IN
Bloomsburg University of Pennsylvania, PA
Boston College, MA
California State University, Long Beach, CA
California State University, Los Angeles, CA
Case Western Reserve University, OH
The Catholic University of America, DC
Clarkson College, NE
Clemson University, SC
The College of New Jersey, NJ
The College of St. Scholastica, MN
College of Staten Island of the City University of
  New York, NY
Columbia University, NY
Concordia University Wisconsin, WI
Creighton University, NE
Daemen College, NY
DePaul University, IL
Drexel University, PA
Duke University, NC
East Carolina University, NC
Emory University, GA
Fairleigh Dickinson University, Metropolitan
  Campus, NJ
Felician College, NJ
Florida Agricultural and Mechanical
  University, FL
Florida Atlantic University, FL
Florida Gulf Coast University, FL
Florida International University, FL
Florida Southern College, FL
George Mason University, VA
The George Washington University, DC
Georgia State University, GA
Goldfarb School of Nursing at Barnes-Jewish
  College, MO
Gwynedd-Mercy College, PA
Indiana University–Purdue University Fort
  Wayne, IN
Indiana University–Purdue University
  Indianapolis, IN
James Madison University, VA
The Johns Hopkins University, MD
Kaplan University Online, FL
Kennesaw State University, GA
Kent State University, OH
La Salle University, PA
Lewis University, IL
Loma Linda University, CA
Long Island University–Brooklyn Campus, NY
Loyola University Chicago, IL
Loyola University New Orleans, LA
Madonna University, MI
Marian University, WI
Marquette University, WI
Maryville University of Saint Louis, MO
McNeese State University, LA
Medical University of South Carolina, SC
Metropolitan State University, MN
MGH Institute of Health Professions, MA
Michigan State University, MI
Molloy College, NY
Monmouth University, NJ
Mount Saint Mary College, NY
Neumann University, PA
Northern Illinois University, IL
Northern Kentucky University, KY
North Park University, IL
Oakland University, MI
The Ohio State University, OH
Otterbein University, OH
Penn State University Park, PA
Purdue University, IN
Quinnipiac University, CT
Regis College, MA
Research College of Nursing, MO
Rhode Island College, RI
The Richard Stockton College of New Jersey, NJ
Rush University, IL
Rutgers, The State University of New Jersey,
  College of Nursing, NJ
The Sage Colleges, NY
St. Catherine University, MN
Saint Louis University, MO
Saint Peter's University, NJ

San Diego State University, CA
Seattle Pacific University, WA
Seton Hall University, NJ
Southern Adventist University, TN
Spalding University, KY
Spring Arbor University, MI
State University of New York Upstate Medical
  University, NY
Stony Brook University, State University of New
  York, NY
Temple University, PA
Texas Woman's University, TX
Thomas Jefferson University, PA
Université de Moncton, NB
Université Laval, QC
The University of Akron, OH
The University of Alabama at Birmingham, AL
University of Alberta, AB
University of Calgary, AB
University of California, Irvine, CA
University of California, Los Angeles, CA
University of California, San Francisco, CA
University of Central Arkansas, AR
University of Central Florida, FL
University of Cincinnati, OH
University of Colorado at Colorado Springs, CO
University of Colorado Denver, CO
University of Delaware, DE
University of Florida, FL
University of Hawaii at Manoa, HI
University of Illinois at Chicago, IL
University of Indianapolis, IN
The University of Iowa, IA
The University of Kansas, KS
University of Kentucky, KY
University of Louisiana at Lafayette, LA
University of Louisville, KY
University of Maryland, Baltimore, MD
University of Massachusetts Boston, MA
University of Massachusetts Dartmouth, MA
University of Medicine and Dentistry of New
  Jersey, NJ
University of Miami, FL
University of Michigan, MI
University of Michigan–Flint, MI
University of Missouri–Kansas City, MO
University of Missouri–St. Louis, MO
University of Nebraska Medical Center, NE
University of New Brunswick Fredericton, NB
University of New Hampshire, NH
The University of North Carolina at
  Chapel Hill, NC
The University of North Carolina at Charlotte, NC
The University of North Carolina at
  Greensboro, NC
University of Oklahoma Health Sciences
  Center, OK
University of Pennsylvania, PA
University of Rochester, NY
University of San Diego, CA
University of Southern Maine, ME
University of South Florida, FL
The University of Tampa, FL
The University of Tennessee, TN
The University of Texas at Arlington, TX
The University of Texas Health Science Center at
  Houston, TX
University of Toronto, ON
University of Vermont, VT
University of Washington, WA
University of Wisconsin–Eau Claire, WI
Ursuline College, OH
Vanderbilt University, TN
Villanova University, PA
Virginia Commonwealth University, VA
Viterbo University, WI
Washburn University, KS
Western Connecticut State University, CT
William Paterson University of New Jersey, NJ
Wilmington University, DE
Winona State University, MN
York College of Pennsylvania, PA

Community Health
Athabasca University, AB

Binghamton University, State University of New
  York, NY
Cedarville University, OH
Hunter College of the City University of New
  York, NY
The Ohio State University, OH
The Sage Colleges, NY
Université de Moncton, NB
The University of British Columbia, BC
University of Hawaii at Manoa, HI
University of Nebraska Medical Center, NE
University of New Brunswick Fredericton, NB
University of Virginia, VA
The University of Western Ontario, ON

Family Health
Albany State University, GA
Alcorn State University, MS
Allen College, IA
Angelo State University, TX
Arizona State University at the Downtown
  Phoenix Campus, AZ
Athabasca University, AB
Austin Peay State University, TN
Azusa Pacific University, CA
Ball State University, IN
Barry University, FL
Baylor University, TX
Belmont University, TN
Binghamton University, State University of New
  York, NY
Boston College, MA
Bowie State University, MD
Brenau University, GA
Briar Cliff University, IA
Brigham Young University, UT
California State University, Dominguez Hills, CA
California State University, Fresno, CA
California State University, Long Beach, CA
California State University, Los Angeles, CA
California State University, Sacramento, CA
Carlow University, PA
Carson-Newman University, TN
Case Western Reserve University, OH
The Catholic University of America, DC
Clarion University of Pennsylvania, PA
Clarke University, IA
Clarkson College, NE
Clemson University, SC
The College of New Jersey, NJ
The College of New Rochelle, NY
The College of St. Scholastica, MN
Colorado State University–Pueblo, CO
Columbia University, NY
Concordia University Wisconsin, WI
Coppin State University, MD
Creighton University, NE
Delta State University, MS
DePaul University, IL
DeSales University, PA
Dominican College, NY
Drexel University, PA
Duke University, NC
Duquesne University, PA
D'Youville College, NY
East Carolina University, NC
Eastern Kentucky University, KY
East Tennessee State University, TN
Emory University, GA
Fairfield University, CT
Fairleigh Dickinson University, Metropolitan
  Campus, NJ
Felician College, NJ
Florida Atlantic University, FL
Florida Gulf Coast University, FL
Florida International University, FL
Fort Hays State University, KS
Franciscan University of Steubenville, OH
Gannon University, PA
Gardner-Webb University, NC
George Mason University, VA
Georgetown University, DC
The George Washington University, DC
Georgia College & State University, GA
Georgia Regents University, GA
Georgia Southern University, GA

Georgia State University, GA
Gonzaga University, WA
Goshen College, IN
Graceland University, IA
Grambling State University, LA
Grand Canyon University, AZ
Hampton University, VA
Hawai'i Pacific University, HI
Holy Names University, CA
Howard University, DC
Hunter College of the City University of New York, NY
Husson University, ME
Idaho State University, ID
Illinois State University, IL
Indiana State University, IN
Indiana University–Purdue University Indianapolis, IN
Indiana University South Bend, IN
Indiana Wesleyan University, IN
Jacksonville University, FL
James Madison University, VA
The Johns Hopkins University, MD
Kaplan University Online, FL
Kennesaw State University, GA
Kent State University, OH
La Salle University, PA
Lehman College of the City University of New York, NY
Lincoln Memorial University, TN
Loma Linda University, CA
Long Island University–Brooklyn Campus, NY
Long Island University–C. W. Post Campus, NY
Loyola University Chicago, IL
Loyola University New Orleans, LA
Malone University, OH
Marshall University, WV
Marymount University, VA
Maryville University of Saint Louis, MO
McNeese State University, LA
Medical University of South Carolina, SC
Mercer University Georgia Baptist College of Nursing, GA
Metropolitan State University, MN
MGH Institute of Health Professions, MA
Michigan State University, MI
Middle Tennessee State University, TN
Midwestern State University, TX
Millersville University of Pennsylvania, PA
Minnesota State University Mankato, MN
Misericordia University, PA
Mississippi University for Women, MS
Missouri State University, MO
Molloy College, NY
Monmouth University, NJ
Montana State University, MT
Mount Carmel College of Nursing, OH
Murray State University, KY
New York University, NY
North Dakota State University, ND
Northern Arizona University, AZ
Northern Illinois University, IL
Northern Kentucky University, KY
Northern Michigan University, MI
North Park University, IL
Northwestern State University of Louisiana, LA
Oakland University, MI
The Ohio State University, OH
Ohio University, OH
Old Dominion University, VA
Olivet Nazarene University, IL
Oregon Health & Science University, OR
Otterbein University, OH
Pace University, NY
Pacific Lutheran University, WA
Patty Hanks Shelton School of Nursing, TX
Penn State University Park, PA
Pittsburg State University, KS
Prairie View A&M University, TX
Purdue University Calumet, IN
Quinnipiac University, CT
Radford University, VA
Regis College, MA
Regis University, CO
Research College of Nursing, MO

Rivier University, NH
Rush University, IL
Rutgers, The State University of New Jersey, College of Nursing, NJ
Sacred Heart University, CT
The Sage Colleges, NY
Saginaw Valley State University, MI
Saint Anthony College of Nursing, IL
Saint Francis Medical Center College of Nursing, IL
St. John Fisher College, NY
Saint Louis University, MO
Saint Xavier University, IL
Salisbury University, MD
Samford University, AL
Samuel Merritt University, CA
San Francisco State University, CA
San Jose State University, CA
Seattle Pacific University, WA
Seattle University, WA
Shenandoah University, VA
Simmons College, MA
South Dakota State University, SD
Southeastern Louisiana University, LA
Southeast Missouri State University, MO
Southern Adventist University, TN
Southern Connecticut State University, CT
Southern Illinois University Edwardsville, IL
Southern University and Agricultural and Mechanical College, LA
Spalding University, KY
State University of New York Downstate Medical Center, NY
State University of New York Institute of Technology, NY
State University of New York Upstate Medical University, NY
Temple University, PA
Tennessee State University, TN
Tennessee Technological University, TN
Texas A&M International University, TX
Texas A&M University–Corpus Christi, TX
Texas Tech University Health Sciences Center, TX
Texas Woman's University, TX
Thomas Jefferson University, PA
Troy University, AL
Union University, TN
Université de Moncton, NB
Université de Montréal, QC
The University of Alabama, AL
The University of Alabama at Birmingham, AL
The University of Alabama in Huntsville, AL
University of Alaska Anchorage, AK
University of Arkansas for Medical Sciences, AR
The University of British Columbia, BC
University of California, Davis, CA
University of California, Irvine, CA
University of California, Los Angeles, CA
University of California, San Francisco, CA
University of Central Arkansas, AR
University of Central Florida, FL
University of Central Missouri, MO
University of Cincinnati, OH
University of Colorado at Colorado Springs, CO
University of Colorado Denver, CO
University of Connecticut, CT
University of Delaware, DE
University of Detroit Mercy, MI
University of Florida, FL
University of Hawaii at Manoa, HI
University of Illinois at Chicago, IL
University of Indianapolis, IN
The University of Iowa, IA
The University of Kansas, KS
University of Kentucky, KY
University of Louisville, KY
University of Maine, ME
University of Mary, ND
University of Mary Hardin-Baylor, TX
University of Maryland, Baltimore, MD
University of Massachusetts Boston, MA
University of Massachusetts Lowell, MA
University of Massachusetts Worcester, MA
University of Medicine and Dentistry of New Jersey, NJ

University of Memphis, TN
University of Miami, FL
University of Michigan, MI
University of Mississippi Medical Center, MS
University of Missouri, MO
University of Missouri–Kansas City, MO
University of Missouri–St. Louis, MO
University of Nebraska Medical Center, NE
University of Nevada, Las Vegas, NV
University of Nevada, Reno, NV
University of New Brunswick Fredericton, NB
University of New Hampshire, NH
University of New Mexico, NM
The University of North Carolina at Chapel Hill, NC
The University of North Carolina at Charlotte, NC
The University of North Carolina Wilmington, NC
University of North Dakota, ND
University of Northern British Columbia, BC
University of Northern Colorado, CO
University of North Florida, FL
University of North Georgia, GA
University of Oklahoma Health Sciences Center, OK
University of Pennsylvania, PA
University of Phoenix–Hawaii Campus, HI
University of Phoenix–Online Campus, AZ
University of Phoenix–Phoenix Main Campus, AZ
University of Phoenix–Sacramento Valley Campus, CA
University of Phoenix–Southern Arizona Campus, AZ
University of Phoenix–Southern California Campus, CA
University of Rhode Island, RI
University of Rochester, NY
University of St. Francis, IL
University of Saint Francis, IN
University of Saint Joseph, CT
University of San Diego, CA
The University of Scranton, PA
University of South Alabama, AL
University of South Carolina, SC
University of Southern Indiana, IN
University of Southern Maine, ME
University of Southern Mississippi, MS
University of South Florida, FL
The University of Tampa, FL
The University of Tennessee, TN
The University of Tennessee at Chattanooga, TN
The University of Texas at Arlington, TX
The University of Texas at Austin, TX
The University of Texas at El Paso, TX
The University of Texas at Tyler, TX
The University of Texas Health Science Center at Houston, TX
The University of Texas Health Science Center at San Antonio, TX
The University of Texas Medical Branch, TX
The University of Texas–Pan American, TX
The University of Toledo, OH
University of Toronto, ON
University of Vermont, VT
University of Virginia, VA
University of Washington, WA
University of Wisconsin–Eau Claire, WI
Ursuline College, OH
Vanderbilt University, TN
Villanova University, PA
Virginia Commonwealth University, VA
Viterbo University, WI
Wagner College, NY
Walden University, MN
Washburn University, KS
Washington State University College of Nursing, WA
Western Carolina University, NC
Western University of Health Sciences, CA
Westminster College, UT
West Texas A&M University, TX
West Virginia University, WV
Wheeling Jesuit University, WV
Widener University, PA
William Paterson University of New Jersey, NJ
Wilmington University, DE

Winona State University, MN
Winston-Salem State University, NC
Wright State University, OH
Yale University, CT

Gerontology

Allen College, IA
Binghamton University, State University of New
  York, NY
Boston College, MA
California State University, Long Beach, CA
Case Western Reserve University, OH
Clemson University, SC
The College of St. Scholastica, MN
College of Staten Island of the City University of
  New York, NY
Columbia University, NY
Concordia University Wisconsin, WI
Creighton University, NE
Delta State University, MS
Duke University, NC
Emory University, GA
Fairleigh Dickinson University, Metropolitan
  Campus, NJ
Florida Agricultural and Mechanical
  University, FL
Florida Atlantic University, FL
Hampton University, VA
Hunter College of the City University of New
  York, NY
James Madison University, VA
The Johns Hopkins University, MD
Marquette University, WI
MGH Institute of Health Professions, MA
Michigan State University, MI
Mississippi University for Women, MS
Mount Carmel College of Nursing, OH
New York University, NY
Oakland University, MI
The Ohio State University, OH
Rush University, IL
The Sage Colleges, NY
St. Catherine University, MN
Saint Louis University, MO
San Diego State University, CA
Seattle University, WA
Seton Hall University, NJ
Spring Arbor University, MI
Texas Tech University Health Sciences Center, TX
Trinity Western University, BC
The University of Akron, OH
The University of Alabama at Birmingham, AL
University of Alberta, AB
University of California, Irvine, CA
University of California, Los Angeles, CA
University of California, San Francisco, CA
University of Hawaii at Manoa, HI
University of Illinois at Chicago, IL
University of Indianapolis, IN
The University of Iowa, IA
The University of Kansas, KS
University of Kentucky, KY
University of Maryland, Baltimore, MD
University of Massachusetts Boston, MA
University of Massachusetts Lowell, MA
University of Massachusetts Worcester, MA
University of Medicine and Dentistry of New
  Jersey, NJ
University of Michigan, MI
University of Mississippi Medical Center, MS
University of Missouri, MO
University of Nebraska Medical Center, NE
University of New Brunswick Fredericton, NB
The University of North Carolina at
  Chapel Hill, NC
The University of North Carolina at
  Greensboro, NC
University of North Dakota, ND
University of Pennsylvania, PA
University of Rhode Island, RI
University of Rochester, NY
University of South Alabama, AL
University of Southern Mississippi, MS
University of South Florida, FL
The University of Texas at Arlington, TX

The University of Texas Health Science Center at
  Houston, TX
The University of Texas Health Science Center at
  San Antonio, TX
The University of Texas Medical Branch, TX
University of Toronto, ON
University of Utah, UT
University of Wisconsin–Eau Claire, WI
Vanderbilt University, TN
Walden University, MN
Wayne State University, MI
Wilmington University, DE

Neonatal Health

Arizona State University at the Downtown
  Phoenix Campus, AZ
Baylor University, TX
Case Western Reserve University, OH
The College of New Jersey, NJ
Creighton University, NE
Duke University, NC
East Carolina University, NC
Indiana University–Purdue University
  Indianapolis, IN
Louisiana State University Health Sciences
  Center, LA
McGill University, QC
McMaster University, ON
The Ohio State University, OH
Regis University, CO
Rush University, IL
St. Catherine University, MN
Saint Francis Medical Center College of
  Nursing, IL
South Dakota State University, SD
Stony Brook University, State University of New
  York, NY
Thomas Jefferson University, PA
The University of Alabama at Birmingham, AL
University of Calgary, AB
University of California, San Francisco, CA
University of Cincinnati, OH
University of Connecticut, CT
University of Florida, FL
University of Indianapolis, IN
The University of Iowa, IA
University of Louisville, KY
University of Missouri–Kansas City, MO
University of Missouri–St. Louis, MO
University of Nebraska Medical Center, NE
University of New Brunswick Fredericton, NB
University of Oklahoma Health Sciences
  Center, OK
University of Pennsylvania, PA
University of Rochester, NY
University of South Alabama, AL
The University of Texas at Arlington, TX
The University of Texas Medical Branch, TX
University of Toronto, ON
University of Washington, WA
Vanderbilt University, TN
Wayne State University, MI
West Virginia University, WV

Occupational Health

The University of Alabama at Birmingham, AL
University of California, Los Angeles, CA
University of California, San Francisco, CA
University of Cincinnati, OH
University of Illinois at Chicago, IL
University of South Florida, FL
University of the Sacred Heart, PR

Oncology

Case Western Reserve University, OH
Columbia University, NY
Creighton University, NE
Duke University, NC
Thomas Jefferson University, PA
Université de Moncton, NB
University of California, Los Angeles, CA
University of Nebraska Medical Center, NE
The University of North Carolina at
  Chapel Hill, NC
University of South Florida, FL
University of Toronto, ON

Pediatric

Arizona State University at the Downtown
  Phoenix Campus, AZ
Azusa Pacific University, CA
Boston College, MA
California State University, Fresno, CA
California State University, Long Beach, CA
California State University, Los Angeles, CA
Case Western Reserve University, OH
The Catholic University of America, DC
Colorado State University–Pueblo, CO
Columbia University, NY
Creighton University, NE
Drexel University, PA
Duke University, NC
Emory University, GA
Florida International University, FL
Georgia Regents University, GA
Georgia State University, GA
Grambling State University, LA
Gwynedd-Mercy College, PA
Hampton University, VA
Indiana University–Purdue University
  Indianapolis, IN
The Johns Hopkins University, MD
Kent State University, OH
Lehman College of the City University of New
  York, NY
Loma Linda University, CA
Marquette University, WI
Medical University of South Carolina, SC
MGH Institute of Health Professions, MA
Mississippi University for Women, MS
Molloy College, NY
New York University, NY
Northern Kentucky University, KY
Northwestern State University of Louisiana, LA
The Ohio State University, OH
Purdue University, IN
Regis College, MA
Rush University, IL
Rutgers, The State University of New Jersey,
  College of Nursing, NJ
St. Catherine University, MN
Saint Louis University, MO
Seton Hall University, NJ
Spalding University, KY
State University of New York Upstate Medical
  University, NY
Stony Brook University, State University of New
  York, NY
Temple University, PA
Texas Tech University Health Sciences Center, TX
Texas Woman's University, TX
Thomas Jefferson University, PA
The University of Akron, OH
The University of Alabama at Birmingham, AL
University of Arkansas for Medical Sciences, AR
University of California, Los Angeles, CA
University of California, San Francisco, CA
University of Central Florida, FL
University of Cincinnati, OH
University of Colorado Denver, CO
University of Florida, FL
University of Hawaii at Manoa, HI
University of Illinois at Chicago, IL
The University of Iowa, IA
University of Kentucky, KY
University of Maryland, Baltimore, MD
University of Michigan, MI
University of Missouri, MO
University of Missouri–Kansas City, MO
University of Missouri–St. Louis, MO
University of Nebraska Medical Center, NE
University of New Brunswick Fredericton, NB
University of New Mexico, NM
The University of North Carolina at
  Chapel Hill, NC
University of Oklahoma Health Sciences
  Center, OK
University of Pennsylvania, PA
University of Rochester, NY
University of San Diego, CA
University of South Alabama, AL
University of South Florida, FL

The University of Tennessee, TN
The University of Texas at Arlington, TX
The University of Texas at Austin, TX
The University of Texas at Tyler, TX
The University of Texas Health Science Center at
  Houston, TX
The University of Texas Health Science Center at
  San Antonio, TX
The University of Texas–Pan American, TX
The University of Toledo, OH
University of Toronto, ON
University of Virginia, VA
University of Washington, WA
Vanderbilt University, TN
Villanova University, PA
Virginia Commonwealth University, VA
Wayne State University, MI
West Virginia University, WV
Wright State University, OH
Yale University, CT

Primary Care

Arkansas State University, AR
Athabasca University, AB
Auburn University Montgomery, AL
Azusa Pacific University, CA
California State University, Los Angeles, CA
California State University, Sacramento, CA
Duke University, NC
Emory University, GA
Florida Southern College, FL
George Mason University, VA
Gonzaga University, WA
Hampton University, VA
The Johns Hopkins University, MD
Kennesaw State University, GA
Kent State University, OH
Loma Linda University, CA
Louisiana State University Health Sciences
  Center, LA
Loyola University Chicago, IL
Madonna University, MI
Marquette University, WI
McGill University, QC
MGH Institute of Health Professions, MA
New York University, NY
The Ohio State University, OH
Queen's University at Kingston, ON
Regis College, MA
Ryerson University, ON
Simmons College, MA
Université de Moncton, NB
Université de Montréal, QC
Université du Québec à Chicoutimi, QC
Université du Québec à Trois-Rivières, QC
Université du Québec en Outaouais, QC
Université Laval, QC
The University of Akron, OH
The University of Alabama at Birmingham, AL
The University of British Columbia, BC
University of Connecticut, CT
University of Indianapolis, IN
University of Manitoba, MB
University of Maryland, Baltimore, MD
University of Massachusetts Worcester, MA
University of Michigan, MI
University of Missouri, MO
University of Nebraska Medical Center, NE
University of New Brunswick Fredericton, NB
The University of North Carolina at
  Chapel Hill, NC
University of North Dakota, ND
University of North Florida, FL
University of Ottawa, ON
University of Pennsylvania, PA
University of San Diego, CA
University of Saskatchewan, SK
University of Toronto, ON
University of Virginia, VA
University of Washington, WA
University of Windsor, ON
Virginia Commonwealth University, VA
Wayne State University, MI

Psychiatric/mental Health

Allen College, IA

Arizona State University at the Downtown
  Phoenix Campus, AZ
Binghamton University, State University of New
  York, NY
Boston College, MA
California State University, Long Beach, CA
California State University, Los Angeles, CA
Case Western Reserve University, OH
The College of St. Scholastica, MN
Columbia University, NY
Creighton University, NE
Delta State University, MS
Drexel University, PA
Eastern Kentucky University, KY
Fairfield University, CT
Fairleigh Dickinson University, Metropolitan
  Campus, NJ
Georgia State University, GA
Gonzaga University, WA
Hunter College of the City University of New
  York, NY
Kent State University, OH
Lincoln Memorial University, TN
Loma Linda University, CA
McNeese State University, LA
MGH Institute of Health Professions, MA
Midwestern State University, TX
Mississippi University for Women, MS
Molloy College, NY
Monmouth University, NJ
Montana State University, MT
New York University, NY
The Ohio State University, OH
Oregon Health & Science University, OR
Regis College, MA
Rivier University, NH
Rush University, IL
Rutgers, The State University of New Jersey,
  College of Nursing, NJ
The Sage Colleges, NY
Saint Francis Medical Center College of
  Nursing, IL
Saint Louis University, MO
Seattle University, WA
Shenandoah University, VA
South Dakota State University, SD
Southeastern Louisiana University, LA
State University of New York Upstate Medical
  University, NY
Stony Brook University, State University of New
  York, NY
The University of Akron, OH
The University of Alabama, AL
The University of Alabama at Birmingham, AL
University of Alaska Anchorage, AK
University of Arkansas for Medical Sciences, AR
University of California, San Francisco, CA
University of Colorado Denver, CO
University of Florida, FL
University of Illinois at Chicago, IL
The University of Iowa, IA
The University of Kansas, KS
University of Kentucky, KY
University of Louisiana at Lafayette, LA
University of Louisville, KY
University of Maryland, Baltimore, MD
University of Massachusetts Lowell, MA
University of Medicine and Dentistry of New
  Jersey, NJ
University of Michigan, MI
University of Mississippi Medical Center, MS
University of Missouri, MO
University of Nebraska Medical Center, NE
University of New Brunswick Fredericton, NB
The University of North Carolina at
  Chapel Hill, NC
University of North Dakota, ND
University of Pennsylvania, PA
University of Rochester, NY
University of Saint Joseph, CT
University of San Diego, CA
University of South Alabama, AL
University of Southern Indiana, IN
University of Southern Maine, ME
University of Southern Mississippi, MS

The University of Tennessee, TN
The University of Texas at Arlington, TX
The University of Texas at Austin, TX
The University of Texas Health Science Center at
  Houston, TX
The University of Texas Health Science Center at
  San Antonio, TX
University of Utah, UT
University of Vermont, VT
University of Virginia, VA
University of Washington, WA
Vanderbilt University, TN
Virginia Commonwealth University, VA
Washington State University College of
  Nursing, WA
Wayne State University, MI
West Virginia Wesleyan College, WV
Winston-Salem State University, NC
Yale University, CT

School Health

The College of New Jersey, NJ
Seton Hall University, NJ
University of Illinois at Chicago, IL

Women's Health

Arizona State University at the Downtown
  Phoenix Campus, AZ
Boston College, MA
California State University, Fullerton, CA
California State University, Long Beach, CA
Case Western Reserve University, OH
Columbia University, NY
Drexel University, PA
Emory University, GA
Florida Agricultural and Mechanical
  University, FL
Georgetown University, DC
Georgia State University, GA
Hampton University, VA
Indiana University–Purdue University Fort
  Wayne, IN
Indiana University–Purdue University
  Indianapolis, IN
Kent State University, OH
Loyola University Chicago, IL
MGH Institute of Health Professions, MA
Northwestern State University of Louisiana, LA
The Ohio State University, OH
Old Dominion University, VA
Regis College, MA
Rutgers, The State University of New Jersey,
  College of Nursing, NJ
Salem State University, MA
San Diego State University, CA
State University of New York Downstate Medical
  Center, NY
Stony Brook University, State University of New
  York, NY
Texas Woman's University, TX
The University of Alabama at Birmingham, AL
University of Cincinnati, OH
University of Colorado Denver, CO
University of Illinois at Chicago, IL
University of Indianapolis, IN
University of Louisville, KY
University of Medicine and Dentistry of New
  Jersey, NJ
University of Missouri–Kansas City, MO
University of Missouri–St. Louis, MO
University of Nebraska Medical Center, NE
University of New Brunswick Fredericton, NB
University of Pennsylvania, PA
University of South Alabama, AL
The University of Texas Health Science Center at
  Houston, TX
Vanderbilt University, TN
Virginia Commonwealth University, VA
Wayne State University, MI
Wesley College, DE
West Virginia University, WV

NURSING ADMINISTRATION

Adelphi University, NY
Allen College, IA
American International College, MA

American Sentinel University, CO
Anderson University, IN
Arkansas State University, AR
Arkansas Tech University, AR
Aspen University, CO
Athabasca University, AB
Aurora University, IL
Austin Peay State University, TN
Azusa Pacific University, CA
Ball State University, IN
Barry University, FL
Bellarmine University, KY
Bellin College, WI
Bethel College, IN
Bethel University, MN
Binghamton University, State University of New
  York, NY
Blessing–Rieman College of Nursing, IL
Bloomsburg University of Pennsylvania, PA
Boise State University, ID
Bradley University, IL
Brandman University, CA
California State University, Dominguez Hills, CA
California State University, Fullerton, CA
California State University, Long Beach, CA
California State University, Los Angeles, CA
California State University, Sacramento, CA
California State University, San Bernardino, CA
Capella University, MN
Capital University, OH
Carlow University, PA
Chatham University, PA
Clarkson College, NE
Clayton State University, GA
Clemson University, SC
The College of New Rochelle, NY
Creighton University, NE
Delta State University, MS
DeSales University, PA
Drexel University, PA
Duke University, NC
East Carolina University, NC
Eastern Mennonite University, VA
East Tennessee State University, TN
Edgewood College, WI
Elms College, MA
Emmanuel College, MA
Endicott College, MA
Excelsior College, NY
Fairleigh Dickinson University, Metropolitan
  Campus, NJ
Felician College, NJ
Ferris State University, MI
Florida Atlantic University, FL
Florida International University, FL
Florida Southern College, FL
Florida State University, FL
Fort Hays State University, KS
Framingham State University, MA
Franklin Pierce University, NH
Gannon University, PA
Gardner-Webb University, NC
George Mason University, VA
The George Washington University, DC
Georgia Southwestern State University, GA
Georgia State University, GA
Goldfarb School of Nursing at Barnes-Jewish
  College, MO
Gonzaga University, WA
Grand Canyon University, AZ
Hampton University, VA
Holy Names University, CA
Hunter College of the City University of New
  York, NY
Idaho State University, ID
Illinois State University, IL
Immaculata University, PA
Indiana State University, IN
Indiana University of Pennsylvania, PA
Indiana University–Purdue University Fort
  Wayne, IN
Indiana University–Purdue University
  Indianapolis, IN
Indiana Wesleyan University, IN
Jacksonville University, FL

James Madison University, VA
Jefferson College of Health Sciences, VA
The Johns Hopkins University, MD
Kean University, NJ
Lamar University, TX
La Roche College, PA
La Salle University, PA
Lehman College of the City University of New
  York, NY
Le Moyne College, NY
Lewis University, IL
Loma Linda University, CA
Long Island University–Brooklyn Campus, NY
Louisiana State University Health Sciences
  Center, LA
Lourdes University, OH
Loyola University Chicago, IL
Madonna University, MI
Mansfield University of Pennsylvania, PA
Marquette University, WI
Marshall University, WV
Marywood University, PA
McGill University, QC
McKendree University, IL
McNeese State University, LA
Mercy College, NY
Metropolitan State University, MN
Middle Tennessee State University, TN
Molloy College, NY
Monmouth University, NJ
Moravian College, PA
Mount Carmel College of Nursing, OH
Mount St. Mary's College, CA
National University, CA
Nebraska Methodist College, NE
Nebraska Wesleyan University, NE
New Mexico State University, NM
New York University, NY
Northern Kentucky University, KY
North Park University, IL
Northwestern State University of Louisiana, LA
Nova Southeastern University, FL
The Ohio State University, OH
Ohio University, OH
Oklahoma City University, OK
Old Dominion University, VA
Otterbein University, OH
Our Lady of the Lake College, LA
Pacific Lutheran University, WA
Penn State University Park, PA
Pittsburg State University, KS
Prairie View A&M University, TX
Purdue University Calumet, IN
Queens University of Charlotte, NC
Regis College, MA
Regis University, CO
Research College of Nursing, MO
Resurrection University, IL
Roberts Wesleyan College, NY
Sacred Heart University, CT
The Sage Colleges, NY
Saginaw Valley State University, MI
St. Ambrose University, IA
Saint Francis Medical Center College of
  Nursing, IL
Saint Joseph's College of Maine, ME
Saint Peter's University, NJ
Saint Xavier University, IL
Salem State University, MA
Samford University, AL
San Diego State University, CA
San Francisco State University, CA
San Jose State University, CA
Seattle Pacific University, WA
Seton Hall University, NJ
Simmons College, MA
South Dakota State University, SD
Southeastern Louisiana University, LA
Southern Nazarene University, OK
Southwest Baptist University, MO
Spalding University, KY
Stevenson University, MD
Tennessee State University, TN
Tennessee Technological University, TN
Texas A&M University–Corpus Christi, TX

Texas A&M University–Texarkana, TX
Texas Tech University Health Sciences Center, TX
Texas Woman's University, TX
Thomas University, GA
Trinity Western University, BC
Troy University, AL
Union University, TN
Université de Moncton, NB
Université de Montréal, QC
Université Laval, QC
The University of Akron, OH
The University of Alabama, AL
The University of Alabama at Birmingham, AL
University of Arkansas for Medical Sciences, AR
The University of British Columbia, BC
University of California, Los Angeles, CA
University of California, San Francisco, CA
University of Central Florida, FL
University of Cincinnati, OH
University of Colorado Denver, CO
University of Detroit Mercy, MI
University of Hartford, CT
University of Hawaii at Manoa, HI
University of Houston–Victoria, TX
University of Illinois at Chicago, IL
University of Indianapolis, IN
The University of Iowa, IA
The University of Kansas, KS
University of Kentucky, KY
University of Louisiana at Lafayette, LA
University of Manitoba, MB
University of Mary, ND
University of Maryland, Baltimore, MD
University of Memphis, TN
University of Michigan, MI
University of Mississippi Medical Center, MS
University of Missouri, MO
University of Mobile, AL
University of Nebraska Medical Center, NE
University of New Brunswick Fredericton, NB
University of New Mexico, NM
University of North Alabama, AL
The University of North Carolina at
  Chapel Hill, NC
The University of North Carolina at Charlotte, NC
The University of North Carolina at
  Greensboro, NC
University of Pennsylvania, PA
University of Phoenix–Bay Area Campus, CA
University of Phoenix–Central Florida
  Campus, FL
University of Phoenix–Cleveland Campus, OH
University of Phoenix–Denver Campus, CO
University of Phoenix–Hawaii Campus, HI
University of Phoenix–Metro Detroit Campus, MI
University of Phoenix–New Mexico Campus, NM
University of Phoenix–North Florida Campus, FL
University of Phoenix–Online Campus, AZ
University of Phoenix–Phoenix Main Campus, AZ
University of Phoenix–Sacramento Valley
  Campus, CA
University of Phoenix–San Diego Campus, CA
University of Phoenix–Southern Arizona
  Campus, AZ
University of Phoenix–Southern California
  Campus, CA
University of Phoenix–South Florida Campus, FL
University of Pittsburgh, PA
University of Puerto Rico, Medical Sciences
  Campus, PR
University of Rhode Island, RI
University of St. Francis, IL
University of San Diego, CA
University of South Alabama, AL
University of Southern Indiana, IN
University of Southern Maine, ME
University of Southern Mississippi, MS
The University of Tennessee, TN
The University of Texas at Arlington, TX
The University of Texas at Austin, TX
The University of Texas at Brownsville, TX
The University of Texas at El Paso, TX
The University of Texas at Tyler, TX
The University of Texas Health Science Center at
  Houston, TX

The University of Texas Health Science Center at San Antonio, TX
The University of Texas Medical Branch, TX
University of Toronto, ON
University of Vermont, VT
University of Virginia, VA
The University of Western Ontario, ON
University of West Florida, FL
University of West Georgia, GA
University of Wisconsin–Eau Claire, WI
Urbana University, OH
Valdosta State University, GA
Vanderbilt University, TN
Virginia Commonwealth University, VA
Walden University, MN
Washburn University, KS
Washington State University College of Nursing, WA
Waynesburg University, PA
Weber State University, UT
Webster University, MO
West Chester University of Pennsylvania, PA
Western Carolina University, NC
Western Governors University, UT
Western Kentucky University, KY
Western Michigan University, MI
Western University of Health Sciences, CA
West Texas A&M University, TX
West Virginia University, WV
West Virginia Wesleyan College, WV
Wheeling Jesuit University, WV
Wilkes University, PA
William Paterson University of New Jersey, NJ
Wilmington University, DE
Winona State University, MN
Wright State University, OH
Xavier University, OH
Yale University, CT

NURSING EDUCATION

Adelphi University, NY
Albany State University, GA
Alcorn State University, MS
Allen College, IA
Alverno College, WI
American International College, MA
American Sentinel University, CO
Anderson University, IN
Andrews University, MI
Angelo State University, TX
Aquinas College, TN
Arkansas State University, AR
Aspen University, CO
Athabasca University, AB
Auburn University, AL
Auburn University Montgomery, AL
Aurora University, IL
Austin Peay State University, TN
Azusa Pacific University, CA
Ball State University, IN
Barry University, FL
Bellarmine University, KY
Bellin College, WI
Belmont University, TN
Bethel College, IN
Bethel University, MN
Binghamton University, State University of New York, NY
Blessing–Rieman College of Nursing, IL
Boise State University, ID
Bowie State University, MD
Bradley University, IL
Brenau University, GA
Briar Cliff University, IA
BryanLGH College of Health Sciences, NE
California Baptist University, CA
California State University, Chico, CA
California State University, Dominguez Hills, CA
California State University, Fresno, CA
California State University, Fullerton, CA
California State University, Long Beach, CA
California State University, Los Angeles, CA
California State University, Sacramento, CA
California State University, San Bernardino, CA
Capella University, MN

Capital University, OH
Cardinal Stritch University, WI
Carlow University, PA
Carson-Newman University, TN
Charleston Southern University, SC
Chatham University, PA
Clarion University of Pennsylvania, PA
Clarke University, IA
Clarkson College, NE
Clayton State University, GA
Clemson University, SC
Cleveland State University, OH
The College of New Rochelle, NY
Colorado State University–Pueblo, CO
Concordia College, MN
Concordia University Wisconsin, WI
Cox College, MO
Creighton University, NE
Daemen College, NY
Delaware State University, DE
Delta State University, MS
DeSales University, PA
Drexel University, PA
Duke University, NC
Duquesne University, PA
D'Youville College, NY
East Carolina University, NC
Eastern Kentucky University, KY
East Tennessee State University, TN
Edgewood College, WI
Elmhurst College, IL
Elms College, MA
Emmanuel College, MA
Endicott College, MA
Excelsior College, NY
Fairleigh Dickinson University, Metropolitan Campus, NJ
Felician College, NJ
Ferris State University, MI
Florida Atlantic University, FL
Florida International University, FL
Florida Southern College, FL
Florida State University, FL
Fort Hays State University, KS
Framingham State University, MA
Franciscan University of Steubenville, OH
Franklin Pierce University, NH
Gardner-Webb University, NC
George Mason University, VA
Georgetown University, DC
Georgia Southwestern State University, GA
Goldfarb School of Nursing at Barnes-Jewish College, MO
Gonzaga University, WA
Graceland University, IA
Grambling State University, LA
Grand Canyon University, AZ
Hampton University, VA
Hawai`i Pacific University, HI
Holy Family University, PA
Holy Names University, CA
Howard University, DC
Husson University, ME
Idaho State University, ID
Immaculata University, PA
Indiana State University, IN
Indiana University of Pennsylvania, PA
Indiana University–Purdue University Fort Wayne, IN
Indiana Wesleyan University, IN
Jacksonville University, FL
Jefferson College of Health Sciences, VA
Kaplan University Online, FL
Kent State University, OH
Lamar University, TX
La Roche College, PA
Lehman College of the City University of New York, NY
Le Moyne College, NY
Lenoir-Rhyne University, NC
Lewis University, IL
Liberty University, VA
Loma Linda University, CA
Long Island University–Brooklyn Campus, NY
Long Island University–C. W. Post Campus, NY

Louisiana State University Health Sciences Center, LA
Lourdes University, OH
Lynchburg College, VA
Mansfield University of Pennsylvania, PA
Marian University, WI
Marshall University, WV
Maryville University of Saint Louis, MO
McKendree University, IL
McNeese State University, LA
Memorial University of Newfoundland, NL
Mercer University Georgia Baptist College of Nursing, GA
Mercy College, NY
MGH Institute of Health Professions, MA
MidAmerica Nazarene University, KS
Middle Tennessee State University, TN
Midwestern State University, TX
Millersville University of Pennsylvania, PA
Millikin University, IL
Minnesota State University Mankato, MN
Minnesota State University Moorhead, MN
Misericordia University, PA
Missouri Southern State University, MO
Missouri State University, MO
Molloy College, NY
Monmouth University, NJ
Moravian College, PA
Mount Carmel College of Nursing, OH
Mount Mercy University, IA
Mount St. Mary's College, CA
Nebraska Methodist College, NE
Nebraska Wesleyan University, NE
Neumann University, PA
New York University, NY
North Dakota State University, ND
Northeastern State University, OK
Northern Illinois University, IL
Northern Kentucky University, KY
Northwestern State University of Louisiana, LA
Northwest Nazarene University, ID
Nova Southeastern University, FL
Oakland University, MI
Ohio University, OH
Oklahoma Baptist University, OK
Oklahoma City University, OK
Old Dominion University, VA
Oregon Health & Science University, OR
Otterbein University, OH
Our Lady of the Lake College, LA
Pace University, NY
Pacific Lutheran University, WA
Patty Hanks Shelton School of Nursing, TX
Pittsburg State University, KS
Point Loma Nazarene University, CA
Prairie View A&M University, TX
Queens University of Charlotte, NC
Ramapo College of New Jersey, NJ
Regis College, MA
Regis University, CO
Research College of Nursing, MO
Resurrection University, IL
Rivier University, NH
Robert Morris University, PA
Roberts Wesleyan College, NY
Sacred Heart University, CT
The Sage Colleges, NY
Saginaw Valley State University, MI
Saint Anthony College of Nursing, IL
St. Catherine University, MN
Saint Francis Medical Center College of Nursing, IL
St. John Fisher College, NY
St. Joseph's College, New York, NY
Saint Joseph's College of Maine, ME
Saint Louis University, MO
Salem State University, MA
Salisbury University, MD
Samford University, AL
San Diego State University, CA
San Jose State University, CA
Seattle Pacific University, WA
Seton Hall University, NJ
South Dakota State University, SD
Southeast Missouri State University, MO

Southern Adventist University, TN
Southern Connecticut State University, CT
Southern Illinois University Edwardsville, IL
Southern Nazarene University, OK
Southern University and Agricultural and
    Mechanical College, LA
South University, FL
Southwest Baptist University, MO
Spalding University, KY
Spring Arbor University, MI
State University of New York Institute of
    Technology, NY
Stevenson University, MD
Temple University, PA
Tennessee State University, TN
Tennessee Technological University, TN
Texas A&M University–Corpus Christi, TX
Texas A&M University–Texarkana, TX
Texas Christian University, TX
Texas Tech University Health Sciences Center, TX
Texas Woman's University, TX
Thomas Jefferson University, PA
Thomas University, GA
Touro University, NV
Towson University, MD
Trinity Western University, BC
Troy University, AL
Union University, TN
Université de Moncton, NB
Université de Montréal, QC
The University of Alabama, AL
The University of Alabama at Birmingham, AL
University of Alaska Anchorage, AK
University of Arkansas, AR
University of Arkansas for Medical Sciences, AR
The University of British Columbia, BC
University of Central Arkansas, AR
University of Central Florida, FL
University of Central Missouri, MO
University of Detroit Mercy, MI
University of Hartford, CT
University of Hawaii at Manoa, HI
University of Houston–Victoria, TX
University of Indianapolis, IN
The University of Iowa, IA
University of Louisiana at Lafayette, LA
University of Louisville, KY
University of Maine, ME
University of Mary, ND
University of Mary Hardin-Baylor, TX
University of Massachusetts Worcester, MA
University of Medicine and Dentistry of New
    Jersey, NJ
University of Memphis, TN
University of Miami, FL
University of Mississippi Medical Center, MS
University of Missouri, MO
University of Missouri–Kansas City, MO
University of Missouri–St. Louis, MO
University of Mobile, AL
University of Nebraska Medical Center, NE
University of Nevada, Las Vegas, NV
University of Nevada, Reno, NV
University of New Brunswick Fredericton, NB
University of New Mexico, NM
University of North Alabama, AL
The University of North Carolina at
    Chapel Hill, NC
The University of North Carolina at Charlotte, NC

The University of North Carolina at
    Greensboro, NC
The University of North Carolina Wilmington, NC
University of North Dakota, ND
University of Northern Colorado, CO
University of North Georgia, GA
University of Oklahoma Health Sciences Center,
    OK
University of Phoenix–Bay Area Campus, CA
University of Phoenix–Central Florida
    Campus, FL
University of Phoenix–Denver Campus, CO
University of Phoenix–Hawaii Campus, HI
University of Phoenix–Metro Detroit Campus, MI
University of Phoenix–New Mexico Campus, NM
University of Phoenix–North Florida Campus, FL
University of Phoenix–Online Campus, AZ
University of Phoenix–Phoenix Main Campus, AZ
University of Phoenix–Sacramento Valley
    Campus, CA
University of Phoenix–San Diego Campus, CA
University of Phoenix–Southern Arizona
    Campus, AZ
University of Phoenix–Southern California
    Campus, CA
University of Phoenix–South Florida Campus, FL
University of Portland, OR
University of Puerto Rico, Medical Sciences
    Campus, PR
University of Rhode Island, RI
University of St. Francis, IL
University of Saint Joseph, CT
University of San Diego, CA
University of Saskatchewan, SK
The University of Scranton, PA
University of South Alabama, AL
University of Southern Indiana, IN
University of Southern Maine, ME
University of South Florida, FL
The University of Texas at Arlington, TX
The University of Texas at Brownsville, TX
The University of Texas at El Paso, TX
The University of Texas at Tyler, TX
The University of Texas Health Science Center at
    Houston, TX
The University of Texas Medical Branch, TX
The University of Toledo, OH
University of Toronto, ON
University of Utah, UT
University of Washington, WA
The University of Western Ontario, ON
University of West Florida, FL
University of West Georgia, GA
University of Wisconsin–Eau Claire, WI
University of Wisconsin–Oshkosh, WI
University of Wyoming, WY
Urbana University, OH
Ursuline College, OH
Valdosta State University, GA
Villanova University, PA
Viterbo University, WI
Wagner College, NY
Walden University, MN
Walsh University, OH
Washington State University College of
    Nursing, WA
Waynesburg University, PA
Weber State University, UT
Webster University, MO

West Chester University of Pennsylvania, PA
Western Carolina University, NC
Western Governors University, UT
Western Kentucky University, KY
Western Michigan University, MI
Westminster College, UT
West Texas A&M University, TX
West Virginia Wesleyan College, WV
Wheeling Jesuit University, WV
Widener University, PA
Wilkes University, PA
William Carey University, MS
William Paterson University of New Jersey, NJ
Wilmington University, DE
Winona State University, MN
Winston-Salem State University, NC
Worcester State University, MA
Xavier University, OH
York College of Pennsylvania, PA
Youngstown State University, OH

NURSING INFORMATICS

American Sentinel University, CO
Austin Peay State University, TN
Chatham University, PA
Duke University, NC
East Tennessee State University, TN
Excelsior College, NY
Fairleigh Dickinson University, Metropolitan
    Campus, NJ
Ferris State University, MI
Georgia State University, GA
Kaplan University Online, FL
Loyola University Chicago, IL
Middle Tennessee State University, TN
Molloy College, NY
National University, CA
New York University, NY
Northern Kentucky University, KY
Nova Southeastern University, FL
Regis College, MA
Tennessee State University, TN
Tennessee Technological University, TN
Thomas Jefferson University, PA
Troy University, AL
The University of Alabama at Birmingham, AL
University of Colorado Denver, CO
University of Illinois at Chicago, IL
The University of Iowa, IA
The University of Kansas, KS
University of Maryland, Baltimore, MD
University of Medicine and Dentistry of New
    Jersey, NJ
University of Michigan, MI
University of Nebraska Medical Center, NE
University of New Brunswick Fredericton, NB
The University of North Carolina at
    Chapel Hill, NC
University of Pittsburgh, PA
University of San Diego, CA
University of Toronto, ON
University of Utah, UT
Ursuline College, OH
Vanderbilt University, TN
Walden University, MN
Xavier University, OH

U.S. AND U.S. TERRITORIES

Alabama

Samford University, Ida V. Moffett School of Nursing, *Birmingham (DNP)*

Troy University, School of Nursing, *Troy (DNP)*

The University of Alabama, Capstone College of Nursing, *Tuscaloosa (DNP)*

The University of Alabama at Birmingham, School of Nursing, *Birmingham (DNP, PhD)*

The University of Alabama in Huntsville, College of Nursing, *Huntsville (DNP)*

Arizona

Arizona State University at the Downtown Phoenix Campus, College of Nursing, *Phoenix (DNP)*

Northern Arizona University, School of Nursing, *Flagstaff (DNP)*

The University of Arizona, College of Nursing, *Tucson (PhD)*

University of Phoenix–Online Campus, Online Campus, *Phoenix (PhD)*

Arkansas

University of Arkansas for Medical Sciences, College of Nursing, *Little Rock (DNP, PhD)*

California

Azusa Pacific University, School of Nursing, *Azusa (PhD)*

Brandman University, School of Nursing and Health Professions, *Irvine (DNP)*

California State University, Fresno, Department of Nursing, *Fresno (DNP)*

California State University, Fullerton, Department of Nursing, *Fullerton (DNP)*

Loma Linda University, School of Nursing, *Loma Linda (PhD)*

National University, Department of Nursing, *La Jolla (DNP)*

Samuel Merritt University, School of Nursing, *Oakland (DNP)*

University of California, Davis, The Betty Irene Moore School of Nursing, *Davis (PhD)*

University of California, Los Angeles, School of Nursing, *Los Angeles (PhD)*

University of California, San Francisco, School of Nursing, *San Francisco (PhD)*

University of San Diego, Hahn School of Nursing and Health Science, *San Diego (DNP, PhD)*

University of San Francisco, School of Nursing and Health Professions, *San Francisco (DNP)*

Western University of Health Sciences, College of Graduate Nursing, *Pomona (DNP)*

Colorado

University of Colorado at Colorado Springs, Beth-El College of Nursing and Health Sciences, *Colorado Springs (DNP)*

University of Colorado Denver, College of Nursing, *Aurora (DNP, PhD)*

University of Northern Colorado, School of Nursing, *Greeley (PhD)*

Connecticut

Fairfield University, School of Nursing, *Fairfield (DNP)*

Quinnipiac University, School of Nursing, *Hamden (DNP)*

Sacred Heart University, Program in Nursing, *Fairfield (DNP)*

Southern Connecticut State University, Department of Nursing, *New Haven (EdD)*

University of Connecticut, School of Nursing, *Storrs (DNP, PhD)*

Yale University, School of Nursing, *New Haven (DNP, PhD)*

Delaware

University of Delaware, School of Nursing, *Newark (PhD)*

District of Columbia

The Catholic University of America, School of Nursing, *Washington (PhD)*

The George Washington University, School of Nursing, *Washington (DNP)*

Florida

Barry University, Division of Nursing, *Miami Shores (PhD)*

Florida Agricultural and Mechanical University, School of Nursing, *Tallahassee (PhD)*

Florida Atlantic University, Christine E. Lynn College of Nursing, *Boca Raton (DNP)*

Florida International University, Graduate Nursing Programs, *Miami (PhD)*

Florida State University, College of Nursing, *Tallahassee (DNP)*

University of Central Florida, College of Nursing, *Orlando (PhD)*

University of Florida, College of Nursing, *Gainesville (PhD)*

University of Miami, School of Nursing and Health Studies, *Coral Gables (PhD)*

University of South Florida, College of Nursing, *Tampa (PhD)*

Georgia

Brenau University, College of Health and Science, *Gainesville (DNP)*

Emory University, Nell Hodgson Woodruff School of Nursing, *Atlanta (PhD)*

Georgia College & State University, College of Health Sciences, *Milledgeville (DNP)*

Georgia Regents University, School of Nursing, *Augusta (DNP, PhD)*

Georgia Southern University, School of Nursing, *Statesboro (DNP)*

Georgia State University, Byrdine F. Lewis School of Nursing and Health Professions, *Atlanta (PhD)*

Mercer University Georgia Baptist College of Nursing, *Atlanta (DNP, PhD)*

University of West Georgia, School of Nursing, *Carrollton (EdD)*

Hawaii

University of Hawaii at Manoa, School of Nursing and Dental Hygiene, *Honolulu (PhD)*

Illinois

DePaul University, Department of Nursing, *Chicago (DNP)*

Illinois State University, Mennonite College of Nursing, *Normal (PhD)*

Loyola University Chicago, Marcella Niehoff School of Nursing, *Maywood (DNP, PhD)*

Rush University, College of Nursing, *Chicago (PhD)*

Saint Francis Medical Center College of Nursing, Baccalaureate Nursing Program, *Peoria (DNP)*

Southern Illinois University Edwardsville, School of Nursing, *Edwardsville (DNP)*

University of Illinois at Chicago, College of Nursing, *Chicago (PhD)*

University of St. Francis, Leach College of Nursing, *Joliet (DNP)*

Indiana

Ball State University, School of Nursing, *Muncie (DNP)*

Indiana State University, Department of Nursing, *Terre Haute (DNP)*

Indiana University–Purdue University Indianapolis, School of Nursing, *Indianapolis (PhD)*

Purdue University, School of Nursing, *West Lafayette (DNP)*

University of Indianapolis, School of Nursing, *Indianapolis (DNP)*

University of Southern Indiana, College of Nursing and Health Professions, *Evansville (DNP)*

Iowa

Allen College, Program in Nursing, *Waterloo (DNP)*

The University of Iowa, College of Nursing, *Iowa City (PhD)*

Kansas

The University of Kansas, School of Nursing, *Kansas City (PhD)*

Wichita State University, School of Nursing, *Wichita (DNP)*

Kentucky

Bellarmine University, Donna and Allan Lansing School of Nursing and Health Sciences, *Louisville (DNP)*

Frontier Nursing University, Nursing Degree Programs, *Hyden (DNP)*

Northern Kentucky University, Department of Nursing, *Highland Heights (DNP)*

University of Kentucky, Graduate School Programs in the College of Nursing, *Lexington (PhD)*

University of Louisville, School of Nursing, *Louisville (PhD)*

Western Kentucky University, School of Nursing, *Bowling Green (DNP)*

Louisiana

Louisiana State University Health Sciences Center, School of Nursing, *New Orleans (DNS)*

Loyola University New Orleans, School of Nursing, *New Orleans (DNP)*

Southeastern Louisiana University, School of Nursing, *Hammond (DNP)*

Southern University and Agricultural and Mechanical College, School of Nursing, *Baton Rouge (PhD)*

Maine

University of Southern Maine, School of Nursing, *Portland (DNP)*

Maryland

The Johns Hopkins University, School of Nursing, *Baltimore (DNP, PhD)*

Salisbury University, Program in Nursing, *Salisbury (DNP)*

University of Maryland, Baltimore, Master's Program in Nursing, *Baltimore (DNP, PhD)*

Massachusetts

Boston College, William F. Connell School of Nursing, *Chestnut Hill (PhD)*

MGH Institute of Health Professions, School of Nursing, *Boston (DNP)*

Northeastern University, School of Nursing, *Boston (DNP)*

Regis College, School of Nursing, Science and Health Professions, *Weston (DNP)*

Simmons College, School of Nursing and Health Sciences, *Boston (DNP)*

University of Massachusetts Amherst, School of Nursing, *Amherst (PhD)*

University of Massachusetts Boston, College of Nursing and Health Sciences, *Boston (DNP, PhD)*

University of Massachusetts Dartmouth, College of Nursing, *North Dartmouth (PhD)*

University of Massachusetts Lowell, Department of Nursing, *Lowell (DNP, PhD)*

University of Massachusetts Worcester, Graduate School of Nursing, *Worcester (PhD)*

Michigan

Grand Valley State University, Kirkhof College of Nursing, *Allendale (DNP)*

Madonna University, College of Nursing and Health, *Livonia (DNP)*

Michigan State University, College of Nursing, *East Lansing (PhD)*

Saginaw Valley State University, Crystal M. Lange College of Health and Human Services, *University Center (DNP)*

University of Michigan, School of Nursing, *Ann Arbor (PhD)*

University of Michigan–Flint, Department of Nursing, *Flint (DAP, DNP)*

Wayne State University, College of Nursing, *Detroit (DNP)*

Minnesota

Capella University, Nursing Programs, *Minneapolis (DNP)*

The College of St. Scholastica, Department of Nursing, *Duluth (DNP)*

Minnesota State University Mankato, School of Nursing, *Mankato (DNP)*

St. Catherine University, Department of Nursing, *St. Paul (DNP)*

University of Minnesota, Twin Cities Campus, School of Nursing, *Minneapolis (DNP, PhD)*

Walden University, Nursing Programs, *Minneapolis (DNP)*

Winona State University, College of Nursing and Health Sciences, *Winona (DNP)*

Mississippi

University of Mississippi Medical Center, Program in Nursing, *Jackson (PhD)*

University of Southern Mississippi, School of Nursing, *Hattiesburg (PhD)*

William Carey University, School of Nursing, *Hattiesburg (PhD)*

Missouri

Goldfarb School of Nursing at Barnes-Jewish College, *St. Louis (PhD)*

Graceland University, School of Nursing, *Independence (DNP)*

Maryville University of Saint Louis, Nursing Program, School of Health Professions, *St. Louis (DNP)*

Missouri State University, Department of Nursing, *Springfield (DNP)*

Saint Louis University, School of Nursing, *St. Louis (DNP, PhD)*

University of Missouri, Sinclair School of Nursing, *Columbia (PhD)*

University of Missouri–Kansas City, School of Nursing, *Kansas City (PhD)*

University of Missouri–St. Louis, College of Nursing, *St. Louis (DNP)*

Montana

Montana State University, College of Nursing, *Bozeman (DNP)*

Nebraska

Creighton University, School of Nursing, *Omaha (DNP)*

University of Nebraska Medical Center, College of Nursing, *Omaha (PhD)*

Nevada

Touro University, School of Nursing, *Henderson (DNP)*

University of Nevada, Las Vegas, School of Nursing, *Las Vegas (DNP, PhD)*

University of Nevada, Reno, Orvis School of Nursing, *Reno (DNP)*

New Jersey

Fairleigh Dickinson University, Metropolitan Campus, Henry P. Becton School of Nursing and Allied Health, *Teaneck (DNP)*

Rutgers, The State University of New Jersey, College of Nursing, *Newark (PhD)*

Seton Hall University, College of Nursing, *South Orange (DNP)*

University of Medicine and Dentistry of New Jersey, School of Nursing, *Newark (DNP)*

William Paterson University of New Jersey, Department of Nursing, *Wayne (DNP)*

New Mexico

New Mexico State University, School of Nursing, *Las Cruces (PhD)*

University of New Mexico, College of Nursing, *Albuquerque (PhD)*

New York

Adelphi University, School of Nursing, *Garden City (PhD)*

Binghamton University, State University of New York, Decker School of Nursing, *Binghamton (DNP, PhD)*

Columbia University, School of Nursing, *New York (PhD)*

Daemen College, Department of Nursing, *Amherst (DNP)*

Hunter College of the City University of New York, Hunter-Bellevue School of Nursing, *New York (DNP)*

Lehman College of the City University of New York, Department of Nursing, *Bronx (DNS)*

Molloy College, Division of Nursing, *Rockville Centre (PhD)*

New York University, College of Nursing, *New York (DNP, PhD)*

Pace University, Lienhard School of Nursing, *New York (DNP)*

The Sage Colleges, Department of Nursing, *Troy (DNS)*

St. John Fisher College, Wegmans School of Nursing, *Rochester (DNP)*

Stony Brook University, State University of New York, School of Nursing, *Stony Brook (DNP)*

University at Buffalo, the State University of New York, School of Nursing, *Buffalo (DNP, PhD)*

University of Rochester, School of Nursing, *Rochester (PhD)*

North Carolina

Duke University, School of Nursing, *Durham (PhD)*

East Carolina University, College of Nursing, *Greenville (PhD)*

Gardner-Webb University, School of Nursing, *Boiling Springs (DNP)*

The University of North Carolina at Chapel Hill, School of Nursing, *Chapel Hill (PhD)*

The University of North Carolina at Greensboro, School of Nursing, *Greensboro (PhD)*

North Dakota

North Dakota State University, Department of Nursing, *Fargo (DNP)*

University of North Dakota, College of Nursing, *Grand Forks (PhD)*

Ohio

Case Western Reserve University, Frances Payne Bolton School of Nursing, *Cleveland (PhD)*

Cleveland State University, School of Nursing, *Cleveland (PhD)*

Kent State University, College of Nursing, *Kent (PhD)*

The Ohio State University, College of Nursing, *Columbus (PhD)*

The University of Akron, College of Nursing, *Akron (PhD)*

University of Cincinnati, College of Nursing, *Cincinnati (PhD)*

The University of Toledo, College of Nursing, *Toledo (DNP)*

Ursuline College, The Breen School of Nursing, *Pepper Pike (DNP)*

Walsh University, Department of Nursing, *North Canton (DNP)*

Wright State University, College of Nursing and Health, *Dayton (DNP)*

Oklahoma

Oklahoma City University, Kramer School of Nursing, *Oklahoma City (DNP, PhD)*

University of Oklahoma Health Sciences Center, College of Nursing, *Oklahoma City (PhD)*

Oregon

Oregon Health & Science University, School of Nursing, *Portland (PhD)*

University of Portland, School of Nursing, *Portland (DNP)*

Pennsylvania

Chatham University, Nursing Programs, *Pittsburgh (DNP)*

Drexel University, College of Nursing and Health Professions, *Philadelphia (Dr NP)*

Duquesne University, School of Nursing, *Pittsburgh (PhD)*

Gannon University, Villa Maria School of Nursing, *Erie (DNP)*

Indiana University of Pennsylvania, Department of Nursing and Allied Health, *Indiana (PhD)*

Penn State University Park, School of Nursing, *University Park (PhD)*

Robert Morris University, School of Nursing and Health Sciences, *Moon Township (DNP)*

Temple University, Department of Nursing, *Philadelphia (DNP)*

Thomas Jefferson University, Department of Nursing, *Philadelphia (DNP)*

University of Pennsylvania, School of Nursing, *Philadelphia (PhD)*

University of Pittsburgh, School of Nursing, *Pittsburgh (PhD)*

Villanova University, College of Nursing, *Villanova (PhD)*

Waynesburg University, Department of Nursing, *Waynesburg (DNP)*

Widener University, School of Nursing, *Chester (PhD)*

York College of Pennsylvania, Department of Nursing, *York (DNP)*

Rhode Island

University of Rhode Island, College of Nursing, *Kingston (PhD)*

South Carolina

Medical University of South Carolina, College of Nursing, *Charleston (PhD)*

University of South Carolina, College of Nursing, *Columbia (PhD)*

South Dakota

South Dakota State University, College of Nursing, *Brookings (PhD)*

Tennessee

East Tennessee State University, College of Nursing, *Johnson City (DNP, PhD)*

Southern Adventist University, School of Nursing, *Collegedale (DNP)*

The University of Tennessee, College of Nursing, *Knoxville (PhD)*

The University of Tennessee at Chattanooga, School of Nursing, *Chattanooga (DNP)*

The University of Tennessee Health Science Center, College of Nursing, *Memphis (DNP)*

Vanderbilt University, Vanderbilt University School of Nursing, *Nashville (DNP, PhD)*

Texas

Baylor University, Louise Herrington School of Nursing, *Waco (DNP)*

Texas Christian University, Harris College of Nursing, *Fort Worth (DNP)*

Texas Tech University Health Sciences Center, School of Nursing, *Lubbock (DNP)*

Texas Woman's University, College of Nursing, *Denton (PhD)*

The University of Texas at Arlington, College of Nursing, *Arlington (PhD)*

The University of Texas at Austin, School of Nursing, *Austin (PhD)*

The University of Texas at Tyler, Program in Nursing, *Tyler (PhD)*

The University of Texas Health Science Center at Houston, School of Nursing, *Houston (PhD)*

The University of Texas Health Science Center at San Antonio, School of Nursing, *San Antonio (PhD)*

The University of Texas Medical Branch, School of Nursing, *Galveston (PhD)*

University of the Incarnate Word, Program in Nursing, *San Antonio (DNP)*

Utah

University of Utah, College of Nursing, *Salt Lake City (PhD)*

Virginia

George Mason University, College of Health and Human Services, *Fairfax (PhD)*

Hampton University, School of Nursing, *Hampton (PhD)*

James Madison University, Department of Nursing, *Harrisonburg (DNP)*

Marymount University, Malek School of Health Professions, *Arlington (DNP)*

Old Dominion University, Department of Nursing, *Norfolk (DNP)*

Radford University, School of Nursing, *Radford (DNP)*

Shenandoah University, Eleanor Wade Custer School of Nursing, *Winchester (DNP)*

University of Virginia, School of Nursing, *Charlottesville (PhD)*

Virginia Commonwealth University, School of Nursing, *Richmond (PhD)*

Washington

Seattle University, College of Nursing, *Seattle (DNP)*

University of Washington, School of Nursing, *Seattle (DNP, PhD)*

Washington State University College of Nursing, *Spokane (PhD)*

West Virginia

West Virginia University, School of Nursing, *Morgantown (DNP, PhD)*

Wisconsin

Concordia University Wisconsin, Program in Nursing, *Mequon (DNP)*

Marquette University, College of Nursing, *Milwaukee (DNP, PhD)*

University of Phoenix–Milwaukee Campus, College of Health and Human Services, *Milwaukee (PhD)*

University of Wisconsin–Eau Claire, College of Nursing and Health Sciences, *Eau Claire (DNP)*

University of Wisconsin–Madison, School of Nursing, *Madison (PhD)*

University of Wisconsin–Milwaukee, College of Nursing, *Milwaukee (DNP, PhD)*

University of Wisconsin–Oshkosh, College of Nursing, *Oshkosh (DNP)*

Wyoming

University of Wyoming, Fay W. Whitney School of Nursing, *Laramie (DNP)*

CANADA

Alberta

University of Alberta, Faculty of Nursing, *Edmonton (PhD)*

University of Calgary, Faculty of Nursing, *Calgary (PhD)*

British Columbia

The University of British Columbia, Program in Nursing, *Vancouver (PhD)*

University of Victoria, School of Nursing, *Victoria (PhD)*

Manitoba

University of Manitoba, Faculty of Nursing, *Winnipeg (PhD)*

Ontario

McMaster University, School of Nursing, *Hamilton (PhD)*

Queen's University at Kingston, School of Nursing, *Kingston (PhD)*

University of Ottawa, School of Nursing, *Ottawa (PhD)*

University of Toronto, Faculty of Nursing, *Toronto (PhD)*

The University of Western Ontario, School of Nursing, *London (PhD)*

Quebec

McGill University, School of Nursing, *Montréal (PhD)*

Université de Montréal, Faculty of Nursing, *Montréal (PhD)*

Université de Sherbrooke, Department of Nursing, *Sherbrooke (PhD)*

Université Laval, Faculty of Nursing, *Québec (PhD)*

Saskatchewan

University of Saskatchewan, College of Nursing, *Saskatoon (PhD)*

POSTDOCTORAL PROGRAMS

U.S. AND U.S. TERRITORIES

Alabama
The University of Alabama at Birmingham, School of Nursing, *Birmingham*

Arkansas
University of Arkansas for Medical Sciences, College of Nursing, *Little Rock*

California
University of California, Davis, The Betty Irene Moore School of Nursing, *Davis*
University of California, Los Angeles, School of Nursing, *Los Angeles*
University of California, San Francisco, School of Nursing, *San Francisco*

Colorado
University of Colorado Denver, College of Nursing, *Aurora*

Connecticut
Yale University, School of Nursing, *New Haven*

Illinois
University of Illinois at Chicago, College of Nursing, *Chicago*

Indiana
Indiana University–Purdue University Indianapolis, School of Nursing, *Indianapolis*

Iowa
The University of Iowa, College of Nursing, *Iowa City*

Kansas
The University of Kansas, School of Nursing, *Kansas City*

Maryland
The Johns Hopkins University, School of Nursing, *Baltimore*

Massachusetts
University of Massachusetts Boston, College of Nursing and Health Sciences, *Boston*

Michigan
University of Michigan, School of Nursing, *Ann Arbor*
Wayne State University, College of Nursing, *Detroit*

Nebraska
University of Nebraska Medical Center, College of Nursing, *Omaha*

New York
Columbia University, School of Nursing, *New York*
University of Rochester, School of Nursing, *Rochester*

North Carolina
The University of North Carolina at Chapel Hill, School of Nursing, *Chapel Hill*

Ohio
Case Western Reserve University, Frances Payne Bolton School of Nursing, *Cleveland*

Oregon
Oregon Health & Science University, School of Nursing, *Portland*

Pennsylvania
Penn State University Park, School of Nursing, *University Park*
University of Pennsylvania, School of Nursing, *Philadelphia*
University of Pittsburgh, School of Nursing, *Pittsburgh*

South Carolina
Medical University of South Carolina, College of Nursing, *Charleston*

Tennessee
Vanderbilt University, Vanderbilt University School of Nursing, *Nashville*

Utah
University of Utah, College of Nursing, *Salt Lake City*

Virginia
University of Virginia, School of Nursing, *Charlottesville*
Virginia Commonwealth University, School of Nursing, *Richmond*

Washington
University of Washington, School of Nursing, *Seattle*

Wisconsin
University of Wisconsin–Madison, School of Nursing, *Madison*

CANADA

British Columbia
The University of British Columbia, Program in Nursing, *Vancouver*
University of Northern British Columbia, Nursing Programme, *Prince George*

Ontario
University of Ottawa, School of Nursing, *Ottawa*
University of Toronto, Faculty of Nursing, *Toronto*
The University of Western Ontario, School of Nursing, *London*

Quebec
McGill University, School of Nursing, *Montréal*
Université de Montréal, Faculty of Nursing, *Montréal*
Université de Sherbrooke, Department of Nursing, *Sherbrooke*
Université Laval, Faculty of Nursing, *Québec*

ONLINE PROGRAMS

ONLINE BACCALAUREATE PROGRAMS

Adventist University of Health Sciences, FL
Albany State University, GA
Alcorn State University, MS
Allen College, IA
Angelo State University, TX
Appalachian State University, NC
Arizona State University at the Downtown
  Phoenix Campus, AZ
Arkansas State University, AR
Arkansas Tech University, AR
Ashland University, OH
Aurora University, IL
Ball State University, IN
Bethel College, KS
Blessing–Rieman College of Nursing, IL
Bluefield State College, WV
Boise State University, ID
Bon Secours Memorial College of Nursing, VA
Brenau University, GA
California State University, Dominguez Hills, CA
Carson-Newman University, TN
Chamberlain College of Nursing, MO
Charleston Southern University, SC
Clarion University of Pennsylvania, PA
Clarkson College, NE
Clayton State University, GA
Cleveland State University, OH
College of Coastal Georgia, GA
The College of St. Scholastica, MN
Colorado Christian University, CO
Colorado Mesa University, CO
Colorado Technical University Online, CO
Columbus State University, GA
Cox College, MO
Creighton University, NE
Cumberland University, TN
Davenport University, MI
East Carolina University, NC
Eastern Illinois University, IL
Eastern New Mexico University, NM
East Tennessee State University, TN
ECPI College of Technology, VA
Ferris State University, MI
Finlandia University, MI
Fitchburg State University, MA
Florida Atlantic University, FL
Florida International University, FL
Fort Hays State University, KS
Francis Marion University, SC
Frostburg State University, MD
Gannon University, PA
Gardner-Webb University, NC
George Mason University, VA
Georgia Southern University, GA
Georgia Southwestern State University, GA
Grand Canyon University, AZ
Great Basin College, NV
Herzing University Online, WI
Howard University, DC
Illinois State University, IL
Indiana State University, IN
Jacksonville State University, AL
Jacksonville University, FL
Kettering College, OH
Lakehead University, ON
Lamar University, TX
Lander University, SC
La Roche College, PA
Laurentian University, ON
Lehman College of the City University of New
  York, NY
Loyola University New Orleans, LA
Marian University, IN
McKendree University, IL
Mercy College, NY
Mercy College of Ohio, OH
Methodist College, IL
Michigan State University, MI
MidAmerica Nazarene University, KS
Middle Tennessee State University, TN

Minnesota State University Moorhead, MN
Minot State University, ND
Mississippi University for Women, MS
Missouri State University, MO
Montana State University–Northern, MT
Morehead State University, KY
Mount Aloysius College, PA
Mount Carmel College of Nursing, OH
Nevada State College at Henderson, NV
Newman University, KS
New Mexico Highlands University, NM
New Mexico State University, NM
Nipissing University, ON
Northeastern State University, OK
Northern Arizona University, AZ
Northwestern State University of Louisiana, LA
Nova Southeastern University, FL
The Ohio State University, OH
Ohio University, OH
Oklahoma Panhandle State University, OK
Our Lady of the Lake College, LA
Penn State University Park, PA
Pittsburg State University, KS
Presentation College, SD
Purdue University Calumet, IN
Queens University of Charlotte, NC
Radford University, VA
Ramapo College of New Jersey, NJ
Rivier University, NH
Robert Morris University, PA
Roberts Wesleyan College, NY
Saint Louis University, MO
St. Petersburg College, FL
Sentara College of Health Sciences, VA
Silver Lake College of the Holy Family, WI
Slippery Rock University of Pennsylvania, PA
South Dakota State University, SD
Southeastern Louisiana University, LA
Southeast Missouri State University, MO
Southern Adventist University, TN
Southern Arkansas University–Magnolia, AR
South University, FL
South University, FL
Southwestern College, KS
Southwestern Oklahoma State University, OK
State University of New York at Plattsburgh, NY
State University of New York College of
  Technology at Delhi, NY
State University of New York Empire State
  College, NY
State University of New York Institute of
  Technology, NY
Stevenson University, MD
Tabor College, KS
Texas A&M Health Science Center, TX
Texas A&M University–Corpus Christi, TX
Texas Tech University Health Sciences Center,
  TX
Texas Woman's University, TX
Touro University, NV
University at Buffalo, the State University of New
  York, NY
The University of Akron, OH
University of Arkansas for Medical Sciences, AR
University of Arkansas–Fort Smith, AR
University of Central Missouri, MO
University of Colorado at Colorado Springs, CO
University of Colorado Denver, CO
University of Delaware, DE
University of Illinois at Chicago, IL
University of Louisiana at Lafayette, LA
University of Louisiana at Monroe, LA
University of Louisville, KY
University of Maine at Fort Kent, ME
University of Mary, ND
University of Maryland, Baltimore, MD
University of Massachusetts Amherst, MA
University of Massachusetts Boston, MA
University of Michigan–Flint, MI
University of Missouri, MO
University of Missouri–St. Louis, MO
University of North Alabama, AL

The University of North Carolina Wilmington,
  NC
University of North Georgia, GA
University of Phoenix–Online Campus, AZ
University of Phoenix–Phoenix Main Campus,
  AZ
University of Phoenix–Sacramento Valley
  Campus, CA
University of Phoenix–Southern Arizona
  Campus, AZ
University of Phoenix–South Florida Campus, FL
University of Phoenix–West Florida Campus, FL
University of St. Francis, IL
University of Saint Francis, IN
University of Saint Mary, KS
University of San Francisco, CA
University of Sioux Falls, SD
University of South Carolina Aiken, SC
University of South Carolina Upstate, SC
University of Southern Indiana, IN
University of Southern Mississippi, MS
University of South Florida, FL
The University of Tennessee at Chattanooga, TN
The University of Texas at Brownsville, TX
The University of Texas at Tyler, TX
University of the Incarnate Word, TX
The University of Toledo, OH
University of Wisconsin–Green Bay, WI
University of Wisconsin–Oshkosh, WI
University of Wyoming, WY
Utica College, NY
Walden University, MN
Western Carolina University, NC
Western Governors University, UT
Western New Mexico University, NM
Wheeling Jesuit University, WV
Wichita State University, KS
Wilmington University, DE

ONLINE ONLY BACCALAUREATE PROGRAMS

Adventist University of Health Sciences, FL
Bluefield State College, WV
Chamberlain College of Nursing, MO
Clarion University of Pennsylvania, PA
Cox College, MO
Eastern Illinois University, IL
Eastern New Mexico University, NM
Florida Atlantic University, FL
Frostburg State University, MD
Herzing University Online, WI
Howard University, DC
Kettering College, OH
La Roche College, PA
Laurentian University, ON
Loyola University New Orleans, LA
Methodist College, IL
Minnesota State University Moorhead, MN
Montana State University–Northern, MT
New Mexico Highlands University, NM
Northeastern State University, OK
Oklahoma Panhandle State University, OK
Slippery Rock University of Pennsylvania, PA
State University of New York College of
  Technology at Delhi, NY
State University of New York Empire State
  College, NY
Stevenson University, MD
Tabor College, KS
Texas Tech University Health Sciences Center,
  TX
University of Arkansas–Fort Smith, AR
University of Louisiana at Monroe, LA
University of North Alabama, AL
University of North Georgia, GA
University of Saint Mary, KS
The University of Tennessee at Chattanooga, TN
The University of Texas at Brownsville, TX
The University of Texas at Tyler, TX
Walden University, MN
Western Governors University, UT
Western New Mexico University, NM

ONLINE MASTER'S DEGREE PROGRAMS

Albany State University, GA
Alcorn State University, MS
Allen College, IA
American International College, MA
Angelo State University, TX
Aspen University, CO
Athabasca University, AB
Austin Peay State University, TN
Ball State University, IN
Baylor University, TX
Bellin College, WI
Benedictine University, IL
Brandman University, CA
California State University, Chico, CA
California State University, Dominguez Hills, CA
California State University, Fullerton, CA
Charleston Southern University, SC
Chatham University, PA
Clarkson College, NE
Clayton State University, GA
Cleveland State University, OH
Cox College, MO
Delta State University, MS
Drexel University, PA
Duke University, NC
Duquesne University, PA
East Carolina University, NC
Eastern Mennonite University, VA
East Tennessee State University, TN
Excelsior College, NY
Fairleigh Dickinson University, Metropolitan Campus, NJ
Felician College, NJ
Ferris State University, MI
Fitchburg State University, MA
Florida Atlantic University, FL
Florida State University, FL
Gardner-Webb University, NC
George Mason University, VA
Georgia College & State University, GA
Georgia Regents University, GA
Georgia Southwestern State University, GA
Gonzaga University, WA
Graceland University, IA
Grand Canyon University, AZ
Hampton University, VA
Howard University, DC
Idaho State University, ID
Indiana State University, IN
Indiana Wesleyan University, IN
Jacksonville State University, AL
Jacksonville University, FL
The Johns Hopkins University, MD
Lamar University, TX
La Roche College, PA
Lewis University, IL
Liberty University, VA
Loyola University Chicago, IL
Loyola University New Orleans, LA
Mansfield University of Pennsylvania, PA
McKendree University, IL
McNeese State University, LA
Medical University of South Carolina, SC
Memorial University of Newfoundland, NL
Mercy College, NY
Michigan State University, MI
Middle Tennessee State University, TN
Midwestern State University, TX
Minnesota State University Moorhead, MN
Missouri State University, MO
National University, CA
Nebraska Methodist College, NE
New Mexico State University, NM
Northeastern State University, OK
Northern Arizona University, AZ
Northern Kentucky University, KY
Northwest Nazarene University, ID
Nova Southeastern University, FL
The Ohio State University, OH
Old Dominion University, VA
Pace University, NY
Penn State University Park, PA
Purdue University Calumet, IN

Ramapo College of New Jersey, NJ
Regis University, CO
Research College of Nursing, MO
Roberts Wesleyan College, NY
Rush University, IL
Sacred Heart University, CT
Saint Francis Medical Center College of Nursing, IL
Saint Joseph's College of Maine, ME
Saint Louis University, MO
Saint Xavier University, IL
Samford University, AL
Seton Hall University, NJ
South Dakota State University, SD
South University, FL
Southwest Baptist University, MO
Spring Arbor University, MI
Spring Hill College, AL
State University of New York Institute of Technology, NY
Stevenson University, MD
Tennessee State University, TN
Tennessee Technological University, TN
Texas A&M University–Corpus Christi, TX
Texas Christian University, TX
Texas Tech University Health Sciences Center, TX
Texas Woman's University, TX
Touro University, NV
Troy University, AL
The University of Alabama, AL
The University of Alabama in Huntsville, AL
The University of Arizona, AZ
University of Arkansas, AR
University of Central Arkansas, AR
University of Central Missouri, MO
University of Cincinnati, OH
University of Colorado at Colorado Springs, CO
University of Colorado Denver, CO
University of Delaware, DE
University of Florida, FL
University of Hawaii at Manoa, HI
University of Indianapolis, IN
The University of Kansas, KS
University of Louisiana at Lafayette, LA
University of Mary, ND
University of Maryland, Baltimore, MD
University of Massachusetts Amherst, MA
University of Medicine and Dentistry of New Jersey, NJ
University of Memphis, TN
University of Michigan–Flint, MI
University of Missouri, MO
University of Missouri–St. Louis, MO
University of Nevada, Las Vegas, NV
University of New Mexico, NM
University of North Alabama, AL
The University of North Carolina at Charlotte, NC
University of North Dakota, ND
University of Northern Colorado, CO
University of Oklahoma Health Sciences Center, OK
University of Phoenix–New Mexico Campus, NM
University of Phoenix–Online Campus, AZ
University of Phoenix–Phoenix Main Campus, AZ
University of Phoenix–Southern Arizona Campus, AZ
University of Phoenix–South Florida Campus, FL
University of Pittsburgh, PA
University of Rochester, NY
University of St. Francis, IL
University of San Francisco, CA
University of Southern Indiana, IN
The University of Texas at Arlington, TX
The University of Texas at Brownsville, TX
The University of Texas at El Paso, TX
The University of Texas at Tyler, TX
The University of Texas Medical Branch, TX
University of Toronto, ON
University of West Florida, FL
University of West Georgia, GA
University of Wisconsin–Oshkosh, WI
University of Wyoming, WY
Vanderbilt University, TN
Walden University, MN
Walsh University, OH

Western Carolina University, NC
Western Governors University, UT
Western University of Health Sciences, CA
West Virginia University, WV
Wheeling Jesuit University, WV
Wilmington University, DE
Wright State University, OH
Yale University, CT

ONLINE ONLY MASTER'S DEGREE PROGRAMS

Albany State University, GA
American International College, MA
Angelo State University, TX
Aspen University, CO
Austin Peay State University, TN
Ball State University, IN
Benedictine University, IL
California State University, Chico, CA
California State University, Dominguez Hills, CA
Charleston Southern University, SC
Chatham University, PA
Clarkson College, NE
Clayton State University, GA
Cleveland State University, OH
Cox College, MO
Delta State University, MS
Duquesne University, PA
Eastern Mennonite University, VA
Excelsior College, NY
Ferris State University, MI
Fitchburg State University, MA
Florida State University, FL
Gardner-Webb University, NC
George Mason University, VA
Georgia College & State University, GA
Georgia Southwestern State University, GA
Gonzaga University, WA
Graceland University, IA
Howard University, DC
Idaho State University, ID
Indiana State University, IN
Jacksonville State University, AL
Lamar University, TX
La Roche College, PA
Lewis University, IL
Liberty University, VA
Loyola University Chicago, IL
Mansfield University of Pennsylvania, PA
McNeese State University, LA
Medical University of South Carolina, SC
Memorial University of Newfoundland, NL
Minnesota State University Moorhead, MN
Missouri State University, MO
National University, CA
Nebraska Methodist College, NE
New Mexico State University, NM
Northeastern State University, OK
Northern Arizona University, AZ
Northwest Nazarene University, ID
Nova Southeastern University, FL
The Ohio State University, OH
Old Dominion University, VA
Pace University, NY
Ramapo College of New Jersey, NJ
Saint Francis Medical Center College of Nursing, IL
Saint Joseph's College of Maine, ME
Saint Louis University, MO
Seton Hall University, NJ
Spring Arbor University, MI
Spring Hill College, AL
Stevenson University, MD
Tennessee Technological University, TN
Texas A&M University–Corpus Christi, TX
Texas Christian University, TX
Texas Tech University Health Sciences Center, TX
Touro University, NV
The University of Alabama, AL
University of Central Arkansas, AR
University of Central Missouri, MO
University of Colorado at Colorado Springs, CO
University of Louisiana at Lafayette, LA
University of Massachusetts Amherst, MA
University of Missouri, MO

University of Nevada, Las Vegas, NV
University of New Mexico, NM
University of North Alabama, AL
University of Northern Colorado, CO
University of Southern Indiana, IN
The University of Texas at Brownsville, TX
The University of Texas at El Paso, TX
The University of Texas at Tyler, TX
The University of Texas Medical Branch, TX
University of West Florida, FL
University of West Georgia, GA
University of Wisconsin–Oshkosh, WI
University of Wyoming, WY
Vanderbilt University, TN
Walden University, MN
Walsh University, OH
Western Governors University, UT
Western University of Health Sciences, CA
West Virginia University, WV
Wheeling Jesuit University, WV

ONLINE DOCTORAL DEGREE PROGRAMS

Allen College, IA
Ball State University, IN
Binghamton University, State University of New York, NY
California State University, Fresno, CA
The Catholic University of America, DC
Chatham University, PA
Concordia University Wisconsin, WI
Drexel University, PA
Duquesne University, PA
George Mason University, VA
Georgia College & State University, GA
Georgia Southern University, GA
Graceland University, IA
Hampton University, VA
Indiana State University, IN
Kent State University, OH
Loyola University New Orleans, LA
Medical University of South Carolina, SC
Mercer University Georgia Baptist College of Nursing, GA
Missouri State University, MO
National University, CA
New Mexico State University, NM
North Dakota State University, ND
Northern Arizona University, AZ
Northern Kentucky University, KY
Old Dominion University, VA
Radford University, VA
Rush University, IL

Saint Francis Medical Center College of Nursing, IL
Samford University, AL
Samuel Merritt University, CA
Southern Adventist University, TN
Southern Connecticut State University, CT
Touro University, NV
Troy University, AL
University at Buffalo, the State University of New York, NY
The University of Alabama, AL
The University of Alabama in Huntsville, AL
The University of Arizona, AZ
University of Colorado at Colorado Springs, CO
University of Florida, FL
University of Hawaii at Manoa, HI
University of Indianapolis, IN
The University of Kansas, KS
University of Massachusetts Boston, MA
University of Michigan–Flint, MI
University of Nevada, Las Vegas, NV
University of Nevada, Reno, NV
University of New Mexico, NM
University of North Dakota, ND
University of Northern Colorado, CO
University of Phoenix–Online Campus, AZ
University of St. Francis, IL
The University of Tennessee, TN
The University of Tennessee at Chattanooga, TN
The University of Tennessee Health Science Center, TN
The University of Texas Medical Branch, TX
University of the Incarnate Word, TX
The University of Toledo, OH
University of West Georgia, GA
University of Wisconsin–Milwaukee, WI
Virginia Commonwealth University, VA
Walden University, MN
Walsh University, OH
Western University of Health Sciences, CA
Winona State University, MN
Wright State University, OH
Yale University, CT

ONLINE ONLY DOCTORAL DEGREE PROGRAMS

Allen College, IA
Ball State University, IN
California State University, Fresno, CA
Chatham University, PA
Concordia University Wisconsin, WI
Drexel University, PA
Duquesne University, PA

George Mason University, VA
Georgia College & State University, GA
Georgia Southern University, GA
Graceland University, IA
Hampton University, VA
Indiana State University, IN
Kent State University, OH
Loyola University New Orleans, LA
Medical University of South Carolina, SC
Mercer University Georgia Baptist College of Nursing, GA
National University, CA
New Mexico State University, NM
Northern Arizona University, AZ
Old Dominion University, VA
Radford University, VA
Rush University, IL
Saint Francis Medical Center College of Nursing, IL
Samford University, AL
Samuel Merritt University, CA
Southern Adventist University, TN
Southern Connecticut State University, CT
Touro University, NV
Troy University, AL
The University of Alabama, AL
The University of Alabama in Huntsville, AL
The University of Arizona, AZ
University of Colorado at Colorado Springs, CO
University of Hawaii at Manoa, HI
University of Indianapolis, IN
University of Michigan–Flint, MI
University of Nevada, Las Vegas, NV
University of Nevada, Reno, NV
University of North Dakota, ND
University of Northern Colorado, CO
University of Phoenix–Online Campus, AZ
University of St. Francis, IL
The University of Tennessee, TN
The University of Tennessee at Chattanooga, TN
The University of Tennessee Health Science Center, TN
The University of Texas Medical Branch, TX
University of the Incarnate Word, TX
University of West Georgia, GA
Virginia Commonwealth University, VA
Walden University, MN
Walsh University, OH
Western University of Health Sciences, CA
Winona State University, MN
Wright State University, OH
Yale University, CT

CONTINUING EDUCATION PROGRAMS

U.S. AND U.S. TERRITORIES

Alabama

Auburn University, School of Nursing, *Auburn University*

Jacksonville State University, College of Nursing and Health Sciences, *Jacksonville*

Samford University, Ida V. Moffett School of Nursing, *Birmingham*

The University of Alabama in Huntsville, College of Nursing, *Huntsville*

University of Mobile, School of Nursing, *Mobile*

University of North Alabama, College of Nursing and Allied Health, *Florence*

Arizona

Arizona State University at the Downtown Phoenix Campus, College of Nursing, *Phoenix*

Grand Canyon University, College of Nursing and Health Sciences, *Phoenix*

University of Phoenix–Online Campus, Online Campus, *Phoenix*

University of Phoenix–Phoenix Main Campus, College of Nursing, *Tempe*

University of Phoenix–Southern Arizona Campus, College of Social Sciences, *Tucson*

Arkansas

Harding University, College of Nursing, *Searcy*

University of Arkansas, Eleanor Mann School of Nursing, *Fayetteville*

University of Arkansas for Medical Sciences, ·College of Nursing, *Little Rock*

California

Azusa Pacific University, School of Nursing, *Azusa*

Brandman University, School of Nursing and Health Professions, *Irvine*

California State University, Bakersfield, Program in Nursing, *Bakersfield*

California State University, Chico, School of Nursing, *Chico*

California State University, Fresno, Department of Nursing, *Fresno*

Dominican University of California, Program in Nursing, *San Rafael*

Pacific Union College, Department of Nursing, *Angwin*

Point Loma Nazarene University, School of Nursing, *San Diego*

San Diego State University, School of Nursing, *San Diego*

San Francisco State University, School of Nursing, *San Francisco*

University of California, Los Angeles, School of Nursing, *Los Angeles*

University of Phoenix–Sacramento Valley Campus, College of Nursing, *Sacramento*

University of Phoenix–Southern California Campus, College of Nursing, *Costa Mesa*

Colorado

University of Colorado at Colorado Springs, Beth-El College of Nursing and Health Sciences, *Colorado Springs*

University of Colorado Denver, College of Nursing, *Aurora*

Connecticut

Fairfield University, School of Nursing, *Fairfield*

Quinnipiac University, School of Nursing, *Hamden*

University of Connecticut, School of Nursing, *Storrs*

University of Hartford, College of Education, Nursing, and Health Professions, *West Hartford*

Delaware

University of Delaware, School of Nursing, *Newark*

Wesley College, Nursing Program, *Dover*

Florida

Florida Agricultural and Mechanical University, School of Nursing, *Tallahassee*

Florida Atlantic University, Christine E. Lynn College of Nursing, *Boca Raton*

Florida Gulf Coast University, School of Nursing, *Fort Myers*

St. Petersburg College, Department of Nursing, *St. Petersburg*

University of Miami, School of Nursing and Health Studies, *Coral Gables*

University of South Florida, College of Nursing, *Tampa*

The University of Tampa, Department of Nursing, *Tampa*

Georgia

Kennesaw State University, School of Nursing, *Kennesaw*

Valdosta State University, College of Nursing, *Valdosta*

Illinois

Lewis University, Program in Nursing, *Romeoville*

Olivet Nazarene University, Division of Nursing, *Bourbonnais*

Rush University, College of Nursing, *Chicago*

Saint Xavier University, School of Nursing, *Chicago*

Southern Illinois University Edwardsville, School of Nursing, *Edwardsville*

University of Illinois at Chicago, College of Nursing, *Chicago*

Indiana

Indiana State University, Department of Nursing, *Terre Haute*

Indiana University Kokomo, Indiana University School of Nursing, *Kokomo*

Indiana University–Purdue University Indianapolis, School of Nursing, *Indianapolis*

Marian University, School of Nursing, *Indianapolis*

Purdue University, School of Nursing, *West Lafayette*

University of Southern Indiana, College of Nursing and Health Professions, *Evansville*

Valparaiso University, College of Nursing, *Valparaiso*

Iowa

Allen College, Program in Nursing, *Waterloo*

Briar Cliff University, Department of Nursing, *Sioux City*

Clarke University, Department of Nursing and Health, *Dubuque*

Grand View University, Division of Nursing, *Des Moines*

Luther College, Department of Nursing, *Decorah*

Mount Mercy University, Department of Nursing, *Cedar Rapids*

St. Ambrose University, Program in Nursing (BSN), *Davenport*

The University of Iowa, College of Nursing, *Iowa City*

Kansas

Pittsburg State University, Department of Nursing, *Pittsburg*

The University of Kansas, School of Nursing, *Kansas City*

Washburn University, School of Nursing, *Topeka*

Kentucky

Bellarmine University, Donna and Allan Lansing School of Nursing and Health Sciences, *Louisville*

Kentucky Christian University, School of Nursing, *Grayson*

Midway College, Program in Nursing (Baccalaureate), *Midway*

Murray State University, Program in Nursing, *Murray*

Northern Kentucky University, Department of Nursing, *Highland Heights*

Spalding University, School of Nursing, *Louisville*

University of Kentucky, Graduate School Programs in the College of Nursing, *Lexington*

University of Louisville, School of Nursing, *Louisville*

Western Kentucky University, School of Nursing, *Bowling Green*

Louisiana

Dillard University, Division of Nursing, *New Orleans*

Louisiana State University Health Sciences Center, School of Nursing, *New Orleans*

McNeese State University, College of Nursing, *Lake Charles*

Nicholls State University, Department of Nursing, *Thibodaux*

Northwestern State University of Louisiana, College of Nursing and Allied Health, *Shreveport*

Our Lady of the Lake College, Division of Nursing, *Baton Rouge*

University of Louisiana at Lafayette, College of Nursing, *Lafayette*

University of Louisiana at Monroe, Nursing, *Monroe*

Maine

Saint Joseph's College of Maine, Master of Science in Nursing Program, *Standish*

University of New England, Department of Nursing, *Biddeford*

University of Southern Maine, School of Nursing, *Portland*

Maryland

The Johns Hopkins University, School of Nursing, *Baltimore*

University of Maryland, Baltimore, Master's Program in Nursing, *Baltimore*

Massachusetts

Anna Maria College, Department of Nursing, *Paxton*

Boston College, William F. Connell School of Nursing, *Chestnut Hill*

Endicott College, Major in Nursing, *Beverly*

Framingham State University, Department of Nursing, *Framingham*

Massachusetts College of Pharmacy and Health Sciences, School of Nursing, *Boston*

Northeastern University, School of Nursing, *Boston*

Regis College, School of Nursing, Science and Health Professions, *Weston*

Salem State University, Program in Nursing, *Salem*

University of Massachusetts Amherst, School of Nursing, *Amherst*

University of Massachusetts Boston, College of Nursing and Health Sciences, *Boston*

University of Massachusetts Dartmouth, College of Nursing, *North Dartmouth*

University of Massachusetts Worcester, Graduate School of Nursing, *Worcester*

Worcester State University, Department of Nursing, *Worcester*

Michigan

Grand Valley State University, Kirkhof College of Nursing, *Allendale*

Madonna University, College of Nursing and Health, *Livonia*

Michigan State University, College of Nursing, *East Lansing*

Northern Michigan University, College of Nursing and Allied Health Science, *Marquette*

Oakland University, School of Nursing, *Rochester*

Saginaw Valley State University, Crystal M. Lange College of Health and Human Services, *University Center*

Wayne State University, College of Nursing, *Detroit*

Western Michigan University, College of Health and Human Services, *Kalamazoo*

Minnesota

Bemidji State University, Department of Nursing, *Bemidji*

Minnesota State University Mankato, School of Nursing, *Mankato*

University of Minnesota, Twin Cities Campus, School of Nursing, *Minneapolis*

Mississippi

University of Mississippi Medical Center, Program in Nursing, *Jackson*

Missouri

Cox College, Department of Nursing, *Springfield*

Missouri State University, Department of Nursing, *Springfield*

Missouri Western State University, Department of Nursing, *St. Joseph*

Saint Louis University, School of Nursing, *St. Louis*

University of Missouri, Sinclair School of Nursing, *Columbia*

University of Missouri–Kansas City, School of Nursing, *Kansas City*

University of Missouri–St. Louis, College of Nursing, *St. Louis*

Nebraska

Clarkson College, Master of Science in Nursing Program, *Omaha*

Nebraska Methodist College, Department of Nursing, *Omaha*

University of Nebraska Medical Center, College of Nursing, *Omaha*

Nevada

University of Nevada, Las Vegas, School of Nursing, *Las Vegas*

New Hampshire

Saint Anselm College, Department of Nursing, *Manchester*

New Jersey

College of Saint Elizabeth, Department of Nursing, *Morristown*

Fairleigh Dickinson University, Metropolitan Campus, Henry P. Becton School of Nursing and Allied Health, *Teaneck*

Monmouth University, Marjorie K. Unterberg School of Nursing, *West Long Branch*

Ramapo College of New Jersey, Master of Science in Nursing Program, *Mahwah*

Rutgers, The State University of New Jersey, College of Nursing, *Newark*

University of Medicine and Dentistry of New Jersey, School of Nursing, *Newark*

New Mexico

New Mexico State University, School of Nursing, *Las Cruces*

New York

Adelphi University, School of Nursing, *Garden City*

Binghamton University, State University of New York, Decker School of Nursing, *Binghamton*

Columbia University, School of Nursing, *New York*

Elmira College, Program in Nursing Education, *Elmira*

Hunter College of the City University of New York, Hunter-Bellevue School of Nursing, *New York*

Lehman College of the City University of New York, Department of Nursing, *Bronx*

Molloy College, Division of Nursing, *Rockville Centre*

New York University, College of Nursing, *New York*

The Sage Colleges, Department of Nursing, *Troy*

State University of New York Downstate Medical Center, College of Nursing, *Brooklyn*

State University of New York Institute of Technology, School of Nursing and Health Systems, *Utica*

State University of New York Upstate Medical University, College of Nursing, *Syracuse*

Stony Brook University, State University of New York, School of Nursing, *Stony Brook*

University of Rochester, School of Nursing, *Rochester*

North Carolina

Queens University of Charlotte, Presbyterian School of Nursing, *Charlotte*

The University of North Carolina at Chapel Hill, School of Nursing, *Chapel Hill*

Winston-Salem State University, Department of Nursing, *Winston-Salem*

Ohio

Case Western Reserve University, Frances Payne Bolton School of Nursing, *Cleveland*

Cleveland State University, School of Nursing, *Cleveland*

Kent State University, College of Nursing, *Kent*

The Ohio State University, College of Nursing, *Columbus*

Otterbein University, Department of Nursing, *Westerville*

Shawnee State University, Department of Nursing, *Portsmouth*

The University of Akron, College of Nursing, *Akron*

University of Cincinnati, College of Nursing, *Cincinnati*

The University of Toledo, College of Nursing, *Toledo*

Urbana University, College of Nursing and Allied Health, *Urbana*

Wright State University, College of Nursing and Health, *Dayton*

Oklahoma

Oklahoma City University, Kramer School of Nursing, *Oklahoma City*

University of Oklahoma Health Sciences Center, College of Nursing, *Oklahoma City*

Oregon

Linfield College, School of Nursing, *McMinnville*

Oregon Health & Science University, School of Nursing, *Portland*

Pennsylvania

Alvernia University, Nursing, *Reading*

Bloomsburg University of Pennsylvania, Department of Nursing, *Bloomsburg*

Carlow University, School of Nursing, *Pittsburgh*

DeSales University, Department of Nursing and Health, *Center Valley*

Drexel University, College of Nursing and Health Professions, *Philadelphia*

Duquesne University, School of Nursing, *Pittsburgh*

Holy Family University, School of Nursing and Allied Health Professions, *Philadelphia*

La Roche College, Department of Nursing and Nursing Management, *Pittsburgh*

La Salle University, School of Nursing and Health Sciences, *Philadelphia*

Marywood University, Department of Nursing, *Scranton*

Moravian College, St. Luke's School of Nursing, *Bethlehem*

Mount Aloysius College, Division of Nursing, *Cresson*

Penn State University Park, School of Nursing, *University Park*

Temple University, Department of Nursing, *Philadelphia*

Thomas Jefferson University, Department of Nursing, *Philadelphia*

University of Pennsylvania, School of Nursing, *Philadelphia*

University of Pittsburgh, School of Nursing, *Pittsburgh*

Villanova University, College of Nursing, *Villanova*

Widener University, School of Nursing, *Chester*

Wilkes University, Department of Nursing, *Wilkes-Barre*

Puerto Rico

Universidad Adventista de las Antillas, Department of Nursing, *Mayagüez*

University of Puerto Rico, Mayagüez Campus, Department of Nursing, *Mayagüez*

University of Puerto Rico, Medical Sciences Campus, School of Nursing, *San Juan*

Rhode Island

Salve Regina University, Department of Nursing, *Newport*

South Carolina

University of South Carolina, College of Nursing, *Columbia*

South Dakota

South Dakota State University, College of Nursing, *Brookings*

Tennessee

East Tennessee State University, College of Nursing, *Johnson City*

Southern Adventist University, School of Nursing, *Collegedale*

Tennessee State University, School of Nursing, *Nashville*

Union University, School of Nursing, *Jackson*

The University of Tennessee, College of Nursing, *Knoxville*

Texas

Lamar University, Department of Nursing, *Beaumont*

Midwestern State University, Nursing Program, *Wichita Falls*

Patty Hanks Shelton School of Nursing, *Abilene*

Tarleton State University, Department of Nursing, *Stephenville*

Texas A&M University–Corpus Christi, College of Nursing and Health Sciences, *Corpus Christi*

Texas Christian University, Harris College of Nursing, *Fort Worth*

The University of Texas at Arlington, College of Nursing, *Arlington*

The University of Texas at Brownsville, Department of Nursing, *Brownsville*

The University of Texas Health Science Center at Houston, School of Nursing, *Houston*

The University of Texas Health Science Center at San Antonio, School of Nursing, *San Antonio*

Virginia

George Mason University, College of Health and Human Services, *Fairfax*

Jefferson College of Health Sciences, Nursing Education Program, *Roanoke*

Old Dominion University, Department of Nursing, *Norfolk*

Shenandoah University, Eleanor Wade Custer School of Nursing, *Winchester*

Washington

Pacific Lutheran University, School of Nursing, *Tacoma*

University of Washington, School of Nursing, *Seattle*

Washington State University College of Nursing, *Spokane*

West Virginia

Fairmont State University, School of Nursing and Allied Health Administration, *Fairmont*

Shepherd University, Department of Nursing Education, *Shepherdstown*

West Virginia University, School of Nursing, *Morgantown*

Wisconsin

Alverno College, Division of Nursing, *Milwaukee*

University of Wisconsin–Eau Claire, College of Nursing and Health Sciences, *Eau Claire*

University of Wisconsin–Madison, School of Nursing, *Madison*

University of Wisconsin–Oshkosh, College of Nursing, *Oshkosh*

Viterbo University, School of Nursing, *La Crosse*

Wisconsin Lutheran College, Nursing Program, *Milwaukee*

CANADA

British Columbia

British Columbia Institute of Technology, School of Health Sciences, *Burnaby*

Thompson Rivers University, School of Nursing, *Kamloops*

Vancouver Island University, Department of Nursing, *Nanaimo*

Manitoba

University of Manitoba, Faculty of Nursing, *Winnipeg*

New Brunswick

Université de Moncton, School of Nursing, *Moncton*

University of New Brunswick Fredericton, Faculty of Nursing, *Fredericton*

Nova Scotia

St. Francis Xavier University, Department of Nursing, *Antigonish*

Ontario

Laurentian University, School of Nursing, *Sudbury*

Ryerson University, Program in Nursing, *Toronto*

University of Toronto, Faculty of Nursing, *Toronto*

University of Windsor, Faculty of Nursing, *Windsor*

York University, School of Nursing, *Toronto*

Quebec

Université de Montréal, Faculty of Nursing, *Montréal*

Université du Québec à Rimouski, Program in Nursing, *Rimouski*

Université Laval, Faculty of Nursing, *Québec*

Saskatchewan

University of Saskatchewan, College of Nursing, *Saskatoon*

In this index, the page locations of the profiles are printed in regular type, the displays are in *italics*, and the two-page descriptions are in **bold** type.

NOTES

NOTES

NOTES

NOTES

NOTES

NOTES

NOTES